Radiography of the Dog and Cat

Guide to Making and Interpreting Radiographs

Radiography of the Dog and Cat

Guide to Making and Interpreting Radiographs

2nd Edition

M.C. Muhlbauer, DVM, MS, DACVR
S.K. Kneller, DVM, MS, DACVR

WILEY Blackwell

Published by John Wiley & Sons, Inc., Hoboken, New Jersey.
Published simultaneously in Canada.

For general information on our other products and services or for technical support, please contact our Customer Care Department within the United States at (800) 762-2974, outside the United States at (317) 572-3993 or fax (317) 572-4002.

Wiley also publishes its books in a variety of electronic formats. Some content that appears in print may not be available in electronic formats. For more information about Wiley products, visit our web site at www.wiley.com.

Library of Congress Cataloging-in-Publication Data
Names: Muhlbauer, Mike C., author. | Kneller, Steve, author.
Title: Radiography of the dog and cat : guide to making and interpreting radiographs / M.C. Muhlbauer, S.K. Kneller.
Description: 2nd edition. | Hoboken, NJ : Wiley-Blackwell, 2024. | Includes bibliographical references and index.
Identifiers: LCCN 2022058867 (print) | LCCN 2022058868 (ebook) | ISBN 9781119564737 (cloth) | ISBN 9781119564959 (adobe pdf) | ISBN 9781119564966 (epub)
Subjects: MESH: Radiography—veterinary | Cat Diseases—diagnostic imaging | Dog Diseases—diagnostic imaging | Diagnosis, Differential | Handbook
Classification: LCC SF757.8 (print) | LCC SF757.8 (ebook) | NLM SF 757.8 | DDC 636.089/607—dc23/eng/20230518
LC record available at https://lccn.loc.gov/2022058867
LC ebook record available at https://lccn.loc.gov/2022058868

Cover Design: Wiley
Cover Images: Courtesy of M.C. Muhlbauer
Set in 9/11pt Meridien LT Std by Straive, Chennai, India

Printed in Singapore
M095395_260923

Contents

About the Companion Website

This book is accompanied by a companion website:

www.wiley.com/go/muhlbauer/dog

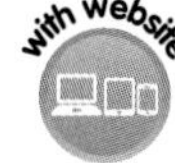

The website includes:

- Review questions
- Figure PowerPoints
- The glossary from the book as a downloadable PDF
- The positioning guide
- Artifact images

Introduction

The purpose of radiography is to lessen uncertainty.

When you perform a radiographic examination, you usually have a question that needs to be answered. There was a reason you made the radiographs. We have created this guide to help you and other veterinary personnel, from student to specialist, answer those questions. We hope it will be a valuable reference for you. It is necessary to know some facts and concepts so that you can make quality radiographs and interpret them correctly. There is also some background information that may be interesting to some of you for deeper understanding. The authors strongly believe that we all retain knowledge that we understand far longer than information that was just memorized. We spent considerable effort in this regard.

We wrote the first edition of this book in two forms: first, we wanted to provide a handy reference guide that you could use "onsite" while reading radiographs, and second, we wanted to provide more in-depth information to help readers understand some of the physics, physiology, anatomy and pathology concepts that are important when using radiography.

In this second edition, we reduce the repetition of material and handle each body system in one part of the book rather than two. We streamlined the subject matter by moving some of the material out of the main text and into the glossary. We've added hundreds of more realistic images and figures to help explain important concepts and demonstrate the radiographic appearances of numerous conditions. Rather than sticking to an outline format, we present the information more as a discussion, which we hope will be easier to read and follow.

Half the magic of radiologists is having high-quality radiographs.

Chapter 1 is all about producing x-rays and safely using x-rays to make quality radiographs. Less and less is taught to veterinary students in this regard, yet we feel that understanding the physics of radiography adds much to the accurate interpretation of radiographs. The more you understand about the principles of radiography and how x-ray equipment works, the more success you will have in making quality radiographs. The basics of current image receptors, both analog (film) and digital, are addressed and helpful tips provided regarding the use and care of radiography equipment.

Chapter 2 is about the radiographs and the various procedures performed in diagnostic radiology. In this chapter, you will find a comprehensive positioning guide with detailed descriptions and illustrations. Many of the artifacts encountered in veterinary radiography are described and illustrated, along with recommendations to deal with them. We provide a "how to" guide for over 25 contrast radiography procedures and list their indications, contraindications, techniques, dosages, and complications. Although the availability of other imaging modalities and endoscopy have reduced the need to perform contrast studies, they still are useful, and we feel a concise reference guide is valuable.

Many people tend to see what they want in a radiograph, whether it is there or not.

It is well known that preconceived expectations are notorious for inventing or overlooking radiographic abnormalities. Valuable information is often available, if one is willing to deliberately and systematically review the images. We encourage you as best you can, to shelve what you know about the patient while you glean the radiographs for useful information. Then review your radiographic findings in light of non-radiographic information. Patient history is not necessary to "read" radiographs, but it is necessary to "interpret" radiographs.

Reading radiographs is an acquired skill and art. Throughout this book we emphasize the systematic approach. Our attitude when looking at a radiograph is try to make "normal" anything that looks "abnormal." In other words, try to explain each radiographic finding as either normal anatomy, a normal variant of anatomy, or an artifact. If you can't explain it as any of these, then your radiographic finding probably is a true abnormality.

> *You must know normal to recognize abnormal.*

Chapters 3, 4, and 5 deal with Thorax, Abdomen, and Musculoskeleton. This is where you go to learn more about "normal" - which includes many of the basic, unique, and sometimes confusing radiographic appearances of numerous structures, and "abnormal" - the radiographic changes that develop during various disease processes. Again, we feel that it is important to understand what is happening to produce the radiograph signs rather than simply trying to memorize the signs. At the end of each chapter, we provide lists of differential diagnoses for numerous radiographic findings because many different diseases present with similar findings.

At the end of the book is an extensive glossary that contains a great many definitions and explanations which cover a variety of radiographic concepts and terms, including those that are older and not used in this book.

What is different about this book?

In this guide, you will once again find language that differs from some of the classic radiography terms which persist from years past. Many of those terms, in our opinion, are confusing or truly inaccurate. We feel that the more we use correct terminology, the better we understand our craft. Rather than sticking with inadequate terms from the past, which were pertinent when radiologists were beginning to understand the radiographic appearances of disease, we hope this to be a fresh approach using simple correlation with physics, physiology, and pathology and based on current advances in diagnostic imaging.

> *It is important to patient care to accurately describe what you see in radiographs.*

Radiopacity is relative. ALL materials block x-rays to some degree, even air. To state that a material is "radiopaque" or "radiolucent" provides little useful information. For example, cystic calculi that are not visible in survey radiographs commonly are called "radiolucent." However, when these same calculi are seen in a pneumocystogram, they are considered "radiopaque," and in a double contrast cystogram, they are visible but again called "radiolucent." The opacity of a material is always relative to the adjacent material. We use the term opacity to describe the characteristic of a material to block or attenuate x-rays, as do other radiography texts in which "radio-" is a given. Remember, it's all about relative opacity and the opacity interfaces between adjacent materials.

Detail in a radiograph, as in a photography, has nothing to do with the subject and everything to do with how the image was created (e.g., type of equipment, exposure technique, method of processing). It is important to determine whether indistinct margins in a radiograph are due to a technical issue or a clinical condition. When you describe indistinct peritoneal serosal margins as "poor abdominal detail" you are stating that the radiograph is a poor quality image due to factors such as a low grade image receptor, over or under exposure, or motion artifact. Nearly always the appearance you are observing is a weak or absent opacity interface due to abdominal fluid or inflammation or lack of intra-abdominal fat. Detail refers to the technical quality of the radiograph while distinction may be technical, but also may be due to opacity interface issues. Pathology may or may not be present in a poor-quality image. In the abdomen, it's all about the opacity interfaces between soft tissue, fat, and gas. It is important to state accurately what you are seeing in the radiograph. When you think in these correct terms, you will find it easier to understand what you are seeing and why you are seeing it.

Periosteal response is a physiologic process to heal bone, not a reaction to disease. Understanding the physiology behind a periosteal response aids in understanding the disease process. For example, periosteal new bone never grows outward from the cortex; it is formed perpendicular to the periosteum to fill the space created by the separation of the periosteum from the cortex. Recognizing a periosteal response and determining whether the lesion is active or inactive, aggressive or non-aggressive, is vital to providing the best patient care. Additional diagnostic tests are required in most situations to establish the etiology, but accurate interpretation of the radiographs often dictates whether there is a need for further diagnostics.

"Sunburst pattern," "ground-glass appearance," and other similar terms rarely are useful by themselves in modern radiography. Classically, a "sunburst" periosteal response was used to describe a bone tumor. However, we now know that osteomyelitis and other diseases can create a similar radiographic appearance. "Ground-glass" appearance is used to describe indistinct or obscured margins, a confusing term at best. Trying to put a label on a specific type of lesion or radiographic appearance often interferes with describing what is actually there.

"Prominent" is not a radiographic sign. If a structure is "prominent" in a radiograph, there is a reason. It may be enlarged or there may be a change in opacity. For example, pulmonary vessels are more "prominent" when enlarged or mineralized or when the lungs are less opaque because they are well-inflated. Abdominal organs become more "prominent" when there is free gas in the abdominal cavity or when opacified by a contrast medium. It is important take that next step and determine why something is "prominent" so you can accurately describe what you are seeing.

Alveolar lung disease is a misnomer. The alveoli are air spaces, not tissue. The walls of the alveoli are part of the lung interstitium. Most lung diseases begin in the interstitium but are not recognized in radiographs until they affect the alveoli. Diseases that produce a mostly cellular response and little fluid result in interstitial thickening, which prevents the alveoli from fully expanding. Diseases that produce more interstitial fluid (edema, pus, hemorrhage) eventually lead to filling of the alveoli, which displaces the air from the alveolar spaces. Don't worry about trying to identify a specific lung pattern, just describe what you are seeing. Lung diseases can involve the parenchyma (the interstitium and air spaces), the airways, or the vasculature. What is important is to recognize the parts of the lung that are predominantly involved. Serial radiographs as needed to monitor the progression of the disease and the response to therapy. This helps provide the best patient care.

More of these discussions are presented throughout this book. We are not just trying to be different or to "buck the system." We have found during our years of teaching veterinary students, interns, residents, and practitioners that some of the classic terminology frequently causes confusion and laborious memorization. We believe a simpler, more straightforward approach will help you make more accurate radiographic diagnoses with less consternation. Enjoy!!!

—mcm and skk

1 X-Rays

Radiography of the Dog and Cat: Guide to Making and Interpreting Radiographs, Second Edition. M.C. Muhlbauer and S.K. Kneller.

Companion website: www.wiley.com/go/muhlbauer/dog

Introduction

X-rays routinely are used to non-invasively examine internal anatomy. The technique is called **Radiography**. The image created using x-rays is called a **radiograph**. Many people confuse the terms "x-ray" and "radiograph." X-rays are a type of energy, whereas radiographs are images.

Radiography is a part of the medical specialty called *Radiology*. Radiology encompasses all of diagnostic imaging, including ultrasound, computed tomography (CT), magnetic resonance imaging (MRI), and scintigraphy. A major advantage of radiography over the other imaging modalities is that a large volume of the patient can be viewed with one image. A major disadvantage is that many structures are superimposed, making interpretation of the images sometimes confusing.

Our goal in radiography is to make images that display the greatest amount of usable information. This requires an understanding of x-rays; what they are, how they are made, and how they can be used safely to "look inside" our patients.

A

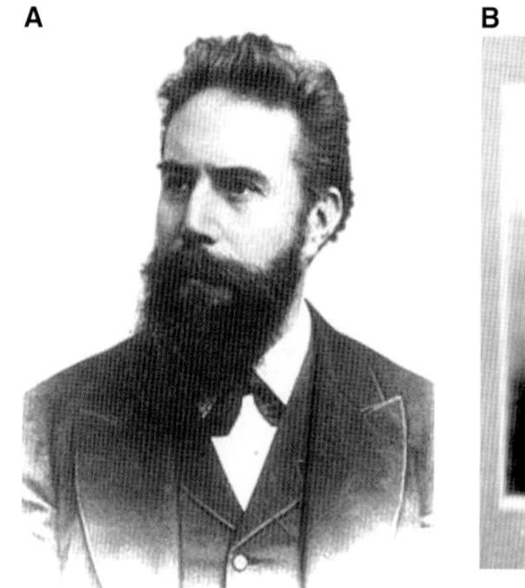

B

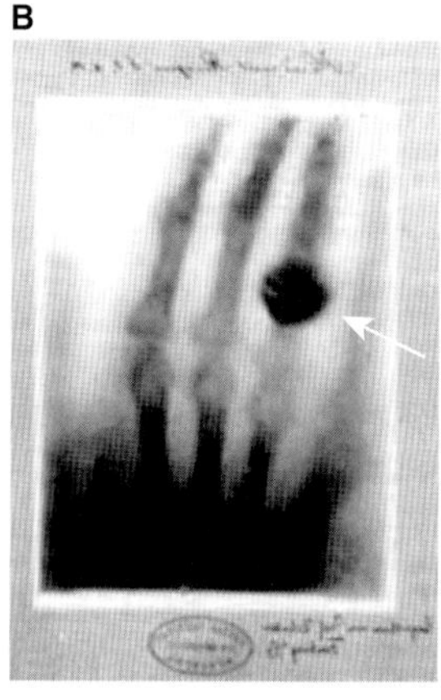

Figure 1.1 Discovery of x-rays. (**A**) Photo of Wilhelm Röntgen, the German physicist who discovered x-rays. Source: JdH/Wikimedia Commons/Public domain. (**B**) Photo of the first radiograph made by Röntgen. It is an image of his wife's hand. The ring on her finger is the first radiographic artifact (arrow). Source: NASA.

X-rays

X-rays were discovered in 1895 by Wilhelm Conrad Röntgen. Röntgen was a German scientist who won the first Nobel Prize in physics for his discovery (Figure 1.1). He used the symbol "X" to name the new rays because they were a type of radiation that was unknown at that time. Radiation is energy that spreads out in all directions as it moves away from its source.

X-rays are a type of electromagnetic radiation (EMR). There are many types of EMR, including radiowaves, microwaves, and visible light (Figure 1.2). EMR behaves both like particles and like waves, sometimes described as a stream of particles that travels in a wave-like pattern. EMR particles are called **photons**. Photons are packets of energy with no mass, no charge, and move at the speed of light. The energy of a photon is directly related to **wavelength**; the shorter the wavelength, the greater the energy. Wavelength is directly related to **frequency**; the higher the frequency, the shorter the wavelength (and the higher the frequency, the greater the energy).

In the EMR spectrum, x-rays are relatively short wavelength, high frequency, and high energy. They are able to penetrate many materials that are opaque to visible light (Box 1.1). X-rays also are **ionizing**, which means they have sufficient energy to remove electrons from atoms and form ions. Ionization can destroy molecules and damage or kill living cells. Adherence to radiation safety guidelines is crucial when working with x-rays (see the Radiation Safety section later in this chapter).

The reason we are able to use x-rays to view internal anatomy is because x-rays pass through some tissues more easily than others. Without differences in tissue transmission, radiography would not be possible. The ability of a tissue to block or *attenuate* x-rays is called **radiopacity** or simply **opacity** ("radio-" is assumed since we are discussing radiography). The greater the opacity, the fewer x-rays will pass through.

Another key point in radiography is that a tissue or object will be visible in a radiograph only if it is adjacent to a material with a different opacity. There must be an **opacity interface**. An opacity interface is the boundary where two materials with different opacities meet. Without opacity interfaces there is no visible image in a radiograph. The greater the difference in opacities between materials, the stronger the opacity interface and the easier it will be to identify structures.

Radiography is possible only because x-rays penetrate some materials more easily than others. An opacity interface must be present to identify a structure in a radiograph.

Box 1.1 Properties of x-rays

- X-rays have no mass or physical form.
- X-rays cannot be detected by human senses; they cannot be seen, heard, or felt.
- X-rays travel in straight lines at the speed of light.
- The path of an x-ray cannot be affected by gravity, electrical fields, or magnetic fields.
- X-rays can penetrate many materials; the degree of penetration depends on the x-ray energy and the type of material.
- X-rays can expose photographic emulsion.
- X-rays are ionizing and can damage or destroy living cells.

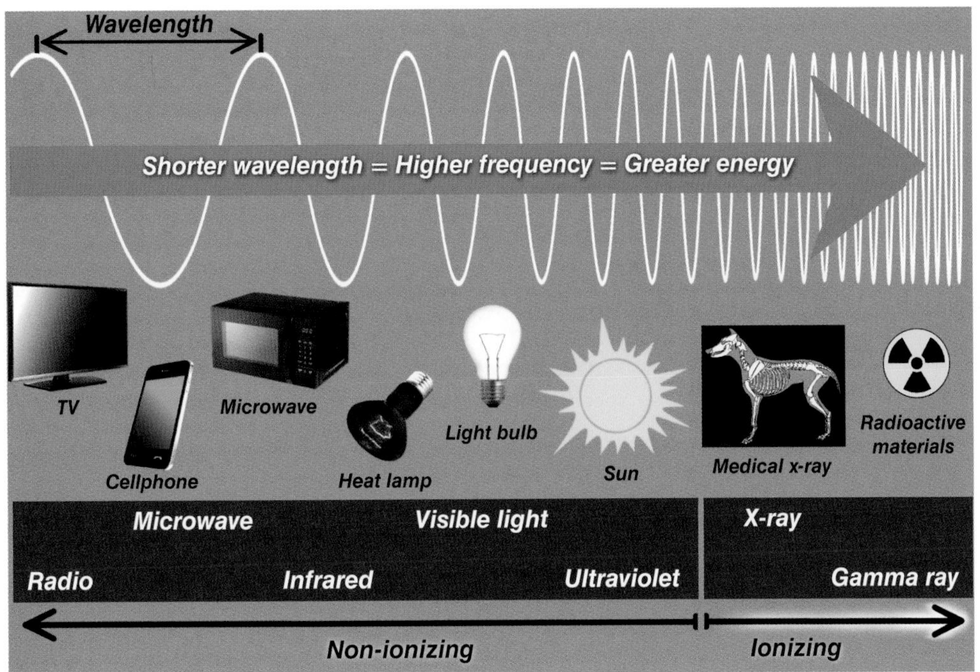

Figure 1.2 Spectrum of electromagnetic radiation (EMR). Different types of EMR are displayed in this image. The type is determined by the energy of the photons. The shorter the wavelength, the higher the frequency, and the greater the energy. High energy EMR can be ionizing. Source: trekandphoto/ Adobe Stock.

As mentioned earlier, our goal is to produce radiographs that provide maximum usable information. Making quality radiographs requires adequate *density, contrast, detail* and minimal *distortion*. Each of these factors is discussed thoroughly later in this chapter. However, a brief introduction may be helpful here.

Density refers to the amount of blackness in the radiograph. The greater the radiographic density, the darker the image. Density is determined by the number of x-rays that are recorded by the image receptor. The more x-rays recorded, the darker that part of the radiograph. In most radiographs there are many levels of density. Each level is displayed as a shade of gray. Each shade of gray corresponds to an opacity. If there is too much density, the radiograph will be too dark. If there is too little density, the radiograph will be too light. In either case we won't be able to differentiate structures in the image.

Contrast refers to the amount of difference between the levels of density in the radiograph. It is the degree of change between the dark areas and the light areas. High contrast means the radiograph is mostly black and white with few shades of gray in between. Some structures will not be visible because there are no shades of gray to display their opacities. Low contrast means there are many shades of gray between white and black. If there is too little contrast, structures with similar opacities will not be distinguished because their individual shades of gray will be too similar and they will visibly blend together.

Detail refers to the sharpness of change from one density to the next in the radiograph. The greater the detail, the sharper the edges of the structures in the image. Detail – or definition – determines how well we can see the borders of structures that are close together. If there isn't enough detail, we won't be able to distinguish the structures as separate.

Distortion occurs when the actual size or shape of an object is misrepresented in the radiograph. It results from poor positioning of the object in relation to the x-ray beam and image receptor.

X-ray production

For medical radiography, x-rays are created inside a glass vacuum tube. This is accomplished by bombarding a metal target with high-speed electrons. Inside the tube are a negatively charged **cathode** and a positively charged **anode** (Figure 1.3). The cathode contains a wire filament which can be heated with an electric current to "boil off" electrons (Figure 1.4). This process is called *thermionic emission* and it is similar to heating the filament in an incandescent light bulb.

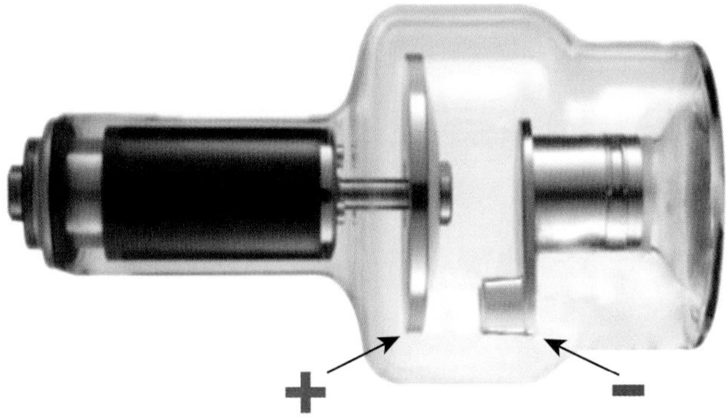

Figure 1.3 X-ray tube. This is a picture of a generic x-ray tube showing the positively charged anode (+) and the negatively charged cathode (–) enclosed in a glass vacuum tube.

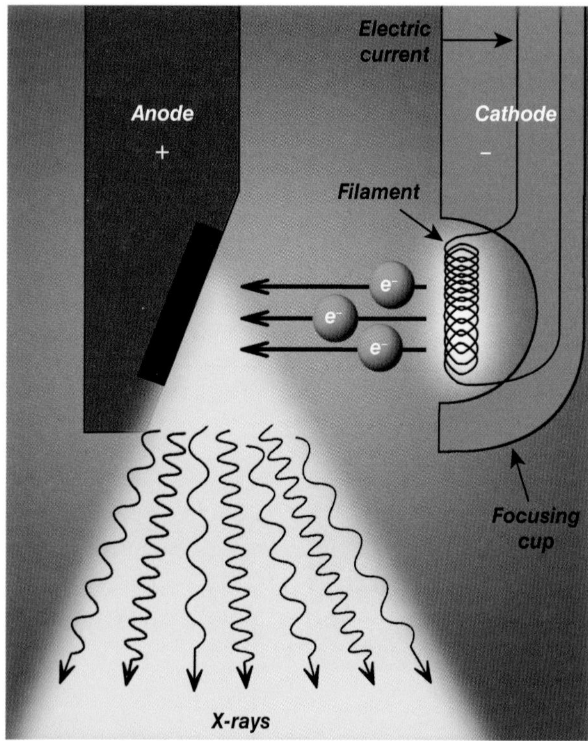

Figure 1.4 X-ray production. This illustration depicts the filament in the cathode being heated to emit a cloud of electrons. The electrons (e^-) are aimed at the anode by the focusing cup and accelerated by a high voltage. The electrons strike a target on the anode (black area) and their kinetic energy is converted into heat and x-rays. The x-rays produced vary in wavelength and energy.

The number of electrons produced is controlled by the strength and duration of the current.

The electrons collect in a "cloud" around the filament and are held in place by the *focusing cup*. The focusing cup concentrates the electrons into a well-defined beam and aims them at the anode. When high voltage is applied across the x-ray tube, a large negative-to-positive gradient is created that rapidly accelerates the electrons from the cathode to the anode. The electrons are traveling at over half the speed of light when they strike the anode.

The anode stops the electrons, converting their kinetic energy into heat and x-rays (about 99% heat and 1% x-rays). Heat is an unwanted by-product of x-ray production and must be dissipated. Methods of heat dissipation will be discussed shortly.

Electron bombardment of the anode produces x-rays with energies that vary from near zero to the maximum energy of the electrons. The variations in energy are due to the way the electrons interact with the anode atoms. There are two types of interactions: *characteristic* and *bremsstrahlung*.

Characteristic x-rays are formed when a high-speed electron from the cathode collides with an atom in the anode target (Figure 1.5). An inner level electron is ejected from the atom, which produces an ion. Ions are unstable, so an outer level electron drops down to fill the void in the inner level. Because the binding energy of an outer electron is greater than that of an inner electron, the outer electron releases some energy in the form of an x-ray. The energy of the x-ray is equal to the difference between the outer level binding energy and the inner level binding energy and therefore is *characteristic* of the type of atom that was ionized. About 20% of medical x-ray production is due to characteristic interactions (Figure 1.7).

Bremsstrahlung x-rays are produced when a high-speed electron from the cathode passes near the nucleus in an anode atom. The positive charge from the nucleus pulls on the electron, slowing it down and altering its direction (Figure 1.6). "Bremsstrahlung" is a German word that means "braking radiation." As it slows down, the electron loses energy which is emitted as an x-ray. The energy of the x-ray depends on how much the electron was slowed down. X-ray energies vary from near zero (the electron barely slowed down) to the total energy of the electron (the electron was completely stopped). About 80% of medical x-ray production is due to Bremsstrahlung interactions (Figure 1.7).

X-ray machine

Basic components of an x-ray machine include the x-ray tube assembly, the collimator, the electrical circuits, the operating console, the table, and the image receptor (Figure 1.8).

X-ray tube assembly

The x-ray tube assembly comprises the x-ray tube and its metal housing (Figure 1.9). The metal housing protects and supports the tube and prevents unwanted x-rays from escaping. It also encases the oil that surrounds the x-ray tube to help dissipate heat and provide electrical insulation. Most x-ray assemblies are mounted so they can be moved horizontally, vertically, and rotated to facilitate making radiographs.

The purpose of an x-ray tube is to convert electricity into x-rays. As described earlier, the **cathode** is the negative terminal in the x-ray tube. It contains the filament and focusing cup. The filament is a coil of thin wire, usually made of tungsten. Tungsten is a very malleable metal with a high melting point (over 3400 °C) and a low rate of evaporation, making it ideal for thermionic emission. The focusing cup generally is made of molybdenum. The point on the anode that is struck by the beam of electrons is called the **focal spot**. Most x-ray machines include two focal spots, a large one and a small one, with a separate filament for each.

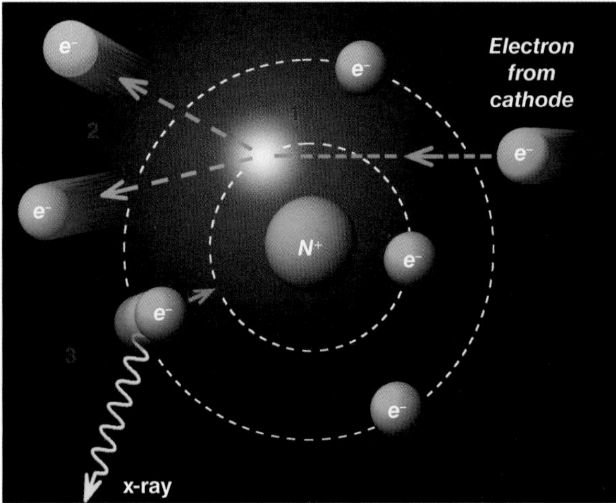

Figure 1.5 Characteristic x-ray production. **1**. A high-speed electron from the cathode (green e⁻) collides with an inner shell electron in an anode atom. **2**. The anode electron is ejected, and the cathode electron continues in a new direction with less energy. **3**. An outer shell electron gives up energy as an x-ray and moves to fill the vacancy in the inner shell (N⁺ = nucleus, e⁻=electron).

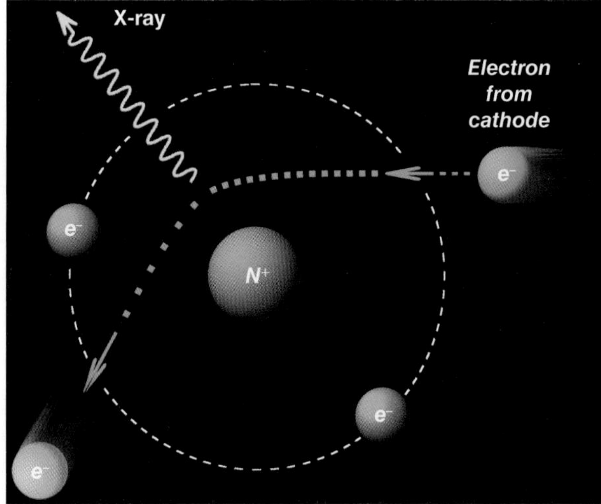

Figure 1.6 Bremsstrahlung x-ray production. A high-speed electron from the cathode (green e⁻) nears the positively charged nucleus (N⁺) in an anode atom. The electron slows down and changes direction. As it slows, the electron loses energy which is emitted as an x-ray. The energy of the x-ray is determined by how much the electron was slowed down.

The **anode** is the positive terminal in the x-ray tube. This is where x-rays are produced. A typical anode consists of a round, flat, metal disc made of molybdenum with a thin rim of tungsten. The high atomic number of tungsten (74) increases the likelihood of electron interactions. The anode rim is the target for the electron beam. It is beveled to create a slope, which is valuable for x-ray beam geometry, as we will discuss later.

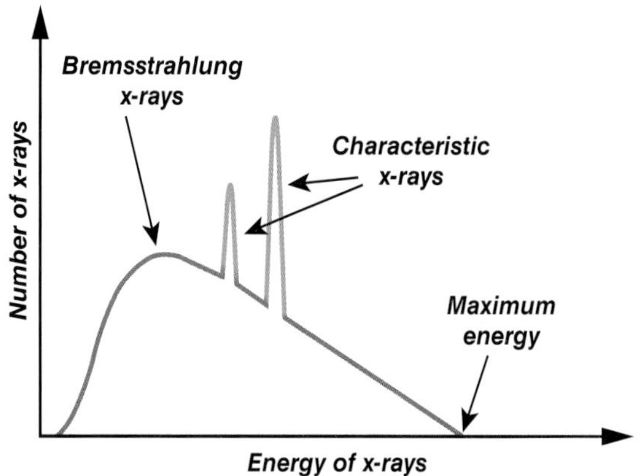

Figure 1.7 Spectrum of x-ray energies. Most of the x-rays used for diagnostic imaging will range in energy from near zero to the maximum energy of the electrons used to produce them. This continuum of energies is due to Bremsstrahlung interactions and is shown in blue in the graph above. A small amount of medical x-rays are characteristic of the material used to produce them, depicted by the green spikes on the graph.

Heat is a major limiting factor in the production of x-rays. To produce an adequate number of electrons, the tungsten filament must be heated to over 2200 °C. To accelerate the electrons, kilovolts of power must be applied across the x-ray tube. To generate x-rays, the target is heated to over 2500 °C during a single exposure. Excessive heating is a primary cause of x-ray tube failure, and the x-ray tube is one of the most expensive parts of an x-ray machine. The most vulnerable part of the tube to heat overload is the focal spot. The larger the focal spot, the greater the heat tolerance. A large focal spot is desirable because more x-rays can be produced; however, the larger the focal spot, the less definition in the radiographs.

Heat is conducted away from the focal spot by the metal in the anode disc, the oil surrounding the x-ray tube, and the protective metal housing. To further dissipate heat, the anode is mounted on a high-speed rotor which spins up to 10,000 rpm during x-ray production. Spinning the anode effectively increases the area of the target that is bombarded by the electron beam and lessens the amount of heating in any one spot.

To avoid overheating, **tube rating charts** are provided by manufacturers. These charts define the maximum *heat units* a particular x-ray tube can tolerate over time before it fails. Heat units (HU) are calculated based on the amount of power that is sent to the x-ray tube (HU = kV × mA). You should never exceed 80% of the maximum heat units with any exposure. **Anode cooling charts** display the minimum time required for the anode to cool down before making another exposure.

X-ray machines that have been idle for more than 6 hours are considered "cold." A cold x-ray tube should be

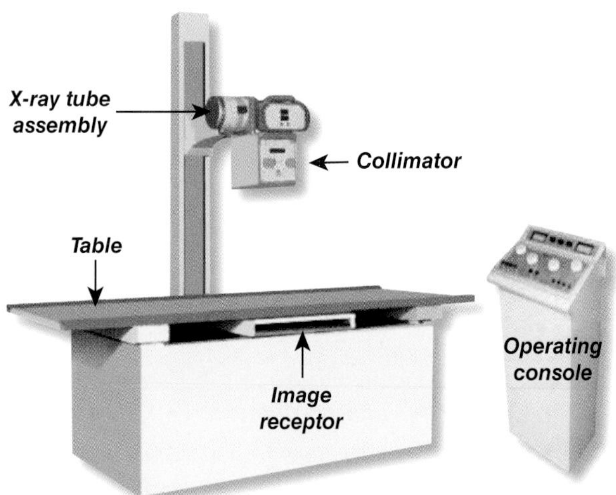

Figure 1.8 Typical x-ray machine. The x-ray tube assembly is mounted above the table, preferably on a slide for horizontal movement and on an adjustable column for vertical movement. The collimator is mounted to the x-ray tube. The image receptor may be positioned atop or underneath the table top. In this picture, the image receptor is secured in a tray under the table, which is aligned with the collimator. The operating console is pictured on the right.

warmed up prior to making a high exposure to avoid damaging the anode. To warm up a cold tube, close the collimator and set a low exposure technique (e.g., 60 kVp, 100 mA, 0.05 seconds). Make two exposures about 30–60 seconds apart. The tube is now warmed up and ready for use (Box 1.2).

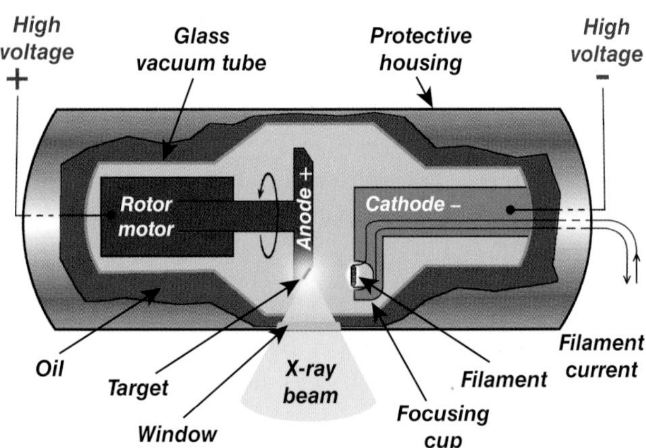

Figure 1.9 X-ray tube assembly. This illustration depicts a cutaway view of an x-ray tube assembly. The glass vacuum x-ray tube is surrounded by oil and encased in a protective metal housing. The anode (+) is mounted on a shaft that is attached to an induction motor. The motor spins the anode to help dissipate heat during x-ray production. The cathode (–) is supplied by a low voltage, high amperage current to heat the filament and produce electrons. The filament is mounted in the focusing cup. The x-ray tube is supplied by a high voltage, low amperage current to accelerate the electrons toward the anode target. X-rays emitted from the target travel in all directions, but the protective housing prevents them from exiting the assembly other than through a small window.

Box 1.2 Prolong the life of your x-ray tube

- Adhere to the tube rating and cooling charts.
- Do not exceed 80% of maximum heat units for any exposure.
- Warm up a cold x-ray tube before making a high exposure.
- Use the lowest mA that is practical.
- Avoid prolonged rotation of the anode.

Collimator

A collimator is an arrangement of x-ray absorbers used to limit the size and shape of the x-ray beam to a specific **field-of-view (FOV)**. The FOV is the area to be irradiated. It is the part of the patient that is exposed to the primary x-ray beam.

Collimators are mounted to the x-ray tube assembly in the path of the x-rays (Figure 1.10). Modern collimators contain adjustable shutters made of lead which can be manipulated to create the desired FOV. The smaller the FOV, the better the definition in the radiograph.

Inside many collimators are a light bulb and an array of mirrors which are used to project a visible light FOV that corresponds to the x-ray beam FOV. This allows the radiographer to accurately configure the area to be irradiated.

Filtration

The purpose of filtration is to absorb low-energy x-rays and remove them from the x-ray beam. Low energy x-rays are

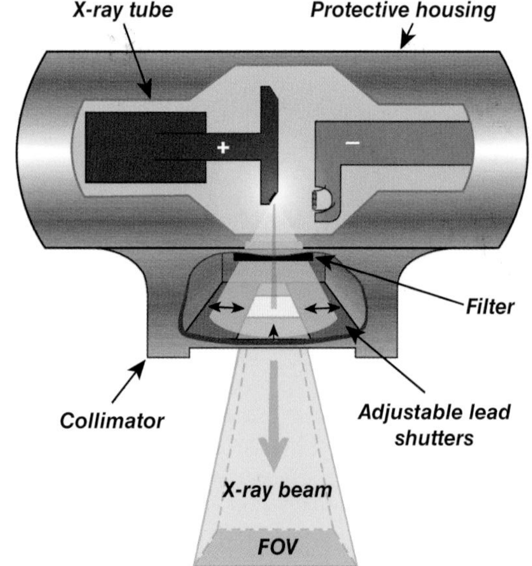

Figure 1.10 Collimator. In this illustration, the collimator is mounted to the x-ray tube assembly in the path of the x-rays. The side of the collimator is cut away to show the adjustable lead shutters inside. The shutters can be moved to change the size and shape of the FOV. The side of the protective housing is cut away to show the x-ray tube. An added filter is visible between the collimator and x-ray tube assembly, in the path of the x-rays.

unable to pass through the patient and therefore provide no useful diagnostic information. They do, however, increase the radiation dose to the patient. All x-ray beams contain low-energy x-rays due to Bremsstrahlung interactions. The National Council on Radiation Protection and Measurements (NCRPM) requires that all x-ray tubes operating above 70 kVp must include filtration that is equivalent to at least **2.5 mm aluminum**. This applies to most veterinary practices. There is some inherent filtration in most x-ray machines, but additional filters usually are needed.

Inherent filtration comes from the x-ray tube glass envelop, the surrounding oil, the glass window in the protective housing, and the collimator. Inherent filtration typically contributes about 1.5 mm aluminum equivalent. **Added filtration** generally consists of aluminum plates that are positioned near the x-ray tube in the path of the x-rays (Figure 1.10). The plates provide the additional 1–2 mm of aluminum required.

In addition to lowering the radiation dose to the patient, filtration also increases the average or **effective energy** of the x-ray beam. Removing the low energy x-rays from the beam is called **beam hardening**. Beam hardening increases the effective energy of the x-rays from about 1/3 of kVp to about 1/2 of kVp. A higher effective energy means the x-ray beam is more uniform in intensity, which can improve radiographic quality.

Selective filtration sometimes is used to make the x-ray beam more intense on one side than the other. This can be helpful when the thickness of the body part varies significantly. Rather than making two different exposures, one for the thick side and another for the thin side, a *compensation filter* can be used (Figure 1.11). A typical compensation filter is a wedge-shaped piece of aluminum that unilaterally absorb x-rays. It makes the x-ray beam less intense on the thin side to prevent overexposing that side of the body part while allowing full exposure on the thicker side. The resulting radiograph is more uniform in density across both thicknesses. The **heel effect** provides a similar benefit and is discussed on page 16.

Compensation filters are attached to the front of the collimator, usually with magnets or Velcro. Some collimators are equipped with an adjustable holder designed to fit a compensation filter. The filter is installed after setting the FOV because the light from the collimator will be blocked by the filter. Compensation filters are less important with digital radiography because computer processing can be used to manipulate the image and adjust for variations in density.

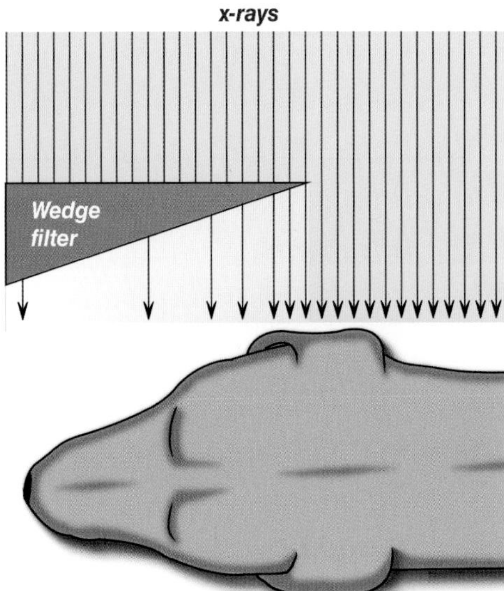

Figure 1.11 Compensation filter. In this illustration, the dog's head varies in thickness from the nose to the ears. A wedge filter is used to reduce the amount of x-rays to the nose while allowing the full intensity of the x-ray beam to reach the thicker skull. This allows the head to be imaged without overexposing the nose or underexposing the skull. The gradual slope of the wedge blends the different x-ray beam intensities together, so there is no sharp demarcation between the lighter and darker areas in the radiograph.

Electrical supply to x-ray machine

The x-ray machine must receive a constant level of power to produce x-rays in a consistent and reliable manner. Fluctuations in power can cause significant variations in x-ray production. The line of incoming electricity should be dedicated to the x-ray machine with no other equipment on the line. Appliances such as a clothes dryer or an air conditioner will pull power away from the x-ray machine. A **line voltage compensator** is a useful device that adjusts for variations in incoming voltage. A voltage compensator is recommended because some power fluctuations are beyond the control of the hospital or clinic (e.g., originate at the power company).

The source of electricity for most x-ray machines is **alternating current** (AC). Alternating current regularly reverses direction, switching the flow of electricity from positive to negative many times per second (Figure 1.12). Depending on the country of origin, AC electricity is either 50 or 60 Hz, which means it cycles from one direction to the other 50 or 60 times per second. **Direct current** (DC) moves in only one direction and does not reverse. X-ray machines use both AC and DC power. However, the high voltage generator in the x-ray machine converts AC to DC, so a separate DC supply is not needed. There are two different electrical circuits in an x-ray machine, the *filament circuit* to produce electrons and the *high voltage generator* to accelerate the electrons.

The **filament circuit** increases the amperage of the incoming AC power to provide enough current to heat the tungsten wire and produce a sufficient number of electrons. The amperage is increased using a *step-down transformer*. A transformer is a device that increases or decreases voltage.

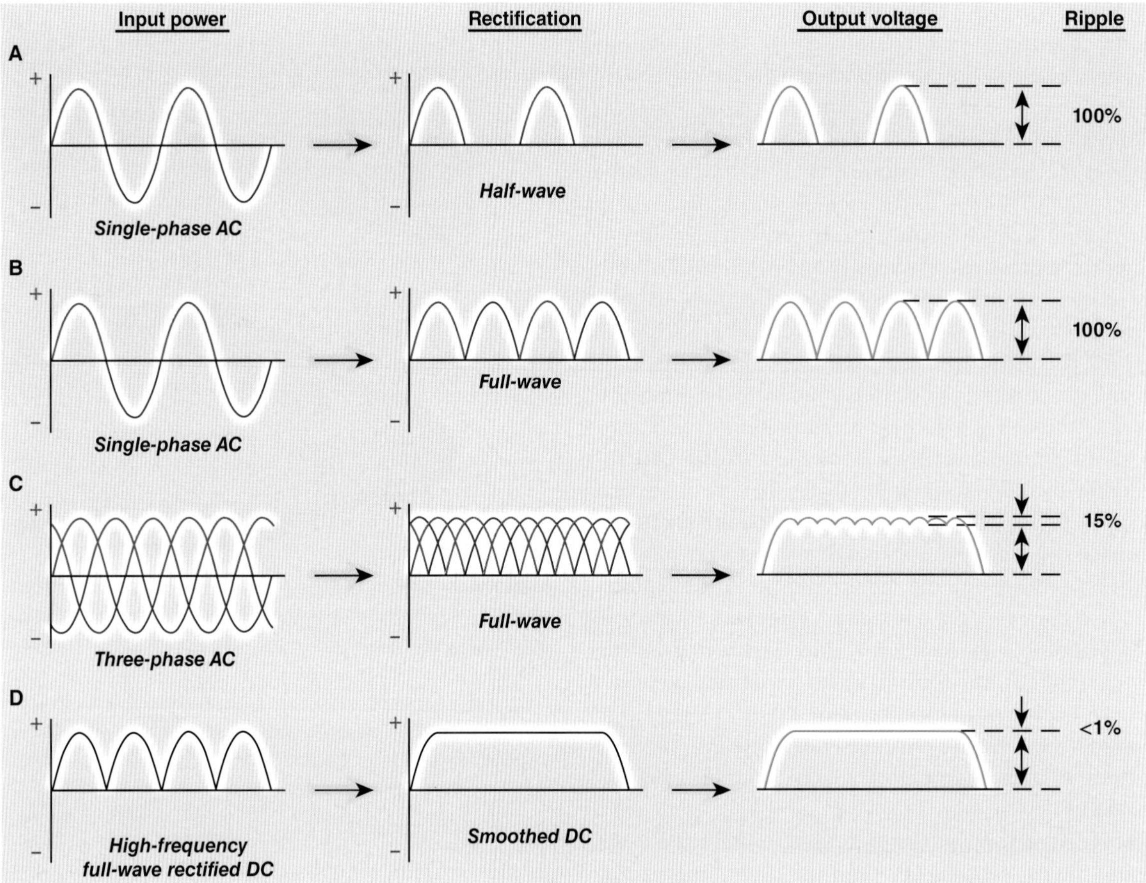

Figure 1.12 High voltage generators. This illustration depicts half-wave and full-wave rectification with single phase, three phase, and high frequency generators. The input power for single-phase generators (**A** and **B**) is a single line of alternating current (AC). AC power oscillates the flow of electricity from a positive direction (+) to a negative direction (–) many times per second. X-ray tubes require a current that moves in one direction only, which means the AC must be rectified to direct current (DC). Half-wave rectifiers (**A**) remove the negative direction of the AC to produce pulses of DC electricity. During each pulse the voltage fluctuates from zero to the maximum and back to zero again, resulting in 100% ripple. Full-wave rectifiers change the negative direction of AC to the positive direction to produce twice the number of DC pulses as half-wave rectifiers. However, the voltage still fluctuates from zero to maximum with each pulse and the ripple is still 100%. Three-phase generators (**C**) utilize three separate lines of input AC power. Each line is slightly out of phase with the other two. All three lines are full-wave rectified to produce overlapping pulses of DC and a more continuous output of voltage than single-phase units. As the voltage begins to drop in one pulse, the next pulse brings it back up to the maximum, resulting in only 15% ripple. High-frequency generators (**D**) utilize either single-phase or three-phase AC input that is full-wave rectified to DC. However, high-frequency generators then "chop" the DC pulses into smaller and smaller pulses and "smooth" them to produce near-constant output voltage with less than 1% ripple.

Voltage and amperage together constitute power, and the power leaving a transformer must be the same as the power coming into it. The equation is W = V × A, where W is power measured in watts, V is voltage, and A is amperage. Any change in voltage must include an opposite change in amperage so the power can remain constant. The step-down transformer, therefore, increases amperage to the filament by decreasing the incoming voltage.

The **high voltage generator** increases the voltage of the incoming AC power to provide the *kilovolts* needed to accelerate the electrons with enough speed to generate x-rays. This is accomplished with a *step-up* transformer. The step-up transformer increases the incoming voltage 500–1000 times, which drops the amperage to only a few milliamps. This means the tube current (current across the x-ray tube) is very low amperage and very high voltage.

The high voltage generator also converts AC to DC. X-ray tubes are designed to use current that flows in one direction only: from the cathode to the anode. Current that flows in the other direction will not produce x-rays and may damage or destroy the x-ray tube. The process of converting AC to DC is called **rectification**. Rectification may be either *half-wave* or *full-wave*, both of which produce a DC output that consists of "pulses" of electricity (Figure 1.12).

Half-wave rectifiers suppress the negative direction of AC, so only the electricity that flows in the positive direction is available. For example, if the input electricity is 60 Hz AC, the half-wave rectifier would produce a DC output to the x-ray tube of 60 pulses/second of electricity (Figure 1.12). As you can see, half-wave rectifiers only use half of the input AC, the other half is wasted. **Full-wave rectifiers,** on the other hand, change the negative direction of AC to the positive direction. Using the same example, a 60 Hz AC input would be converted to a DC output with 120 pulses/s, which is twice the electrical output of a half-wave rectifier.

A sidenote that may be interesting: because x-ray tubes only operate when current flows in one direction, a simple x-ray tube that receives only AC power actually is *self-rectified*. The problem with a self-rectified tube is that the anode is likely to get hot enough to emit its own free electrons and then the current would flow in the reverse direction and destroy the cathode.

Because rectification produces DC output in pulses, the amount of electricity going to the x-ray tube can fluctuate greatly. This fluctuation in power is called **ripple** (Figure 1.12). Specifically, ripple is the percent variation in voltage, from minimum to maximum, that is received by the x-ray tube. The smaller the ripple, the more constant the voltage and the more uniform and intense the x-ray beam. The amount of ripple depends on the type of high voltage generator. Currently, there are three basic types of generators: *single-phase, three-phase,* and *high-frequency*.

Single-phase generators receive a single source of AC power. The AC is rectified to produce a DC output with 100% ripple (Figure 1.12). 100% ripple means the x-rays are produced in bursts instead of continuously. The intermittent production of x-rays leads to longer exposure times, higher radiation doses, and a lower x-ray beam intensity (only about 70% of peak output). The shortest exposure time with a single-phase generator is 1/120 second (~8 ms).

Three-phase generators receive three separate lines of AC power. Each line is superimposed on the other and 120° out of phase with the other two (Figure 1.12). All lines are full-wave rectified so each line of 60 Hz AC produces 120 pulses of DC. The three lines are combined so together they produce 360 pulses/s of DC power. Because the lines are out of phase with each other, as the voltage in one pulse begins to drop another pulse brings it back up to the maximum so the voltage never falls to zero. The x-ray tube receives more constant power with a ripple that is only about 15%. Some three-phase generators include extra rectification to produce DC with 720 pulses/s and only 4% ripple. These are called three-phase, 12-pulse generators. Exposure times with three-phase generators can be as short as 1/1000 second (1 ms), and the x-ray beam intensity is about 95% of peak output.

High-frequency generators supply near-constant voltage to the x-ray tube. The input power may be single-phase or three-phase AC which is then full-wave rectified (Figure 1.12). High-frequency generators then use high-speed switches called *inverters* to effectively "chop" the DC pulses into smaller and smaller pulses. Inverters can produce DC with up to 25,000 pulses/s. All of these pulses are then "smoothed" using additional rectifiers and capacitors so the x-ray tube receives voltage with less than 1% ripple. High-frequency generators enable shorter exposure times, lower radiation doses, and help extend the life of the x-ray tube. The x-ray beam intensity may be over 99% of peak output. In addition, many high-frequency generators are more compact, about 1/10 the size of a three-phase generator.

Operating console

The x-ray machine operating console includes controls to turn the equipment on and off and to adjust the mA, kVp, and the length of time the x-rays are being produced.

The **mA** (*milliamperes*) control regulates the quantity of x-rays produced. It determines the amount of current that is sent to the filament and therefore the number of electrons that are emitted. The higher the mA, the more electrons and the more x-rays. The mA control has no effect on the energy or penetrating power of the x-rays. Most x-ray machines provide fixed settings for mA (i.e., 100 mA, 200 mA, 300 mA).

The **kVp** (*kilovolt peak*) control primarily regulates the energy or quality of the x-rays. It regulates the amount of voltage that is sent to the x-ray tube which determines the speed of the electrons. The higher the kVp, the greater the kinetic energy of the electrons and the greater the energy of the x-rays.

The kVp control also contributes to the number of x-rays produced. Higher kVp means electrons are more quickly removed from the cloud, which allows more electrons to be emitted from the filament. More electrons leads to more x-rays.

The kVp control on most operating consoles displays continuously variable units of *kilovoltage* (kV). Voltage can be thought of as the "force" that moves the electrons from the cathode to the anode. Thousands of volts are required to accelerate the electrons with enough energy to create useful x-rays. The maximum speed of the electrons is determined by the maximum or **peak kilovoltage,** which is called **kVp**. It is important to realize that kVp determines the peak energy of the x-rays and not the total energy or the individual energy of the x-rays. This is because not all of the electrons will be moving at maximum speed (due to the sine wave distribution of the voltage, as shown in Figure 1.12). The slower electrons produce less energetic the x-rays. In addition, remember that many of the x-rays produced at the anode will be less than maximum energy due to Bremsstrahlung. Therefore, the average or effective energy of most x-ray beams is only about 1/3 of kVp. The effective energy can be increased to about 1/2 of kVp with high-efficiency generators and beam hardening (filtration).

The **exposure switch** is a manual control that is used to start the production of x-rays. The **timer** is an automatic control that stops x-ray production. The exposure switch typically operates in two stages: a *prep stage* and an *exposure stage*. The **prep stage** prepares the x-ray tube by rotating the anode and initiating the heating of the filament. It is important to make sure the anode is rotating at full speed before making an exposure, but it is equally important to avoid prolonged rotation as this will shorten the life of the x-ray tube. During the **exposure stage,** x-rays are being produced. The exposure stage is terminated automatically by the timer. There are a variety of timer mechanisms and most include a meter or digital display with units in fractions of a second (S) or milliseconds. In each case, the radiographer begins the exposure and the timer automatically stops it.

X-ray table

The x-ray machine table supports the patient during radiography. X-ray tables are made of strong materials with low x-ray attenuation, such as carbon fibers. Tables should be uniform in thickness and opacity and able to support at least 300 lb (136 kg). A slightly elevated rim or edge around the table top helps prevent liquids from spilling onto the floor or into the equipment under the table. Many x-ray tables include a built-in tray designed to hold a grid and various types and sizes of cassettes. The tray should be aligned with the x-ray tube so the two can be moved simultaneously.

Floating tables help facilitate patient positioning. Most floating table tops can easily be locked, unlocked, and moved in multiple horizontal directions. The tray under a floating table generally remains aligned with the x-ray tube while the tabletop is being moved. Tables that are height adjustable also facilitate patient positioning, especially given the variety of patient sizes commonly encountered in a veterinary practice.

Image receptors

Image receptors record the x-rays that pass through an object or patient. The x-rays received are used to form a **latent** image. The latent image is invisible and must be converted to a visible image for interpretation. Methods of conversion will be discussed shortly.

An image receptor must record all of the different x-ray intensities that emerge from a patient and accurately translate them into acceptable levels of radiographic density (visible shades of gray). The minimum number of x-rays a receptor can receive and still adequately darken the radiograph (produce a visible shade of gray) is known as its **sensitivity**. The more sensitive the system, the fewer x-rays are needed. An image receptor must also display each level of density (shade of gray) with enough contrast so one can be distinguished from the next. This is called the **dynamic range** or **latitude** of the receptor. Wide latitude receptors are able to form many shades of gray over a large range of x-ray intensities, which means they can display many different levels of opacity. Narrow latitude receptors form fewer shades of gray over a smaller range of x-ray intensities. Narrow latitude means fewer levels of opacity can be displayed. The amount of radiographic **detail** an image receptor can provide determines how well we can discriminate the edges of structures that are close together.

Currently, there are two basic types of image receptors: *film:screen* and *digital*. Both types are used with conventional x-ray machines.

Film:screen image receptors

The image receptors in traditional film radiography utilize special photographic film coupled with phosphorescent sheets called **screens**. The screens convert x-rays into visible light. X-ray film is much more sensitive to light than to x-rays so the screens act to *intensify* the effect of the x-rays on the film. This means fewer x-rays are needed to adequately expose the film when using an intensifying screen. In a typical film radiograph, over 95% of the film exposure is due to light from an intensifying screen and less than 5% is from the x-rays themselves. Intensifying screens enable lower x-ray exposures, less radiation dose, and longer life of the x-ray tube.

An **intensifying screen** consists of a thin polyester base coated on one side with phosphors. The phosphor layer is covered with a thin protective coating. The amount of light emitted by the phosphors is directly proportional to the amount of x-rays received by the screen. Most phosphors are either a *rare earth* material that emits a green light or *calcium tungstate* which emits blue light. Modern x-ray films are orthochromatic, which means the film is more sensitive to a specific color of light. It is important to match the phosphor emission color with the film absorption color.

X-ray film consists of a thin, flexible, polyester sheet coated on one or both sides with an emulsion that contains silver halide crystals. The emulsion is covered with a thin protective layer. The plastic base is transparent and often tinted blue to reduce eye strain.

Silver halide crystals become structurally altered when struck by light from an intensifying screen or from direct interaction with an x-ray. The altered crystals form the latent image. The latent image is then *processed* to become visible. Processing converts the altered silver halide crystals to black metallic silver. Film processing is discussed further below.

Both the intensifying screens and the x-ray film commonly are enclosed in a protective, light-proof container called a **cassette** (Figures 1.13 and 1.15). A cassette may contain one screen for use with single emulsion x-ray film or two screens for double emulsion film. It is important to load the cassette with the correct type of film. Cassettes are available in a variety of sizes that correspond to different film sizes. Most cassettes swing open on a hinge, making it easy to remove and load the film. Screens usually are permanently mounted in the cassette, often on a flexible foam pad to maintain close, uniform contact with the film. The back of the cassette frequently is made of a radiation absorbing material to block backscatter radiation.

Cassettes can last for a long time with proper care. They should be regularly inspected for damaged hinges, loose screens, light leaks, etc. (Box 1.3). Do not store cassettes in prolonged heat as this will damage the intensifying screens. Numbering each cassette is useful to help identify problems that may arise. Use a permanent marker to write the number on an inconspicuous part of a screen, such as near the ID label or in a corner (Figure 1.14). Write the same number on the outside of the cassette. If an artifact appears in a radiograph, you'll know which cassette to inspect for a possible cause.

A

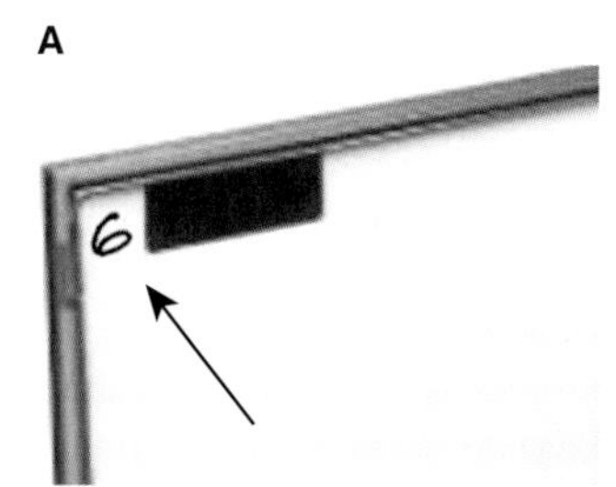

B

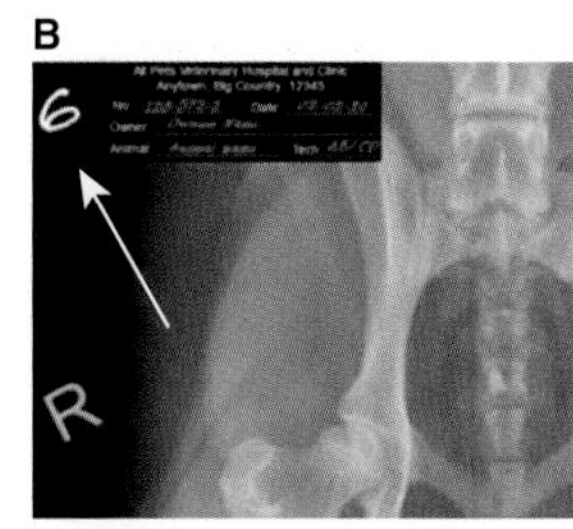

Figure 1.14 Numbered cassette. **A**. The number "6" is written on an intensifying screen (arrow) in the corner of an open cassette. **B**. In a radiograph made using this cassette, the number "6" is visible in the corner (arrow). Numbering the cassettes helps identify those with problems.

Film processing

The process of converting the invisible latent image into a visible radiograph involves immersing the film in different chemicals for specific periods of time. Film processing may be performed manually or automatically in a machine. With manual film processing, the chemical solutions are stored in dip tanks and the technician transfers the film from one tank to another, paying special attention to the time intervals (Box 1.4). With automatic processors, the film quickly moves from one solution to the next without human intervention. Automatic processors operate at higher temperatures to speed up the chemical reactions and shorten the processing time. The chemicals used in automatic processors differ from those used for manual processing in that they are specifically designed to work at high temperatures. Whether manual or automatic, film processing involves five basic steps:

Box 1.3 Caring for intensifying screens

1. Screens should be cleaned at least monthly with a gentle, antistatic cleaner and a soft, lint-free cloth. Stand the cassette on end while the screens are drying so dust doesn't collect on them.
2. Handle the screens carefully. They are coated with a thin protective layer but can easily be scratched. Scratches in screens are permanent.
3. Periodically inspect each screen for dirt, stains, scratches, etc., as these can produce radiographic artifacts. Use a UV light or a "black light" in a darkened room to see the damaged areas.

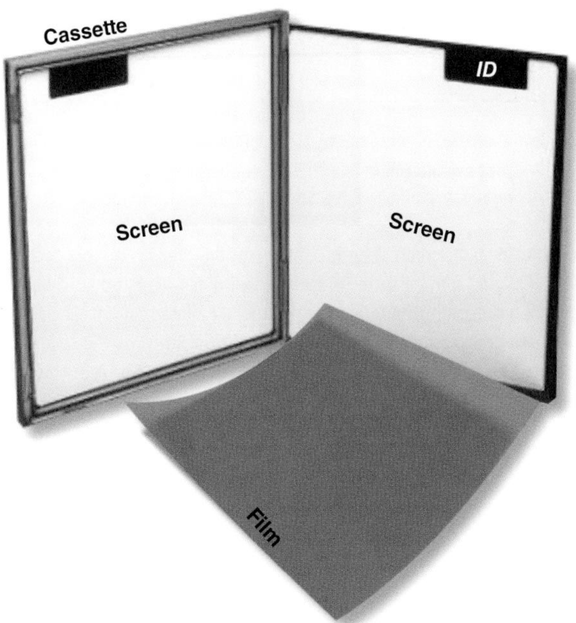

Figure 1.13 Film:screen image receptor. In this picture, the cassette is open and standing on end with a sheet of x-ray film in front. Intensifying screens are mounted inside the cassette, one on each side. The rectangular cutouts along the upper edge of each screen are for labeling the radiograph for identification (ID).

1. Develop.
2. Rinse.
3. Fix.
4. Wash.
5. Dry.

The **developer** is a chemical that converts the silver halide crystals to black metallic silver. The altered crystals are converted more quickly than the unaltered crystals, but given enough time the developer will eventually change all of the crystals to black. Therefore, the time the film spends in contact with the developer must be carefully controlled. Development is stopped by **rinsing** the film with water to dilute and remove the chemicals. Automatic processors incorporate rollers to squeeze the rinse water and chemicals away from the film.

The **fixer** is a chemical that dissolves any undeveloped silver halide crystals so they can be washed from the film. Fixer also "hardens" the film emulsion to help preserve the image. After an appropriate length of time in the fixer, the film is **washed** with water to remove the dissolved crystals and any chemicals. Automatic processors again use rollers to squeeze away the wash water and chemicals. The film is then **dried** for viewing and storage. Film radiographs should always receive a final viewing after they are dry, as the appearance of the radiograph may differ between wet and dry.

Film processing can significantly affect the quality of the radiograph. It is critical to maintain the developer and fixer at proper concentrations and temperatures per the manufacturer's recommendations. Pay special attention to film immersion times and sequences. Be careful to avoid rough handling of film and splashing of chemicals. All processing equipment should be periodically inspected to ensure peak performance and proper chemical replenishment rates.

Disposal of processing chemicals must be in accordance with environmental protection rules and regulations. Companies and special equipment are available for reclaiming silver from fixer and washer solutions and from x-ray film that is no longer needed. Reclaimed silver can be both environmentally and financially rewarding.

Film fog

Silver halide crystals can be altered by conditions other than light from intensifying screens or x-ray interactions. These include exposure to ambient light, heat, pressure, chemicals, and aging. Crystals that are altered by conditions other than those caused by x-rays add density to the radiograph, but do not provide any useful information. Unwanted blackening of x-ray film is called *fog*. Fog makes it more difficult to identify structures in the image (Figure 1.16 and 1.36). Many of the causes of x-ray film fog can be avoided if we know about them. See the Artifacts section in Chapter 2 for figures depicting film fog.

Light fog is caused by exposing unprocessed x-ray film to visible light. Light fog can be avoided by storing unused film in light-proof containers. Also, make sure the darkroom is light-proof, and the safelight is the correct color and intensity (see safelight test in the Artifacts section of Chapter 2). Static electricity is a common cause of light fog and can be minimized by electrically grounding darkroom personnel, controlling the humidity, and carefully handling the x-ray film.

Heat fog is caused by prolonged exposure of unprocessed x-ray film to temperatures above 70 °F (20 °C). Avoid heat fog by storing unused film in a controlled environment.

Pressure fog is caused by physically compressing unprocessed x-ray film. Pressure fog can result from storing boxes of unused film flat instead of upright. Over time the weight of the top sheets will fog the bottom sheets. Pressure fog also

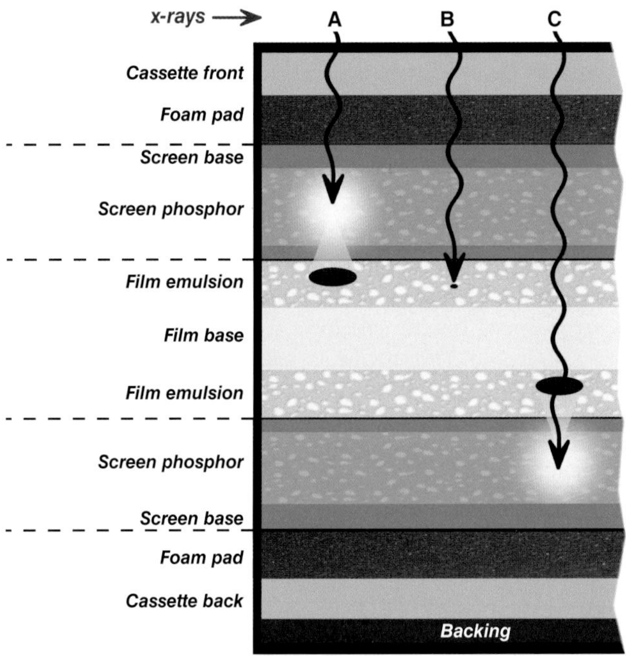

Figure 1.15 Film:screen system. This illustration depicts a cross-sectional view of a loaded film cassette. A sheet of x-ray film (colored light blue) is sandwiched between two intensifying screens (colored green). The film is coated with emulsion on both sides. Three x-rays, labeled A, B, and C, are depicted interacting with the film:screen system. **X-ray A** strikes a phosphor in the top screen causing it to emit light in all directions. The light that hits the film alters some silver halide crystals in the upper film emulsion, which will produce a black area when the film is developed (depicted by the black oval). **X-ray B** passes through the top screen without interacting with any phosphors and strikes the film directly. It alters fewer silver halide crystals than light from the screen (thus, a smaller black oval will be produced when the film is developed). **X-ray C** passes through all of the upper layers to strike a phosphor in the bottom screen. The light emitted from the screen travels in all directions and alters some of the silver halide crystals in the bottom film emulsion. This is the advantage of double emulsion x-ray film: it increases the likelihood of x-ray detection so fewer x-rays are needed to produce acceptable radiographic density. The backing in the cassette is designed to block backscatter x-rays from exposing the film.

Box 1.4 TIPS for manual film processing

- Keep the developer and fixer tanks covered to reduce evaporation and chemical breakdown.
- An aquarium heater in the water bath is helpful to maintain proper temperature.
- Thoroughly mix both the developer and fixer solutions prior to each use.
- Agitate the film for a second or two while it is immersed to ensure good contact with the chemicals and to dislodge any air bubbles.
- Do not allow the solution clinging to the film to drain back into the tank for more than 2 seconds; used solution will weaken the remaining chemicals.
- Make sure the darkroom has an exhaust fan that is in use whenever the room is occupied; this is an OSHA requirement in the United States.

A

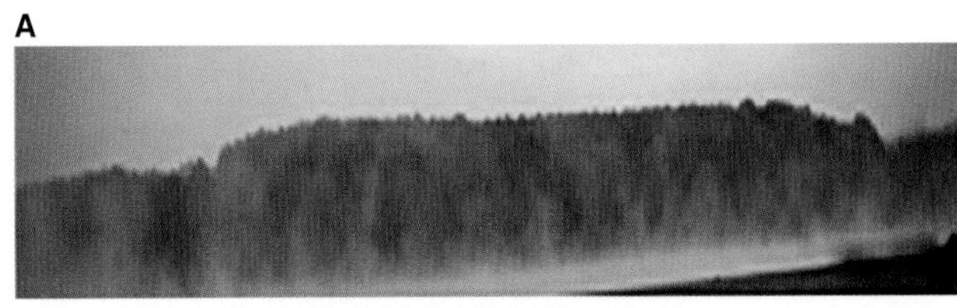

B

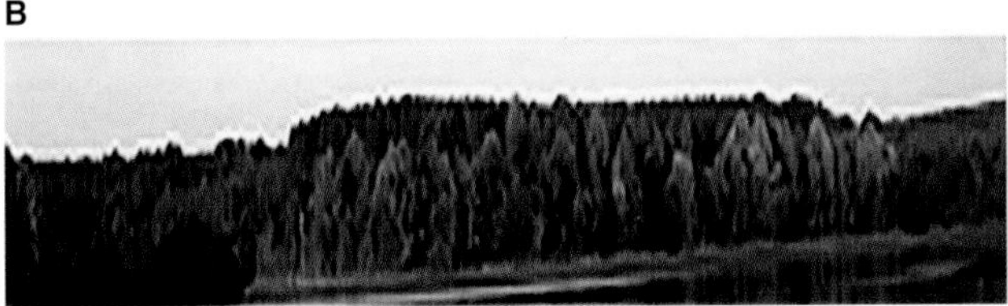

Figure 1.16 Fog. Two photographs of a lakeshore depicting the appearance of structures with fog (**A**) and without fog (**B**).

is caused by bending or creasing the film (Figure A23) or by sliding it across a table or countertop.

Chemical fog is caused by exposing unprocessed x-ray film to the vapors from cleaning solutions, ammonia, formaldehyde, spare developer, and others. Avoid chemical fog by storing unused film away from these and similar agents and making sure your fingers are clean and dry before handling the film.

Aging fog occurs with expired x-ray film. Over time, the unused film will "self-process" and become darker. Aging fog can be avoided by paying attention to expiration dates and not using expired film for radiography.

Characteristics of film:screen systems

The thickness of the emulsions and the sizes of the *grains* in a film:screen image receptor determine its sensitivity and the amount of radiographic detail it can provide. **Grains** are the silver halide crystals in the film emulsion and the phosphors in the intensifying screens. Both sensitivity and detail are directly related to the sizes of the grains, but they are inversely related to each other. The larger the grains, the more sensitive the system, but the less detail it will provide. The smaller the grains, the better the detail, but more x-rays will be needed to adequately darken the image.

Sensitivity in film radiography sometimes is called **speed**. Speed is a term from the early days of radiography when the x-ray machine controls for mA and kVp were limited and setting the exposure time was the most variable factor. Film:screen systems that could accommodate short exposure times and still produce acceptable density in a radiograph were called *high speed*. Systems that required longer exposure times were called *slow speed*. The term "speed" has persisted even though modern x-ray machines allow intricate mA and kVp manipulations in addition to exposure times.

The **sensitivity** and **detail** of a film:screen system is built-in. The only way to change it is to switch to a system with different size grains or a different emulsion thickness. A film:screen system with larger grains can produce acceptable radiographic density with fewer x-rays. When fewer x-rays are needed, shorter exposure times are possible and larger body parts can be imaged. However, radiographic detail will suffer because larger grains are more visible in the film radiograph, resulting in a "mottled" or "grainy" appearance. A film:screen system with smaller grains produces better detail, however, higher x-ray exposures will be needed to adequately darken the radiographs. High detail film:screen systems generally are limited to imaging smaller body parts.

Digital image receptors

Digital image receptors convert x-rays into electronic signals. The signals are then digitized and sent to a computer. The computer transforms the digital image into an analog radiograph so it can be viewed and interpreted by humans. Newer technologies are constantly evolving and digital systems are continuing to improve. The currently available systems may be broadly classified as either *CR* (*computed radiography*) or *DR* (*digital radiography*). DR systems can be further divided into three general categories: (1) those that directly convert x-rays into electronic signals, (2) those that indirectly convert x-rays into electronic signals, and (3) CCD, which stands for *charged coupling device*. Whether CR or DR, all-digital image receptors incorporate four basic steps:

1. Capture the x-rays to form a latent image.
2. Translate the latent image into electronic signals.
3. Convert the signals to digital data for the computer.
4. Process the data to form an analog image.

Computed radiography

A computed radiography (CR) image receptor captures x-rays using an imaging plate with *photostimulable storage phosphors* (PSP). The imaging plate is enclosed in a cassette that is similar in size, look, and feel to the cassettes used in film radiography (Figure 1.17). CR and film:screen sometimes are called "cassette radiography."

When exposed to x-rays, PSP temporarily stores captured x-ray energy to form a latent image. After exposure, the CR cassette is manually transferred to a machine that removes the imaging plate and scans it with a laser beam (Figure 1.18). The laser light stimulates the PSP to release the stored x-ray energy as light, a process known as *photostimulation*. The amount of light emitted is proportional to the captured x-ray energy. A light guide collects the emitted light and sends it to a photomultiplier tube (PMT). The PMT converts the light into electronic signals, amplifies the signals, and sends them to an analog-to-digital converter (ADC). The ADC digitizes the signals and sends them to a computer for processing. While it is scanning the imaging plate, the laser removes most of the latent image. Any remaining latent image is erased by exposing the plate to bright light, making the cassette immediately ready for re-use. With proper care, CR cassettes can be used thousands of times.

CR imaging plates are always "on," meaning they are always sensitive to nearby radiation. Nearby radiation includes that coming from the environment (background radiation) and scatter from radiographing other patients. CR cassettes should not be stored near the x-ray machine and any cassettes that haven't been used for several days should be placed in the CR reader and erased prior to use.

CR image receptors have been around since the mid-1980s and closely emulate traditional film:screen systems. They are compatible with most existing x-ray facilities and often utilize the same exposure techniques as for film radiography. CR cassettes are portable, enabling them to be used with multiple radiography facilities and different x-ray machines as well as for positional radiography and both table-top and under-the-table techniques. The initial cost of a CR system often is lower than many DR systems. Compared to DR, however, CR requires more user intervention, which means it takes longer to complete a radiographic study and patient throughput is slower.

Digital radiography

Digital radiography (DR) image receptors capture x-rays using either a *photoconductor* or a *scintillator*. A photoconductor translates x-ray energy directly into electrical charge as a one-step process. A scintillator is a crystalline structure that converts x-ray energy into visible light and then channels that light through thin crystals to a photodiode. The photodiode converts the light into electrical charge. This is a two-step process that indirectly converts x-ray energy into electrical charge. Whether formed directly or indirectly, the electrical charge is proportional to the energy of the x-rays and forms the latent image.

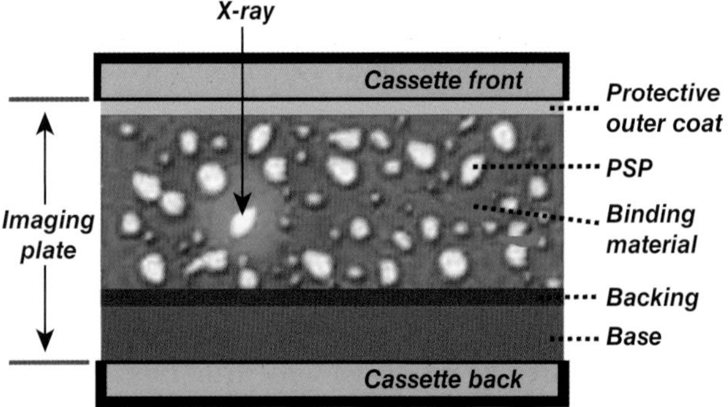

Figure 1.17 CR image receptor. This illustration depicts a cross-sectional view of a CR cassette. The typical CR imaging plate is about 0.3 mm thick and composed of a stiff base material coated with a layer of photostimulable phosphors (PSP). The PSP grains are held in a polymer binding material. They absorb and temporarily store x-ray energy. The surface of the imaging plate is protected by a tough plastic coating. The backing material between the base and the PSP layer is designed to block backscatter x-rays.

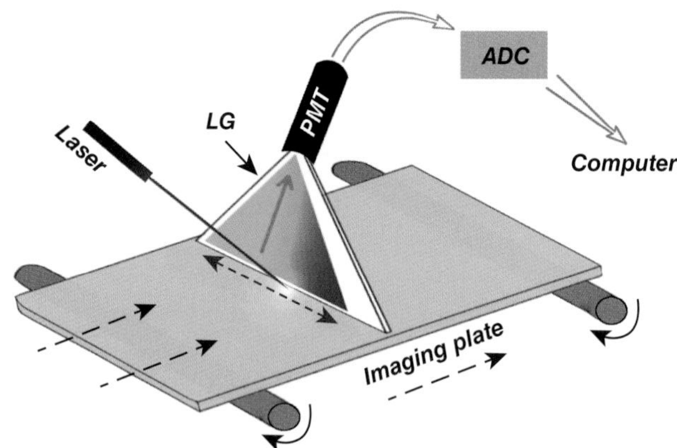

Figure 1.18 CR read-out. This illustration depicts a CR imaging plate inside the CR reader. The plate is transported along rollers as a laser beam sweeps back and forth scanning the latent image. The red laser light stimulates the phosphors to release their stored energy as blue light. The blue light is captured in a light guide (LG) and channeled to a photomultiplier tube (PMT). The PMT converts the light into electronic signals and sends them to an analog-to-digital converter (ADC). The ADC digitizes the signals and sends them to a computer for processing and analog display.

Transistors are used to convert electrical charge into electrical signals. Each transistor contains a detector element that corresponds to a pixel in the digital radiograph. A group of thin-film transistors called a *TFT array* produces the electronic signals, which are then digitized by an ADC and forwarded to a computer (Figure 1.19).

A **charged coupling device** (CCD) is a type of indirect DR image receptor. A CCD uses a scintillator to convert x-rays to light which is collected by an optical system. The optical system may consist of mirrors, lenses, prisms, or fiber optics. It captures the light and sends it to an array of CCD sensors. CCD sensors both convert the light into electrical charge and convert the electrical charge into electronic signals, without the need for photodiodes or a TFT array. CCD sensors are incorporated in many digital cameras.

As opposed to CR systems, DR image receptors convert captured x-rays into electronic signals without the need for user intervention (Figure 1.20). In addition, DR systems are linked directly to a computer which further reduces the time needed to complete a radiography study. Compared to CR and film radiography, DR systems enable faster patient throughput and shorter turnaround times. DR image receptors can be permanently mounted under the x-ray table, or they can remain portable for tabletop use and positional radiography (Figure 1.21).

Characteristics of digital systems

Unlike film:screen systems, digital image receptors do not have a fixed sensitivity. They are able to capture many more of the incident x-rays and successfully convert them into acceptable radiographic density. How accurately and

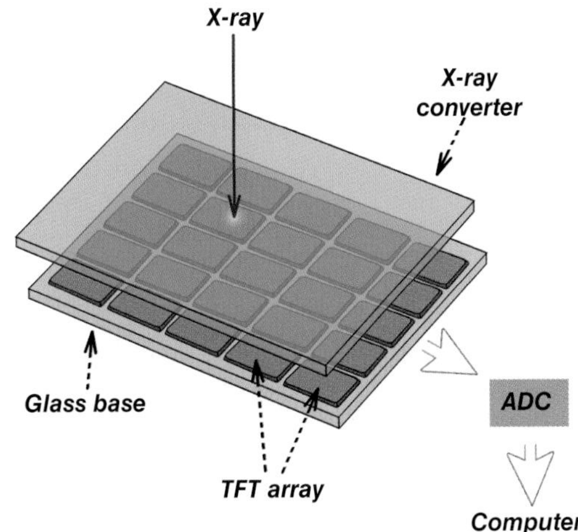

Figure 1.19 DR image receptor. This illustration depicts the key components in a DR image receptor. The x-ray converter either directly or indirectly translates x-ray energy into an electrical charge. It is layered over a thin film transistor array which is mounted on a glass base. The TFT array converts electrical charge to electronic signals and sends them to an analog-to-digital converter, where they are digitized and sent to a computer.

efficiently a digital receptor does this is described by various measurements including the *modulator transfer function* and the *detective quantum efficiency*, both of which are briefly discussed below.

Not all parts of a digital image receptor can convert x-rays into electronic signals. This means that digital sensitivity is affected not only by the number of x-rays that reach the receptor but also where they land. The area of the receptor that is sensitive to x-rays in relation to the total area of the receptor is called the **fill factor**. The larger the fill factor, the fewer x-rays will be needed to produce adequate density.

Modulator transfer function (**MTF**) measures how accurately a digital receptor transfers the different x-ray intensities into different levels of radiographic density. The higher the MTF, the more different opacities can be displayed. MTF ranges from 0 (no structures in the patient are visible) to 1 (all structures are visible). An MTF of 0.5 means the receptor can display 50% of the differences in opacity as different radiographic densities.

Detective quantum efficiency (**DQE**) measures how efficiently a digital receptor captures the x-rays it receives and converts them into acceptable radiographic density. The higher the DQE, the fewer x-rays are needed. For example, a DQE of 0.4 means the receptor can utilize 40% of the x-rays it receives. DQE is the ratio of input SNR to output SNR (SNR is signal-to-noise ratio). The higher the DQE, the better the radiographic detail.

The **exposure index** (**EI**) is a measure of the amount of x-rays the digital image receptor actually received during the making of a particular radiograph. EI was standardized in 2018 and can be used to compare the sensitivities of different digital systems. EI is especially valuable to determine whether the exposure used was too high. In these cases, EI can be used to limit **dose creep**. Dose creep refers to the unnecessarily high radiation doses that frequently are encountered in digital radiography (dose creep is discussed later in this chapter).

EI is directly related to the x-ray exposure dose. With most digital radiography systems, it should be in range of 1700–2100. If the exposure is doubled, the EI increases by 300. If the exposure is cut in half, the EI decreases by 300. Here's how EI can be used: suppose a particular radiographic study resulted in an EI of 2500. An EI of 2500 is above the desired range of 1700–2100. This means the exposure used was too high and the radiograph should be overexposed. However, most digital systems can still display a good quality radiograph from an overexposure, so the image may appear acceptable. But the radiation dose to the patient and nearby personnel was too high. Overexposures need to be discussed with staff and prevented whenever possible. Any future

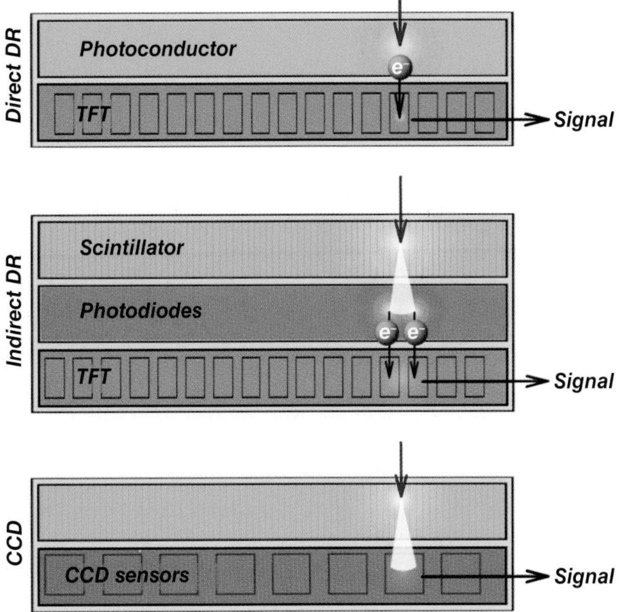

Figure 1.20 Types of DR image receptors. These illustrations highlight the different methods of converting x-ray energy into electronic signals, which are then sent to be digitized and processed by a computer. **Direct DR systems** (**A**) capture x-ray energy using a photoconductor which directly translate the energy into electrical charge (e^-). The TFT array converts the electrical charge to electronic signals. **Indirect DR systems** (**B**) use a scintillator to convert captured x-ray energy into visible light. The thin, needle-shaped crystals in the scintillator channel the light to photodiodes, where it is converted into electrical charge (e^-). Electrical charge is then converted to electronic signals by the TFT array. CCD (**C**) also uses a scintillator to convert captured x-ray energy to light, but special sensors then convert both the light into electrical charge and the electrical charge into electronic signals.

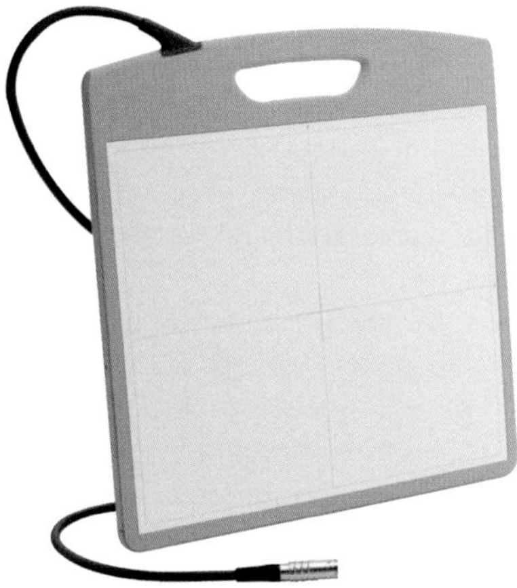

Figure 1.21 DR image receptor. This picture depicts a type of portable DR image receptor that can be positioned under the x-ray table or table-top and can be used for positional radiography. It is shown with a cable to link it to a computer, but some models are available as wireless units.

images of this patient should be made using lower exposure. To bring an EI of 2500 into the desired range, we would cut the mAs in half (which reduces the EI by 300 to an EI of 2200) and cut the mAs in half again (which reduces the EI another 300 to an EI of 1900, which is in the desired range).

Sensitivity number (**S-number**) is inversely proportional to x-ray exposure. As exposure increases, the S-number decreases. For most radiographic studies, the S-number should be between 200 and 300. For example, a radiograph made with an S-number of 100 is below the desired range of 200–300. This means the exposure used was too high (about twice what was needed). Future radiographs should be made with half the mAs, which would make the S-number 200 and in the acceptable range. Another example: a radiograph made with an S-number of 1200 is above the desired range of 200–300, which means the exposure was too low. Future exposures should be higher. Doubling the mAs reduces the S-number to 600 and doubling the mAs again decreases the S-number to 300, which is in the desired range.

The amount of **radiographic contrast** a digital receptor can display is determined by its **pixels**. "Pixel" is short for *picture element*. Pixels are the smallest pieces of a digital radiograph. Each pixel can appear as any of several different shades of gray, depending on its pixel number. Pixel numbers are **binary numbers**. Binary is a "base 2" numbering system that is used by computers, as opposed the "base 10" numbering system we humans use in our everyday lives (i.e., a decimal system). Each digit in a binary number is called a **bit**. "Bit" is short for binary digit, and it is the smallest unit of digital data. Each bit is a digit in a binary number and is assigned a value of either 0 or 1. The position of each bit in the binary number represents an exponent of 2. In the decimal system, the position of each digit represents an exponent of 10.

In digital radiography, the contrast in an image can be adjusted after the radiograph has been acquired. This is a tremendous advantage over film radiography. Digital contrast can be optimized using the large amount of data in each pixel. Computer processing and user manipulations determine the best shades of gray for the pixels to display. However, for a computer to produce quality radiographs, it requires a properly calibrated image receptor and correct input from the user. The method of receptor calibration usually is built into each manufacturer's system. Calibrations should be done per the manufacturer recommendations prior to radiography to correct any defects, imperfections, and non-uniformities in the image receptor.

Geometry of the x-ray beam

It is essential to understand the effects of x-ray beam geometry and how to use them to make quality radiographs. The radiographic appearance of an object is greatly influenced by its position and orientation relative to the x-ray beam and to the image receptor.

Focal spot

The focal spot is the source of x-rays. It is the point on the anode target that is struck by the high-speed stream of electrons. The focal spot, however, is not a tiny dot without length or width; it has dimensions. X-rays are emitted from all parts of the focal spot and travel in straight lines in all directions. The x-rays coming from one side of the focal spot overlap with those coming from the other side. This overlap makes the edges of objects appear blurry in the radiograph (Figure 1.22). Edge-blurring is called **geometric unsharpness**. Geometric unsharpness reduces radiographic detail, making it more difficult to distinguish two objects that are close together. Edge-blurring sometimes is called *penumbra*, which is an astronomy term used to describe the fuzzy-edged shadow cast by the moon during a partial eclipse. The term *umbra* refers to the more sharply defined center part of the shadow.

The degree of geometric unsharpness depends on the ratios of the distances between the focal spot, the object, and the image receptor and on the size of the focal spot. These ratios are explained in greater detail when we discuss distortion later in this chapter. The size of the focal spot may be altered by changing its physical size or its effective size. The smaller the focal spot, the less geometric unsharpness and the better the radiographic detail.

The **physical size of a focal spot** is fixed by the x-ray tube manufacturer. Most x-ray tubes are equipped with two focal spots; a small one and a large one (Figure 1.23). A small focal spot typically is about 0.5–1.0 mm in size and a large

A

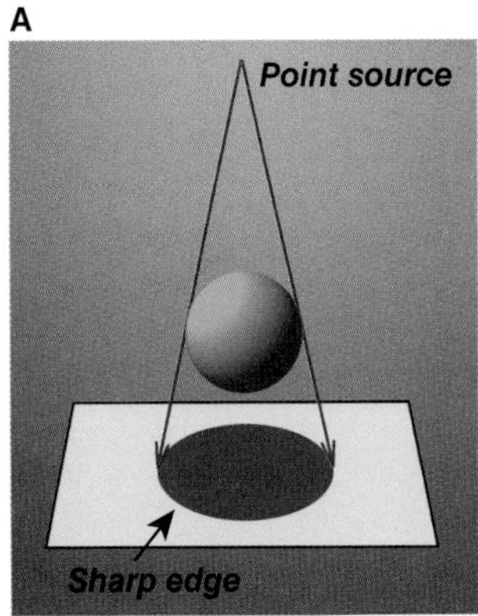

B

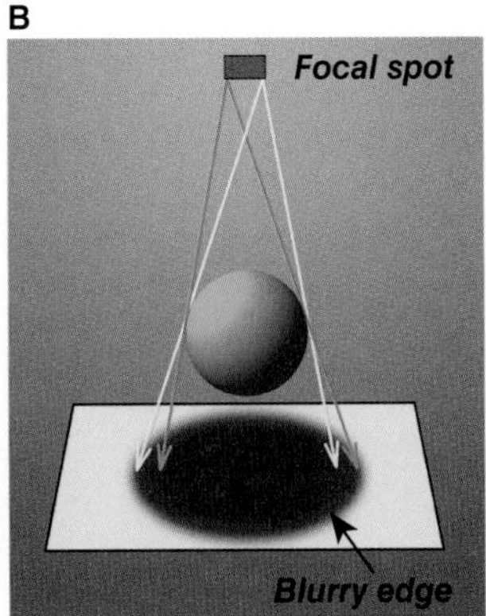

Figure 1.22 Geometric unsharpness. If x-rays originated from a point source, as shown in illustration **A**, the margin of the object would appear sharp in the image below. However, x-rays originate from a focal spot with dimensions, as shown in illustration **B**. X-rays coming from one side of the focal spot (orange arrows) overlap with those coming from the other side (yellow arrows), which causes the object margin to appear blurred in the image below.

focal spot is about 1.0–2.0 mm. The small focal spot produces better radiographic detail than the large focal spot, but it is less tolerant of heat. Fewer and less energetic x-rays can be produced at the small focal spot, which generally limits its use to body parts measuring less than 10–12 cm thick. The large focal spot is more heat tolerant and allows greater x-ray exposures, shorter exposure times, and imaging of larger body parts, but there is less radiographic detail.

The **effective size of the focal spot** can be altered using the *line focus principle*. The line focus principle states that viewing a sloped surface at an angle reduces its apparent size. This is why the anode disc is beveled. Tilting the anode target makes the focal spot appear smaller (Figure 1.24).

The effective focal spot size also can be reduced by moving the x-ray tube further away from the image receptor. With increased distance, the focal spot more closely resembles a point source. The greater the distance, the better the radiographic detail. However, as you increase the distance, the x-ray exposure must be increased exponentially to maintain radiographic density. If you double the distance, you will need four times the x-ray exposure due to the *inverse square law*.

Inverse square law

The inverse square law occurs because x-rays diverge as they move away from the focal spot, spreading out over larger and larger areas (Figure 1.25). This means that there are fewer x-rays per unit area (less x-ray beam intensity) as you move further away from the source. The decrease in x-ray beam intensity is inversely proportional to the square of the distance from the focal spot: $I = 1/D^2$, where "I" is the intensity of the x-ray beam and "D" is the distance from the focal spot.

Heel effect

Because the target is angled to create a smaller effective focal spot, the bottom of the anode is thicker. The thicker bottom commonly is called the "heel" of the anode. The heel absorbs some of the x-rays produced at the focal spot. Absorption results in fewer x-rays being emitted from the anode side of the x-ray tube and more x-rays coming from the cathode side. The heel effect can produce as much as a 40% difference in x-ray beam intensity between the anode side and the cathode side of the x-ray tube (Figure 1.26). This difference is useful when imaging body parts that vary in thickness or opacity. The thicker or more opaque end of the body part is positioned toward the cathode side where the x-ray beam is more penetrating. Remember, the word "cathode" has more letters than the word "anode" and more x-rays come from the cathode side than the anode side. The heel effect is most noticeable when using a:

1. Large FOV.
2. Lower x-ray exposure.
3. Short distance between the x-ray tube and the image receptor.

Distortion

Distortion occurs when an object's actual size or shape is misrepresented in the radiograph. It is caused by equal or unequal magnification of the object. Equal magnification makes an object appear overall larger in the radiograph than its actual size. Unequal magnification causes *foreshortening* or *elongation* distortion which are described below. Any form of

A

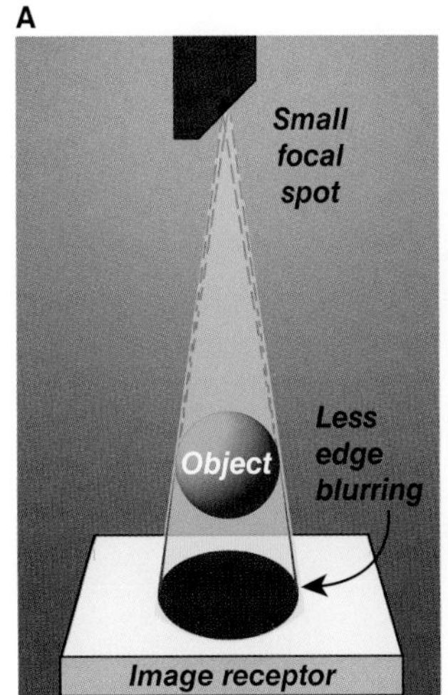

B

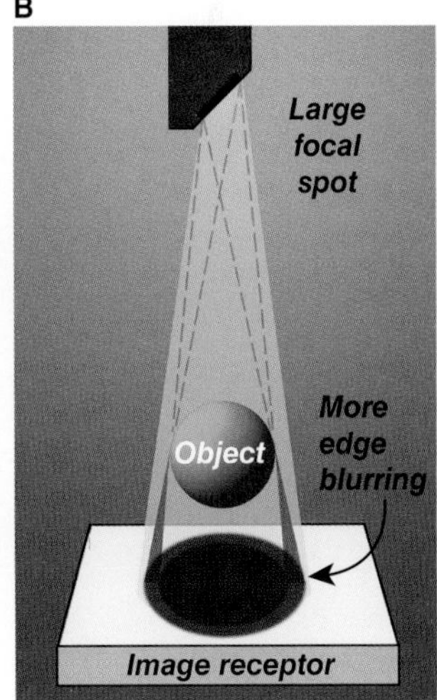

Figure 1.23 Physical size of the focal spot. These illustrations depict the effect of focal spot size on edge sharpness. The anode is shown in red at the top of each image. (**A**) With a small focal spot there is less overlap of the x-rays and less blurring of the object margin in the image below. (**B**) With a larger the focal spot there is greater overlap of x-rays and more geometric unsharpness.

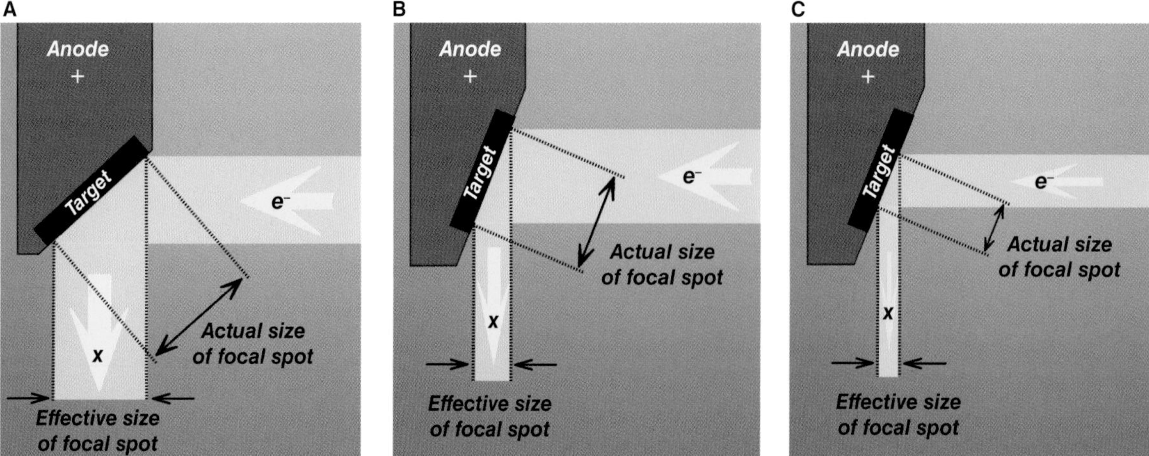

Figure 1.24 Line focus principle. These illustrations depict variations in the effective size of the focal spot due to the slope of the anode target and the size of the electron beam (e^-). The steeper the slope, the smaller the effective size of the focal spot. The actual size of the focal spot is determined by the size of the electron beam. (**A**) 45° slope. (**B**) 20° slope. (**C**) The actual size of the focal spot is smaller because the stream of electrons is smaller (due to using a smaller filament). x = x-rays.

magnification also causes geometric unsharpness. There are three distances that are important in distortion:

1. Distance between the focal spot and the image receptor: the **source-to-image distance** or **SID**.
2. Distance between the focal spot and the object: the **source-to-object distance** or **SOD**.
3. Distance between the object and the image receptor, the **object-to-image distance** or **OID**.

It is the ratio between any two of these distances that is important when dealing with magnification and geometric unsharpness (Figure 1.27). To minimize magnification, we want the object to be as close to the image receptor as possible (OID as short as practical). The degree of magnification is determined by the ratio of SID to SOD (SID/SOD is called the *magnification factor*). The closer the ratio is to 1.0, the less magnification (Figure 1.28).

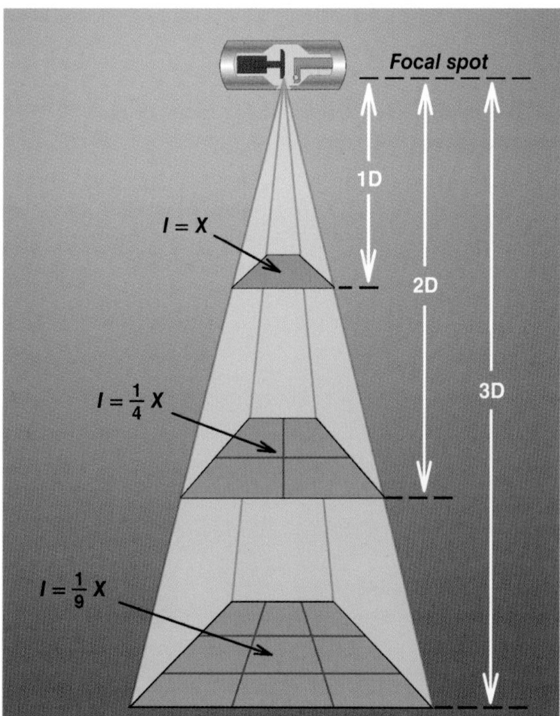

Figure 1.25 Inverse square law. This illustration depicts the divergence of x-rays as they move further from the focal spot. The x-rays spread out over a larger and larger area as the distance (*D*) increases. The intensity (*I*) of the x-ray beam is inversely proportional to the square of the distance from the focal spot: $I = 1/D^2$. Doubling the distance decreases the x-ray beam intensity to 1/4 *x*.

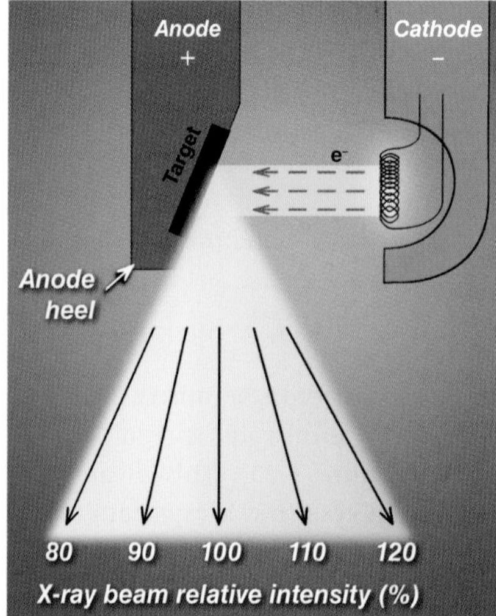

Figure 1.26 Heel effect. More x-rays are emitted from the cathode side of the x-ray tube than from the anode side because some of the x-rays produced are absorbed in the anode heel. There is a gradual loss of x-ray beam intensity moving from cathode side to anode side.

A

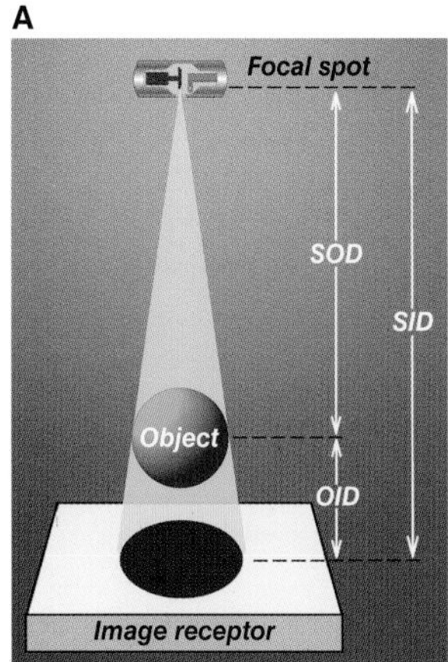

B

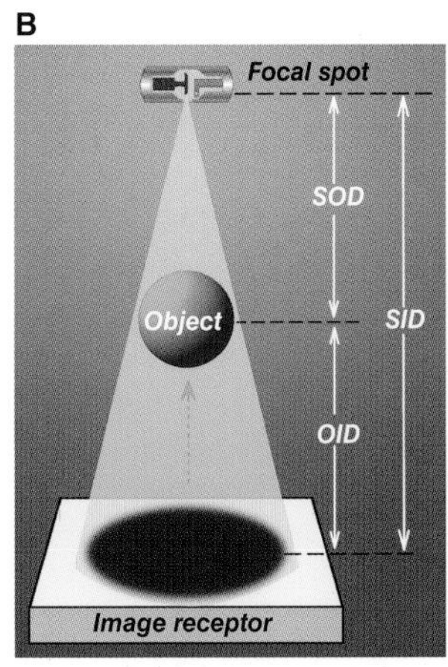

C

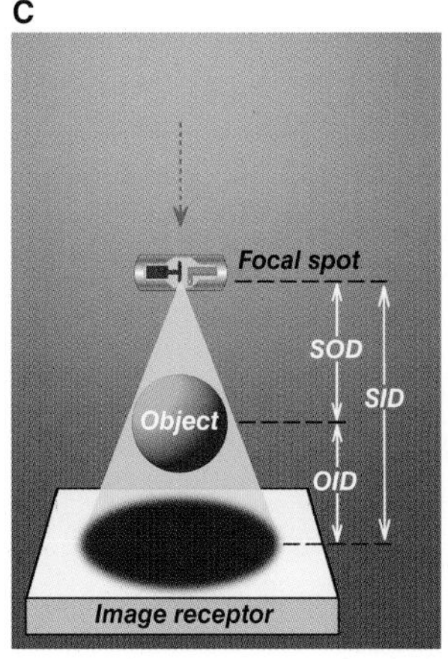

D

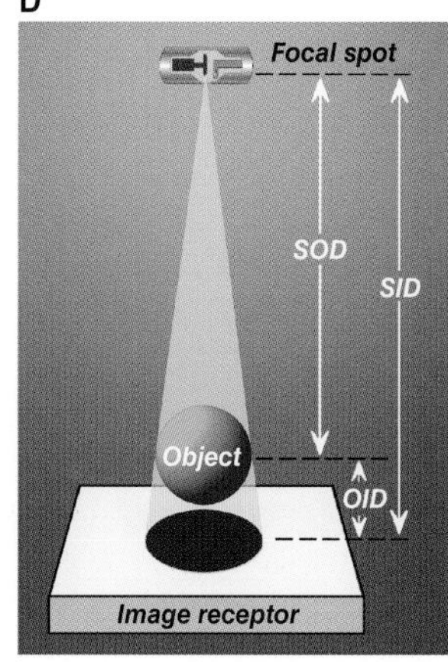

Figure 1.27 Magnification. (**A**) Source-to-image distance (SID), source-to-object distance (SOD), and object-to-image distance (OID) are illustrated. (**B**) Increasing the OID (moving the object further away from the image receptor) while maintaining the same SID creates magnification distortion and geometric unsharpness. (**C**) Shortening the SID (moving the x-ray tube closer to the image receptor) while maintaining the same OID also creates magnification. (**D**) Shortening the OID (placing the object closer to the image receptor, such as using a table-top-technique instead of under the table) and using the same SID will lessen magnification.

Sometimes magnification is desired. Here is an example: suppose we want to make a radiograph that displays the magnification of a paw. We position the patient's foot on a cardboard box or foam block to move it further away from the image receptor, increasing the OID. This will cause magnification and geometric unsharpness. To minimize the edge-blurring, we use the small focal spot and move the x-ray tube further away, increasing the SID. Because the SID is longer, the x-ray exposure needs to be increased due to the inverse square law, so we increase the mAs.

Both **elongation distortion** and **foreshortening distortion** occur when the position of an object is oblique to the x-ray beam or image receptor. Oblique positioning makes the OID longer on one side of the object than the other. When one side is magnified more than the other the shape of the object is distorted. Unequal magnification also can occur if the image receptor is obliquely positioned in relation to the object or x-ray beam. Foreshortening distortion makes an object appear overall shorter in the radiograph than its actual size (Figure 1.29). Elongation distortion makes an object appear overall longer than its actual size (Figures 1.30 and 1.31).

Elongation also occurs in objects that are off-center to the x-ray beam. Because x-rays diverge, objects nearest the center of the beam will be imaged more accurately than objects at the periphery of the beam. All peripheral objects in a radiograph suffer some degree of elongation distortion. For example, when imaging the spine only the vertebrae and intervertebral disc spaces in the center of the image are accurately depicted for size and shape. The peripheral vertebrae are more elongated than actual, which may be mistaken for narrowed intervertebral disc spaces. Another example is the appearance of the cardiac silhouette at the periphery of an abdominal radiograph. Due to elongation distortion the cardiac silhouette is distorted and may appear longer than actual, which may be mistaken for cardiomegaly.

To minimize distortion, position the object of interest as close to the image receptor as practical (minimize the OID), align the object with the center of the x-ray beam, and collimate the FOV as small as practical. When interpreting radiographic findings, be aware of distortion artifacts.

A

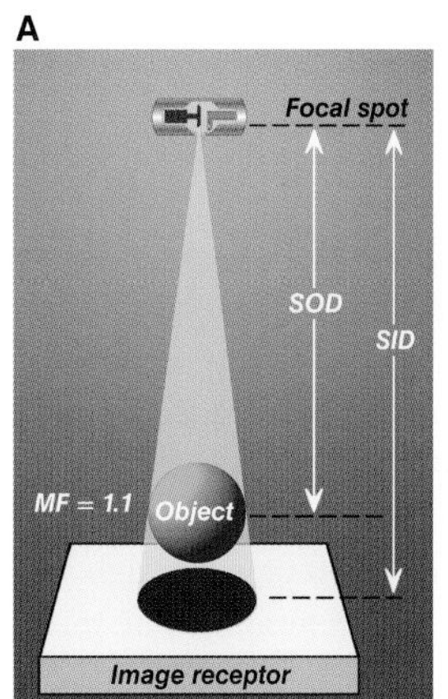

B

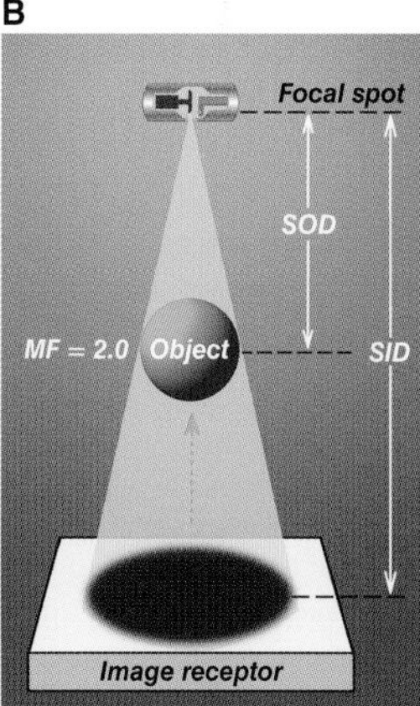

Figure 1.28 Magnification factor. Illustration **A** depicts an object close to the image receptor with little magnification. The SID and SOD are similar resulting in a magnification factor (MF) near 1.0. In illustration **B**, the object is further from the image receptor, resulting in magnification and geometric unsharpness. The object appears twice as large in the image as actual size (magnification factor is 2.0).

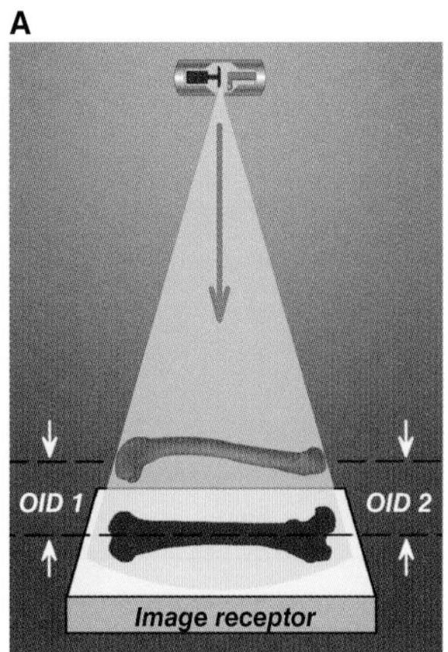

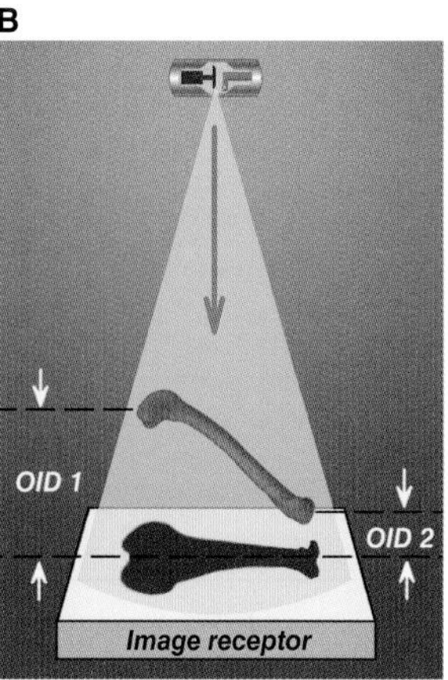

Figure 1.29 Foreshortening distortion. **A**. The long axis of the bone is parallel with the image receptor and perpendicular to the x-ray beam and therefore its size and shape are accurately represented in the image below. **B**. The bone is tilted in relation to the image receptor and oblique to the x-ray beam so that it appears shorter than actual and abnormal in shape due to unequal magnification.

X-ray interactions with matter

Each x-ray that enters a material will result in one of three possible outcomes: (1) it may be *transmitted*, passing through the material unchanged, (2) it may be *absorbed* and completely disappear inside the material, or (3) it may be *scattered*, becoming a secondary x-ray that travels in a new direction with less energy (Figure 1.32). Transmitted and absorbed x-rays are valuable to make radiographs. Scatter x-rays provide no useful diagnostic information, degrade image quality, and expose the patient and nearby personnel to unnecessary radiation.

Transmitted x-rays that reach the image receptor and are recorded produce useful blackened areas in a radiograph (i.e., radiographic density). The more transmitted x-rays, the darker that part of the image. The likelihood of an x-ray being transmitted is affected by its energy. The higher the energy, the more penetrating the x-ray. Recall that x-ray energy is controlled by kVp, so the higher the kVp, the more transmitted x-rays and the darker the radiograph. The likelihood of x-ray transmission also is affected by the opacity of the material. The greater the opacity, the fewer x-rays will pass through. Higher opacity materials appear lighter in radiographs. The mAs also will affect the number of transmitted x-rays because mAs affects the overall quantity of x-rays produced. The higher the mAs, the greater the number of transmitted x-rays.

Absorbed x-rays never reach the image receptor and therefore produce no radiographic density. The more absorbed x-rays, the lighter or brighter that part of the image. In medical radiography, x-ray absorption primarily occurs via the *photoelectric effect*.

The **photoelectric effect** is similar to characteristic x-ray production (Figure 1.5) except it is an x-ray instead of a high-speed electron that collides with an atom. The x-ray transfers all of its energy to an inner level electron, ejecting the electron and ionizing the atom (Figure 1.33). The ejected electron travels a short distance before losing its energy to other atoms along its path. Both the ionization of the atom and the energy from the ejected electron can damage or destroy living cells. Ionized atoms are unstable so a higher energy outer level electron drops down to fill the void in the inner level. The outer level electron loses energy in the form

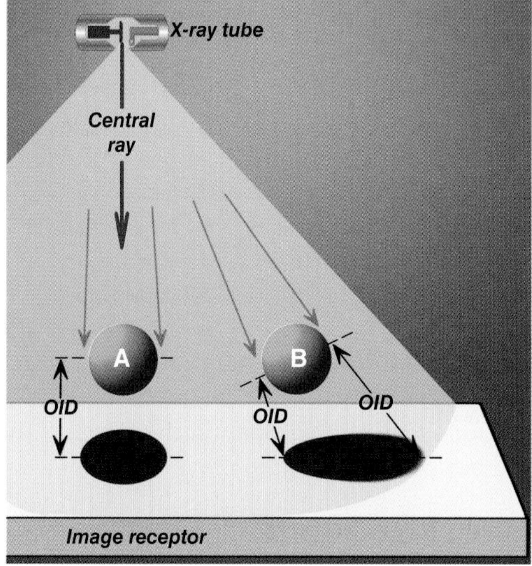

Figure 1.30 Elongation distortion. Object **A** is aligned with the central ray (red arrow) resulting in an accurate depiction of its size and shape in the image below. Object **B** is off-center, peripheral to the central ray, making it appear longer and more ovoid than actual in the image below.

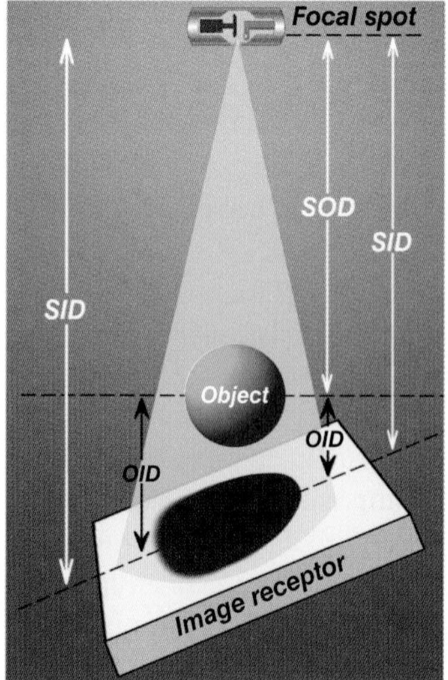

Figure 1.31 Elongation distortion. In this illustration the image receptor is tilted in relation to the x-ray beam and object resulting in unequal magnification. The OID is longer on one side than the other, which distorts the shape of the object and causes geometric unsharpness on that side.

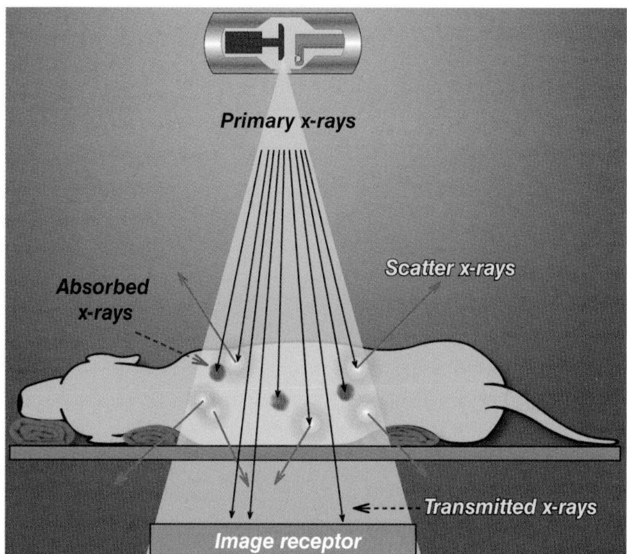

Figure 1.32 X-ray interactions. X-rays produced in the x-ray tube are called *primary* x-rays. Primary x-rays that pass through the patient unchanged are *transmitted* x-rays. Primary x-rays that interact with atoms in the patient may either be *absorbed* (lose all of their energy and completely disappear) or be *scattered* (become a secondary x-ray that travels in a new and unpredictable direction, as shown by the red arrows).

of an x-ray. This new x-ray is a *secondary* x-ray because it was not produced in the x-ray tube (primary x-rays are emitted from the tube). The energy of the secondary x-ray is equivalent to the difference between the outer level and inner level binding energies. In most cases, the secondary x-ray is absorbed without further damage to cells.

The likelihood of x-ray absorption via the photoelectric effect depends on the size of the atoms (i.e., atomic number) and the energy of the x-rays (i.e., kVp). The larger the atomic number, the greater the chance of x-ray absorption. Doubling the atomic number increases the probability of x-ray absorption by a factor of 8. The higher the kVp, the less the chance of x-ray absorption because the x-rays are more penetrating. Doubling the x-ray energy decreases the probability of absorption by a factor of 8.

The photoelectric effect is a major cause of x-ray attenuation up to about 70 kVp. Above 70 kVp the probability of x-ray absorption decreases, except at the **K-edge**. At the K-edge there is a sudden increase in absorption. K-edge refers to the binding energy of an inner level electron (the inner level of an atom is called the *K-shell*). X-rays with energy that is slightly greater than the binding energy of an inner level electron (just above the K-edge) are more likely to be absorbed (Figure 1.34).

The K-edge can be quite useful when imaging materials with a high atomic number, particularly positive contrast media (e.g., barium, iodine). Materials with high atomic numbers contain more K-shell electrons and therefore are more likely to absorb x-rays with a certain energy. The K-edge is not nearly as useful in soft tissues because these materials are composed of elements with smaller atomic numbers and fewer K-shell electrons (e.g., carbon, hydrogen, oxygen, nitrogen). The K-edges of barium and iodine are around 35 keV which is about the effective energy of a 70 kVp x-ray beam. This is one reason why barium and iodine are such ideal positive contrast agents for medical radiography. When performing a positive contrast study try to keep the kVp as close to 70 as practical to enhance x-ray absorption. The greater the x-ray absorption, the greater the contrast.

Scatter x-rays are secondary radiation. During most radiographic procedures, about 95% of scatter comes from the patient and the rest from the x-ray table, image receptor, floor, or any other material that happens to be in the x-ray beam FOV.

Scatter x-rays result from the incoherent or coherent interactions of primary x-rays. Most scatter is caused by **incoherent scattering**, which is also called the *Compton effect, inelastic scattering*, or *modified scattering*. Incoherent scattering occurs throughout the range of x-ray energies used in medical imaging (40–125 kVp). An x-ray collides with an atom, ejecting an electron and ionizing the atom (Figure 1.35). The x-ray energy is transferred to the ejected electron and to a secondary x-ray. The secondary x-ray travels in a completely random

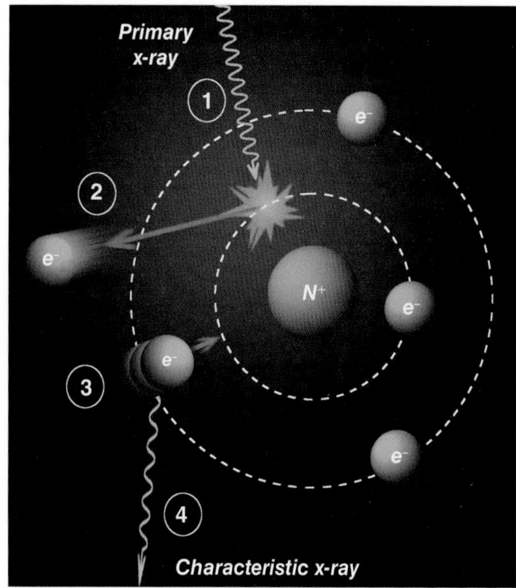

Figure 1.33 Photoelectric absorption. **1**. A primary x-ray collides with an atom in the patient. The x-ray transfers all of its energy to an inner shell electron and completely disappears. **2**. The electron now has enough energy to escape the atom and is ejected. **3**. An outer shell electron drops down to fill the void in the inner shell. **4**. The outer shell electron emits excess energy as a new x-ray. The energy of the secondary x-ray is less than that of the primary x-ray (note the longer wavelength). N^+ = nucleus; e^- = electrons.

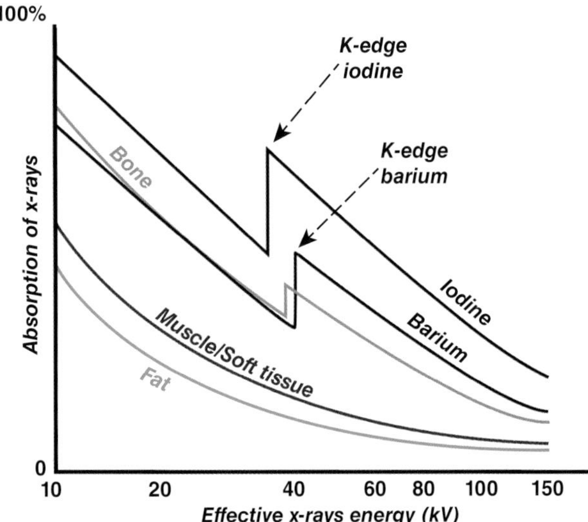

Figure 1.34 K-edge absorption. This graph depicts the relative abilities of fat, soft tissue, bone, barium, and iodine to absorb or attenuate x-rays. The differences in attenuation are highest with lower x-ray energies (lower kV). Radiographic contrast between the different tissues is greatest with lower energy x-rays. As x-ray energy increases, the x-rays are more penetrating and less likely to be absorbed. There is less contrast between tissues when using higher energy x-rays. However, at the K-edges of iodine, barium, and to a lesser extent bone, there is a sudden increase in x-ray absorption. At these parts of the graph there is a significant difference in attenuation between tissues which can be used to maximize radiographic contrast.

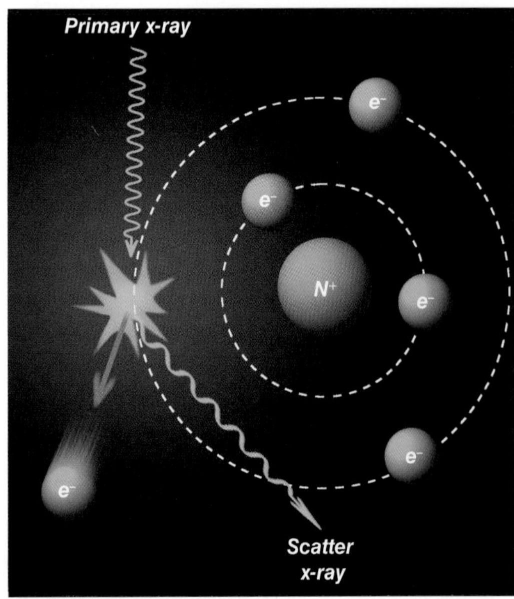

Figure 1.35 Incoherent scattering. A primary x-ray collides with an atom, ejecting a loosely bound outer level electron. The x-ray energy is transferred to the electron and to a secondary x-ray. The scatter x-ray travels in a new and unpredictable direction with less energy (longer wavelength) than the primary x-ray.

Box 1.5 To lessen the amount of scatter fog, minimize the x-ray interactions with tissue

- Make the FOV as small as practical
- Use grid when body part is thicker than 10–12 cm
- Use air gap when grid is not available

direction, anywhere from 0° to 180° from the original x-ray's path. Most incoherent scattering tends to be in the forward direction, but it is wholly unpredictable. If the secondary x-ray travels back toward the x-ray tube it is called **back-scatter** radiation.

Coherent scattering occurs with low-energy x-rays, less than 10 kVp. It is also called *elastic, unmodified, classical, Rayleigh* scattering, or the *Thompson effect*. Coherent scattering usually is not significant in medical imaging, but it is mentioned here because even very low energy x-rays can interact with atoms in the body. This type of scattering occurs when an x-ray collides with a firmly bound electron in an atom and creates a secondary x-ray. The electron is not ejected and the atom is not ionized. The secondary x-ray continues in a new direction with the same energy.

Scatter x-rays are a major cause of poor quality radiographs. Most of the x-rays emerging from the patient are scatter (50%–90%). Unfortunately, an image receptor cannot distinguish between scatter and transmitted x-rays. Scatter increases radiographic density, but does not represent anything inside the patient. Scatter causes a diffuse, unwanted darkening of the radiograph which is called **fog**. Fog reduces contrast and visible detail. We discussed earlier some of the causes of film fog as it pertains to film:screen radiography. Scatter fog is a much bigger problem and affects both film and digital systems. In addition to reducing image quality, scatter x-rays also expose the patient and nearby personnel to unnecessary radiation. Though less energetic than primary x-rays, many scatter x-rays retain sufficient energy to ionize atoms and damage cells.

The primary contributor to the amount of scatter radiation is the volume of tissue being irradiated (Box 1.5). Tissue volume is determined by the **field-of-view** (FOV) and the **thickness of the body part**. The larger the FOV, the more scatter (Figures 1.36 and 1.37). The thicker the body part, the more scatter. Some of the most effective and practical methods to limit the amount of scatter include making the FOV as small as possible and using a grid whenever body part thickness exceeds 10–12 cm.

Grids

A **grid** is one of the most effective and practical methods of minimizing scatter fog and enhancing radiograph quality.

Grids are devices that are placed between the patient and the image receptor to absorb scatter x-rays (Figures 1.38

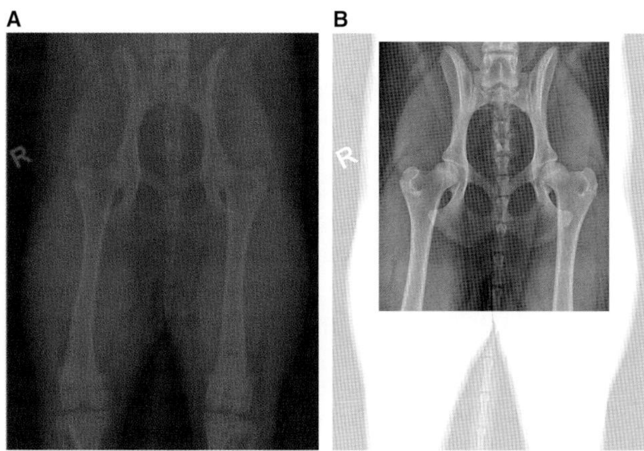

Figure 1.36 Scatter fog. **A**. VD view of a dog pelvis depicting the effect of scatter fog. There is an overall increase in radiographic density with poor contrast and less visible detail due detail. **B**. VD view of the same dog made with a smaller FOV. The radiograph is better quality due to less scatter fog.

and 1.39). A grid consists of alternating strips of an x-ray absorbing material, typically lead, and a non-absorbing material such as carbon fiber or aluminum. The strips may be arranged in a parallel or cross-hatched pattern, or they may be focused toward the x-ray tube so they align with the x-ray beam. A focused grid is more likely to absorb x-rays that are not aligned with the primary beam (scatter x-rays) and less likely to absorb x-rays that are aligned with the beam (transmitted x-rays). Focused grids must be positioned in the center of the x-ray beam and used at a specific distance from the focal spot (Figure 1.40).

Grids are most useful when larger volumes of tissue are irradiated. They should be used whenever body part thickness exceeds 10–12 cm. The effectiveness of a grid (the amount of scatter radiation it can absorb) is affected by its *grid ratio* and the *grid frequency* (Figure 1.41).

The **grid ratio** is the height of a lead strip divided by the distance between two strips. The higher the ratio, the more scatter will be absorbed (Figure 1.42). High ratio grids can absorb up to 90% of scatter radiation. Unfortunately, high ratio grids also absorb as much as 30% of transmitted x-rays. A grid ratio must be high enough to remove most of the scatter but not so high that there aren't enough transmitted x-rays to make a quality radiograph. In most practice situations, a grid ratio of 8 : 1 is appropriate for x-ray exposures in the range of 70–90 kVp.

Grid frequency is the number of lead strips per unit distance. Frequency generally is expressed as *lines per cm (lpc)* or *lines per inch (lpi)*. The higher the grid frequency, the more scatter will be absorbed. Low-frequency grids (40–50 lpc or 100–120 lpi) generally are used in x-ray systems with a moving grid (see Bucky-Potter mechanism below). Medium frequency grids (50–60 lpc or 120–150 lpi) are suitable for most veterinary practices and can be used in stationary grid holders. High-frequency grids (more than 60–70 lpc or 150–170 lpi) may be preferred for some digital imaging systems to help reduce grid artifacts.

Because the grid is physically located between the patient and the image receptor, its lead strips sometimes are visible in the radiograph. The strips appear as thin, parallel, white lines that are regularly-spaced across the entire radiograph (see Artifacts in Chapter 2). These lines are called **grid lines**. They tend to be less noticeable with higher frequency grids. Grid lines can be blurred using a Bucky-Potter mechanism, which makes them less distracting in the radiograph.

The grid was invented in 1913 by a German radiologist named Gustav Bucky. Shortly thereafter, an American radiologist named Hollis Potter designed a device to blur the grid

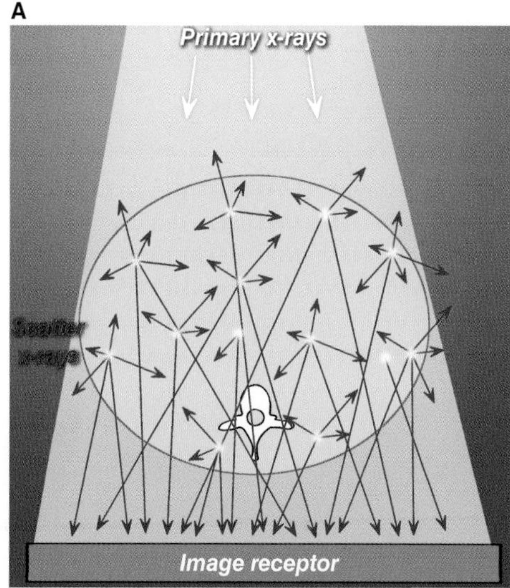

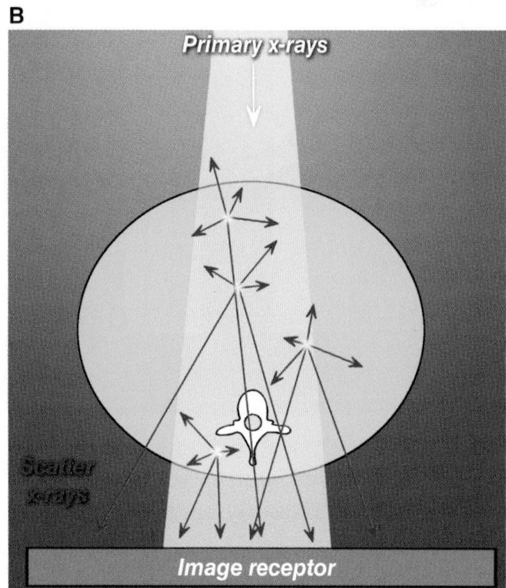

Figure 1.37 Scatter and FOV. These illustrations depict the amount of scatter radiation created by using a larger FOV (**A**) and a smaller FOV (**B**) with the same body part thickness. The size of the FOV is a primary determinant of the amount of scatter radiation produced.

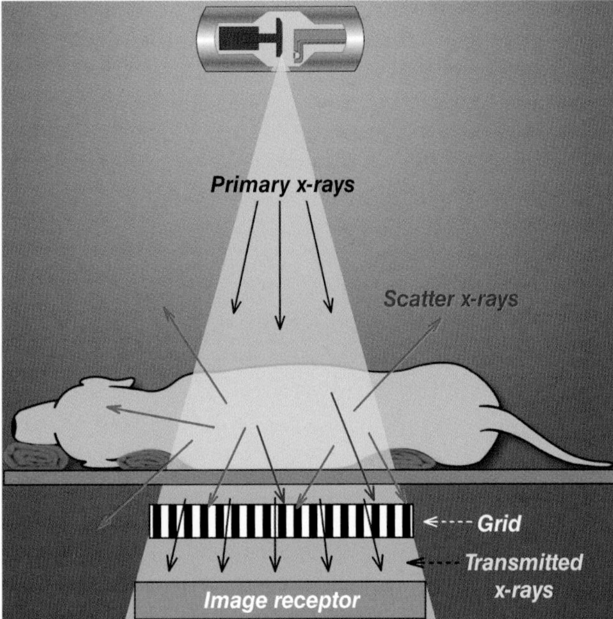

Figure 1.38 Grid. This illustration depicts a grid positioned between a patient and the image receptor. The purpose of the grid is to block unwanted scatter x-rays (red arrows) from reaching the image receptor while allowing transmitted x-rays (black arrows) to pass through.

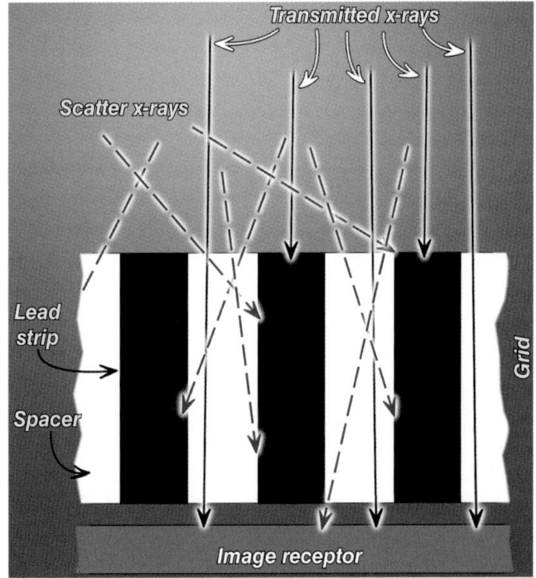

Figure 1.39 Grid close up. This illustration depicts the method by which a grid reduces scatter fog. Scatter x-rays travel in various directions and most are not incident to the image receptor. Many scatter x-rays are absorbed by the lead strips in the grid, but some will pass through the spacers to reach the receptor. Transmitted x-rays travel in straight lines incident to the receptor. These ideally pass through the spacers, but some will strike a lead strip and be absorbed.

lines. The device, now known as the **Bucky-Potter mechanism** or the *Potter-Bucky diaphragm*, moves the grid during the x-ray exposure, oscillating it at right angles to the lead strips. The speed at which the grid moves determines the shortest exposure time possible to avoid grid lines. Moving the grid during exposure is most valuable when using a low ratio grid or a low-frequency grid. However, the movement may startle some patients and create movement artifacts in the radiograph.

Ideally, all transmitted x-rays pass through a grid to reach the image receptor. Unfortunately, the grid absorbs many of them. The amount of transmitted x-rays that reach the grid compared to the number that pass through the grid is called the **grid factor** (also known as the *Bucky factor*). The grid factor determines the additional x-ray exposure needed when using a grid compared to not using a grid. For example, a grid factor of 2 means that for every two x-rays that reach the grid, one is absorbed and one passes through. A grid factor of 2 means the x-ray exposure must be doubled when using the grid, usually twice the mAs. The grid factor increases as the grid ratio or grid frequency increases. In digital radiography, software is available to compensate for scatter fog which may reduce the need for a grid.

Air gap

The air gap technique takes advantage of the fact that scatter x-rays are lower energy and more divergent than transmitted x-rays. Moving the image receptor further away from the patient creates a space that allows more of the scatter x-rays to dissipate in the air gap or miss the receptor (Figure 1.43). A 10–15 cm spacing between patient and image receptor has been shown to be effective in reducing scatter fog. The tradeoff with using an air gap is the object-to-image distance (OID) is increased which results in magnification and geometric unsharpness.

Radiographic density

Density in a radiograph is the amount of black in the image. The darker areas in the radiograph are high density and the whiter areas are low density. Each shade of gray represents a level of density.

The term "density" may be a source of confusion. In the early days of radiology, "density" was used to describe both the physical density of the material being imaged (i.e., its weight per unit volume) and the concentration of black metallic silver on the film (Box 1.6). Physical density was called *subject density* and it produced the whiter areas in the radiograph. The amount of black in the film image was called *radiographic density*. However, subject density is only one factor to consider when evaluating the lighter areas in a radiograph. The ability of a

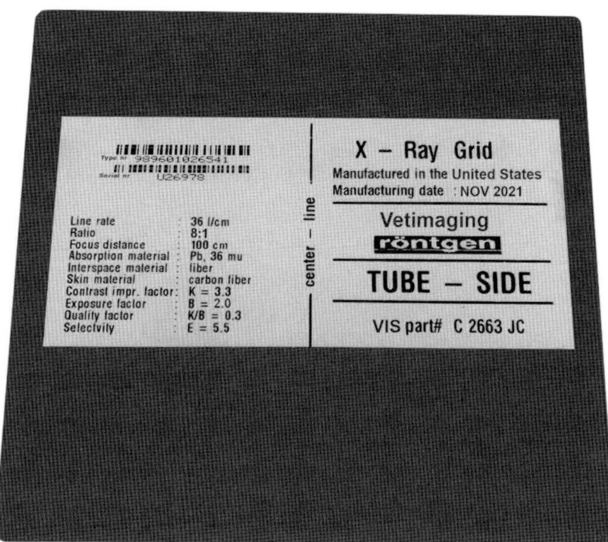

Figure 1.40 Grid. A picture of the front of a grid depicting a typical label that lists the characteristics of the grid including type, composition, ratio, frequency, focal distance, and others.

material to attenuate x-rays is based on more than its physical density alone. Therefore, the more correct term for subject density is radiopacity or simply opacity. Opacity is the ability to attenuate x-rays. Opacity produces the whiter areas in the radiograph and density is the blacker areas. Opacity and density are inversely related: the greater the opacity of a material, the less density it will produce in the radiograph.

Box 1.6 Density in film radiography

In film radiography, radiographic density sometimes is called *optical density* or *transmitted density* because with film, the amount of density is determined by the amount of light that can be seen through the film. A film radiograph with high density permits little light to shine through.

The levels of density in a radiograph are determined by the number of x-rays that are recorded by the image receptor. The number recorded depends on the number that reach the receptor and the **sensitivity** of the receptor. Sensitivity is the minimum quantity of x-rays a receptor must receive to form acceptable levels of density. The number of x-rays that reach the image receptor is determined the number produced (mAs), their energy (kVp), and the opacities of the objects and tissues being imaged. The SID also affects the number because a shorter SID will result in more x-rays reaching the image receptor than a longer SID due to the inverse square law (see Box 1.7, SID and density).

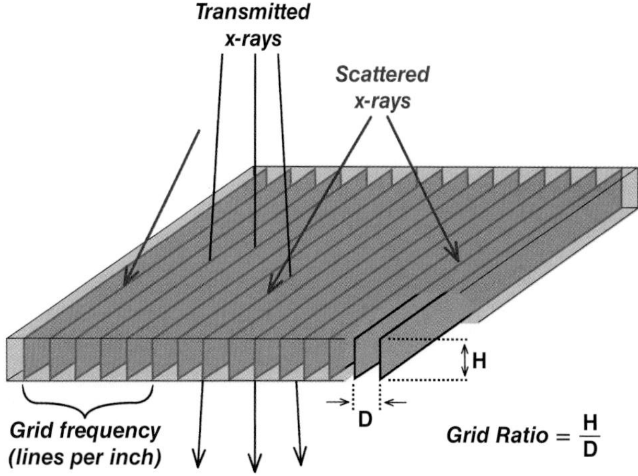

Figure 1.41 Grid. This illustration depicts a cutaway view of a parallel grid with alternating lead and carbon fiber strips. Grid frequency is the number of lead strips per inch. Grid ratio is the height of a lead strip (H) divided by the space between two strips (D).

The larger the quantity of x-rays produced, the more will reach the receptor. Recall that the number of x-rays produced is determined by the **mA** control and the **exposure time**, which together are called **mAs** (*milliamp-seconds*).

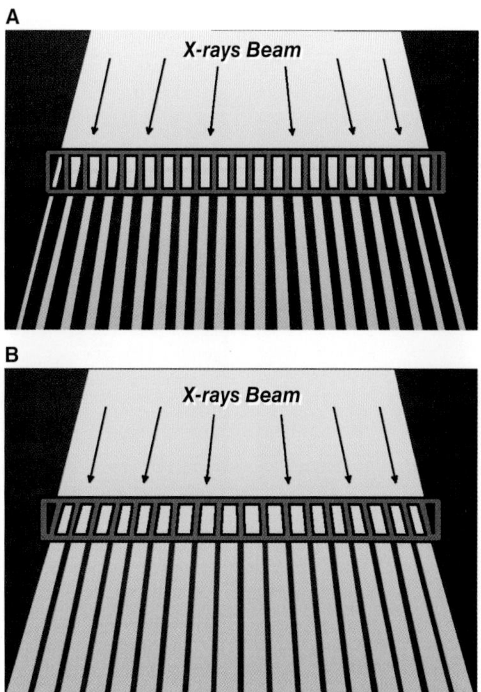

Figure 1.42 Focused grid. These illustrations depict (**A**) a parallel grid with vertical strips and (**B**) a focused grid with strips aligned to the x-ray beam. The grids are colored blue and the black streaks below each grid depict areas where the primary x-rays are absorbed by the strips. The parallel grid absorbs significantly more of the primary x-rays than the focused grid.

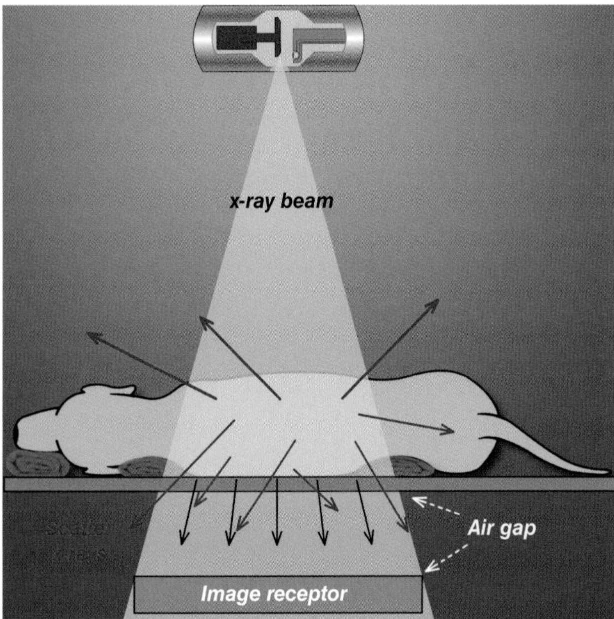

Figure 1.43 Air gap technique. Scatter x-rays (red arrows) are more divergent than transmitted x-rays (black arrows). An air gap is present between the patient and the image receptor to allow more scatter x-rays to miss the receptor.

A

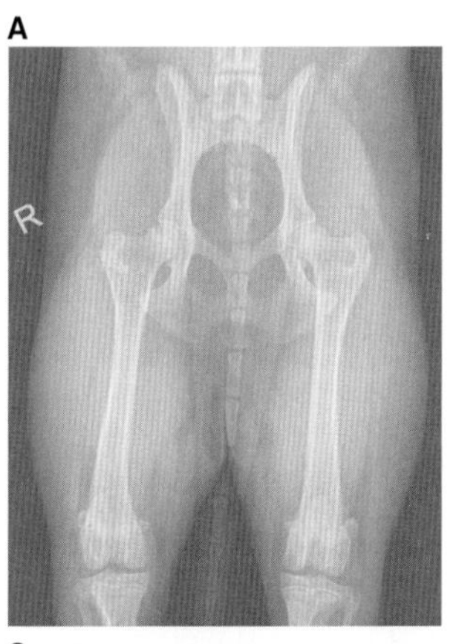

B

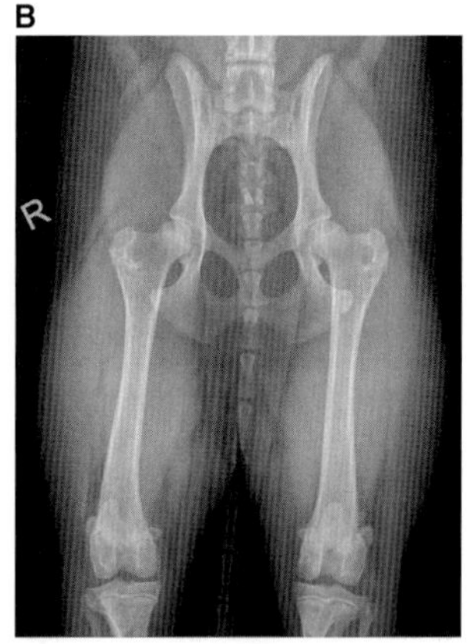

C

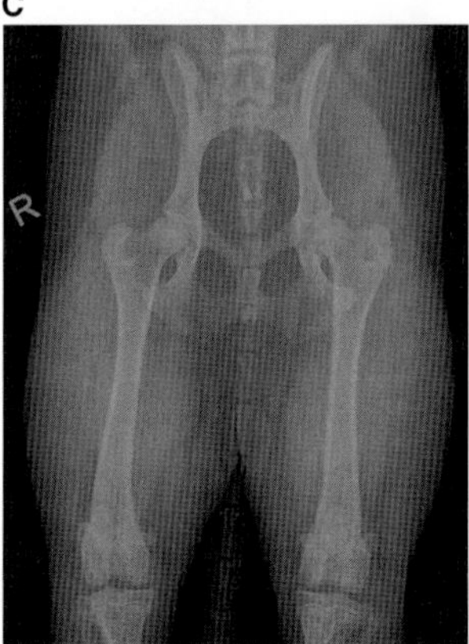

Figure 1.44 Density, mAs, and kVp. VD views of a dog pelvis depicting levels of radiographic density. Radiograph **A** is underexposed; it is too light. We need to increase the mAs or kVp. In radiograph **B** the mA was increased and in radiograph **C** the kVp was increased. Both **B** and **C** are satisfactory density, but there is more contrast in **B** than in **C**.

The kVp control also affects the number of x-rays, but primarily determines the energy of the x-rays.

When you need to increase or decrease the density in a radiograph, **mAs** is the first adjustment to consider (Figure 1.44). To make the radiograph darker, double the mAs (double either the mA or the exposure time, not both). To make the radiograph lighter, reduce the mAs by 50% (cut the exposure time in half). Adjusting the mAs less than by a factor of 2 usually doesn't cause a visible change in the image.

The higher the energy of the x-rays, the more will reach the receptor. As **kVp** increases the x-rays become more penetrating and more will be transmitted. Sometimes you need to adjust the kVp rather than the mAs to produce acceptable radiographic density. This is particularly true when the exposure time needs to be shortened. A short exposure time is desirable because it helps minimize motion artifacts. A **20% increase** in kVp will darken the radiograph as much as doubling the mAs; a **16% decrease** in kVp will lighten the image as much as halving the mAs.

The greater the **opacity** of the material being imaged, the fewer x-rays will reach the receptor, and the less density will be produced. More opaque materials appear whiter in the radiograph. As an x-ray beam passes through a patient, it encounters objects and tissues with many different opacities. The x-rays that exit the patient exhibit many different x-ray intensities (numbers of x-rays per unit area). The emerging x-ray intensities can differ by 1000-fold or more. To effectively record all of these different intensities, an image receptor needs a wide *dynamic range*.

Box 1.7 SID and density

The SID is inversely related to radiographic density. The longer the SID, the less the density. The shorter the SID, the greater the density. The standard SID in most veterinary practices is 100 cm (40 in.). In some situations the SID needs to be altered, such as when performing mobile radiography or when using a low output x-ray machine. Changing the SID often requires an adjustment in the x-ray exposure to maintain the same density in the radiograph. The following formula is helpful:

$$\left(\frac{\text{SID1}}{\text{SID2}}\right)^2 = \frac{\text{mAs1}}{\text{mAs2}}$$

For example, if the SID must be shortened from 100 to 70 cm and the mAs at 100 cm was 3.0, the mAs at 70 cm must be reduced to 1.5 to achieve the same radiographic density, as shown below:

$$\left(\frac{100\,\text{cm}}{70\,\text{cm}}\right)^2 = \frac{3\,\text{mAs}}{X\,\text{mAs}}$$

$$2.0 = \frac{3}{X}$$

$$1.5\,\text{mAs} = X$$

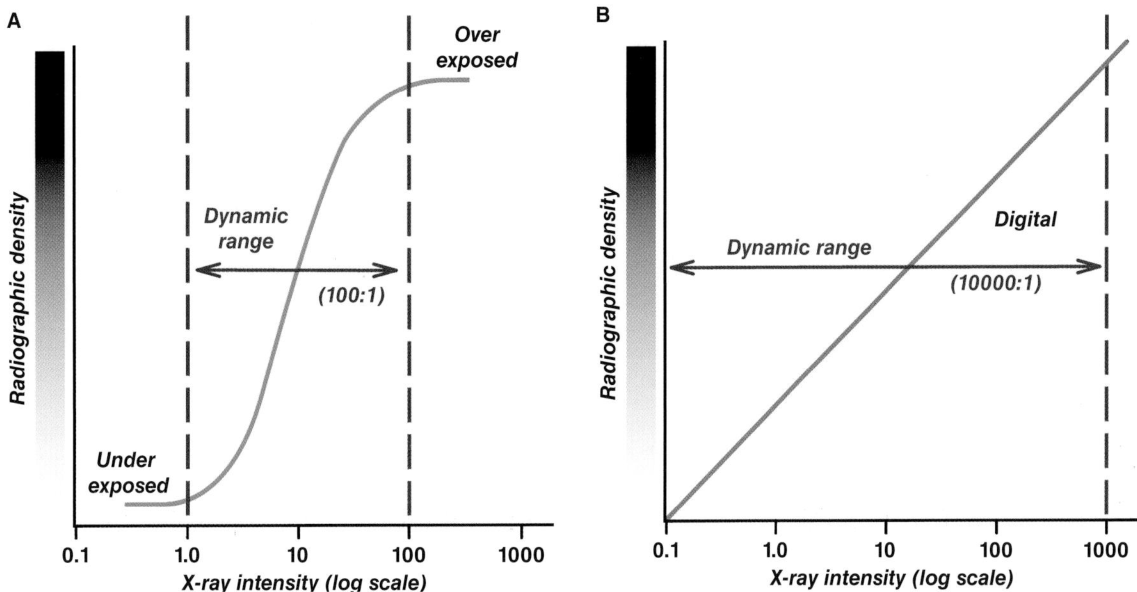

Figure 1.45 Dynamic range of film vs. digital. Characteristic curves for a film:screen image receptor (**A**) and a digital image receptor (**B**). Radiographic density is along the vertical axes. These are the visible shades of gray, from minimum to maximum, that the image receptor can produce. X-ray intensity is along the horizontal axes and represents the amount of x-rays the image receptor received. X-ray intensity is displayed as a logarithmic scale because the amounts of x-rays emerging from the patient can vary by a 1000-fold or more and log numbers are easier to work with when dealing with such magnitudes. The curve for the film:screen image receptor (**A**) is flat along the left bottom, which means no significant density can be formed with this amount of x-rays. This part of the film radiograph would appear too light or underexposed. The top right part of the film:screen curve again is flat, which means no more density can be formed above this amount of x-rays. This part of the film radiograph would be too dark or overexposed. The part of the curve with slope is the area where an image with acceptable density can be formed. The slope is the *dynamic range*. The dynamic range for the film:screen system is 100 : 1, as shown between the two red dotted lines. Notice that the film:screen characteristic curve does not begin at 0. This is because in all x-ray film there is some inherent radiographic density due to the tint in the base and some unexposed emulsion that typically remains. The curve for the digital image receptor (**B**) is linear because digital systems can accept a much wider range of x-ray intensities and still form visible shades of gray. The dynamic range of this digital image receptor is 10,000 : 1, which is 100 times greater than the film:screen system in (**A**).

Dynamic range refers to all of the different quantities of x-rays – minimum to maximum – that an image receptor can receive and still form acceptable levels of density. The wider the dynamic range, the more different shades of gray the receptor can display. The more shades of gray, the more different opacities it can display. The dynamic range of an image receptor is described by a *characteristic curve*. **Characteristic curves** are useful to illustrate and compare the capabilities of different image receptors (Figure 1.45).

The dynamic range of digital radiography systems is much wider than the range in film:screen systems, which is why digital receptors are able to produce acceptable radiographs over a wide range of x-ray exposures. A typical film:screen system, for example, has a dynamic range of about 100, whereas the dynamic range of many digital systems is over 10,000.

Sometimes it is useful to have a graph that displays all of the different levels of density and the areas in the radiograph associated with each density. Such a graph is called a **histogram** (Figure 1.46). Histograms reveal the number of pixels with each shade of gray in the image. The wider the histogram, the more shades of gray. The histogram must fit within the dynamic range of the image receptor or parts of the radiograph will be too light or too dark.

Opacity

The only reason we can see anything in a radiograph is because of differences in opacity. It is the **relative opacity** of one material compared to an adjacent material that allows us to distinguish it or not distinguish it. Differences in opacity are determined by the sizes of the atoms in the materials, how tightly the atoms are packed together (Table 1.1) and the thickness of each material.

In medical radiography, the opacity of each tissue or object is categorized into one of five different groups. Every shade of gray you see in a radiograph is either **gas**, **fat**, **fluid/soft tissue**, **mineral**, or **metal** opacity. When in doubt, the opacity is decided by comparing it to the opacity of a known material. A material may be known by its anatomical shape and location (Figure 1.47).

Gas opacity materials attenuate very few x-rays and produce the most radiographic density (Figure 1.48). Gas is the

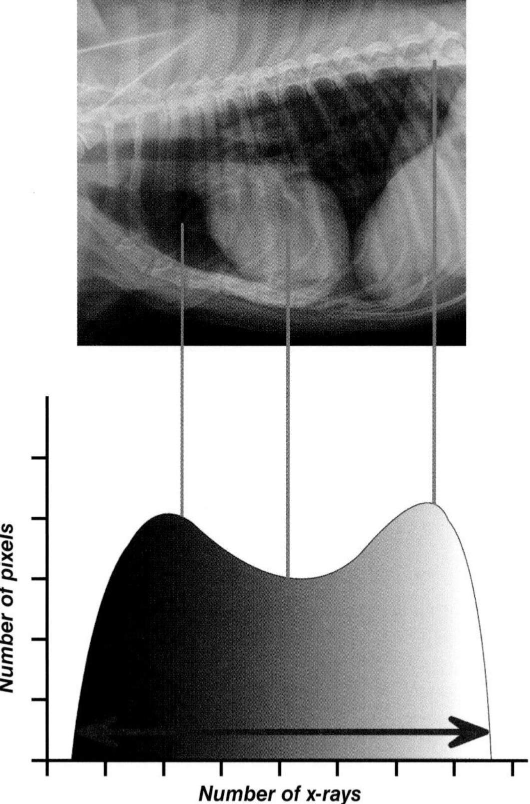

Figure 1.46 Histogram. The histogram displays all of the different radiographic densities (visible shades of gray) in the radiograph. Each shade of gray is determined by the number of x-rays the image receptor receives. The number of pixels with each shade of gray is represented by the height of the graph. On the left side of the graph, lower opacity tissues such as lung allow more x-rays to pass through to the image receptor. These appear as darker areas in the radiograph. Higher opacity tissues such as spine attenuate more x-rays so fewer pass to the image receptor. These appear as lighter areas in the radiograph. To display all of the dark and light areas, the width of the histogram (red double-headed arrow) must fit within the dynamic range of the image receptor. Shades of gray that fall outside the dynamic range will not be visible in the radiograph.

material that appears darkest or blackest in a radiograph. Examples include lungs, any collection of gas inside the body, and the air outside the body.

Fat opacity materials attenuate more x-rays than gas and produce shades of gray that are lighter than gas but darker than fluid/soft tissue. Examples include fascial planes, omentum, falciform ligament, mediastinal fat, retroperitoneal fat, and lipomas.

Fluid/soft tissue opacity materials attenuate more x-rays than fat and produce lighter shades of gray than fat, but not as white as bone. The soft tissues and fluids in the body are the same relative opacity. Examples include muscles, organs, cartilage, blood, urine, and body cavity effusions.

Mineral opacity materials attenuate more x-rays than soft tissue/fluid and produce whiter areas in the radiograph. Examples include skeletal structures, many types of calculi,

Table 1.1 Relative opacities of various materials

Material	EAN	SG	Relative Opacity
Air	7.6	0.001	0.01
Foam rubber	5.0	0.15	0.8
Lung	7.4	0.32	2.4
Plastic[a]	5.8	0.05–1.06	0.03–6.1
Cellulose (wood, fabric)	7.0	0.20–1.50	1.4–10.5
Fat	6.0	0.91	5.5
Solid rubber	5.0	1.10	5.5
Ice	7.5	0.93	7.0
Water	7.5	1.00	7.5
Seawater	7.5	1.03	7.7
Muscle	7.6	1.04	7.8
Blood	7.6	1.06	7.9
Graphite	6.0	2.30	13.8
PVC	13.9	1.30	18.1
Diamond	6.0	3.50	19.5
Bone	13.8	1.85	25.5
Glass	10.3	2.50	25.8
Calcium	20.0	1.55	31.0
Aluminum	13.0	2.70	35.1
Concrete	17.0	2.30	39.0
Barium	53.0	3.50	122.0
Stainless steel	25.8	7.85	202.5
Zirconium	40.0	6.49	259.6
Iodine	56.0	4.93	276.0
Lead	82.0	11.34	930.0
Tungsten	74.0	19.25	1424.0
Gold	79.0	19.30	1524.7

The opacity of a material is its ability to attenuate x-rays. The more opaque the material, the fewer x-rays will pass through. The opacity of a material is affected by the sizes of its atoms (atomic number) and how tightly the atoms are packed together (specific gravity). The higher the atomic number (Z), the greater the opacity. As the atomic number increases, the likelihood of x-ray absorption grows exponentially (Z^3). In medical imaging, we frequently deal with materials that are made of a number of different elements, each with its own atomic number. Soft tissues in the body, for example, contain hydrogen, oxygen, carbon, nitrogen, and others. When dealing with composite materials, we use an approximate or effective atomic number (EAN). Specific gravity (SG) is a comparison of the number of atoms in a given volume of a material to the same volume of water. The larger the specific gravity, the more tightly the atoms are packed together. The higher the specific gravity, the greater the opacity because more atoms in the path of the x-rays and more x-rays are likely to be attenuated. Specific gravity has a greater effect on opacity than atomic number. Consider the opacities of air and muscle. Air attenuates far fewer x-rays than muscle, yet the effective atomic number for each is the same. They both are composites of hydrogen, oxygen, carbon, and nitrogen. However, the atoms in muscle are 1000 times more tightly packed together than in air. In this table, the relative opacity for various materials is calculated by multiplying EAN × SG. These are approximate values for illustration purposes only.

[a] Polystyrene and polyethylene.

and dystrophic mineralization. Although they are all mineral opacity, the relative opacity in different parts of bones differ, particularly in cortical and cancellous bone (Figure 1.49).

Metal opacity materials attenuate a large number of the x-rays used in medical imaging and produce the lightest, whitest areas in a radiograph. Examples include foreign objects, body markers, orthopedic implants, and positive contrast media such as barium and iodine compounds.

Categorizing a material as one of these five opacities does not mean it will produce the same shade of gray in every radiograph. It means that the material appears as one of these opacities relative to a known material. The actual gray shade a material will produce in a radiograph depends on its thickness, summation of other materials, and the intensity of the x-rays.

The **thicker** the material, the more atoms in the path of the x-rays and more x-rays are more likely to be attenuated. As thickness increases, opacity increases. A thick piece of material is more opaque than a thin piece of the same material (Figure 1.50). The thicker piece will attenuate more x-rays and appear lighter in the radiograph than the thinner piece, even though both are part of the same material with the exact same composition. The thicker material will be relatively more opaque than the thinner piece.

Thickness also can affect the relative opacities of two different materials with different compositions. Consider a thick piece of fat and a thin piece of bone (Figure 1.51). Fat is inherently less opaque than bone, but thick fat may produce the same shade of gray in a radiograph as thin bone because they both will attenuate the same number of x-rays and therefore appear as similar opacities in the radiograph.

Similar to alterations in thickness, **summation** can lead to an increase or decrease in the relative opacity of a material.

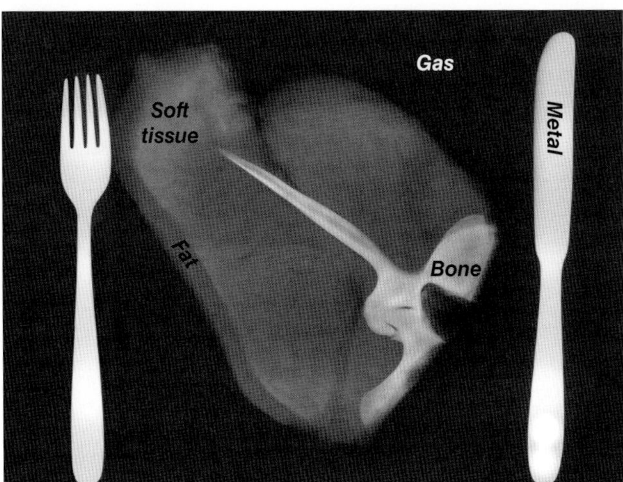

Figure 1.47 Five opacities. In this radiograph, all five relative opacities are represented by structures that are readily identified. Gas opacity in the surrounding air; fat opacity in the fascial planes and along the edge of the steak; soft tissue opacity in the steak muscle; mineral opacity in the bone, and metal opacity in the eating utensils.

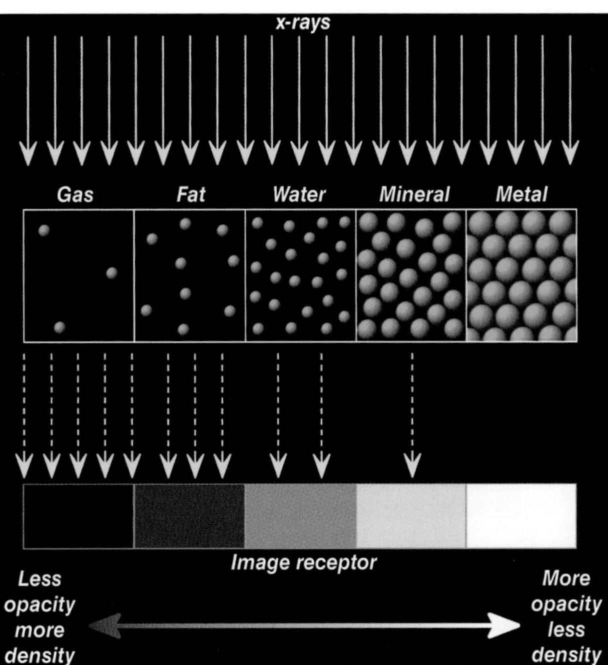

Figure 1.48 Five relative opacities. This illustration depicts equal thicknesses of gas, fat, water, mineral, and metal. The opacity of each is determined by the sizes of the atoms and how tightly they are packed together. The greater the opacity, the greater the x-ray attenuation and the fewer transmitted x-rays (dotted arrows). The fewer x-rays that reach the image receptor, the less the radiographic density. Opacity is inversely related to density.

Summation occurs when two or more materials in different planes overlap. The resulting opacity is the sum of all of the superimposed opacities (Figure 1.52). For example, soft tissue summated with gas will appear darker (less opaque), whereas soft tissue summated with soft tissue will appear lighter (more opaque). Because radiographs are two-dimensional images of three-dimensional structures, there is a lot of summation in most images. Summation can alter the opacity of a material to the point that it resembles the opacity of a different material in the radiograph. When this occurs, we differentiate the materials based on their location, shape or pattern in the radiograph (Figure 1.53).

So far, we have determined that the opacity of a material, and conversely the amount of radiographic density it will produce, is affected by its composition, thickness, and summation with other materials. The appearance of a material in the radiograph (shade of gray it will produce) is also affected by the **x-ray beam intensity**. The greater the number or energy of the x-rays, the more will pass through the material to reach the image receptor. A material will appear whiter in a radiograph made with low exposure and darker with high exposure. However, the intensity of the x-ray beam affects all materials in the field of view and all parts of the radiograph. Even though a specific material may appear lighter or darker based on x-ray beam intensity, its relative opacity compared to the other materials remains the same (Figure 1.54).

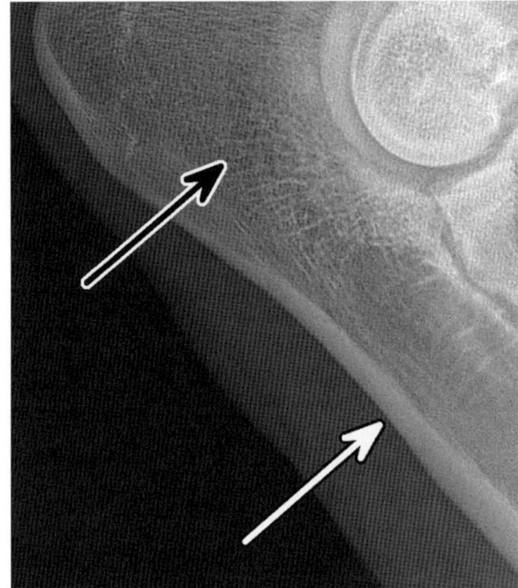

Figure 1.49 Relative opacity. Close up lateral view of a bone depicting the opacity of cortical bone (white arrow) compared to cancellous bone (black arrow). Both are mineral opacity, but cancellous is a mixture of bone and soft tissue, whereas cortical is mostly bone.

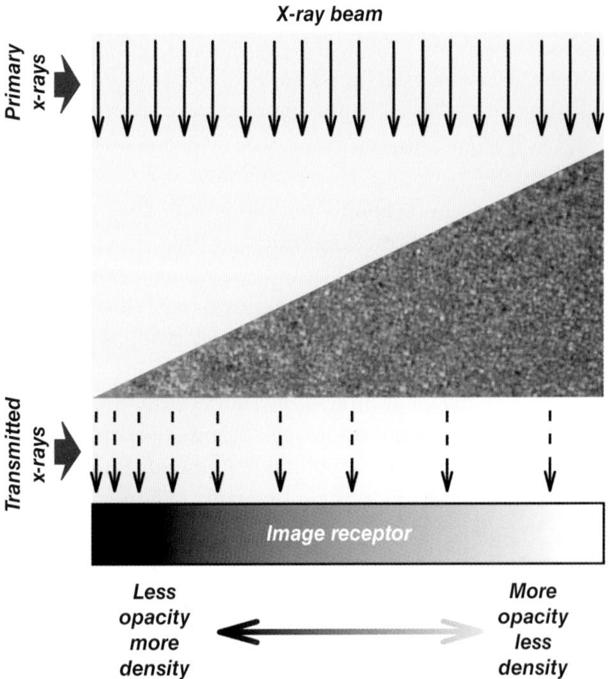

Figure 1.50 Thickness. An x-ray beam passing through a wedge-shaped piece of material will penetrate the thin part more easily than the thick part. The image receptor will receive more transmitted x-rays from the thin side than the thick side and will form more radiographic density on the thin side than on the thick side. The opacity of the thicker part is greater than the opacity of the thinner part, even though it is the same material with exactly the same composition throughout.

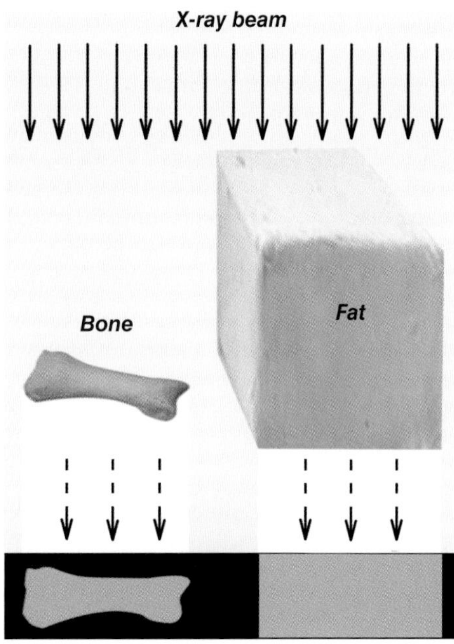

Figure 1.51 Thickness and contrast. This illustration depicts an x-ray beam passing through a thin piece of bone (**A**) and a thick piece of fat (**B**). The opacity of fat is inherently less than that of bone, but because it is very thick, the fat will attenuate an amount of x-rays equivalent to the thin bone. Both the bone and the fat produce the same radiographic density in the image below.

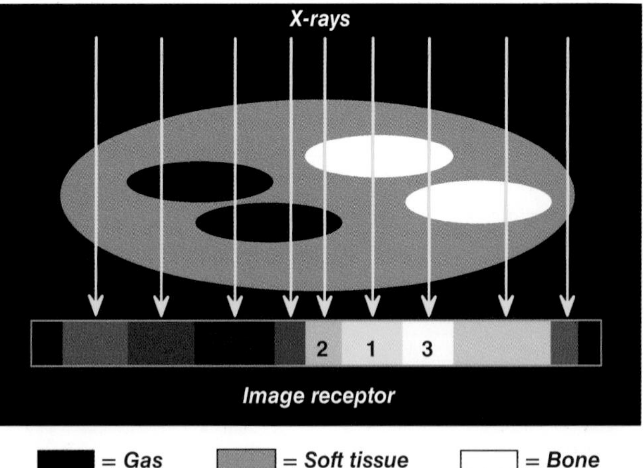

Figure 1.52 Summation. This illustration depicts x-rays passing through a structure that contains gas, soft tissue, and bone opacity materials. The opacity of each material and the amount of density it produces in the radiographic image varies due to summation. Bone, for example, appears as one shade of gray when summated with soft tissue (**1**), a darker shade when summated with gas (**2**), and a lighter shade when summated with bone (**3**).

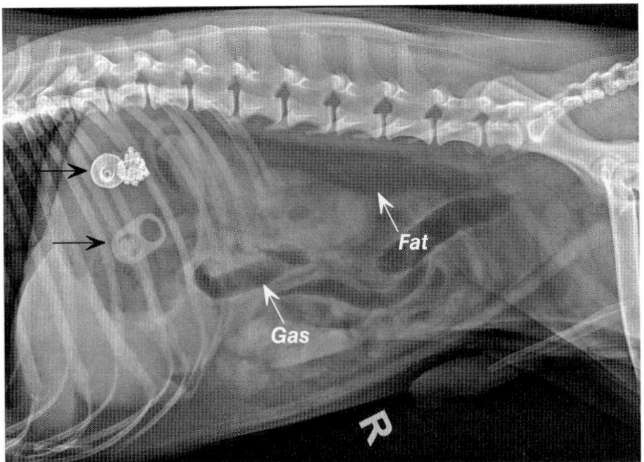

Figure 1.53 Relative opacity. Lateral view of a dog abdomen depicting similar radiographic densities of materials with different opacities. An area of bowel gas and an area of retroperitoneal fat produce the same shade of gray (white arrows), but they are readily distinguished based on their locations and adjacent structures. Gas is inherently less opaque than fat, but summation with soft tissue results in a radiographic density that is similar to fat. There are two metal opacity objects in the stomach (black arrows). Both are metal, but they differ in radiographic density. The density of the earring (closer to the spine) is clearly metal opacity. The density of the pop tab is similar to bone or soft tissue, but we recognize the shape and know it is metal.

The terms "radiolucent" and "radiopaque" have long been used to describe the opacity of materials, but they are actually misnomers. For example: mineral opacity calculi will appear white in urine and black in contrast medium (Figure 1.55). These calculi could be described as both "radiopaque" and "radiolucent". Soft tissue opacity calculi will not be visible in urine (commonly called "radiolucent"), will appear black in contrast medium (also "radiolucent"), and will appear white when surrounded by gas ("radiopaque"). All materials are "radiopaque" to some degree and any material may appear "radiolucent" adjacent to a more opaque material. Labeling a radiographic finding as radiolucent or radiopaque does not convey nearly as much useful information as descriptions such as "mineral opacity", "gas opacity", "increased in opacity", "decreased in opacity", "more opaque than", "less opaque than", etc. For example, diamonds are less opaque than cubic zirconia (Figure 1.56).

Radiographic contrast

Contrast is the amount of difference between the dark areas and the light areas in a radiograph. It is the degree of change from one density (shade of gray) to the next. The **level of contrast** is determined by the number of shades of gray that are displayed. The more grays between black and white, the lower the contrast because there is less difference between one shade and the next. A high contrast radiograph is mostly black and white with few shades of gray in between. High contrast sometimes is called *short scale* and low contrast sometimes is also called *long scale* (Figure 1.57).

The goal in making radiographs is to balance contrast with density so all areas of interest are visible. If contrast is too low, there will be no visible distinction between similar radiographic densities and we won't be able to distinguish structures. If contrast is too high, some opacities will not be visible because the shade of gray needed to display them is not available (some adjacent shades of gray will be grouped together). The key factors that determine the level of contrast in a radiograph are the:

1. Latitude of the image receptor.
2. Energy of the x-rays (kVp).
3. Differences in opacities in the subject (patient).
4. Amount of fog.

Latitude is the range of x-ray intensities, from minimum to maximum, that an image receptor can receive and still form acceptable radiographic contrast. The latitude of a

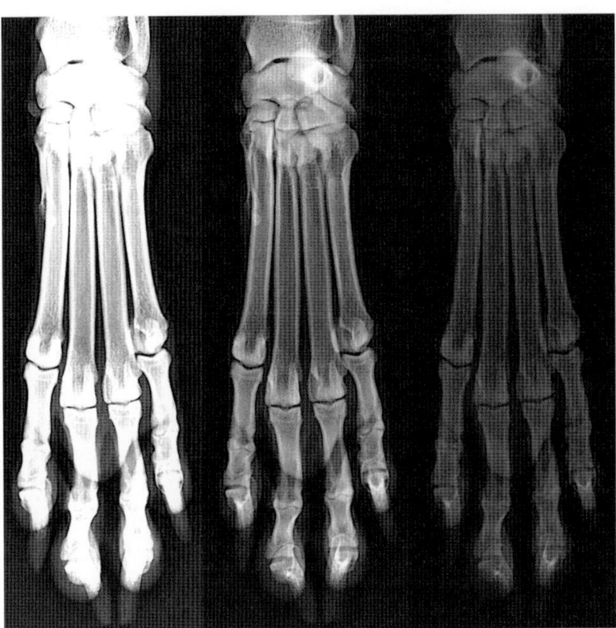

Figure 1.54 Exposure and opacity. Three radiographs of the same dog foot made with increasing x-ray exposures. As exposure increases, the overall opacity of the structures decreases, but relative opacity remains constant. Notice that any point in one radiograph is a different shade of gray compared to the same point in another radiograph, but its *relative* opacity to other points in the foot remains the same. We recognize the different parts of the foot in each image because of the differences in relative opacity. It would be incorrect to describe any particular shade of gray as "bone" or "soft tissue" just because it is a certain level of radiographic density. We know it is soft tissue or bone because of its relative opacity to the tissue next to it.

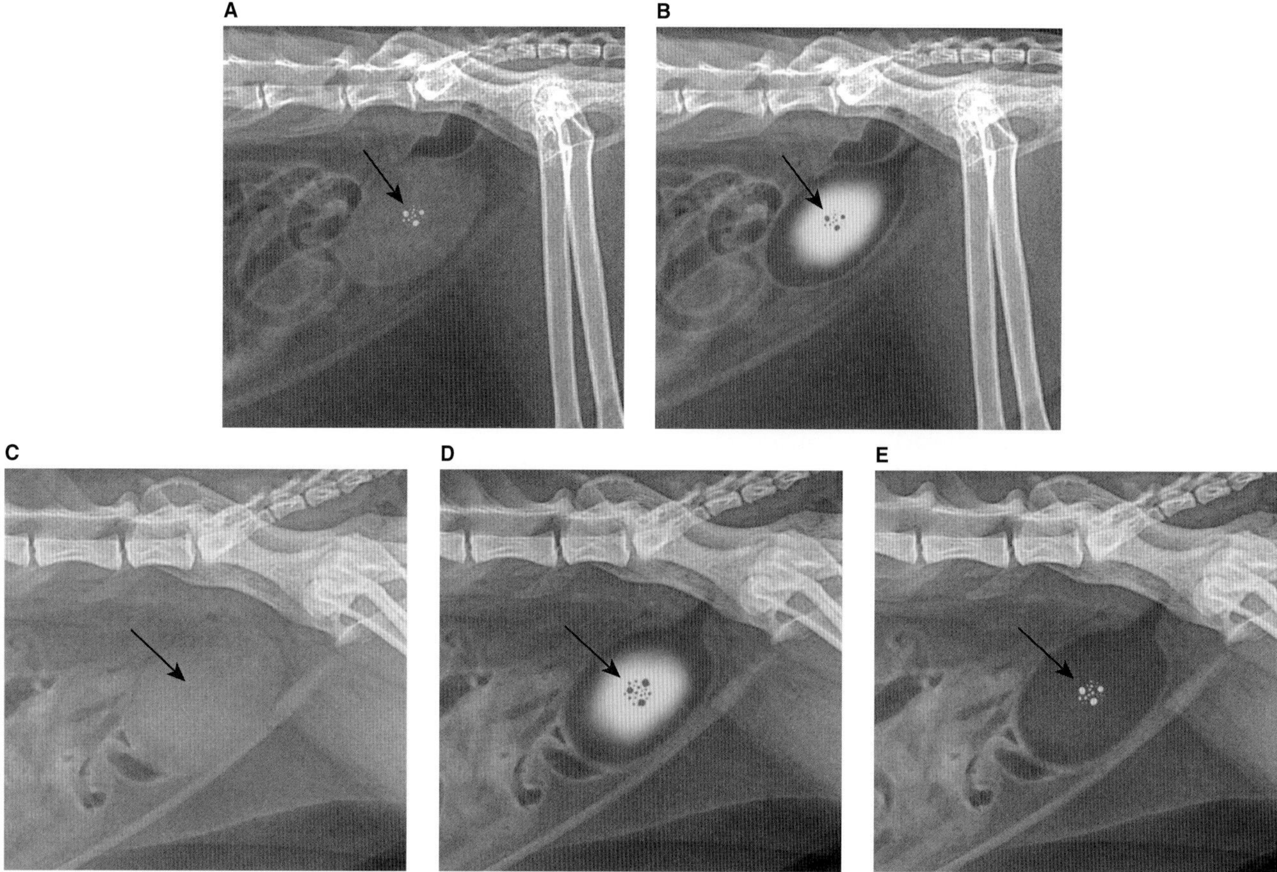

Figure 1.55 Radiolucent vs. radiopaque. Lateral views of a dog abdomen depicting mineral opacity and soft tissue opacity calculi in the urinary bladder. (**A**) Mineral opacity calculi in urine appear white or "radiopaque". (**B**) The same mineral opacity calculi in contrast medium appear black or "radiolucent". (**C**) Soft tissue opacity calculi in urine are not visible, but they commonly are called "radiolucent". (**D**) The same soft tissue opacity calculi in a thin layer of positive contrast medium appear black or "radiolucent". (**E**) The same soft tissue opacity calculi surrounded by gas appear white or "radiopaque". As you can see, the words radiolucent and radiopaque are not stand-alone descriptors and convey less meaningful information than terms such as mineral opacity and soft tissue opacity.

receptor is represented by a characteristic curve (Figure 1.58). Latitude is inversely related to contrast: the wider the latitude, the less the contrast. Wide latitude receptors are able to form many shades of gray over a large range of x-ray intensities, which means they can display many different levels of opacity. Wide latitude is low contrast so there will be less distinction from one density to the next and less contrast between one opacity and the next. Narrow latitude receptors form fewer gray shades over a smaller range of x-ray intensities, which means fewer different levels of opacity can be displayed. Narrow latitude is high contrast so the radiograph will be more black and white. The latitude of the image receptor needs to be wide enough to display all of the structures of interest (levels of opacity) and narrow enough so there is adequate contrast to identify each structure in one radiograph. X-ray exposures that fall outside the latitude of an image receptor will result in little or no radiographic contrast.

In **film radiography**, the latitude of the image receptor is built-in and cannot be changed. The only way to increase or decrease contrast is to switch to a film:screen system with a different emulsion formulation. Contrast in film radiography also is affected by processing. Over-development or under-development of the film can significantly and permanently reduce contrast.

In **digital radiography**, the latitude of the image receptors is very wide. Digital receptors are able to form acceptable contrast over a broad range of x-ray exposures.

The **higher the kVp, the lower the contrast**. Higher energy x-rays are more penetrating, which means there is less differential absorption between different materials. When there is less difference in x-ray attenuation, the different shades of gray that result from passing the x-ray beam through tissues of different opacities will be more similar in the radiograph and less distinguishable (Box 1.8). To quote a common expression used in medical radiography: "kVp kills contrast."

Radiographic contrast can be altered to a certain degree by manipulating kVp and mAs. To increase contrast and maintain radiographic density, decrease the kVp by 16% and

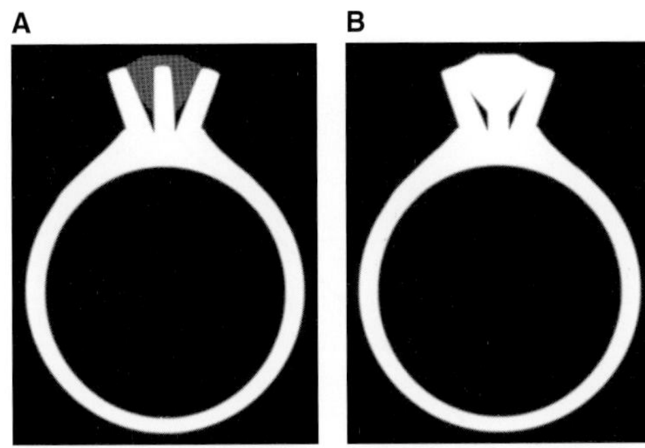

Figure 1.56 Diamond vs zirconium. The above images depict close-up radiographs of two similar engagement rings, one containing a diamond (**A**) and the other a cubic zirconium crystal (**B**). The relative opacity of the zirconium crystal is much greater than that of a diamond and it appears whiter in a radiograph. Diamonds are made of carbon which is essentially soft tissue opacity.

double the mAs. In most cases, you will need to repeat this adjustment more than once to make a visible difference in the radiograph (which may result in very large changes in kVp and mAs). To decrease contrast and maintain density, increase kVp 20% and cut the mAs in half. Again, repeat these adjustments as needed to achieve the desired effect. You may wonder why we say increase kVp by 20% and decrease it by 16%. If you do the math, you will see that we end up changing the kVp by nearly the same number each way. Some simply say change the kVp by 15% up or down.

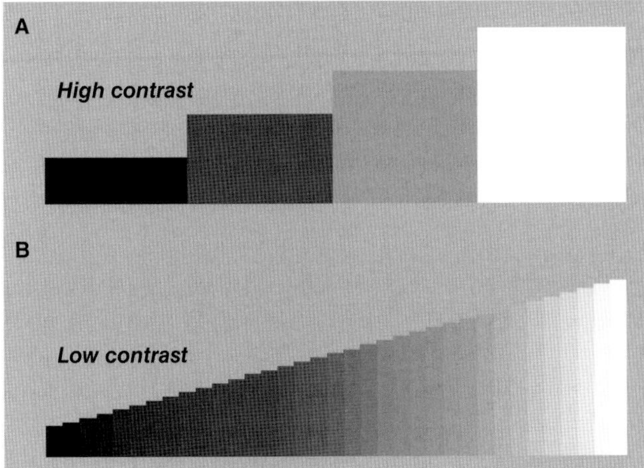

Figure 1.57 Contrast. (**A**) High contrast. There is a big difference moving from one shade of gray to the next and fewer steps between black and white. There are only a few gray shades available so only a few different levels of opacity can be displayed. (**B**) Low contrast. There is little distinction from one gray shade to the next and many steps between black and white. There are more shades of gray available to display more different levels of opacity. In this illustration, roughly 10 different shades of gray in the low contrast example are grouped into each shade of gray in the high contrast example. None of the 10 shades that are displayed in the low contrast image can be distinguished from each other in the high contrast image.

Always try to keep the exposure time as short as possible. In general, kVp above 70 results in relatively low radiographic contrast. Higher kVp techniques can be useful to help distinguish tissues with similar opacities because more shades of gray are available, such as imaging the lungs, abdomen, and thicker body parts. Lower kVp techniques (below 70) generally result in more radiographic contrast because there are fewer shades of gray. X-ray exposures near 70 kVp take advantage of the K-edges of bone and positive contrast agents to optimize their radiographic contrast (Figure 1.36).

Fog can significantly reduce radiographic contrast, as we discussed with scatter x-rays.

Displayed contrast

A tremendous advantage of digital radiography over film radiography is the ability to change contrast after the image has been acquired. In film radiography, contrast may be altered slightly by adjusting the intensity of the light that is transmitted through the film using variable intensity view-boxes and "hotlights." Digital contrast, however, can be optimized using the numerous shades of gray available in each pixel. Post-processing in digital radiography allows us to evaluate both thin and thick structures in the same radiograph.

The amount of contrast a digital receptor can display is determined by the number of shades of gray available to each pixel, which is called **bit depth**. Bit depth (represented by "*N*") is inversely related to contrast. As bit depth increases (*N* gets larger), the number of gray shades available to each pixel increases exponentially (2^N). For example, a pixel with a bit depth of 4 can display any of 2^4 or 16 different shades of gray. A pixel with bit depth of 8 can display any of 2^8 or 256 different shades (Figure 1.59). Recall that a bit is a digit in a binary number. Each shade of gray a pixel can display is represented by a binary number (Table 1.2). As bit depth increases, pixel numbers grow larger and larger and commonly are expressed in **bytes**. A byte is 8 bits which means a byte represents 2^8 or 256 shades of gray. A kilobyte (Kb) is 2^{10} shades and a megabyte (Mb) is 2^{20} shades.

Box 1.8 Radiographic contrast

With high contrast, it is easier to see the differences, but there is less to see.

With low contrast, there are more things to see, but it is more difficult to see the differences.

The computer automatically configures each pixel to display the best contrast by using a *look-up table*.

A **look-up table** (LUT) is a set of algorithms designed to optimize radiographic contrast for the specific body part

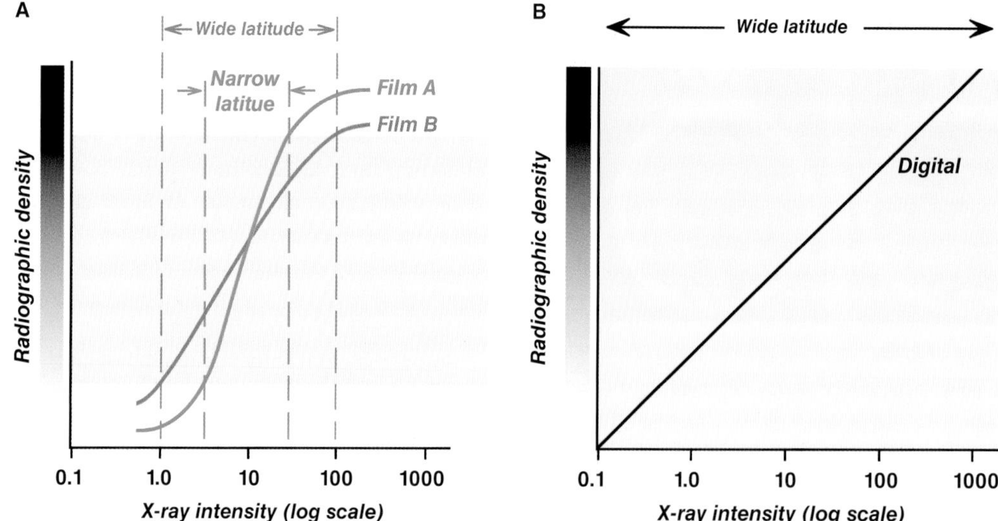

Figure 1.58 Latitude and contrast. These illustrations depict characteristic curves for film radiography (**A**) and digital radiography (**B**). Along the vertical axis (*x*-axis) of each graph are the acceptable levels of radiographic density (visible shades of gray). The horizontal axes (*y*-axes) is a logarithmic scale displaying the amount of x-rays the image receptor receives (the different x-ray intensities emerging from the patient). The yellow region across each graph depicts the shades of gray the image receptor can form. The slope of each curve represents the level of contrast the receptor can produce; the steeper the slope, the bigger the difference from one gray shade to the next. Latitude ranges from the minimum amount of x-rays the receptor needs to make any discernible shades of gray to the maximum amount of x-rays, above which no more contrast can be made. Any amount of x-rays below or above the latitude of a receptor will result in little or no contrast. **Film A** is narrow latitude. It can form contrast over the range of x-ray intensities between the two green dotted lines. The slope of the green curve is steep, which means small changes in the amount of x-rays will produce big changes in density and lots of contrast between shades of gray. **Film B** is wide latitude. It can form contrast over the range shown between the two blue dotted lines. The slope of the blue curve is not as steep as the green curve, which means more different levels of density can be formed over a larger range of x-ray intensities. There is less distinction from one gray shade to the next.

being imaged (e.g., thorax, abdomen, spine, extremity). The user selects the body part and the computer compares the histogram of the just acquired radiograph with its table of stored histograms. It "looks up" and selects the best histogram using specific pixel values of interest to properly display the radiograph. The LUT process permanently alters the raw data to improve contrast in the final radiograph. After computer processing, the user can use computer software to further alter the displayed contrast by *leveling* and *windowing* the image.

Leveling makes all of the pixels lighter or darker, effectively decreasing or increasing the radiographic density. **Windowing** allows the user to select a certain range of pixel values (shades of gray) from the numerous values available to increase or decrease contrast (Table 1.3). The range of selected values is called the **window width**. Any pixel values outside the window width will either be all white or all black. Window width is inversely related to contrast; the wider the window, the more shades of gray (less contrast). The narrower the window, the more black and white the image. The *window center* is the part of the radiograph where contrast will be focused. Leveling and windowing do not permanently alter the data; any changes made can be undone.

Radiographic detail

Detail is the sharpness of change from one radiographic density (one shade of gray) to the next. It determines how clear the edges appear when two structures are close together.

Radiographic detail is not the same as *opacity interface*. Detail refers to the quality of the radiographs whereas *opacity interface* relates to issues with the patient. Key factors that affect radiographic detail are listed below and in Box 1.9.

1. Motion.
2. Geometric unsharpness.
3. Noise.
4. Image receptor characteristics.

Motion during x-ray exposure is a major cause of poor detail in veterinary radiology. Motion may result from a struggling patient, an unstable x-ray tube, or inadvertent bumping of the image receptor. Motion leads to blurry margins in the radiograph. To minimize motion artifacts, use as short an exposure time as practical and appropriate patient restraint. Keep in mind that sedation may be less stressful to the patient than struggling with it.

Periodically inspect all equipment to make sure it is secure.

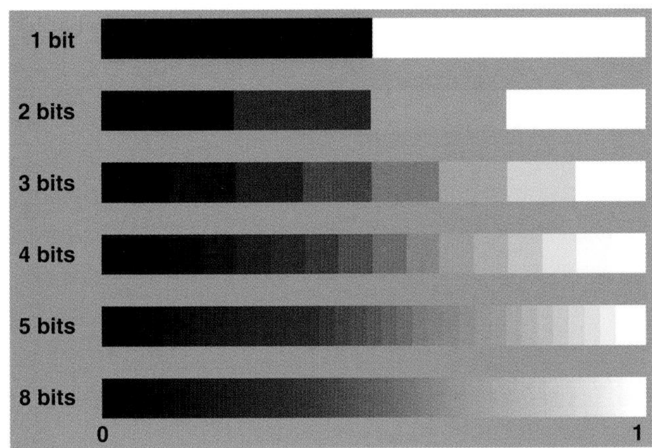

Figure 1.59 Bit depth. This illustration depicts the number of different shades of gray each pixel in an image is able to display as determined by its number of bits. An image made with 1-bit pixels would display the highest contrast because there are only 2^1 gray shades available: black or white. An image made with 4-bit pixels could display up to 2^4 or 16 different shades of gray. With 8 bit pixels, any of 2^8 or 256 shades of gray could be displayed.

Avoid hand-holding of portable x-ray tubes or image receptors. Not only does this lead to poor-quality radiographs, but it exposes the operator to more radiation than necessary.

Minimize geometric unsharpness to maximize detail. Use the small focal spot whenever practical (Figure 1.23) and the longest source-to-image distance (SID) that is feasible (Figures 1.27 and 1.28). Position the body part of interest as close to the image receptor as practical and align the x-ray beam, body part, and image receptor to minimize distortion (Figures 1.29–1.31).

Table 1.2 Pixel numbers with 4-bit depth[a]

Pixel Number	Pixel Value	Shade of Gray
0 0 0 0	0	
0 0 0 1	1	
0 0 1 0	2	
0 0 1 1	3	
0 1 0 0	4	
0 1 0 1	5	
0 1 1 0	6	
0 1 1 1	7	
1 0 0 0	8	
1 0 0 1	9	
1 0 1 0	10	
1 0 1 1	11	
1 1 0 0	12	
1 1 0 1	13	
1 1 1 0	14	
1 1 1 1	15	

[a] A pixel with bit depth of 4 means it can display any of 16 different shades of gray. Each value of gray is represented by a 4-bit (4 digit) pixel number (a binary number).

Noise diminishes radiographic detail. Noise is random variations in density that produce a "mottled" or "grainy" pattern in the radiograph. The mottling does not represent anything in the patient and makes the edges of structures less distinct. The more noise, the less detail.

Noise is present in all radiographs. It ranges from non-distracting to severe enough to obscure all detail and render the radiograph useless. The mottled pattern created by noise tends to be more noticeable in underexposed and high-contrast radiographs. The cause of noise may be inherent in the image receptor itself or it may be due to the naturally uneven manner in which x-rays strike the image receptor. The latter is called *quantum noise* or *quantum mottle*.

Inherent noise or "background" noise occurs in all imaging systems and cannot be eliminated. In film radiography, it is associated with the sizes of the silver crystals and phosphors; the bigger the grains, the more noise. In digital radiography, inherent noise results from random electrical currents. These currents may be generated by thermal activity within the system or they may be caused by interference from other electronics in the area (e.g., fluorescent lights, nearby motors).

Quantum noise is caused by unequal numbers of x-rays striking the image receptor. In physics, a *quantum* refers to a discrete amount of energy. The term quantum commonly is used to describe an x-ray photon, thus the name "quantum noise." The patchy pattern created by quantum noise is similar to that created by the first few drops of rain that fall on a paved walkway. In some areas, there are clusters of raindrops (x-rays) and in others there are only a few. The variation is due to the non-uniform nature in which the raindrops emerge from the raincloud or the x-rays emerge from the patient. Quantum noise becomes less noticeable as more and more x-rays strike the image receptor (more raindrops hit the pavement).

To assess the amount of detail an image receptor can provide, we look at the minimum distance between two lines that allow them to be distinguished as separate in the radiograph. This can be accomplished using a test pattern that contains progressively thinner and more numerous lines (Figure 1.60). The more lines that can be discriminated over a certain distance, the better the detail. The number of visible lines typically is expressed as line pairs per millimeter (lpm) or line pairs per inch (lpi). The human eye can discriminate about 10–14 lpm. Film:screen systems can resolve about 7–10 lpm. Many current digital systems are capable of about 5–6 lpm, but some can resolve 10 lpm. Although detail in digital imaging systems typically is less than in film radiography, the wide dynamic range and latitude of digital

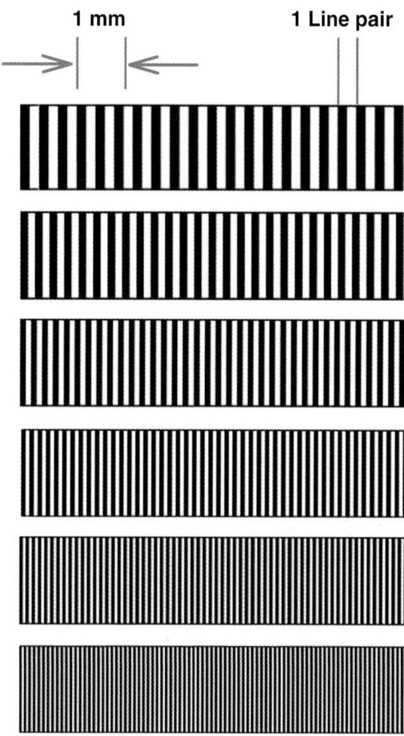

Figure 1.60 Line-pairs. Pictured here is a test pattern that can be used to evaluate the level of radiographic detail an image receptor can provide. The more line pairs that can be resolved over a distance of 1 mm, the better the detail. In this example, the top test pattern resolves 2 line pairs per mm. A line pair consists of a black line and a white line (the white lines are the spaces between the black lines). Radiographic detail is expressed as line pairs per millimeter or lpm.

receptors more than makes up for the difference. Digital detail likely will continue to improve **with advancing technology**.

Radiographic detail is also affected by **line spread** (Figure 1.61). Line spread refers to the lateral diffusion of light that occurs in image receptors that convert x-rays to visible light as an intermediate step (i.e., film:screen systems and indirect digital systems). The light emitted by a phosphor or scintillator spreads out to produce an area of light that is larger than the size of the x-ray itself. The more line spread, the less detail. Line spread does not occur in direct digital radiography or in film radiography where no screens are used.

Box 1.9 Maximize radiographic detail

- Use smallest focal spot that is practical.
- Make SID and SOD as long as feasible.
- Make OID as short as possible.
- Position central ray in middle of area of interest.
- Make area of interest parallel to image receptor.
- Use shortest exposure time practical.
- Utilize appropriate patient restraint.

Displayed radiographic detail

The radiographic detail provided by a film:screen image receptor cannot be changed. Detail is limited by the sizes of the silver crystals in the film and the phosphors in the screen. The larger the grains, the more noise mottling and the less detail.

The amount of detail in a digital system is determined by **spatial resolution**. Spatial resolution is affected by pixel size, pixel pitch, and the signal-to-noise ratio. Pixel size is not a permanent, fixed, or defined number. There is no standard physical size to a pixel. Pixel size is determined by the size of the FOV and the size of the matrix used to display the digital image. A matrix is a rectangular array arranged in rows and columns (Figure 1.66). The FOV determines the overall length and width of the matrix. The size of the matrix (number of pixels it contains) is determined by its number of rows and columns. The smaller and more numerous the pixels, the better the detail (Box 1.10). Pixels generally are considered to be square-shaped therefore they are measured along one side. Pixel size and pixel pitch usually are expressed as length in microns (μ).

Pixel pitch is the distance between two adjacent pixels. Pitch is measured from the middle of one pixel to the middle of the next. The shorter the pixel pitch, the better the detail (Figure 1.62). In current digital radiography systems, the distance between pixels is about the same as the pixel size and the two generally are considered to be equivalent. Pixel pitch in current systems is around 100–150 μ. The human eye can distinguish about 25 μ. The width of a human hair is about 40 μ. Smaller pixel pitches are possible, but they would lead to much higher x-ray exposures.

Signal-to-noise ratio (SNR) affects the detail in digital radiographs. SNR is a comparison of the amount of useful information generated by a digital image receptor to the amount of non-useful information. In other words, it is the number of electronic signals produced by x-rays compared to the amount of noise. The higher the SNR, the better the detail. Low SNR most often is due to an insufficient amount of x-rays reaching the image receptor. Many digital imaging systems automatically try to compensate for low exposures by amplifying the few electronic signals. Unfortunately, amplification also increases noise.

The type of **monitor** used for viewing digital radiographs contributes greatly to visible detail. The monitor must be able to display the same size matrix and number of shades of gray that the digital receptor provides, otherwise some detail will be lost.

The Art of radiography. The quality of a radiograph is affected by four characteristics: **density**, **detail**, **distortion**, and **contrast**. There are multiple technical factors that

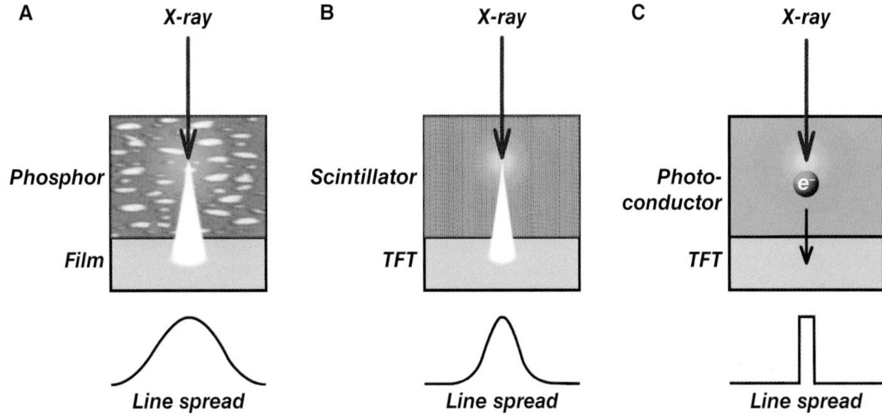

Figure 1.61 Line spread. These illustrations depict light being emitted by (**A**) a phosphor and (**B**) a scintillator in response to an x-ray interaction. The light spreads as it travels to the film or TFT array. Light spread is less with the scintillator due to the linear crystals that channel the light to reduce lateral diffusion. **C**. Image receptors that convert x-rays directly to electronic signals eliminate line spread.

influence these four characteristics, including mAs, kVp, focal spot size, SID, and others. In Table 1.4, we summarize the effects on radiographic quality caused by increasing or decreasing various factors. As you can see, altering a particular factor may increase one characteristic of radiographic quality while decreasing another. Often there is a compromise. Knowing how to adjust different factors is part of the Art of radiography. The more skilled you are at image acquisition, the better the radiographic quality and the more diagnostic the images. The Art of radiography also includes proper

Box 1.10 Pixel size and radiographic detail

Increasing the matrix size (number of rows and columns) while maintaining the same FOV (length and width of the matrix) will reduce the sizes of the pixels and increase radiographic detail.

$$\text{Pixel size} = \frac{\text{FOV}}{\sqrt{\text{Matrix size}}}$$

For example: a FOV that is 20 × 20 mm will produce a radiograph that is 400 mm^2. If the radiograph is displayed with a resolution of 512 × 512 (a matrix size of 512 rows × 512 columns), there will be 262,144 pixels in the image (512 × 512). The size of each pixel is calculated as follows:

$$\frac{400}{\sqrt{(512 \times 512)}} = \frac{400}{512} = 0.78\,\text{mm} = 780\,\mu$$

If we double the resolution, increasing the matrix size to 1024 × 1024, the number of pixels increases to 1,048,576, which means the size of each pixel must decrease by half to fit in the same FOV:

$$\frac{400}{\sqrt{(1024 \times 1024)}} = \frac{400}{1024} = 0.39\,\text{mm} = 390\,\mu$$

If we double the resolution again, to 2048×2048, pixel size decreases by another 50%:

$$\frac{400}{\sqrt{(2048 \times 2048)}} = \frac{400}{2048} = 0.19\,\text{mm} = 190\,\mu$$

Smaller and more numerous pixels leads to greater radiographic detail.

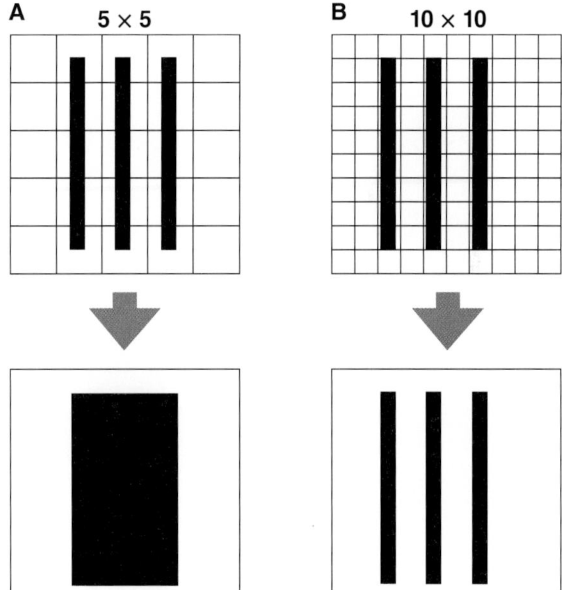

Figure 1.62 Pixel pitch. In this illustration, a 3-line test pattern is used to evaluate detail with two different matrix sizes. Each square in each matrix represents one pixel. To display the 3 lines as separate structures the sizes of the pixels must be smaller than the spaces between the lines. In matrix **A**, the resolution is 5 × 5 and the pixel pitch is larger than the spaces between the lines, which means there aren't enough pixels to distinguish the individual lines as separate. The test pattern is displayed as one thick line in the image below. In matrix **B**, the resolution is doubled to 10 × 10, which reduces both pixel size and pixel pitch. This allows a column of pixels between each line. The test pattern is displayed as three separate lines in the image below.

Table 1.3 Radiograph quality[a]

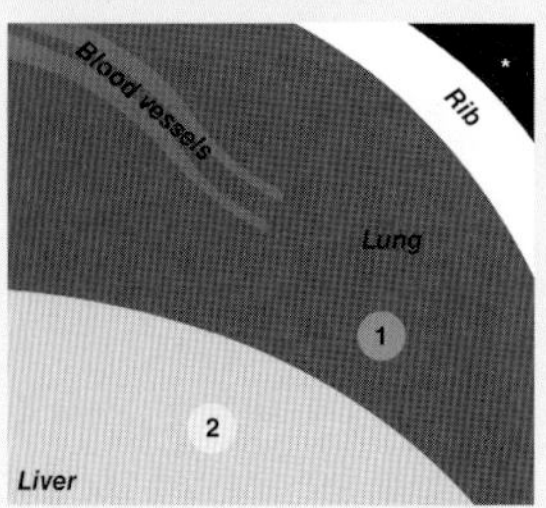

This illustration depicts structures in a close-up VD view of the thorax. Included are soft tissue opacity blood vessels, liver, and lung nodules. Nodule 1 is in the lung field and nodule 2 is summated with the liver. The rib is mineral opacity. The lung is gas opacity and there is gas opacity outside the rib (*)

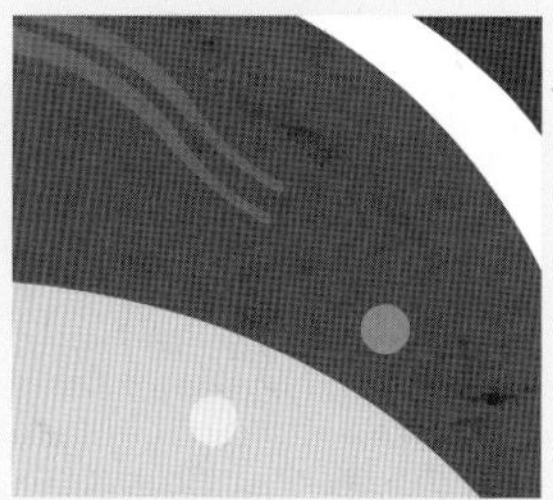

Good quality
Good detail the margins of the structures are distinct and well-defined
Good contrast all structures are displayed with acceptable density and contrast so they are visible in the image

High contrast
High contrast narrow latitude The visible structures are mostly black and white. There are not enough shades of gray to display all of the different opacities in the thorax.

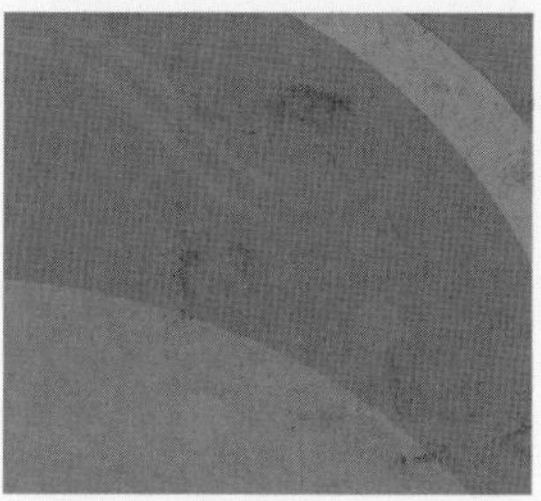

Low contrast
Wide latitude There are many shades of gray between black and white, but little distinction from one shade to the next. Structures with different opacities are visible but not very distinct.

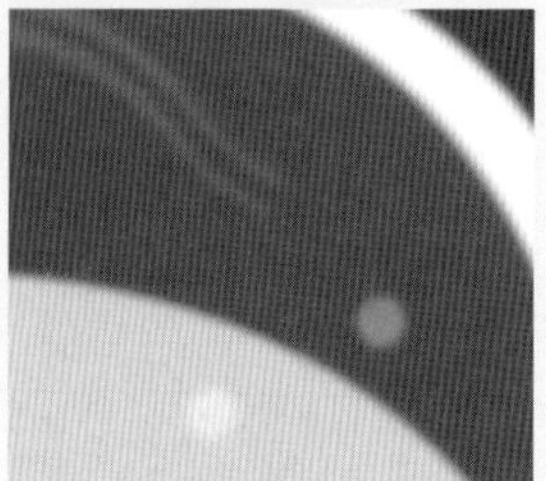

Poor detail
The margins of structures are indistinct, the edges appear hazy and ill-defined

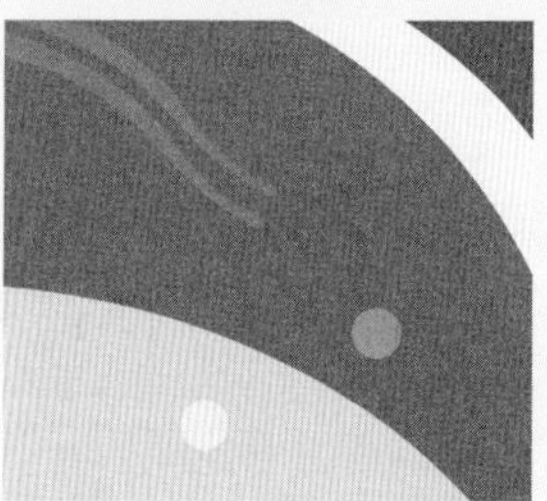

Noise
The background in the image appears mottled or grainy, which makes the margins of structures less distinct.

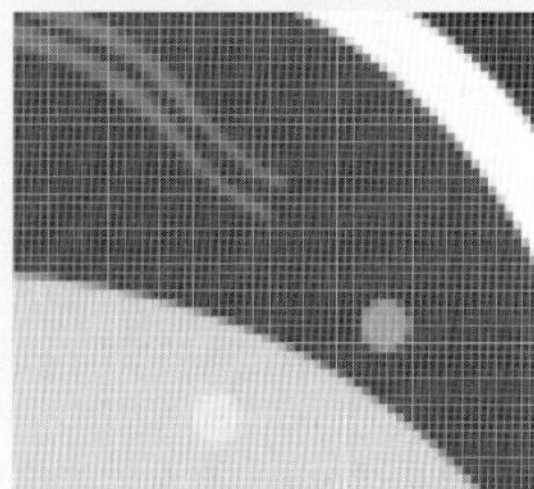

Large pixels
Detail is less because the image is displayed with large pixels. The image is "pixilated," making the margins of structures appear irregular and indistinct

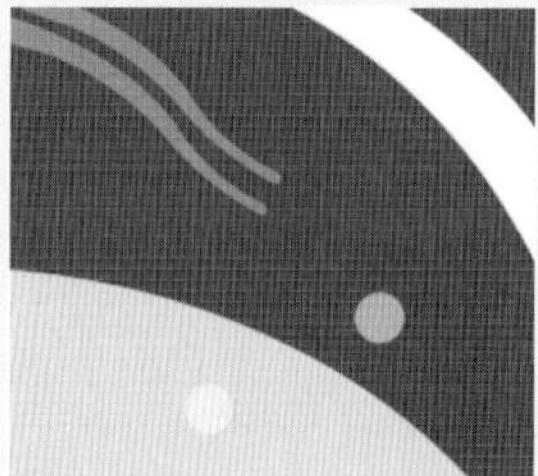

Small pixels
Detail is better because the image is displayed using smaller pixels. The matrix is larger, which means more pixels are available.

[a] In this table are several illustrations that depict the same area in a thoracic radiograph. The structures in this area are labelled in the first image (upper left corner). A good quality radiograph, with adequate density, contrast and detail, is depicted in the upper right corner. Poor quality radiographs due to unacceptable contrast, detail, noise, and pixel size are depicted in the remaining images.

Table 1.4 Table of compromise for radiography[a]

Factor	Increase Decrease	Effect on Radiograph Quality			
		Density	Detail	Distortion	Contrast
mAs	↑	↑	—	—	—
	↓	↓	—	—	—
kVp	↑	↑	—	—	↓
	↓	↓	—	—	↑
SID with static OID	↑	↓	↑	↓	—
	↓	↑	↓	↑	—
OID with static SID	↑	↓	↓	↑	↑
	↓	↑	↓	↓	↓
Sensitivity of image receptor	↑	↑	↓	—	—
	↓	↓	↑	—	—
Focal spot size	↑	—	↓	↑	—
	↓	Limits exposure	↑	↓	—
Fog grid (reduce fog)	↑	↑	↓	—	↓
	↓	↓	↑	—	↑
Pixel size	↑	—	↓	—	—
	↓	—	↑	—	—
Noise	↑	—	↓	—	—
	↓	—	↑	—	—
Latitude	↑	—	—	—	↓
	↓	—	—	—	↑

[a]This table lists various technical factors that can affect radiographic quality. For example: increasing or decreasing mAs affects radiographic Density. Increasing or decreasing kVp affects both Density and Contrast. Increasing OID with static SID will decrease Density and increase Contrast due to an air gap (object will be further away from the image receptor) and will increase magnification distortion.

patient positioning and accurate interpretation of the images, which are discussed in the next chapter.

Technique chart

A chart of reliable x-ray exposures is essential to making consistent quality radiographs. A technique chart must be customized to the individual radiography system, whether digital or film. Technique charts commonly are **kVp variable**, which means the mAs is fixed according to the body part being imaged and the kVp is adjusted for thickness. A variable mAs chart can be made if the kVp settings are limited.

Prior to creating your technique chart, all equipment should be installed, properly calibrated, and in good working order. The x-ray machine should be connected to a dedicated line of electricity with a voltage compensator to minimize fluctuations in power. Set your **source-to-image distance**. The standard SID in most veterinary practices is 100 cm (40 in.). A shorter SID may be needed if the x-ray machine is low output, perhaps 75 cm (30 in.). Low output units such as portable x-ray machines may limit the flexibility of a technique chart.

The **grid** you plan to use should be installed or otherwise available. Grids are recommended when body part thickness exceeds 10–12 cm. When using a grid, the x-ray exposure needs to be increased from the non-grid technique. Some digital imaging systems incorporate software to compensate for scatter radiation, which may reduce the need for a grid.

With film radiography, make sure the **processing equipment**, whether manual or automatic, is installed and in optimal condition. The chemicals should be relatively fresh, well-mixed, and at the proper temperatures. However, brand new chemicals sometimes are "hot" and it may be preferable to make your technique chart about 2 weeks after changing chemistry, depending on how often it is changed.

The first step in the creation of your technique chart is to make a **mAs table**. Begin by listing all of the available mA settings across the top and all of the available exposure times down the left side. Then multiply each mA setting by each exposure time to determine all of the possible mAs settings (Table 1.5). This table will be used to choose the shortest exposure times available to help reduce motion artifacts.

The next step is to make some **test radiographs**. Select an animal that is typical of the type of patient seen at your clinic or hospital. In general, a medium-sized dog that is not overweight is a good candidate. Select a dog less than 20 kg (50 lb), perhaps with thickness of about 15 cm at its widest part. Make three lateral views of the abdomen. We image the abdomen because it contains many soft tissue opacity structures.

Make one abdominal radiograph using 5 mAs, another with 10 mAs, and the third with 20 mAs. Use your mAs chart to select the shortest exposure time for each. To select a kVp, measure the width of animal's abdomen in centimeters and

Table 1.5 mAs table[a]

mA	50 mA	100 mA	200 mA	300 mA
Time (seconds)				
1/60 (0.016)	0.83	1.67	3.33	5.00
1/30 (0.033)	1.67	3.33	5.00	10.0
1/20 (0.050)	2.50	5.00	10.0	15.0
1/15 (0.066)	3.33	6.67	13.3	20.0
1/10 (0.100)	5.00	10.0	20.0	30.0
2/10 (0.200)	10.0	20.0	40.0	60.0
3/10 (0.300)	15.0	30.0	60.0	90.0
4/10 (0.400)	20.0	40.0	80.0	120
1/2 (0.500)	25.0	50.0	100	150
3/5 (0.600)	30.0	60.0	120	180
4/5 (0.800)	40.0	80.0	160	240
1 (1.000)	50.0	100	200	300

[a] For this particular x-ray machine, the available mA settings are listed across the top of the table and the available exposure times are listed down the left side. Times are displayed as both fractions and decimals. Multiplying each mA by each time gives all of the possible mAs settings for this particular x-ray machine.

the SID in inches. The kVp is calculated from these two factors. It should be twice the abdomen thickness plus the SID. For example, if the abdomen is 15 cm and the SID is 40 in., the kVp would be 70; $(2 \times 15) + 40 = 70$. Use this kVp for all three radiographs.

After all three radiographs have been made, select the one with the best radiographic density (Figure 1.63). The mAs used to make this radiograph will be the **base mAs** for the technique chart. Be sure to dry completely all hand-processed film radiographs before reviewing them.

If all of the radiographs are underexposed (too light), either the kVp or the mAs needs to be increased. If there is too much contrast in the radiographs (too black and white), increase the kVp. If the contrast is acceptable, increase the mAs. If increasing the mAs makes the exposure time exceed 1/30 second, increase the kVp instead. If all of the test radiographs are overexposed (too dark), cut the exposure time in half to reduce the mAs by 50%.

Variable kVp chart

The third step in creating your technique chart is to determine the **variable kVp** settings for different thicknesses and body parts. Let's begin with abdomen. Suppose from our test radiographs we determined that the exposure needed to make an acceptable lateral view of a 15 cm thick abdomen was 10 mAs and 70 kVp. We can then determine the exposure needed for every other thickness of abdomen. For each 1 cm decrease in abdomen thickness, we subtract 2 kVp. For each 1 cm increase in thickness, we add 2 kVp. We can do this up to 80 kVp. Above 80 kVp, we add 3 kVp for each 1 cm increase in thickness until we get to 100 kVp. Over 100 kVp, we add 4 kVp for each 1 cm increase in thickness.

For **thoracic** radiography we use the same kVp settings as for abdomen, but decrease the mAs by half. The thoracic cavity is mostly air-filled and generally requires less exposure. Lower mAs means shorter exposure times which is important to minimize cardiac and respiratory motion blur. Make a lateral thoracic radiograph of your test animal to confirm this thoracic technique is satisfactory. If needed, increase or decrease kVp to darken or lighten the test image. Then extrapolate the rest of the kVp values for the other thicknesses (Table 1.6).

For **orthopedic** imaging we use the same kVp settings as for abdomen, but double the mAs. Make a lateral view of the lumbar spine of your same test animal to confirm this

A

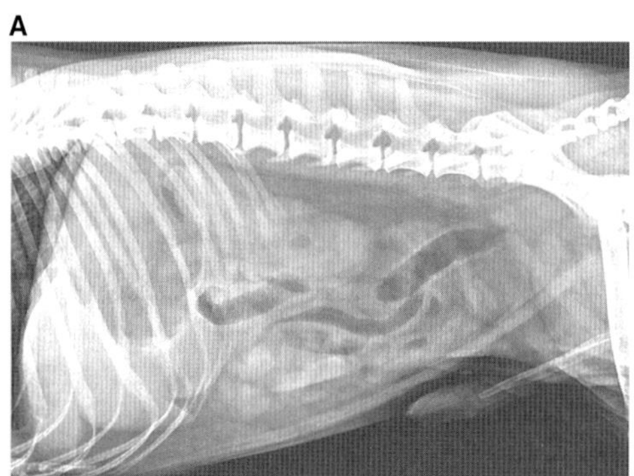

B

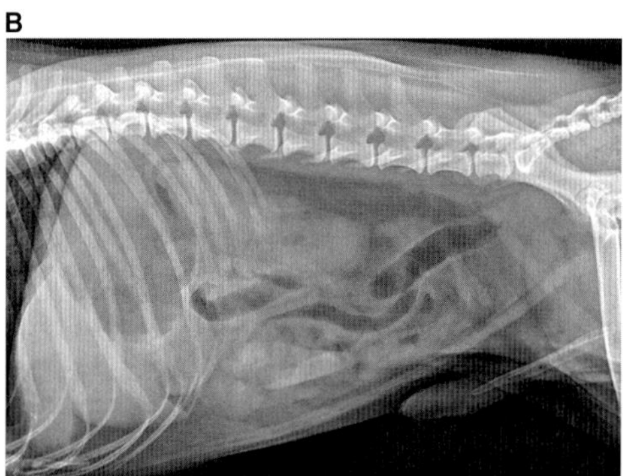

C

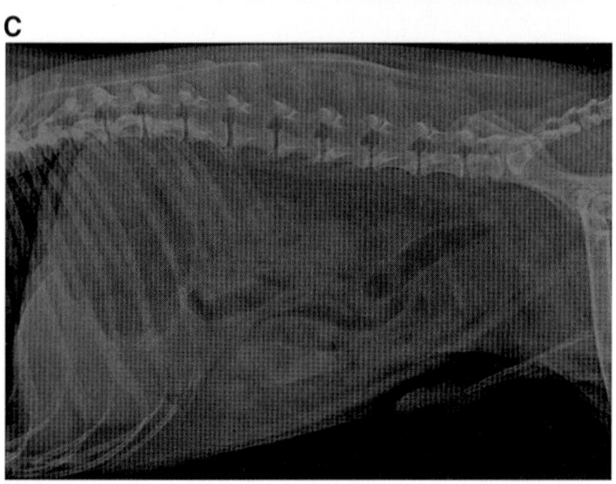

Figure 1.63 Test radiographs. Three lateral views of a dog's abdomen depicting (**A**) too little radiographic density due to underexposure, (**B**) acceptable density, and (**C**) too much density due to overexposure.

Table 1.6 Variable kVp chart.[a]

Thickness	Thorax		Abdomen		Skeleton	
cm	kVp	mAs	kVp	mAs	kVp	mAs
1	50	2.5	42	5.0	36	5
2	52	2.5	44	5.0	38	5
3	54	2.5	46	5.0	40	5
4	56	2.5	48	5.0	42	5
5	58	2.5	50	5.0	44	5
6	60	2.5	52	5.0	46	5
7	62	2.5	54	5.0	48	5
8	64	2.5	56	5.0	50	5
9	66	2.5	58	5.0	52	5
10	68	2.5	60	5.0	54	5
			Grid			
11	70	5.0	62	10	56	10
12	72	5.0	64	10	58	10
13	74	5.0	66	10	60	10
14	76	5.0	68	10	62	10
15	78	5.0	70	10	64	10
16	80	5.0	72	10	66	10
17	83	5.0	74	10	68	10
18	86	5.0	76	10	70	10
19	89	5.0	78	10	72	10
20	92	5.0	80	10	74	10
21	95	5.0	83	10	76	10
22	98	5.0	86	10	78	10
23	101	5.0	89	10	80	10
24	105	5.0	92	10	67	20
25	109	5.0	95	10	69	20
26	113	5.0	98	10	71	20
27	117	5.0	86	20	73	20
28	121	5.0	89	20	75	20
29	125	5.0	92	20	77	20
30	110	10	95	20	79	20

[a] This chart was made for a particular x-ray machine. It displays the mAs and kVp settings needed to image a wide range of body part thicknesses. The test radiographs were made using a 15 cm thick patient. A grid is used when body part thickness exceeds 10 cm. Notice the mAs is doubled when using the grid. In this example chart, the kVp used for thorax was increased 20% over the abdomen technique because the test radiograph for thorax was underexposed. The kVp for musculoskeletal radiographs was decreased 16% from abdomen technique because the test radiograph of the spine was overexposed.

technique is acceptable. Then extrapolate the rest of the kVp values. Double the mAs again if the radiograph needs to be darker or decrease kVp by 16% if the image needs to be lighter. Try to keep the kVp below 80 to take advantage of the K-edge of bone and enhance contrast (Table 1.6).

Adjustments to the technique chart

Patients presented for veterinary radiography vary significantly in size, shape and conformation. In addition, the reasons that bring them into the clinic or hospital often necessitate adjustments to the exposure technique (e.g., fluid or gas in a body cavity). The mAs or kVp suggested by the technique chart may need to be altered for a particular patient, particularly with film radiography (Boxes 1.11 and 1.12). The choice of which factor to adjust often is based on experience and equipment limitations.

Changes to mAs typically are made to increase or decrease radiographic density. If you don't like a radiograph that is well positioned with good detail and is not fogged, think density first. If the radiograph is too light, double the mAs. If it is too dark, cut the mAs in half. Altering the mAs by less than a factor of 2 probably won't make a visible change in the radiograph. Changing the mAs can be repeated as needed to achieve the desired density. If you correct the density and the radiograph still is not acceptable, then consider changing the contrast.

Adjustments to kVp alter the penetrating abilities of the x-rays and affect the radiographic contrast. The minimal change to kVp to produce a visible difference in the radiograph is either a 20% increase or a 16% decrease. These adjustments also can be repeated as needed to achieve the desired result. To increase the contrast in a radiograph, but maintain the same radiographic density, decrease the kVp 16% and double the mAs. Do this at least twice. To decrease contrast and maintain density, increase kVp 20% and cut mAs in half. Again, do this at least twice.

Box 1.11 Conditions that typically require higher exposures

1. Obesity.
2. Pleural or peritoneal effusion.
3. Positive contrast studies.
4. Overlying bandaging or cast material.

When using a low-power x-ray machine, a good rule of thumb is to increase kVp when the radiograph is too light (if possible), and decrease the mAs when it is too dark. This allows you to use the shortest exposure time possible.

Box 1.12 Conditions that typically require lower exposures

1. Emaciation.
2. Immature animals.
3. Pneumothorax.
4. Negative contrast studies.
5. Compression radiography.

CHAPTER 1

Radiograph storage and distribution

Radiographs are part of the medical record and must be safeguarded. Film radiographs must be physically stored in a safe environment where they are protected from theft, abuse, chemicals, and extremes in temperature and humidity for the legal life of the records. Digital radiographs must be stored in computer files with reliable backup copies both onsite and offsite.

Federal laws in the United States mandate that all radiographs be securely maintained and readily accessible both for the short term and the long term. All states in the US have enacted laws that govern the retention of medical records. In general, veterinarians are required to keep records at least 5 years past their last contact with the patient. Consult your local governmental guidelines and malpractice statutes of limitations for specific requirements.

Radiographs usually are regarded as the property of the hospital or clinic. However, in the US most state laws guarantee that your clients have access to them. It is a good idea to have a written policy regarding the release of any radiographs. The policy should state whether the originals will be loaned out or if copies will be made and how the radiographs will be tracked to ensure their safe return. Signed documents are recommended.

Most veterinary practice laws require specific medicolegal documentation be attached to all radiographs (Box 1.13). This information must be permanently embedded in the emulsion of film radiographs using photo flashing equipment, lead markers, or lead-based writing tape (Figure 1.64). Body markers also should be visible (e.g., Right and Left markers). In some practices, each technologist has his or her own R and L body markers with their initials on them. Digital radiographs must be saved in a format that securely attaches the required information to the image file. This most often is done using DICOM.

DICOM is an acronym that stands for **D**igital **I**maging and **C**ommunication **I**n **M**edicine. It is a worldwide standardized method for storing and transmitting digital radiographs. DICOM is not a type of image, rather it is a type of file format. With DICOM, various types of data can be permanently attached to the radiographic image, including patient information, the type of digital equipment that was used to make the radiograph, pixel information, facts about transmission, image compression, and more. The data is protected and cannot be altered without destroying the file. A major advantage with DICOM is its worldwide acceptance. Radiographs created on one type of digital imaging system can be viewed on a different system without loss of quality. Radiographs saved in DICOM format typically are stored, retrieved, transmitted, and viewed using a PACS.

Box 1.13 Required information on all radiographs

- Name of veterinarian or hospital/clinic.
- Name of animal.
- Name of owner.
- Date radiograph was made.
- Initials of persons making the radiograph.

PACS is an acronym that stands for **P**icture **A**rchiving and **C**ommunications **S**ystem. It refers to a network of hardware and software designed to securely store and transmit radiographs (Figure 1.65). Most PACS can handle multiple imaging modalities in addition to radiography, such as ultrasonography, computed tomography and magnetic resonance imaging. The PACS provides individual points of access to the images and associated data and to both short term and long term archives. Another name for a PACS is DIMS which stands for Digital Image Management System.

Within a PACS network is a group of two or more computers that are connected to each other. Linked computers that are close together (e.g., in the same building) is called a *local area network* or LAN. Computers that are further apart and linked by telephone lines, cables, or radio waves across

A

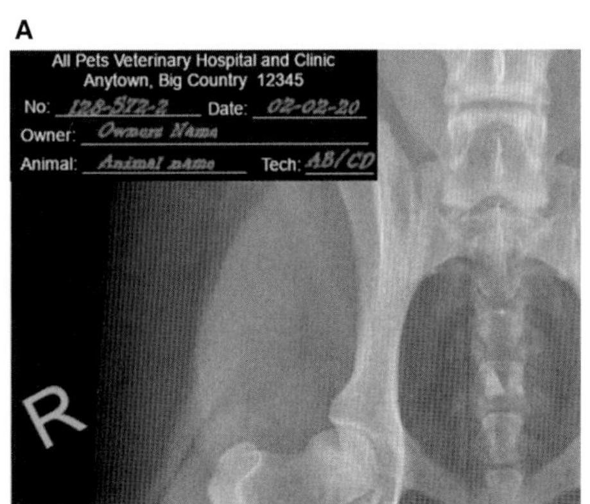

B

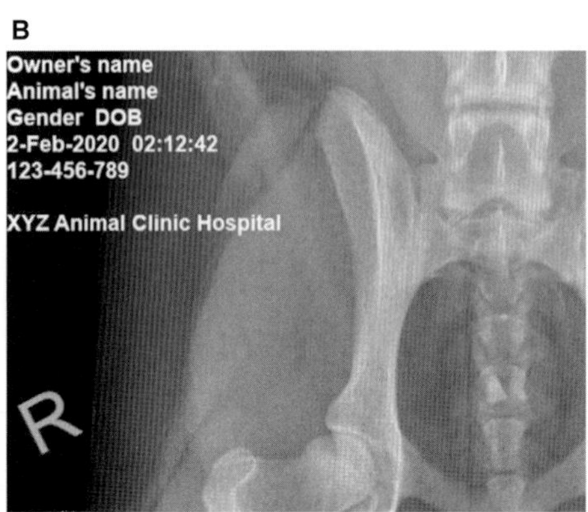

Figure 1.64 Radiograph identification. **A**. Film: photo flash. **B**. Digital. Identifying information should be clearly visible and permanent in each radiograph.

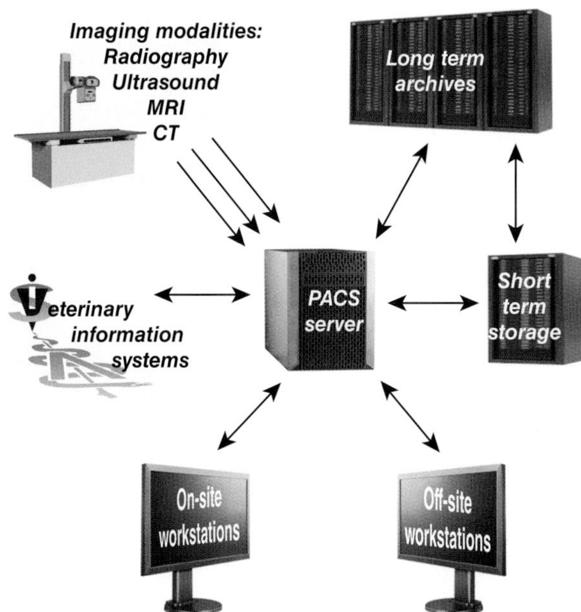

Figure 1.65 PACS. This illustration depicts the various components of a typical PACS. Each component is linked to a central server in a geometric arrangement called *star topology*. Other types of topology are also possible. Imaging modalities send radiographs and other data to the server, which in turn communicates with the hospital information system, onsite and offsite workstations, and both long-term and short-term storage archives.

a city, country, or the world is called a *wide area network* or WAN.

The **server** computer in a PACS manages the resources, runs the operations, and stores the data. The **client** computers request information from one or more servers and are part of the *workstations*. Workstations are used to display, process, and review radiographs and to link them with patient information and other data. A workstation may either be onsite, physically located in the hospital or clinic, or offsite, set up in a location that is remote from the medical facility. Many workstations are equipped with a diagnostic grade monitor, PACS viewing software, and a teleradiology service.

A great benefit of a PACS is the ease of transmitting digital radiographs, medical reports, and patient information among its various components and to the hospital medical systems (e.g., Hospital Information System, Radiology Information System, Electronic Medical Records). There are many complex components that need to operate well together for a PACS to function properly. Software and network connections must be compatible with multiple users, various storage sites, and the practice management system. It is essential to have good technical support and to train your technicians and staff so they have a basic understanding of the PACS. A well-managed PACS is mostly invisible, operating behind the scenes to minimize the need for repeated input of data, providing ready access to the radiographs, speeding up the turnaround times for radiographic studies, and improving patient care. A PACS is only as good as its weakest link.

Digital radiographs contain vast amounts of information, which makes for very large file sizes (Box 1.14 and Figure 1.66). The larger the file, the more computer memory is needed and the longer it takes to process and transmit the data. In addition, the files must be backed up, which doubles or triples the amount of storage space required. To make file sizes more manageable they usually are **compressed**.

Various computer algorithms are used to compress digital radiographs. Some of these are proprietary and therefore not compatible with other applications. It is important to determine whether your PACS is using a DICOM compliant algorithm. If not, the type of compression you are using may lock you in with your current PACS vendor. There are two basic types of compression: *lossless* and *lossy*.

Lossless compression is reversible, which means the original radiograph can be reconstructed from the compressed data without any loss of image quality. The amount of compression or the *compression ratio* with the lossless method is about 2 : 1.

Lossy compression is not reversible. The original radiograph cannot be completely reconstructed from the compressed file, so there will be some loss of image quality. The clinical significance of the lost quality varies with the type of algorithm used. The compression ratio with the lossy method is greater than with the lossless method and can be as high as 20 : 1.

As mentioned earlier, back-up copies of digital radiographs must be safely stored both onsite and offsite. The back-ups need to be readily accessible at all times, either through a direct link to your PACS or via a network. **Onsite storage** requires something in addition to just backing up to the computer hard drive. **Reliable redundancy is crucial.** Backup copies must be dependable so they can be used to replace your data should it be lost for whatever reason. Many options are available to make spare copies of your data onsite, including extra computer hard drives, portable

Box 1.14 File size of a digital radiograph

The file size of a digital radiograph is calculated by multiplying the total number of pixels in the image by the pixel bit depth. For example: a radiograph made on a 12-bit digital system with a 1024 × 1024 resolution results in a file size of 1.5 Mb.

The total number of pixels in the image is

1024 × 1024 = 1,048,576 pixels

1,048,576 × 12-bit = 12,582,912 bits

12,582,912 bits ÷ 8 = 1,572,864 bytes

1,572,864 bytes ÷ 1024 = 1536 Kb

1536 Kb ÷ 1024 = 1.5 MB

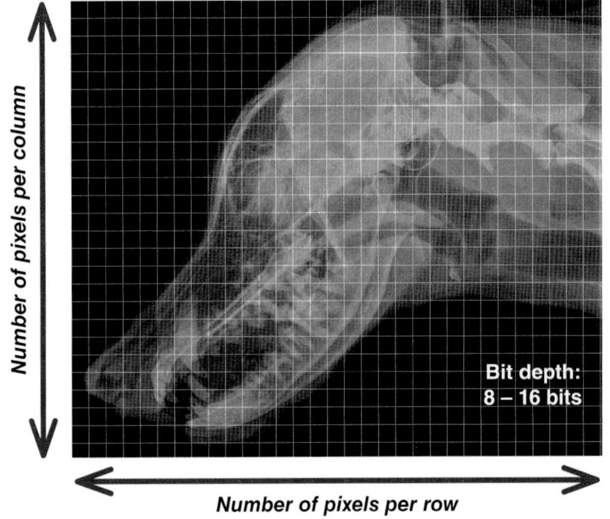

Matric size (R × C)	Number of Pixels	Radiograph size in Mb
512 × 512	262,144	0.25 – 0.50
1024 × 1024	1,048,576	1.0 – 2.0
2048 × 2048	4,194,304	4.0 – 8.0

Figure 1.66 File size of digital radiographs. A matrix is superimposed on a lateral view of a dog's head. The file size of the radiograph is determined by multiplying the total number of pixels in the matrix by the bit depth of the digital imaging system. In this example, three different matrix sizes are listed (512, 1024, and 2048). The total number of pixels in each matrix is determined by multiplying the number of pixels in a row (R) by the number of pixels in a column (C). The file sizes of radiographs made using digital systems ranging from 8–16 bit depth are listed in megabytes.

external disc drives, optical drives, flash storage, tape, and others. A redundant array of independent disks (RAID) can be configured to mirror the data on the computer so that if one hard drive fails the data remains safe on the others. Portable media can be used off-line while not connected to the network and also can be transferred off-site.

Offsite storage means the back-up data is moved away from the medical facility. This commonly includes sending it to one or more remote servers, known as *cloud* storage. **Cloud storage** may provide some advantages, including technical support and a large amount of storage space, the latter usually is expandable to meet future needs. Radiographs stored in the cloud often are easily shared with clients, colleagues, radiologists, and other specialists. When selecting a cloud storage platform, be sure your data is stored in a vendor-neutral and DICOM compliant format.

Radiographs are stored for different lengths of time in different locations. Initially, they are sent to the PACS server, where they are stored for a few months up to 2 years, depending on whether the facility is in-patient or out-patient. A copy typically remains in the digital system where the radiographs were made for a few days. The server sends copies to be archived in long-term storage. In the archives, the radiographs that are not being actively used are stored for the legal life of the study.

Radiation safety

Exposure to x-radiation can damage or destroy living cells and increase the risk of developing cancer. Although the health risk is relatively small, there is no "safe dose" of radiation. Any amount of exposure can cause damage (Box 1.15). The level of health risk depends on the dose of radiation received, the time over which the dose was received, and the body parts exposed. The higher the dose and the shorter the time to receive that dose, the greater the risk. Some body parts are more sensitive to radiation damage than others (Table 1.7).

We are exposed to radiation every day, from both natural and man-made sources (Figure 1.67). **Natural radiation** is ever-present, coming from outer space, the earth, and even our own bodies. Cosmic radiation originates in the sun and stars and continuously impacts the earth. It is more intense at higher elevations. Radiation from the earth originates in the low levels of radon, uranium, radium, and others that are ubiquitous in the soil, water, and vegetation. We frequently ingest this type of radiation with our food and water and also inhale it, the latter primarily as radon. Radiation within our bodies comes from isotopes of carbon and potassium present since birth. The average dose of natural radiation to persons living in the United States is about 0.3 rem/year.

Man-made radiation mostly comes from medical procedures such as diagnostic imaging and radiation therapy. It also comes from consumer products such as televisions, smoke detectors, building materials, airport x-ray security systems, and to a lesser extent from the fallout of nuclear weapons, nuclear accidents, and the fuel used in nuclear reactors. The average dose of man-made radiation to persons living in the United States is about 0.3 rem/year.

Box 1.15 Radiation safety

- Any amount of x-ray exposure can damage cells.
- There is no threshold dose of x-rays below which it is certain that an adverse effect cannot occur.
- The effects of radiation are cumulative and may not become apparent until later in life.
- Any exposure to x-rays should be As Low As Reasonably Achievable (**ALARA**).

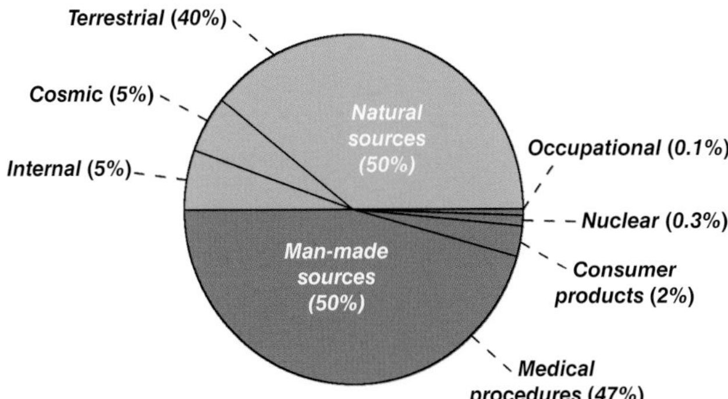

Figure 1.67 Sources of radiation exposure. The average dose of radiation received by persons living in the United States is around 0.6 rem/year. About half of this dose comes from natural sources and half from man-made sources (this illustration is modified from NCRP Report No. 160.) The dose can be much higher for persons receiving radiation therapy.

Biologic effects of radiation

Radiation is one of the most thoroughly investigated causes of disease. More is known about the effects of x-rays on cells and organ systems than is known about many other health risks. The damage caused by x-rays is due to ionization. When electrons are lost chemical bonds can break and molecules can fall apart. Ionization can directly or indirectly injure or kill cells.

Direct cellular damage occurs when vital molecules in the cell wall or in the DNA are destroyed by ionization. Indirect damage results from the free radicals that are generated by the ionization of water. Most living cells are nearly 80% water. Free radicals are highly reactive molecules that can severely alter cell functions. The susceptibility of a cell to the damaging effects of x-rays is known as *radiosensitivity*.

Radiosensitivity is relative (Table 1.7). Some cells are more sensitive to radiation than others. The most radiosensitive cells are those with high rates of division, high rates of metabolism, and immature or non-specialized cells. When a cell is damaged by ionizing radiation there are three possible outcomes:

1. The damage may be completely repaired and the cell returns to normal function.
2. The damage may kill the cell or make it unable to reproduce, either of which results in complete loss of cell function. This is known as **deterministic** damage and becomes clinically evident when enough cells lose function and cause the organ to fail.
3. The damage may be poorly repaired, resulting in mutation of the cell and possible future malignancy. This is known as **stochastic** damage and clinical signs are less predictable. The severity of a mutation is not dependent on the dose of radiation received; any dose can lead to the development of cancer.

Measuring radiation exposure

Several different measurements are used to describe the effects of radiation on living tissue. The *exposure dose* is the amount of radiation energy delivered to an area. The *absorbed dose* is the amount of energy deposited in tissue. The *effective dose* is the amount of biological damage that was caused by the absorbed dose. When dealing with x-rays, each of these dose measurements is equivalent. They are all affected by the x-ray beam intensity, the distance from the source of x-rays, and time during which the tissue is irradiated. We currently are measuring radiation doses using units from two different systems (Table 1.8): the *British system* with its "conventional units" and the *System International* (SI).

The **exposure dose** is a measurement of the amount of ionizations a given intensity of x-rays can cause in air. The conventional unit of measure is the Roentgen (R). The SI unit is coulomb/kilogram (C/kg). Specifically, 1 R is the amount of x-ray energy needed to create 1.6×10^{12} ion pairs/g in dry air at 0 °C. This amount of energy is very small in everyday life, but at the cellular level it is quite large, able to cause thousands of trillions of ionizations. The conversion

Table 1.7 Relative radiosensitivity of various tissues in the body

Level of Radiosensitivity	Tissue
High	• Lymphoid organs, thymus • Bone marrow, blood • Spleen • Testes, ovaries • Small intestine
Fairly high	• Skin, hair follicles • Cornea • Oral cavity, esophagus • Rectum • Urinary bladder, ureters • Vagina, uterine cervix
Moderate	• Optic lens • Stomach • Growing cartilage and bone • Fine vasculature
Fairly low	• Mature cartilage and bones • Salivary glands • Lungs, kidneys, liver • Pancreas • Thyroid, adrenal, pituitary glands • connective tissue
Low	• Muscle, • brain, spinal cord, nerves

factor to change conventional units to SI units is $1\ R = 2.58 \times 10^{-4}$ C/kg.

The **absorbed dose** relates the exposure dose to the amount of damage the x-rays could cause in living tissue. The conventional unit of measure is the rad, which is short for **r**adiation **a**bsorbed **d**ose. The SI unit is the gray (Gy). Specifically, 1 rad = 100 ergs of energy/g of material and 1 Gy = 1 J of energy/kg. The conversion factor to change conventional units to SI units is 100 rad = 1 Gy.

The **effective dose** is a measure of the biological effects of different types of radiation. It is sometimes called the **dose equivalent**. Some forms of radiation are more damaging than others and the effective dose can be greater than the absorbed dose. However, with x-rays the effective dose and the absorbed dose are equivalent. The conventional unit of measure is the rem, which is short for **r**oentgen **e**quivalent in **m**an. The SI unit is the sievert (SV). The conversion factor for changing conventional units to SI is 1 rem = 0.01 SV.

In the United States, the Nuclear Regulatory Commission (NRC) has set limits for the **maximum allowable radiation doses** a person can receive in a year (Table 1.9). These limits are in addition to any exposure received from natural and other man-made sources of radiation, which is about 0.6 rem/year. People who work with radiation and are occupationally exposed are allowed up to 5 rem (0.05 Sv) per year. This includes medical personnel. Occupational workers who are pregnant or under the age of 18 are allowed only 10% of the annual dose limit or 0.5 rem (0.005 Sv) per year. Non-medical personnel and the general public are allowed no more than 2% of the whole body occupational dose in a year (0.1 rem or 0.001 Sv). In a veterinary practice, no one under the age of 18 or pregnant should be exposed to x-rays.

Table 1.8 Units of radiation measurement

Measurement	Conventional Unit	SI Unit
Exposure dose	Roentgen (R)	Coulomb/kg (C/kg)
Absorbed dose	rad (r)	Gray (Gy)
Effective dose	rem	Sievert (Sv)
Radioactivity	Curie (Ci)	Becquerel (Bq)
	Conversions	
Exposure dose	1 C/kg = 3876 R, 1 R = 258 μC/kg	
Absorbed dose	1 Gy = 100 rad	
Effective dose	1 Sv = 100 rem	
Radioactivity	1 mCi = 37 mBq	

In this table, System International (SI) units and conventional units are listed along with the conversion factors needed to move between systems.

Table 1.9 Maximum allowable radiation exposures per year[a]

Tissue	Dose Limit
Whole body (10 mm)	5 rem (0.05 Sv)
Lens of the eye (3 mm)	15 rem (0.15 Sv)
Skin of whole body or any extremity (0.07 mm)	50 rem (0.50 Sv)
Any organ	50 rem (0.50 Sv)
Declared pregnant	0.5 rem (0.005 Sv)
Declared under 18	0.5 rem (0.005 Sv)
General public (non-radiation workers)	0.1 rem (0.001 Sv)

[a] This table lists the maximum allowable radiation exposures per year for various body parts. Whole body refers to deep exposure, which is 10 mm tissue depth. The lens of the eye is 3 mm tissue depth. Skin is considered shallow exposure, 0.07 mm tissue depth.

Protection from x-rays

X-rays cannot be detected by human senses and the damage caused by x-rays is not immediately apparent. Not only is protection from radiation a good idea, it is required by law. Per the US federal government; all reasonable efforts must be made to keep exposure to ionizing radiation as low as practical. Law also requires that all individuals working with radiation receive proper training in the safe use of any device that produces radiation.

The guiding principle of radioprotection is **ALARA**, which stands for **As Low As Reasonably Achievable**. Exposures to ionizing radiation must be as far below dose limits as practical while accomplishing the desired diagnostic or therapeutic goal. The three major tenets of ALARA are *time, distance,* and *shielding*.

Time: minimize the amount of time spent near x-rays. The damaging effects of radiation are cumulative. The more time spent in the presence of x-rays, the greater the health risk. Radiology personnel should be on rotating shifts to avoid any individual receiving excessive exposure. Only persons necessary to the imaging procedure should be in the x-ray room during an exposure. When possible, avoid manual restraint of patients during radiography. Minimize the need to repeat radiographs by ensuring the x-ray machine settings are correct and the patient is properly positioned. Every repeat radiograph increases the exposure to x-radiation by another 100%.

Distance: maximize the distance from x-rays. The greater the distance from the source of x-rays, the lower the exposure. Recall the inverse square law; doubling the distance reduces the x-ray beam intensity by a factor of four (Figure 1.28). Distance is perhaps the most effective way to reduce x-ray exposure. Just taking two steps back, away from the x-ray machine, can reduce your exposure by 75% or more. Try to avoid manual restraint of patients whenever possible.

Shielding: use a barrier to block exposure to x-rays. A barrier made of a material that absorbs x-rays and placed in the path of the x-rays will decrease exposure. Shielding should be used to protect against both primary and secondary or scatter radiation. Lead is a commonly used material because of its large, densely packed atoms (high atomic number and high weight per volume). Other materials such as concrete and certain metals also are used for shielding. Different materials attenuate x-rays to different degrees.

The attenuating ability of material often is compared to lead and expressed as **lead equivalents**. A lead equivalent is the thickness of lead that would block the same amount of x-rays as the thickness of the material being used. Shielding materials are assessed by **half-value layer**. The half-value layer (HVL) is the thickness of a material that would be needed to reduce the x-ray beam intensity by half. HVL, however, is dependent on x-ray energy. The higher the energy of the x-rays, the thicker the material needed (Table 1.10). For example: the HVL of lead for a 50 kVp x-ray beam is 0.06 mm. The HVL needed for a 100 kVp beam is 0.27 mm, more than four times the thickness needed for the 50 kVp beam.

Three types of shielding are used in radiography: *structural, equipment,* and *personal.* **Structural shielding** is embedded in the walls and doors of the x-ray room. In the United States, structural shielding must limit radiation exposure to persons outside the x-ray room to less than 1 mGy/year (less than 0.02 mGy/week). **Equipment shielding** surrounds the x-ray tube. There must be enough shielding to prevent the emission of x-rays other than through the tube window. Mobile shields are commercially available and provide protection to those behind the shield. It is important to know the rating of the shielding material you are depending on. Some are meant for secondary radiation, while others may protect against primary radiation (up to a stated limit of energy).

Personal shielding is protective clothing. Personal shielding includes protective aprons, gloves, glasses and thyroid shields (Figure 1.68). These are essential components of radiation safety. Protective clothing is designed to protect against scatter radiation, NOT primary x-rays. Protection against primary x-rays would require much thicker and heavier equipment. Personal shielding should provide at least 0.25 mm lead equivalents. Lead aprons, thyroid shields and gloves typically supply 0.25–0.50 mm lead equivalents. Lead glasses generally provide 0.75 mm lead equivalents of shielding (eyes are radiosensitive). The life expectancy of lead aprons and gloves is about 10 years, depending on their use and storage. Periodically inspect and radiograph all items for cracks in the shielding material. Personal shielding ONLY is protective when it is worn. Modern radiation protective clothing is much more functional than in the past and gets easier to use with practice.

Table 1.10 Approximate HVLs of lead and concrete[a]

X-ray Energy (kVp)	HVL Lead (mm)	HVL Concrete (mm)
50	0.06	4.32
100	0.27	15.10
150	0.30	22.32

[a] This table lists the approximate half-value layers (HVLs) of lead and concrete for various x-ray energies.

Radiation safety controls are designed to provide a safe working environment. Physical safety controls include shielding around the x-ray room and equipment, making sure protective clothing is available to all radiology personnel, and restricting access to radiation areas.

Administrative safety controls include radiation warning signs that are clearly posted at all radiology facilities (Figure 1.69). All radiology personnel must receive documented training and must be monitored on a regular basis for radiation exposure. Protocols for normal operating procedures and emergency situations should be written down, readily available, and strictly followed. This is the job of the radiation safety officer.

All organizations that are licensed to use x-rays must have a **Radiation Safety Officer** (RSO). The RSO is the point of contact for all activities associated with the use of x-rays and ensures that radiation safety protocols are in place and that people adhere to them. The RSO makes sure all individuals that use the x-ray equipment are appropriately trained, supervised, and formally authorized. He or she is responsible for knowing the appropriate governmental radiation safety regulations and ensures that all rules and procedures for the safe use of x-rays are observed. Lack of knowledge is indefensible according to most government agencies. The RSO must keep accurate records of the use and maintenance of the x-ray equipment and ensure that it is protected from unauthorized access or removal. In the US, veterinary x-ray machines may be inspected every 3 years by the state department of health. These inspections frequently are random and unannounced.

Dose creep

There is a tendency among radiographers to use higher than necessary x-ray exposures to avoid repeat radiographs. Digital image receptors are far more forgiving of too many x-rays than too few x-rays. The higher the x-ray exposure, the greater the signal-to-noise ratio (SNR) and the less the chance of a poor quality radiograph. Increases in exposure usually start small and may initially go unnoticed. Over time, however, the exposures gradually get higher and higher, which is

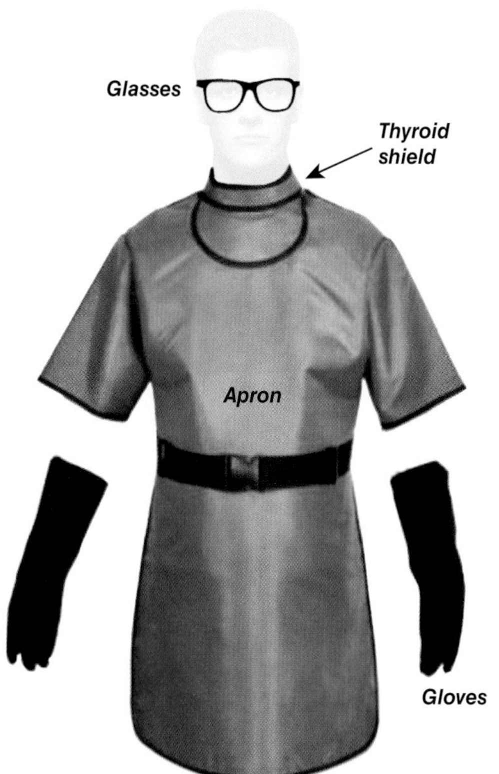

Figure 1.68 Radiation protective clothing. This image depicts the typical appearance of a lead apron, lead gloves, thyroid shield, and protective glasses.

why the problem is called *dose creep*. Dose creep is not an issue in film radiography because a higher than needed exposure results in a visibly overexposed radiograph. Dose creep is a growing problem in digital radiography and can lead to significant increases in radiation exposure to the patient and nearby personnel and a shortened life of the x-ray tube.

In general, there is an optimum x-ray exposure that produces a good balance between radiograph quality and radiation dose. Regular monitoring of the exposure techniques used at a hospital or clinic can help identify these optimum exposures. Monitoring can be done using the EI and S-numbers as discussed earlier with digital image receptors. The Optimum EI and S-numbers will differ between different digital systems and different clinical procedures. You will need to determine the acceptable EI and S-numbers for your particular radiography facility.

Dose creep is less likely to occur with higher quality digital image receptors because they typically produce less noise and a higher SNR at standard exposures. Digital noise reduction software also can be used to increase the SNR, especially at low exposures. Automatic exposure control timers (AEC timers) and anatomical programming software can help standardize x-ray exposures with less user input. Control of dose creep is best managed when exposure records are accurately maintained and periodically reviewed.

Dosimetry

In the US, federal law requires that any individual who is likely to receive more than 10% of any annual occupational dose limit be monitored for radiation exposure. The Occupational Safety and Health Administration (OSHA) standard 1910.1096 states, "Every employer shall supply appropriate personnel monitoring equipment, such as film badges, pocket chambers, pocket dosimeters, or film rings, and shall require the use of such equipment." Other countries and jurisdictions have similar regulations about monitoring x-ray exposure.

Monitoring typically involves a personal radiation detection device called a **dosimeter**. Dosimeters are attached to the users clothing. They must be worn outside of protective clothing to accurately measure the radiation dose. Whole-body dosimeters commonly are attached somewhere between the neck and the waist.

Dosimeters generally are worn for a specific period of time and then processed. Most are examined about every 3 months to determine what dose of radiation the user received. The two most common types of dosimeters currently in use are *film badges* and *thermoluminescent dosimeters* (Figure 1.70).

Film badges, as the name implies, measure exposure to x-rays using a piece of radiation-sensitive film. The film is packaged in a tightly sealed envelope that prevents light, moisture and chemicals from affecting it. The envelope is enclosed inside a plastic holder called a "badge." Inside the badge are a series of filters that differentially attenuate x-rays. The filters are used to calculate the energy of the x-rays based on the amount of radiographic density under each one. The film is double-coated so the emulsion on one side contains large grains which are sensitive to low x-ray exposures and

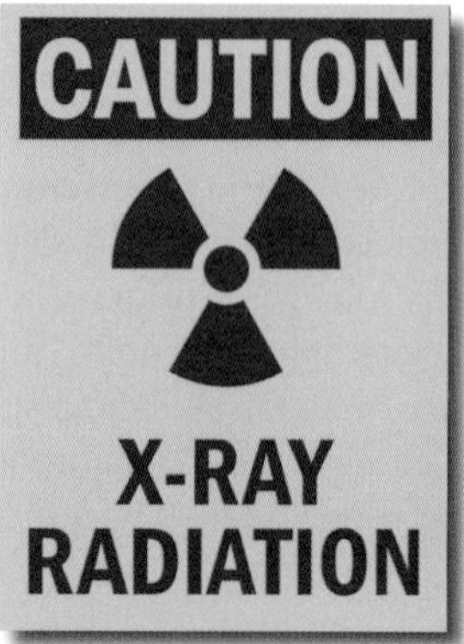

Figure 1.69 Radiation warning sign. This is an example of a standard international sign used to warn people about onsite radiation. It typically is yellow with purple lettering and includes the symbol for radiation.

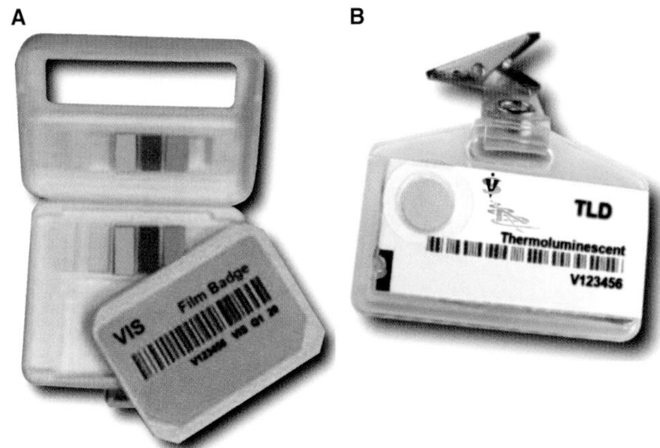

Figure 1.70 Types of dosimetry. Pictured are a film Badge (**A**) and a Thermoluminescent dosimeter (**B**). The plastic badge is propped open with the envelope containing the film sitting outside it. The series of filters is visible.

the other side contains small grains to detect high exposures. The film must be sent to a lab for processing. If the large grain emulsion is overexposed, the film was exposed to higher x-ray intensity and the user's exposure dose is computed using the small grain emulsion. Film badges are simple, inexpensive, and very reliable. They provide a permanent record of exposure and are quite accurate for x-ray exposure doses greater than 0.1 rem. In addition, different x-ray energies can be distinguished. The disadvantages of film badges include: the film can only be processed once, the film is susceptible to heat and pressure fogging, and the film must be sent away for processing, which is more time-consuming than using an onsite reader.

A **thermoluminescent dosimeter** (TLD) contains phosphors that absorb x-ray energy. When heated, the phosphors release the captured energy as light, which is called thermoluminescence. The amount of light released is proportional to the amount of x-rays absorbed. Instead of reading the amount of darkening in a piece of film, a TLD reader measures the amount of light emitted by the phosphors. TLDs are able to measure a greater range of x-ray exposure doses than film badges. The exposure dose is easily obtained and can be read onsite. TLDs can be reused many times, but each exposure dose can be read out only once, so TLDs do not provide a permanent record of exposures.

2 Radiographs

Radiography of the Dog and Cat: Guide to Making and Interpreting Radiographs, Second Edition. M.C. Muhlbauer and S.K. Kneller.

Companion website: www.wiley.com/go/muhlbauer/dog

CHAPTER 2

Introduction – plan for success

The quality of your radiographs reflects a level of excellence in your practice. Proper patient preparation, restraint, and positioning are essential for making good quality radiographs. Patients in distress must be stabilized prior to radiography. Radiation safety protocols should always be in effect (see ALARA in the Radiation Safety section of the previous chapter).

The patient's hair coat should be clean and dry. Examine the patient's body for any cutaneous or subcutaneous nodules, masses, or other structures which may mimic lesions in the radiograph. Remove collars, harnesses, leashes, clothing, etc., before making radiographs. Move any medical monitoring equipment and positioning devices out of the field of view.

Whenever practical, empty the GI tract and urinary bladder prior to abdominal radiography. Remove known large volumes of pleural or peritoneal fluid prior to thoracic or abdominal radiography.

Patient movement is a major cause of poor-quality radiographs in veterinary medicine. Motion artifacts often require repeat radiographs, which wastes time, money, and exposes both the patient and nearby personnel to more radiation. Adequate patient restraint is crucial to minimize stress to both the patient and the radiographer.

Non-manual restraint is recommended whenever possible. This means avoid holding the patient with your hands. Instead, use positioning devices such as foam wedges, towels, sandbags, V-troughs, and tie-downs (e.g., rope, tape, gauze) to help maintain the proper alignment of the body part being imaged (Figures 2.1 and 2.2). When sedation/anesthesia is used, note the agents in the radiography file for future reference and good medical record keeping. Patient sedation frequently is less stressful than struggling with the animal and often yields superior radiographs.

Orthogonal views

Radiographs are two-dimensional pictures of three-dimensional objects. With rare exceptions, at least two orthogonal views are necessary for accurate evaluation of a body part. The term "orthogonal" means perpendicular or 90° to each other (e.g., lateral and VD radiographic views). When an orthogonal view is not possible, try to make a second view at an alternative angle to the first view or from the opposite side. This often is more beneficial than no second view at all.

At least two views are important because a structure can appear normal in one view and abnormal in the other (Figure 2.3). Two views also help us understand the positions of structures in relation to each other, such as a foreign object relative to an organ.

Standard radiographic views are those that are essential to a complete radiographic study. Typically, this means a lateral view and either a ventrodorsal/dorsoventral view or a dorsopalmar/dorsoplantar view of the body part of interest. **Supplemental** views frequently are added to further evaluate a specific structure or to help clarify a radiographic finding.

Radiographic views are named according to the **direction** in which the x-ray beam passes through the body. For example, in a ventrodorsal view, the x-rays enter the ventral

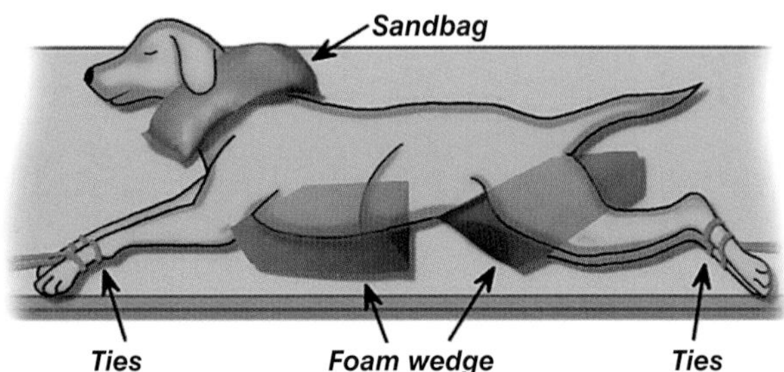

Figure 2.1 Positioning devices. Whenever feasible, use non-manual animal restraint during radiography. Common positioning devices include sandbags, ties (e.g., rope, gauze, tape), and foam wedges or towels.

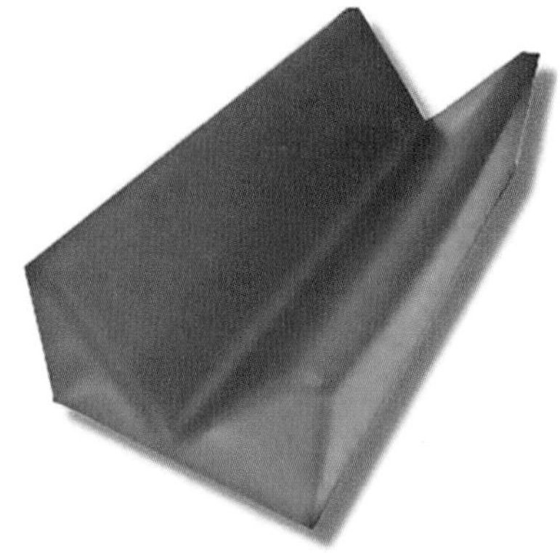

Figure 2.2 V-trough. A padded V-shaped positioning device can be used to help maintain the alignment of the patient's spine and sternum and keep the pelvis straight during radiography.

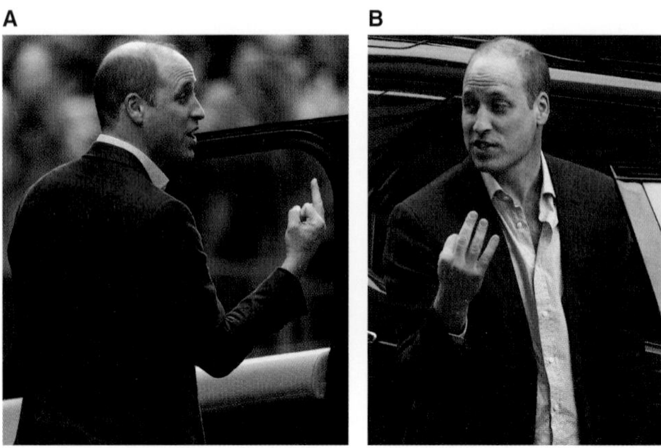

Figure 2.3 The importance of two views. A body part can appear one way from one perspective and quite different in the orthogonal view. Source: (A) Reuters/Peter Nicholls. (B) Reuters/Hannah Mckay.

surface and exit the dorsal surface. In a dorsopalmar view, the x-rays enter the dorsal side and exit the palmar side. In a right-to-left lateral view, the x-rays enter the right side and exit the left side. In many cases, the name of a lateral view has been shortened and it is simply called either a right lateral view or a left lateral view. In these cases, the name is based on the side that is closest to the image receptor. For example, a lateral view made with the patient lying on its right side (right side is close to the image receptor) is called a right lateral view.

When imaging the extremities, the lateral side of the limb usually is closest to the image receptor and the x-ray beam passes from the medial side to the lateral side. Commonly, this is simply called a lateral view of the limb being imaged.

Procedure for making radiographs

Plan for success. As much as practical, prepare the radiography room, equipment, and the patient prior to performing the procedure. Select the appropriate technique chart to use for the body part of interest (e.g., thorax, abdomen, skeleton). Create the ID for the radiographs. Make a label for film radiography or enter the information into the digital system. The radiograph ID should include the following information:

1. Patient name and owner name.
2. Date the radiograph is being made.
3. Hospital name or name of veterinarian.
4. Initials of technicians making the radiograph.

Select the appropriate body markers to indicate the patient's right or left side and which view was made (e.g., VD, DV). Calibration markers may be needed to provide a reference for making measurements from the radiograph. Position markers are used to indicate the direction of gravity, which is helpful to determine whether the patient was standing or recumbent at the time of radiography. All markers should be placed in the field-of-view (FOV) so they will be visible in the radiograph, but away from the area of interest.

Make sure nothing is superimposed on the body part being imaged (e.g., positioning devices, IV lines, ECG leads).

Measure the thickest portion of the body part. Measurements tend to be most accurate when made while the patient is in position for radiography because the thickness of some parts will vary between standing and lying down. Use a **grid** when body part thickness exceeds 10 cm (12 cm for thorax).

Set the technique on the x-ray machine prior to final patient positioning to minimize the length of time the animal must remain in position and lessen its stress. Use the small focal spot whenever feasible to maximize radiographic detail. Make the exposure time as short as practical to minimize motion artifact.

Center the x-ray beam on the body part of interest. Collimate the FOV as small as practical to include the entire body part. The smaller the FOV, the less scatter radiation, and the higher the quality of the radiograph. Commonly, the FOV is made too large for the thorax and too small for the abdomen. Pay attention to the landmarks for the body part of interest, as described in the positioning guide in this chapter.

When the body part is too large to fit in one view, divide the anatomy over two overlapping images. The FOV for the first radiograph should extend from the cranial landmark caudally (for abdomen, this would be from the diaphragm caudally, as shown in Figures 2.4 and 2.5). The FOV for the second radiograph should extend from the caudal landmark cranially (for abdomen, this would be from the pelvic inlet cranially). The two radiographs will overlap in the middle.

With many patients it may be useful to make the lateral radiograph first because positioning an animal in lateral recumbency tends to be less stressful than dorsal recumbency and may improve compliance with subsequent radiographs.

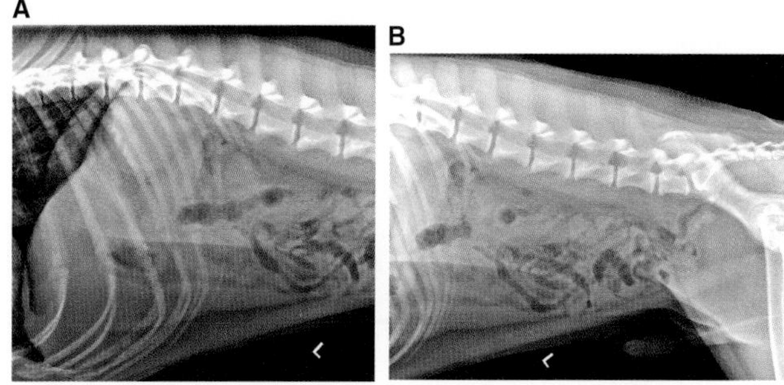

Figure 2.4 Lateral views of a large dog abdomen. The abdomen is too large to be imaged in its entirety in one radiograph, so the anatomy is divided over two overlapping views as shown in (**A**) and (**B**).

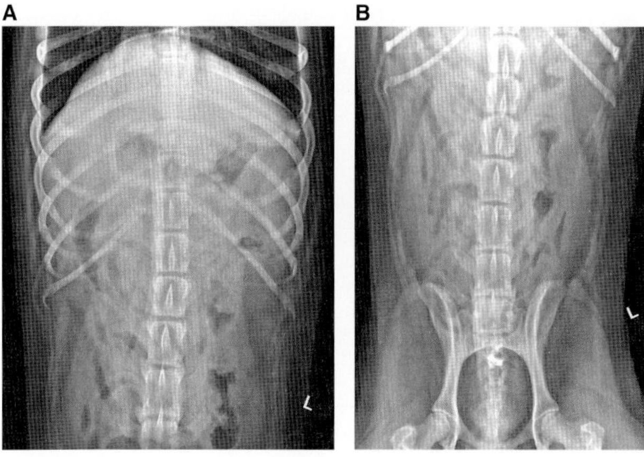

Figure 2.5 Ventrodorsal views of a large dog abdomen. The abdomen is too large to be imaged in its entirety in one radiograph, so the anatomy is divided over two overlapping views as shown in (**A**) and (**B**).

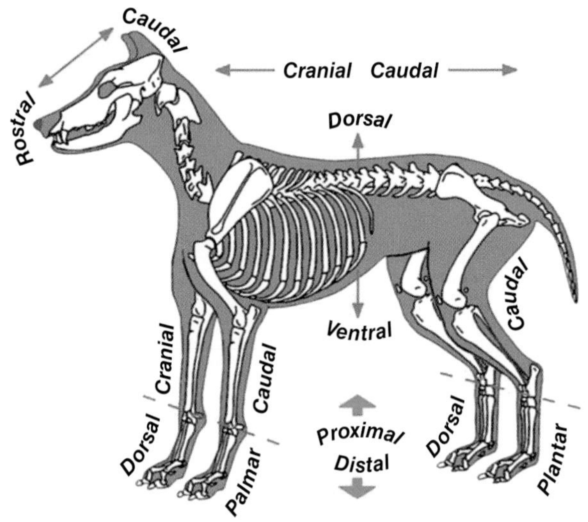

Figure 2.6 Anatomical nomenclature. This illustration depicts the correct veterinary terms used to describe the direction of the x-ray beam and the locations of radiographic findings.

Nomenclature

It is important to use correct veterinary terminology when communicating your radiographic findings (Figure 2.6; Table 2.1). This includes accurately describing the radiographic views and the locations of the radiographic

Table 2.1 Veterinary nomenclature and their meanings

Term	Meaning and anatomical direction
Cranial	Toward the head
Caudal	Toward the tail
Dorsal	Toward the back or spine
Ventral	Toward the front or sternum
Lateral	Away from midline of the body
Medial	Toward midline of the body
Median	On the midline of the body
Rostral	Toward the nose
Proximal	Toward the point of origin or nearer the center of the body
Distal	Toward the point of insertion or away from the center of the body
Superficial	Toward the surface of the body
Deep	Away from the body surface or below the body surface
Ipsilateral	On the same side of the body
Contralateral	On the opposite side of the body
Palmar	Bottom or caudal part of the manus (front paw with carpus)
Plantar	Bottom, sole, or caudal part of the pes (rear paw with tarsus)
Recumbency	Lying down
Anatomical planes	
Transverse planes	Divide body into cranial and caudal sections and divide limbs into proximal and distal sections.
Dorsal planes	Divide body into dorsal and ventral sections
Sagittal planes	Divide body into right and left sections
Median plane	Sagittal plane on midline (divides body into equal right and left halves)
Anatomical movements	
Flexion	Decrease the angle of the joint
Extension	Increase the angle of the joint
Abduction	Move limb away from midline
Adduction	Move limb toward midline
Supination	Rotate palmar side to face up or cranial
Pronation	Rotate palmar side to face down or caudal
Radiographic views	
Ventrodorsal (VD)	X-rays pass from ventral to dorsal
Dorsoventral (DV)	X-rays pass from dorsal to ventral
Lateral (L)	X-rays pass from one side of the body to the other through the axial plane
Right lateral (RL)	Patient lying on right side, right side is closest to image receptor
Left lateral (LL)	Patient lying on left side, left side is closest to image receptor
Craniocaudal (CrCa)	X-rays pass from cranial to caudal
Caudocranial (CaCr)	X-rays pass from caudal to cranial
Dorsopalmar or dorsoplantar (DP)	X-rays pass from dorsal to palmar/plantar
Oblique (O)	X-ray beam enters the body at an angle other than 90°.
20° CrM-CaLO	20° craniomedial to caudolateral oblique, which means the central ray enters cranially and medially at 20° off perpendicular and exits the caudal, lateral side.

abnormalities. For descriptive purposes, the body may be divided into three imaginary anatomical planes: *sagittal, dorsal,* and *transverse* (Figure 2.7).

The **sagittal plane** divides the body into right and left sections. The *mid-sagittal* or *median* plane divides the body into equal right and left halves. The **dorsal plane** (also called *frontal* or *coronal* plane) divides the body into dorsal and ventral sections. The **transverse plane** (also called *axial* or *cross-sectional* plane) divides the body into cranial and caudal sections. The transverse plane divides the limbs into proximal and distal parts.

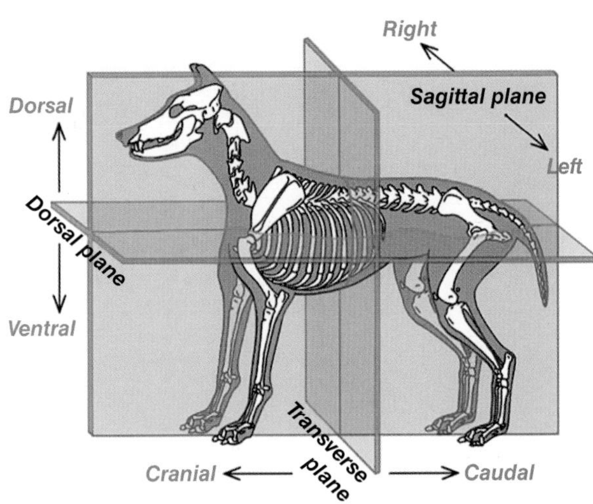

Figure 2.7 Anatomical planes. This illustration depicts the three imaginary planes used to describe anatomy. The sagittal plane divides the body into right and left. The dorsal plane divides the body into dorsal and ventral. The transverse plane divides the body into cranial and caudal.

Positioning guide

Figure 2.8 Thorax lateral view.

A

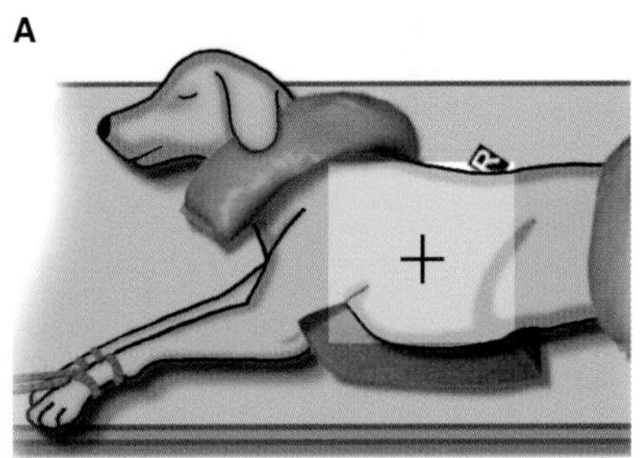

B

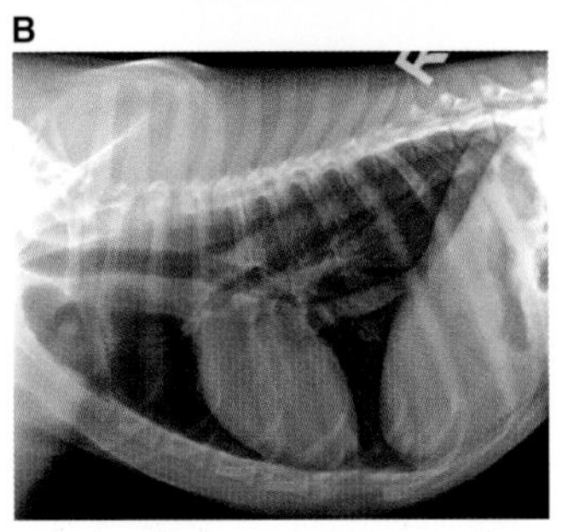

A. *Positioning*

- Patient is in lateral recumbency; both right and left lateral views are recommended for a complete study.
- Thoracic limbs are pulled cranially; avoid overstretching the patient.
- Sternum and spine are aligned in the same horizontal plane, parallel with the image receptor. Place a foam wedge (pictured) or a towel under the sternum to correct rotation.
- Measure the thickest part of the thorax, usually over the liver.
- X-ray beam is centered on the heart or caudal edge of the scapula (+).
- Field-of-view (FOV) is collimated to include the entire bony thorax from thoracic inlet to last ribs.
- Make exposure at peak inspiration.

B. *Radiograph*

- Right lateral view of the thorax.

Figure 2.9 Thorax ventrodorsal (VD) view.

A. *Positioning*

- Patient is in dorsal recumbency
- Thoracic limbs are pulled cranially (avoid overstretching the patient).
- Sternum and spine are superimposed in the same vertical plane, perpendicular to the image receptor.
- Head and neck are in line with the spine.
- Measure the thickest part of the thorax, usually over the liver.
- X-ray beam is centered on the heart or at the caudal edge of the scapula (+).
- Collimate the FOV to include the thoracic inlet, outer edges of the ribs, and the last ribs.
- Make exposure at peak inspiration.

B. *Radiograph*

- Ventrodorsal (VD) view of the thorax.

A

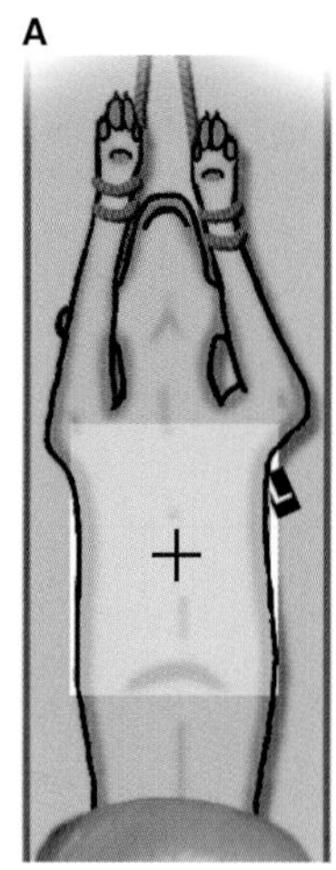

B

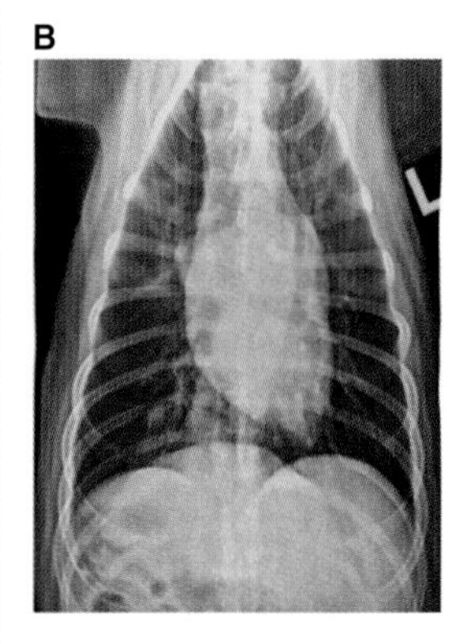

Figure 2.10 Thorax dorsoventral (DV) view.

A. *Positioning*

- Patient is in ventral (sternal) recumbency.
- Elbows and stifles are slightly abducted and pelvic limbs are in a crouching position for the patient's comfort.
- Sternum and spine are superimposed in the same vertical plane, perpendicular to the image receptor.
- Head and neck are in-line with the spine.
- Measure the thickest part of the thorax, usually over the liver.
- X-ray beam is centered on the heart or at the caudal edge of the scapula (+); NOTE: A common error is centering the x-ray beam too far caudally and missing the cranial thorax.
- Collimate the FOV to include the entire boney thorax from the thoracic inlet to the last ribs.
- Make exposure at peak inspiration.

B. *Radiograph*

- Dorsoventral (DV) view of the thorax.

A

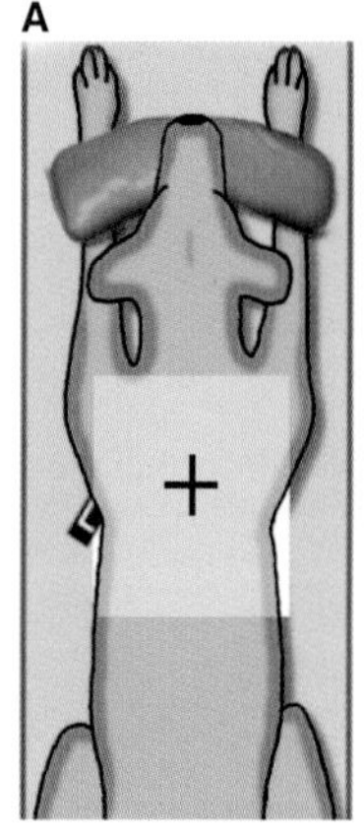

B

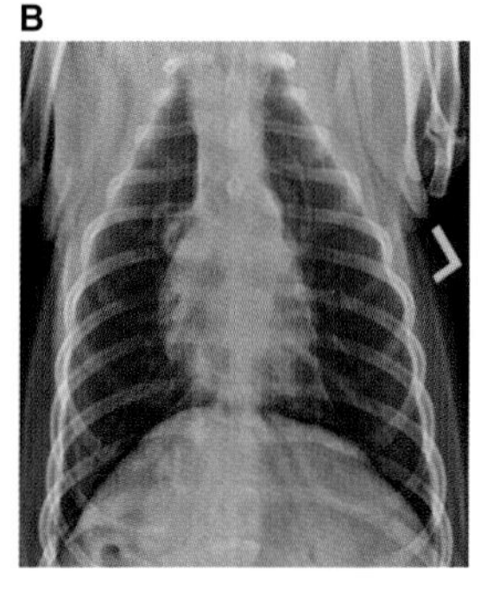

Figure 2.11 Thorax VD view with limbs pulled caudal (human view).

This is a supplemental radiograph of the thorax made in addition to the standard lateral and VD/DV views.

A. *Positioning*

- Patient is positioned for VD view of the thorax as described in Figure 2.9.
- Thoracic limbs are pulled caudally instead of cranially.

B. *Radiograph*

- VD view of the thorax with the limbs pulled caudally to eliminate superimposition of the scapula and associated musculature on the cranial thorax.

A

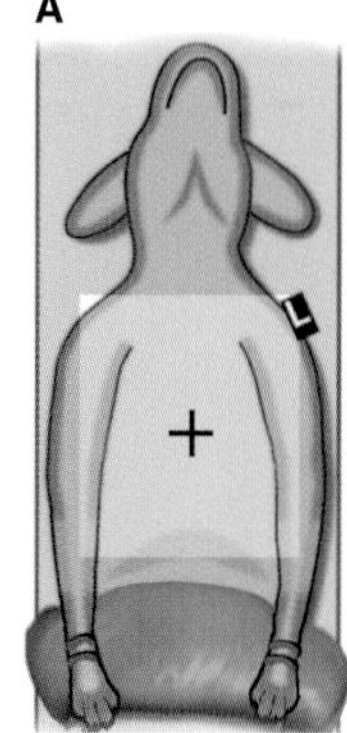

B

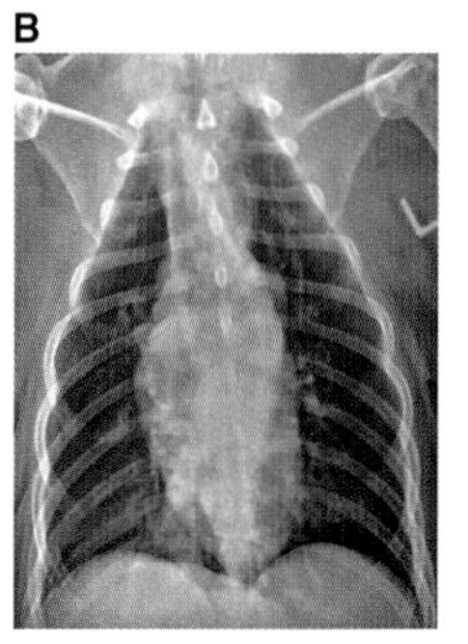

Figure 2.12 Thorax VD oblique view.

This is a supplemental radiograph of the thorax made in addition to the standard lateral and VD/DV views.

A. *Positioning*

- Patient is positioned for a VD thorax view as described in Figure 2.9.
- Sternum is rotated to the right or left to better visualize the area of interest by eliminating superimposition of the heart, spine, and sternum.
- X-ray beam is centered on the area of interest (+).
- Collimate the FOV as for the VD view.
- Make exposure at peak inspiration.

B. *Radiograph*

- VD oblique view of the thorax (**B**), the sternum is rotated to the right, which enhances visualization of the left lung (the heart follows the sternum); notice the thoracic dorsal spinous processes project to the left in this view.
- To name an oblique view, we describe the path of the x-rays. For example, a D15R-VLO view means the x-rays passed through the thorax from Dorsal 15° Right to Ventral Left Obliquely. In simple terms, the patient was in sternal recumbency (DV view) and rotated 15° to the left.

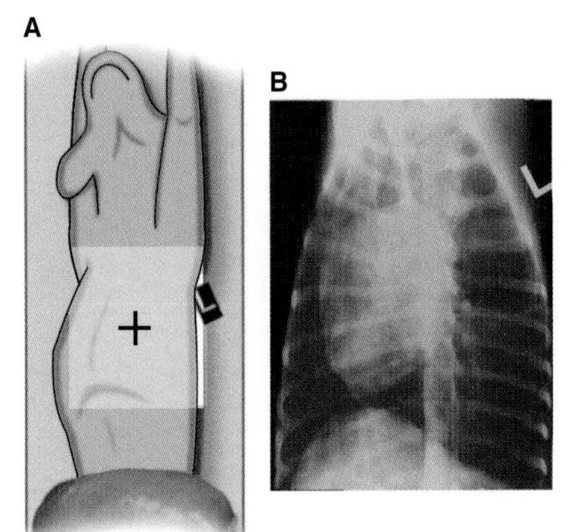

Figure 2.13 Thorax VD tangential view.

This is a supplemental radiograph of the thorax made in addition to the standard lateral and VD/DV views.

A. *Positioning*

- Patient is positioned for a VD thorax view as described in Figure 2.9.
- Sternum is rotated to the right or left, whichever makes the area of interest perpendicular to the x-ray beam.
- X-ray beam is centered on the area of interest (+).
- Collimate the FOV as small as feasible to the size of the area of interest. This view is not made to image the entire thorax, rather it is intended to focus on a specific site or lesion.

B. *Radiograph*

- VD tangential view of the thorax (white arrows point to rib fractures).

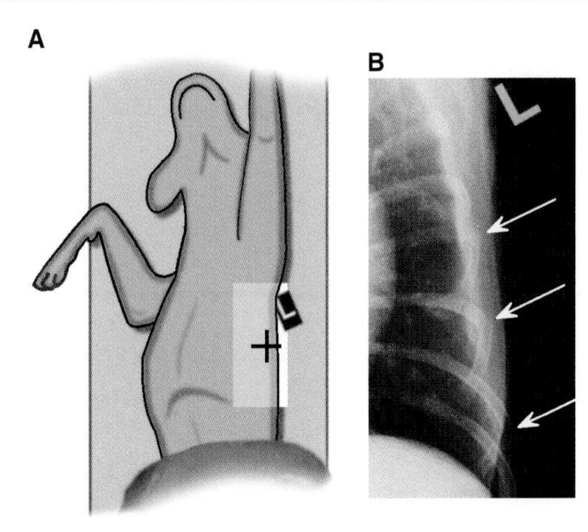

NOTES:

Figure 2.14 Thorax craniodorsal–caudoventral view (skyline view).

This supplemental radiograph of the thorax is made in addition to the standard lateral and VD/DV views.

A. *Positioning*

- Patient is in ventral (sternal) recumbency with the thoracic limbs extended.
- Head and neck are hyperextended; avoid excessive tension on the neck as this can distort the shape of the trachea.
- Thickness is measured from the thoracic inlet to the ventral thorax.
- Increase the x-ray exposure: double the mAs or increase the kVp by 20% over what is listed in your technique chart for this thickness of thorax.
- X-ray beam is centered on the thoracic inlet (+).
- Collimate the FOV as small as feasible to include the boney thorax at the thoracic inlet.

B. *Radiograph*

- Skyline view of the thoracic inlet; arrow points to the trachea.

A

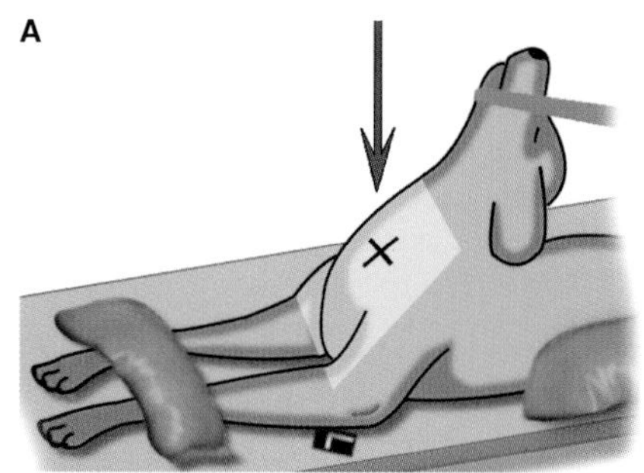

B

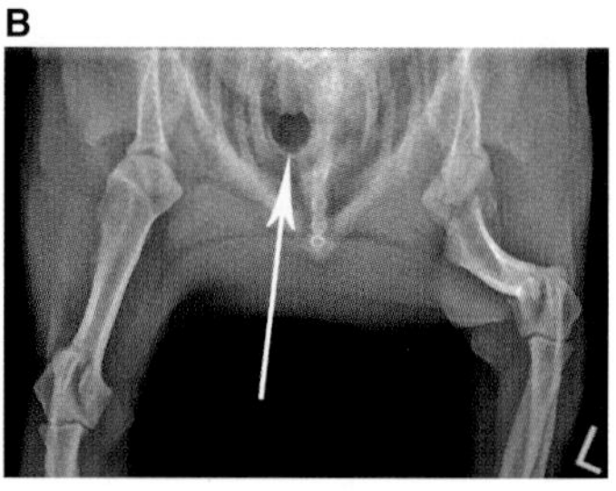

Figure 2.15 Horizontal beam radiography.

A and C. *Positioning*

- Patient is standing, held erect, or recumbent, depending on the purpose of the study.
- **A:** the dog is in right lateral recumbency with the image receptor along its dorsum for a horizontal beam VD view.
- **C:** the dog is in dorsal recumbency with the image receptor alongside its body for a horizontal beam lateral view.
- X-ray beam is directed across the table, perpendicular to the image receptor, and centered on the area of interest.
- Set the source-to-image distance (SID) to the standard SID for your practice, typically 100 cm or 40 in.
- Measure the thickest part of the body part being imaged.
- Collimate the FOV to the size of the area of interest.

B and D. *Radiographs*

- **B:** horizontal beam VD view of the thorax. The dependent (down) lung is partially collapsed and increased in opacity and the heart "falls" toward the dependent side due to the effects of gravity and the collapsed lung.
- **D:** horizontal beam lateral view of the thorax. A small volume of abnormal pleural gas is visible between the cardiac silhouette and the sternum (arrow). Gas rises to the uppermost part of the thoracic cavity. The dorsal lungs are dependent, partially collapsed, and increased in opacity.

A

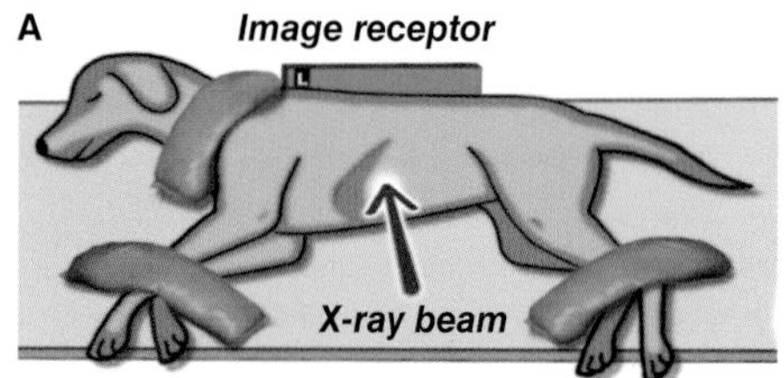

B

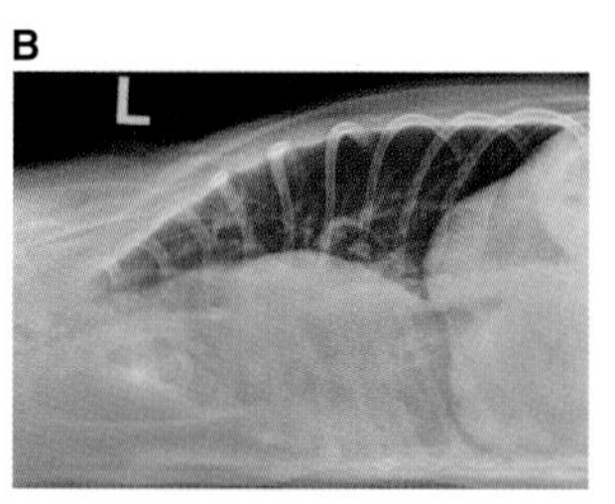

C

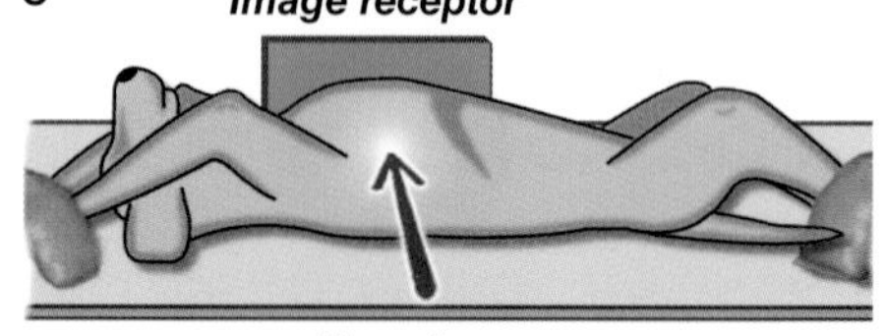

D

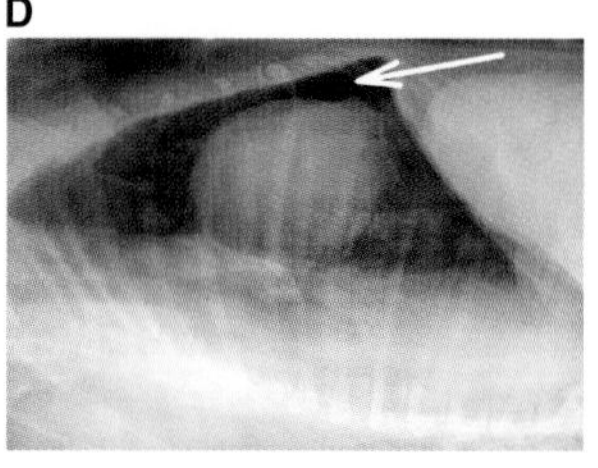

Abdominal radiographs

Figure 2.16 Abdomen lateral view.

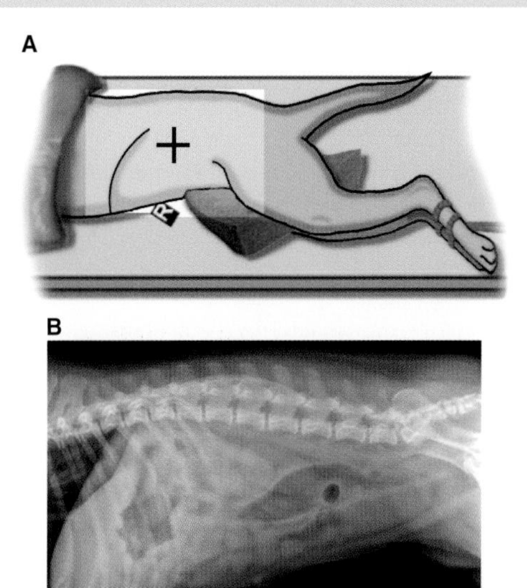

A. ***Positioning***

- Patient is in right or left lateral recumbency.
- Pelvic limbs are pulled caudally; avoid overstretching the patient.
- Place foam wedges or small towels between the pelvic limbs and under the sternum as needed to correct rotation (Figures 2.8 and 2.60).
- Both ilial wings should be superimposed in the same vertical plane, perpendicular to the image receptor.
- Measure the thickest part of the abdomen, usually over the liver.
- X-ray beam is centered caudal to the last rib, midway between the diaphragm and the pelvic canal (+), in the area of the umbilicus.
- Collimate the FOV to include the diaphragm, spine, pelvic inlet, and ventral body wall.
- Make exposure at end expiration.

B. ***Radiograph***

- Right lateral view of the abdomen.

Figure 2.17 Abdomen ventrodorsal (VD) view.

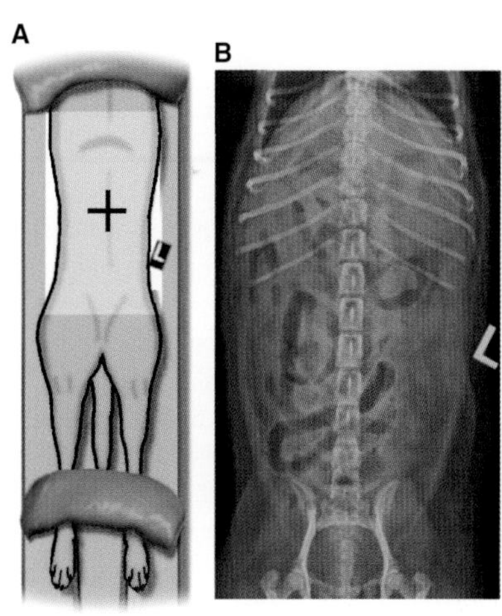

A. ***Positioning***

- Patient is in dorsal recumbency.
- Sternum and spine are superimposed in the same vertical plane, perpendicular to the image receptor.
- Make both ilial wings equal distance from the receptor (or table top) and do the same with the right and left lumbar transverse processes.
- Measure the thickest part of abdomen, usually over the liver.
- X-ray beam is centered near the last rib, midway between the diaphragm and the pelvic canal (+), in the area of the umbilicus.
- Collimate the FOV to include the diaphragm, greater trochanters, and lateral body walls.
- Make the exposure at end expiration.
- The standard VD view may create inguinal skin folds in some patients, which appear as linear artifacts.

B. ***Radiograph***

- **B:** ventrodorsal (VD) view of the abdomen.

NOTES:

Figure 2.18 Abdomen dorsoventral (DV) view.

A. ***Positioning***

- Patient is in ventral (sternal) recumbency.
- Elbows and stifles are slightly abducted and the pelvic limbs are in a crouching position for the patient's comfort.
- Sternum and spine are superimposed in the same vertical plane, perpendicular to the image receptor.
- Measure the thickest part of abdomen, usually over the liver.
- X-ray beam is centered near the last rib, midway between the diaphragm and the pelvic canal (+).
- Collimate the FOV to include the diaphragm, greater trochanters, and lateral body walls.
- Make the exposure at the end of expiration.

B. ***Radiograph***

- Dorsoventral (DV) view of the abdomen. This view is not routinely made because it leads to visceral crowding and less distinct intra-abdominal margins.

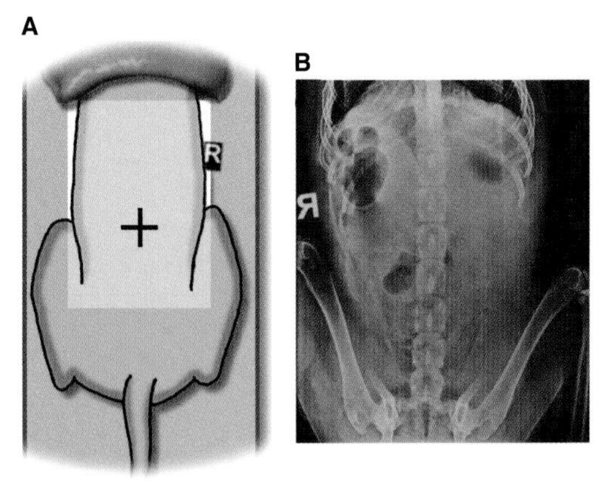

Figure 2.19 Abdominal compression.

This is a supplemental radiograph of the abdomen made in addition to the standard lateral and VD views.

A. ***Positioning***

- Patient may be in position for either a lateral or VD view (Figure 2.16 or 2.17).
- A low-opacity paddle, such as a plastic or wooden spoon, is used to gently compress the abdomen and displace the moveable viscera (e.g., intestines) away from structures that are more fixed in position (e.g., urinary bladder, kidney).
- Decrease the x-ray exposure to compensate for the reduced abdominal thickness. In most cases, cut the exposure time in half.
- X-ray beam is centered on the structure being investigated.
- Collimate the FOV to include the structure; this FOV will be smaller than the one used for the standard view.

B and C. ***Radiographs***

- **B:** lateral view of the abdomen without compression. The margins of the urinary bladder and uterus are not identified.
- **C:** lateral view of the same dog abdomen with compression; the intestines are displaced cranially and dorsally away from the uterus (**u**) and urinary bladder (**b**). Notice that the x-ray exposure was decreased for compression radiography.

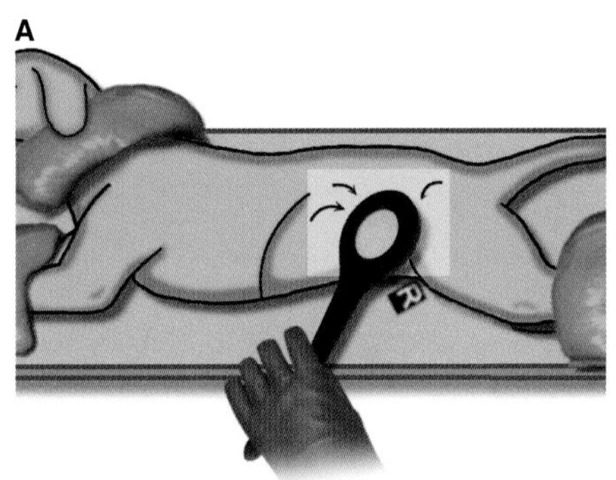

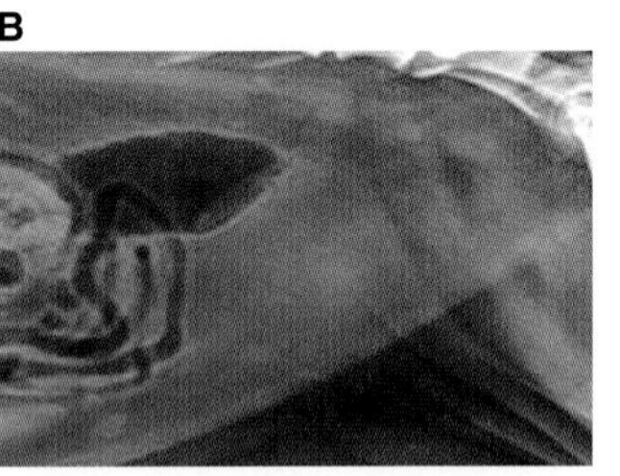

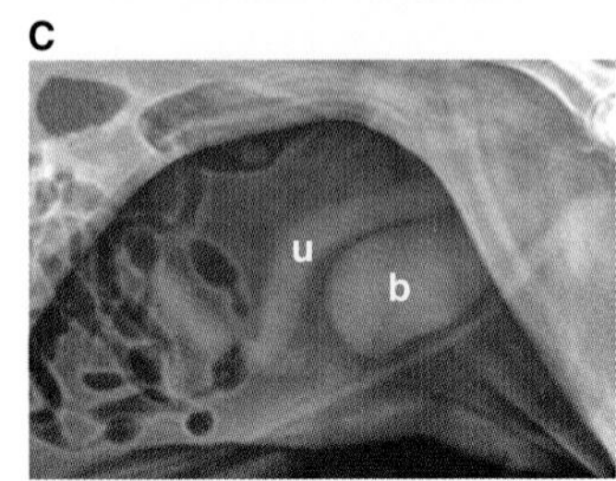

Figure 2.20 Abdomen lateral view of urethra.

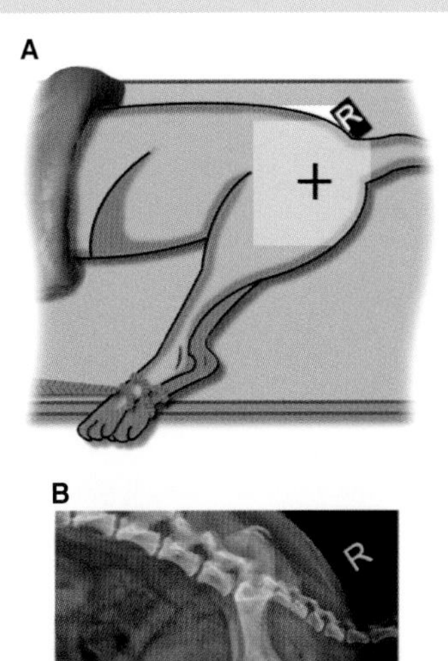

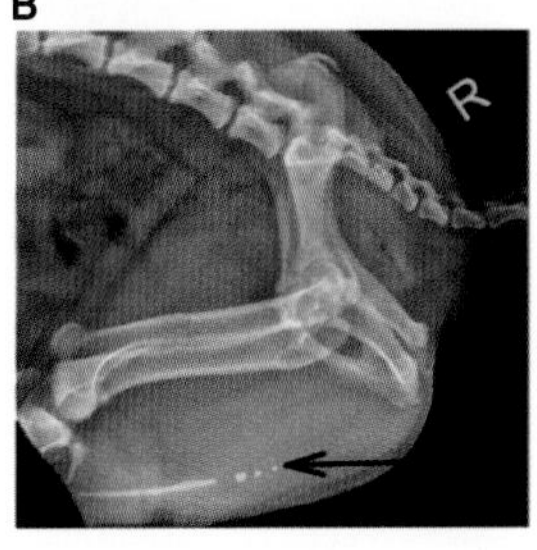

This is a supplemental radiograph of the abdomen made in addition to the standard lateral and VD views. It is used to evaluate the penile urethra in male dogs.

A. *Positioning*

- Patient is in right or left lateral recumbency.
- Pelvic limbs are pulled cranially to eliminate superimposition.
- X-ray beam is centered on the mid-portion of the urethra (+).
- Collimate the FOV to include the urinary bladder and the entire urethra.

B. *Radiograph*

- Lateral view of the urethra. Mineral opacity calculi are visible in the urethra just proximal to the os penis (arrow).

Appendicular skeleton

Figure 2.21 Shoulder lateral view (medial-to-lateral view).

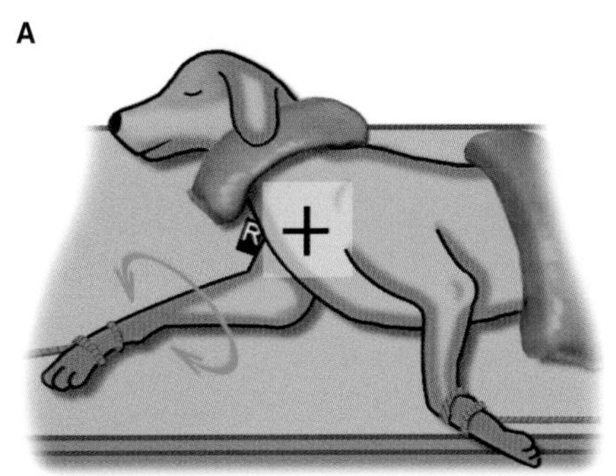

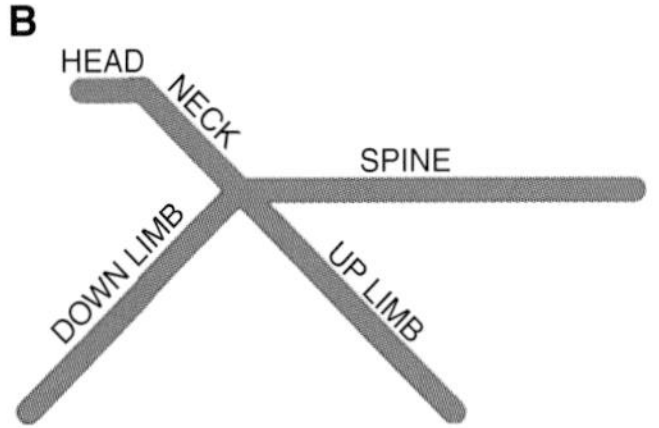

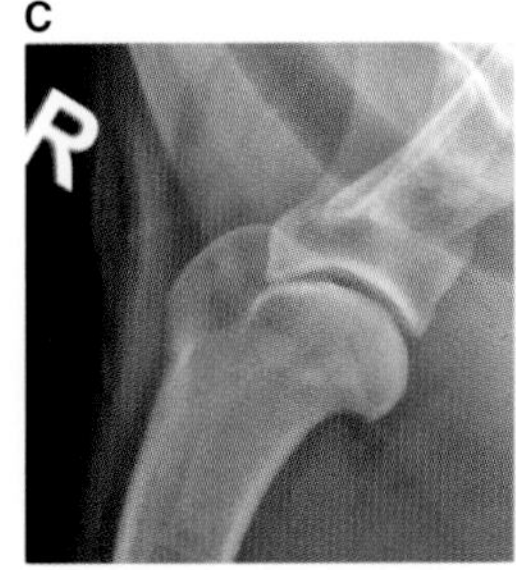

A and B. *Positioning*

- Patient is in lateral recumbency with the limb of interest down (closest to the image receptor) and fully extended.
- The head and neck are extended to eliminate superimposition of the cervical spine on the scapulohumeral joint.
- The opposite (up) limb is pulled caudally out of the FOV. Avoid pulling the limb too far caudally as this will superimpose the two shoulders.
- Limb thickness is measured at the shoulder, between the dependent thoracic wall and about the level of the sternum.
- X-ray beam is centered on the scapulohumeral joint (+). Palpate the thoracic inlet and then move your fingers cranially until you feel the scapulohumeral joint.
- Collimate the FOV to include the distal third of the scapula and the proximal third of the humerus.
- As needed, the lateral view can be repeated with the limb **pronated** or **supinated** (green arrow) to view more of the humeral head. This is particularly useful when searching for osteochondrosis lesions on the humeral head.
- Diagram **B** illustrates the correct alignment of the head, neck, spine, and thoracic limbs. The neck is angled about 135° in relation to the thoracic spine. The down limb is perpendicular (90°) to the line of the neck and the up limb is in a straight line with the neck.

C. *Radiograph*

- Lateral view of the right scapulohumeral joint.

Figure 2.22 Shoulder cranioproximal–craniodistal view (skyline view).

This supplemental radiograph of the shoulder is made in addition to the standard lateral and caudocranial views.

A. *Positioning*

- Patient is in ventral (sternal) recumbency (Figure 2.10).
- Limb of interest is moved caudally to flex both the shoulder and the elbow (dashed arrow).
- Turn the patient's head toward the opposite limb.
- X-ray beam is centered on the bicipital groove (+).
- Collimate the FOV to include the proximal humerus and adjacent soft tissues.

B. *Radiograph*

- Skyline view of the right shoulder highlighting the humeral bicipital groove (arrow), the latter is also called the intertubercular groove.

A

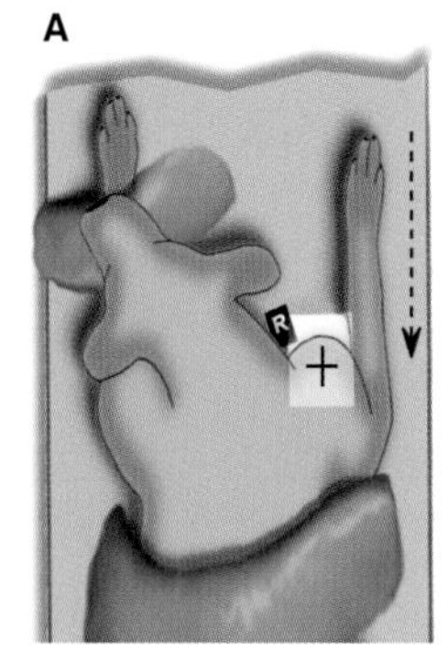

B

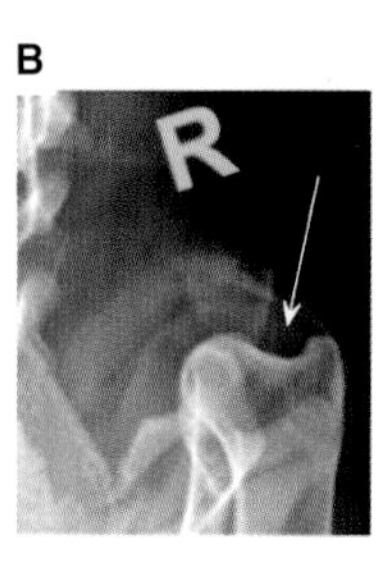

Figure 2.23 Scapula lateral view.

A. *Positioning*

- Patient is in lateral recumbency with the limb of interest down (closest to the image receptor).
- Head and neck are mildly flexed.
- Push the down limb dorsally to move the scapula dorsal to the spine (arrow **1**) and pull the up limb ventrally (arrow **2**) to eliminate superimposition.
- Limb thickness is measured laterally across the scapula.
- X-ray beam is centered on the scapula (+).
- Collimate the FOV to the size of the scapula and adjacent soft tissues.
- Alternatively, this view can be made with the limb of interest up and pushed dorsally while pulling the down limb ventrally; however, the up limb will be magnified.

B. *Radiograph*

- Lateral view of the right scapula, which is visible dorsal to the thoracic spine.

A

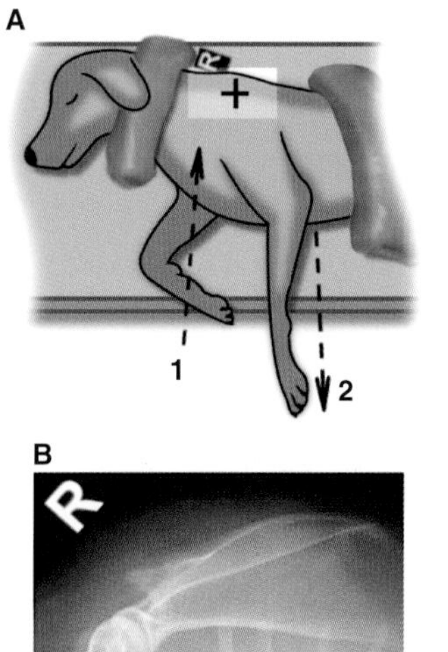

B

R

NOTES:

Figure 2.24 Shoulder (or scapula) caudocranial (CrCa) view.

A. *Positioning*

- Patient is in dorsal recumbency with the limb of interest fully extended.
- Sternum is rotated about 30° toward the opposite limb.
- Limb thickness is measured from ventral to dorsal across the scapula.
- X-ray beam is centered on the scapulohumeral joint (+) or on the scapula, depending on the purpose of the study. Palpate the scapular spine to help locate the center point.
- Collimate the FOV for the scapulohumeral joint to include the distal third of the scapula and the proximal third of the humerus. For the scapula, collimated to include the entire scapula and any swelling in the adjacent soft tissues.
- Collimate the FOV to the area of interest.
    - For the scapulohumeral joint, include the distal third of the scapula and the proximal third of the humerus.
    - For the scapula, include the entire scapula and the adjacent soft tissues.

B and C. *Radiographs*

- **B:** caudocranial view of the left scapulohumeral joint.
- **C:** caudocranial view of the left scapula.

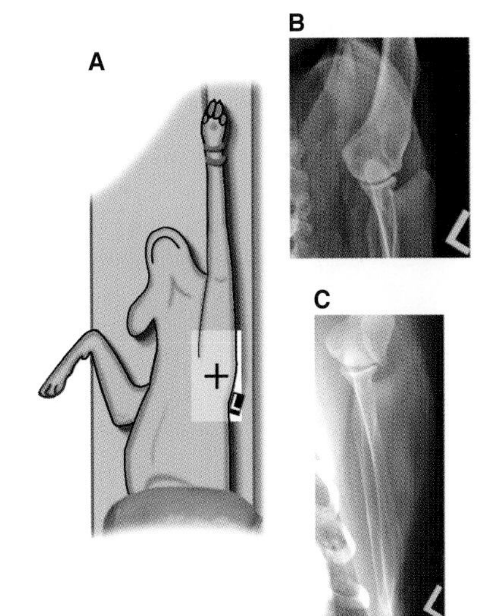

Figure 2.25 Elbow lateral view (medial-to-lateral view).

A. *Positioning*

- Patient is in lateral recumbency with the limb of interest down, closest to the image receptor, and mildly extended.
- The "up" limb is pulled caudally to eliminate superimposition.
- Limb thickness is measured at the level of the elbow.
- X-ray beam is centered on the elbow joint (+).
- Collimate the FOV to include the distal third of the humerus and the proximal third of the antebrachium.

B. *Radiograph*

- Lateral view of the right elbow.

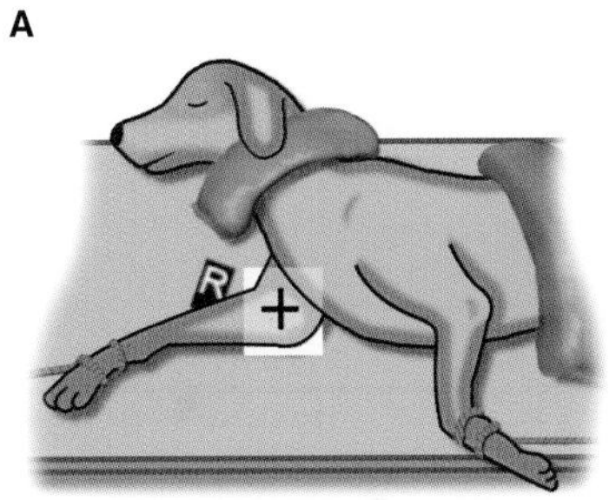

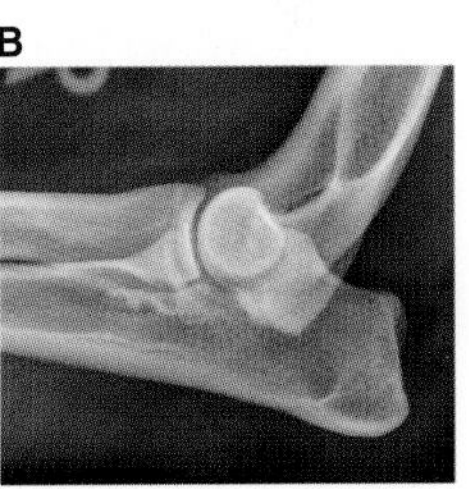

Figure 2.26 Elbow flexed lateral view (flexed medial-to-lateral view).

A. *Positioning*

- Patient is positioned for a lateral elbow view (Figure 2.25) with the elbow extremely flexed (dashed arrow). Flexion should be greater than 90° to eliminate superimposition of the humeral medial epicondyle on the ulna.

B. *Radiograph*

- Flexed lateral view of the right elbow.

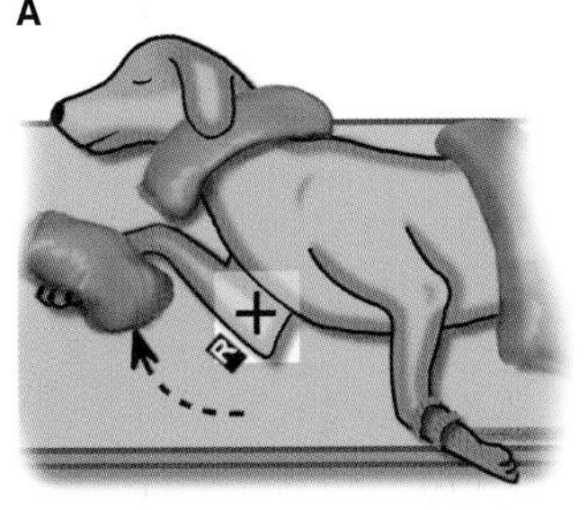

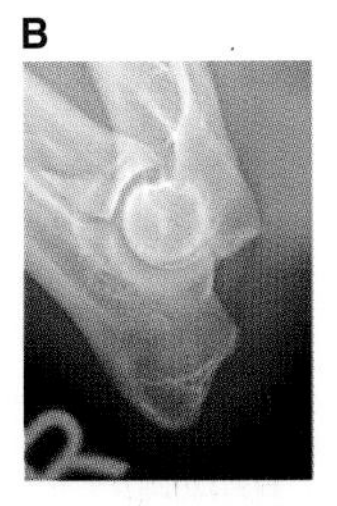

Figure 2.27 Elbow craniocaudal (CrCa) view.

A and B. *Positioning*

- Patient is in ventral (sternal) recumbency with the limb of interest fully extended.
- Turn the patient's head toward the opposite limb.
- Gently push or pull on the animal's muzzle or head to maneuver its body and correct any elbow rotation, as illustrated by the gloved hand in image **B**.
- Limb thickness is measured at the level of the elbow.
- X-ray beam is centered on the elbow joint (+).
- Collimate the FOV as small as feasible to include the distal third of the humerus and the proximal third of the antebrachium.
- To better visualize the elbow joint space, angle the x-ray beam approximately 20° craniodistal-to-caudoproximal as shown by the red arrow in image **B**.

C. *Radiograph*

- Craniocaudal view of the right elbow.

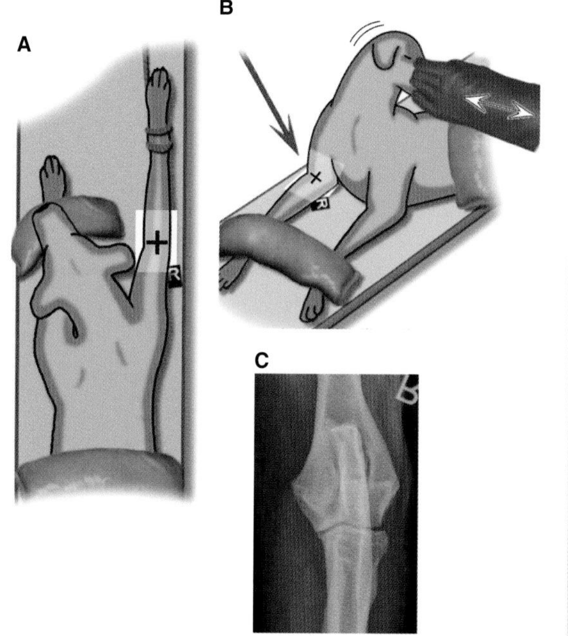

Figure 2.28 Elbow craniolateral–caudomedial oblique (CrLCaMO) view.

A. *Positioning*

- Patient is positioned for a craniocaudal elbow view (Figure 2.27).
- The limb of interest is in a neutral, slightly pronated position. It is not fully extended. Allow the limb to relax so the elbow rotates slightly inward to eliminate superimposition of the olecranon on the medial coronoid process.
- X-ray beam is centered on the elbow (+).

B. *Radiograph*

- Craniolateral-caudomedial oblique view (CrLCaMO) of the right elbow. The x-rays pass through the joint in a cranial-lateral to caudal-medial direction to produce a tangential view of the medial coronoid process (MCP).

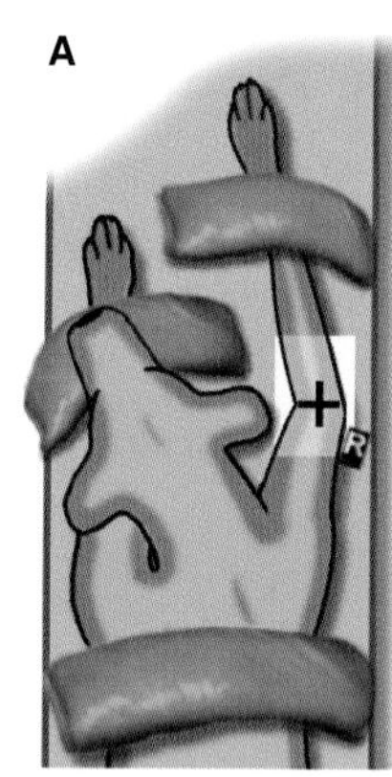

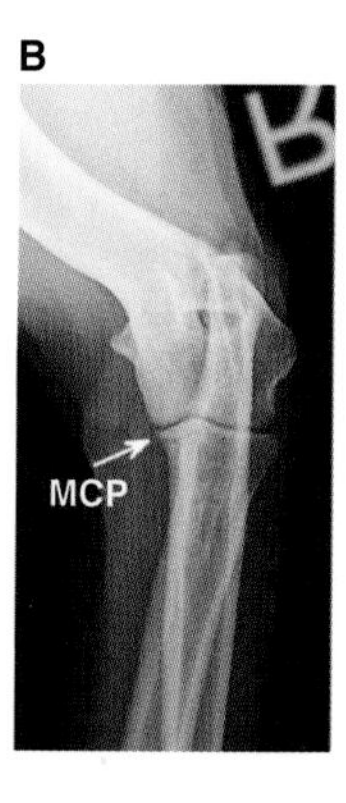

NOTES:

Figure 2.29 Carpus and manus lateral and lateral oblique views.

A. *Positioning*

- Patient is in lateral recumbency with the limb of interest down, closest to the image receptor, and extended. The carpus may be more easily extended by pushing on the elbow rather than pulling on the foot.
- The "up" limb is pulled caudally to eliminate superimposition.
- Limb thickness is measured at the level of the carpus.
- X-ray beam is centered on the carpus (+).
- Collimate the FOV to include the distal third of the antebrachium and the proximal third of the metacarpus.
- As needed, the lateral view can be repeated with the limb slightly **supinated** or **pronated** to visualize more of the bony margins in the carpus (green dashed arrow).

B and C. *Radiographs*

- **B:** lateral view of the right carpus (medial-to-lateral view).
- **C:** lateral oblique view of the right carpus. The limb was pronated (rotated inward) about 45° so the x-ray beam passed through the carpus from the dorsal and lateral side to the palmar and medial side; a dorsopalmar-to-lateromedial oblique view (DPLMO).

A

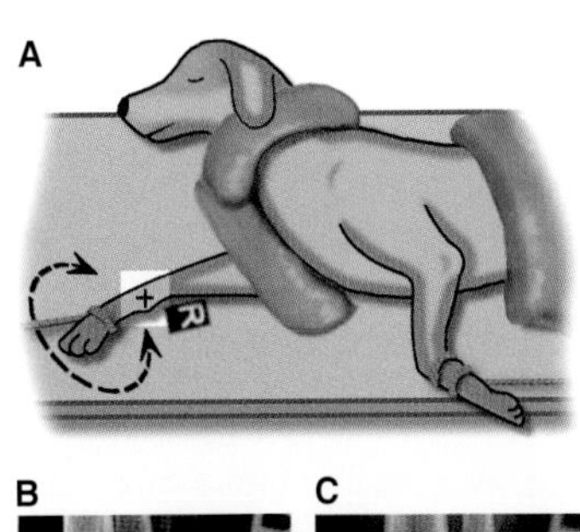

B

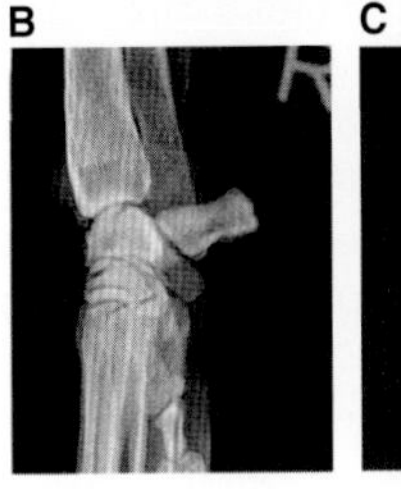

C

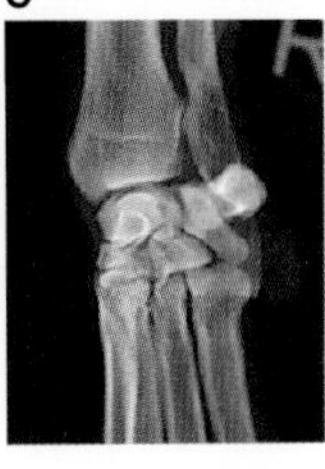

Figure 2.30 Carpus and manus dorsopalmar (DP) view.

A. *Positioning*

- Patient is in ventral (sternal) recumbency.
- The limb of interest is extended. The carpus may be more easily positioned by pushing the elbow rather than pulling the foot.
- Turn the patient's head toward opposite limb.
- Limb thickness is measured at the distal antebrachium.
- X-ray beam is centered on the carpus (+).
- Collimate the FOV to include the distal third of the antebrachium and the proximal third of the metacarpus.

B. *Radiograph*

- Dorsopalmar (DP) view of the right carpus.

C. *Skyline view*

- To better visualize the dorsal aspects of the carpus, the limb can be flexed and the x-ray beam directed perpendicular to the image receptor (1) or slightly angled from proximal to distal (2). A flexed dorsoproximal-to-dorsodistal view enhances visualization of the dorsal border of the distal radius or intercarpal bones or proximal metacarpus, depending on the degree of carpal flexion and the angle of the x-ray beam (particularly useful when looking for chip fractures).

A B

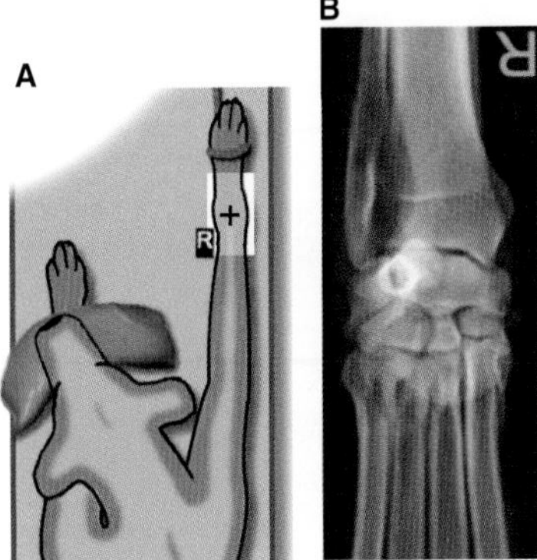

C

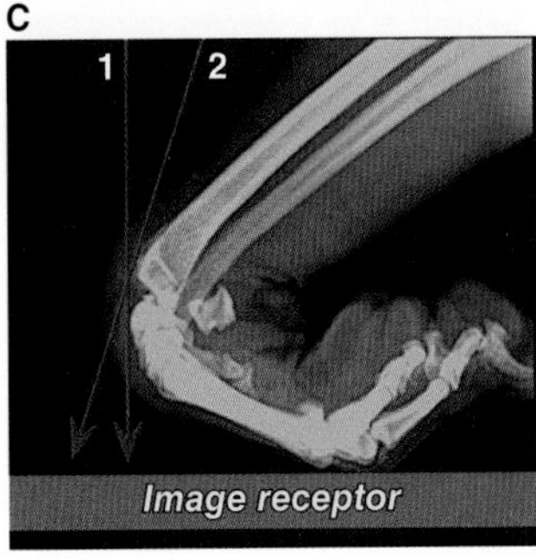

NOTES:

Figure 2.31 Stress radiography.

These supplemental views are used to assess joint laxity. They are made in addition to the standard orthogonal views.

A and B. *Positioning*

- Patient may be in ventral, dorsal, or lateral recumbency with the joint of interest closest to the image receptor.
- The bones proximal and distal to the joint are stabilized and a force is applied to the joint using something like a wooden or plastic stick.
  - **A:** a lateral-to-medial force is applied to the elbow while the carpus is stabilized using rope ties.
  - **B:** a medial-to-lateral force is applied to the carpus while the manus is stabilized with a rope tie.
- X-ray beam is centered on the joint of interest.
- Collimate the FOV as small as feasible to include the adjacent one-third of the long bones proximal and distal to the joint.
- Make the x-ray exposure while the force is being applied to the joint.

C and D. *Radiographs*

- **C:** craniocaudal view of the elbow without stress.
- **D:** craniocaudal view of the same elbow made while a lateral-to-medial force was applied (black arrow). Widening of the medial aspect of the elbow joint (white arrow) and malalignment between the humerus and antebrachium indicate joint laxity.

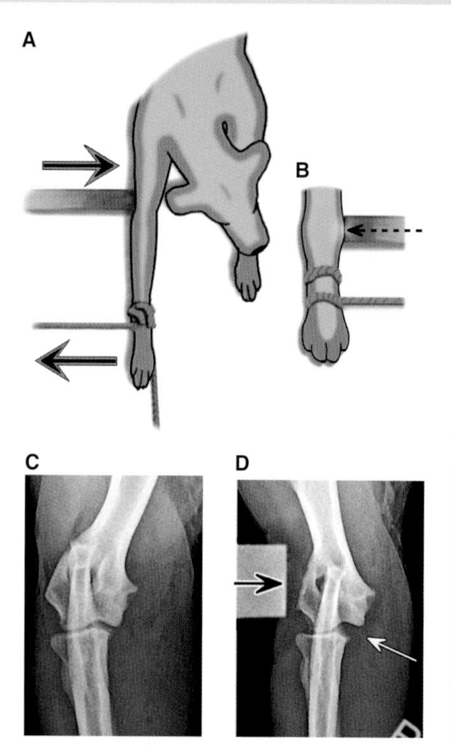

Figure 2.32 Digits mediolateral view.

A and B. *Positioning*

- Patient is positioned for a lateral view of the manus or pes (Figure 2.29 or 2.46).
- Digits may be separated using either a compression technique or traction.
  - **A:** a low opacity paddle (e.g., plastic or wooden spoon) is used to gently compress the foot.
  - **B:** tape or gauze is wrapped around the digits and used to gently pull them apart.
- X-ray beam is centered on the digits.
- Collimate the FOV to include the digits and the distal half of the metacarpus or metatarsus.

C. *Radiograph*

- Close up lateral view of the left digits (mediolateral view). The foot was gently compressed with a wooden spoon to separate the digits and eliminate superimposition.

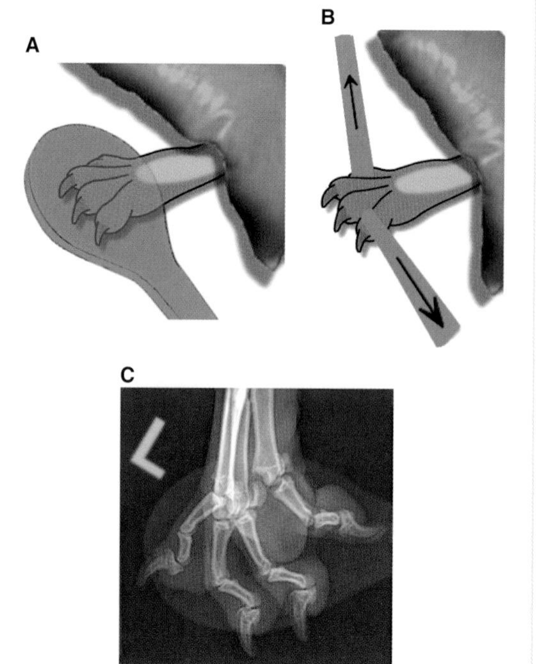

Figure 2.33 Digits dorsopalmar or dorsoplantar (DP) view.

A. *Positioning*

- Patient is positioned for DP view of manus or pes (Figure 2.30 or 2.43).
- A low opacity paddle (e.g., plastic or wooden spoon) is used to gently hold the paw in position and to softly compress and separate the digits. Wrapping a tie around the foot can distort the anatomy.
- X-ray beam is centered on the digits.
- Collimate the FOV as small as feasible to include distal half of the metacarpus or metatarsus.

B. *Radiograph*

- Close up dorsopalmar view of the left digits.

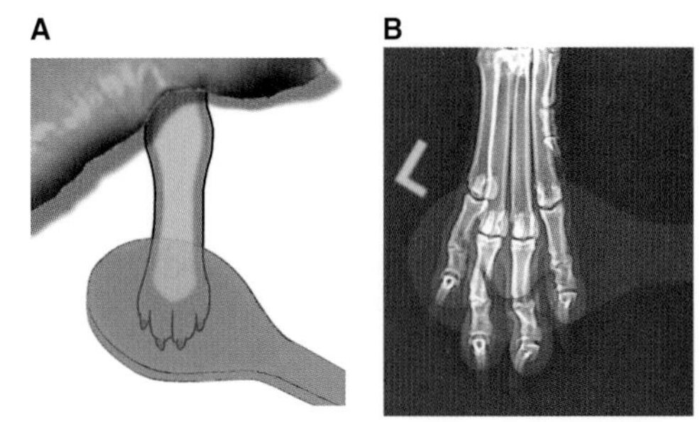

Figure 2.34 Pelvis lateral view.

A, B, and C. *Positioning*

- Patient is in right or left lateral recumbency.
- The pelvic limbs are in a neutral position with the down limb moved slightly cranial to the up limb.
- The ilial wings are superimposed in the same vertical plane, perpendicular to the image receptor.
- A foam wedge or towel between the stifles is used to correct pelvic rotation as shown in B and C.
    - **B:** viewing the dog from the caudal aspect, the dotted lines represent the dorsal and sagittal planes. The dorsal plane naturally rotates in lateral recumbency, making the pelvis oblique to the x-ray beam.
    - **C:** a rolled towel between the stifles corrects the rotation of the pelvis and spine.
- Pelvis thickness is measured at the iliac crests.
- X-ray beam is centered on the greater trochanters (+).
- Collimate the FOV to include the iliac crests, ischiatic tuberosities and proximal half of each femur.

D and E. *Radiographs*

- **D:** lateral oblique view of the pelvis (due to patient rotation). Notice the ilial wings are not aligned. Note: sometimes an oblique view is desirable to view each hemipelvis with less summation.
- **E:** true lateral view of the pelvis. The ilial wings are superimposed and the intervertebral disc spaces and coxofemoral joint space are more distinct.

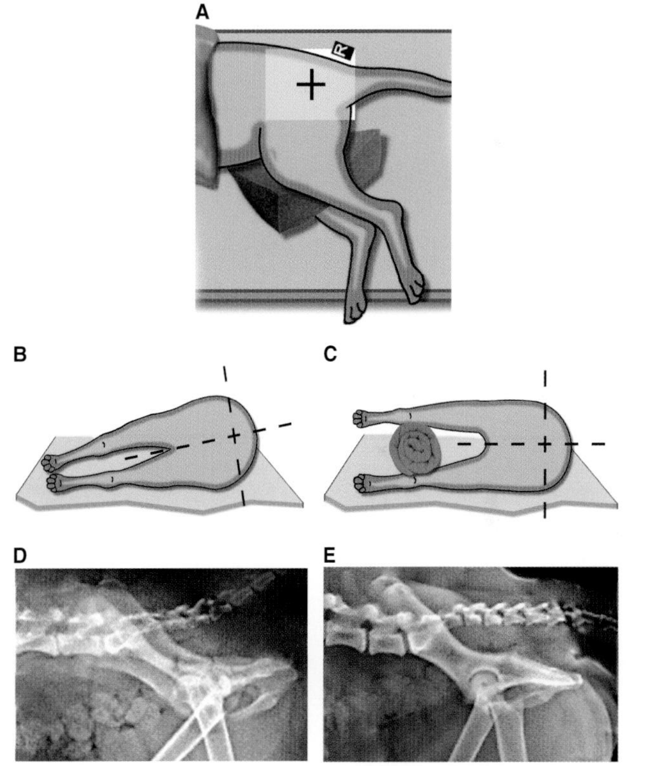

NOTES:

Figure 2.35 Pelvis extended ventrodorsal (VD) view.

A. ***Positioning***

- Patient is in dorsal recumbency. A padded V-trough can be used to simplify positioning and to make the patient more comfortable. Notice that the edge of the trough is cranial to the pelvis to avoid superimposition and magnification artifacts.
- The pelvic limbs are extended and parallel. If extending the pelvic limbs is difficult, try temporarily binding the stifles together with a piece of gauze or tape (as shown in **A**) and then extend both limbs while bound together.
- Rotate the stifles inward (toward each other) to center each patella in the middle of its femur.
- Pelvic thickness is measured across the iliac crests.
- X-ray beam is centered at level of greater trochanters (+).
- Collimate the FOV to include the ilial crests and both stifles.

B. ***Radiograph***

- Extended VD view of the pelvis.

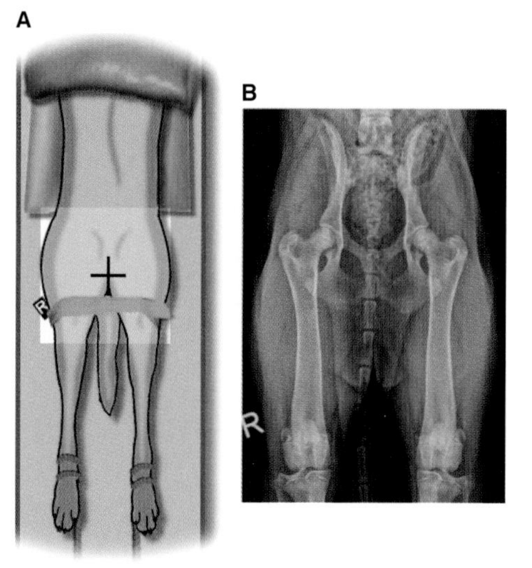

Figure 2.36 Pelvis flexed ventrodorsal (VD) view (frog-leg view).

A. ***Positioning***

- Patient is in dorsal recumbency and in a padded V-trough, similar to Figure 2.35.
- Pelvic limbs are allowed to naturally flex and abduct.
- Pelvic thickness is measured at the level of the iliac crests.
- X-ray beam is centered at the level of the greater trochanters (+).
- Collimate the FOV as small as feasible to include the iliac crests, proximal half of each femur, and the ischiatic tuberosities.

B. ***Radiograph***

- Flexed VD view of the pelvis.

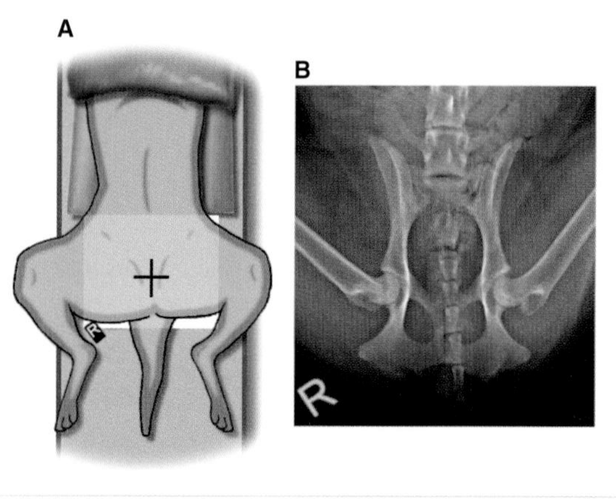

NOTES:

Figure 2.37 Pelvis half-axial VD view.

This is a supplemental radiograph of the pelvis made in addition to the standard orthogonal views. It is used to assess hip laxity.

A and B. *Positioning*

- Patient is in dorsal recumbency as described in Figure 2.35.
- Pelvic limbs are parallel and in a neutral position.
- **A:** a rolled towel is placed between the thighs, proximal to the stifles, to act as a fulcrum. When the tarsi are adducted (black arrows) the hips are distracted (red arrows). The tarsi can be temporarily bound together while making the radiograph.
- **B:** the pelvic limbs are neither extended (E) nor flexed (F). The neutral position (N) results in less 'twisting' of the hip muscles and joint capsules than the extended VD view, making it easier for a "loose" hip to subluxate.
- Pelvic thickness is measured at the iliac crests.
- X-ray beam is centered at the level of greater trochanters (+).
- Collimate the FOV to include the iliac crests and the stifles.
- Make the exposure while the tarsi are adducted.

C and D. *Radiographs*

- **C:** extended VD view of the pelvis (made without a fulcrum). The coxofemoral joints are highlighted and appear normal.
- **D:** half-axial VD view of the same pelvis. The rolled towel fulcrum is visible between the femurs. Distraction causes both coxofemoral joints to subluxate (each femoral head is displaced laterally and there is cranial wedging of the joint spaces), indicating excessive hip laxity.

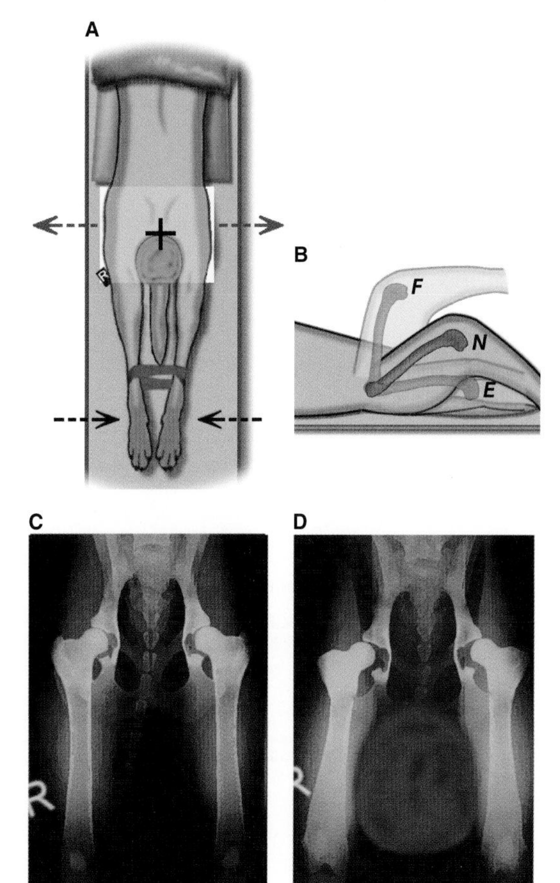

Figure 2.38 Pelvis dorsal acetabular rim view.

This is a supplemental radiograph of the pelvis made in addition to the standard orthogonal views. It is used to evaluate coxofemoral fit and acetabular depth.

A. *Positioning* (A)

- Patient is in ventral (sternal) recumbency.
- The pelvic limbs are moved cranially, flexing the hips.
- The tarsi are elevated about 5 cm. In illustration **A**, the tarsus is resting on a sandbag.
- X-ray beam is centered at the level of the greater trochanters (red arrow). The x-ray beam passes through the long axis of the pelvis, from cranial to caudal.
- Collimate the FOV to include the ilial crests, proximal third of each femur, and the ischiatic tuberosities.

B. *Radiograph*

- Dorsal acetabular rim view of pelvis. The black arrows point to the right dorsal acetabular rim. The white dashed circle indicates the left femoral head. The white arrow points to the left ischiatic tuberosity.

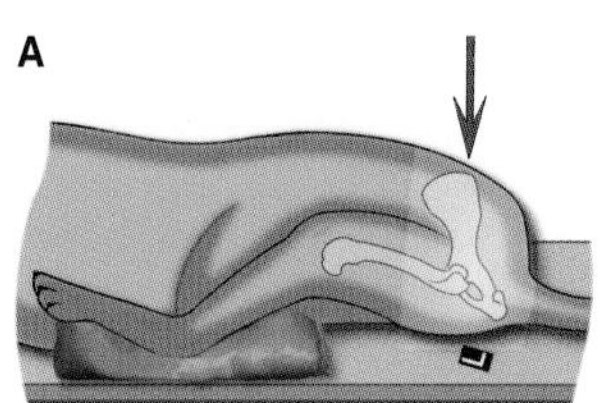

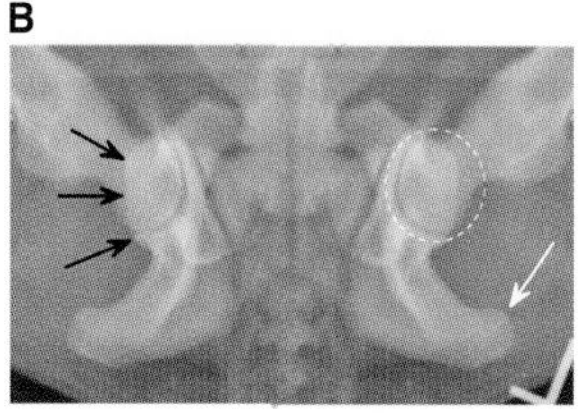

Figure 2.39 Stifle lateral view.

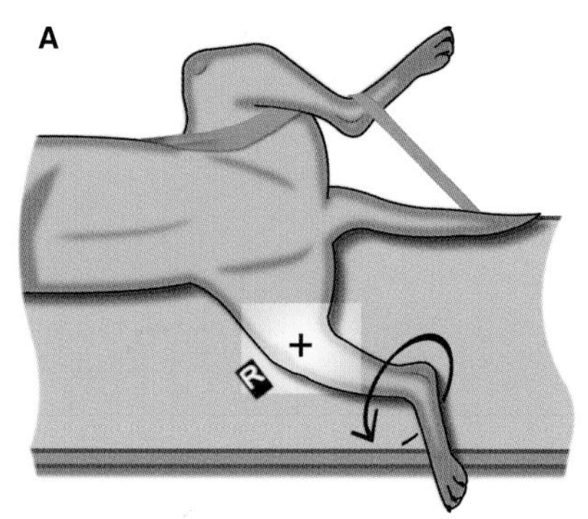

A. *Positioning*

- Patient is in lateral recumbency.
- Limb of interest is down (closest to the image receptor) and in a neutral position. The angle of the stifle should be about 120°.
- The opposite (up) pelvic limb is flexed and abducted to eliminate superimposition (up limb may be secured with tape, as shown).
- To make a true lateral view, you may need to slightly rotate the patella toward the image receptor to superimpose the femoral condyles (arrow at tarsus).
- Stifle thickness is measured at the distal femur.
- X-ray beam is centered on the stifle (+).
- Collimate the FOV to include the distal third of the femur and the proximal third of the tibia.
- For surgical planning the stifle may need to be flexed 90° instead of a neutral 120°.

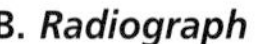

B. *Radiograph*

- Lateral view of the right stifle.

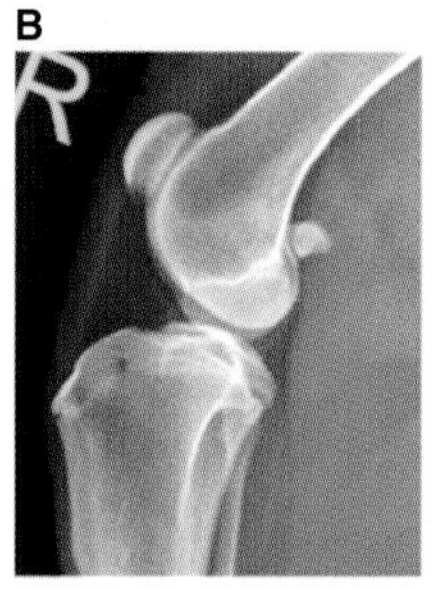

Figure 2.40 Stifle caudocranial view.

A. *Positioning*

- Patient is in ventral (sternal) recumbency.
- The limb of interest is extended and the opposite limb is flexed.
- Rotate the pelvis slightly toward the limb of interest.
- Rotate the limb of interest inward as needed to center the patella on the distal femur.
- Stifle thickness is measured at the distal femur. Note: the thickness of the limb often is greater than in the lateral view.
- X-ray beam is centered on the stifle (+). Angle the beam about 10° caudodistal-to-cranioproximal to better visualize the joint space.
- Collimate the FOV to include the distal third of the femur and the proximal third of the tibia.
- NOTE: the craniocaudal view of the stifle (patient in dorsal recumbency) results in more magnification and less detail.

B. *Radiograph*

- Caudocranial (CaCr) view of the right stifle.

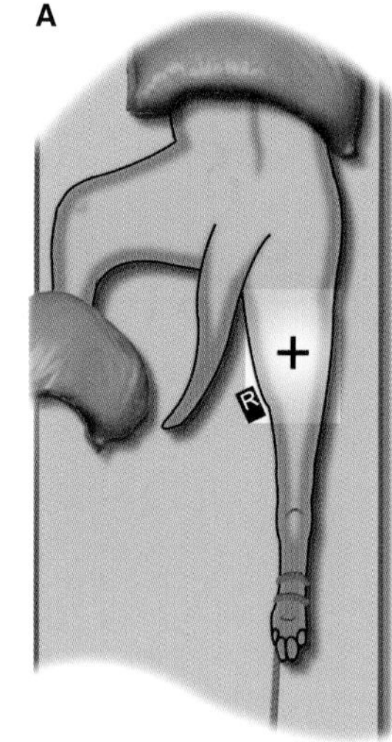

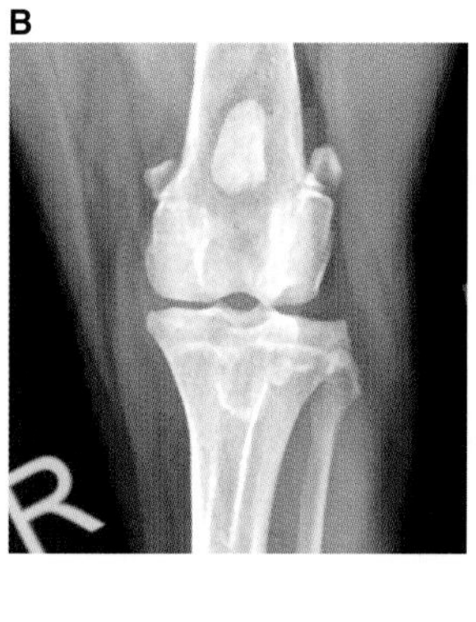

NOTES:

Figure 2.41 Stifle flexed lateral view with tibial compression.

This is a supplemental radiograph of the stifle made in addition to the standard orthogonal views.

A. *Positioning*

- Patient is positioned for a lateral view of the stifle (Figure 2.39).
- Stifle is flexed 90° and the tarsus is maximally flexed (curved arrow). Try to make the metatarsus parallel with the femur.
- Stifle thickness is measured at the distal femur.
- X-ray beam is centered on the stifle (+).
- Collimate the FOV to include the distal third of the femur and the proximal third of the tibia.
- Make the x-ray exposure while both the stifle and the tarsus are flexed.

B and C. *Radiographs*

- **B:** lateral view of the stifle (without tibial compression). The proximal tibia and distal femur appear to be in normal alignment.
- **C:** flexed lateral view made with the tarsus flexed. The proximal tibia is cranially displaced in relation to the distal femur. In many cases, this tibial compression view is as sensitive and specific for the diagnosis of cranial cruciate ligament injury as palpation for a cranial drawer sign.

A

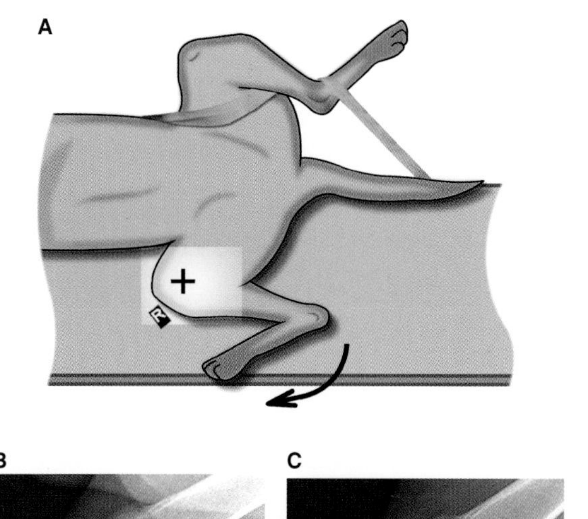

B

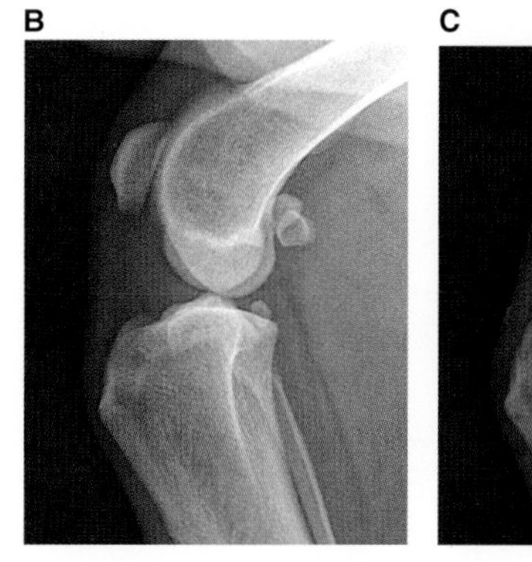

C

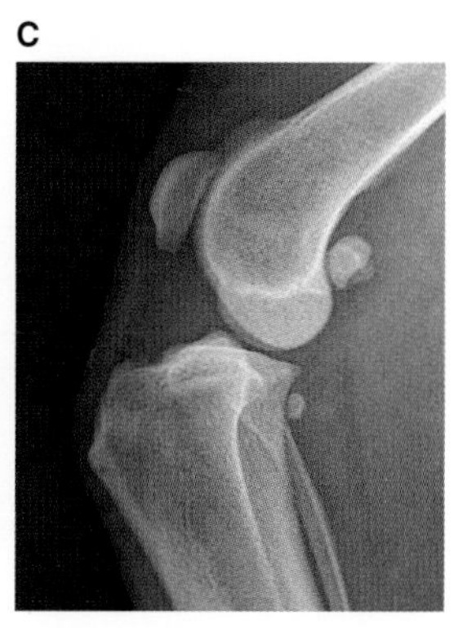

Figure 2.42 Stifle cranioproximal–craniodistal view (skyline view of stifle).

This is a supplemental radiograph of the stifle made in addition to the standard orthogonal views. It is used to examine the patella and patellar groove.

A. *Positioning*

- Patient is in ventral (sternal) recumbency with both pelvic limbs extended caudally.
- The stifle of interest is then flexed and pushed cranially, but the tarsus remains extended.
- Angle the x-ray beam about 10° off perpendicular (caudoproximal-to-craniodistal, as shown by the red arrow) to better visualize the patellar groove.
- Stifle thickness is measured at the distal femur.
- X-ray beam is centered on the cranial aspect of the stifle.
- Collimate the FOV to include the distal third of the femur and the patella.

B. *Radiograph*

- Skyline view of the left stifle.

A

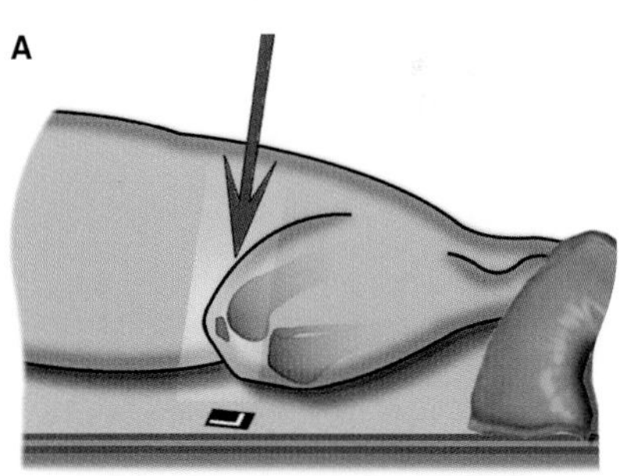

B

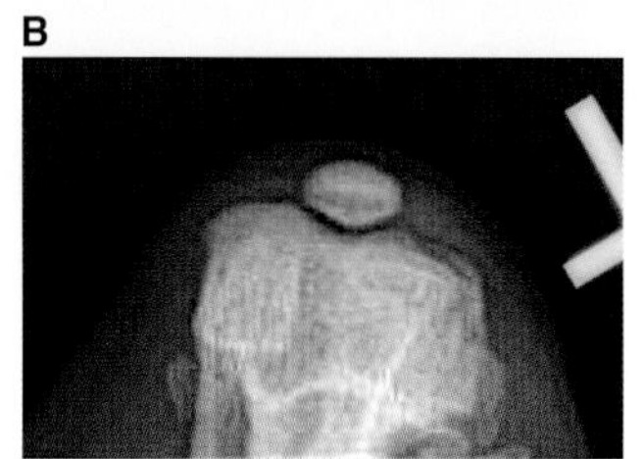

Figure 2.43 Tarsus mediolateral view.

A. ***Positioning***

- Patient is in lateral recumbency.
- Limb of interest is down (closest to the image receptor) with the tarsus in a neutral position.
- The tarsus may be more easily positioned by pushing the stifle rather than pulling the foot.
- The opposite (up) limb is moved out of the FOV.
- Tarsal thickness is measured at the distal crus.
- X-ray beam is centered on the tarsus (+).
- Collimate the FOV to include the distal third of the tibia and the proximal third of the metatarsus.

B. ***Radiograph***

- Lateral (mediolateral) view of the right tarsus.

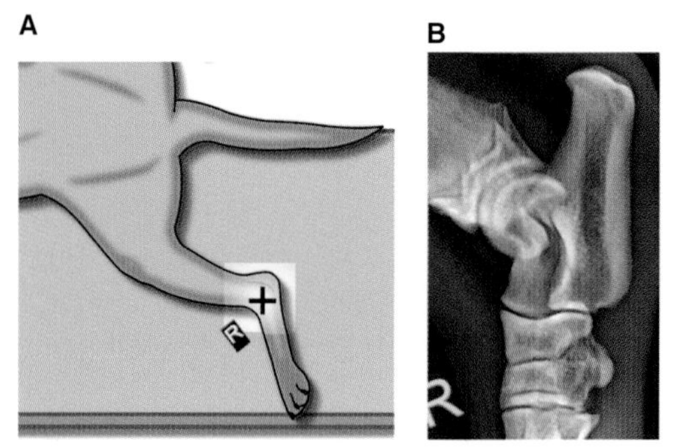

Figure 2.44 Tarsus dorsoplantar (DP) view.

A. ***Positioning***

- Patient is in ventral (sternal) recumbency.
- Limb of interest is extended cranially and moved slightly laterally, away from the body. The tarsus may be more easily positioned by pushing the stifle rather than pulling the foot.
- Tarsal thickness is measured at the distal crus.
- X-ray beam is centered on the tarsus (+).
- Collimate the FOV to include the distal third of the tibia and the proximal third of the metatarsus.
- As needed, the DP view can be repeated with the tarsus slightly rotated to the right or left to visualize more of the bony margins (arrow).

B–D. ***Radiographs***

- **B:** dorsoplantar view of the right tarsus.
- **C:** dorsolateral-to-plantaromedial oblique (DLPMO) view of the tarsus (the limb was rotated outward about 45°).
- **D:** dorsomedial-to-plantarolateral oblique (DMPLO) view of the tarsus (the limb was rotated inward about 45°).
- Notice the "R" marker is positioned on the lateral side in each radiograph.

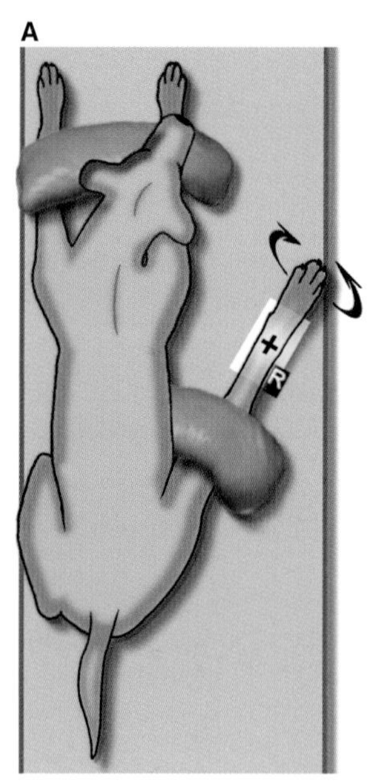

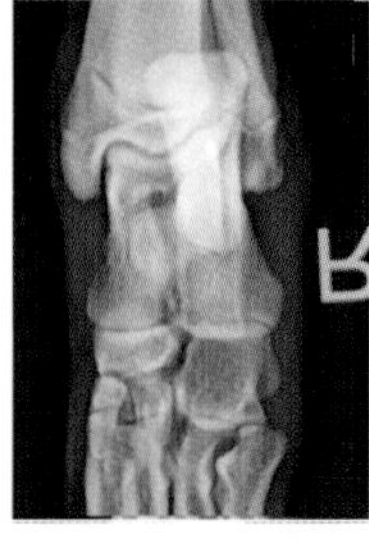

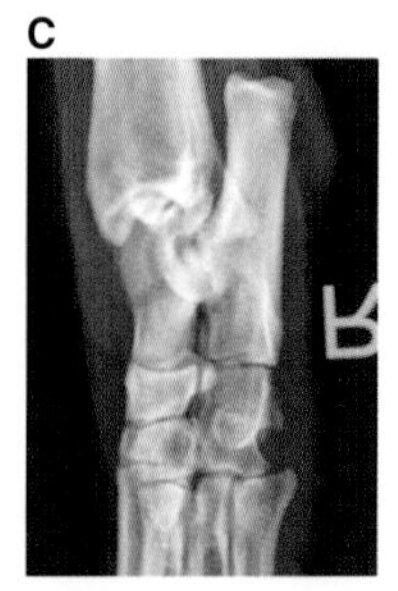

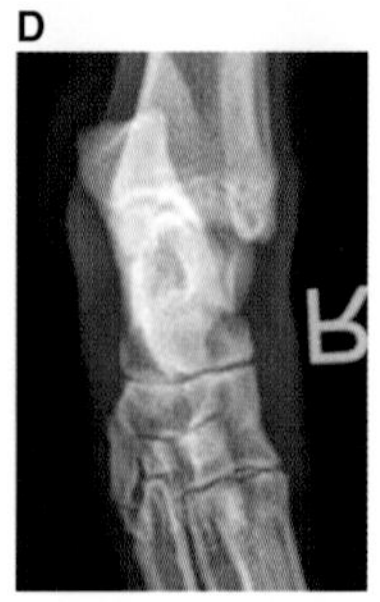

NOTES:

Figure 2.45 Tarsus flexed dorsoplantar view.

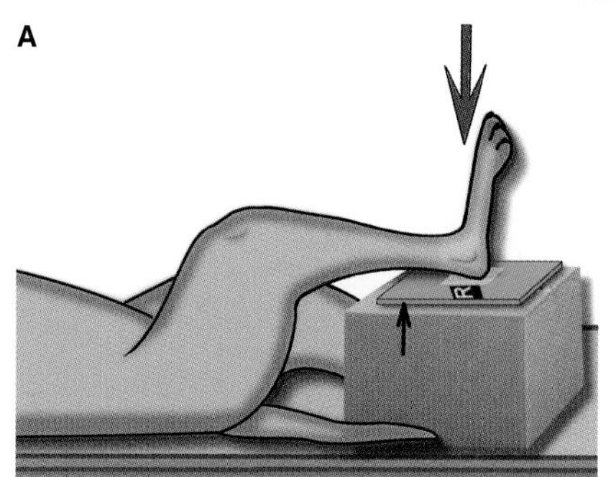

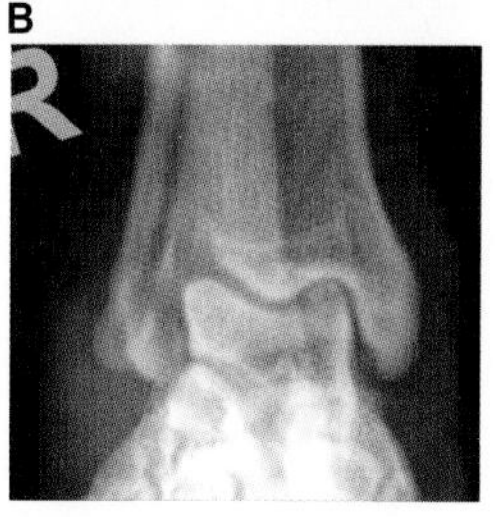

This is a supplemental radiograph of the tarsus made in addition to the standard orthogonal views. It is used to visualize the tibiotarsal joint without superimposition of the calcaneus.

A. *Positioning*

- Patient is in dorsal recumbency.
- The tarsus of interest is elevated atop a small cardboard box or similar device. The tarsus is flexed with the toes pointing up toward the x-ray tube.
- If feasible, place the image receptor on top of the box and under the tarsus to minimize magnification distortion.
- Adjust the source-to-image distance (SID) as needed.
- Tarsal thickness is measured at the distal crus.
- X-ray beam (red arrow) is centered on the tibiotarsal joint.
- Collimate the FOV to include the distal third of the tibia and the plantar border of the foot.

B. *Radiograph*

- Flexed dorsoplantar view of the right tarsus.

Figure 2.46 Tarsus plantaroproximal–plantarodistal view of calcaneus (skyline view of calcaneus).

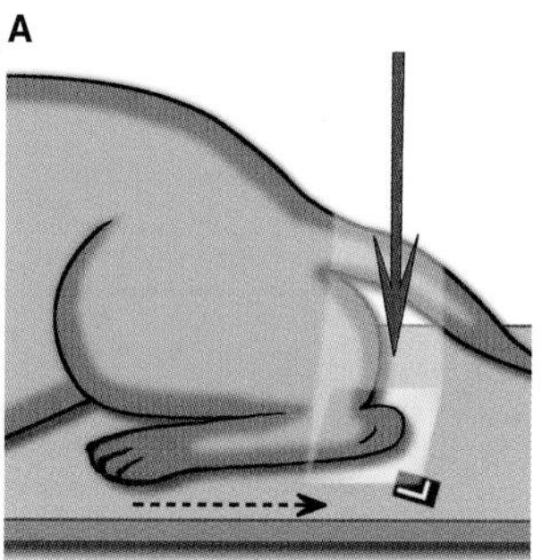

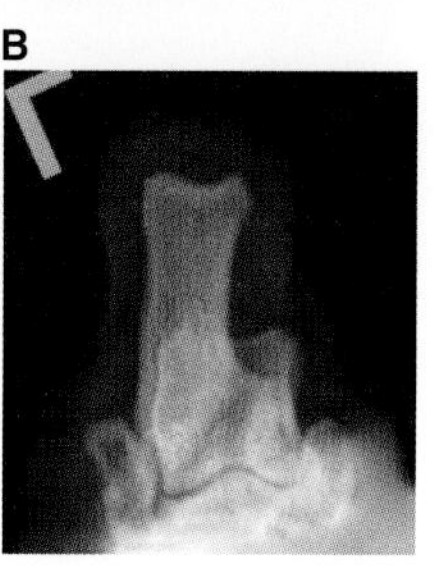

This is a supplemental radiograph of the tarsus made in addition to the standard orthogonal views. It is used to evaluate the calcaneus.

A. *Positioning*

- Patient is in ventral (sternal) recumbency.
- Both pelvic limbs are in a crouching position under the animal.
- Slide the limb of interest caudally until the calcaneus is caudal to the ischium (black dotted arrow) to eliminate superimposition.
- X-ray beam (red arrow) is centered on the calcaneus.
- Collimate the FOV to include the calcaneus and adjacent soft tissues.

B. *Radiograph*

- Skyline view of the left calcaneus.

NOTES:

Axial skeleton

Figure 2.47 Head lateral view.

A and B. *Positioning*

- Patient is in lateral recumbency with the side of interest down, closest to the image receptor.
- The head and neck are extended.
- As needed, elevate the nose with a foam wedge or similar to make the median plane of the head parallel to the image receptor.
- Align the patient's eyes in a vertical plane perpendicular to the image receptor and do the same with the mandibles. If you can open the mouth and visualize the hard palate, this may help in positioning: if you align the hard palate, you align the skull.
- Thickness of the head is measured mid-way between the level of the eyes and the level of the ears.
- X-ray beam (red arrow) is centered at the level of the eyes (+).
- Collimate the FOV to include the entire head, from the tip of the nose to the first cervical vertebra.
- To better visualize the nasopharynx, open the mouth to rotate the mandibular rami away from the nasopharynx. This view is helpful when looking for evidence of a mass or foreign object in the nasopharynx. Increase the x-ray exposure for this view by doubling the mAs (or increase the kVp 20%).

C. *Radiograph*

- Right lateral view of the head.

A

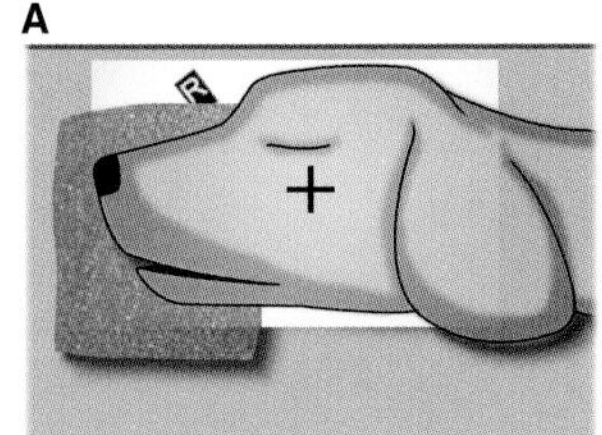

B

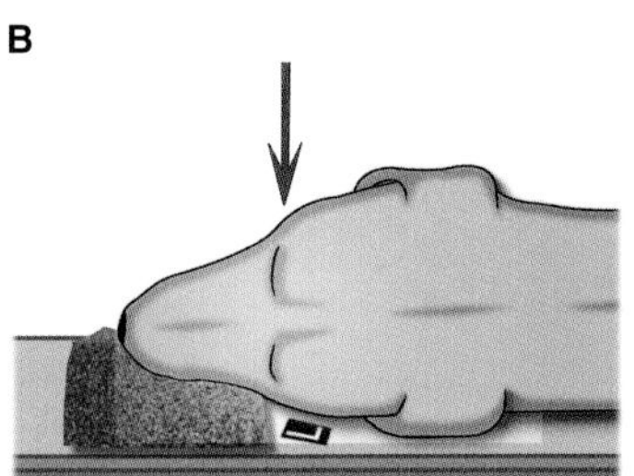

C

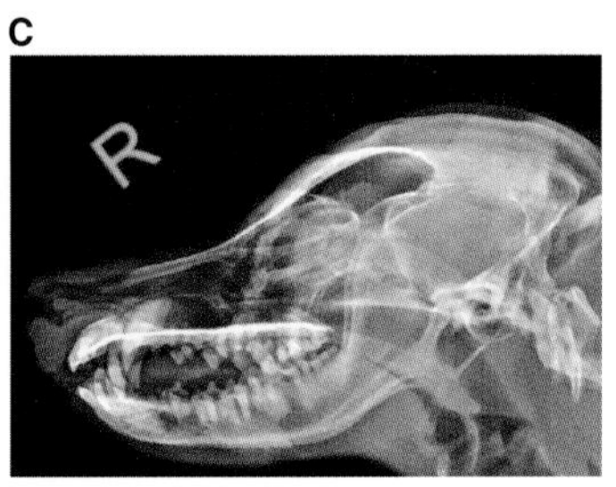

Figure 2.48 Head dorsoventral (DV) view.

A and B. *Positioning*

- Patient is in ventral (sternal) recumbency.
- The head and neck are extended with the mandibles resting on the top table or on top of the image receptor.
- The hard palate should be parallel with the table top.
- The eyes should be level, aligned in the same horizontal plane. The same with the right and left zygomatic arches.
- Thickness of the head is measured mid-way between the level of the eyes and the level of the ears.
- X-ray beam is centered on midline at the level of the eyes (+).
- Collimate the FOV to include the entire head, from the tip of the nose to the first cervical vertebra.
- A ventrodorsal (VD) view of the head can be made with the patient in dorsal recumbency but may be more difficult to position with symmetry than a DV view.

C. *Radiograph*

- DV view of head.

A

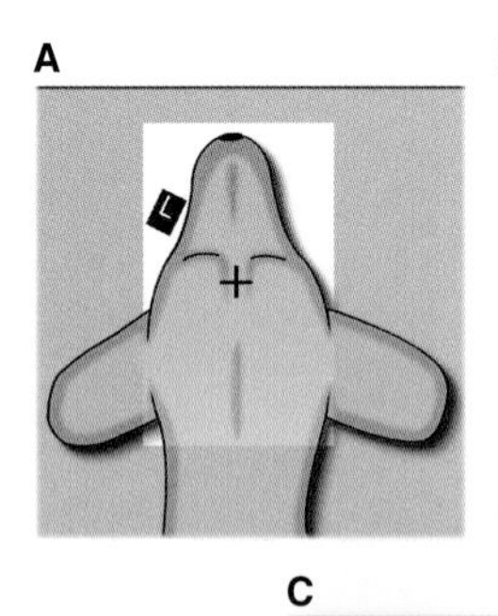

B

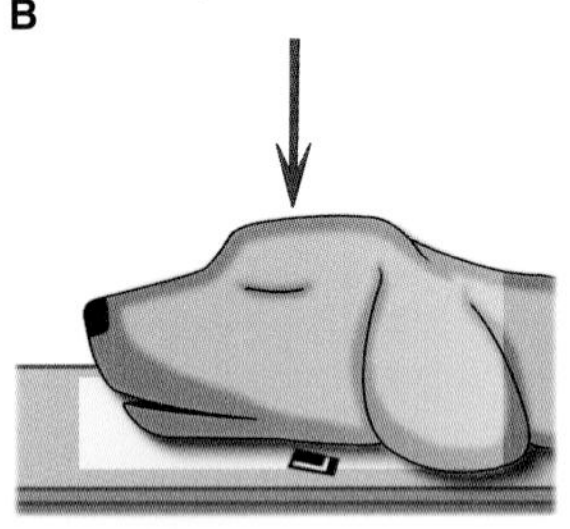

C

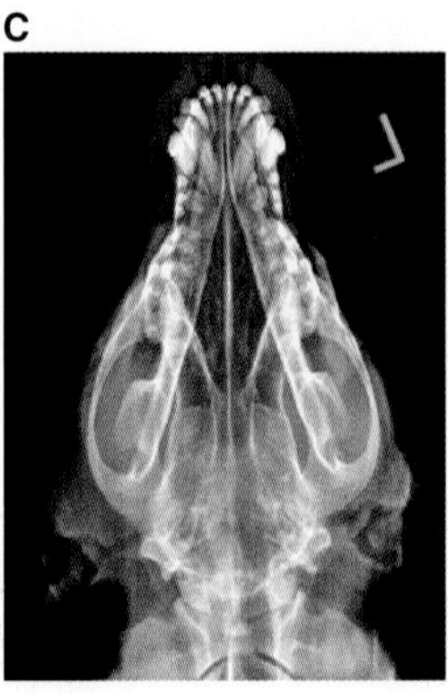

Figure 2.49 Head lateral oblique view.

This is a supplemental radiograph of the head made in addition to the standard lateral and DV views. It is used to better isolate and evaluate a part of the skull.

A. *Positioning*

- Patient is in lateral recumbency with the side of interest closest to the image receptor.
- The head is propped up, resting obliquely on a foam wedge or similar (the side of interest is against the wedge).
- Thickness of the head is measured mid-way between the level of the eyes and the level of the ears.
- <u>Both</u> "Right" and "Left" markers are recommended to avoid confusion. The side of interest will be projected dorsally in the radiograph.
- X-ray beam is centered on the area of interest (e.g., frontal sinus, mass on head).
- Collimate the FOV to include the entire head, from the tip of the nose to the first cervical vertebra.

B. *Radiograph*

- Lateral oblique view of head. The right frontal sinus and the right nasal passage are projected dorsal to the left. The left hemimandible is ventral to the right.

A

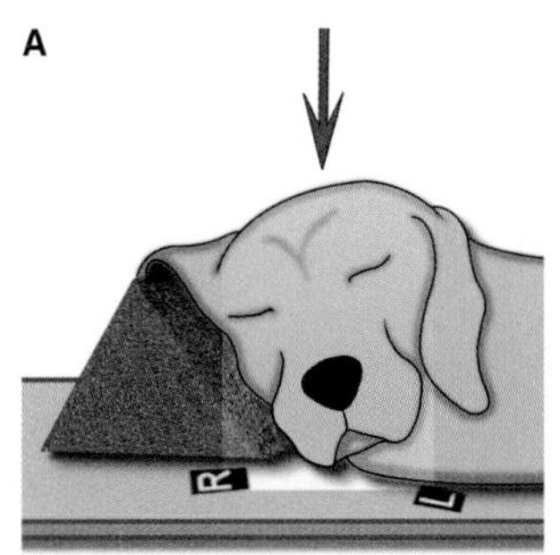

B

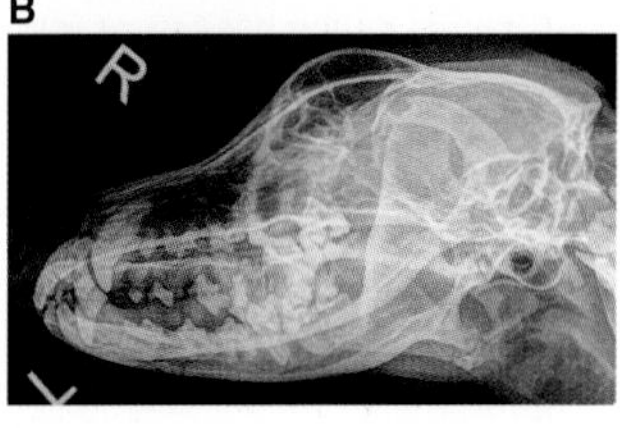

Figure 2.50 Head open-mouth lateral oblique view.

This is a supplemental radiograph of the head made in addition to the standard lateral and DV views. It is used to evaluate a mandible or maxilla.

A and B. *Positioning*

- Patient is in lateral recumbency with the head resting obliquely against a foam wedge; the side of interest adjacent to the wedge and closest to the image receptor.
- Open the mouth and move the tongue and endotracheal tube away from the area of interest. If needed, support the mouth open with an oral speculum or other device, but be careful not to superimpose the device on the area of interest.
  - **A:** positioning to evaluate the right hemimandible.
  - **B:** positioning to evaluate the left maxilla.
- Thickness of the head is measured at the level of the eyes.
- Both "Right" and "Left" markers are recommended to help avoid confusion.
- X-ray beam is centered on the area of interest (the mandible in illustration **A** and the maxilla in **B**).
- Collimate the FOV as small as feasible to include the entire area of interest. Remember: the smaller the FOV, the better the radiographic detail.

C and D. *Radiographs*

- **C:** open-mouth lateral oblique view of the mandible. The right mandibular dental arcade is projected dorsal to the left.
- **D:** open-mouth lateral oblique view of the maxilla. The left maxillary dental arcade is ventral to the right.

A

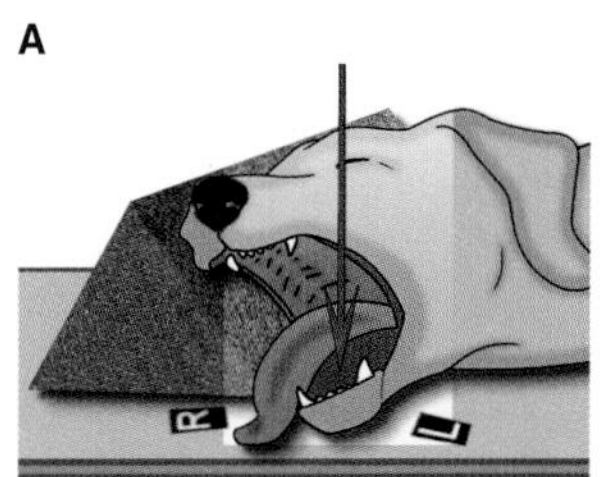

B

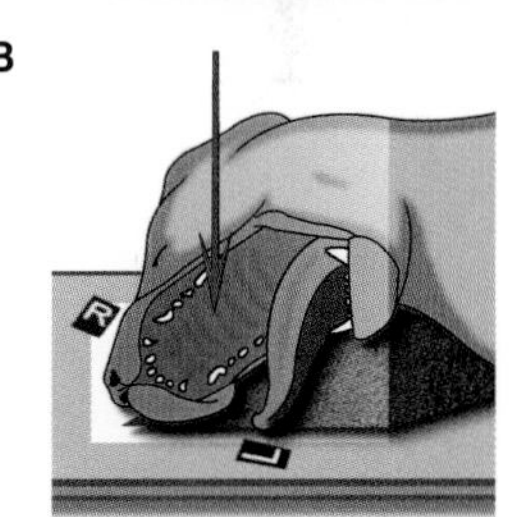

C

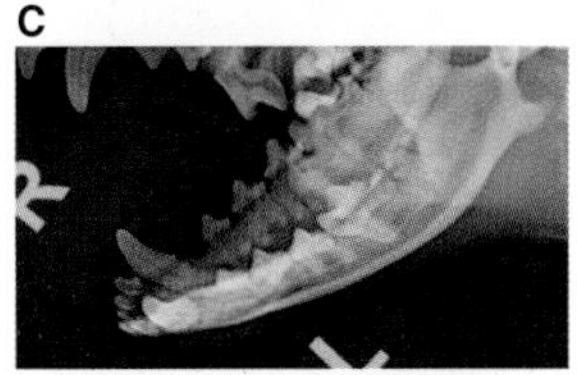

D

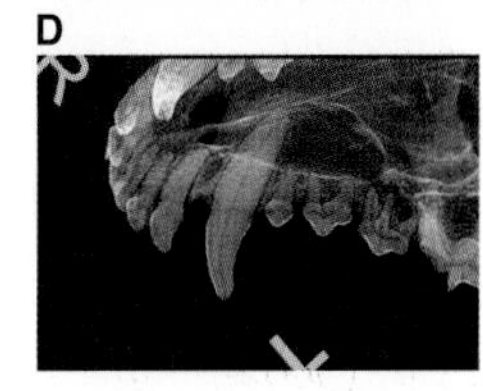

CHAPTER 2

Figure 2.51 Head open mouth ventrodorsal (VD) view.

This is a supplemental radiograph of the head made in addition to the standard lateral and DV views. It is used to evaluate the maxilla and nasal cavities without superimposition of the mandible.

A. *Positioning*

- Patient is in dorsal recumbency.
- Head is extended with the mouth fully open. The mouth may be held open using tape or gauze (as shown in **A**), an oral speculum, or another device. Be sure the positioning device is not in the area of interest.
- Move the tongue and endotracheal tube away from the area of interest.
- Thickness of the head is measured at the level of the eyes, between the hard palate and the medial canthus of the eye.
- X-ray beam is angled about 20° rostroventral to caudodorsal (red arrow) to make it parallel with the mandible. Center the beam in the middle of the hard palate.
- Collimate the FOV as small as practical to include the tip of the nose, the tip of the mandible, and the lateral soft tissues.

B. *Radiograph*

- Open mouth VD view of the maxilla.

A

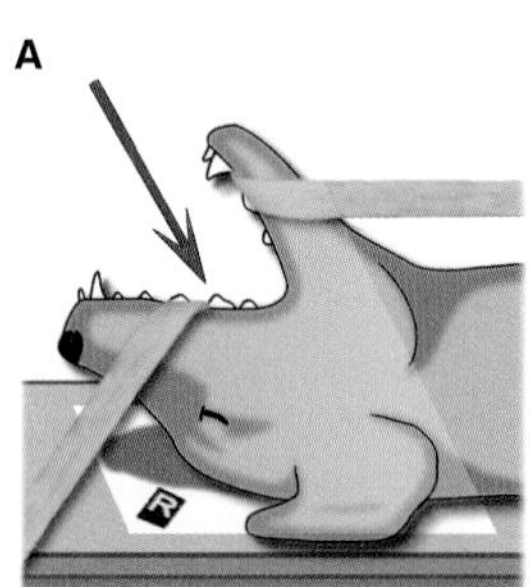

B

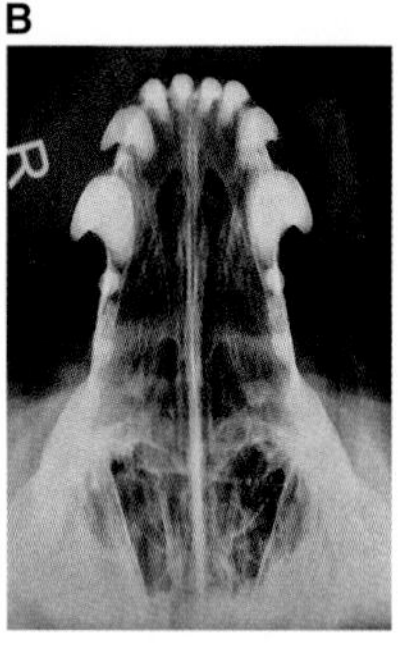

Figure 2.52 Head rostrocaudal view.

This is a supplemental radiograph of the head made in addition to the standard lateral and DV views. It is used to evaluate the frontal sinuses.

A and B. *Positioning*

- Patient is in dorsal recumbency.
- The head is flexed with the nose pointing up, toward the x-ray tube.
- Thickness of the head is measured from the medial canthus of the eye to the caudal part of the head.
- X-ray beam is centered on midline, just dorsal to the eyes and between the frontal sinuses (red arrow in **A**).
- Collimate the FOV as small as feasible to include the top of the head, the tip of the nose, and the width of skull.
- When properly positioned, the collimator light will project a shadow of the frontal sinuses as two humps above the head (arrows point to the two humps in **B**). The nose may need to be tipped about 10° dorsally, depending on the patient conformation.

C. *Radiograph*

- Rostrocaudal view of the head, tightly collimated to the frontal sinuses. This view sometimes called a "frog-eye" view.

A

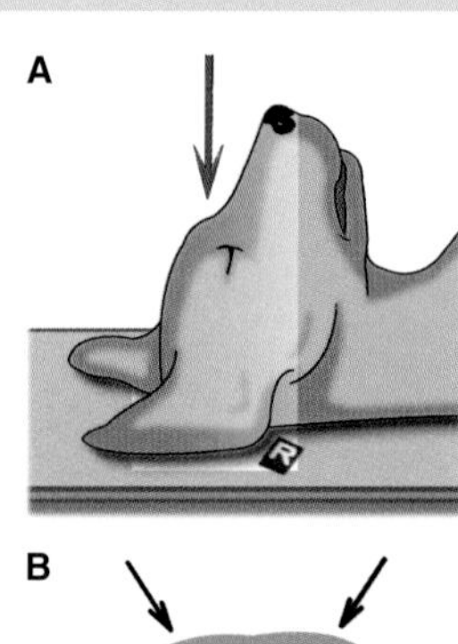

B

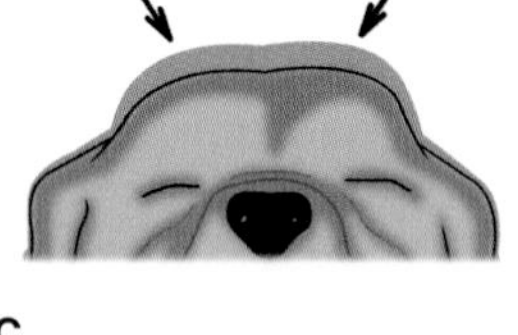

C

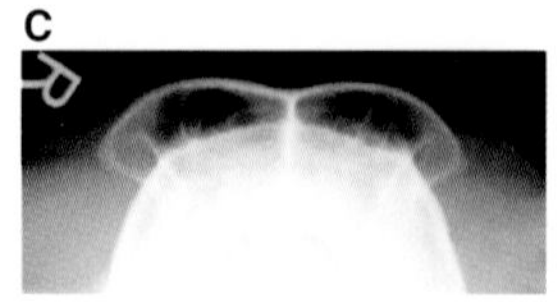

NOTES:

Figure 2.53 Head rostrocaudal flexed view.

This is a supplemental radiograph of the head made in addition to the standard lateral and DV views. It is used to evaluate the foramen magnum.

A. *Positioning*

- Patient is in dorsal recumbency.
- The head is flexed with nose tipped toward the sternum, about 20° past vertical.
- Thickness of the head is measured from the medial canthus of the eye to the caudal part of the head.
- X-ray beam is centered between the eyes (red arrow).
- Collimate the FOV as small as feasible to include the top of the head, the tip of the nose, and the width of the skull.
- Increase the x-ray exposure by doubling the mAs (or increase kVp 20%) to better penetrate the skull and visualize the foramen magnum.

B. *Radiograph*

- Rostrocaudal flexed view of the head. The arrow points to the foramen magnum.

A

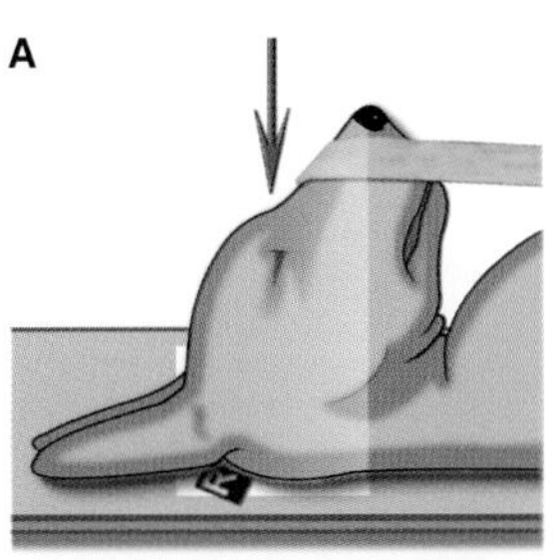

B

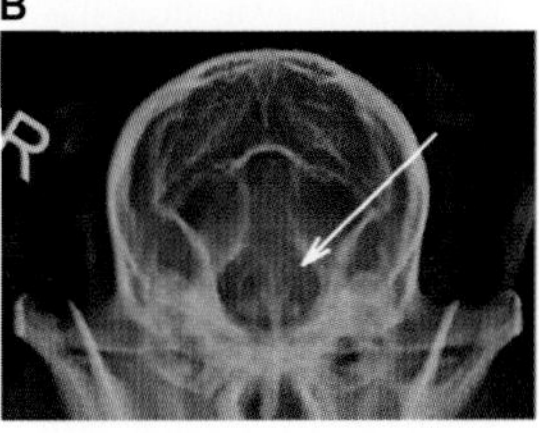

Figure 2.54 Feline head extended rostrocaudal view.

This is a supplemental radiograph of the feline head made in addition to the standard lateral and DV views. It is used to evaluate the tympanic bullae in cats. This view is also called a VD 10° dorsal oblique view of the head.

A. *Positioning*

- Cat is in dorsal recumbency with the mouth closed and the nose pointing up, toward the x-ray tube. The nose is tilted dorsally about 10° off vertical (dotted arrow).
- Thickness of the head is measured from the corner of the mouth to the caudal part of the head.
- X-ray beam is centered on midline at the level of the ears (red arrow) and directed so that it passes between the tympanic bullae.
- Collimate the FOV as small as feasible to include the tip of the nose, the first cervical vertebra, and the width of the skull.

B. *Radiograph*

- Extended rostrocaudal view of the feline head. The arrows point to the tympanic bullae. The endotracheal is visible between the bullae as a thin white line.

A

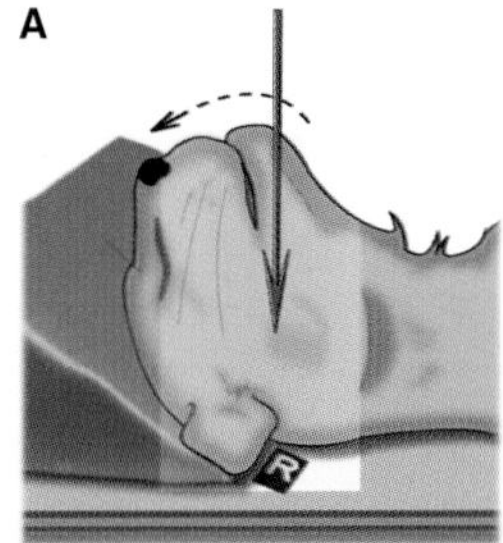

B

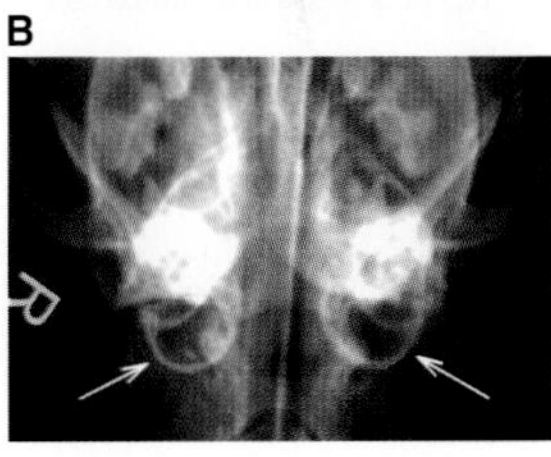

NOTES:

Figure 2.55 Head open-mouth rostrocaudal view.

This supplemental radiograph of the head is made in addition to the standard lateral and DV views. It is used to evaluate the odontoid process and canine tympanic bullae.

A, B, and C. *Positioning*

- Patient is in dorsal recumbency with the nose pointed up, toward the x-ray tube.
- Open the mouth and move the tongue and endotracheal tube away from the area of interest. The mouth may be held open using gauze or tape (as shown in A and B) or an oral speculum or other device positioned away from the area of interest.
  - **A:** to image the odontoid process (dens), tilt the nose dorsally about 45° past vertical (curved arrow).
  - **B:** to image the tympanic bullae, tilt the nose about 20° past vertical.
  - **C:** when the head is in the correct position, the collimator light projects the shadows of the nose and the two frontal sinuses as 3 humps of equal height (sometimes described as the "sun setting between two mountains").
- Thickness of the head is measured from the medial canthus of the eye to the caudal part of the head.
- X-ray beam is centered in the middle of the mouth, directed at the uvula (red arrows in **A** and **B**).
- Collimate the FOV as small as feasible to include the area of interest.

D and E. *Radiographs*

- **D:** open-mouth 45° rostrocaudal view of the head. The arrow points to the dens.
- **E:** open-mouth 20° rostrocaudal view, tightly collimated to the tympanic bullae (arrows).

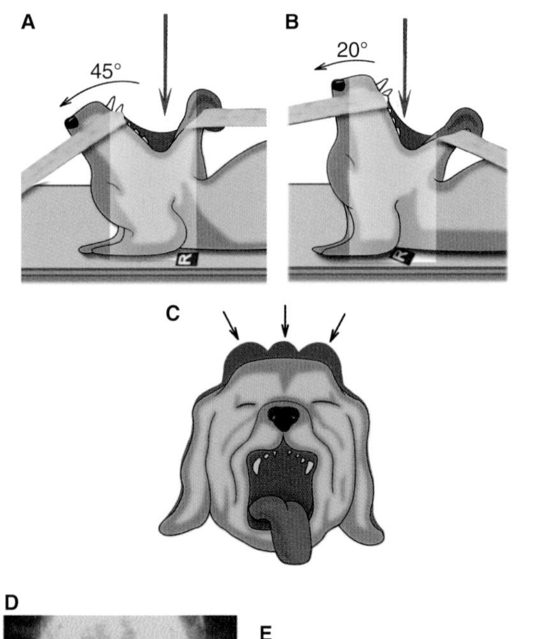

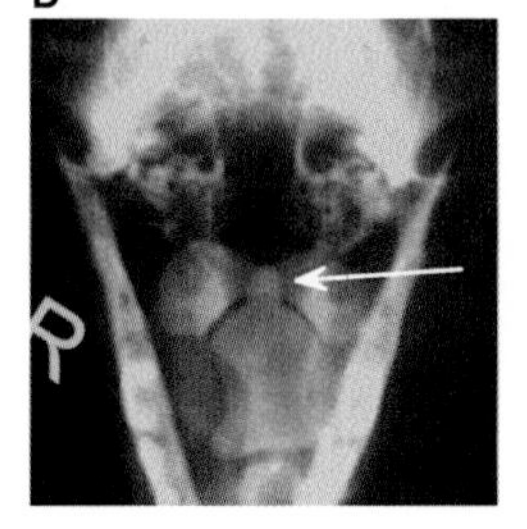

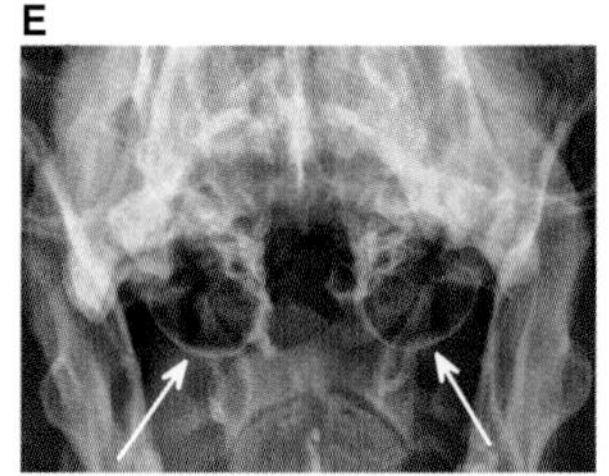

Figure 2.56 Intra-oral view of the maxilla.

This supplemental radiograph of the head is made in addition to the standard lateral and DV views.

A. *Positioning*

- Patient is in ventral (sternal) recumbency.
- The image receptor is placed inside the patient's mouth. Insert the receptor corner first to image the caudal part of the maxilla.
- Thickness of the maxilla is measured from the medial canthus of the eye to the hard palate.
- X-ray beam is centered on midline, halfway between the eyes and the to reduce superimposition of the frontal bones and image the more caudal aspect of the maxilla, angle the beam 20° rostrodorsal-to-caudoventral (dashed arrow).
- Collimate the FOV as small as feasible to include all of the maxilla that will fit on the image receptor.

B. *Radiograph*

- Intraoral view of the rostral maxilla and nasal cavities.

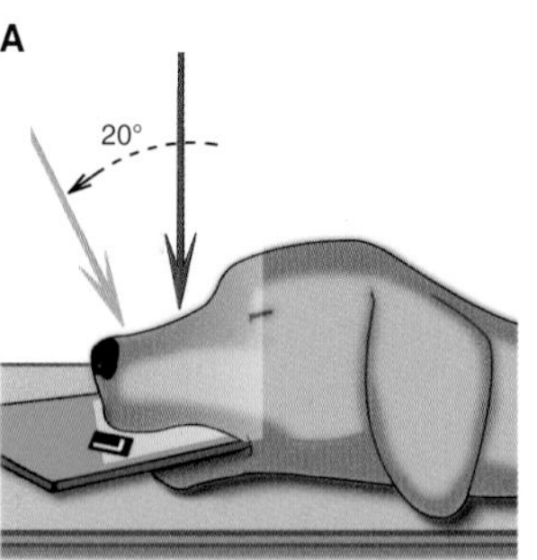

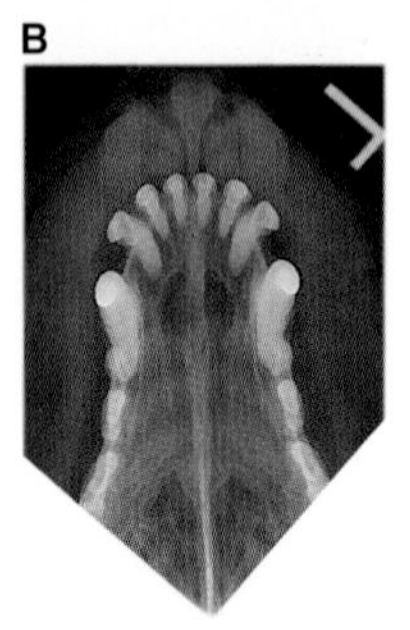

Figure 2.57 Intra-oral view of the mandible.

This supplemental radiograph of the head is made in addition to the standard lateral and DV views.

A. *Positioning*

- Patient is in dorsal recumbency.
- The image receptor is placed inside the patient's mouth; insert the corner of the receptor first to image the more caudal mandible.
- Measure the thickness of the mandible from the corner of the mouth to the ventral border of the mandible.
- X-ray beam is centered on midline, in the middle of the mandible. Angle the beam about 20° rostroventral-to-caudodorsal to better visualize the rostral mandible (red arrow).
- Collimate the FOV as small as feasible to include as much of the mandible as will fit on the image receptor.

B. *Radiograph*

- Intraoral view of the rostral mandible.

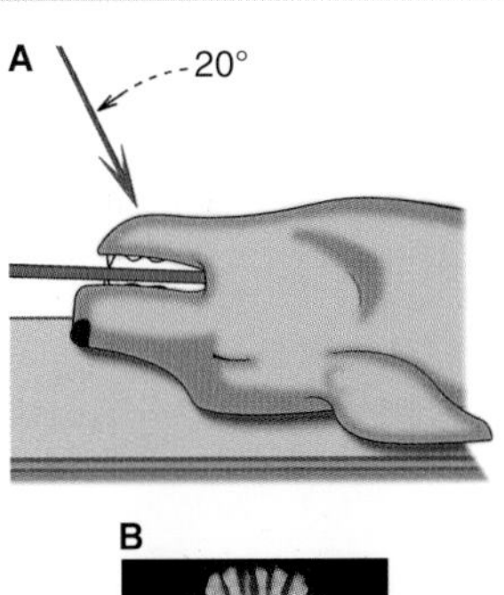

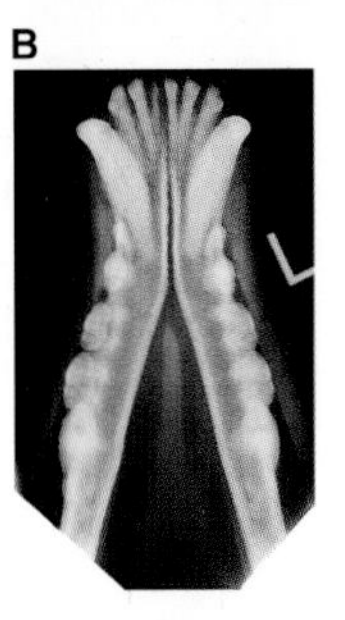

Figure 2.58 Head lateral oblique view for temporomandibular joint (TMJ).

This supplemental radiograph of the head is made in addition to the standard the lateral and DV views.

A, B, and C. *Positioning*

- Patient is in right or left lateral recumbency.
- The patient's head and neck are extended with the head resting on a foam block or towel and the nose tilted as needed.
- **A** and **B:** to image a TMJ with minimal distortion, position it closest to the image receptor and tilt the patient's nose up, toward the x-ray tube. In dogs, tilt the nose up about 20°. In cats, tilt it up about 10°. As can be seen in B, the x-ray beam (arrow) is well-aligned with the "down" TMJ. The "up" TMJ will be less visible in the radiograph.
- **C:** to magnify a TMJ, position it up, closest to the x-ray tube, and tilt the patient's nose downward. The x-ray beam (arrow) will align with the "up" TMJ. Tilting the nose downward to image a TMJ is not recommended in cats because there will be too much distortion in the radiograph.
- Thickness of the head is measured at the level of the eyes.
- X-ray beam is centered on the TMJ, about the middle of the masseter muscle (arrows in **A**, **B**, and **C**).
- Collimate the FOV as small as feasible to include the TMJ (the smaller the FOV, the better the radiographic detail).

D. *Radiograph*

- Lateral oblique view of the head. The white arrow points to the dependent (down) TMJ, which was well-aligned with the x-ray beam. The black arrow points to the "up" TMJ which was not aligned with the x-ray beam and is indistinct in the radiograph. In cats, the down TMJ often is more ventral in position than in dogs.

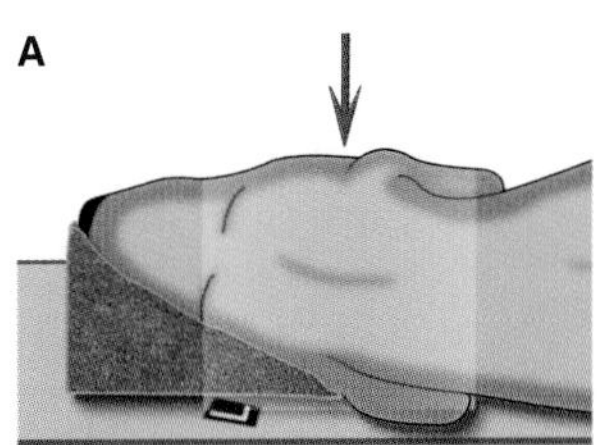

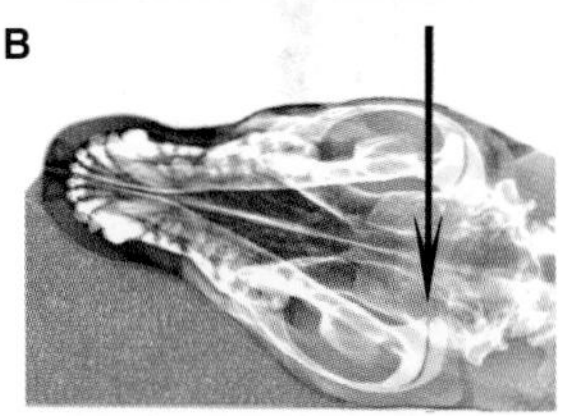

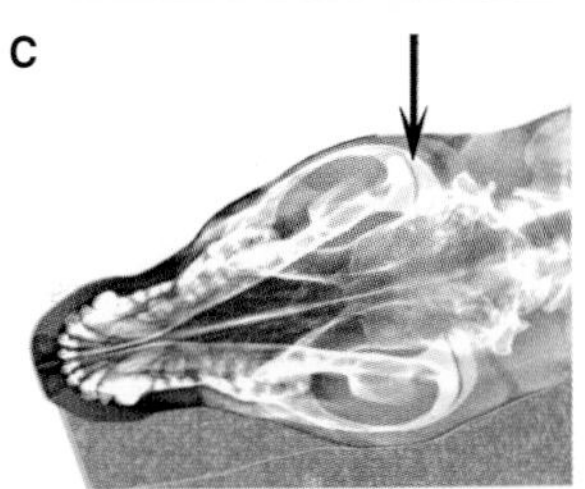

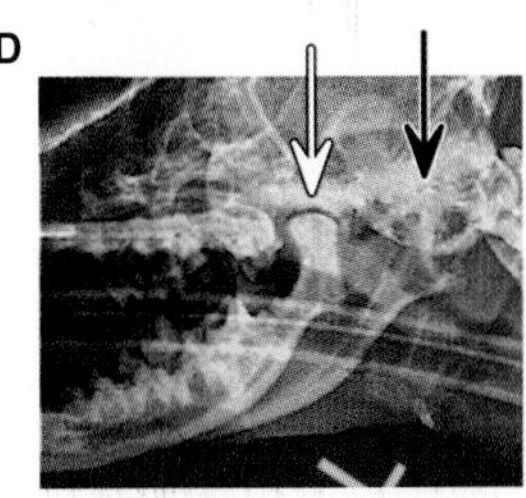

Figure 2.59 Bisecting angle view of tooth.

This supplemental radiograph of the head is made in addition to the standard lateral and DV views. It is used when a parallel view of the tooth is not possible.

A, B, and C. *Positioning*

- Patient is in ventral (**A**) or dorsal (**B**) recumbency with its mouth open.
- Place the image receptor (IR) inside the patient's mouth, as close to the tooth as possible.
- The bisecting line (B-line) is an imaginary line that equally divides (bisects) the angle between the long axis of the tooth (white dashed line) and the plane of the image receptor.
- Make the x-ray beam (red arrow) perpendicular to the B-line and center it on the tooth.
- Collimate the FOV as small as feasible to include the entire tooth.

D. *Radiograph*

- Bisecting angle view of a mandibular canine tooth, tightly collimated to maximize radiographic detail.

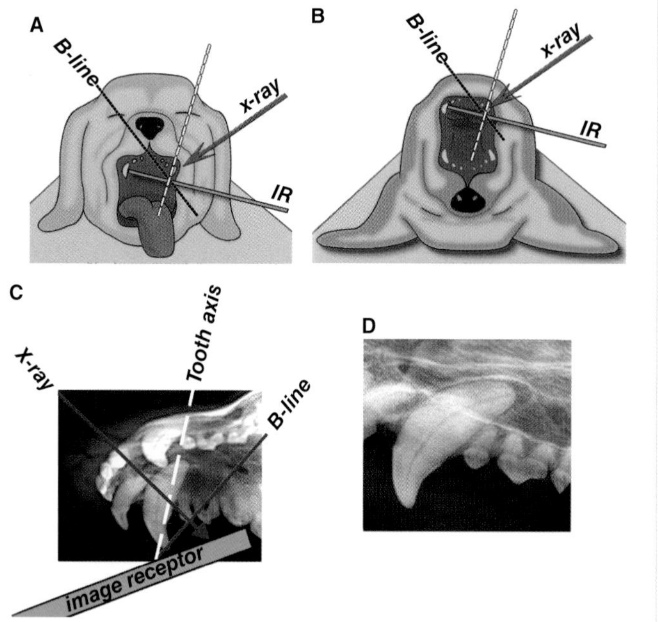

Figure 2.60 Spine positioning.

- **A:** without support, the cervical and lumbar regions of the spinal column normally sag while the patient is in lateral recumbency. Poor positioning of the spine can easily mimic or mask vertebral and intervertebral abnormalities.
- **B:** Small rolled towels (shown in the illustration), foam wedges, or similar low opacity materials placed under the patient's nose, neck, and mid-lumbar spine will help support the sagging areas and improve the alignment of the vertebrae.

A

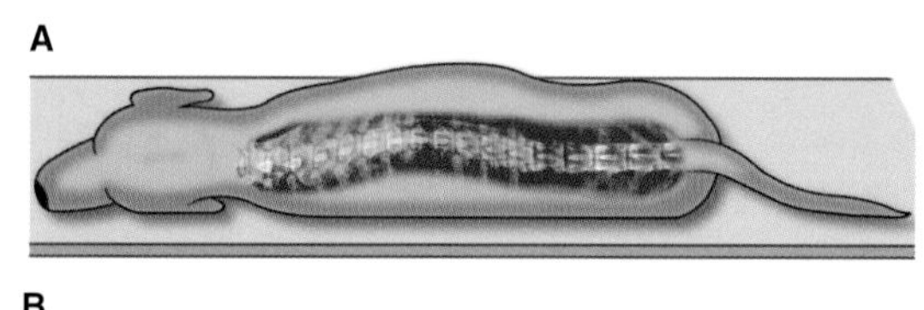

B

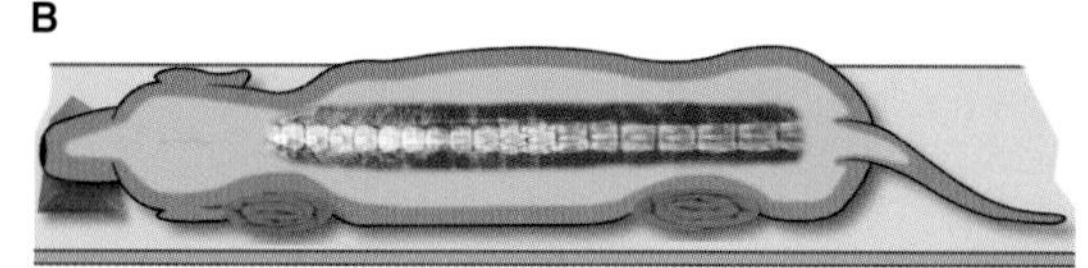

Figure 2.61 Cervical spine lateral view.

A. *Positioning*

- Patient is in lateral recumbency.
- The head and neck are extended. A sandbag may be used to maintain the position of
the head.
- A foam wedge or small towel under the neck eliminates sagging of the spine (Figure 2.60).
- Move the thoracic limbs <u>caudally</u> to eliminate superimposition.
- Thickness of the cervical spine is measured at the thoracic inlet.
- X-ray beam is centered on C3–4.
- Collimate the FOV as small as feasible to include the base of the skull and the first 2–3 thoracic vertebrae.

B. *Radiograph*

- Lateral view of the cervical spine.

A

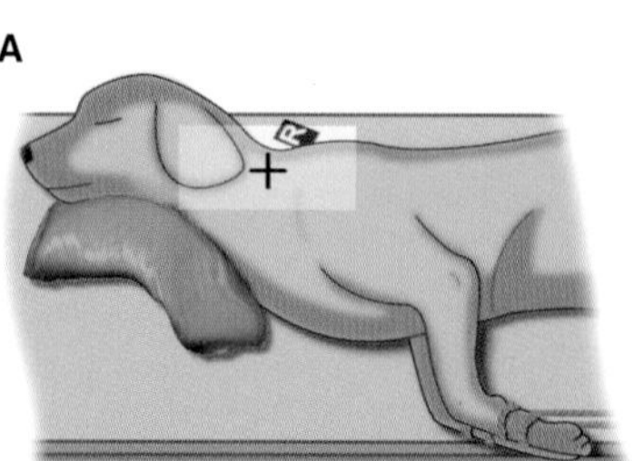

B

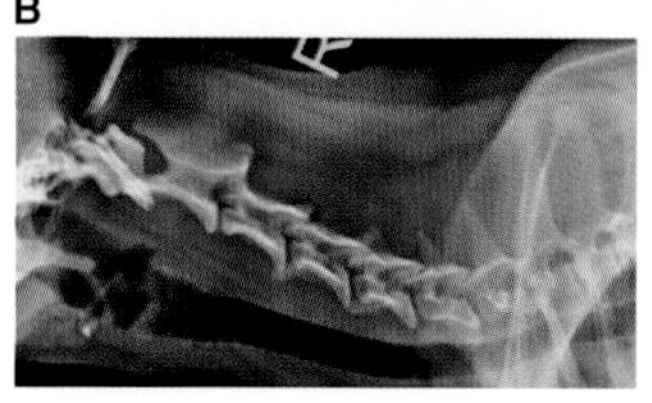

Figure 2.62 Cervical spine ventrodorsal (VD) view.

A and B. *Positioning*

- Patient is in dorsal recumbency with the head and neck extended.
- The thoracic limbs are pulled caudally.
- Thickness of the cervical spine is measured across the thoracic inlet.
- X-ray beam is centered on C3–4 (+).
- **B:** to enhance visualization of the intervertebral disc spaces, angle the x-ray beam about 20° caudoventral-to-craniodorsal.
- Collimate the FOV as narrow as feasible to include the width of the cervical spine, from the base of the skull to the first 2–3 thoracic vertebrae.

C. *Radiograph*

- Ventrodorsal (VD) view of the cervical spine.

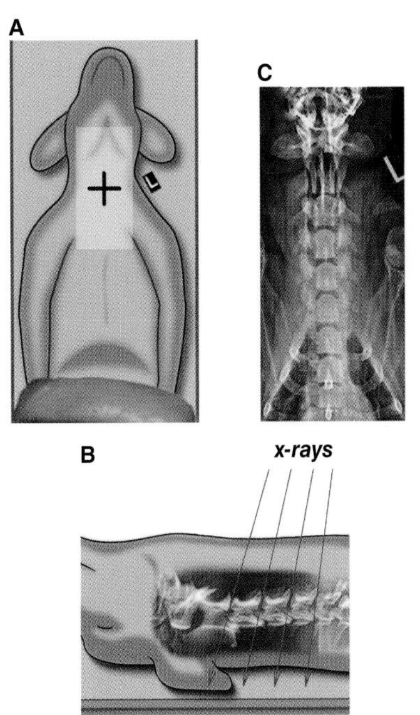

Figure 2.63 Thoracic spine lateral view.

A. *Positioning*

- Patient is in lateral recumbency.
- Sternum and spine are aligned in the same horizontal plane and parallel with the image receptor. Place a foam wedge or towel under the sternum to correct rotation.
- Slightly flex the pelvis to help straighten the thoracic spine.
- Measure the thickest part of thorax, typically over the liver.
- X-ray beam is centered on T5–7 (+).
- Collimate the FOV as narrow as feasible to include the width of the thoracic spine from the last 2–3 cervical vertebrae to the first 2–3 lumbar vertebrae.

B. *Radiograph*

- Lateral view of the thoracic spine.

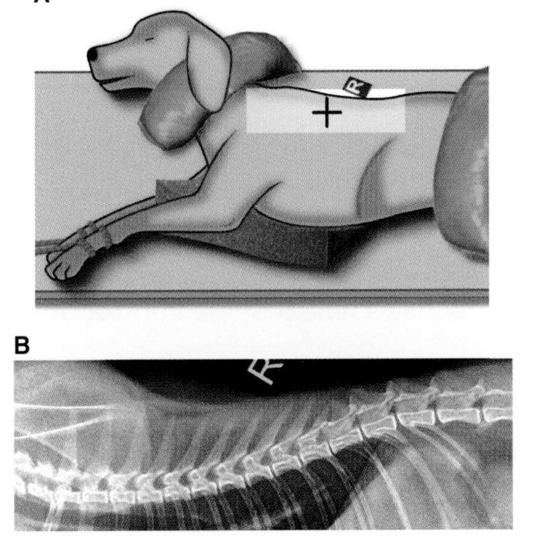

NOTES:

Figure 2.64 Thoracic spine ventrodorsal (VD) view.

A. ***Positioning***
- Patient is in dorsal recumbency with the thoracic limbs extended.
- Spine and sternum are straight and superimposed in the same vertical plane, perpendicular to the image receptor.
- Measure the thickest part of the thorax, usually over the liver.
- X-ray beam is centered on T5–7 (+).
- Collimate the FOV as narrow as feasible to include the width of the thoracic spine from the last 2–3 cervical vertebrae to the first 2–3 lumbar vertebrae.

B. ***Radiograph***
- Ventrodorsal (VD) view of the thoracic spine.

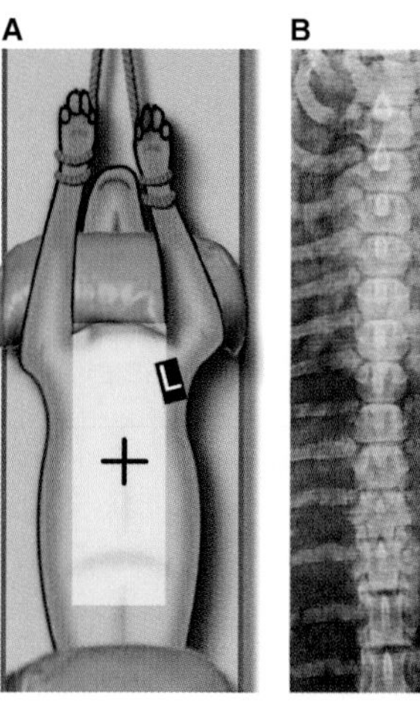

Figure 2.65 Lumbar spine lateral view.

A. ***Positioning***
- Patient is in lateral recumbency.
- Place foam wedges or towels between the stifles and under the sternum to correct rotation (Figures 2.35 and 2.59) and under the lumbar region to eliminate sagging of the spine (Figure 2.60).
- Measure the thickest part of the abdomen, usually over the liver.
- X-ray beam is centered on L3–4 (+).
- Collimate the FOV as narrow as practical to include the width of the lumbar spine from the last 2–3 thoracic vertebrae to the end of the sacrum.

B. ***Radiograph***
- Lateral view of the lumbar spine of a cat.

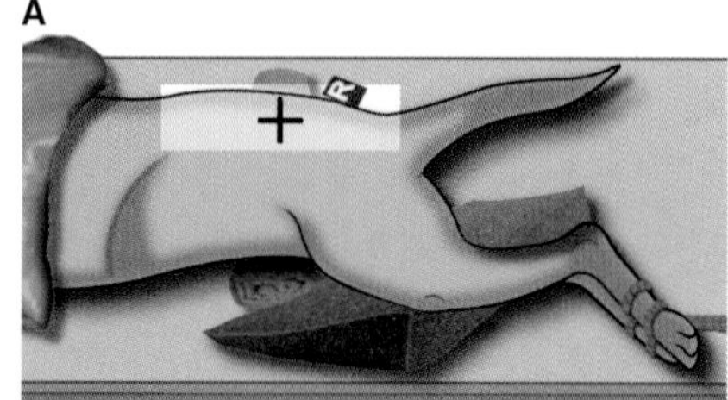

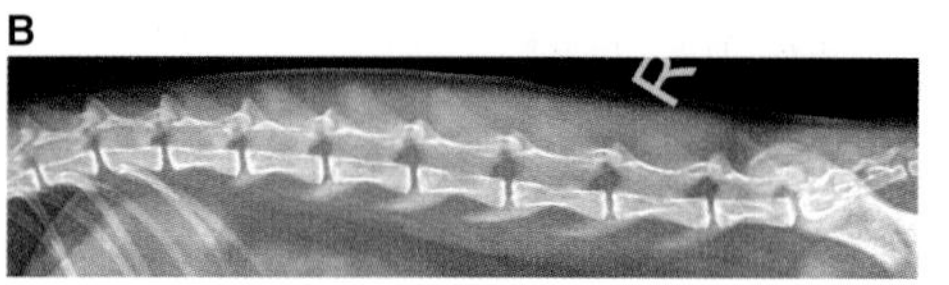

Figure 2.66 Lumbar spine ventrodorsal (VD) view.

A. ***Positioning***
- Patient is in dorsal recumbency with the pelvic limbs extended.
- Spine and sternum are straight and superimposed in the same vertical plane, perpendicular to the image receptor.
- Both ilial wings should be equal distance from table top. The right and left vertebral transverse processes should be equal distance from the table top.
- Measure the thickest part of the abdomen, usually over the liver.
- X-ray beam is centered on L3–4 (+).
- Collimate the FOV as narrow as practical to include the width of the lumbar spine from the last 2–3 thoracic vertebrae to the end of the sacrum.

B. ***Radiograph***
- Ventrodorsal (VD) view of the lumbar spine.

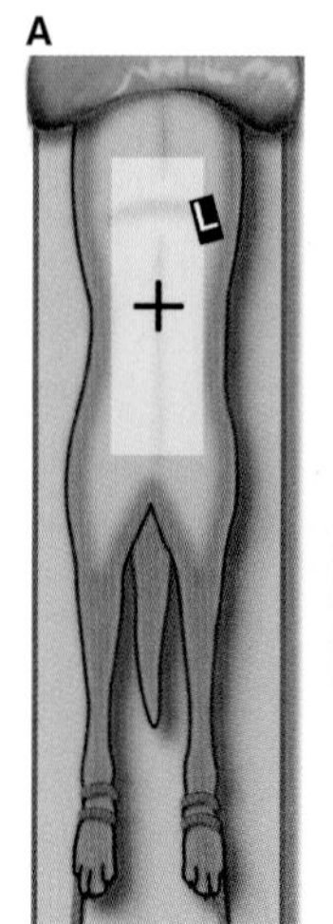

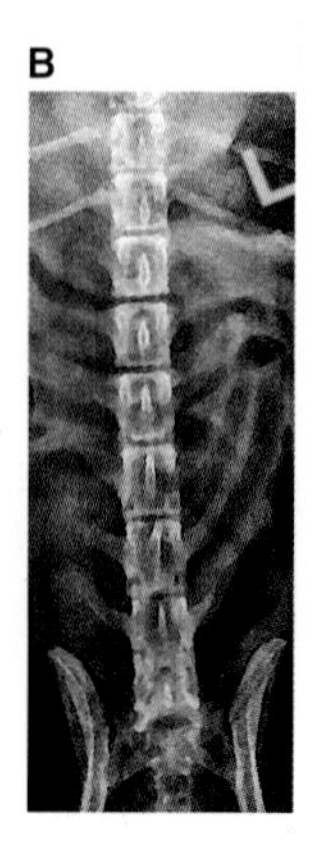

Artifacts

An artifact is something seen in a radiograph that is not present in the patient. It is a variation between the *image* of the patient and the *reality* of the patient.

Artifacts can vary greatly in appearance, but they mostly cause abnormal darkening or lightening in part or all of the radiograph. Dark artifacts may be called *plus density* artifacts because they increase radiographic density. Light artifacts may be called *minus density* artifacts.

Artifacts can degrade radiograph quality and mimic or mask abnormalities. It is important to understand the conditions under which artifacts occur so you can take steps to prevent them and recognize their presence when interpreting radiographs.

Film radiography artifacts most often occur in the darkroom or in the cassette. They are more common with manual processing than with automatic processors. Most film artifacts are permanent and cannot be removed. If the artifact is severe enough, the radiograph must be repeated to correct the problem.

Dark or plus density film artifacts result from conditions that alter the silver halide crystals prior to finished processing. Essentially, they overexpose part or all of the radiograph. Light or minus density film artifacts result from conditions that prevent exposure, interfere with development, or remove emulsion from the film.

Digital radiography has reduced the occurrence of many film artifacts because digital systems are much more tolerant of errors in exposure. However, digital radiography has not eliminated artifacts. Technical errors still occur, including malpositioning, motion, double exposures, and various computer-related problems. Many of these are discussed in the following pages.

Motion artifacts are a frequent and major cause of poor detail in both film and digital radiography. They usually result from voluntary or involuntary movements by the patient during x-ray exposure. Sometimes they are due to movement of the x-ray tube or image receptor caused by loose equipment or inadvertently bumping into the equipment.

Dark or plus density artifacts

1. Causes in both film and digital radiography:
   - a. Overexposure or double exposure.
   - b. Scatter fog.
   - c. Negative Mach band.
2. Causes limited to film radiography:
   - a. Overdevelopment.
   - b. Light fog (e.g., light leak in darkroom, cassette, film storage container; static electricity).
   - c. Pressure fog (e.g., rough handling of film, improper storage of film).
   - d. Chemical fog (e.g., processing solutions, cleaning agents).
   - e. Age fog (expired film).
   - f. Dirt or stain on the viewbox that causes uneven lighting behind the film.
3. Causes limited to digital radiography:
   - a. Processing error (LUT error).
   - b. Calibration error.
   - c. Halo artifact (*überschwinger* artifact).

Light or minus density artifacts

1. Causes in both film and digital radiography:
   - a. Underexposure.
   - b. Grid lines.
   - c. Superimposition of objects outside the patient:
     1) Collar, harness
     2) ID/vaccination tags.
     3) Wet/dirty hair coat.
     4) Skin nodules, masses, defects.
     5) ECG leads.
     6) Tissue drains.
     7) Blanket/sweater.
     8) Bandaging or casting material.
     9) Stretcher.
     10) Positioning devices (e.g., sandbags).
   - d. Objects inside the patient:
     1) Microchip.
     2) Foreign objects (e.g., metal projectiles).
     3) Sutures.
     4) Implants.
   - e. Debris in or on the cassette (e.g., dust, hair, contrast agent).
   - f. Damaged image receptor.
   - g. Positive Mach band.
2. Causes limited to film radiography:
   - a. Underdevelopment.
   - b. Film exposed to fixer before developer.
   - c. Film not in contact with developer (e.g., air bubbles on film, film stuck to side of tank).
   - d. Contaminated developer with fixer.
3. Causes limited to digital radiography:
   - a. Processing error (LUT error).
   - b. Calibration error.
   - c. Dead pixels.

Figure A1. Artifacts

Appearances:

- Abnormal blackening or whitening in part or all of a radiograph.
- Artifacts can present in a variety of shapes, sizes, patterns, and densities.
- Artifacts may be focal, multifocal, or diffuse.
- Figure A1 is an example of a good-quality film radiograph that can be used for comparison with the various artifacts described and pictured below (Figures A2 through A38). NOTE: the radiographic images are enhanced to better illustrate the artifact being described.

Causes:

1. Image acquisition errors (e.g., motion, wrong exposure, scatter radiation).
2. Equipment errors (e.g., damaged or dirty image receptor, poor grid alignment, faulty data cable, poor calibration).
3. Image processing errors (e.g., darkroom problem, computer problem).

Remedies:

1. Understand the conditions that produce artifacts and take steps to prevent their occurrence.
2. Be aware of how artifacts look in radiographs. When artifacts are present, take them into account when interpreting the radiographs.

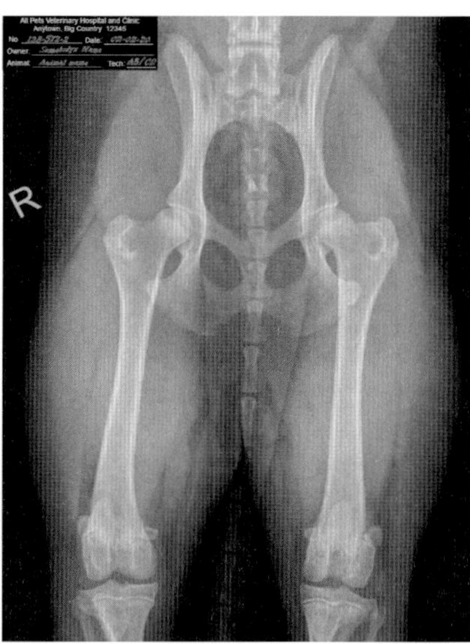

Figure A1 VD view of a dog pelvis. This is a good-quality radiograph that can be used as a comparison with the artifacts presented below. The pelvis is slightly rotated to the right and the pelvic limbs are slightly shifted to the right. Radiograph identification is photo-flashed into the upper left corner of the image.

Figure A2. Mottling (film and digital)

Other names:

1. Noise, quantum mottle, graininess.

Appearance:

1. Generalized grainy, sand-like or speckled pattern throughout the radiograph (Figure A2).

Causes:

1. Insufficient x-rays recorded by the film or digital image receptor due to either underexposure or low receptor sensitivity.
2. Film radiography: the larger the grain size (sizes of the silver crystals and phosphors), the more sensitive (faster speed) the film:screen system, and the more mottling in the images.
3. Digital radiography: low signal-to-noise ratio (low SNR).

Remedies:

1. Increase the x-ray exposure (double the mAs or increase kVp 20%).
2. Switch to a film:screen system with smaller grains (lower sensitivity).
3. Computer software may be available to increase the SNR.

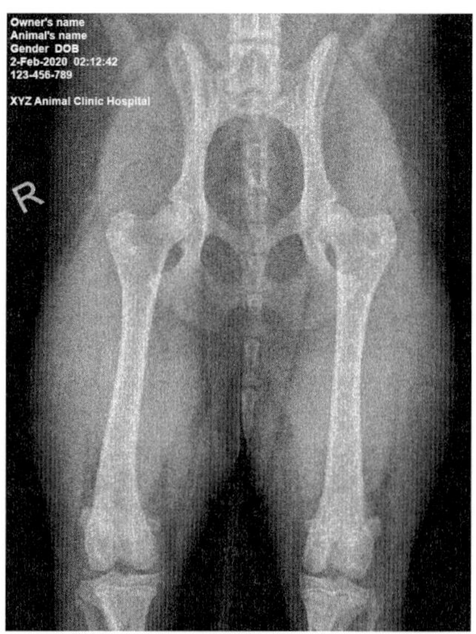

Figure A2 Quantum mottle.

Figure A3. Overexposure (film and digital)

Appearance:

1. The entire image is too dark; radiographic density overall is too high (Figure A3).
2. Film radiograph: if a photo-flash was used to label the radiograph, the area with the film ID will not be overexposed.
3. Digital radiography: clipping/saturation artifact usually is concurrent with overexposure (see Figure A23).

Causes:

1. Too many x-rays recorded by the image receptor due to:
   a. User input error (wrong exposure selected).
   b. SID too short.
   c. X-ray machine malfunction (i.e., surge in power supply).
2. If a film radiograph is all black (no visible image), it is more likely the film was completely exposed to light rather than too many x-rays.
3. Digital radiography: in addition to too many x-rays, a digital image that is too dark may result from using the wrong LUT to display pixel values which may be due to:
   a. User input error (i.e., wrong body part selected).
   b. Field-of-view (FOV) too large.
   c. Computer error.

Remedies:

1. Repeat the study with proper exposure and FOV as small as practical.
2. Film radiographs can be viewed with a high-intensity light source ("hot light") to enhance the image.
3. Digital radiographs: reprocess the raw data with the correct LUT.

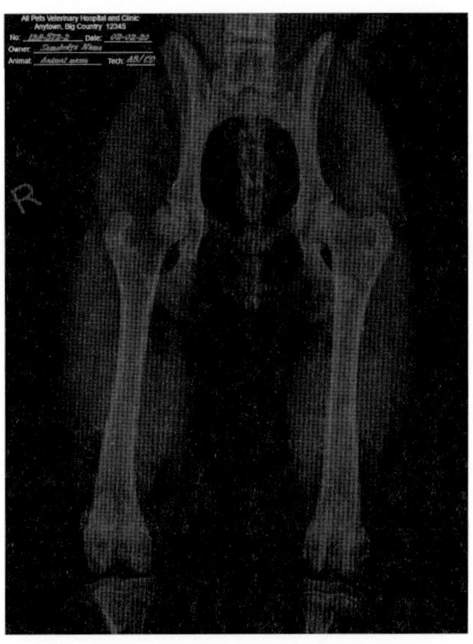

Figure A3 Overexposed film radiograph. Notice the identification label in the upper left corner is not overexposed because the ID was added via photo-flash after the x-ray exposure.

Figure A4. Overdevelopment (film)

Appearance:

1. The entire film is too dark; radiographic density overall is too high (Figure A4).
2. Area with photo-flash ID labeling also is too dark because all exposures, either from x-rays or photo-flash light, have been overdeveloped.

Cause:

1. Developer was too warm or too concentrated.
2. Film was immersed in developer for too long a time.
3. Localized dark areas in the film (spots of increased radiographic density) may result from developer splashed on the film prior to processing.

Remedies:

1. Maintain proper temperature and concentration of developer.
2. Pay attention to immersion times and thoroughly rinse film after development.
3. Make sure the automatic processor is functioning properly.

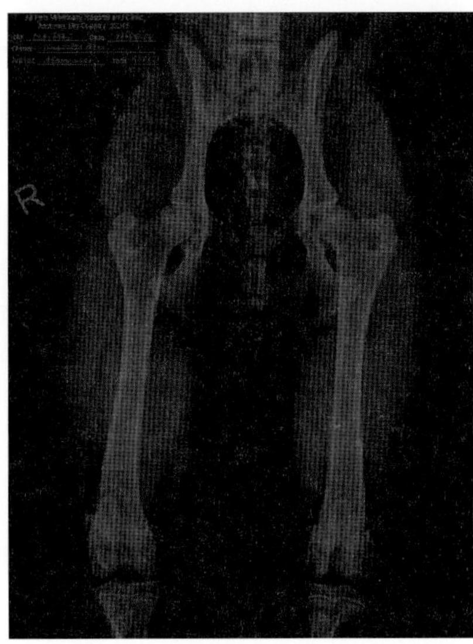

Figure A4 Overdeveloped film radiograph. The identification label in the upper left corner also is too dark because all exposed parts of the film are overdeveloped.

Figure A5. Underexposure (Film and Digital)

Appearance:

1. The entire image is too light; radiographic density overall is too low (Figure A5).
2. Film radiography: if photo-flash was used to label the radiograph, the area with the film ID will <u>not</u> be underexposed.
3. Digital radiography: quantum mottling usually is concurrent with underexposure due to low SNR (see Figure A2).

Causes:

1. Too few x-rays recorded by the film or digital image receptor due to:
   a. User input error (wrong exposure selected).
   b. Source-to-image distance (SID) too long.
   c. X-ray machine malfunction (e.g., drop in incoming line voltage).
2. Wrong film:screen combination (film type not matched to screen type).
   NOTE: If a film radiograph is completely clear (i.e., a transparent sheet with no visible image), it is likely the x-ray machine malfunctioned (no exposure was made) or the film was placed in fixer before developer.
3. Digital radiography: in addition to too few x-rays, a digital image that is too light may result from using the wrong LUT used to display pixel values, either due to user input error (wrong body part selected) or computer error.

Remedies:

1. Repeat the study with proper exposure.
2. Digital radiography: reprocess the raw data with the correct LUT.

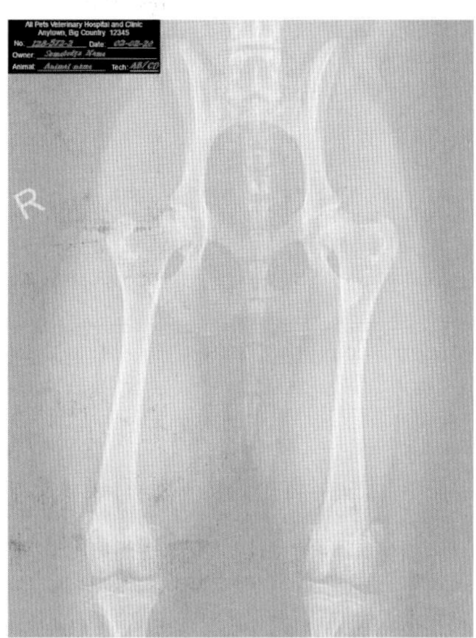

Figure A5 <u>Underexposed film radiograph</u>. Notice the area with the identification label is not underexposed because the ID was added via photo-flash after x-ray exposure.

Figure A6. Underdevelopment (film)

Appearance:

1. The entire film is too light; radiographic density overall is too low (Figure A6).
2. Area with photo-flash ID labeling also is too light because all exposures, whether from x-rays or photo-flash light, have been underdeveloped.

Cause:

1. Developer was too cold or too weak (exhausted chemicals).
2. Film was immersed in developer for insufficient length of time.

Remedies:

1. Maintain proper temperature and concentration of developer.
2. Pay attention to immersion times.
3. Make sure automatic processor is functioning properly.

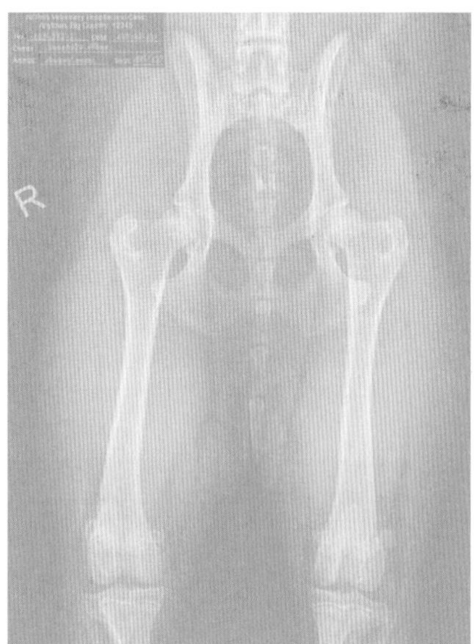

Figure A6 <u>Underdeveloped film radiograph</u>. The area with the identification label also is too light.

Figure A7. Uneven development (film)

Appearance:

1. Non-uniform, mottled streaking in part or all of the film radiograph (Figure A7).
2. Ill-defined, patchy, lighter areas in the film (minus density artifacts).

Cause:

1. Uneven contact between the film and the developer chemicals due to insufficient mixing (stirring) of the developer solution.

Remedies:

1. Maintain proper temperatures and replenishment rates of processing chemicals.
2. Manual processing:
   a. Thoroughly mix solutions prior to each use.
   b. Agitate film for a few seconds after each immersion to evenly coat the film and remove air bubbles.
   c. Thoroughly rinse and dry each film prior to viewing and storage.

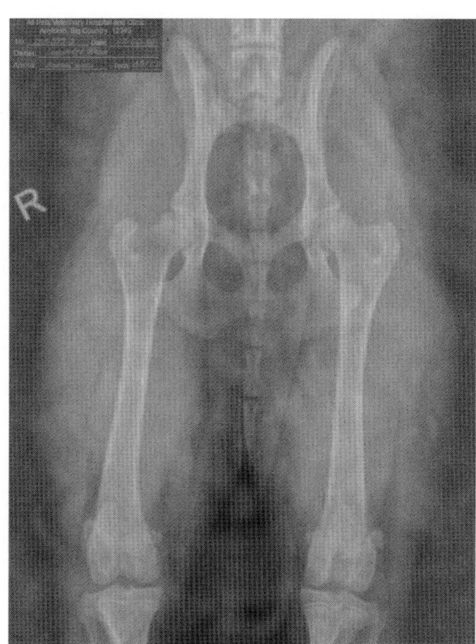

Figure A7 Uneven development. Film radiograph that was processed in developer that was insufficiently mixed.

Figure A8. Yellowish stains (film)

Appearance:

1. Cloudy, sticky residue on film with a sulfur smell.
2. Yellow-brown discoloration of film that commonly appears dichroic or multi-colored in reflected light (Figure A8).

Cause:

1. Dried fixer on the film due to insufficient rinsing.
2. Prolonged adherence of fixer will stain the film a yellowish-brown.

Remedies:

1. Thoroughly rinse and dry each film radiograph prior to viewing and storage.
2. If the film is not yet stained yellow, try rinsing it again or running it through the automatic processor again.

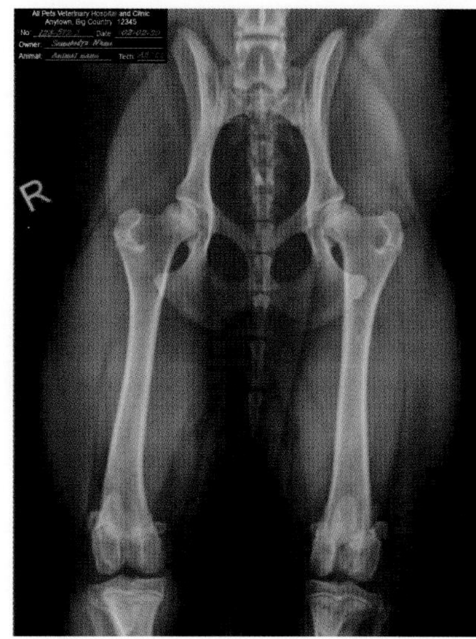

Figure A8 Yellow stains on film. Film radiograph stained by retained fixer.

CHAPTER 2

Figures A9–10. Fog (film and digital)

Appearance:

1. Hazy darkening or graying in the radiograph that reduces contrast and visible detail.
2. Fog can be diffuse throughout the entire image (Figure A9) or localized (Figure A10).

Causes:

1. Scatter radiation is a common cause and increases with:
   a. Thicker body part.
   b. Larger field-of-view (FOV).
   c. Higher kVp.
   d. No grid.
2. Scatter fog also can result from a previous exposure (e.g., the film or CR cassette was near the x-ray machine during an earlier radiographic study).

Causes unique to film radiography

1. Light fog: film was exposed to visible light prior to development:
   a. Light leak in darkroom, cassette, or storage area.
   b. Film not completely in processor before lights turned on.
   c. Film was exposed to light prior to finished development (e.g., darkroom door was opened).
   d. Safelight with wrong filter or too bright lightbulb.
   e. Static electricity (localized light fog, see Figure A22).
2. Pressure fog: film was exposed to excessive pressure prior to development:
   a. Rough handling of film (Figure A23).
   b. Improper storage of film (laying boxes of unused film flat instead of on-end results in the weight of the upper sheets, eventually fogging the lower sheets).
3. Heat fog: prolonged exposure of unused film to heat (temperature above 24 °C or 75 °F).
4. Chemical fog: exposure of unused film to chemicals (e.g., cleaning agents, hydrogen peroxide, formaldehyde).
5. Age fog: film is expired; over time, unused film will eventually undergo "self-development" and become fogged.

Remedies:

1. Repeat the study with less scatter radiation:
   a. Collimate the FOV as small as practical; this will have the greatest impact on reducing the amount of scatter fog.
   b. Use a grid whenever body part thickness exceeds 10 cm.
   c. Lower the kVp: decrease kVp 16% and double mAs; repeat as often as needed to achieve desired contrast.
2. Shield unused film and cassettes from scatter radiation.

Remedies unique to film radiography:

1. Correct any light leaks.
2. Perform a Safelight test (see Figure A11).
3. Ensure proper storage of unused x-ray film:
   a. Temperature: 10–24 °C (50–75 °F).
   b. Humidity: 30%–60%.
   c. Store boxes of unused film on-end instead of flat.
   d. No nearby chemicals.

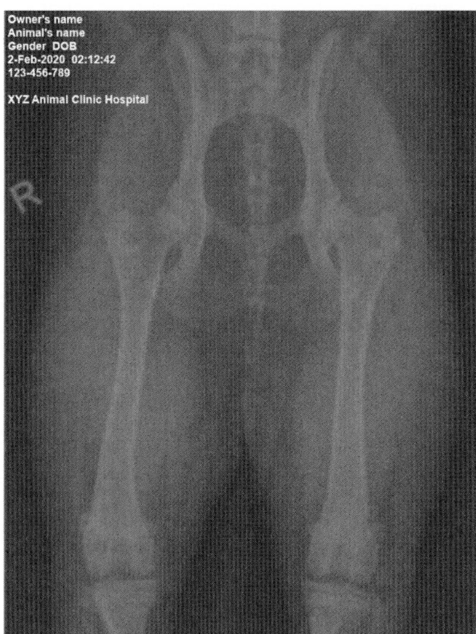

Figure A9 Diffuse scatter fog. Digital radiograph made without a grid.

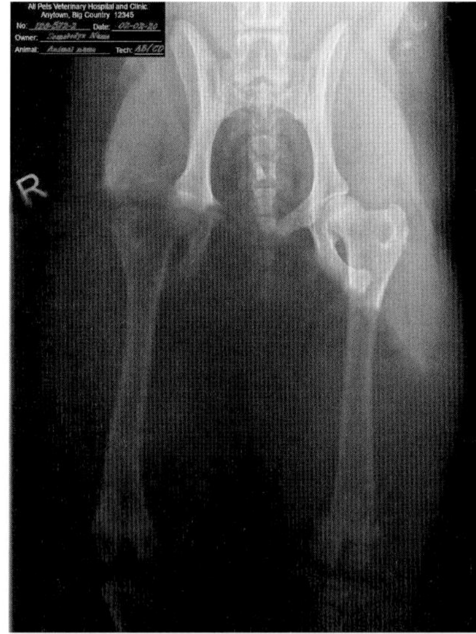

Figure A10 Localized light fog. Film radiograph that was exposed to light along the bottom and left side of the film.

Figure A11. Safelight test (film)

Do this test to evaluate the amount of light fog caused by your safelight:

1. Darkroom should be completely dark with the safelight turned off.
2. Place a piece of unexposed film on the countertop.
3. Cover half of the film with a piece of cardboard.
4. Turn on the safelight.
5. Leave the film exposed for 2 min.
6. Process the film.
7. The two halves of the film should be equal in density; if not, there is safelight fog (Figure A11).

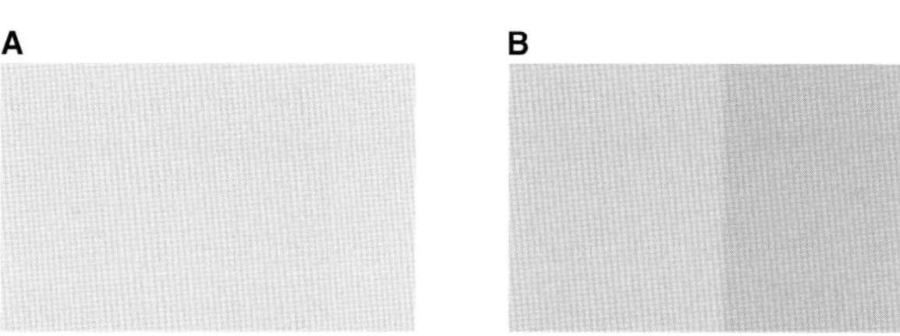

Figure A11 Safelight test. **A**. Passed: safelight does not produce significant light fog. **B**. Failed: the part of the film that was exposed to the safelight is darker than the covered part due to light fog. Fog may be due to either a wrong safelight filter or the safelight bulb is too bright (wattage too high).

Figure A12. Clipping artifact (digital)

Other names:

1. Saturation artifact; pixel burnout; pixel dropout.

Appearance:

1. There are black areas in the digital radiograph where tissues should be visible (Figure A12); the black areas cannot be brightened enough to restore missing information.
2. Usually occurs in the thinner, less opaque, or peripheral parts of the patient (e.g., extremities, lungs); more opaque tissues such as bone often are visible, but the soft tissues are lost.

Causes:

1. Overexposure: pixels are overwhelmed by too many x-rays and incapable of responding to windowing and leveling.
2. Computer processing error (e.g., LUT error, problem with contrast enhancement software).
3. Damaged or otherwise non-functional pixels.

Remedy:

1. Repeat the study with proper exposure and correct LUT settings.
2. If clipping artifact remains, image receptor may need to be repaired or replaced.

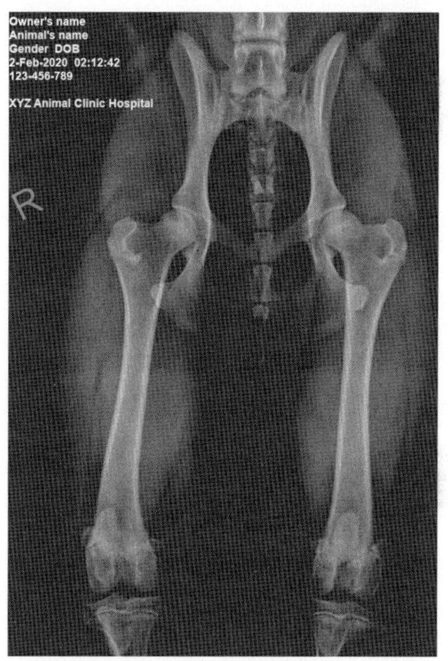

Figure A12 Clipping artifact in a digital radiograph.

NOTES:

Figures 13–14. LUT errors (digital)

Appearance:

1. Poor quality radiograph with incorrect levels of contrast, brightness, and/or detail (Figures A13 and A14).
2. Other artifacts may be concurrent (e.g., overexposure, underexposure, clipping).

Cause:

1. Computer used wrong look-up table (LUT) to display pixel values due to:
   a. User selected wrong body part, such as entering "thorax" for a pelvic radiograph (thorax typically is a low contrast study, so pelvic radiographs will be displayed with insufficient contrast, as depicted in Figure A13).
   b. Computer malfunction.

Remedies:

1. Re-process the raw data using appropriate LUT settings.
2. Repeat the study with correct LUT settings.

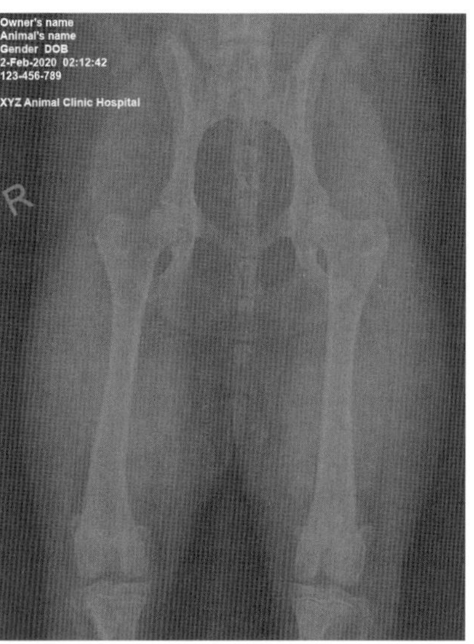

Figure A13 LUT error. Digital radiograph of dog pelvis with too low contrast and density due to LUT error (user selected "thorax" instead of "pelvis").

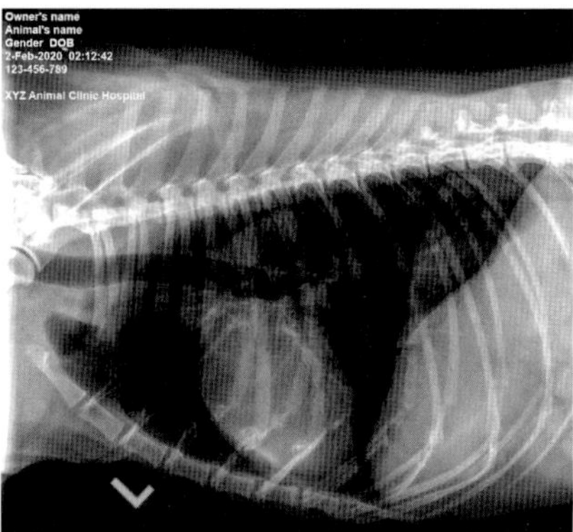

Figure A14 LUT error. Digital radiograph of dog thorax with too high contrast and density due to LUT error (user selected "pelvis" instead of "thorax").

Figure A15. Pixelated image (digital)

Appearance:

1. Digital radiograph appears grainy with poor detail (Figure A15).

Causes:

1. Pixel size is too large due to:
   a. Computer processing error.
   b. Excessive magnification by user.
   c. Low-quality monitor with insufficient resolution.

Remedies:

1. Adjust image processing algorithm.
2. View image with higher quality monitor

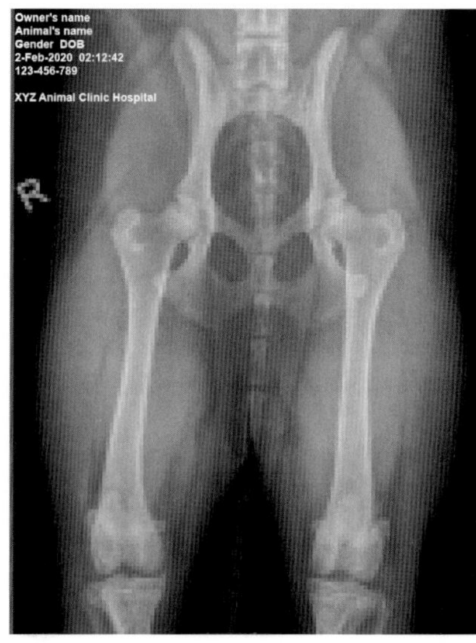

Figure A15 Pixelated. Digital radiograph displayed with large pixels, resulting in a grainy image with poor detail.

Figure A16. Planking artifact (digital)

Appearance:

1. Broad, dark bands across the entire radiograph (Figure A16).

Cause:

1. Overexposure; x-ray saturation of the digital image receptor reveals the plank-like arrangement of the receptor components.

Remedy:

1. Repeat the study with proper exposure.

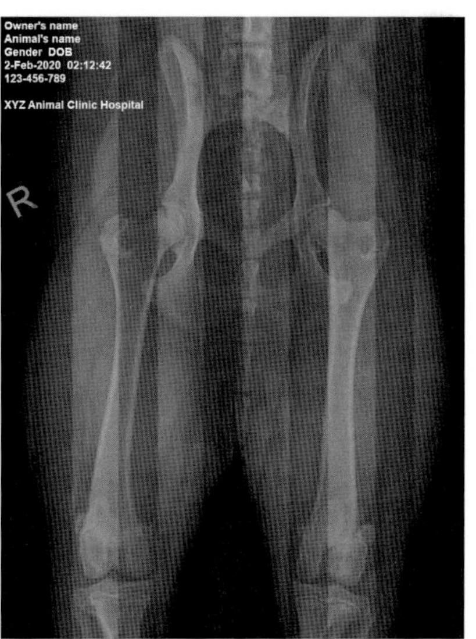

Figure A16 Planking artifact. Digital radiograph with dark bands due to overexposure.

Figures A17–18. Moiré pattern or Aliasing (digital)

Appearance:

1. A series of repeating dark and light lines that run across the entire digital radiograph (Figures A17 and A18); the thickness and orientation of the lines do not correspond to grid lines.
2. The term "moiré" describes a repeating wavy or rippled pattern in an image (it was originally used to describe the appearance of silk fabrics).

Causes:

1. Inadequate sampling of the x-ray data by the computer leads to distortion of the grid lines; a moiré pattern is more prevalent with low-frequency grids.
2. Faulty data cable (cable is damaged or loose).

Remedy:

1. If the artifact is severe enough, repeat the study.
2. Use a high-frequency grid.
3. Make sure the Bucky mechanism is functioning properly.
4. Increase the computer sampling rate.
5. Inspect and tighten the data cables.

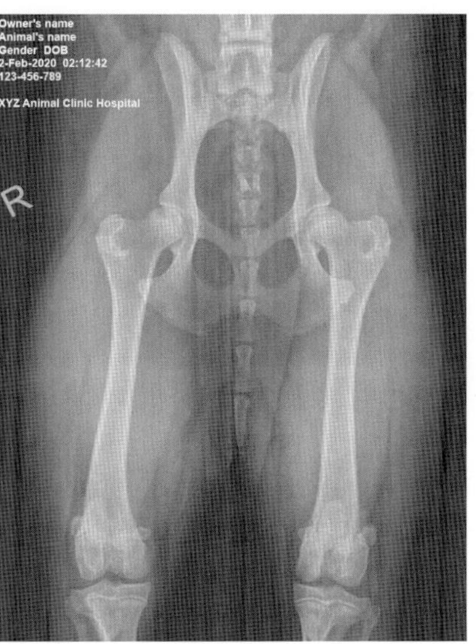

Figure A17 Moiré pattern. Digital radiograph with numerous repeating lines running vertically across the entire image due to computer error and insufficient sampling of grid lines.

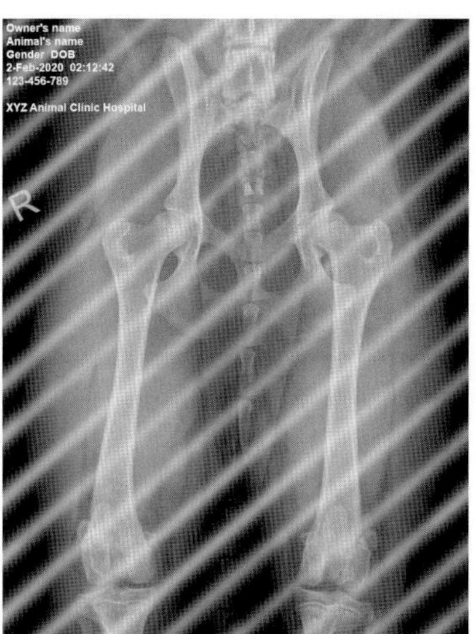

Figure A18 Moiré pattern. Digital radiograph with repeating lines due to a loose data cable.

Figure A19. Motion blur (film and digital)

Appearance:

1. Unsharp margins or a streak-like appearance associated with the edges and outlines of structures in the film or digital radiograph (Figure A19).

Causes:

1. Voluntarily or involuntarily movements by the patient (e.g., struggling, tachypnea) during x-ray exposure. Motion is a major cause of poor quality radiographs in veterinary radiology.
2. X-ray tube movement during exposure (e.g., loose equipment; equipment bumped by personnel or patient, hand holding the x-ray tube).

Remedies:

1. Repeat the study with proper patient restraint.
2. Use the shortest exposure time practical.
3. Secure all imaging equipment.

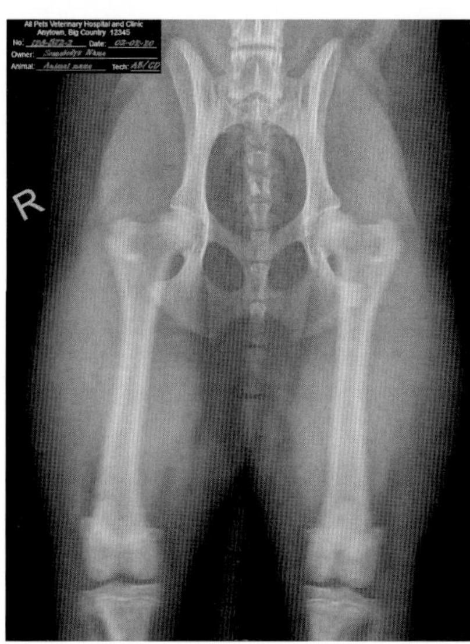

Figure A19 Motion blur. Radiograph with reduced detail in the pelvic limbs due to movement during exposure.

Figure A20. Double exposure (film and digital)

Appearance:

1. Two images of the same body part in one radiograph (Figure A20).
2. Margins usually are blurry (may resemble motion artifact).
3. Film: the image will be too dark (overexposed).
4. Digital: radiographic density often is the same as it would be with a single exposure because the computer performs an automatic correction.

Causes:

1. Two exposures were made of the same body part, one immediately following the other.
2. Patient moved during a long exposure time.

Remedy:

1. Repeat the study using a shorter exposure time and proper patient restraint.

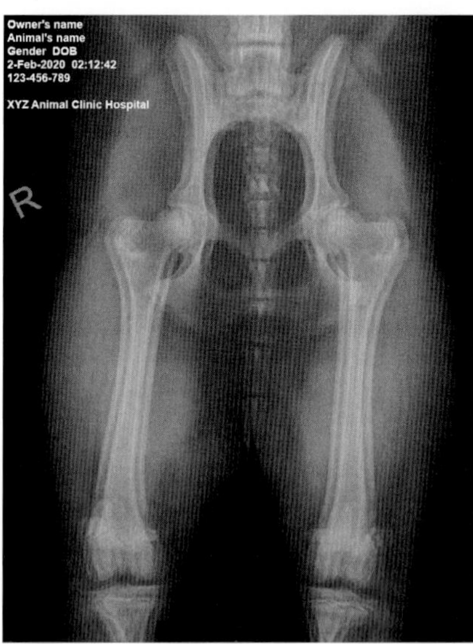

Figure A20 Double exposure in a digital radiograph.

NOTES:

Figure A21. Ghost image (film and digital)

Other names:
1. Phantom image; image lag; ghosting artifact.

Appearance:
1. Two images are visible in the same film or digital radiograph. Often it is the orthogonal view of the same body part, but sometimes a different body part is visible (Figure A21).

Cause:
1. Persistence of a latent image from a previous study.
2. Film radiography: a piece of film that was previously exposed, but not processed, was inadvertently used again (i.e., user forgot to change to a new cassette).
3. Digital radiography: image receptor was not completely erased (e.g., failure of erasure mechanism in CR reader) or was reused too quickly (receptor had not lost all of its charge from the previous exposure).

Remedy:
1. Repeat the study with unused film or a "clean" digital imaging plate.

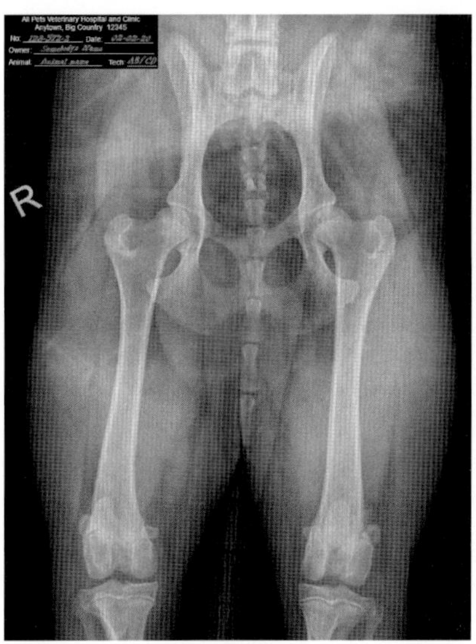

Figure A21 Ghost image. A lateral view of a thorax is faintly visible in this VD view of a pelvis.

Figure A22. Static electricity (film)

Appearances:
1. Localized black areas (plus density artifacts) that can present in a variety of patterns in a film radiograph (Figure A22). They may appear as:
   a. Irregular branching black lines that resemble "lightning" or "trees."
   b. Multiple, tiny black spots or smudges.
   c. Linear dark areas that are somewhat mottled and inhomogeneous.

Cause:
1. Static electricity exposes undeveloped film to visible light (i.e., static electricity is a type of light fog).
2. Static electricity can be generated by rapidly opening a film packet or it can be directly transferred from the user to the film.

Remedies:
1. If the artifact is severe enough, repeat the study.
2. Maintain relative humidity at 30%–60% in the radiology department.
3. Handle film gently, avoid friction, slowly unwrap film from its packaging.
4. Ground yourself before handling film.
5. Use an antistatic cleaner with film cassettes.

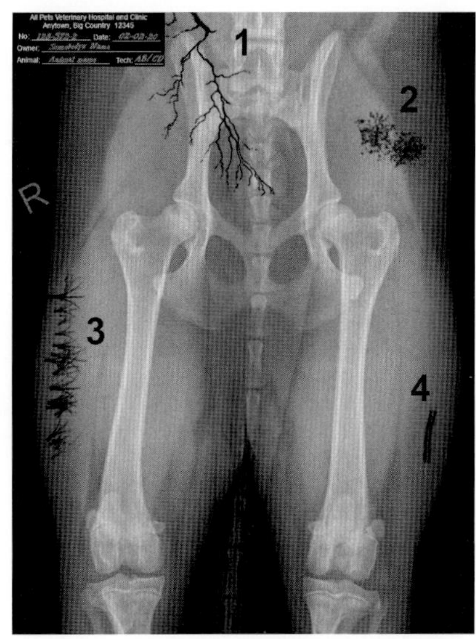

Figure A22 Static electricity artifacts. Film radiograph depicting light fog as a **1**. Lightning pattern. **2**. Multiple tiny spots and smudges. **3**. Tree-like branching. **4**. Linear pattern.

Figure A23. Rough handling of film

Appearances:

1. Localized plus density artifacts; dark or black spots, lines, or regions in a film radiograph (Figure A23). These artifacts are a type of pressure fog.
2. Crimping marks are common and appear as thin, crescent-shaped, dark lines in the radiograph (sometimes called "thumbnail" or "fingernail" marks).
3. Abrasion marks appear as fine black lines or dark hazy smudges.
4. Some of the dark patterns may resemble fingerprints.

Causes:

1. Bending, flexing, or creasing the film prior to development creates crimping marks due to pressure (Figure A23 **B**). Note that these artifacts are <u>not</u> made by "digging" a thumbnail into the film as the name "thumbnail artifact" might suggest.
2. Pushing or sliding undeveloped film across the darkroom table or countertop causes abrasion damage and pressure fog.
3. Touching undeveloped film with dirty or contaminated fingers (e.g., developer on fingers) can create a fingerprint pattern in the developed film. (Note: white fingerprints in a film radiograph may be caused by transferring fixer to the undeveloped film or by leaving skin oil on the film that blocks contact with the developer.)

Remedy:

1. If the artifact is severe enough, repeat the study.
2. Careful handling of x-ray film.
3. Keep fingers clean and dry.

A

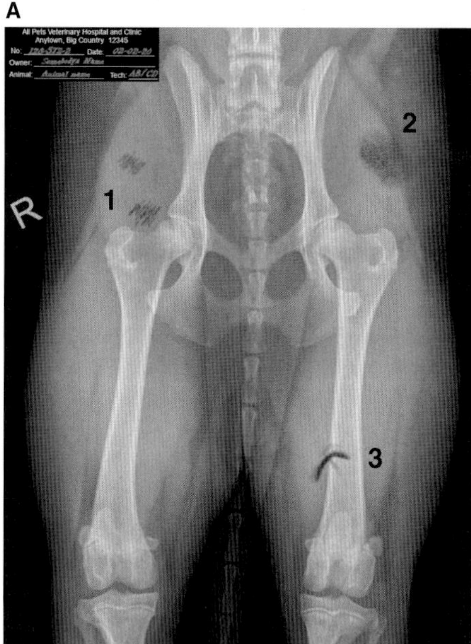

B

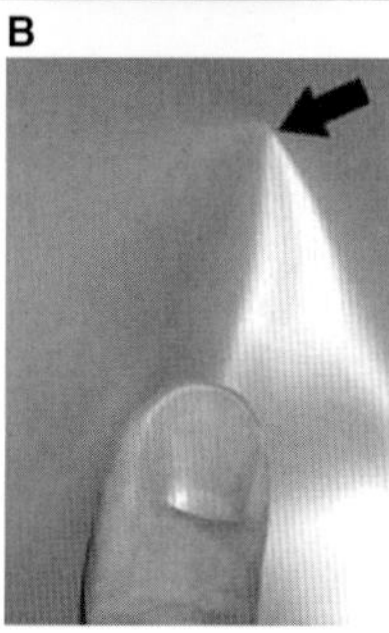

Figure A23 <u>Localized plus density artifacts</u>. (**A**) Film radiograph depicting various types of pressure fog: **1**. Abrasion marks. **2**. Fingerprints. **3**. Crimping mark. (**B**) The crimping mark seen in radiograph A is caused by bending the undeveloped piece of film as indicated by the arrow.

NOTES:

Figure A24. Local white areas in film

Appearance:

1. Localized minus density artifacts; lighter or whiter spots, lines, or regions in a film radiograph (Figure A24).
2. The edges of these artifacts tend to be sharp and well-defined because their causes are located immediately adjacent to the film, which means there is little or no magnification distortion or edge blurring.

Causes:

1. A high opacity material such as contrast medium or a metallic object is present on the surface of the cassette, table top, or patient.
2. Debris is present in the cassette (dust, hair, etc.). The debris blocks emitted light from reaching the film. NOTE: debris in a cassette is very close to the film so the artifact will be sharply-defined with very distinct margins.
3. Debris on a roller in the automatic processor can produce white lines across the radiograph or can scratch and remove film emulsion. Artifacts generated by automatic processors usually repeat in multiple studies.
4. Water spot on the film.
5. Poor contact between the developer chemicals and the film due to:
   a. Film stuck to the side of the dip tank or to another piece of film; latter sometimes is called a "kissing artifact" because both pieces of film will have the same lighter area where they were in contact with each other.
   b. Air bubbles on the film during development.
6. Fixer splashed on film prior to development.
7. Physical scratches in film; wet film is especially vulnerable to loss of emulsion, which can result from rough handling.
8. Cracked or permanently stained intensifying screen (no light is emitted from the damaged part of the phosphorescent screen).

Remedies:

1. If artifact is severe, repeat the study (with a new cassette if needed).
2. In the darkroom, inspect the open cassette with a blacklight, looking for damage or debris on the intensifying screen; clean the cassette as needed.
3. Damaged screens will need to be replaced, but in the interim you should label any damaged cassettes and make note of the locations of any problem areas that produce artifacts.
4. Inspect and clean the automatic processor.
5. Be careful when handling and processing x-ray film.

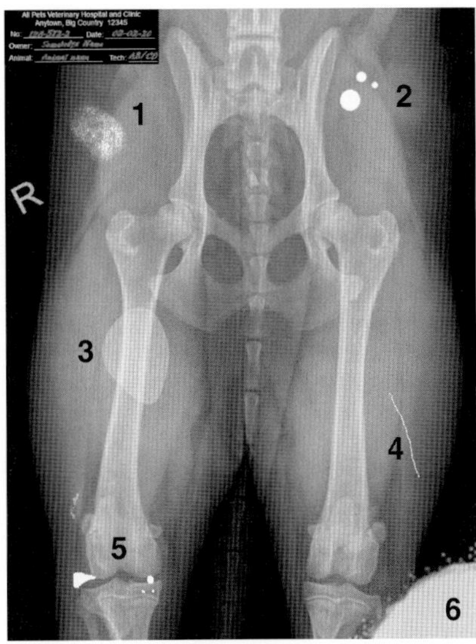

Figure A24 Localized minus density artifacts. Film radiograph depicting various light area artifacts: **1**. Fingerprint due to fixer on fingers. **2**. Well-defined round spots caused by air bubbles clinging to film during development or fixer splashed on film prior to development. **3**. Well-defined larger white area representing either a water spot on the film or a "kissing" artifact. **4**. Scratch in the film emulsion. **5**. Either debris in a cassette (located between the screen and the film) or pieces of metallic material on the table top or patient's hair. Debris inside the cassette will produce an artifact with sharp margins. **6**. A damaged intensifying screen (e.g., cracked screen) or a stain in the corner of a screen that prevents light emission from this area.

NOTES:

Figure A25. Local white areas in digital

Appearance:

1. Localized minus density artifacts; brighter or whiter spots, lines, or regions in a digital radiograph (Figure A25).

Causes:

1. A high opacity material such as contrast medium or a metallic object is present on the table or on the surface of the image receptor.
2. Dust, dirt, hair, etc. in the CR cassette can block emitted light from reaching the imaging plate. NOTE: debris in a cassette is very close to the imaging plate so the artifact will be displayed with very sharp, well-defined edges in the radiograph.
3. Dead pixels; the affected pixels cannot display any shade of gray due to a physically damaged image receptor or a calibration error.
4. Causes of parallel white lines across the entire digital image include:
   a. Poor calibration.
   b. Faulty or loose data cable.
   c. Damaged imaging plate.
   d. Defective laser scanner (CR system).
   e. Dust or debris on the light guide (CR system).

Remedies:

1. If the artifact is severe, repeat the study after cleaning or repairing the image receptor (remove any debris).
2. Calibrate or re-calibrate the image receptor.
3. Severely damaged digital receptors will need to be replaced.
4. Inspect and tighten all data cables.

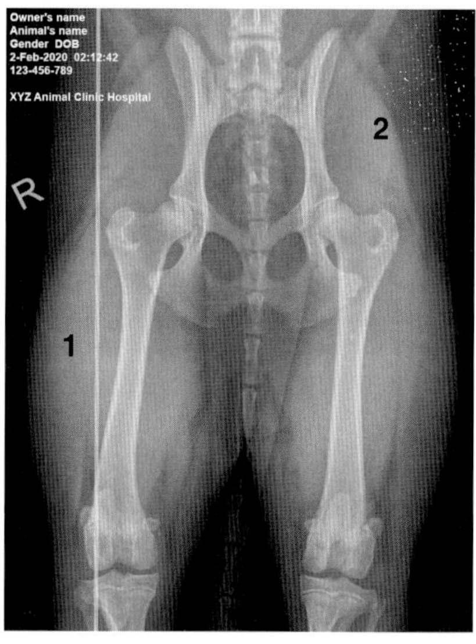

Figure A25 Localized minus density artifacts. Digital radiograph depicting: **1**. White line caused by debris on a light guide in a CR reader. **2**. Dead pixels.

Figure A26–27. Superimposition of objects outside the patient (film and digital)

Appearance:

1. Objects external to the patient can create superimposition artifacts that appear as lighter, brighter, or whiter lines, streaks, or distinct shapes in the radiograph (Figure A26).

Causes:

1. High opacity materials on the patient or next to the patient that are in the field-of-view, such as:
   a. Patient's collar, harness, leash, etc.
   b. Medical devices (e.g., ECG leads, IV tubing).
   c. Positioning aids (e.g., sandbags, lead gloves).
   d. Wet or dirty patient hair coat.
   e. Contrast agent or medication on the patient's skin or hair coat.
   f. Skin folds (Figure A27).
   g. Cutaneous nodule or mass (e.g., nipple, lipoma, engorged tick).
   h. Mineralization on or in the skin.

Remedy:

1. If the artifact is severe enough (and removable), repeat the radiograph after correcting the cause of the artifact (e.g., move it out of the field-of-view, clean it up).

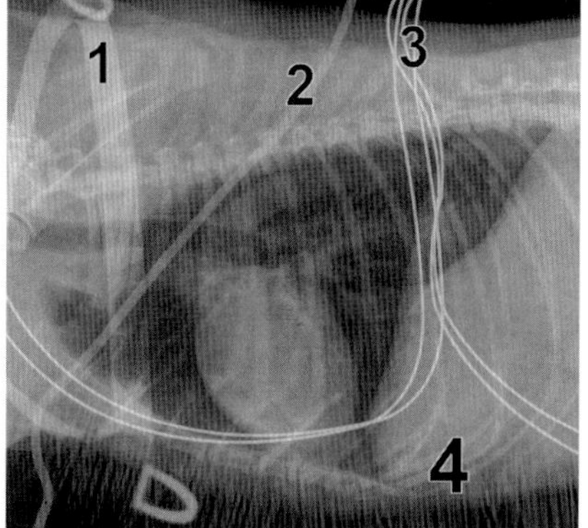

Figure A26 Superimposition artifacts. Radiograph of the thorax depicting superimposition of external structures: **1**. Harness with dorsal and ventral metal D-rings; **2**. IV tubing; **3**. ECG leads; **4**. Wet or dirty haircoat along the patient's ventrum.

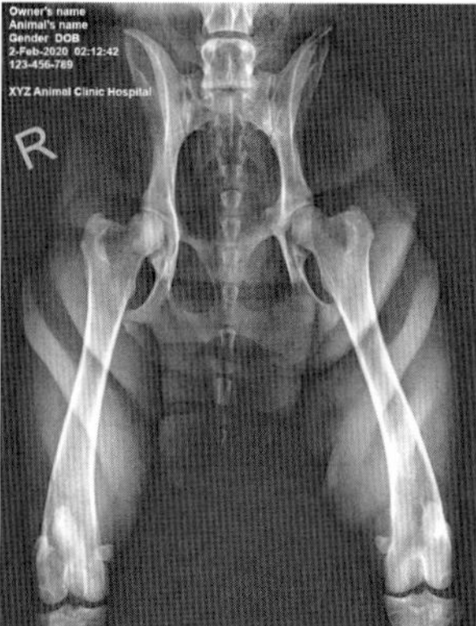

Figure A27 Skin folds. VD radiograph of a Shar-pei dog with visible skin folds superimposed on the pelvic limbs. Also present in this digital radiograph is clipping artifact. Notice that the peripheral soft tissues and the distal part of the tail are not visible.

Figure A28–29. Backscatter (film and digital)

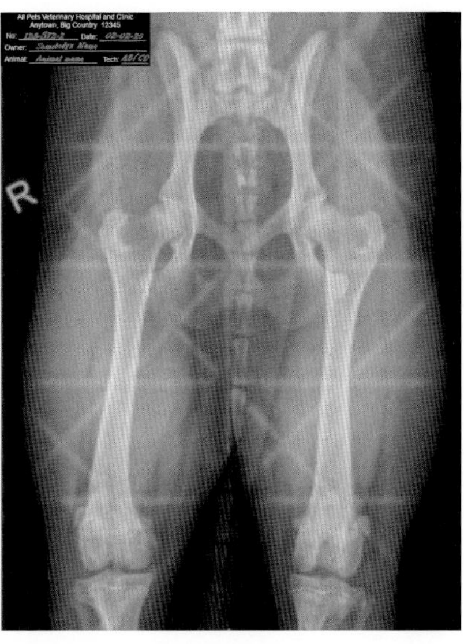

Figure A28 Backscatter. Visible in this VD view of a pelvis are the support structures in the back of the cassette. They appear as multiple crossing white lines. The lines are due to backscatter but may also be caused by a cassette that was installed upside down.

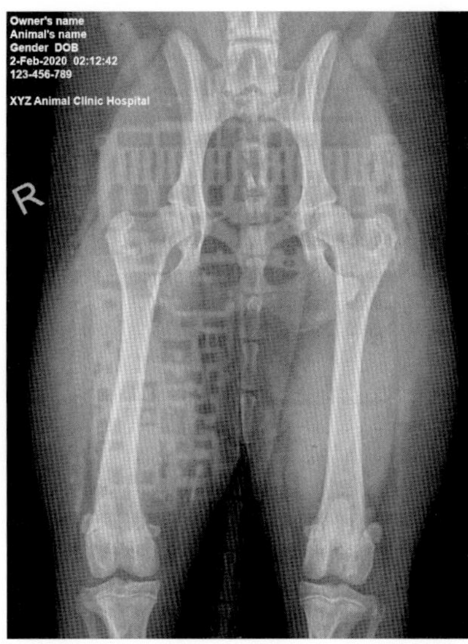

Figure A29 Backscatter. In this VD view of a pelvis, the electronics inside the digital image receptor are visible due to backscatter.

Appearance:

1. Shapes of objects or structures located behind the film or digital image receptor are visible in the radiograph.
2. The support structures in the back of the cassette may appear as radiating white lines (Figure A28).
3. The electronics inside a wireless digital image receptor may be visible (Figure A29).

Causes:

1. Backscatter refers to x-rays that pass through the patient and image receptor to interact with the floor, wall, table, or other structure and produce secondary x-rays that travel back toward the x-ray tube.
2. Backscatter adds an image of the structures located behind the receptor to the radiograph of the patient.
3. The back of a cassette may also be visible in the patient's radiograph if the cassette was installed upside down.

Remedies:

1. If the artifact is severe enough, repeat the study with less kVp; lower energy x-rays are less likely to result in backscatter.
2. Make sure the image receptor is properly installed and positioned.
3. Add shielding behind the film or digital image receptor:
   a. For an immediate fix, place a lead apron behind the image receptor to provide temporary shielding.
   b. Long-term shielding usually requires the manufacturer to install additional shielding to the back of the cassette or behind the image receptor.

NOTES:

Figure A30. Gridlines (film and digital)

Appearance:

1. Parallel, evenly-spaced white lines that extend across the entire film or digital radiograph (Figure A30).

Cause:

1. Undesirable absorption of transmitted x-rays by the grid due to:
   a. Stationary grid.
   b. Grid ratio too low.
   c. Grid frequency too low.
   d. Failure of the Bucky mechanism to move the grid.
   e. Digital: failure of grid suppression software.

Remedies:

1. Change to a higher ratio grid.
2. Change to a higher frequency grid.
3. Ensure that the Bucky mechanism is functioning properly.
4. Digital: add or correct grid-line removal software.

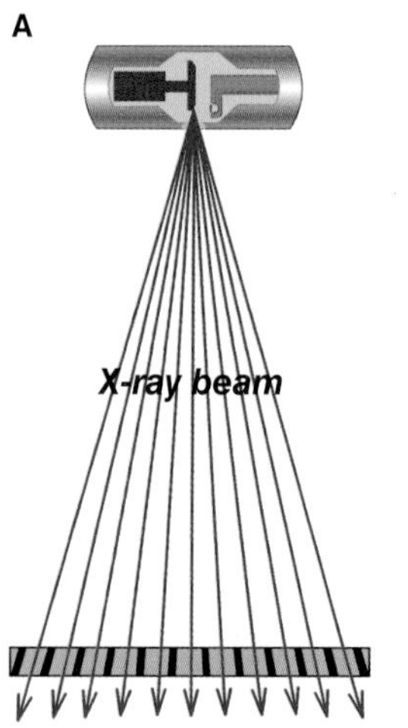

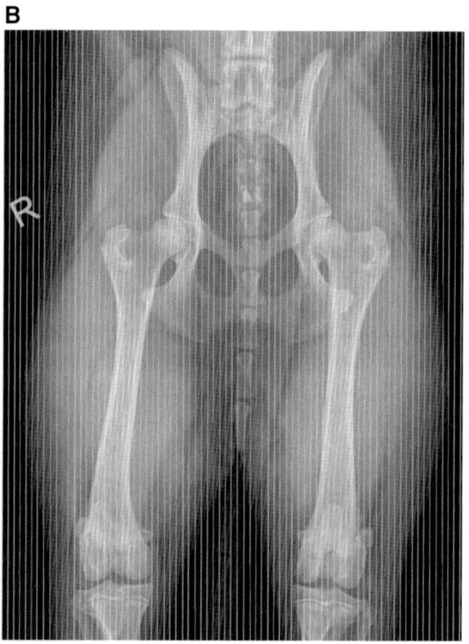

Figure A30 Gridlines. (**A**) Grid is properly positioned in relation to the x-ray beam. (**B**) Radiograph with visible parallel white lines.

Figure A31–A34. Grid cutoff (film and digital)

Off-center grid cutoff

Appearance:

1. Parallel white lines across one side of the film or digital radiograph; one side of the image is too light (underexposed) and the other side is too dark (overexposed) (Figure A31).

Cause:

1. Grid is laterally misaligned with the center of the x-ray beam resulting in increased absorption of transmitted x-rays along one side.
2. Cutoff is more severe with cross-hatched grids, which must be perfectly aligned with the central ray.

Remedy:

1. Repeat the study after correcting the grid position.

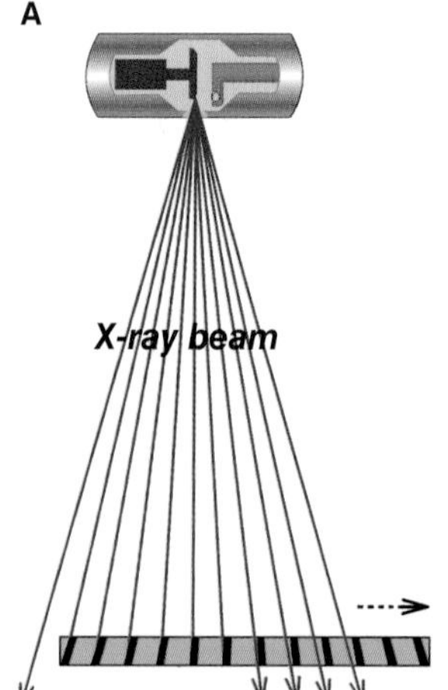

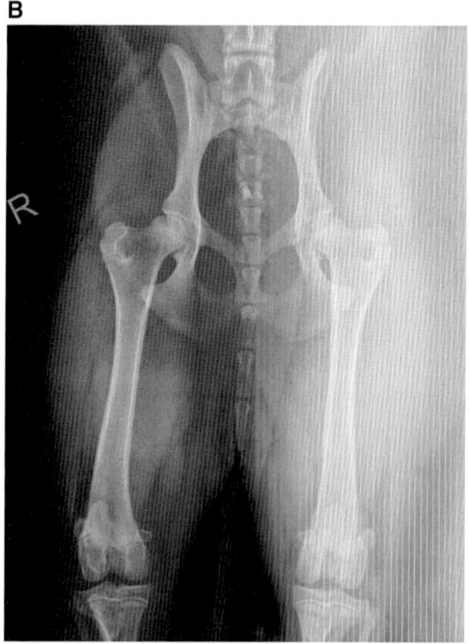

Figure A31 Grid cutoff. **A**. Grid is off-center in relation to the x-ray beam (grid is moved to the right). **B**. Radiograph with parallel white lines on one side of the image due to an off-center grid.

Figure A31–A34. Grid cutoff (film and digital) (*Continued*)

Off-level grid cutoff

Appearance:

1. Parallel white lines across the entire film or digital radiograph; image is overall too light (underexposed) (Figure A32).

Causes:

1. Grid is tilted in relation to the center of the x-ray beam resulting in increased absorption of transmitted x-rays.
2. Cutoff also will occur when the x-ray beam is angled in relation to the grid.

Remedy:

1. Repeat the study after correcting the alignment between the grid and the x-ray beam.

A

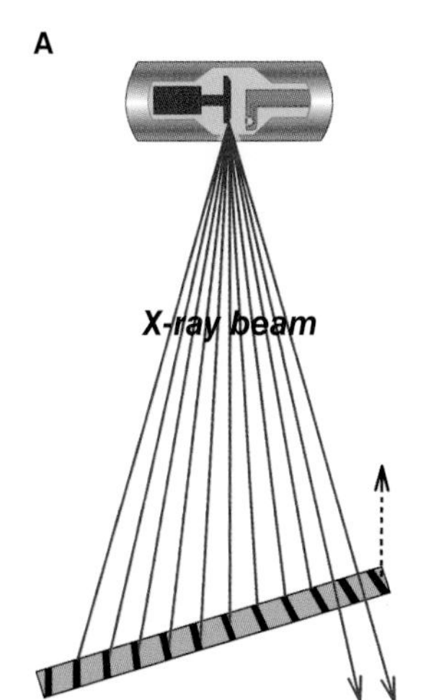

B

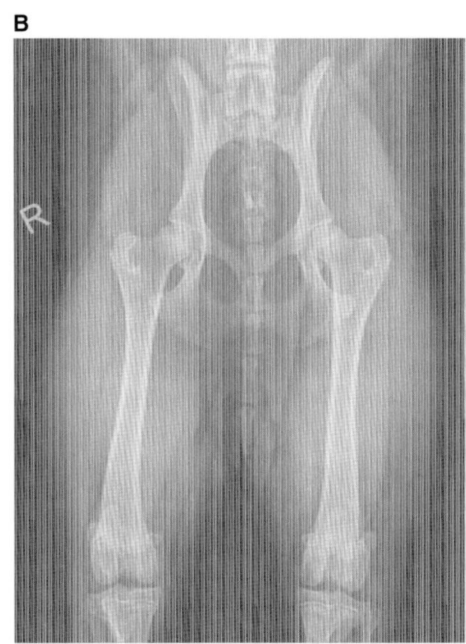

Figure A32 Grid cutoff. (**A**) Grid is tilted in relation to the x-ray beam (right side is closer to the x-ray tube). (**B**) Radiograph with parallel white lines across the entire image due to an off-level grid.

Off-focus grid cutoff

Appearance:

1. Parallel white lines along both sides of the film or digital radiograph; the edges of the image are too light or underexposed (Figure A33).

Cause:

1. The distance between the grid and the focal spot is not within the recommended range, which means the lead strips are not properly aligned with the x-ray beam and there is increased absorption of transmitted x-rays at the periphery.
2. The distance at which cutoff occurs is determined by SID/grid ratio.

Remedy

1. Repeat the study after correcting the distance between the grid and the x-ray tube or focal spot.

A

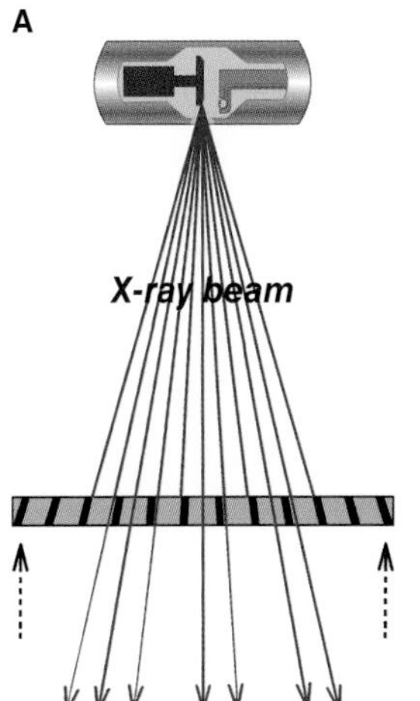

B

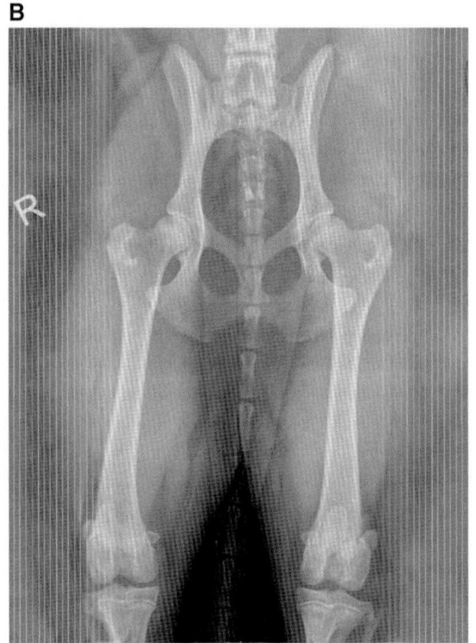

Figure A33 Grid cutoff. (**A**) Grid is too close to the x-ray tube (the source-to-grid distance is too short for this focused grid). (**B**) Radiograph with parallel white lines on either side of the image due to an off-focus grid.

Figure A31–A34. Grid cutoff (film and digital) (*Continued*)

Upside-down grid cutoff

Appearance:
1. Parallel white lines that span the entire film or digital radiograph, especially at the edges of the image where there will be severe grid cutoff (Figure A34).
2. Radiograph is overall too light (underexposed).

Cause:
1. Grid is installed upside down, which greatly increases absorption of the transmitted x-rays, especially peripherally.

Remedy:
1. Repeat the study after correcting the grid position.

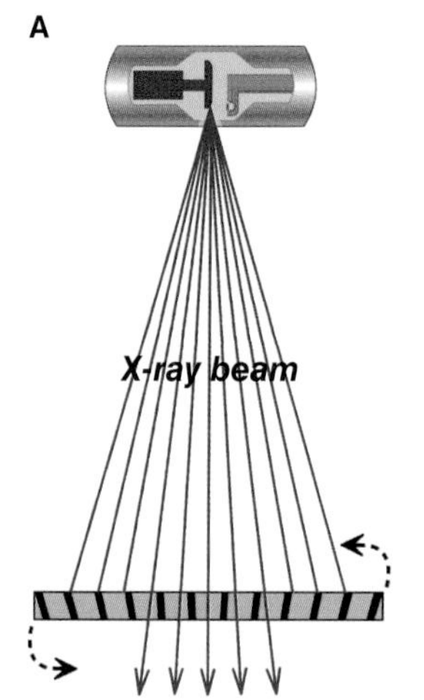

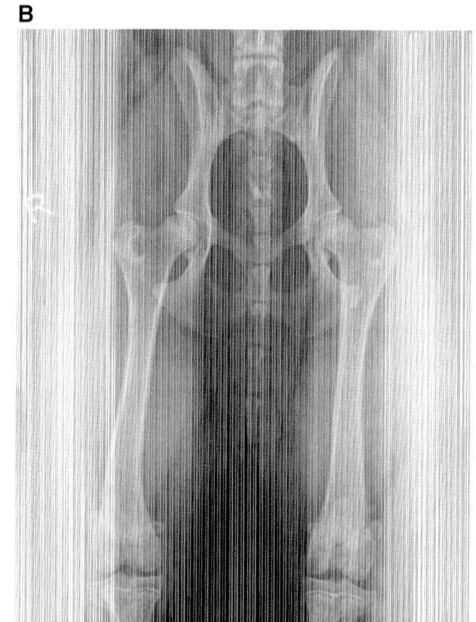

Figure A34 Grid cutoff. (**A**) Grid is upside down in relation to the x-ray beam. (**B**) Radiograph with parallel white lines that are more numerous on either side of the image due to an upside down grid.

Figure A35. Halo effect (digital)

Other names:
1. Rebound artifact, *überschwinger* artifact.

Appearance:
1. A local plus density artifact in a digital radiograph.
2. A dark zone or black rim is seen adjacent to a high opacity structure such as metallic object (Figure A35).
3. Halo artifacts can mimic osteolysis and may be mistaken for loosening or infection near an implant.

Cause:
1. Computer edge-enhancement error; edge-sharpening algorithms commonly are used to enhance digital radiographic contrast and image detail, but frequently create this artifact near high opacity objects.

Remedies:
1. Repeat the study with corrected computer settings.
2. Turn off the edge-enhancement algorithm and view the digital image as raw data.

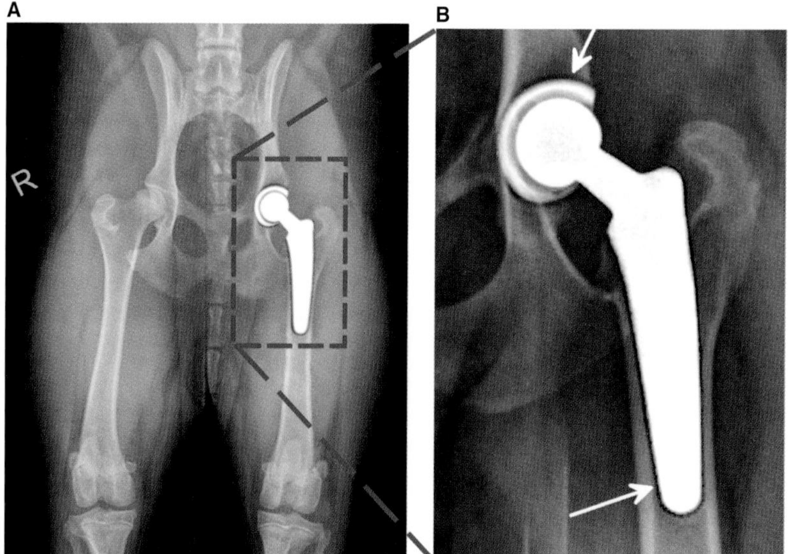

Figure A35 Halo artifact. (**A**) VD view of the pelvis and (**B**) a close-up of the hip implant. The white arrow points to the dark "halo" adjacent to the metal implant.

Figure A36. Radiofrequency or "zipper" artifact (digital)

Appearance:

1. Multiple, repeating, dark lines in a digital radiograph (Figure A36).
2. The size and pattern of the lines vary with the severity of the cause and often occur only intermittently. Zipper artifacts seldom are seen in every radiographic study.

Causes:

1. Interference from a nearby radiofrequency (RF) source (e.g., computer equipment, cell phones, Bluetooth devices, microwaves, fluorescent lights, electric motors, others).
2. Loose or damaged data cable.
3. Patient making rapid, minor movements against the image receptor (i.e., patient is trembling or shaking).

Remedies:

1. If the artifact is severe enough, repeat the study.
2. Identify the source of the RF interference (sometimes difficult, especially when the artifact occurs intermittently).
3. Inspect and tighten data cables.
4. Move the patient slightly further away from the image receptor.
5. Add RF shielding to the radiology room.

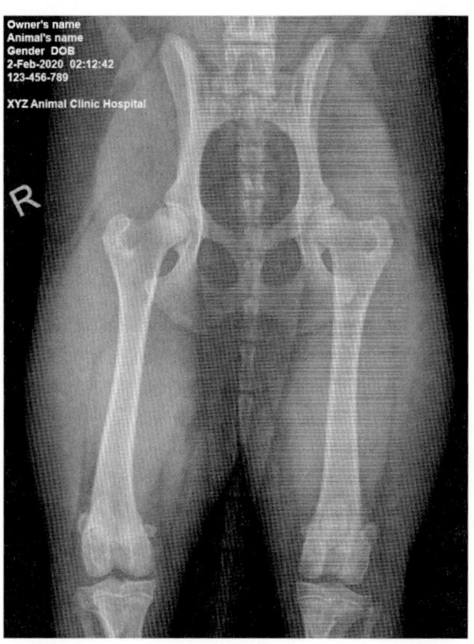

Figure A36 Radiofrequency artifact VD view of a pelvis depicting multiple, thin, black, repeating lines caused by interference from nearby electrical equipment.

Figure A37. Border detection error or Cropping artifact (digital)

Appearance:

1. Plus density artifact in a digital radiograph in which an edge of the field-of-view is seen in the area of interest (Figure A37).

Cause:

1. Computer error with automatic border detection software caused by:
   a. Imaging receptor and field-of-view (FOV) not properly aligned.
   b. User attempting to divide the digital image receptor for multiple x-ray exposures (create more than one radiograph in the final image).
   c. Area of interest is positioned off-center.
   d. Presence of a high opacity structure (e.g., bone, metal) which the computer mistakes for the edge of the field-of-view.

Remedies:

1. Turn off automatic border detection software and view the digital image as raw data.
2. Repeat the study after improving alignment between the field-of-view and the digital image receptor.

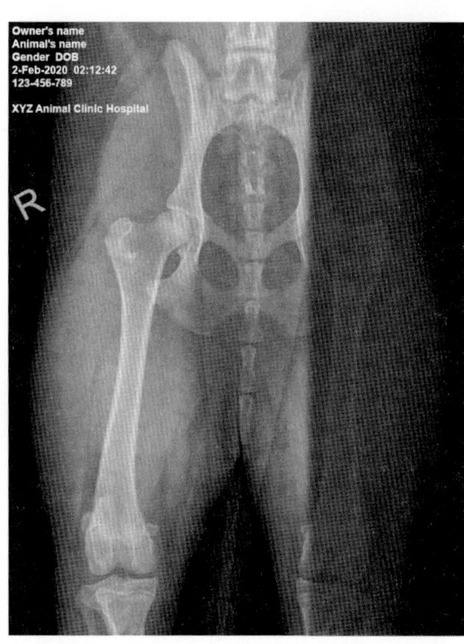

Figure A37 Cropping artifact. Digital radiograph depicting darkening along the left side of the patient due to a border detection error.

CHAPTER 2

Figure A38. Edge enhancement or Mach band/Mach line (film and digital)

Appearance:

1. The edges of objects appear darker or lighter in the radiograph than actual. For example, in the gray-scale image below, the edge of a shade of gray appears lighter next to a darker shade (white arrow) and darker next to a lighter shade (black arrow) (Figure A38).
2. Mach bands can be mistaken for bone fractures, osteosclerosis, osteolysis, free gas, and other abnormal radiographic findings. A Mach line may be mistaken for a cavitary lung lesion.

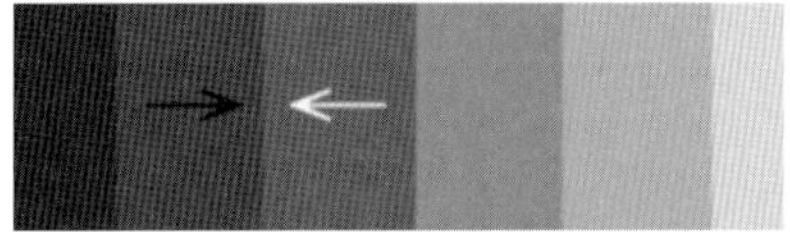

A

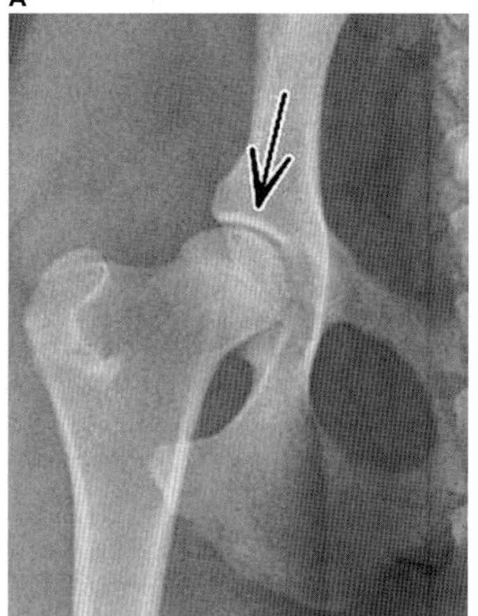

B

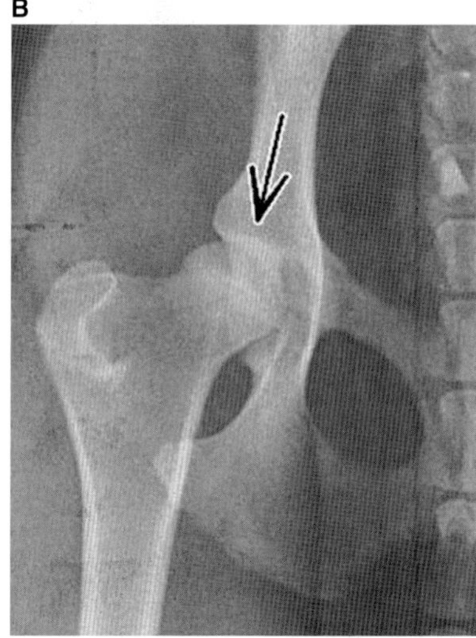

Figure A38 Mach band. Close up VD views of a dog pelvis. **A**. The concave cranial aspect of the acetabulum appears sclerotic next to the darker joint space (arrow) due to a positive Mach band. **B**. When the joint space is made whiter, the Mach band and apparent sclerosis are less evident (arrow).

Cause:

1. A Mach line is an optical illusion. It may be caused by an abrupt change from one shade of gray to the next or it may be caused by the curved edge of a structure. A curved structure such as a blood vessel, bronchus, rib, or costal cartilage can falsely increase or decrease the adjacent opacity.
2. Negative Mach bands are darker than actual and occur along convex edges and where a darker edge meets a lighter edge.
3. Positive Mach bands are lighter than actual and occur along concave edges and where a lighter edge meets a darker edge.

Remedies:

1. Mach lines are not real and seldom repeat in serial radiographs. When in doubt, make another radiograph with the subject at a slightly different angle to the x-ray beam.
2. Knowledge of the edge enhancement artifact does not eliminate it. The illusion occurs inside the retina. But knowing about Mach bands helps prevent mistaking them for true abnormalities.

Contrast radiography

Radiographic contrast studies are performed to enhance visualization of a specific organ or structure of interest. A gas or metal opacity **contrast medium** is introduced into a lumen or potential space to create an opacity interface where none exists. The different types of contrast media frequently used in veterinary radiography, as well as their advantages and disadvantages, are discussed below. Detailed descriptions of numerous contrast procedures are provided on the subsequent pages. Representative normal radiographs are included with each study description. Abnormalities are discussed with each body part in Chapters 3–5.

Indications for contrast radiography

1. To obtain needed information that is not available in survey radiographs.
2. To better evaluate the size, shape, and position of an organ or structure that is not adequately seen in survey radiographs.
3. To examine the luminal contents, mucosal margin, or inner wall of a hollow viscus.
4. To provide some assessment of organ function.
5. To aid in determining appropriate therapy, such as whether surgery is indicated.

The ideal contrast medium

1. Sufficiently alters the opacity of the organ or structure of interest to make it visible in radiographs.
2. Persists long enough to make radiographs.
3. Carries a low risk of harm to the patient.
4. Is successfully eliminated from the body.

Types of contrast media

In veterinary radiography, we use both positive and negative contrast agents. **Negative contrast agents** are gases. The most commonly used gases are atmospheric air (room air), carbon dioxide, nitrous oxide, and oxygen. Room air, of course, is readily available, but it is less soluble than the other gases and therefore carries a greater risk of gas embolism.

Positive contrast media contain either barium or iodine. They may be administered enterally or parenterally to assess the position, size, shape, margination, and internal architecture of an organ. They also provide a non-invasive means of detecting leakage from an organ. Positive contrast media are metal opacity and most opaque in radiographs when the kVp is close to 70 (see discussion about K-edge in Chapter 2).

Both negative and positive contrast agents sometimes are used together to create a **double contrast study**. Typically, this is accomplished by filling the organ of interest with gas and then adding a small amount of positive contrast medium to coat the mucosal surface. Double contrast studies tend to provide better visualization of the mucosa than either a positive or negative contrast study alone.

Barium contrast media contain barium sulfate, a chalky-white, crystalline powder that is micropulverized and placed in suspension. The barium sulfate usually is combined with carboxymethylcellulose to enable it to remain in suspension and more efficiently coat the mucosal surfaces. Barium sulfate powder is available by itself (e.g., USP $BaSO_4$), but it is difficult to mix evenly and tends to quickly fall out of suspension. The commercially available premixed preparations generally are preferred because they tend to produce better contrast studies that are easier to interpret. Notice that a barium contrast medium is a suspension, not a solution. Barium never is injected intravenously.

Barium contrast agents (or simply "barium") most often are used to study the alimentary tract. They may be administered orally or per-rectum. Barium is not absorbed in the GI tract and is eliminated in the feces. A variety of concentrations of barium are available to provide a thin or thick suspension to fill or coat different parts of the GI tract. The concentration needed for a particular study is discussed with each specific procedure later in this chapter. Concentrations may be listed as a percentage weight-to-volume (w/v), a weight-to-weight (w/w) ratio, or as specific gravity. Many commercial barium preparations include additional ingredients to provide therapeutic benefits to the patient's alimentary tract, including a protective coating action, additives to help reduce GI gas, and compounds that help bind irritating or harmful substances (e.g., bile acids, toxins, and bacteria).

Iodinated contrast media contain compounds that are composed of benzene rings with three iodine atoms plus various side chains. They are water-soluble and either **ionic** or **non-ionic**. Ionic compounds split into two ions when placed in solution. Non-ionic agents do not disassociate in solution. The osmolality of most ionic contrast media is high, about 5–8 times that of serum. This is particularly true of the older or "first generation" ionic agents. High osmolar agents are *hypertonic,* and they are quickly diluted and absorbed in the body. Ionic agents are irritating and much more likely to cause an adverse reaction than non-ionic agents. Non-ionic agents are less than three times the osmolality of serum. Ionic agents should not be used in very young or debilitated patients due to their hypertonicity. They are occasionally used for alimentary and cystourethral studies in adult animals, but in general, ionic contrast agents are not recommended.

Non-ionic contrast media are more available to veterinarians today than in the past, greatly reducing the need to use ionic agents. Non-ionic agents may be administered intrathecally, intravenously, orally, or intra-articular. They are used in numerous radiographic contrast studies, including angiography, myelography, urography, and to study the alimentary tract.

Iodinated contrast media are available in a variety of concentrations, expressed as milligrams of iodine per milliliter of solution or **mgI/ml** (Table 2.2). The higher the concentration, the greater the opacity. With some iodinated agents, a higher concentration makes them more viscous (thick and sticky) and resistant to flow. In these cases, the viscosity may be reduced by warming the contrast medium to body temperature. The mgI/ml needed for a particular contrast study is discussed with each specific procedure later in this chapter. When the concentration exceeds what is needed, the contrast medium can be diluted with sterile water or saline.

About 98% of an iodinated contrast medium is eliminated from the body via the kidneys. The remainder is removed by the small intestine and the biliary system. Clearance from the central nervous system is slower than from the vascular system due to the blood–brain barrier. Iodinated compounds that are used to study the hepatobiliary system are designed to be preferentially excreted in the bile.

Contrast medium in the urine can inhibit bacterial growth, increase urine specific gravity, and affect the appearance of the urine sediment. These are not contraindications to a contrast study, but keep them in mind if laboratory testing is to follow radiography. Also, intravenous iodinated contrast agents will temporarily increase the level of iodine in the blood, which may inhibit the uptake of I-131 by the thyroid gland. Decreased iodine uptake means radioisotope therapy may be less effective.

Adverse effects related to contrast media

Unwanted reactions to contrast media range from a mild inconvenience to a life-threatening emergency situation. It is important to be aware of the risk factors and the signs of an adverse reaction before administering a contrast agent. A successful outcome depends on prevention and early treatment. A problem can arise during the contrast study or after the study is completed; some adverse effects may be delayed 30 minutes or longer after dosing.

Adverse effects of gas

A potentially serious complication from a negative contrast study is a *gas embolism*. Gas emboli are more likely to occur when the study involves an organ that is bleeding, such as

Table 2.2 Iodinated contrast media[a]

Name	Type	Osmolality		mgI/ml
Isopaque-370 (metrizoate)	Ionic	2100	High	370
Hypaque-76, *Gastrografin* (diatrizoate)	Ionic	2000	High	370
Conray-60 (iothalamate)	Ionic	1800	High	325
Hypaque-50, *Renografin*-60 (diatrizoate)	Ionic	1550	High	300
Omnipaque-350 (iohexol)	Non-ionic	884	Low	350
Isovue-370 (iopamidol)	Non-ionic	796	Low	370
Ultravist-370 (iopromide)	Non-ionic	774	Low	370
Oxilan-350 (ioxilan)	Non-ionic	695	Low	350
Optiray-300 (ioversal)	Non-ionic	651	Low	300
Iomeron-350 (iomeprol)	Non-ionic	618	Low	350
Hexabrix (ioxaglate)	Ionic	580	Low	320
Isovist (iotrolan)	Non-ionic	320	Low	300
Visipaque-320 (iodixanol)	Non-ionic	290	Low	320
Serum	**—**	**300**	**—**	**—**

[a] In this table, the common trade names of various iodinated contrast agents are listed in order of decreasing osmolality. The key component of each agent is shown in parenthesis. A concentration in mgI/ml is given for each agent, but other concentrations frequently are available from the manufacturer. Some of the contrast media listed are discontinued in the United States.

pneumocystography in a patient with hematuria. The risk of gas embolism is less when using a soluble gas such as carbon dioxide, nitrous oxide, or oxygen. Symptoms of gas embolism often develop quickly and may include dyspnea, tachycardia, altered mentation, hypotension, and abnormal heart sounds (the latter has been described as a "rumbling" heart sound). The severity of the clinical signs depends on the size and extent of the embolism. Sudden death has been reported.

Treatment of a suspected gas embolism must begin immediately. The goal is to prevent embolization of the pulmonary outflow tract. Place the patient in left lateral recumbency and elevate its caudal body in an effort to trap the gas in the right ventricle. The patient may need to remain in this position for up to 60 minutes to allow the gas to be absorbed. Additional treatments such as fluid therapy and oxygen therapy may be needed.

Adverse effects of barium

Barium in the alimentary tract generally is safe because it is not irritating and not absorbed or metabolized. Barium in the esophagus, stomach, or intestines may physically obscure visualization of the mucosal surfaces during endoscopy or surgery. Barium also can block the propagation of ultrasound waves, which can complicate an ultrasonography examination. When practical, a barium contrast study should be avoided when one of these other procedures is planned.

Although a barium contrast study can be performed to investigate a possible rupture in the esophagus, stomach, or bowel, it should be performed with caution. Barium outside the alimentary tract is irritating and inflammatory. The severity of a reaction to barium depends on the amount and location. Reactions to small amounts of barium in the peritoneal cavity or mediastinum often are no more severe than reactions to equal amounts of ingesta without barium. A large amount of barium, however, can become life-threatening. Patients that survive may develop extensive adhesions and chronic granulomas.

Keep in mind that a rupture along the alimentary tract is likely to leak gas as easily, if not easier, than liquids. When leakage is suspected, make plain radiographs (without contrast) to detect free gas. Use horizontal beam radiography if needed (Figure 2.15). If free gas is detected, the diagnosis is confirmed. If no free gas is seen, then the leakage most likely is absent or very small. At this point, the risk of using barium is as low as using an iodinated contrast agent, and barium is more likely to demonstrate a leak. Iodinated contrast media may be preferred when a GI contrast study is needed during the first few days after GI surgery because there is already free gas in the abdominal cavity.

Barium in the trachea or lungs may or may not cause problems. Again, it depends on the volume. Small amounts of barium usually are benign and mostly cleared by the bronchial cilia or alveolar macrophages. Some barium may localize in the tracheobronchial lymph nodes or in the alveoli where it can persist for long periods of time, but rarely is it clinically significant. A large volume of barium in the respiratory tract, however, can lead to airway obstruction, hypoxia, and respiratory distress. In these cases, as much barium as possible should be removed using endotracheal suction. Sometimes barium is aspirated during oral administration or secondary to vomiting or inadvertently deposited in the respiratory tract due to incorrect placement of an orogastric or nasogastric tube. Rarely, an esophageal fistula is the cause of in barium in the trachea, lungs, or mediastinum.

Adverse effects of iodinated compounds

Ionic contrast media are much more likely to induce an adverse reaction than non-ionic agents. Adverse effects range from mild to severe (Table 2.3). Warming an ionic agent to body temperature and injecting it as slowly as possible reduces risk, but the increased availability and affordability of non-ionic compounds has virtually eliminated the need to use ionic contrast media.

Adverse reactions to non-ionic agents are uncommon. Most are mild and transient, requiring no specific therapy (e.g., tachycardia, nausea, vomiting). Rarely, more severe reactions can occur (e.g., bronchospasm, hypotension). Fatal reactions are extremely rare (less than 0.001%). Unfortunately, the likelihood of an adverse reaction cannot be predicted, even by administering a small test dose to the patient. It is important to be prepared to treat any adverse effects. Keep emergency supplies readily available (e.g., IV fluids, oxygen, antihistamines, corticosteroids, epinephrine, atropine, valium). Patients at increased risk include those with a history of sensitivity to the contrast agent and those with a preexisting condition (e.g., renal disease, hypovolemia, diabetes mellitus).

Table 2.3 Adverse effects of IONIC contrast agents[a]

Mild

1. Bitter taste; patient may be reluctant to accept oral dosing.
2. Nausea, brief retching or vomiting.
3. Peripheral vasodilation and skin erythema.
4. Osmotic diuresis or osmotic diarrhea.
5. Local irritation at the injection site.
6. General discomfort.

Moderate

1. Persistent vomiting.
2. Facial swelling.
3. Laryngeal edema.
4. Dehydration; due to osmotic diuresis or diarrhea.
5. Tachycardia or bradycardia.
6. Hypertension; due to osmotic hypervolemia.

Severe

1. Cardiac arrhythmias.
2. Hypotension; due to bradycardia, vasodilation, osmotic diarrhea.
3. Pulmonary edema; due to hypertonic contrast agent inadvertently deposited in lungs.
4. Vascular collapse; due to damaged capillaries and desiccated red blood cells caused by hypertonic agents; may lead to thromboemboli and hemorrhage.
5. Acute renal failure; due to direct tubular toxicity or renal vasoconstriction or hypotension.
6. Cerebral edema, seizures, syncope; due to increased permeability of the blood–brain barrier.
7. Death.

[a] This table lists the physiologic changes and clinical signs that may result from the administration of an ionic contrast agent. Adverse effects are more likely to occur with intravenous and intra-thecal routes than with oral dosing.

Procedures in contrast radiography

Although many radiographic contrast studies are less frequently performed in modern veterinary medicine, they still are useful. Endoscopy and advanced imaging modalities such as ultrasonography, computed tomography, and magnetic resonance imaging often yield superior anatomic detail and frequently are less invasive. However, a contrast study can provide valuable diagnostic information, especially when the other modalities are unavailable due to cost, time constraints, travel distance, or other. In the following pages, you will find indications, contraindications, and step-by-step procedures for performing many different radiographic contrast studies. Some of the contraindications to performing contrast radiography are listed in Box 2.1.

Box 2.1 Contraindications for contrast radiography

- Diagnosis is evident in survey radiographs.
- Patient is debilitated, compromised, or in distress.
- Patient has a known sensitivity or allergic reaction to the contrast agent.
- Infection or other disease is present that may be disseminated during performance of a contrast study.
- Any contraindication to sedation or anesthesia in a contrast study that requires chemical restraint.
- Inexperience with an invasive or potentially dangerous contrast procedure.
- A less invasive imaging modality is available and likely to provide similar or superior information (e.g., ultrasonography, endoscopy, CT, MRI).

When performing a contrast study, it is important to proceed in an accurate and systematic manner, paying special attention to the type and volume of contrast medium, the x-ray exposure settings, patient positioning, and appropriate imaging intervals. Proper patient preparation is essential, including an empty GI tract and empty urinary bladder when required, adequate patient hydration, and a clean and dry hair coat. Patient sedation or anesthesia is recommended whenever practical. A plan of action should be in place for any medical emergencies that may arise.

Any procedure may need to be modified, depending on the specific reason for the study, the type of equipment available, and the status of the patient. The experience of the radiographer is important. During some contrast studies, a new or unexpected radiographic finding leads to a modification of the procedure.

The patient body conformation can alter the recommended dose of a contrast medium because dosage is based on ideal body weight. Patients that are overweight or have a large amount of fluid in a body cavity may require a lower dose.

Always make **survey radiographs** prior to beginning a contrast study, even if radiographs were made only a few days earlier. Things can change. Survey radiographs are valuable to:

1. Determine whether the contrast study is needed.
2. Confirm proper preparation of the patient.
3. Establish correct settings for kVp and mAs.
4. Detect abnormalities that may become masked by the contrast medium.
5. Provide a baseline from which to compare and interpret the contrast study.

The **x-ray exposure** used to make survey radiographs usually needs to be adjusted for the contrast radiographs. In most cases, the exposure is doubled for a positive contrast study and cut it in half for a negative contrast study. Doubling the exposure may be accomplished by using twice the mAs or increasing the kVp by 20%. Try to keep the time as short as possible and the kVp as close to 70 as practical. Reducing the exposure usually is accomplished by decreasing the exposure time by half. Alternatively, the kVp can be reduced by 16%.

Alimentary tract contrast studies

Positive, negative, and double contrast radiographic studies of the alimentary tract are used to evaluate the esophagus, stomach, small intestine, and large intestine. Appropriate laboratory testing is recommended beforehand to determine whether the patient's clinical signs could be related to a condition that may not be evident in radiographs (e.g., GI parasites, uremia, Addison's disease, etc.). The following procedures are discussed in this section:

1. Esophagography
2. Gastrography
3. Upper GI study
4. Colonography

Prior to beginning a contrast study, the patient should be properly prepared, especially if it is an elective procedure. The **GI tract should be empty** of ingesta. Retained ingesta can mask or mimic disease and may affect GI function in ways that influence the study. A 12-hour fast allows the stomach to empty and an 18- to 24-hour fast usually empties the intestines. Prior to fasting, make sure withholding food is not detrimental to the patient. Water should be allowed during fasting. **Drugs** that affect GI motility should be discontinued 24–72 hours prior to contrast radiography. When sedation or anesthesia is required, try to use drugs that produce less effects on GI motility.

Fasting does not necessarily ensure that a patient's GI tract will be empty. Be prepared to complete the cleansing procedure with **enemas**. When needed, enemas should be administered 2–4 hours prior to contrast radiography. An enema can be made from isotonic saline or a mild soap and water solution. Enemas that are slightly below body temperature will help reduce the volume of residual bowel gas. The commercially available phosphate enemas are not recommended because they can be toxic, particularly in cats and small dogs.

Barium is the preferred contrast medium for most positive contrast studies of the alimentary tract. Non-ionic iodinated media can be used, but they do not yield as good mucosal definition. Ionic contrast agents are <u>not</u> recommended because they are irritating to the mucosa and their hypertonicity can lead to fluid imbalances, particularly in young, debilitated, and hypovolemic patients. Ionic agents are rapidly diluted and pass through the GI tract much more quickly than barium.

Esophagography and swallowing studies

The use of contrast radiography to investigate problems with swallowing often depends on the severity of the clinical signs. Patients with mild signs of dysphagia and no abnormalities in survey radiographs most likely will require dynamic imaging, such as fluoroscopy of the throat and esophagus, to determine the cause of the swallowing dysfunction. Patients with abnormal but inconclusive radiographic findings, particularly those associated with the esophagus, may benefit from an esophagram. However, extra care must be taken with a dysphagic patient to avoid aspiration.

A **positive contrast esophagram** (Figure 2.67) is more likely to yield useful diagnostic information than a negative contrast study. Even to simply identify or locate the

A

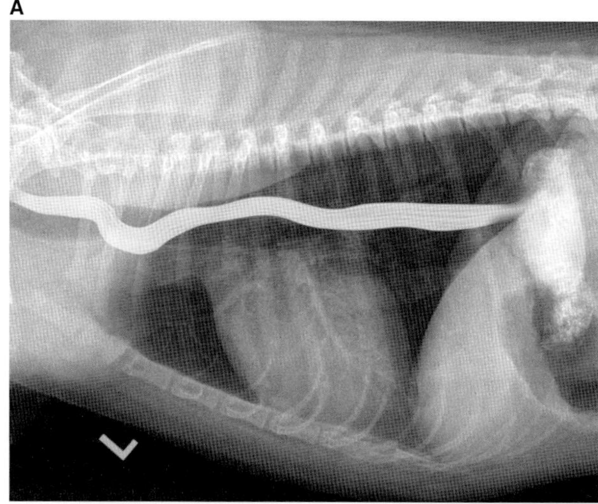

B

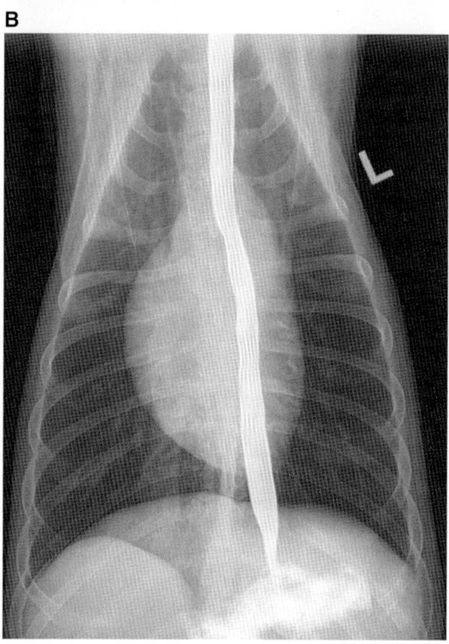

Figure 2.67 Normal esophagram. Lateral view (**A**) and VD view (**B**) of a dog thorax depicting barium in the esophagus. The thin, curvilinear filling defects in the barium are caused by mucosal folds.

esophagus, gas is less reliable than a small amount of a positive contrast medium. Barium is the preferred contrast agent. Non-ionic iodinated contrast media sometimes are substituted for barium such as when endoscopy or surgery is planned to follow radiography; however, iodinated compounds taste bitter, and patients may be reluctant to accept oral dosing. In addition, they do not coat the mucosa as well as barium and esophageal leaks are more difficult to detect with iodinated media than with barium. Ionic compounds are not recommended for esophagography because they can cause severe pulmonary edema should aspiration occur.

An esophagram will provide some information about esophageal motility, but fluoroscopy is more effective for this purpose. Some patients with a swallowing dysfunction have difficulty with liquids, while others have problems with solid foods. To obtain a diagnosis, the patient may need to be dosed with multiple consistencies of contrast medium rather than just a liquid alone. In these cases, use the liquid medium first, followed by soft food mixed with contrast medium, and then a dry, solid food (kibble) mixed with medium.

An esophagram may or may not be indicated in a patient with a large, gas-distended esophagus (i.e., megaesophagus). In such a patient the oral administration of contrast medium carries a high risk of aspiration because esophageal motility obviously is abnormal. A horizontal beam lateral view (without adding contrast) may yield diagnostic information by redistributing the esophageal gas. If findings are still equivocal, try administering a small volume of barium with the patient standing and repeat the horizontal beam lateral view.

Indications for esophagram

1. Evaluate the esophageal mucosa (e.g., esophagitis, neoplasia).
2. Examine questionable findings from survey radiographs (e.g., suspected foreign material).
3. Evaluate for possible esophageal stricture.
4. Investigate the cause of regurgitation, gagging, persistent vomiting, or vomitus containing red blood.
5. Determine the position of the esophagus relative to a cervical, mediastinal, or pulmonary mass.

Procedure for esophagram

1. Empty the stomach prior to radiography with a 4–6 hour fast.
2. Sedation/anesthesia is not recommended due to its effects on esophageal motility and increased risk of aspiration.
3. Make and evaluate survey thoracic and cervical radiographs.
4. Increase x-ray exposure from survey radiographs.
5. Warm the contrast medium to body temperature prior to administration.
6. **Barium paste** (45% to 100% w/v) is used if the purpose of the esophagram is to evaluate the mucosa rather than esophageal motility, size, or content. Barium paste is thick, enabling it to adhere to the mucosa. Placing the paste on the roof of the patient's mouth and holding its mouth shut usually works well. Do not use paste if the esophagram is part of an upper GI study because paste does not mix well with liquid barium; it clumps in the stomach.
   a. Dose is 5–10 ml; several doses may be required for complete evaluation.

7. **Liquid barium suspension** (20%–30% w/v) is used if the purpose of the esophagram is to assess size, content, and patency. Barium is administered orally using a syringe placed in the buccal pouch. If oral administration is complicated or contraindicated, a bolus of barium can be infused via an oroesophageal or nasoesophageal tube. Position the tube just cranial to the suspected lesion. If the esophagus is greatly dilated, a much larger volume of barium may be needed to fully opacify the lumen. Bear in mind that administering large volumes increases the risk of aspiration.
   a. Dog dose: 15–30 ml; additional doses may be given if the initial esophagram is unsatisfactory.
   b. Cat dose: 5–7 ml.
8. **Non-ionic iodinated contrast media** (300 mgI/ml):
   a. Dog dose: 10–15 ml.
   b. Cat dose: 5–10 ml.
9. **Barium mixed with food** can be used if the findings with liquid barium are equivocal. Mix 20 ml of liquid barium suspension (20%–30% w/v) with half a cup of wet food or 1 cup of dry kibble.
10. Allow the patient to swallow two to three times to ensure coating of the esophagus and then make lateral and DV oblique views centered on the cranial thorax. DV is preferred over VD because it is quicker and safer to place the patient in ventral recumbency rather than on its back. Rotating the patient 15°–30° to make an oblique view eliminates superimposition of the spine and sternum.
11. Collimate the FOV to include the pharynx and the stomach.
12. If more radiographs are needed to evaluate a suspected lesion, additional doses of contrast medium can be administered.

A

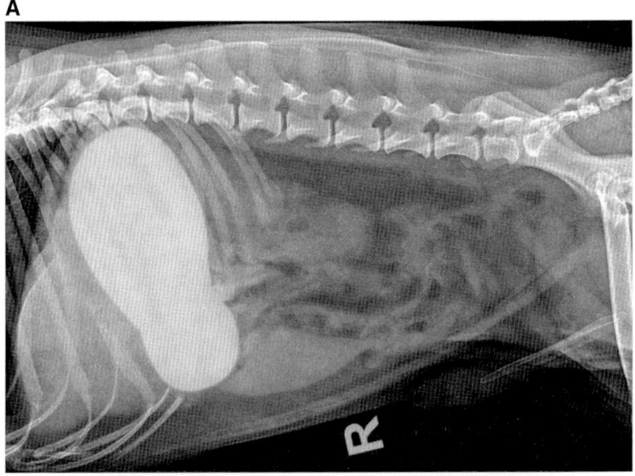

B

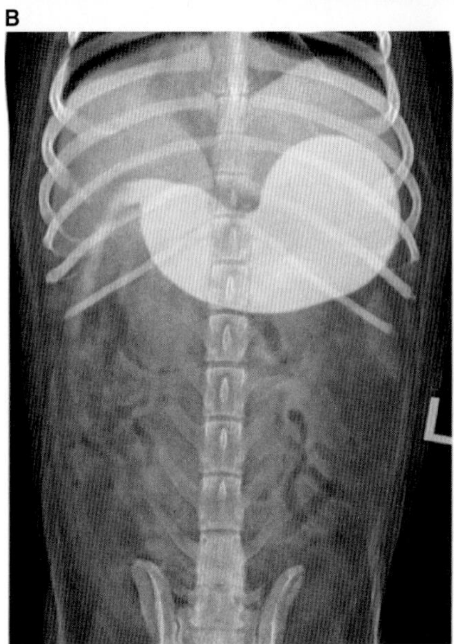

Figure 2.68 Normal gastrogram. Lateral view (**A**) and VD view (**B**) of a dog abdomen depicting positive contrast medium in the stomach.

Gastrography

In many patients, questionable findings associated with the stomach can be resolved by making four view survey radiographs (without contrast). Positioning the patient for right lateral, left lateral, VD, and DV views of the cranial abdomen takes advantage of gravity to redistribute fluid and gas within the stomach. If survey radiographs remain inconclusive, a gastrogram may be useful.

A **negative contrast gastrogram** can be used to simply identify the stomach or to outline some of its contents. A **positive contrast gastrogram** (Figure 2.68) provides more anatomical and functional information. If no abnormalities are evident in a positive contrast gastrogram, be prepared to continue with an upper GI study. A **double contrast gastrogram** enhances visualization of the stomach mucosa, but it is a more difficult procedure to perform. Glucagon is reported to improve the study by decreasing GI motility, allowing the stomach to distend and delaying gastric emptying, but its efficacy is controversial and it is contraindicated in some patients.

Indications for gastrography

1. Identify the stomach; determine its location and orientation.
2. Examine the stomach contents.
3. Evaluate the shape, wall thickness, and mucosal margins of the stomach.
4. Assess gastric emptying (e.g., suspected gastric outflow problem).
5. Investigate the cause of clinical signs such as chronic or persistent vomiting, hematemesis, cranial abdominal pain, anorexia, chronic weight loss, melena, or chronic bloating.

Procedure for gastrogram

1. Empty the GI tract, including the colon. A 12–24 hour fast and cleansing enemas may be required.
2. Make and evaluate survey abdominal radiographs.
3. Drugs that affect GI motility should be discontinued 24 hours prior (e.g., anticholinergics, opioids).

4. Adjust the x-ray exposure from survey radiographs:
   a. Decrease exposure for a negative gastrogram.
   b. Increase exposure for a positive gastrogram.
5. For positive contrast studies, intubate the stomach as described in Box 2.2. Intubation is preferred because oral dosing often results in excess gas in the stomach, which compromises the study.
6. Warm the contrast medium to room temperature prior to administration.
7. Carefully monitor the size of the cranial abdomen during infusion or make test radiographs to assess gastric filling.
8. Make DV, VD, right lateral, and left lateral views centered on the stomach immediately after administering the contrast agent.

Box 2.2 Procedure for orogastric intubation.

1. Position the patient is in ventral recumbency.
2. The length of orogastric tube needed is measured from the corner of the patient's mouth to the tenth rib.
3. Lubricate the tube prior to insertion.
4. Using a mouth speculum, pass the tube into the patient's stomach.
5. Confirm proper tube placement by palpating the patient's neck; you should feel two "tubes," the trachea and the orogastric tube in the esophagus.
6. Proper tube placement also is confirmed by adding 3–15 ml of water to the orogastric tube. If the patient coughs, the tube is in the trachea and must be repositioned.
7. After administering the contrast medium, clear the orogastric tube with air.
8. Block the opening of the tube before withdrawing it.

Negative contrast gastrogram

1. Without gastric intubation, a small volume of gas can be added to the stomach by allowing the patient to drink some carbonated beverage (about 5 ml/kg). Commercially available effervescent tablets or granules also can be used for this purpose.
2. Larger volumes of gas generally are administered via gastric intubation. Gas is added to the stomach by pumping room air or manually blowing into the orogastric tube. The volume of gas needed depends on the purpose of the study:
   a. 2 ml/kg to simply locate the stomach or outline some of the gastric contents.
   b. 20 ml/kg to moderately distend the stomach. Note: this dose of air is an estimate; the cranial abdomen should be carefully monitored for visible distention.
   c. Additional air may be added to the stomach as needed because some will be lost due to regurgitation.

Positive contrast gastrogram

1. Infuse a volume of contrast medium into the stomach sufficient for moderate distention:
   a. Dose of liquid barium suspension (20%–30% w/v):
      1) Small and medium-size dogs: 8–12 ml/kg.
      2) Large dogs: 5–7 ml/kg.
      3) Cats: 8–10 ml/kg.
   b. Dose of iodinated contrast media (300 mgI/ml); dilute the agent with water if the concentration is greater than 300 mgI/ml:
      1) Dogs: 2.0–3.0 ml/kg.
      2) Cats: 1.0–2.0 ml/kg.

Double contrast gastrogram

1. Infuse a small volume of concentrated barium suspension (60%–100% w/v) into the stomach followed by sufficient gas to moderately distend the stomach, estimated dosages:
   a. Small and medium dogs: 2 ml/kg barium followed by 20 ml/kg of room air.
   b. Large dogs: 1 ml/kg barium followed by 20 ml/kg of room air.
   c. Cats: 6 ml concentrated barium followed by 20 ml/kg of room air.
2. Carefully roll the patient 2–3 times to coat the gastric mucosa.

Upper gastrointestinal study (upper GI)

An upper GI study is essentially a continuation of a positive contrast gastrogram. The upper GI tract includes the stomach and small intestine.

Indications for upper GI study

1. Inconclusive gastrogram.
2. Investigate the cause of vomiting that is acute, persistent, recurrent, or unresponsive to therapy.
3. Evaluate animals with blood in vomitus (hematemesis) or feces (melena).
4. Examine questionable findings in survey radiographs (e.g., a suspected obstruction).
5. Evaluate the size, shape, position, and mucosal margins of the stomach and small intestine.
6. Investigate the cause of anorexia, acute abdominal pain, or chronic weight loss.
7. Differentiate intra-abdominal masses that may originate from the GI tract vs. other organs.
8. Postoperative assessment of GI tract integrity.
9. An upper GI study provides some information about GI motility, but there are many physiologic and pathologic conditions that can affect GI transit times (Figure 2.69). These are discussed further in Chapter 4: GI tract.

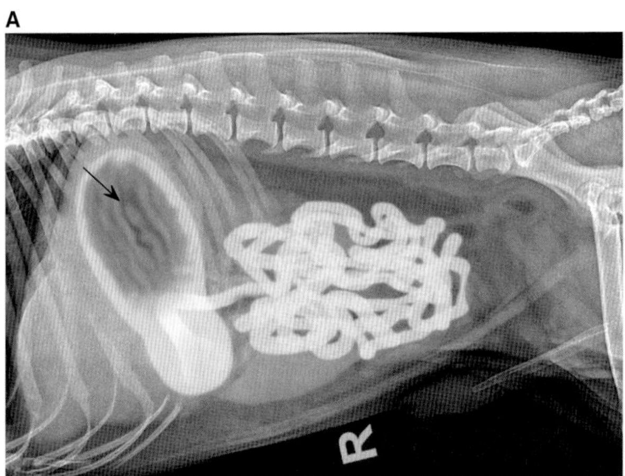

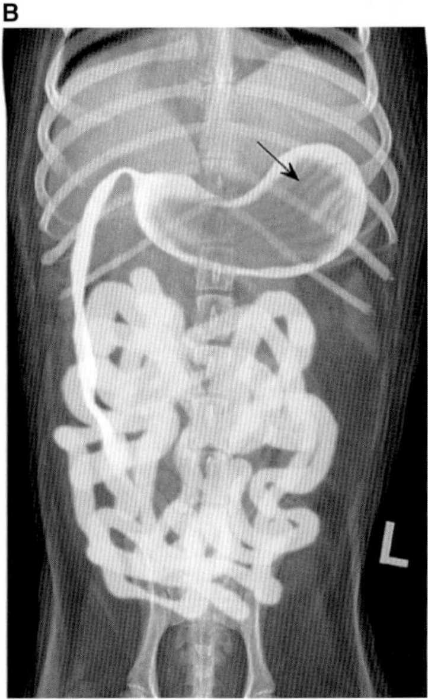

Figure 2.69 Normal upper GI study. Lateral view (**A**) and VD view (**B**) of a dog abdomen depicting positive contrast medium in the stomach and most of the small intestine. These radiographs ae a continuation of the positive contrast gastrogram depicted in Figure 2.68. There is less barium in the stomach allowing visualization of the rugal folds (black arrow).

Table 2.4 Imaging sequence for a barium upper GI study

Time	Views
5 min	VD, DV, right and left lateral
15 min	VD, DV, right and left lateral
30 min	VD and a lateral
60 min	VD and a lateral
Every 30–60 min until barium is out of stomach and in colon	VD and a lateral

Table 2.5 Average GI transit times for barium in dogs and cats

	Dog	Cat
Stomach begins to empty	1–15 min	1–10 min
Contrast in duodenum	1–15 min	1–10 min
Contrast in jejunum	30 min	15–20 min
Jejunum fills with contrast	40–60 min	20–60 min
Contrast in ileum	60 min	30–60 min
Contrast in colon	90–120 min	30–60 min
Stomach empty	1–4 h	30–60 min
Small intestine empty	3–5 h	1–3 h

Procedure for upper GI study

1. Perform a positive contrast gastrogram.
2. Make serial abdominal radiographs as shown in Table 2.4. Four views are made initially (gastrogram) and then lateral and VD views are made at the suggested time intervals until the contrast medium is in the colon and most of it has cleared the stomach and small intestine. The goal is to identify the stages of opacification as listed in Table 2.5.
3. A gastric or intestinal lesion or foreign object may be masked initially and become visible after the majority of the contrast has passed. The time sequence may need to be shortened or lengthened depending on the transit time of the contrast agent.
4. An initial delay in gastric emptying is common in stressed patients due to anxiety, fear, rage, pain, etc. In most cases, emptying will proceed normally after the patient is allowed to calm down for about 30 minutes. Delayed emptying after 30 minutes suggests pathology.
5. Any time there is a questionable radiographic finding, make the opposite lateral view and a DV view.
6. Average GI transit times for barium in dogs and cats are listed in Table 2.5.

Technical errors that can ruin an upper GI study

1. Poor patient preparation: ingesta in the GI tract can alter transit times and mimic or mask disease.
2. Insufficient volume of contrast medium: underdosing or patient vomiting may result in an inadequate amount of contrast medium to accurately evaluate the GI tract. Oral dosing may delay delivery, allowing some contrast medium to pass into the small intestine before the stomach is full, compromising the gastrogram.
3. Improper placement of orogastric tube: a tube that is kinked in the pharynx or esophagus may inhibit delivery of the contrast medium. A tube that is wrongly inserted into the trachea can lead to the deposition of contrast medium in the lungs.

4. Inadequate number or sequence of radiographs: some parts of the GI tract will not be adequately evaluated and assessment of GI transit times may be compromised. Normal physiology may be mistaken for pathology without serial radiographs to prove otherwise, such as mistaking normal peristalsis for abnormal narrowing.

Large intestine (colonography)

The large intestine includes the cecum, ascending colon, transverse colon, descending colon, rectum, and anal canal. Contrast radiography is used most often to evaluate the colon (Figure 2.70) and includes:

1. Pneumocolon.
2. Barium enema.
3. Double contrast enema.

Pneumocolon is the simplest procedure and ranges from merely infusing a syringe full of gas via the rectum to cleaning out the large intestine and completely filling it with gas. Pneumocolon most often is used to identify the colon when its position is unclear in survey radiographs. Little is expected from this procedure; however, simply differentiating a normal colon from a peritoneal gas pocket or an abnormally distended small intestine can be very helpful. When there is abundant gas in the intestinal tract, barium provides more accurate identification because there is less chance of confusing barium with other materials in the abdomen and GI tract. If other metal opacity materials are present, they should be identified in the survey radiographs. Infusing a small amount of barium via the rectum is quicker than performing an upper GI study.

A **barium enema** provides a more complete evaluation of the large intestine. Barium is the preferred contrast medium due to its superior coating action and better mucosal definition. However, if a perforation is suspected in the large intestine and a contrast study is deemed necessary, a non-ionic iodinated agent can be used.

A **double contrast enema** is a more labor-intensive contrast procedure, but provides the best visualization of the mucosal margins and may reveal small lesions that were masked by barium alone. Lesions may be masked because a barium enema completely fills the colon so that the only part of the mucosa that is visible is the thin border on either side, the remainder is obscured by barium. With a double contrast enema, the majority of the bowel lumen is filled with gas, and the mucosa is coated with just a small amount of barium. This allows a more complete evaluation of the colonic mucosa.

Indications for pneumocolon or a limited barium enema

1. Identify the position of the large intestine.
2. Differentiate gas-filled or fluid-filled small intestine from large intestine.
3. Distinguish the colon from free abdominal gas.
4. Investigate inability to pass an endoscope.

A

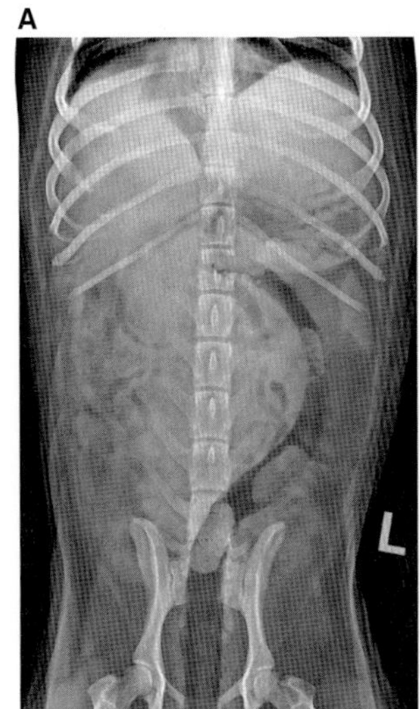

B

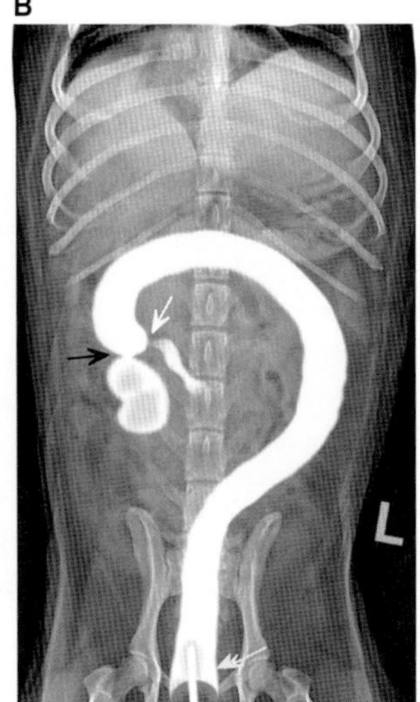

C

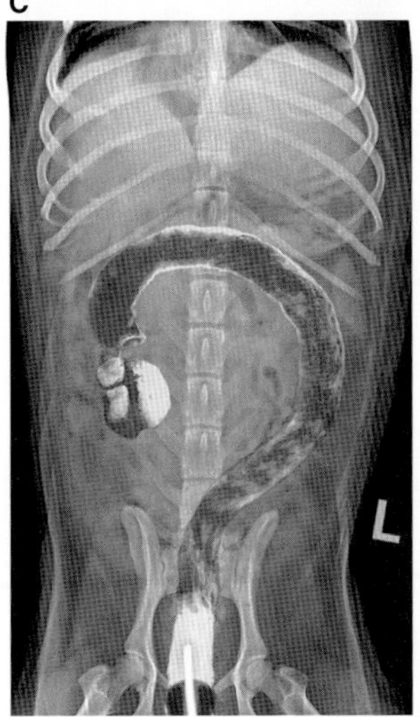

Figure 2.70 Normal colonography. VD views of a dog abdomen depicting a pneumocolon (**A**), barium enema (**B**), and a double contrast enema (**C**). In the barium enema (radiograph **B**) barium outlines the cecocolic junction (black arrow) and the ileocolic junction (white arrow). The balloon tip catheter is visible in the rectum (yellow arrow).

Indications for full barium or double contrast enema

1. Assess the size, shape, and mucosal margins of the colon (oral administration of barium will not distend the colon sufficiently for complete evaluation).
2. Investigate unexplained clinical signs of large bowel disease (e.g., tenesmus, abnormal shaped feces).
3. Aid in the diagnosis of large bowel diseases:
   a. Partial or complete obstruction.
   b. Ileocolic intussusception, cecal inversion.
   c. Mucosal damage, perforated bowel.
   d. Fistula; diverticulum; perineal hernia.
4. Postoperative evaluation of the large intestine.
5. Endoscopy is not available or limited.

Complications associated with colonography

1. Perforation of the colon, either due to faulty technique or a diseased bowel wall. Carefully inspect survey radiographs for evidence of free gas in the abdominal cavity

before proceeding with colonography. Barium in the peritoneal cavity is inflammatory, the severity of which depends on the volume deposited.

2. Inadvertent filling of the distal small intestine during a barium enema may obscure visualization of the large intestine (Figure 2.71).
3. Colon spasms can mimic pathology (e.g., infiltrative disease, stricture). Spasms may result from infusion of a cold barium solution or irritation of the colon wall caused by insertion of the catheter, a rectal examination, or prior enemas.
4. Gas embolism following pneumocolon is a rare complication. Patients with mucosal damage or portosystemic shunt are at increased risk.
5. Inadequate dosing: insufficient filling of the colon is a common problem that can mimic or mask lesions.

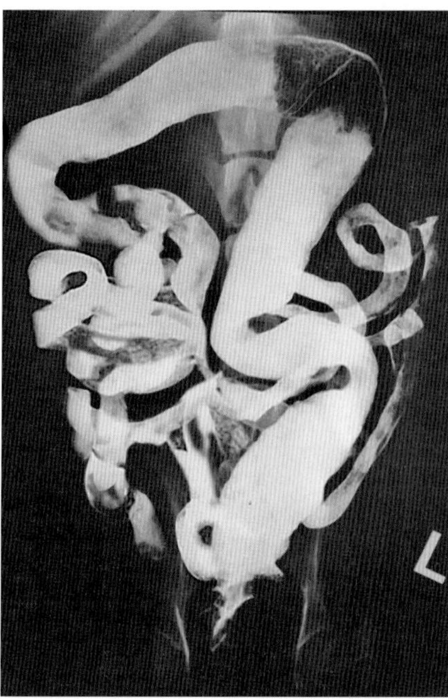

Figure 2.71 Barium enema. VD view of a dog abdomen depicting barium in both the large and small intestine. Inadvertent filling of the small bowel creates superimposition artifacts that obscure parts of the large intestine.

Procedure for pneumocolon or limited barium enema

1. No special patient preparation is required.
2. Insert a soft tip catheter or the tip of a dose syringe into the patient's rectum and slowly infuse room air:
   a. Dog dose: 1–3 ml/kg.
   b. Cat dose: 20–30 ml.
3. Make lateral and VD abdominal radiographs.
4. If the position of the colon remains unclear with a pneumocolon, repeat the study using barium.

Procedure for full barium enema

1. The GI tract should be emptied: 24–36 hour fast, oral laxatives, and cleansing enemas as needed.
2. The patient must be properly hydrated.
3. Make and evaluate survey abdominal radiographs.
4. General anesthesia or deep sedation is recommended to eliminate straining, which may expel the barium.
5. Position the patient in ventral recumbency (for a DV view) and elevate the pelvis using a towel or foam pad.
6. Insert a balloon-tipped catheter into the rectum and advance it just cranial to the anal sphincter.
7. Inflate the balloon to completely occlude the anal canal. Tape the catheter to the animal's tail.
8. Contrast medium is barium (15%–20% w/v):
   a. Dog dose: 10–15 ml/kg.
   b. Cat dose: 7–10 ml/kg.
9. Fill an enema bag or other 500 ml container with the appropriate dose and connect it to the catheter.
10. Warm the barium to body temperature prior to administration.
11. Increase the x-ray exposure over survey radiographs.
12. Allow the barium to flow with gravity into the colon. Alternatively, barium can be slowly infused using large dose syringes.
13. After half the dose is in the colon, make a DV view to assess the degree of filling. If the large bowel is not sufficiently distended, continue to add barium and monitor with additional radiographs.
14. When the large bowel is satisfactorily filled, cap the catheter to prevent leakage of barium. Rarely, a purse-string suture in the anus may be required to keep the barium in the colon. Don't forget to remove the suture prior to withdrawing the catheter.
15. Make DV, VD, right lateral, left lateral, and VD oblique views of the abdomen. Each view is important because gravity greatly affects the distribution and appearance of contrast medium in a hollow viscus. **After completing the lengthy preparations for a barium enema, don't fail to make ALL the views.**
16. If needed, gentle abdominal compression can be used to displace the overlying bowel (Figure 2.19).
17. When finished, place the patient in left lateral recumbency and elevate its cranial half to allow the barium to drain back into the enema bag. Place the bag on the floor for quicker emptying. Gently massaging the patient's abdomen may speed the process.
18. Deflate and remove the catheter unless a double contrast enema is planned.
19. The rectum and anal canal may not be adequately examined with a barium enema. Radiographs made during evacuation of the contrast medium may yield useful information as the barium opacifies these areas during its exit.

Procedure for double contrast barium enema

1. Perform a barium enema as described.
2. After draining the barium from the colon, leave the catheter in place and position the patient in ventral recumbency.
3. Slowly infuse 10 ml/kg of gas (typically room air), a volume sufficient to re-distend the colon.
4. Periodically make DV radiographs to assess the degree of colon distention.
5. When the colon is sufficiently distended, rotate the patient several times to reduce the pooling of barium and evenly coat the mucosa.
6. Make DV, VD, right lateral, left lateral, and VD oblique views of the abdomen.
7. Place the patient in left lateral recumbency between radiographs to trap any gas emboli in the right atrium, should emboli occur.
8. When finished, deflate the catheter balloon and allow gas to escape. Gently massaging the patient's abdomen may help empty the colon if needed.

Urogenital contrast studies

Radiographic contrast studies used to evaluate the kidneys, urinary bladder, urethra, and uterus. Barium is never used for these studies, only iodinated contrast media. During contrast radiography of the urinary tract, the patient may urinate and contaminate the FOV with urine that contains contrast medium. This can create artifacts in the radiographs. The following urogenital procedures are discussed in this section:

1. Excretory urography (EU)
2. Cystography
3. Urethrography
4. Vaginography

Excretory urography

Intravenous injection of an iodinated contrast medium is used to evaluate the kidneys, ureters, and urinary bladder (Figure 2.72). Other names for excretory urography (EU) include *intravenous urography* or *intravenous pyelography* (*IVP*).

Indication for excretory urography (EU)

1. Evaluate abnormal size or shape of the kidney(s).
2. Determine the location of the kidney(s), either when not identified in survey radiographs or in relation to an intra-abdominal mass.
3. Investigate the cause of abnormal urine (e.g., hematuria, pyuria, crystalluria) or abnormal urination (e.g., dysuria, stranguria, incontinence).
4. Evaluate the integrity of a kidney or ureter.
5. Examine the ureters for suspected ectopic location.
6. Investigate inability to catheterize the urinary bladder.
7. Provide a crude measurement of renal function.
8. Postoperative assessment of the urinary tract.

A

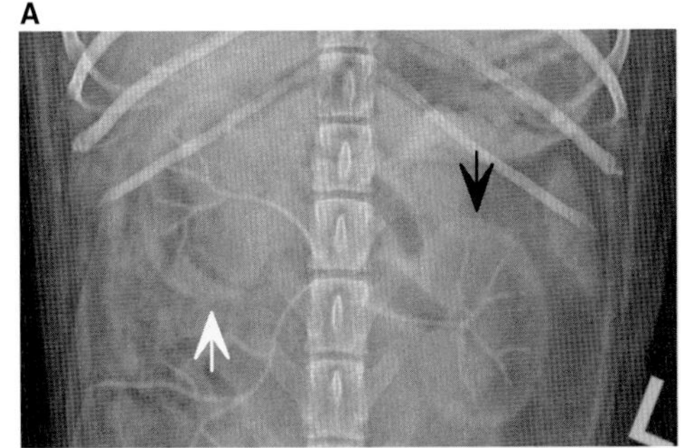

B

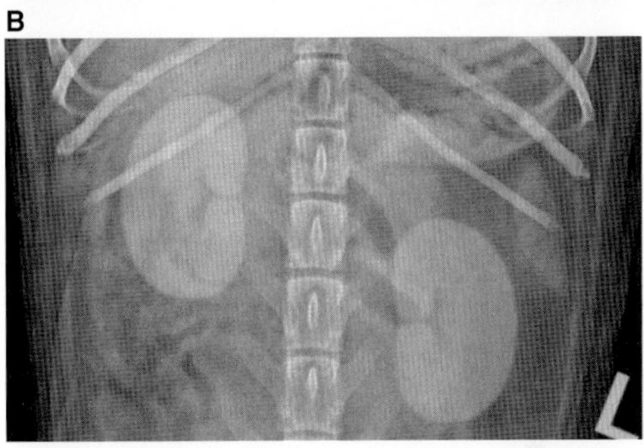

C

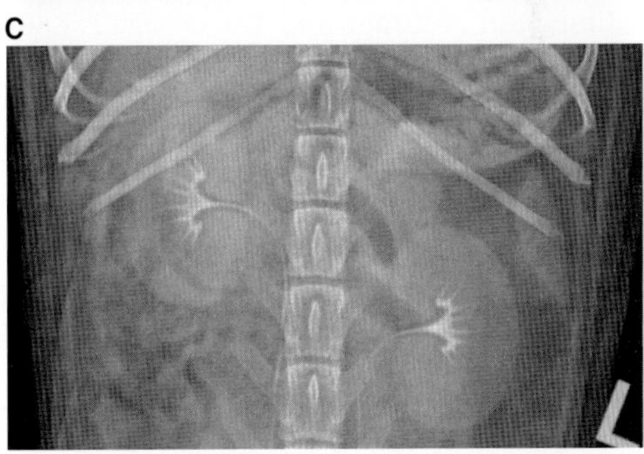

D

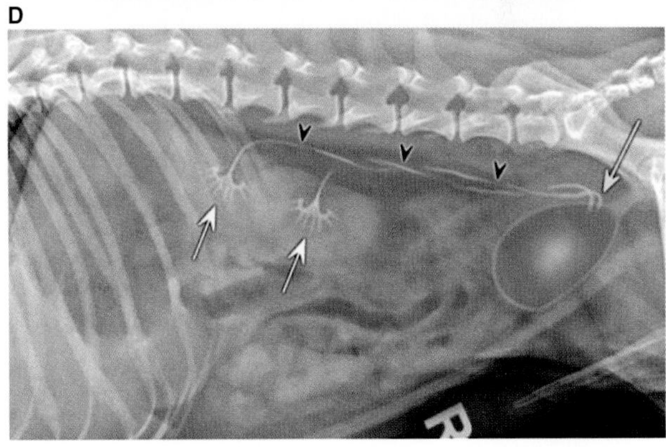

Figure 2.72 Normal excretory urogram. VD views of a dog abdomen (**A–C**) depicting the normal appearance of the right (white arrow) and left (black arrow) kidneys during the vascular phase (**A**), nephrogram phase (**B**), and pyelogram phase (**C**) of an excretory urogram. The lateral view (**D**) depicts the pyelogram phase with positive contrast medium in the renal collecting systems (white arrows) and ureters (black arrowheads). A concurrent negative contrast cystogram is visible which enhances visualization of the ureterovesicular junctions (yellow arrow). Positive contrast medium entering the gas-filled urinary bladder produces a double contrast cystogram.

Contraindications to excretory urography

1. Anuria.
2. Severe dehydration.
3. Urethral obstruction.
4. Uremia is not a true contraindication, but decreased glomerular filtration may prevent opacification of the urinary tract, resulting in an ineffective study.

Procedure for excretory urography

1. Empty the GI tract: 12–24 hour fast and cleansing enemas as needed.
2. Sedation/anesthesia is recommended to aid in patient positioning, to minimize adverse reactions, and to simplify the application of abdominal compression.
3. The patient should be well hydrated and renal function should be known prior to EU.
4. Make and evaluate survey abdominal radiographs.
5. Place an intravenous (IV) catheter in a peripheral vein. A jugular vein can be used if neither a cephalic nor saphenous vein is available.
6. Contrast agent is 0.45 ml/kg of sterile, non-ionic, iodinated medium (400 mgI/ml). The dosage is 880 mgI/kg. If uremia is present, increase the dose by 10%–50%. An adequate dose of contrast agent is critical to making a meaningful study.
7. Warm the contrast medium to body temperature prior to administration.
8. Increase the x-ray exposure over survey radiographs.
9. With the patient positioned for a VD view of the abdomen, inject the contrast medium as rapidly as possible (i.e., inject it as a bolus).
10. In large dogs, use two catheters for rapid bolus injection; equally divide the total dose of contrast medium between the two catheters and inject simultaneously.
11. Immediately at the end of injection begin making abdominal radiographs as described in Table 2.6. The right lateral view may be preferred to better separate the kidneys.

Table 2.6 Serial radiographs for excretory urography

Phase	Time	Views	Structures
Vascular	15 s	VD	Renal vasculature
Nephrogram	1 min	VD, R Lat	Renal parenchyma
Pyelogram	5 min	VD, R Lat	Renal collecting system
Compression	10 min	VD, VD oblique	Distal ureters, vesicoureteral jct
Ureteral	15 min	VD, R Lat	Ureters, urinary bladder
Bladder	40 min	VD, Lat	Urinary bladder filled

Modifications to EU procedure

1. If evaluation of the vascular phase is not important, the contrast medium can be injected more slowly, which reduces the likelihood of an adverse reaction. In this case, begin making radiographs 1 minute after injection.
2. If an ectopic ureter is suspected, a concurrent pneumocystogram may enhance visualization of the ureterovesicular junction (Figure 2.72).
3. **Compression radiography** sometimes is used to increase filling of the renal collecting systems and ureters. This technique involves tightly wrapping the patient's caudal abdomen with an elastic bandage or "belly band" to temporarily restrict the flow of urine. Compression is applied for 1–2 minutes after making the 5-minute radiographs. Lateral, VD, and VD oblique views are made immediately after removing the compression. The VD oblique views are made by rotating the patient 20° to the right and then 20° to the left to reduce superimposition artifacts and better visualize the ureters. Compression tends to be most successful when the patient is sedated or anesthetized. It may be useful to investigate suspected ectopic ureters, but it is not done with a concurrent pneumocystogram. Abdominal compression should not be performed in patients with an intra-abdominal mass or full urinary bladder.

Cystography

Contrast radiography of the urinary bladder may be performed with negative contrast media, positive contrast media, or both (Figure 2.73). The choice of which type of agent to use depends on the purpose of the study. During cystography, the urinary bladder should be only moderately distended because full distention will stretch the bladder wall and may hide mucosal lesions. Chronic cystitis or fibrosis can significantly limit distensibility; the volume a diseased bladder can hold may be less than 20% of a normal bladder.

Pneumocystography is the simplest procedure. It involves replacing urine in the bladder with gas, typically room air. Pneumocystography may be contraindicated in patients with hematuria due to the risk of gas embolism. In these patients, carbon dioxide or nitrous oxide is safer than room air because these gases are more rapidly absorbed should they enter the bloodstream. A pneumocystogram is an effective method to examine bladder wall thickness but generally is not as reliable as positive contrast cystography to locate the urinary bladder or to assess bladder wall integrity. Gas in the bladder may help identify larger masses, but it is less reliable for smaller lesions.

Positive contrast cystography is preferred over pneumocystography to diagnose a ruptured urinary bladder or urethral leakage and to identify abnormal communications between the bladder and adjacent structures. With positive contrast cystography, the bladder lumen often is highly opacified, which may obscure smaller lesions and calculi.

Because of this, positive contrast agents usually are diluted for cystography.

Double contrast cystography provides the best evaluation of the bladder mucosa and is more reliable in the detection of smaller and less opaque lesions, including soft tissue opacity calculi. In a double contrast cystogram, the bladder lumen is distended with gas, and there is a thin layer or "pool" of positive contrast medium in the dependent portion. Although it is a more time-consuming procedure, a double contrast cystogram is more likely to demonstrate smaller mucosal lesions, masses, and calculi.

A

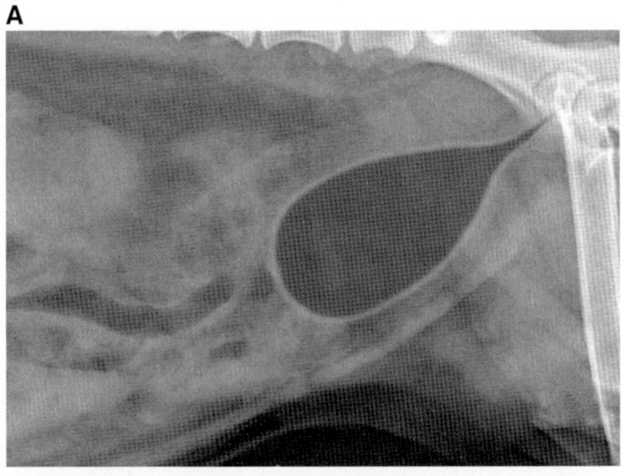

B

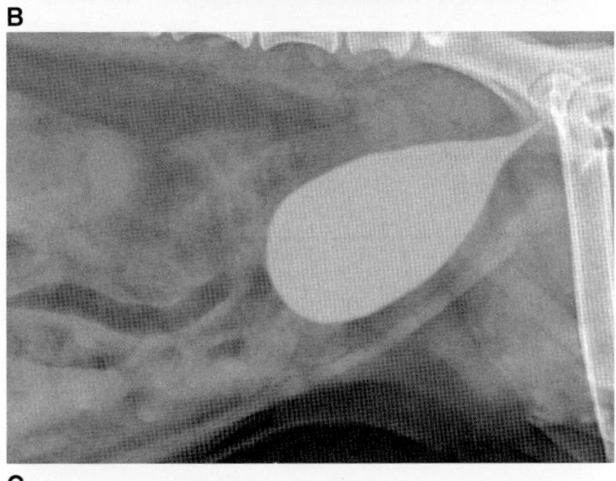

C

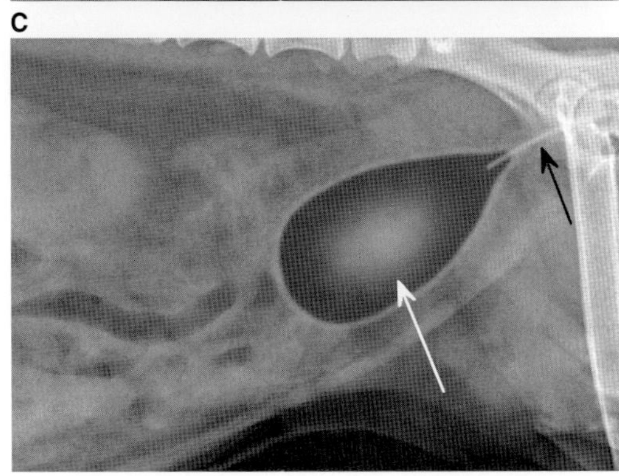

Figure 2.73 Cystography. Lateral views of a dog abdomen depicting a pneumocystogram (**A**), a positive contrast cystogram (**B**), and a double contrast cystogram (**C**). In the double contrast study, a catheter is visible in the neck of the urinary bladder (black arrow) and a small puddle of positive contrast medium is visible in the center of the bladder lumen (white arrow).

Indications for cystography

1. Determine the location of the urinary bladder, either when the bladder is not visible in survey radiographs or to distinguish it from a caudal abdominal mass.
2. Investigate a urinary bladder that palpates or appears in radiographs as abnormal.
3. Evaluate the integrity of the urinary bladder.
4. Investigate the cause of abnormal urine (e.g., hematuria, pyuria, crystalluria) or abnormal urination (e.g., stranguria, pollakiuria, incontinence).
5. Aid in the diagnosis of chronic or recurrent cystitis.
6. Examine the urinary bladder for suspected neoplasia.
7. Identify an abnormal communication between the urinary bladder and an adjacent structure.

Procedure for cystography

1. Evacuate the colon and rectum with cleansing enemas.
2. Make and evaluate survey abdominal radiographs.
3. Sedation/anesthesia is recommended.
4. Patient is in lateral recumbency. During pneumocystography, left lateral recumbency is recommended to trap gas emboli in the right atrium, should emboli occur.
5. Aseptically catheterize and empty the urinary bladder; submit urine for analysis as needed.
6. Flush and remove any blood clots and/or debris from the bladder lumen.
7. Contrast agent is either gas (typically room air) or sterile iodinated medium (100 mgI/ml). Most iodinated agents need to be diluted with sterile saline or sterile water to make this low concentration.
8. The dose of contrast medium is a volume that is sufficient to moderately distend the urinary bladder. The doses listed below are based on the volume a normal bladder is expected to hold. Keep in mind that chronic bladder disease may limit distensibility to 1 ml/kg or less.
   a. Dogs: estimated dose is 5–10 ml/kg.
   b. Cats: estimated dose is 2–5 ml/kg.
9. Warm the contrast agent to body temperature prior to administration.
10. Reduce the x-ray exposure for pneumocystography and increase the exposure for a positive contrast cystogram.
11. To reduce straining caused by urinary bladder distention, 3–5 ml of 2% lidocaine can be infused into the bladder lumen prior to adding the contrast medium. Lidocaine generally is not needed in patients that are anesthetized or heavily sedated.
12. Carefully monitor the administration of the contrast agent and stop when the bladder feels firm and adequately distended, as evidenced by external palpation or back pressure on the syringe plunger.
13. After infusion, make lateral and VD oblique views of the caudal abdomen.
14. When evaluating bladder wall integrity, make the radiographs during infusion, near the end of contrast

administration. Leakage must be detected quickly because the contrast agent will rapidly dissipate in the abdominal cavity.

15. Additional contrast medium can be added as needed to maintain adequate bladder distention.

Procedure for double contrast cystography

1. Perform a negative contrast cystogram as described.
2. Add a small volume of warm, undiluted, iodinated contrast medium (300 mgI/ml) to the bladder lumen:
   a. Dose in small dogs (less than 12 kg): 1–3 ml.
   b. Dose in large dogs (more than 12 kg): 5–10 ml.
   c. Dose in cats: 0.5–1.0 ml.
3. Gently roll the patient 360° to coat the entire bladder.
4. Make lateral and VD oblique views of the caudal abdomen.
5. Infuse additional gas as needed to maintain bladder distention during radiography.
6. If a positive contrast cystogram was done first, remove most of the contrast agent from the bladder before adding gas. Infuse the dose of gas slowly to minimize formation of bubbles, which can complicate interpretation of the study.

Urethrography

Positive or negative contrast media used to evaluate the urethra. Positive contrast urethrograms are much easier to interpret than negative contrast studies (Figure 2.74). In general, the urethra is larger and better visualized with a moderately distended urinary bladder. The bladder may be distended with urine, sterile saline, or contrast medium. The urethra in cats and female dogs may be more difficult to catheterize than in male dogs and therefore is discussed separately below.

Indications for urethrography

1. Evaluate the size, shape, and position of the urethra.
2. Investigate the cause of abnormal urination (e.g., stranguria, hematuria, dysuria).
3. Assess urethral integrity.
4. Examine the urethra for suspected obstruction.
5. Investigate difficulty or inability to catheterize the urethra.
6. Aid in the diagnosis of prostatic disease.
7. Evaluate a congenital urethral anomaly.

Procedure for urethrography

1. Evacuate colon and rectum with cleansing enemas.
2. Make and evaluate survey abdominal radiographs. With male dogs, include a flexed lateral view of the urethra (Figure 2.20).
3. Sedation/anesthesia is recommended.
4. Patient is in lateral recumbency. Male dogs are positioned for the lateral urethral view.
5. Contrast agent is sterile, non-ionic, iodinated medium (100 mgI/ml). Most agents must be diluted with sterile saline or sterile water to make this low concentration.
   a. Dog dose: 10–20 ml.
   b. Cat dose: 5–10 ml.
6. Warm the contrast medium to body temperature prior to administration.
7. Increase the x-ray exposure over survey radiographs.

A

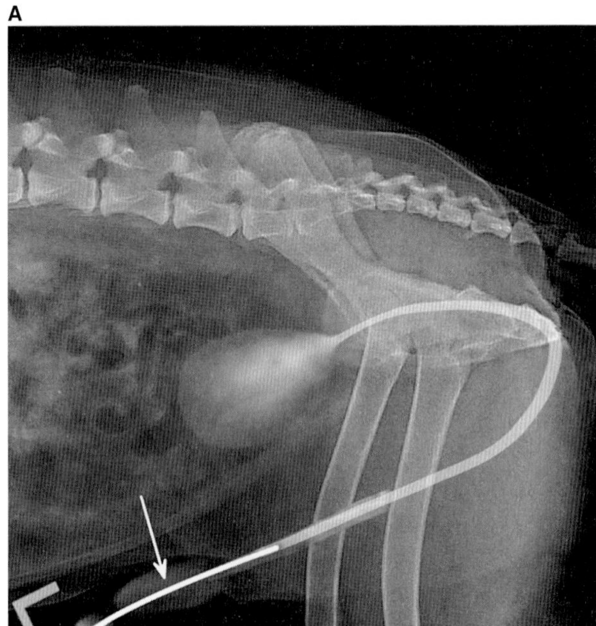

B

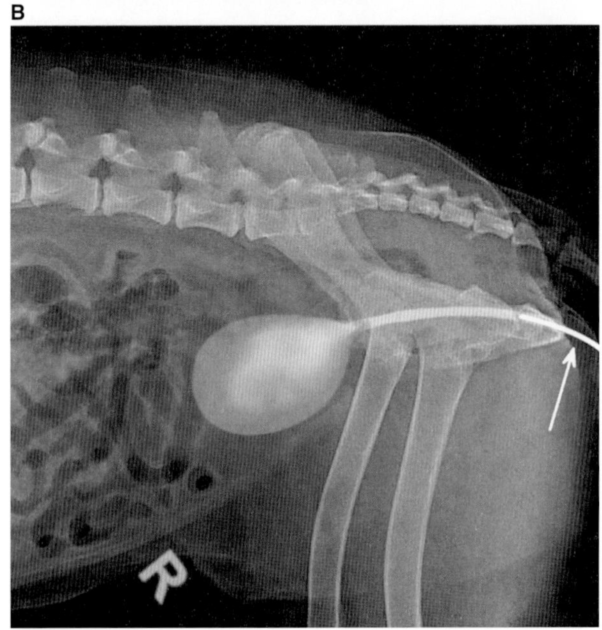

Figure 2.74 Normal retrograde urethrography. Lateral views of the caudal abdomen of a male dog (**A**) and a female dog (**B**) depicting a catheter in the distal urethra (arrows) and positive contrast medium filling the urethra and entering the urinary bladder.

Male dogs

1. Infuse 2 ml of 2% lidocaine into the urethra as needed to reduce straining and urethral spasms.
2. Prefill the lumen of a balloon tip catheter (e.g., Swan Ganz, Foley) with contrast medium to avoid injecting air bubbles.
3. Insert the catheter just inside the urethra, so the tip is in the most distal portion of the urethra. Inflate the balloon enough to prevent leakage of contrast medium. If the purpose of the study is to evaluate the prostatic urethra only, the catheter can be advanced to the level of the ischial arch.
4. Rapidly infuse the contrast medium retrograde into the urethra.
5. Make a lateral view of the urethra during infusion of the final 2–3 ml of contrast medium. The pressure inside the urethra during infusion helps distend it.
6. Infuse additional doses of contrast agent while making VD and VD oblique views.
7. Urethrography can be performed with cystography by positioning the tip of the catheter at the level of the ischial arch or further distally prior to infusion.

Female dogs and all cats

1. Retrograde urethrography can be performed in cats and female dogs using a technique similar to that just described for male dogs:
   a. Insert a balloon tip catheter into the distal urethra and inflate the balloon.
   b. Infuse 5–10 ml of undiluted contrast medium.
   c. Make a lateral radiograph near the end of infusion.
   d. Repeat contrast infusion for VD and oblique views.
2. Alternatively, a retrograde urethrogram can be done after positive contrast cystogram by infusing 5–10 ml of undiluted contrast medium while withdrawing the catheter (make lateral radiograph while infusing).
3. A voiding or antegrade urethrogram (Figure 2.75) also can be done after positive contrast cystogram (bladder is filled via either excretory urography or catheterization). Gently compress the abdomen over the urinary bladder using a low-density plastic paddle or wooden spoon and make lateral radiograph during voiding (use caution to avoid rupturing the bladder).
4. The female urethra may be adequately visualized during vaginography.

Vaginography

Positive contrast radiography used to evaluate the vagina, cervix, and urethra (Figure 2.76).

Indications for vaginography

1. Determine size, shape, and position of female urethra.
2. Assess integrity of female urethra.
3. Examine vagina for suspected mass, tear, or stricture.
4. Investigate urogenital abnormality (e.g., ectopic ureter, rectovaginal fistula).

A

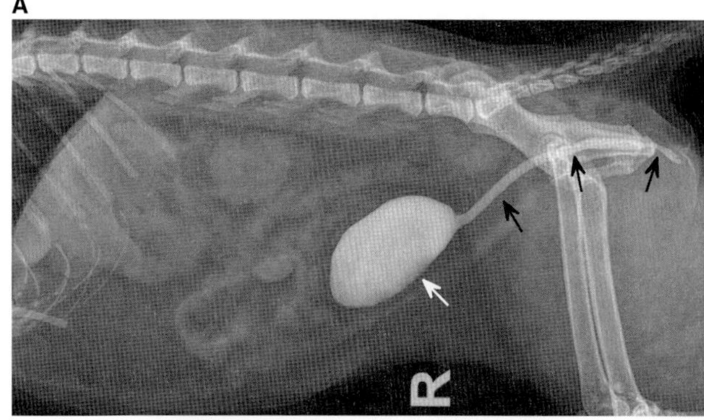

B

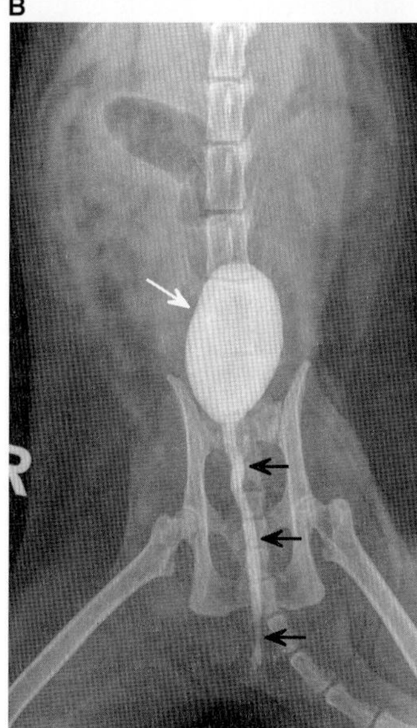

Figure 2.75 Normal antegrade urethrography. Lateral view (**A**) and VD view (**B**) of a cat abdomen depicting positive contrast medium in the urinary bladder (white arrows) and urethra (black arrows).

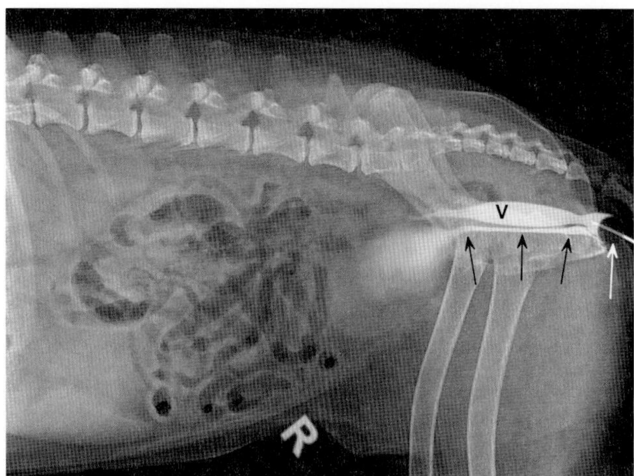

Figure 2.76 Vaginography. Lateral view of a dog caudal abdomen depicting a balloon tip catheter inserted into the vagina (white arrow). Positive contrast medium fills the vagina (V) and the urethra (black arrows) and enters the urinary bladder.

Procedure for vaginography

1. Make and evaluate survey radiographs.
2. General anesthesia is required.
3. Patient is in lateral recumbency.
4. Aseptically catheterize and empty the urinary bladder. Save a urine sample for analysis if needed.
5. Remove the urinary catheter and insert a balloon tip catheter (e.g., Swan Ganz, Foley) into the vestibule. If the tip of catheter (the part distal to the balloon) is too long and enters the vagina, it may be necessary to cut the tip to make it shorter.
6. Inflate the catheter balloon to prevent leakage of contrast medium. If needed, a plastic clamp can be used to tightly seal the vaginal orifice around the catheter.
7. Contrast agent is a volume of sterile, non-ionic, iodinated medium (300 mgI/ml) sufficient to fill the vagina:
   a. Dog estimated dose: 10–30 ml.
   b. Cat estimated dose: 5–10 ml.
8. Warm the contrast medium to body temperature prior to administration.
9. Increase the x-ray exposure over survey radiographs.
10. Infusion of the contrast solution will fill the vagina first and then reflux into the urethra and urinary bladder.
11. Make a lateral view of the pelvis and caudal abdomen near the end of infusion while the vagina is distended with contrast medium. Administer additional doses for the VD and VD oblique views.

Cardiovascular contrast studies

Iodinated contrast media can be used to evaluate the heart, blood vessels, and lymphatics. Barium is <u>never</u> used in these procedures. Gas has been used to evaluate the pericardium, but it is <u>never</u> injected intravenously. The following procedures are discussed:

1. Angiocardiography
2. Pneumopericardiography
3. Lymphography
4. Venous portography

Angiocardiography

Radiographic contrast studies to evaluate the heart and vascular system range from simply injecting contrast medium into a peripheral blood vessel and making sequential radiographs (*non-selective* angiocardiography) to the use of highly specialized equipment and precise injection techniques (*selective* angiocardiography). **Non-selective angiocardiography** can be performed by most veterinary professionals using good quality x-ray equipment and a method for rapidly producing multiple radiographs (Figures 2.77 and 2.78).

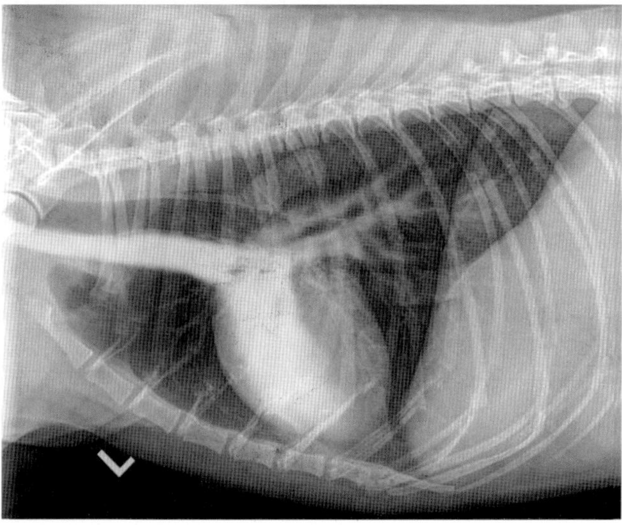

Figure 2.77 <u>Non-selective angiocardiogram</u>. Lateral view of a dog thorax depicting positive contrast medium injected into a jugular vein. The cranial vena cava, right heart, and main pulmonary arteries are beginning to opacify.

Selective angiocardiography requires specialized training, custom catheters, a power injector, a rapid film recording device, and fluoroscopy. In a selective study, an intravascular catheter is advanced to a point close to a suspected lesion, and contrast medium is rapidly injected under high pressure. These procedures typically are limited to teaching hospitals and larger specialty practices.

Indications for non-selective angiocardiography

1. Evaluate size and shape of cardiac chambers.
2. Differentiate some types of feline cardiomyopathy.
3. Investigate suspected right-to-left shunt.
4. Identify intra-cardiac mass (e.g., tumor, thrombus).
5. Evaluate cause of pericardial effusion.
6. Examine aorta, main pulmonary arteries, and cranial or caudal vena cava for displacement or blockage.

Procedure for non-selective angiocardiography

1. Make and evaluate survey thoracic radiographs.
2. General anesthesia is recommended, although well-monitored sedation may be used.
3. Patient is in lateral recumbency.
4. Contrast agent is sterile iodinated medium (300 mgI/ml), non-ionic is recommended:
   a. <u>Dose</u> in dog or cat: 400 mgI/kg.
   b. Maximum volume per injection is 90 ml.
   c. Maximum dose per patient is 1000 mgI/kg.
   d. Contrast agent may be diluted with sterile saline or sterile water to create sufficient volume to opacify all parts of the area of interest.

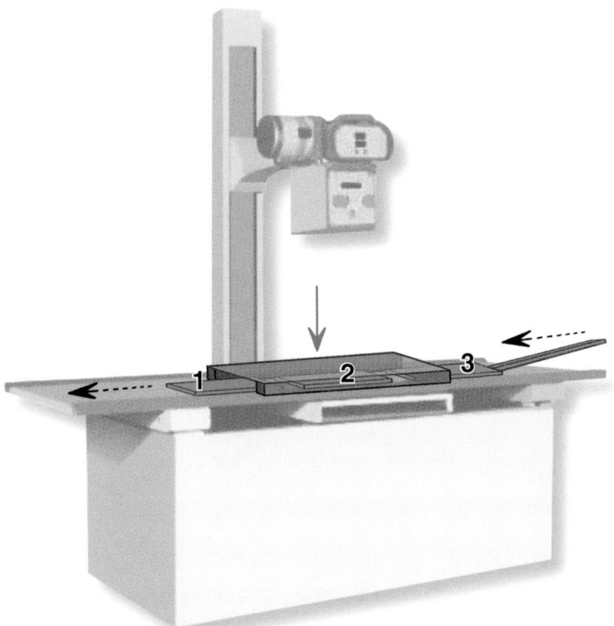

Figure 2.78 Cassette tunnel for rapidly producing multiple radiographs. This illustration depicts a cassette tunnel and three imaging cassettes sitting on an x-ray table. The cassettes are colored green and numbered 1, 2, and 3. The cassettes are sliding under the tunnel in the direction of the black dotted arrows. The cassette tunnel consists of a wooden platform supported on either side by a thin strip of wood. The patient rests on the platform (blue arrow). The tunnel is just tall enough and wide enough to allow cassettes to pass through, under the patient. Behind cassette number 3 is a wooden stick or "push pole" which is used to quickly move the next cassette into position. With a cassette tunnel, multiple x-ray exposures can be made quickly without moving the patient.

5. Place an indwelling 14–18 gauge catheter in a peripheral vein:
   a. Use a cephalic or jugular vein to evaluate the cranial vena cava and heart.
   b. Use a saphenous or lateral metatarsal vein to evaluate the caudal vena cava.
6. Warm the contrast agent to body temperature prior to administration.
7. Increase the x-ray exposure over survey radiographs.
8. Make a test injection and a test radiograph to ensure correct catheter placement.
9. Rapidly inject the contrast medium as a bolus; total injection time should be 1–3 seconds.
10. Make a lateral view immediately at the end of injection followed by serial radiographs every 1–3 seconds.
11. A cassette tunnel (Figure 2.78), rapid film changer, or high-speed digital radiography system usually is needed to make multiple radiographs over such a short period of time.
12. As needed, inject additional doses of contrast medium to make more lateral views; total dose not to exceed 1000 mgI/kg.
13. Reposition the patient for VD/DV views and inject doses of contrast medium as needed to make the number of VD views required. Again, the total dose not to exceed 1000 mgI/kg.

Pneumopericardiography

Injecting gas into the pericardial sac is rarely performed due to the availability of echocardiography. It has been used to investigate the cause of pericardial effusion and to better visualize epicardial, pericardial, and heart base masses (Figure 2.79).

Procedure for pneumopericardiogram

1. Make and evaluate survey thoracic radiographs.
2. Patient sedation/anesthesia is recommended.
3. Patient is in left lateral recumbency to trap gas emboli in right atrium, should emboli occur.
4. Aseptically place an indwelling catheter into the pericardial sac at the right fifth or sixth intercostal space.
5. Remove as much pericardial fluid as possible.
6. Contrast medium is gas, typically is room air. Carbon dioxide or nitrous oxide may be preferred because they are better absorbed and carry less risk of gas embolism. The dose of gas is about 80% of the volume of fluid extracted from the pericardial sac.
7. Decrease the x-ray exposure from survey radiographs.
8. After injecting the dose of gas, make right lateral, left lateral, DV, and VD views. Horizontal beam radiographs may also be helpful.
9. Return the patient to left lateral recumbency when finished.

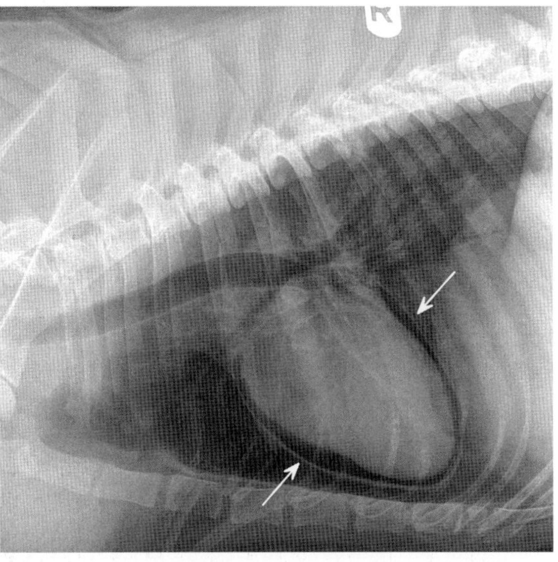

Figure 2.79 Normal pneumopericardiogram. Lateral view of a dog thorax depicting gas injected into the pericardial sac (arrow).

Lymphography

Positive contrast radiography used to evaluate the lymphatic vessels and lymph nodes (Figure 2.80). The lymphatic system is part of the circulatory system. Cells and tissues throughout the body are bathed in lymphatic fluid. The fluid is transported in fragile, low-pressure vessels that connect to lymph nodes. The lymph nodes filter the fluid at known locations in the body. Lymphography is used to evaluate the flow of lymphatic fluid. The procedure may be useful in patients with a suspected lack of lymphatic flow, either due to blockage or rupture. Lymphography, however, is difficult to perform. It requires expert skill, experience, and considerable patience. Even in normal patients, there often is inconsistent flow and lymph vessels are easily ruptured during the procedure.

Peripheral lymphography can be performed by catheterizing a small lymphatic vessel in a distal limb or by directly injecting a palpable lymph node with contrast medium (Figure 2.80). Injection into deeper lymph nodes may be useful to evaluate the cisterna chyli and the thoracic duct (i.e., *mesenteric lymphography*).

Procedure for peripheral lymphography

1. Make and evaluate survey radiographs of the limb of interest.
2. Use chemical restraint to avoid patient movement.
3. Patient is in lateral recumbency.
4. Aseptically inject 0.25–1.5 ml of blue dye into an interdigital space to help identify a peripheral lymphatic vessel. A blue dye is a dilute vegetable dye such as methylene blue or Evan's blue.
5. Wait 10–20 minutes for the dye to be absorbed.
6. Surgically expose a blue stained lymphatic vessel. The lymphatics commonly are found along the dorsal aspect of the metatarsus or metacarpus. Sometimes they are more visible proximally, near the saphenous vein in the tarsus or near the accessory cephalic vein in the carpus.
7. Preplace two sutures around the lymphatic vessel and cannulate the vessel with a 25- to 30-gauge needle.
8. Attach an extension tube prefilled with heparinized saline to the needle.
9. Contrast agent is 0.5 ml/kg of sterile, non-ionic iodinated media (200 mgI/ml).
10. Warm the contrast medium to body temperature prior to administration.
11. Increase the x-ray exposure over survey radiographs.
12. Injection can be made by hand or via an infusion pump, but avoid excessive pressure as this can rupture the lymphatic vessel.
13. Alternatively, non-diluted contrast agent can be injected directly into a peripheral lymph node, such as the popliteal lymph node when investigating pelvic limb lymphedema. However, opacification of the lymphatics tends to be less consistent and less visible with the technique.

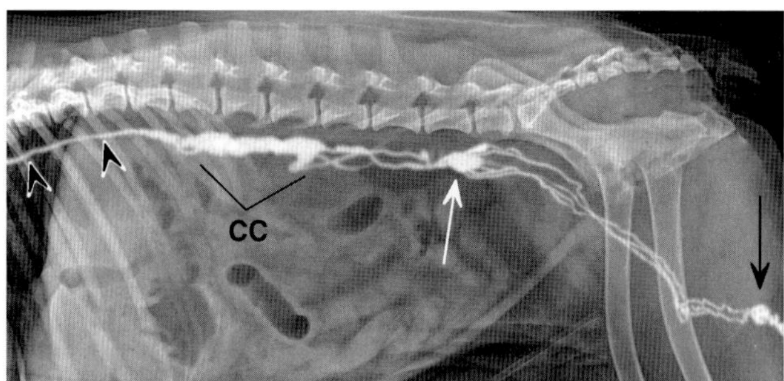

Figure 2.80 Normal lymphogram. Lateral view of a dog abdomen depicting positive contrast medium injected into a popliteal lymph node (black arrow). The contrast medium migrates through the lymphatic vessels to the medial iliac lymph nodes (white arrow) and then cranially into the cisterna chyli (CC) and thoracic duct (black arrowheads).

14. Immediately after injection begin making orthogonal views of the limb and any associated lymphatic draining regions (e.g., abdomen, pelvis, thorax).
15. The number of radiographs needed depends on the rate of lymphatic filling.

Procedure for mesenteric lymphography

1. Make and evaluate survey radiographs of the thorax and abdomen.
2. Patient anesthesia is required.
3. Perform exploratory laparotomy to isolate a lymph node near the cecum.
4. Inject the lymph node with 0.5–1.0 ml of blue dye to improve visualization of the lymphatics.
5. Cannulate a mesenteric lymphatic vessel with a 22-gauge catheter. Alternatively, the cisterna chyli itself can be cannulated directly.
6. Contrast agent is 1.0 ml/kg of a sterile, non-ionic, iodinated medium (300 mgI/ml).
7. Warm the contrast medium to body temperature prior to administration.
8. Increase the x-ray exposure over survey radiographs.
9. Make lateral abdominal radiographs every 5–10 minutes until there is adequate filling of the thoracic duct.

Venous portography

Positive contrast radiographic evaluation of the portal venous system is called **portography** and involves injecting an iodinated contrast agent into a mesenteric vein (*venous portography*) or into the spleen (*splenoportography*). Venous portography is more likely to yield a diagnosis than splenoportography and is associated with lower morbidity (Figure 2.81).

Indications for venous portography

1. Investigate a suspected portosystemic vascular shunt.
2. Differentiate intra-hepatic from extra-hepatic portosystemic shunts.

Procedure for venous portography

1. Make and evaluate survey abdominal radiographs.
2. General anesthesia is required because laparotomy is performed.
3. Patient is in lateral recumbency.
4. Contrast agent is 1 ml/kg of non-ionic iodinated contrast medium (400 mgI/ml).
   a. Maximum volume per injection is 90 ml.
   b. Total dose should not exceed 1000 mgI/kg.
5. Warm the contrast medium to body temperature prior to administration.
6. Increase the x-ray exposure over survey radiographs.
7. Perform exploratory laparotomy to look for a portosystemic venous shunt. If no shunt is identified, place an 18–20 gauge catheter in a jejunal vein.
8. If the patient must be moved for imaging, attach an extension tubing to the catheter and leave the end of the tubing outside the abdomen.
9. In radiography, make a small test injection and a test lateral view to document proper catheter placement.
10. Rapidly inject the full dose of contrast as a bolus, but avoid excessive pressure as this may dislodge the catheter or rupture the vein.
11. At the end of the injection, make a lateral view of the abdomen. Make additional radiographs as needed until the portal vascular system or the caudal vena cava is visualized. The number of images depends on the size and location of the shunt.
12. Reposition the patient for VD views and inject additional doses of contrast as needed; total dose not to exceed 1000 mgI/kg.

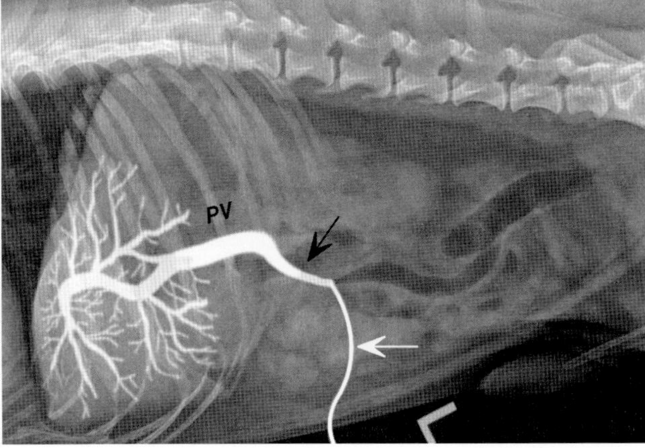

Figure 2.81 Normal portogram. Lateral view of a dog abdomen depicting positive contrast medium injected through a catheter (white arrow) into a jejunal vein (black arrow) to create a venous portogram. The contrast agent flows to the portal vein (PV) and then into liver where it opacifies the intra-hepatic branches.

Procedure for splenoportography

1. Make and evaluate survey abdominal radiographs.
2. General anesthesia is required.
3. Patient is in lateral recumbency.
4. Contrast agent is non-ionic iodinated contrast medium (400 mgI/ml):
   a. Dose in dogs and cats: 1 ml/kg.
   b. Maximum volume per injection is 90 ml.
   c. Total dose should not exceed 1000 mgI/kg.
5. Warm the contrast medium to body temperature prior to administration.
6. Increase the x-ray exposure over survey radiographs.
7. Aseptically inject the contrast agent directly into the spleen, either percutaneously or via laparotomy.
8. If available, ultrasound guidance is recommended for percutaneous injection.
9. Make lateral and VD views of the abdomen shortly after injection. Make additional radiographs as needed to evaluate portal circulation.

Neurologic contrast studies

Positive contrast radiographic studies of the spine to evaluate the spinal canal, spinal cord, and intervertebral discs. **These studies are performed only if there is intent to do surgery, should a surgical lesion be found.** Only sterile, non-ionic, iodinated contrast media are used for these studies. Ionic agents or barium are never used.

Discography

Discography is a positive contrast evaluation of an intervertebral disc (Figure 2.82), specifically to evaluate the integrity of the annulus fibrosis. Discography involves injecting contrast medium into the nucleus pulposus. It has been used most often to investigate disease at the cauda equina because, unlike in other parts of the spinal column, a needle can be positioned relatively accurately at the lumbosacral junction without using fluoroscopy.

Indications

1. Evaluate the integrity of the annulus fibrosis by visualizing the size, shape, and position of the nucleus pulposus.
2. Investigate a suspected Schmorl's node.

Procedure for discography

1. Make and evaluate survey spinal radiographs.
2. Note any congenital anomalies or degenerative changes along the spine that may interfere with needle placement.
3. General anesthesia is required.
4. Patient is in lateral recumbency.

5. Contrast agent is 0.25–3.0 ml of sterile, non-ionic, iodinated medium (300 mgI/ml); the dose should not exceed 3.0 ml.
6. Warm the contrast agent to body temperature prior to administration.
7. Increase the x-ray exposure over survey radiographs.
8. From a lateral approach, ventral to the transverse vertebral process, aseptically insert a spinal needle into the intervertebral disc of interest. At the lumbosacral junction, use a dorsal approach to aseptically insert the needle through the interarcurate ligament and through the spinal canal into the disc.
9. Slowly inject contrast medium into the disc. If resistance is encountered, reposition the needle tip.
10. A normal disc will accommodate about 0.2–0.3 ml. Abnormal discs may accept a much larger volume, depending on the severity of the lesion.
11. Immediately after injection, make lateral, flexed lateral, extended lateral, and DV/VD views centered on the disc of interest.

A

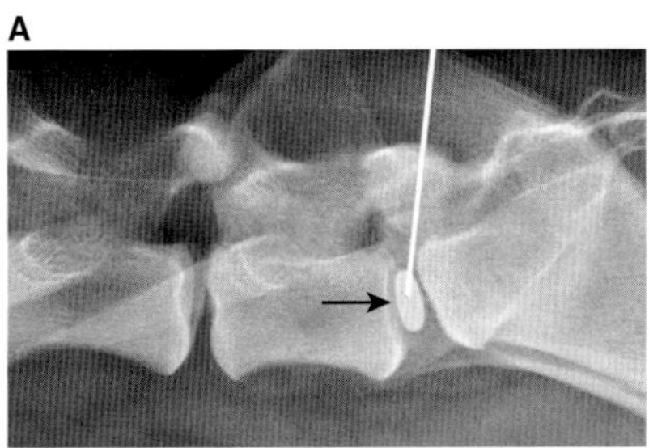

B

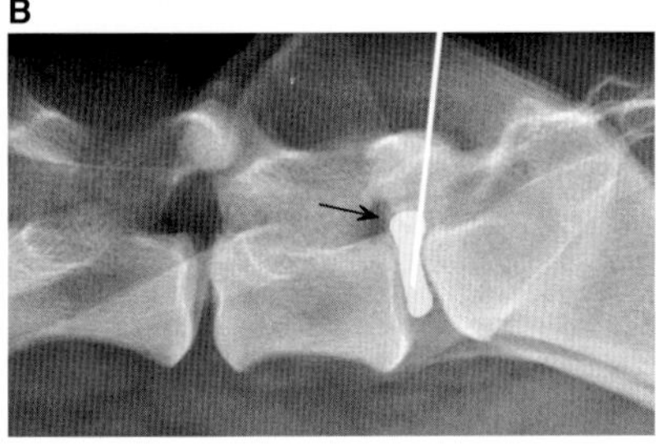

Figure 2.82 Discography. **A**. Lateral view of a dog lumbosacral junction depicting injection of contrast medium into a normal disc at L7–S1 (black arrow). **B**. Lateral view depicting dorsal rupture of the annulus fibrosis with protrusion of intervertebral disc material at the lumbosacral junction (black arrow).

Epidurography

Positive contrast study used to evaluate the epidural space (Figure 2.83). Epidurograms can be difficult to interpret because the epidural space is not a well-defined compartment.

Indications for epidurography

1. Examine the cauda equina and proximal spinal nerve roots for evidence of compression or displacement.

Procedure for epidurography

1. Make and evaluate survey spinal radiographs.
2. General anesthesia is required.
3. Patient may be in sternal or lateral recumbency.
4. Contrast agent is sterile, non-ionic, iodinated medium (250–300 mgI/ml):
   a. Dose in cats, small and medium dogs: 2–4 ml.
   b. Dose in large dogs: 4–8 ml.
5. Warm the contrast agent to body temperature prior to administration.
6. Increase the x-ray exposure over survey radiographs.
7. At the sacrocaudal junction, aseptically insert a 22-gauge spinal needle from a dorsal approach to the floor of the spinal canal. Insertion can be made at the lumbosacral junction, but try to avoid this site because a lesion may be present here. In some patients, however, it is necessary to inject at the LS junction.
8. Slowly inject the contrast medium into the epidural space.
9. Remove the needle and immediately make lateral, flexed lateral, extended lateral, and VD/DV views centered on the lumbosacral junction.

A

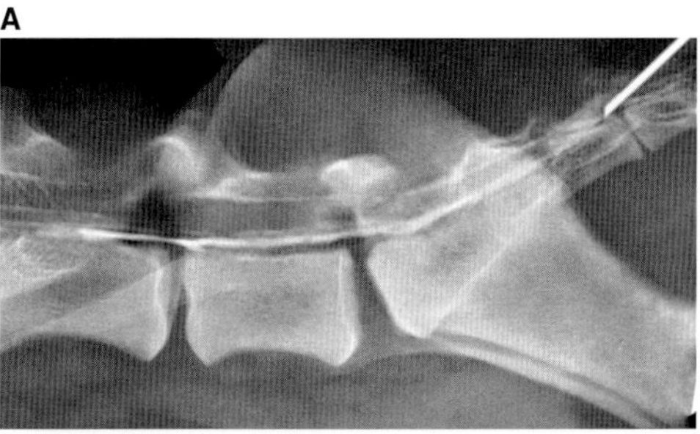

B

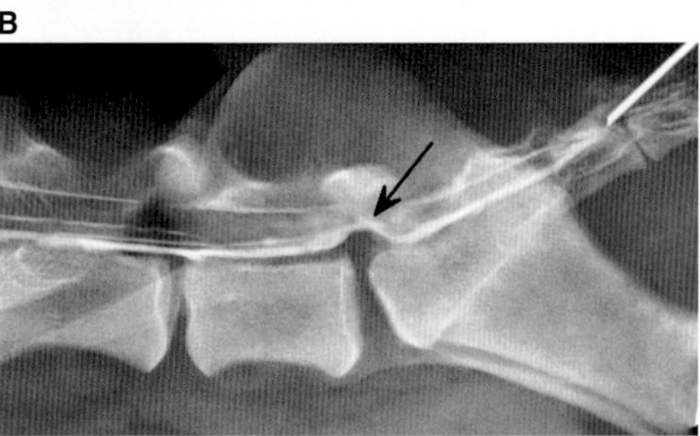

Figure 2.83 Epidurography. Lateral views of a dog lumbosacral junction depicting the injection of contrast medium into the epidural space at the sacrocaudal junction. **A**. Normal epidurogram. **B**. Disc protrusion at the LS junction displaces the ventral contrast column dorsally (black arrow).

Myelography

A myelogram is a positive contrast evaluation of the spinal canal (Figure 2.84). It is used to examine the subarachnoid space and spinal cord.

Indications for myelography

1. Examine suspected spinal lesion(s) seen in survey radiographs.
2. Investigate the cause of spinal pain, paresis, or paralysis when no lesion is evident in survey radiographs.
3. Myelograms generally provide limited information regarding conditions such as nerve root lesions, meningopathies, and disseminated myelopathies.

Complications associated with myelography

1. Increase in severity of clinical signs related to spinal disease. This is more likely to occur when injecting cold contrast media or using a rapid rate of infusion.
2. Seizures during recovery from anesthesia. This adverse effect occurs much less frequently with the newer contrast agents.
3. Inadvertent injection into the central canal. This error can lead to paresis or paralysis, depending on the quantity of contrast medium deposited. It occurs more often when lumbar puncture is performed cranial to L5.
4. Apnea due to rapid infusion in the cervical region.
5. Death if the cervical spinal cord is penetrated.

A

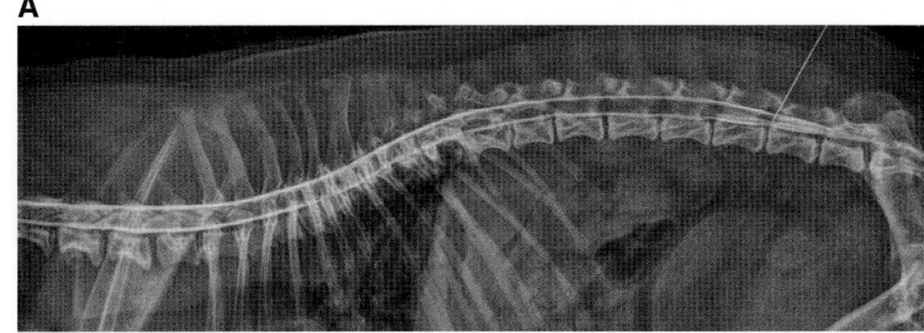

B

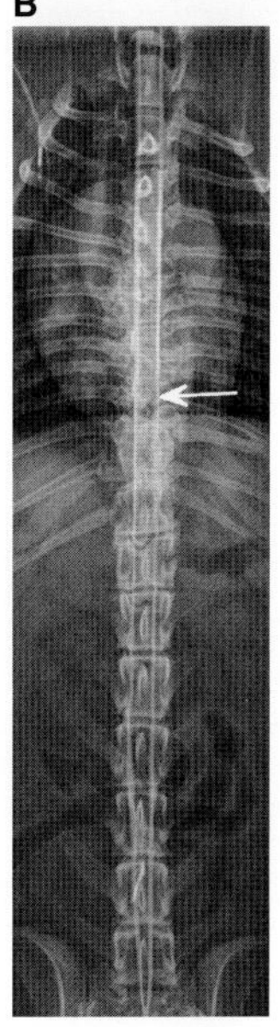

Figure 2.84 Normal myelogram. Lateral view (**A**) and VD view (**B**) of a dog depicting positive contrast medium in the subarachnoid space. The spinal needle is visible at L5–6. Columns of contrast medium outline the spinal cord (white arrow in **B**). Notice the FOV is tightly collimated to the vertebral column.

Procedure for myelography

1. Make and evaluate survey spinal radiographs.
2. General anesthesia is required.
3. Contrast agent is 0.45 ml/kg of sterile, non-ionic, iodinated medium (400 mgI/ml). The dose can be reduced to 0.30 ml/kg if only the cervical or lumbar region is being imaged.
4. Warm the contrast agent to body temperature prior to administration. This is especially important with myelography. Warming helps lower the viscosity of the solution, which improves mixing with cerebrospinal fluid and helps minimize the likelihood of an adverse reaction.
5. Increase the x-ray exposure over survey radiographs.
6. Use a spinal needle to inject the contrast agent into either the cervical or lumbar subarachnoid space (Figure 2.85). The choice of where to inject depends on the location of the suspected lesion.
7. To reduce the odds of inadvertently injecting the contrast agent into the epidural space, insert the needle with a slight caudal-to-cranial angle rather than perpendicular (Figure 2.85). Use a needle with a short bevel and aim the bevel ventrally (Figure 2.86).

Cervical myelogram

1. The patient is in either lateral or sternal recumbency with its head flexed and its nose parallel to the table top (lateral position) or perpendicular to the table (sternal position). In lateral recumbency, a radiograph can be made to check needle placement without moving the patient. In sternal recumbency, it often is easier to accurately insert the needle, but the patient cannot be moved to check needle placement (a horizontal beam lateral view can be made in sternal recumbency if needed).
2. From a dorsal approach at the atlantooccipital junction, aseptically insert a 20- or 22-gauge spinal needle (with stylet) into the subarachnoid space. Larger gauge needles tend to track more accurately through the tough cervical tissues. The site for needle insertion is the center of a triangle formed by the two transverse processes of the first cervical vertebra and the caudal sagittal crest of the skull (Figure 2.87).
3. Slowly advance the needle until a "pop" is felt as the needle penetrates the strong atlantooccipital ligament and enters the cisterna magna. The patient may jerk slightly when the dura is penetrated.
4. Remove the stylet from the needle and check for cerebrospinal fluid (CSF) flowing into the needle hub. Collect some CSF for analysis.
5. If there is no CSF flow, replace the stylet in the needle and reposition the needle. Check periodically for CSF flow. Rarely, the needle will be in the correct location without CSF flow.
6. Needle placement requires considerable practice and "feel." Each patient is different. The "pop" may be very

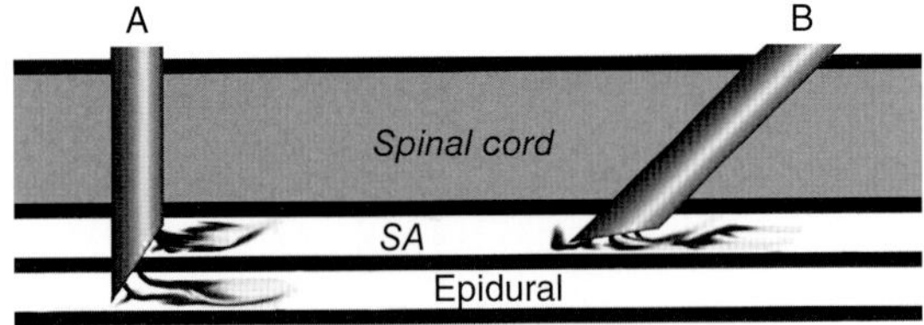

Figure 2.85 Spinal needle insertion. A spinal needle that is inserted perpendicular to the spinal canal, as shown in **A**, is more likely to extend into the epidural space. A needle that is angled caudal-to-cranial, as shown in **B**, is more likely to remain in the subarachnoid space (SA).

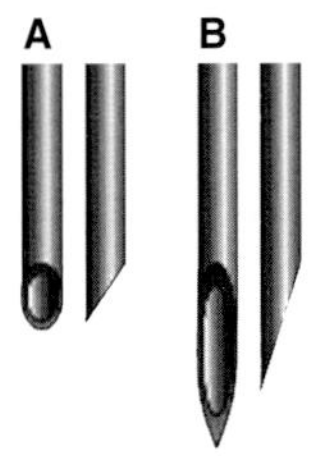

Figure 2.86 Spinal needles for myelography. Short-bevel spinal needles, as depicted in **A** (e.g., *Pitkin* needles), are less likely to extend into the epidural space than long-bevel needles, as shown in **B**. However, longer bevel needles should be inserted more cautiously because they tend to be "sharper" and penetrate more easily.

evident in some patients and in others it may not be felt at all, particularly in small dogs.

7. Always proceed cautiously when inserting a spinal needle. Avoid rapid movements or advancing the needle too far as puncture of the brainstem can cause paralysis or death.
8. When needle placement is in doubt, make a small test injection of contrast medium (0.5–1.0 ml) and a test lateral view, being careful not to move the needle while waiting for the results.
9. After correct needle placement, slowly inject the dose of contrast medium, no faster than 1 ml/s.
10. Immediately after injection make a lateral view. The needle can remain in place or be removed for this initial radiograph. If the needle remains in place, be careful not to move the patient's head/neck or the needle. In small patients, the needle may not be adequately supported by the surrounding tissues and you may have to hold it in place.
11. Remove the needle prior to making the VD view and any additional radiographs. Sometimes a DV or oblique views are needed as well as extended and flexed lateral views.
12. Elevate the cranial end of the patient as needed to improve caudal flow of the contrast medium. If the contrast does not flow well, flexing and straightening the head may help, but be very careful not to increase the severity of the patient's clinical signs.

Lumbar myelogram

1. The patient is in either lateral or sternal recumbency with the lumbar spine flexed.
2. Using a dorsal approach between the fifth and seventh lumbar vertebrae (ideally, L5–6 in dogs and L6–7 in cats), aseptically insert a 22-gauge spinal needle with stylet past the vertebral lamina and into the spinal canal. If the needle cannot be inserted here, move to the next cranial site (L4–5 in dogs or L5–6 in cats).
3. Once in the spinal canal, gently advance the needle through the spinal cord until it touches bone. The bone is the ventral part of the spinal canal and the patient's pelvic limbs may jerk slightly when the dura is penetrated.
4. Withdraw the needle slightly and remove the stylet to check for CSF flow. There will be significantly less CSF flow from the lumbar region than the cervical region. A lack of lumbar CSF flow does not necessarily mean that the needle is not in the correct position. Blood in the needle hub indicates the needle is too deep, located in the venous sinus rather than in the subarachnoid space, and should be further withdrawn.
5. Perform a small test injection and make a test lateral view to confirm correct needle placement.
6. As with cervical myelography, needle placement requires practice. The "pop" described with cervical myelography may or may not be felt in the lumbar region.
7. Slowly inject the dose of contrast agent over a period of 5–10 seconds.

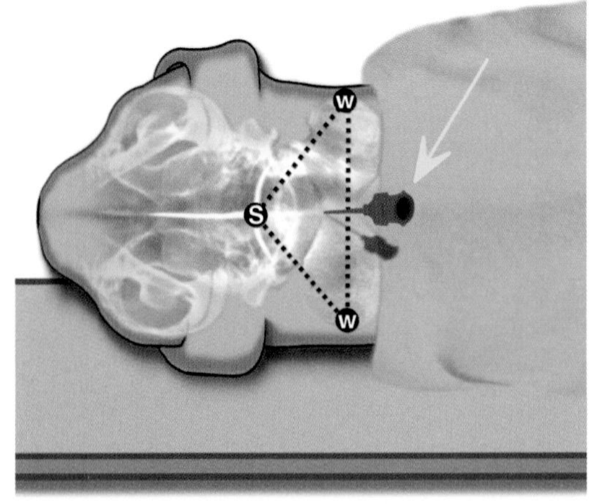

Figure 2.87 Cisternal tap. This illustration depicts a dorsal view of a dog's head with the patient in lateral recumbency. The head is flexed with the nose pointing away. The landmarks for cervical puncture include the sagittal crest (S) and the wings of the atlas (W). The spinal needle (yellow arrow) is inserted in the center of a triangle made by these landmarks.

8. Immediately following injection make a lateral view. The needle can remain in place for the lateral view if the patient is not moved.
9. Remove the needle prior to making the VD view and any other radiographs.
10. Elevate the patient's caudal end and lower its cranial end as needed to improve cranial flow of contrast.

Myelogram artifacts and technical errors

1. In a normal myelogram, the contrast medium is evenly distributed in the subarachnoid space to produce thin, smooth, well-defined contrast columns on either side of the spinal cord (Figures 2.84, 2.88, 2.89).
2. Air bubbles may be introduced into the subarachnoid space if there was gas in the syringe during injection. Bubbles typically appear as round, 1–3 mm, filling defects that change in size and position in serial radiographs (Figure 2.90).
3. Uneven or heterogeneous opacification indicates poor distribution of the contrast medium, which may result from an insufficient dose, high viscosity, or injecting too slowly.
4. Contrast medium that leaked or was injected into the epidural space can obscure the myelogram and severely compromise its interpretation (Figure 2.89). Compression of the jugular veins may be attempted to increase pressure in the choroid plexus in the hope of increasing CSF production to help "wash out" epidural contrast medium.
5. Contrast medium in the spinal cord or in the central canal may result from an inadvertent injection or severe spinal cord disease (e.g., spinal cord malacia, hydromyelia). In the spinal cord, contrast appears as persistent, patchy, irregular areas of increased opacity. The prognosis for patient survival depends on the volume of contrast in the cord. Contrast medium in the central canal appears as a linear, uniform opacity in the center of the spinal cord (Figure 2.90). A canal less than 2 mm wide is normal size, whereas a canal wider than 2 mm wide is likely distended due to a faulty injection. Opacification of a normal central canal may be due to leakage through the needle tract made during spinal puncture.
6. Leakage of contrast medium into the soft tissues dorsal to the spine (at the site of needle insertion) is a frequent occurrence and rarely compromises interpretation of the radiographs (Figure 2.89).

A

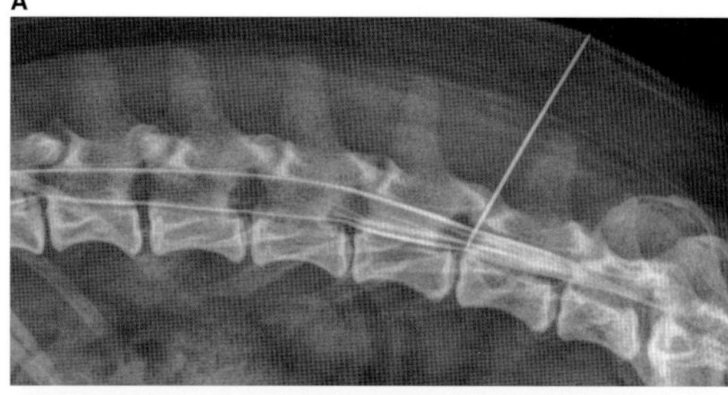

B

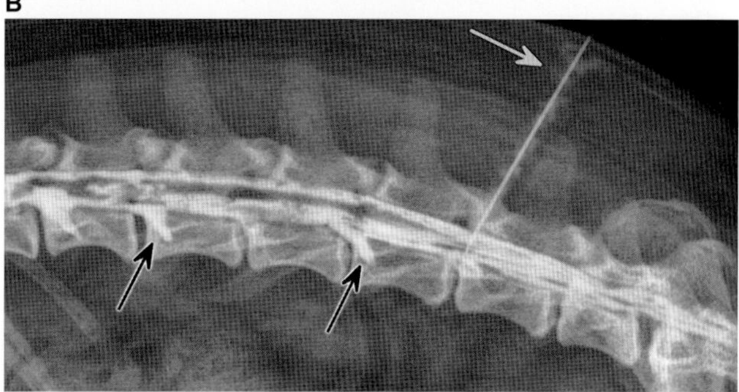

Figure 2.89 Epidural spillage. (**A**) Lateral view of a dog lumbar spine depicting a normal myelogram injected at L5–6. (**B**) Lateral view of a lumbar myelogram depicting leakage of contrast medium into the epidural space. Epidural spillage outlines the exiting nerve sheaths (black arrows). Some contrast medium has leaked into the dorsal soft tissues along the needle track (white arrow).

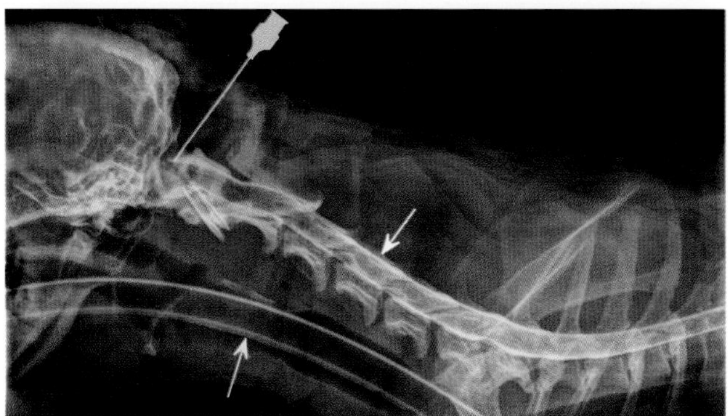

Figure 2.88 Cervical myelogram. Lateral view of a dog cervical spine depicting contrast medium injected at the cisterna magna and filling the subarachnoid space. The spinal cord is outlined by the contrast columns (white arrow). The yellow arrow points to the endotracheal tube.

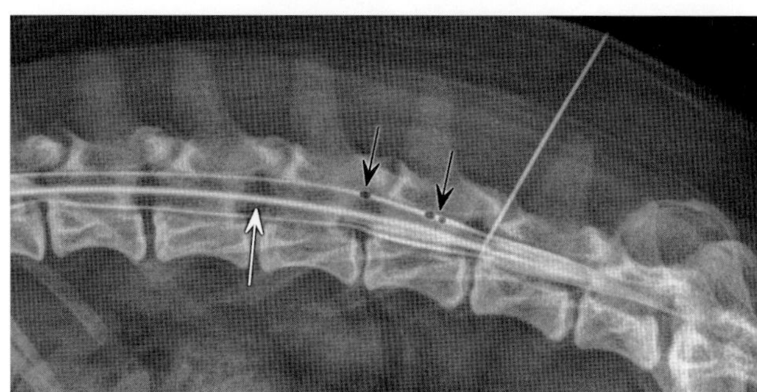

Figure 2.90 Filling of the central canal. Lateral view of a dog lumbar spine depicting a myelogram with contrast medium in the central canal (white arrow). The spinal needle is visible at L5–6. Tiny air bubbles are present in the dorsal subarachnoid space (black arrows).

Head contrast studies

Positive contrast radiography used to evaluate the ear canals, nasal cavities, and salivary glands. Non-ionic iodinated agents are preferred. Barium is not used and ionic media are not recommended because they are irritating and rapidly absorbed. Procedures described here include:

1. Dacryocystorhinography
2. Otic canalography
3. Rhinography
4. Sialography

Dacryocystorhinography

Iodinated contrast media can be used to evaluate the nasolacrimal ducts (Figure 2.91).

Indications for dacryocystorhinography

1. Investigate cause of chronic, recurring, or intractable conjunctivitis and dacryocystitis.
2. Assess cause of abnormal drainage of tears.
3. Evaluate obstruction of nasolacrimal duct.
4. Examine size or course of nasolacrimal duct (nasal or paranasal mass or disease can alter duct).

Procedure for dacryocystorhinography

1. Make and evaluate survey skull radiographs.
2. General anesthesia is required.
3. Patient is in lateral recumbency with the side of interest up and the nose tilted down.
4. Contrast agent is 0.5–2.0 ml of non-ionic iodinated medium (300 mgI/ml), volume depends on the size of the animal.
5. Cannulate either the superior or inferior lacrimal puncta with a 23–27 gauge lacrimal needle.
6. Flush the duct with sterile saline.
7. Warm the contrast medium to body temperature prior to administration.
8. Increase the x-ray exposure over survey radiographs.
9. Slowly infuse the contrast agent until several drops appear in the external nares. Keep the patient's nose tilted down to prevent contrast medium from flowing retrograde into the nasal cavity.
10. Immediately after infusion, make lateral, VD/DV, and oblique views of the nasal region.

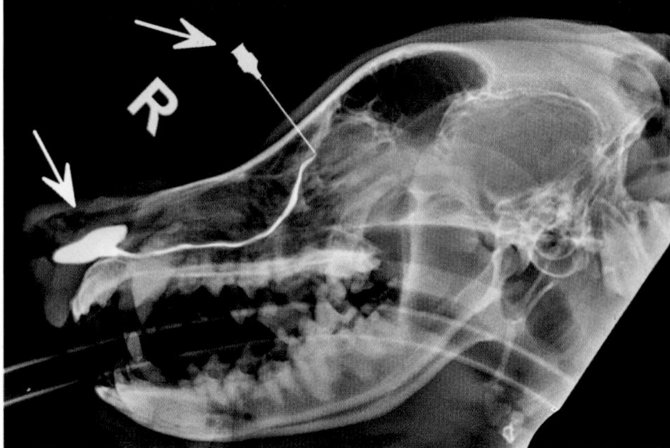

Figure 2.91 Normal dacryocystorhinogram. Lateral view of a dog head depicting contrast medium infused into the lower lacrimal puncta (yellow arrow points to the needle). Contrast medium flows rostrally in the lacrimal duct, where it pools in the nares (white arrow).

Otic canalography

Positive contrast radiographic evaluation of an external auditory canal can be used to assess the integrity of the tympanic membrane (Figure 2.92).

Procedure for otic canalography

1. Make and evaluate survey radiographs of the head.
2. Patient sedation/anesthesia is recommended.
3. Patient is in lateral recumbency with the affected side up.
4. Contrast agent is 2–5 ml of non-ionic iodinated medium (300 mgI/ml).
5. Warm the contrast agent to body temperature prior to administration.
6. Increase the x-ray exposure over survey radiographs.
7. Infuse the contrast medium into the ear canal.
8. When finished, block the ear canal with a cotton ball, soft foam earplug, or similar to prevent contrast from leaking out and contaminating the hair, skin, or x-ray table. Keep the side of interest up as much as possible when not making radiographs.
9. Make VD and open-mouth rostrocaudal views of the head.

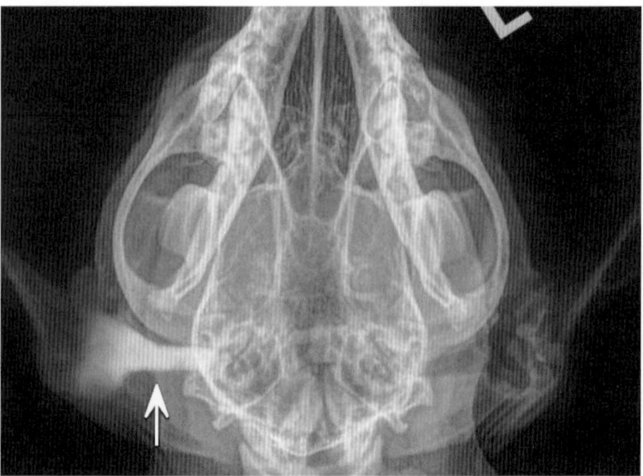

Figure 2.92 Normal otic canalogram. DV view of a dog head depicting contrast medium in the right external auditory canal (white arrow).

Rhinography

Positive contrast radiography can be used to evaluate the nasal cavity (Figure 2.93).

Indications for rhinography

1. Investigate a suspected obstruction in the nasal cavity or nasopharynx.
2. Explore the cause of nasal discharge, reverse sneezing, pharyngeal discharge, or upper airway obstruction.

Procedure for rhinography

1. Make and evaluate survey radiographs of the head.
2. General anesthesia and intubation are required.
3. Patient may be in lateral recumbency with the side of interest down (closest to the image receptor) or in dorsal recumbency with the head flexed and the nose pointing upward.
4. Contrast agent is 1 ml per 5 kg bodyweight of non-ionic, iodinated medium (300 mgI/ml). Barium can be used for rhinography (20%–30% w/v), but iodinated agents are preferred.
5. Warm the contrast medium to body temperature prior to administration.
6. Increase the x-ray exposure over survey radiographs.
7. In lateral recumbency, elevate the patient's nose about 15° to encourage the contrast agent to flow caudally. In dorsal recumbency, the nose is pointed upward.
8. Infuse the dose of contrast medium into the ventral nasal meatus.
9. Make lateral and open-mouth VD views of the nasal passages and nasopharyngeal region. Horizontal beam radiography can be used, especially if the patient is in dorsal recumbency.

A

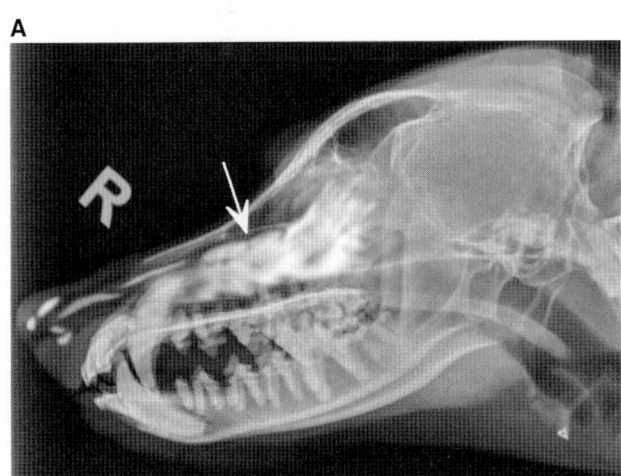

B

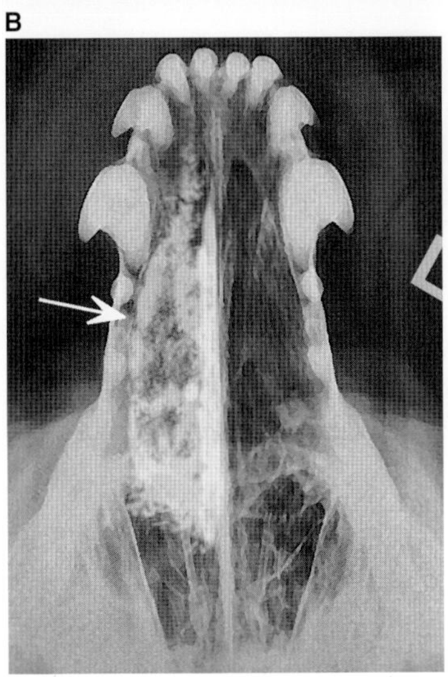

Figure 2.93 Normal rhinogram. Lateral view (**A**) and open mouth VD view (**B**) of a dog head depicting positive contrast medium in the right nasal cavity (arrow).

Sialography

Positive contrast radiography used to evaluate the salivary ducts and salivary glands (Figure 2.94).

Indications for sialography

1. Evaluate a suspected salivary mucocele.
2. Investigate a suspected rupture of a salivary gland or salivary duct.
3. Examine a salivary duct for possible obstruction.

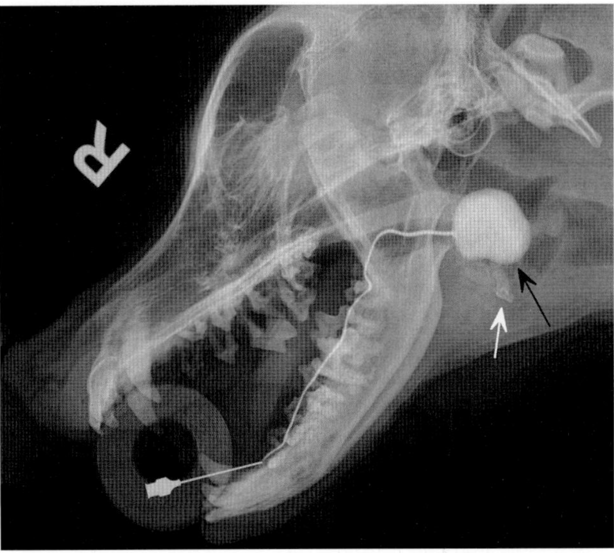

Figure 2.94 Normal sialogram. Lateral view of a dog head depicting positive contrast medium injected into the duct of the mandibular salivary gland. The needle is visible at the rostral end of the mandible. The duct runs caudally and parallel with the horizontal ramus of the mandible to the angle of the jaw and then curves ventrally to the salivary gland (black arrow). The basihyoid bone (white arrow) sometimes is mistaken for extravasation of contrast medium. The patient's mouth is held open by a roll of tape.

Procedure for sialography

1. Make and evaluate survey radiographs of the head and neck.
2. General anesthesia is required.
3. Avoid use of atropine or other parasympatholytic agents because they inhibit salivary secretion, making it difficult to cannulate the salivary duct.
4. Patient is in lateral recumbency with the affected side up.
5. Contrast agent is sterile, non-ionic iodinated medium (300 mgI/ml):
   a. Dose in cats and small dogs: 0.1–0.3 ml.
   b. Dose in large dogs: 0.5–1.0 ml.
6. Aseptically cannulate the salivary duct using a 23–27 gauge lacrimal needle.
7. Warm the contrast agent to body temperature prior to administration.
8. Increase the x-ray exposure over survey radiographs.
9. Slowly infuse the dose of contrast medium.
10. Immediately after infusion make lateral views centered on the area of interest; VD and oblique views may be needed to complete the study.

Miscellaneous contrast studies

1. Arthrography
2. Fistulography
3. Peritoneography
4. Pleurography
5. Tracheobronchography

Arthrography

Injecting an iodinated contrast agent into a joint enhances visualization of the synovial surfaces (Figure 2.95). Gas can be used, but negative contrast arthrograms are much more difficult to interpret. Double contrast arthrograms are not recommended because gas bubbles create numerous artifacts. Barium is not used for arthrography.

Indications for arthrography

1. Investigate cause of lameness and joint pain.
2. Evaluate abnormalities associated with joint soft tissues (e.g., articular cartilage, meniscal cartilage, bursae, intra-articular ligaments and tendons).
3. Examine joints for osteochondrosis lesions.
4. Determine whether fragments (free or attached) are present within a joint.

Procedure for arthrography

1. Make and evaluate survey radiographs, including comparison radiographs of the contralateral joint.
2. Chemical restraint is recommended to avoid patient movement.
3. Contrast agent is 1–4 ml of sterile, non-ionic, iodinated medium (200 mgI/ml), a volume equal to the amount of joint fluid removed. Most iodinated media must be diluted with sterile saline to make this low concentration. Higher concentrations are too opaque and may mask lesions.
4. Warm the contrast agent to body temperature prior to administration.
5. Increase the x-ray exposure over survey radiographs.
6. Perform aseptic arthrocentesis and remove as much joint fluid as possible. Submit the fluid for analysis.
7. Leave the needle in the joint and inject 0.2 mg of epinephrine to improve the quality and duration of the arthrogram.
8. Make a small test injection and a test radiograph to document correct needle placement.
9. Slowly inject the contrast medium into the joint; injection time should be 10–20 seconds.

A

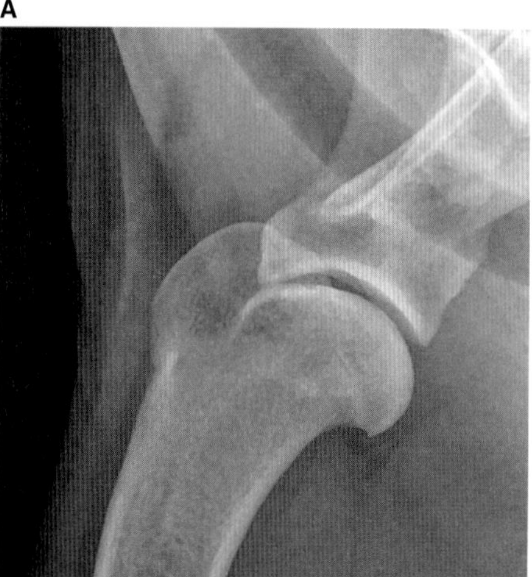

B

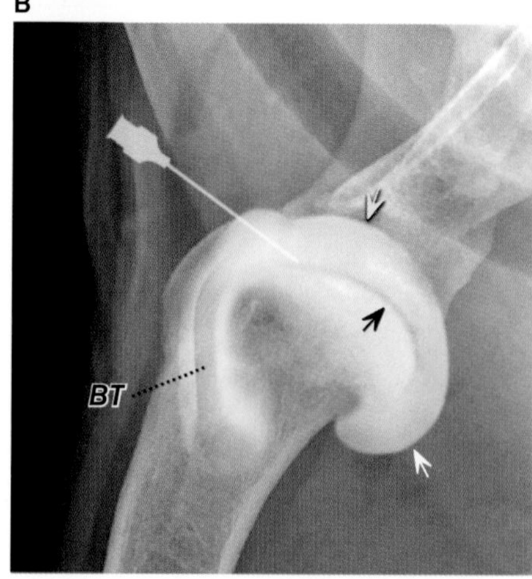

Figure 2.95 Normal arthrogram. Lateral radiograph of a normal dog shoulder (**A**) and a positive contrast arthrogram of the same shoulder (**B**). In the arthrogram, contrast medium in the scapulohumeral joint outlines the caudal joint pouch (white arrow), the medial joint pouch (yellow arrow), the articular cartilage along the humeral head (black arrow), and the bicipital tendon (BT).

10. After injection, remove the needle and manipulate the joint to ensure uniform filling and coating.
11. Immediately make lateral, caudocranial, and lateral oblique views of the joint. Flexed lateral and rotated views may enable detection of lesions not otherwise demonstrated, particularly when imaging larger joints. During flexion the width of contrast medium in the joint typically becomes thinner.
12. Repeat the radiographs in 10–15 minutes, after the contrast has been partially absorbed, to see subtle lesions that may have been masked earlier.

Fistulography

Positive contrast agents can be used to investigate a fistulous tract, sinus cavity, or draining wound (Figure 2.96). Large sinuses or cavities may not be adequately examined due to pooling of contrast medium. Gas can be used to make a negative contrast or double contrast fistulogram, but these studies are more difficult to interpret. Fistulography is performed only if surgical intervention is planned, should a surgical lesion be found.

Indications for fistulography

1. Investigate origin, depth, and extent of a draining wound that has not responded to medical or surgical treatment.
2. Aid in detecting suspected foreign material or sequestered bone fragment not visible in survey radiographs.
3. Evaluate abnormal communication between two hollow structures.

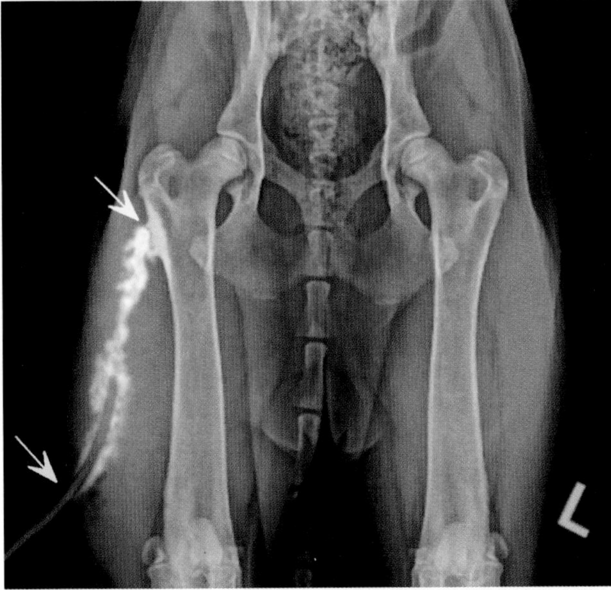

Figure 2.96 Fistulogram. VD view of a dog pelvis depicting a catheter (yellow arrow) inserted into a draining tract in the lateral aspect of the right thigh. Contrast medium outlines the tract and extends to the right proximal femur (white arrow), where there is a local periosteal response caused by osteomyelitis.

Procedure for fistulography

1. Make and evaluate survey radiographs of the area of interest.
2. Clean and shave the area of interest. Removing the hair makes it easier to wipe away superficial contrast medium and avoid superimposition artifacts.
3. Contrast agent is 10–20 ml of non-ionic, iodinated medium (300 mgI/ml), a volume sufficient to fill the tract and/or cavity. It is a good idea to have more than anticipated contrast medium available.
4. Gently insert a sterile catheter into the sinus or fistula, being careful not to create a new tract.
5. A balloon tip catheter or a purse-string suture around the catheter can be used to minimize leakage.
6. Warm the contrast medium to body temperature prior to administration.
7. Increase the x-ray exposure over survey radiographs.
8. Immediately after infusion, make orthogonal views centered on the area of interest.
9. Metal opacity body markers or sterile needles inserted into the skin can help identify landmarks around a draining tract.
10. Infuse additional doses of contrast medium if more radiographs are needed.
11. When dealing with long tracts, advance the catheter as far as possible (gently) and infuse contrast while slowly withdrawing the catheter.

Pleurography

A positive contrast agent infused into the pleural space to enhance visualization of the parietal and visceral pleural surfaces (Figure 2.97). Gas is not recommended because it causes a pneumothorax and negative contrast pleurograms are more difficult to interpret. Barium is never used in these procedures and ionic agents should be avoided because they are highly irritating and rapidly diluted.

Pleurography rarely is performed due to the risk to the patient's health and the availability of less invasive imaging modalities or endoscopy. Pleurography is contraindicated in patients with severe pleural effusion or infection because fluid in the pleural space dilutes the contrast agent, rendering the study useless, and infection may be disseminated during the procedure.

Indications for pleurography

1. Differentiate pleural and extrapleural masses from pulmonary masses.
2. Examine a mediastinal or heart base mass.
3. Investigate suspected pleural adhesions.
4. Assess diaphragm integrity.
5. Other imaging modalities are unavailable.

Procedure for pleurography

1. Make and evaluate survey thoracic radiographs.
2. General anesthesia is recommended.

3. Patient is in lateral recumbency.
4. Contrast agent is non-ionic iodinated medium (300 mgI/ml). Lidocaine can be mixed with the agent prior to injection (0.5–1.0 ml per 10 ml of contrast) to reduce adverse reactions to pleural injection (e.g., muscle tremors, tachypnea, and tachycardia). Lidocaine is not needed if the patient is anesthetized.
   a. Dose for cat or small dog: 0.5–1.0 ml/kg.
   b. Dose for large dog: 0.25–0.5 ml/kg.
5. Aseptically place an indwelling catheter into the pleural space. Prefill the needle and extension set with contrast medium to avoid air bubbles.
6. Warm the contrast medium to body temperature prior to administration.
7. Make a test injection (about 0.5 ml); if the patient coughs, reposition the catheter.
8. Increase the x-ray exposure over survey radiographs.
9. Slowly infuse the contrast solution into the pleural space over a period of 20–30 seconds; STOP injection immediately if there are signs of respiratory distress.
10. Remove the needle and gently roll the patient several times to distribute the contrast agent throughout the pleural space.
11. Make VD, DV, right and left lateral thoracic radiographs. If there is a specific location of interest in the thorax, horizontal beam radiography may add information.
12. Contrast medium normally is absorbed via the pleura and lymphatics within 30 minutes.

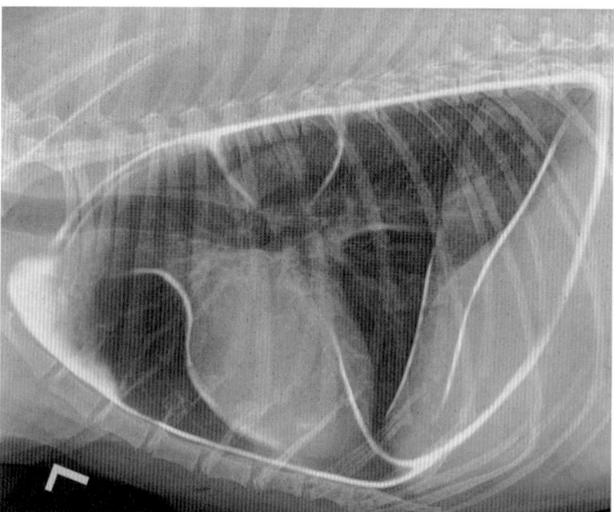

Figure 2.97 Normal pleurogram. Lateral view of a dog thorax depicting positive contrast medium in the pleural space, outlining the pleural edges.

Peritoneography (celiography)

Infusion of a positive or negative contrast agent into the peritoneal cavity can be used to evaluate the diaphragm and peritoneal surfaces, particularly in the peripheral abdomen

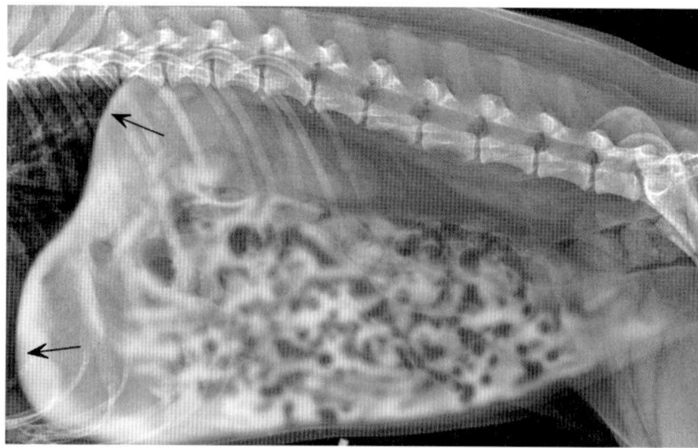

Figure 2.98 Peritoneogram. Lateral view of a dog abdomen depicting positive contrast medium in the peritoneal cavity. Contrast medium outlines the caudal border of the diaphragm (black arrows).

where there are fewer summation and superimposition artifacts. The preferred contrast agent for peritoneography is a non-ionic, iodinated medium (Figure 2.98). Barium is never used and ionic agents should be avoided because they are highly irritating and rapidly diluted. Gas can be used to make a pneumoperitoneogram (Figure 2.99), but should not be administered to patients where diaphragm integrity is in doubt. Peritoneography also is contraindicated in patients with severe peritoneal effusion or infection.

Indications for peritoneography

1. Evaluate the integrity of the diaphragm or body wall.
2. Investigate suspected congenital or acquired hernias.
3. Improve visualization of an intra-abdominal mass.
4. Other imaging modalities are unavailable.

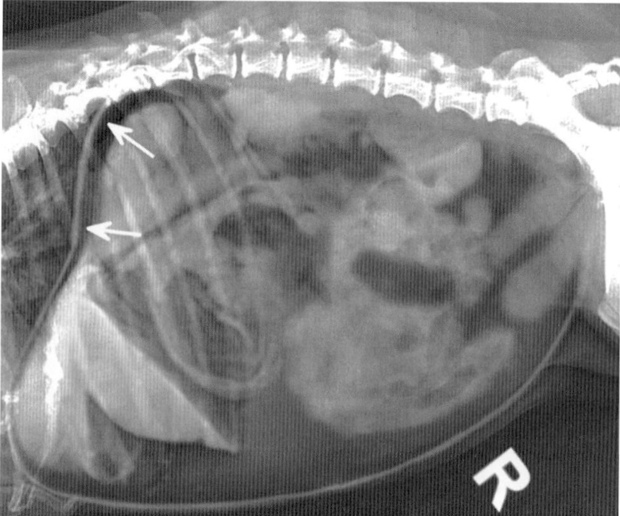

Figure 2.99 Pneumoperitoneogram. Lateral view of a dog abdomen depicting free gas in the peritoneal cavity. The caudal border of the diaphragm is outlined by gas (white arrows).

Procedure for peritoneography

1. Make and evaluate survey abdominal radiographs.
2. GI tract and urinary bladder should be empty.
3. Anesthesia/sedation is recommended.
4. Patient is in lateral recumbency.
5. Insert a needle or catheter into the peritoneal cavity, lateral to midline and caudal to the umbilicus.
6. Perform a test aspiration to be sure no organ or vessel has been punctured.
7. If peritoneal fluid is present, remove as much as feasible prior to infusing contrast medium.
8. Adjust the x-ray exposure from survey radiographs:
   a. Decrease exposure for a negative peritoneogram.
   b. Increase exposure for a positive peritoneogram.
9. Positive contrast peritoneogram: slowly infuse non-ionic iodinated medium (300 mgI/ml) and carefully roll the patient 360° to distribute it throughout the peritoneal space. To outline the diaphragm, elevate the caudal part of the patient for 5 minutes:
   a. Dose in dogs and cats: 1.1 ml/kg; dose may be doubled (2.2 ml/kg) if peritoneal fluid persists.
10. Pneumoperitoneogram: patient is in left lateral recumbency to trap gas emboli in the right atrium, should emboli occur. Slowly infuse nitrous oxide or carbon dioxide until the abdomen is fully distended. Room air is not recommended because it is less soluble and carries a greater risk of gas embolism. If room air is used remove as much of it as possible after making the radiographs.
11. Monitor heart rate and respiration during procedure.
12. Make VD, DV, right and left lateral views of the abdomen.
13. Horizontal beam radiography may aid in evaluation; position the area of interest "up" with a negative contrast peritoneogram and "down" with a positive contrast peritoneogram.

Tracheobronchography

Positive contrast agents used to coat the surfaces of the trachea (*tracheography*) and bronchi (*bronchography*), thus enhancing their visualization in radiographs (Figure 2.100). Tracheobronchography has been used to investigate abnormal airway dilations, stenoses, obstructions, and abnormal communications. Types of contrast media used for this procedure include iodinated agents, barium liquids and powders, and an older agent called tantalum powder.

Procedure for tracheobronchography

1. Make and evaluate survey thoracic radiographs.
2. General anesthesia is required.
3. Animal is in lateral recumbency with the side of interest down (closest to the image receptor); only the dependent lung is studied.
4. Contrast medium most often used is 1–4 ml of sterile barium suspension (50%–60% w/v).

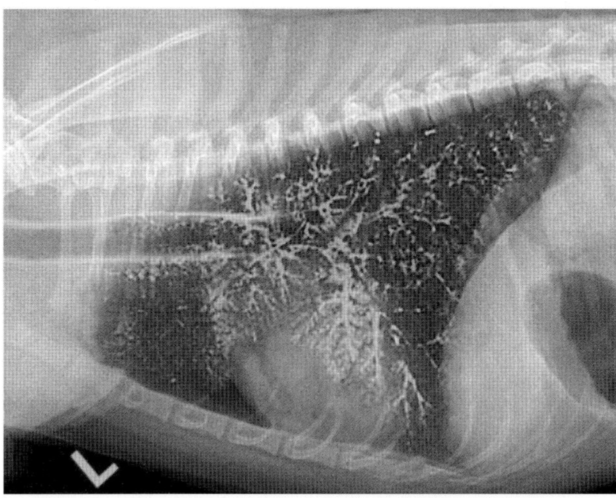

Figure 2.100 Tracheobronchogram. Lateral view of a dog thorax depicting positive contrast medium in the trachea and bronchial tree.

5. Small amounts of barium generally are well tolerated in the lungs; mild reactions sometimes occur but usually subside within a few days.
6. Most barium is eliminated by the mucociliary transport system; some barium may collect and persist in regional lymph nodes or alveoli.
7. Barium is not well cleared from a diseased lung.
8. Insert a catheter through the endotracheal tube to the tracheal or bronchial lesion (if available, fluoroscopic or endoscopic guidance is recommended).
9. Warm barium suspension to body temperature prior to administration.
10. Increase the x-ray exposure over survey radiographs.
11. After infusion make lateral, VD, and VD oblique radiographs, keeping the lung of interest dependent (down) as much as possible.
12. Radiographs made during inspiration and expiration may aid in diagnosis.

Reading radiographs

Reading radiographs is an acquired skill that combines careful observation with a knowledge of anatomy and an understanding of disease processes and radiographic principles. A systematic approach is essential. There are three basic steps to reading radiographs:

1. Evaluation of the images.
2. Detection of the abnormalities.
3. Interpretation of the findings.

Evaluation of radiographs

Proper viewing conditions are important when reading radiographs. Your reading room should be comfortable and free of distractions so you can give your full attention to studying the images. The ambient light should be low but not total darkness. Try to arrange the lighting in the room so there are no reflections on the radiographic images.

Film radiographs are viewed on lightboxes. Using multiple boxes can expedite the reading process. The light from the box should be evenly diffused and relatively cool (heat can distort the film). A high-intensity light source or spot illuminator (commonly called a "hot light") is useful to enhance darker areas in a film radiograph. Keep a magnifying glass nearby to help evaluate subtle radiographic findings.

Digital radiographs are viewed on monitors, either color or monochrome (grayscale). Poor-quality monitors are a major weak link in digital radiography. The resolution, brightness, and contrast of any monitor used for viewing radiographs in a clinical setting must be adequate to view all of the information available in a digital radiographs. Minimum standards for radiographic monitors have been established and are available elsewhere. Monitors must be calibrated on a regular basis to ensure peak performance. Important characteristics of diagnostic monitors include contrast ratio, luminance (brightness), and contrast resolution.

Contrast ratio is the difference between the lightest part and the darkest part of the screen image. It is the difference between a completely white pixel and a totally black background. The higher the contrast ratio, the better the image contrast and the easier it is to see features in a radiograph. Most diagnostic monitors offer contrast ratios of at least 10,000 : 1.

Luminance refers to the brightness of the monitor. It determines the appearance of the screen image in ambient light (the amount of background light in the room or environment). The monitor should be able to maintain adequate luminance at all times with a deviation of no less than 15% between all parts of the screen. Monitors that are too dim or too bright will not display the lighter shades of gray. The ambient light in your reading room should be as consistent as possible, especially if the monitor is not auto-calibrating.

Contrast resolution is a measure of the amount of detail in the screen image. It refers to the number of shades of gray that can be visibly distinguished. Contrast resolution is determined by the monitor's pixel bit depth. The bit depth for most diagnostic monitors is at least 8–10, which means the monitor can display 256–1024 shades of gray. The human eye can discriminate between 700 and 900 simultaneous shades of gray under optimum conditions (about 9–10 bits). Monitors that display more than 10 bits exceed that capability, but digital radiographs can be leveled and windowed to make those other gray shades visible and enhance different parts of the image. Remember, digital radiographs made with 16 bits contain over 65,000 shades of gray.

Other considerations in the selection of a diagnostic monitor include overall size, display noise, geometric distortion (due to monitor concavity or convexity), and veiling glare, the latter caused by stray light which can "fog" the displayed image.

A step-by-step method of evaluating radiographs is crucial to avoid missing valuable information. A number of items need to be systematically considered, evaluated, and "checked off" before you interpret your radiographic findings. The method should be written down as a **checklist** and posted in the reading room for quick reference (Tables 2.7–2.9). Checklists are particularly valuable during busy practice situations.

Checklists vary between individuals and most are developed and refined over time. All checklists should include three basic steps:

1. Confirm the radiographs are the correct patient and date.
2. Verify that the radiographic quality is adequate.
3. Carefully examine all parts of the anatomy.

First, make sure the radiographs you are evaluating belong to the patient of interest and that they are current and depict the correct body part. Unless you are investigating a specific condition, such as hip dysplasia, orthogonal views are needed for a complete examination.

Next, make sure the radiographs are of adequate quality. Poor quality radiographs can mimic or mask lesions. All borders of the body part of interest should be visible in each radiograph. Determine whether the exposure technique provides adequate radiographic density, contrast, and detail. Evaluate patient positioning to see whether there is rotation, motion artifact, or distortion due to off-centering or poor alignment with the image receptor. Make note of any light or dark artifacts in the images. Determine whether patient preparation was adequate (e.g., empty GI tract). Always review poor-quality radiographs before disposing of them because occasionally a lesion will be apparent in a poorly positioned or improperly exposed radiograph.

It is important to recognize radiation safety errors and explain them to your staff so they can be corrected. Hands should never be in the FOV, whether wearing gloves or not. Collimation borders should be visible in all radiographs. Make sure the x-ray exposure wasn't too high, particularly with digital systems.

ALL parts of the patient's anatomy must be scrutinized before your radiographic evaluation is complete. The method you use is not important, as long as you followed it every time. Here are three examples of systematic approaches commonly used to read radiographs:

1. Cranial-to-caudal or left-to-right or top-to-bottom method: begin at one end of the radiograph and proceed toward the opposite end.
2. Inventory method: examine each anatomical structure or organ system in a predetermined order for the body part being imaged (i.e., abdomen, thorax, skeleton).

Table 2.7 Checklist for radiograph evaluation

Correct patient and date
Correct body part, verify right vs. left
Orthogonal views
Radiographic density
Radiographic contrast
Radiographic detail
Centered on area of interest
Entire body part is included
Collimation is appropriate
Positioning is acceptable (absence of rotation)
Proper patient preparation (e.g., empty GI tract)
Artifacts/technical errors
Radiation safety
Patient factors
Patient age
Patient body condition (obese, emaciated)
Phase of respiration (inspiration/expiration)
Thorax
Extrathoracic soft tissues
Thoracic limbs
Caudal cervical region and thoracic inlet
Thoracic wall including spine, sternum, ribs
Diaphragm and cranial abdomen
Pleura and pleural space
Mediastinum
Esophagus
Trachea and mainstem bronchi
Cardiac silhouette
Aorta
Main pulmonary artery
Caudal vena cava
Lungs
Pulmonary arteries and veins
Bronchi
Lung parenchyma
Abdomen
Extra-abdominal soft tissues
Caudal thoracic cavity
Diaphragm
Body wall (dorsal, ventral and lateral)
Spine, ribs, pelvis
Pelvic limbs
Peritoneal space
Retroperitoneal space
Liver
Gall bladder
Spleen
Stomach
Pancreas
Small intestine
Large intestine
Kidneys
Adrenal glands
Urinary bladder
Prostate/uterus
Pelvic canal
Musculoskeletal
Bones (periosteum, cortex, medulla)
Soft tissues (swelling, atrophy, etc.)
Joints (alignment, degenerative changes)
Contralateral limb (comparative anatomy)

3. Method of circles: begin in the center of the radiograph and work outward in ever-expanding circles. Alternatively, begin at the periphery and work inward in ever-tightening circles.

To help with your deliberate, consistent, and systematic method of radiographic evaluation, display the images the same way every time. Position the cranial aspect of the patient toward your left or on top. The patient's right side in the image should be on your left. The proximal part of a limb should be toward your right or on top.

It is important to confirm that the right and left sides of the patient are correctly labeled. Do not automatically trust

Table 2.8 Checklist for good quality thoracic radiographs

- Centered on the heart.
- Collimation edges are visible and include entire bony thorax from thoracic inlet to last ribs.
- Thoracic limbs are pulled cranially.
- Thorax is not overly stretched.
- Right/left body markers are visible and not in the area of interest.
- No superimposition artifacts (e.g., collar, ECG leads, sandbags, IV tubing, gloves).
- Take into account any rotation in lateral view:
  - Costochondral junctions at the same level.
  - Ribs do not extend above the spine.
- Take into account any rotation in VD/DV view:
  - Sternebrae and vertebrae are superimposed.
  - Dorsal spinous processes do not extend beyond the lateral borders of the vertebrae.
  - Distance from spine to lateral thoracic wall is equal on both sides.
  - Right and left ribs are same length.
  - If rotated, the direction of rotation is toward the side with the heart, sternum, and shorter ribs ("the heart follows the sternum").
- Lungs are well inflated:
  - Cranial lung borders extend to first ribs.
  - Cardiac silhouette and diaphragm are separated by lung, with little or no contact.
  - Caudal vena cava is horizontal (lateral view) or parallel with the spine.
  - Lumbophrenic angles are open and caudal to T11–12 (lateral view).
  - Costophrenic angles are open and caudal to tenth rib (VD/DV view).
  - Diaphragm cupula is caudal to T8.
- Exposure is correct:
  - Background (outside of animal where there is only air) is black.
  - Heart and lungs are adequately exposed.
  - Lateral view: cranial thoracic vertebrae are faintly visible through the shoulders; ribs are faintly visible over the cardiac silhouette.
  - VD view: vertebrae and intervertebral spaces are faintly visible over the cardiac silhouette, more distinct cranial to the heart.

body markers. Look at the positions of the caudal vena cava, spleen, gas in the stomach fundus, the shape of the cardiac silhouette, and other landmarks to help verify the patient's right or left side.

Keep in mind the patient's age and body condition while you are reading the radiographs because these can affect the appearance of many structures. For example:

1. Immature animals have open physes, less distinct peritoneal serosal margins, more opaque lungs, and relatively large hearts and livers.
2. Aged animals are likely to have increased interstitial lung opacity and degenerative joint disease.

Table 2.9 Checklist for good quality abdominal radiographs

- Centered on the mid-abdomen.
- Collimation edges are visible and include entire abdomen, diaphragm to greater trochanters.
- Pelvic limbs are pulled caudally.
- Abdomen is not overly stretched.
- Right/Left body markers are visible and not in area of interest.
- No superimposition artifacts (e.g., ECG leads, sandbags, IV tubing, gloves).
- Take into account any rotation on lateral view:
  - Lumbar transverse processes lie within the vertebral bodies (processes do not extend ventral to the vertebrae).
  - Ilial wings are superimposed.
- Take into account any rotation on VD/DV view:
  - Lumbar dorsal spinous processes are centered on the vertebral bodies (do not extend beyond lateral edges of vertebrae).
  - Distance from spine to lateral body wall is equal on both sides.
- Exposure is correct:
  - Background (only air) is black.
  - Lumbar spine is underexposed, but vertebral trabeculae are faintly visible.

3. Patients with little body fat may have indistinct peritoneal serosal margins and lungs that appear hyperinflated.
4. Obese patients frequently have a wide mediastinum, large cardiac silhouette, and indistinct peritoneal serosal margins, the latter due to scatter fog.

Rest is an important part of reading radiographs that often is overlooked. The mind as well as the eyes need an occasional break while reviewing multiple radiographs. Try the 20-20-20 rule: for every 20 minutes of close screen or viewbox work, take 20 seconds to stare at something at least 20 ft away. A desirable viewing distance (reader to screen) is about 60 cm with the screen at eye level and appropriately angled.

Detection of radiographic abnormalities

To find an abnormality, one must look for it. To identify an abnormality, one must know about it. The ability to detect lesions in radiographs requires detailed knowledge of normal radiographic anatomy and its normal variations. What is "normal" can vary significantly among the many different breeds of dogs and cats. Reference materials such as textbooks, trusted websites, anatomical models, and a file of normal radiographs can be very helpful. A "normal radiographs" file can be made with film radiographs by physically placing normal studies in a folder and noting their location in the patient's record. With digital radiographs, normal images can be simply copied into a file. An easily accessible "normal file" also is a convenient reference source to help explain radiographic findings to pet owners.

When reading radiographs, always prepare for unexpected findings, including abnormalities not suggested by the patient's history or clinical data. Do not stop your evaluation after finding a lesion. Finish your systematic evaluation of the entire radiograph.

Examine each anatomical structure for abnormal size, shape, position, number, or opacity. Most actual abnormalities will be visible in more than one radiograph. If an abnormal finding does not repeat, it may be an artifact. As a general rule, whenever you find a suspected abnormality in a radiograph try to prove that it is a normal variation or an artifact. If you cannot prove one of these, then the abnormal finding is probably an actual lesion. This approach will help avoid many errors in diagnosis. Comparison radiographs of the contralateral side or limb also can be useful, provided the suspected disease or condition is unilateral.

Abnormal size: a structure that is larger than expected may be due to hypertrophy, hyperplasia, neoplasia, inflammation, infection, obstruction, or edema. A structure smaller than expected may be due to hypoplasia, atrophy, fibrosis, hypovolemia, or loss of tissue due to trauma or surgery.

Abnormal shape usually is accompanied by abnormal size. The border of an abnormally shaped structure may be smooth or irregular and its margin may be well-defined or ill-defined. An indistinct margin may be due to disease in the adjacent tissues, such as inflammation or fluid accumulation. Superimposition of adjacent structures can mimic abnormal shapes.

Abnormal position of a structure may be caused by a mass effect pushing the structure away from its normal location or an adhesion pulling on the structure. Loss of support can allow a structure to become displaced (e.g., hernia, body wall rupture, reduced size of an adjacent organ). Twisting or rotation along its axis may alter the position of an organ. A structure may develop in an ectopic location. Surgery can result in the absence or altered position of a structure.

Abnormal number: fewer than expected may be due to aplasia, surgical removal, or loss secondary to trauma. An increase in number may represent a congenital anomaly (e.g., supernumerary teeth or digits) or it may be due to surgery, such as a renal transplant.

Abnormal opacity: greater than expected opacity may be due to increased fluid (e.g., inflammation, effusion), mineralization, foreign material, or contrast medium. A structure that is less opaque than expected may be due to loss of mineral or an increase in gas or fat.

Evidence of **abnormal function** sometimes is seen in survey radiographs or in a contrast radiography study. Abnormal GI motility or renal function, for example, maybe evident.

When the radiographic appearance of a structure is not as expected, it is an abnormality. An abnormality in a radiograph may be called a radiographic *sign*, a *Roentgen sign*, a radiographic *finding*, or a radiographic *change*. The terms frequently are used interchangeably. A radiographic sign may represent a true abnormality, a normal variation, or an artifact. Recognizing the difference is a crucial part of radiographic interpretation.

Interpretation of radiographic findings

Patient history is not necessary to evaluate radiographs, but it is needed to interpret the findings. A definitive diagnoses seldom is made from radiographs alone. The purpose of radiography is to lessen uncertainty. Radiographs can help rule in or rule out some if not all of the possible causes for the patient's clinical signs. All radiographic findings must be carefully considered along with the results of your physical examination and laboratory testing. In the light of this information, a prioritized list of differential diagnoses can be formulated, ranked from most likely to least likely. A written report should be provided for each radiographic study and included in the patient record.

If one has never heard of a disease, one cannot diagnose it. Consultation with board-certified radiologists is a valuable source of learning (i.e., teleradiology). A radiologist can provide expert opinion, make recommendations for additional diagnostic tests and help guide treatment. Diplomates of the American College of Veterinary Radiology (ACVR) and the European College of Veterinary Diagnostic Imaging (ECVDI), both in private practice and in veterinary teaching hospitals, provide these services.

3 Thorax

Radiography of the Dog and Cat: Guide to Making and Interpreting Radiographs, Second Edition. M.C. Muhlbauer and S.K. Kneller.

Companion website: www.wiley.com/go/muhlbauer/dog

Introduction

Air-filled lungs provide an excellent opacity interface to visualize intra-thoracic soft tissues. The ratio of gas to soft tissue in normally inflated lungs is greater than 10:1. To take full advantage of the gas-to-soft tissue opacity interface, make thoracic radiographs at peak inspiration. Fully inflated lungs not only enhance the visibility of intra-thoracic structures, they also separate the structures to reduce summation and superimposition artifacts (Figures 3.1 and 3.2). Poor lung inflation can mimic or mask disease. At the end of this chapter there are extensive lists of differential diagnoses for numerous radiographic findings regarding the thorax.

Procedure for making thoracic radiographs

1. As needed, clean and dry the patient's hair coat and skin prior to radiography.
2. Remove any collars, harnesses, or coverings and move any monitoring equipment out of the field-of-view (e.g., ECG leads, IV tubing).
3. Note any cutaneous or subcutaneous growths on the patient that may create artifacts in the radiographs.
4. **Measure** the widest part of the thorax, usually over the liver at the level of the xyphoid or 12th rib.
5. **Center** the x-ray beam on the heart. Landmarks include the caudal edge of the scapula or between the fourth and sixth intercostal spaces or at the point of maximum heartbeat intensity.

A

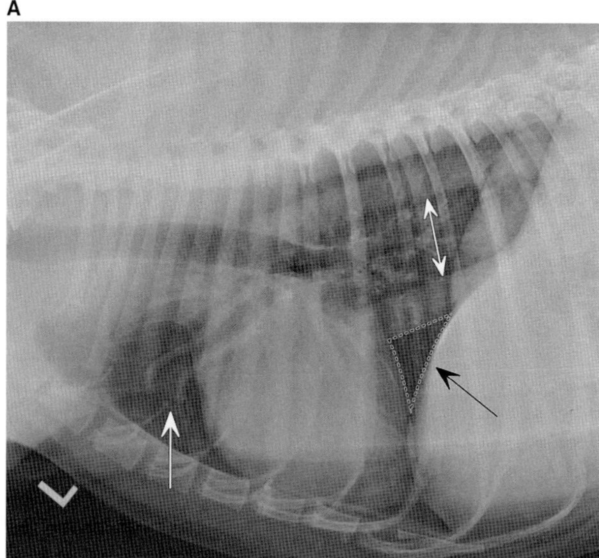

B

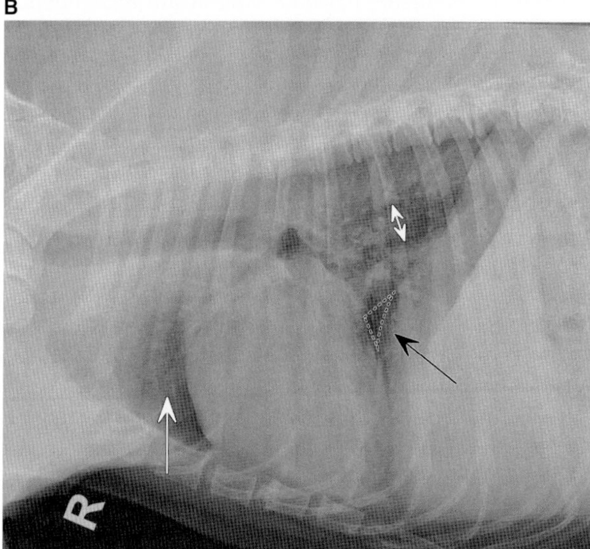

Figure 3.1 Inspiration vs. Expiration. Lateral views of a dog thorax made during inspiration (**A**) and expiration (**B**). Fully inflated lungs provide the gas-to-soft tissue opacity interfaces needed to identify the intra-thoracic structures. The cranial lobar blood vessels are better visualized during inspiration than expiration (white arrow). During inspiration, there is a better separation between the aorta and caudal vena cava (white double-headed arrow) and between the heart and diaphragm (black arrow and dotted triangle). The caudal vena cava is more parallel with the spine during inspiration.

6. **Collimate** the field-of-view (FOV) as small as practical to include the entire bony thorax (ribs, spine, sternum) from the thoracic inlet to the last ribs. Collimation reduces scatter radiation and improves radiographic detail.
7. Move the thoracic limbs cranially to eliminate superimposition. **Avoid overstretching** the patient as this will distort the shape of the thorax, especially with cats and small dogs (Figure 3.3).
8. Align the **spine and sternum** in the same plane.
9. Use body markers to indicate **R**ight or **L**eft. Place the markers away from the area of interest.
10. Make the **x-ray exposure** at peak inspiration. If the patient is panting, try temporarily holding its mouth closed and then allowing it to take a deep breath just prior to making the exposure.

A

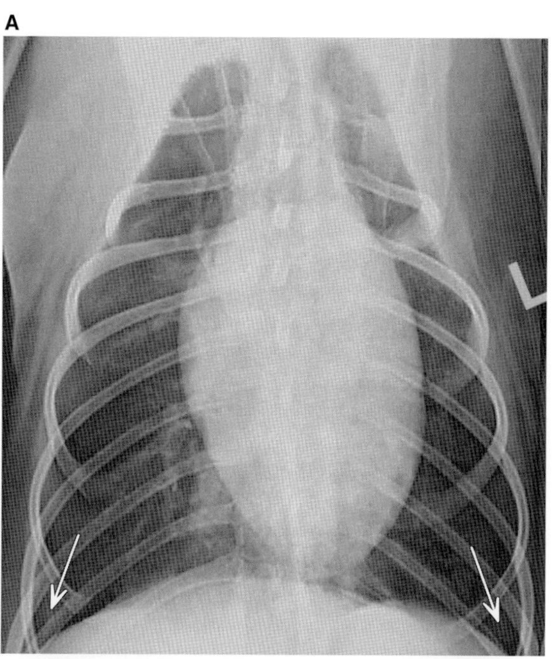

B

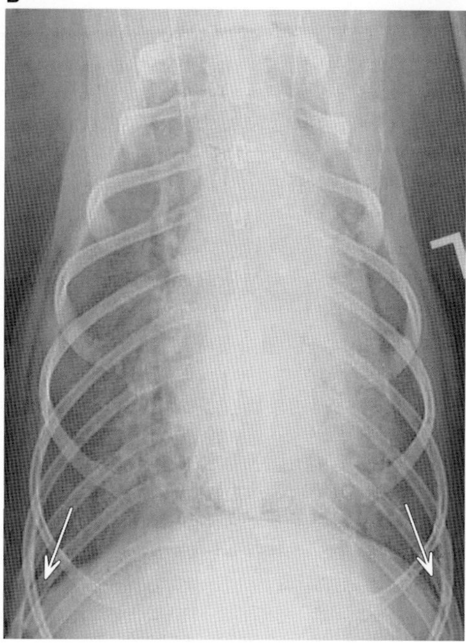

Figure 3.2 Inspiration vs. Expiration. VD views of a dog thorax made during inspiration (**A**) and expiration (**B**). Fully inflated lungs separate the cardiac silhouette and diaphragm and enhance the opacity interface. The costophrenic angles (white arrows) are wider and sharper during inspiration.

11. Use the **shortest exposure time** practical to minimize the effects of respiratory and cardiac motion. If your x-ray equipment is not capable of a short exposure time, make the exposure at the end of expiration when there is a slight pause in the patient's breathing.
12. **High kVp** and **low mAs** techniques generally are preferred for thoracic radiography because there are more shades of gray in low contrast radiographs. Many gray shades are needed to visualize the fine pulmonary structures.
13. In a **properly exposed** thoracic radiograph, both the individual thoracic vertebrae and the peripheral pulmonary vessels should be visible. Film radiographs that are slightly underexposed or overexposed usually require only minor changes in kVp, typically a 10% increase or decrease. More severe errors in exposure often can be corrected by doubling or halving the mAs. Digital radiographs are much more forgiving of errors in exposure.
14. **External body markers** placed on skin growth, nipple, or subcutaneous swelling can be used to identify the structure in a radiograph. Extra-thoracic structures are a common cause of false lung lesions. Use a small amount of positive contrast medium or a commercially available skin marker to indicate the structure (Figure 3.134).

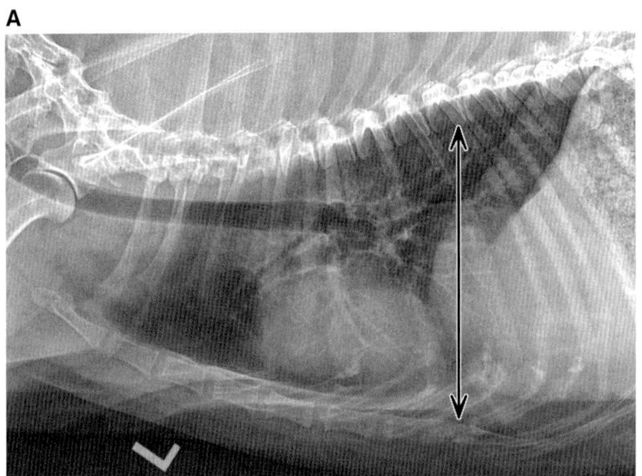

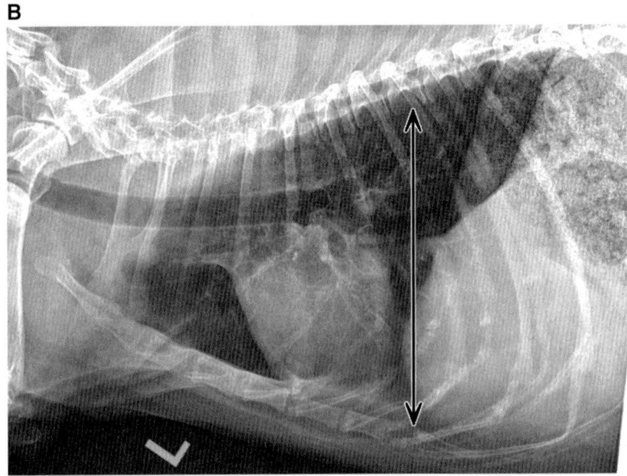

Figure 3.3 Stretching the patient. Two lateral views of the same 10-year-old, 22-kg dog. In radiograph **A**, the patient is hyperextended resulting in dorsoventral narrowing of the thorax (double-headed arrow), less inflated lungs, a narrowed trachea, and distortion of the cardiac silhouette. In radiograph **B**, the patient is in a more neutral and relaxed position, allowing the lungs to expand and producing a truer representation of the trachea and cardiac silhouette.

Radiographic views of the thorax

Orthogonal views are necessary for complete evaluation. Standard orthogonal views of the thorax include a left or right lateral view (preferably both) and a ventrodorsal (VD) or dorsoventral (DV) view.

1. **Lateral views** (Figure 2.8): either a right or left lateral view can be made, but both laterals are recommended because unilateral lung lesions may not be visible when that lung is dependent. This is because in lateral recumbency the "down" lung collapses, which reduces the opacity interface and may hide a lesion (see "Nodular lung lesions" later in this chapter). Lung collapse can occur in less than 5 minutes of recumbency.
2. Right lateral view is preferred over left lateral to visualize lesions in the left lung.
3. Left lateral view is preferred over right lateral to visualize lesions in the right lung and to evaluate the cranial pulmonary blood vessels.
4. **VD view** (Figure 2.9) often is preferred over a DV view to facilitate patient positioning, particularly with cats. The mediastinum, caudal vena cava, and accessory lung lobe tend to be better visualized in a VD view than in a DV. Small volumes of pleural fluid may be easier to detect in a VD view.
5. **DV view** (Figure 2.10) may be preferred over a VD view to position patients that are in distress (e.g., shock, severe dyspnea). The dorsal parts of the thoracic cavity tend to be better visualized in a DV view than in a VD (e.g., dorsal lungs, caudal pulmonary vessels, esophagus, hilar region). Small volumes of pleural gas may be easier to detect in a DV view.
6. **Altering the x-ray exposure** can be used to enhance visualization of certain areas, more so with film radiography than with digital radiography. Doubling the mAs increases density and contrast to enhance visualization of skeletal and mineralized structures. Cutting the exposure time in half may improve visualization of peripheral soft tissues or aid in detection of small volumes of free gas.
7. **Expiratory radiographs** can be used to increase lung opacity and decrease lung volume, which may aid in the detection of small volumes of gas or fluid in the pleural

space and cavitary lesions in the lungs. Comparing expiratory with inspiratory radiographs may be useful to evaluate suspected tracheal collapse syndrome or lung emphysema.

8. **Oblique views** are made with the patient rotated (Figure 2.11) and can be used to displace overlying structures away from an area of interest. For example, the heart and spine are rotated away from the esophagus in a VD oblique view.
9. **Tangential beam** views are made with the x-ray beam centered on a peripheral lesion in the thoracic wall or pleural space (Figure 2.12). The FOV is tightly collimated to isolate the lesion and enhance its visibility.
10. "**Human view**" is a VD view made with the thoracic limbs pulled caudally (Figure 2.13). It is used to eliminate superimposition of the scapula and shoulder muscles on the cranial lung lobes and mediastinum.
11. **Skyline view** is a craniodorsal-to-caudoventral view of the thoracic inlet (Figure 2.14). It is used to visualize the trachea in cross-section, which often aids in the evaluation of suspected tracheal collapse syndrome, tracheal stenosis, or tracheal hypoplasia.
12. **Horizontal beam radiography** (Figure 2.15) can be used to detect small volumes of gas or fluid in the thoracic cavity. It also can be used to reposition intra-thoracic fluid or gas to better visualize lungs or pleural space. Pleural fluid flows with gravity into the dependent part of the thoracic cavity. Gas rises to the highest or uppermost part.

Radiographs of the **pharynx or larynx** are useful to examine the upper respiratory tract, which may be helpful in determining the etiology of lower respiratory disease. Whenever practical, remove the endotracheal tube and any superimposed monitoring equipment prior to imaging the cervical region. Measure the thickest part of the neck, usually near the head, and center the x-ray beam on the larynx. Collimate the FOV to the area of interest and use the small focal spot. The lateral view is made with the mouth closed and the head and neck in a neutral position, about a 135° angle between the spine and the mandibles. Align the transverse processes of C1 in the same plane and elevate the sternum as needed to correct rotation. The VD/DV view is made with the head and neck extended. If needed, rotate the patient slightly to the left or right to eliminate superimposition of the skull and spine.

Patient factors

The patient's age, body type, body condition, phase of respiration, and position at the time of radiography can significantly affect the radiographic appearance of thoracic structures. Conditions outside the thoracic cavity may affect the appearance of the intra-thoracic structures, including abdominal distention that limits lung inflation (Figure 3.4). Some of these effects are described below and discussed in more detail with each specific structure later in this chapter.

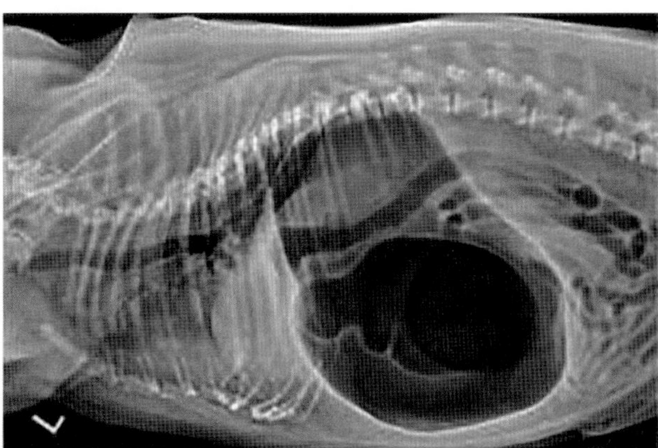

Figure 3.4 Distended abdomen. Lateral view of a dog depicting abdominal distention due to gastric bloat. The distended abdomen limits expansion of the thoracic cavity which results in poor lung inflation.

Immature animals

1. Lungs are more opaque than in adults due to higher water content.
2. Tracheal diameter is relatively smaller than in adults.
3. Cardiac-to-thoracic ratio is larger than in adults (the heart appears relatively larger in immature animals than in adults).
4. Cranial mediastinum is more opaque due to the thymus, which may be visible in dogs up to 6–12 months of age and in cats up to two years of age.

Aged animals

1. Bone spurs commonly form at the edges of the sternebrae and vertebrae (e.g., spondylosis deformans).
2. Costal cartilages normally grow larger, mineralize, and become more irregular as an animal ages.
3. Cartilaginous discs between the sternebrae may mineralize, particularly in large breed dogs.
4. Tracheal and bronchial walls frequently increase in opacity due to mineralization or fibrosis.
5. Remnants of previous disease may increase lung opacity and make pleural fissure lines more visible.
6. In older cats, the cardiac silhouette often is more horizontal (inclined toward the sternum) and the aorta appears more wavy or tortuous.

Obese animals

1. Thoracic wall is thickened due to subcutaneous fat.
2. Widened cranial mediastinum due to fat deposits.
3. Trachea may be displaced due to mediastinal fat.

4. Pericardial fat gives the appearance of a large cardiac silhouette. Cardiac shadow may be dorsally displaced away from the sternum by excess fat.
5. Margins of cranial mediastinal soft tissues may be more visible due to surrounding fat.
6. Lungs are more opaque due to summation of overlying fat and because lungs cannot fully expand. Lung margins may not extend all the way to the ribs.
7. Fat between lung lobes can create "reverse" pleural fissure lines that are wide centrally and taper peripherally.

Emaciated animals

1. Thoracic cavity and lungs tend to be less opaque due to less overlying tissue and greater lung inflation.
2. Cardiac shadow may appear small due to loss of pericardial fat and greater lung inflation.
3. Cranial mediastinal structures may be more visible against inflated lungs due to a thin mediastinum.
4. Diaphragm may be more caudal in position due to reduced abdominal content and expanded lungs.

Breed conformation

1. In dogs with a narrow, deep thorax the cardiac silhouette is more upright and narrow and may be dorsally separated from the sternum.
2. In dogs with a wide, shallow thorax the cardiac silhouette is wider and more rounded, and the trachea is closer to the spine.
3. In athletic animals (e.g., greyhounds) the cardiac-to-thoracic ratio is relatively large.
4. In heavily-muscled animals the lungs may appear more opaque due to superimposition of overlying tissue.
5. In brachycephalic and chondrodystrophic breeds the cranial mediastinum is wider and the thoracic trachea is slightly curved or bent. The aortic arch is relatively large in these breeds. Mineralization of the tracheal rings, bronchial walls, costal cartilages, and costochondral junctions occurs at a younger age in chondrodystrophic breeds.

Effects of positioning

1. As little as five degree rotation of the patient can significantly alter the apparent size, shape, and position of the intra-thoracic structures, including the cardiac shadow, trachea, lung lesions, and others (Figure 3.5).
2. Lungs frequently appear more opaque in lateral views than in VD/DV views. Suspected increases in lung opacity should be confirmed in orthogonal views.
3. The dependent lungs are less inflated, more perfused, and more opaque than the non-dependent lungs due to the effects of gravity. This means the opacity interface is weak in the dependent lungs, and the margins of soft tissue structures will be less distinct.
4. Stretching or hyperextending the patient during radiography can distort the thorax and alter the appearance of the intra-thoracic structures (Figure 3.3).

A

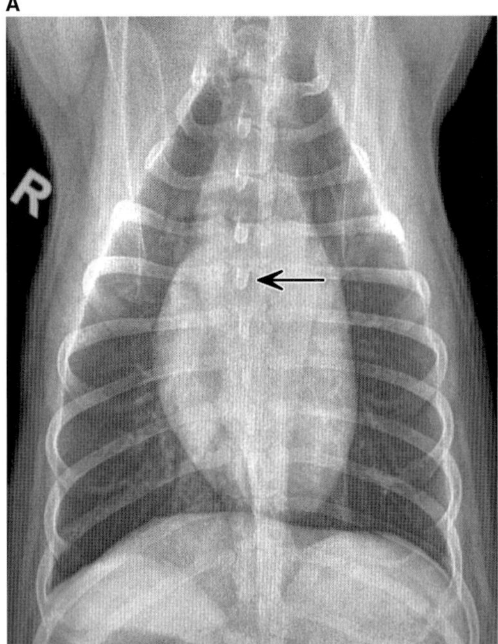

B

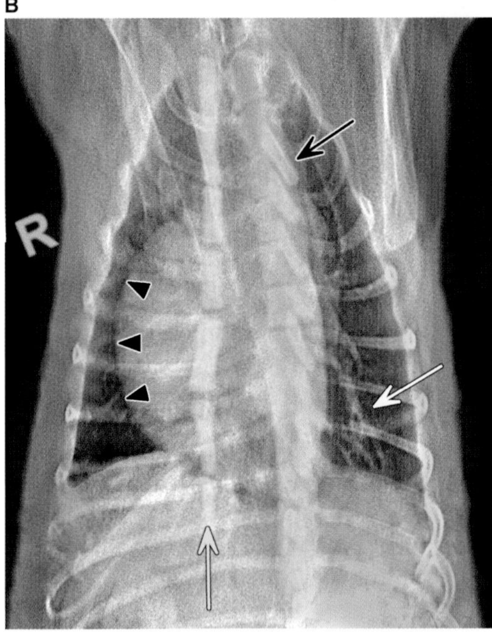

Figure 3.5 Patient rotation artifacts. **A**. A properly positioned VD view of a dog thorax: the spine and sternum are superimposed, the dorsal spinous processes are centered in the vertebral bodies (black arrow), and the right and left ribs are equal length. **B**. A VD view made with the patient rotated to the right: the appearance of the thorax is distorted. The sternum is right of the spine (yellow arrow) and most of the cardiac shadow is right of midline (the heart follows the sternum). The right cardiac border is closer to the right thoracic wall (black arrowheads) which may be mistaken for right heart enlargement. The right ribs are longer than the left and the dorsal spinous processes project lateral to the vertebral bodies (black arrow). The left caudal pulmonary vessels, which normally are superimposed on the cardiac silhouette, are visible spine (white arrow) and may be mistaken for enlarged vessels or lung disease.

Thoracic wall

Normal radiographic anatomy

The thoracic wall is composed of bones, soft tissues, and fat. The bony thorax includes the ribs, vertebrae, and sternebrae. Soft-tissue structures are skin, muscle, blood vessels, nerves, and pleura.

The average number of **ribs** in both dogs and cats is 26 or (13 pair). The head of each rib articulates with the cranial aspect of the same numbered thoracic vertebra (Figure 3.6). For example, the third rib attaches to the cranial end of the third thoracic (T3) vertebra. The ribs in chondrodystrophic dogs (e.g., Bassett Hound, Dachshund) normally curve inward and indent the lungs at the costochondral junctions (Figure 3.12). Inward curving ribs may be mistaken for pleural fluid.

The gaps between ribs are the **intercostal spaces**. Comparing the right and left sides, the intercostal spaces (ICS) are relatively symmetrical; however, the symmetry may temporarily be lost due to oblique positioning or muscular contractions. Each ICS is numbered according to its cranial rib (e.g., the third ICS is caudal to the third rib).

The **sternum** contains 8–9 sternebrae, which are similar in appearance to the vertebrae. The first sternebra is the *manubrium*, which is the longest. The last sternebra is the *xyphoid*, which can vary significantly in size and shape. Located between the sternebrae are cartilaginous discs. These discs are similar in appearance and function to intervertebral discs. Two or more sternebrae may be fused or malaligned due to a congenital or developmental abnormality. Congenital abnormalities usually are asymptomatic and may be differentiated from pathology of the sternum by the lack of soft tissue swelling and absence of a periosteal response.

Costal cartilages extend from the distal end of each rib to the sternum. Cartilages from the first 8 ribs join the intersternebral discs. Cartilages from the caudal ribs attach at the xyphoid or merge together. Mineralization of the costal cartilages normally begins at a few months of age. Mineralization has been described as heterogenous, mottled or granular and frequently becomes more sclerotic and irregular over time (Figure 3.7). Mineralized costal cartilages can become quite large, especially in chondrodystrophic and large breed dogs. Large mineralizations may be mistaken for lesions in the lungs or thoracic wall. Costal cartilage mineralization sometimes occurs in short segments, appearing as transverse lines of increased and decreased opacity. These lines may be mistaken for fractures. Carefully inspect the costal cartilages when interpreting radiographic findings to avoid an erroneous diagnosis.

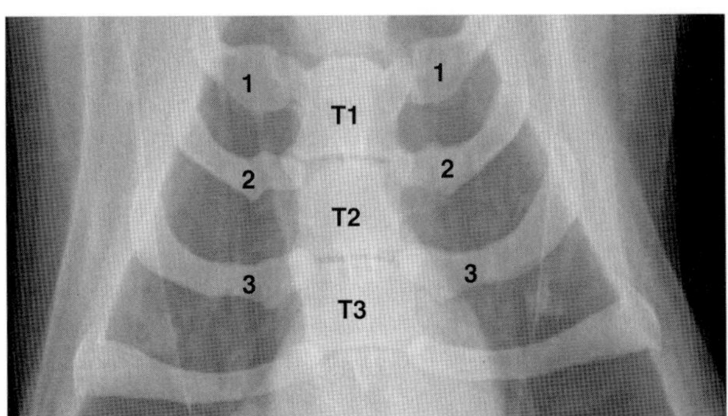

Figure 3.6 Rib articulations. VD view of a dog thorax depicting numbered ribs and the corresponding numbered thoracic vertebrae.

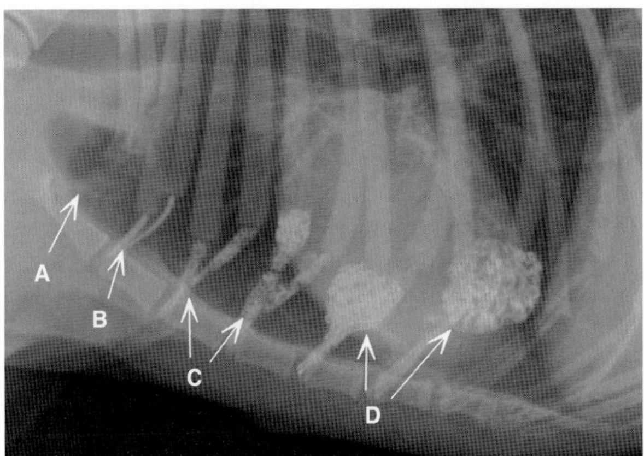

Figure 3.7 Costochondral junctions. Lateral view of a dog thorax depicting various appearances of costal cartilages. **A**. Soft tissue opacity cartilage that is not mineralized. **B**. Uniform mineralization of cartilage. **C**. Heterogenous mineralizations, common in older dogs. **D.** Large mineralizations at multiple costochondral junctions.

Thickened thoracic wall

The normal thickness (width) of the thoracic wall varies with the patient body condition. The wall is thicker in obese and heavily muscled patients and thinner in lean animals. Abnormal thickening usually is *extracostal* (outside the ribs) and may be unilateral or bilateral, focal or diffuse. Focal thickening is due to a mass (see thoracic wall mass below), whereas diffuse thickening may result from subcutaneous accumulation of fat, gas, or fluid (Figure 3.8).

Subcutaneous fat may represent obesity or a large lipoma. Obesity is bilateral and lipomas tend to be unilateral. The extracostal muscles may be outlined and displaced by fat, appearing as thin, curved, soft tissue opacity lines that resemble the shapes of the ribs.

Subcutaneous emphysema may be unilateral or bilateral, typically producing a mixed pattern of gas and soft tissue opacities. Emphysema may result from a penetrating wound or migration of gas from a ruptured trachea or pneumomediastinum. Superimposition of subcutaneous gas may compromise evaluation of the thoracic cavity and

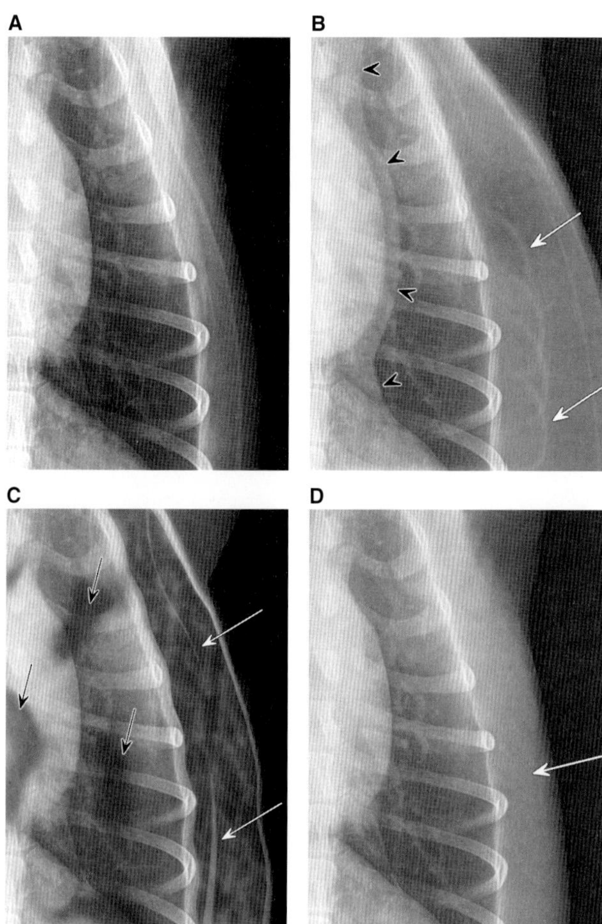

Figure 3.8 Diffuse thickening of the thoracic wall. VD views of a dog thorax depicting thickening of the thoracic wall. **A**. Normal thoracic wall for comparison. **B**. Subcutaneous fat due to obesity causes diffuse thickening of the thoracic wall. The extracostal muscles are displaced and outlined by fat to create curved, soft tissue opacity lines (white arrows) that conform to the shapes of the ribs. Notice the lungs are more opaque than in image A due to summation of overlying fat. Pericardial fat surrounds the cardiac silhouette (black arrowheads). **C**. Subcutaneous emphysema creates a mixed pattern and outlines the extracostal muscles (white arrows). Summation of emphysema may be mistaken for gas in the thoracic cavity (black arrows). **D**. Subcutaneous fluid produces uniform soft tissue opacity thickening of the thoracic wall (white arrow) and obscures the fascial planes and extracostal muscles. The type of fluid cannot be determined from radiographs. Compared to image A, the thoracic cavity is overall increased in opacity due to summation of the subcutaneous fluid.

may mask or mimic free gas in the mediastinum or pleural space.

Subcutaneous fluid may be unilateral or bilateral and can obscure the margins of the extracostal muscles. Fluid may represent edema, inflammation, hemorrhage, or it may be iatrogenic (i.e., fluid therapy). Summation of subcutaneous fluid may increase the opacity of the thoracic cavity.

Thoracic wall mass

Masses in the thoracic wall can involve any osseous or soft tissue structure. They produce localized, defined areas of thickening. The margins of a mass may be well-defined or indistinct, depending on the opacity interface. Masses that are walled-off and surrounded by a different opacity may be well-visualized, provided they are large enough to be distinguished. Adjacent inflammation or other fluid accumulation can obscure the margins of soft tissue opacity masses.

A mass in the thoracic wall may not be physically palpable or radiographically visible until quite large. Large masses can displace the adjacent ribs and widen the intercostal spaces. The ribs near a mass should be carefully examined for evidence of a periosteal response, osteolysis, and/or expansile remodeling.

A thoracic wall mass that grows inward, toward the thoracic cavity, can produce a bulge that displaces the adjacent lung. The bulge creates an **extra-pleural sign**. The extra-pleural sign helps differentiate masses that originate outside the pleura from those that originate in the lung or pleural space (Figure 3.9). The edges of an extra-pleural mass gradually taper toward the inner chest wall, forming angles greater than 90°. Pulmonary and pleural masses form acute angles (less than 90°) with the chest wall. Pleural effusion is absent with

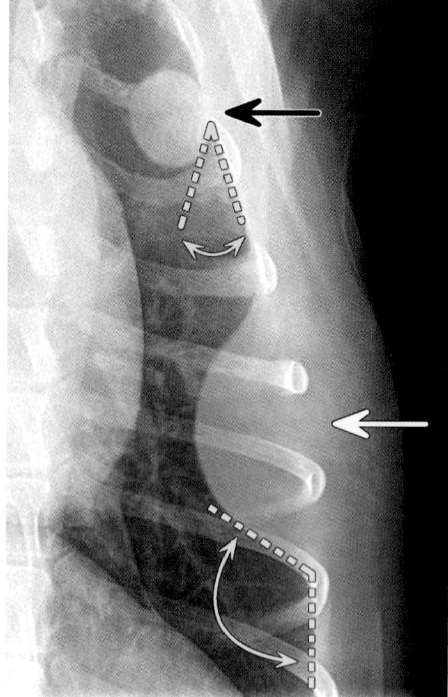

Figure 3.9 Extra-pleural sign. VD view of a dog thorax depicting a mass in the thoracic wall (white arrow) and a pulmonary nodule located near the thoracic wall (black arrow). The margins of the thoracic wall mass gradually taper cranially and caudally to form angles greater than 90° with the inner chest wall. The margins of the lung mass form acute angles less than 90° with the chest wall.

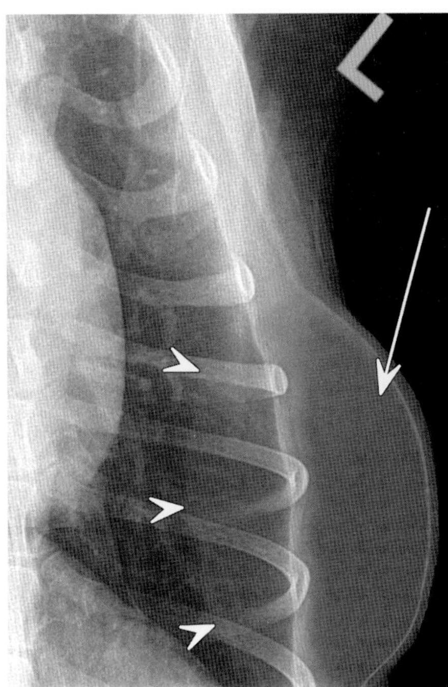

Figure 3.10 Thoracic wall lipoma. VD view of a dog thorax depicting a well-defined, fat opacity mass in the left thoracic wall (white arrow). There is no extra-pleural sign because the lipoma does not bulge into the thoracic cavity (notice the small pulmonary vessels that are visible through the lipoma and extend to the chest wall). Part of the lipoma is superimposed on the lung to create an area of faintly increased opacity (white arrowheads).

extra-pleural masses (unless the pleura is damaged), but fluid is common with masses that originate in the pleural space.

The opacity of a thoracic wall mass provides clues to its etiology. **Gas** opacity may result from a penetrating wound or infection with a gas-producing bacteria. Herniation of a gas-filled GI structure can produce a defined area of gas opacity. A **fat** opacity mass may represent a lipoma (Figure 3.10) or contents in a hernia. Lipomas can become very large, often with well-defined margins. Indistinct margins suggest fluid adjacent to the lipoma (e.g., inflammation, edema) or a dissecting lipoma (or liposarcoma). **Soft tissue** opacity masses include tumors, abscesses, granulomas, seromas, and hematomas. **Mineral** opacity in a mass may be foreign material or dystrophic mineralization, the latter occurring in long-standing abscesses, granulomas, or tumors.

A paracostal hernia can create an extra-pleural mass that is mixed in opacity due to the presence of displaced viscera, gas-filled bowel, and fat (Figure 3.26).

Abnormal bony thorax

Congenital skeletal abnormalities are common in dogs and cats. Most are benign and asymptomatic. It is important to recognize benign conditions because they can alter the shape of the thorax, distort the positions of intra-thoracic structures, and vary the locations of landmarks used during surgical and advanced imaging procedures. Benign conditions often can be differentiated from pathology by a lack of soft tissue swelling and an absence of active bone remodeling. Poor patient positioning also can alter the appearance of the bony thorax, such as making the curvature of the spine appear abnormal and distorting the sizes and shapes of the ribs.

Vertebral abnormalities

Congenital spinal abnormalities such as transitional vertebrae and hemivertebrae occur frequently in dogs and cats. **Transitional vertebrae** can affect the number of vertebrae and ribs (Figures 5.202 and 5.203). **Hemivertebrae** can alter the curvature of the spine, as well as cause narrowing of the intercostal spaces and crowding of the ribs (Figure 3.11). Spinal abnormalities are discussed further in Chapter 5: Musculoskeletal.

A

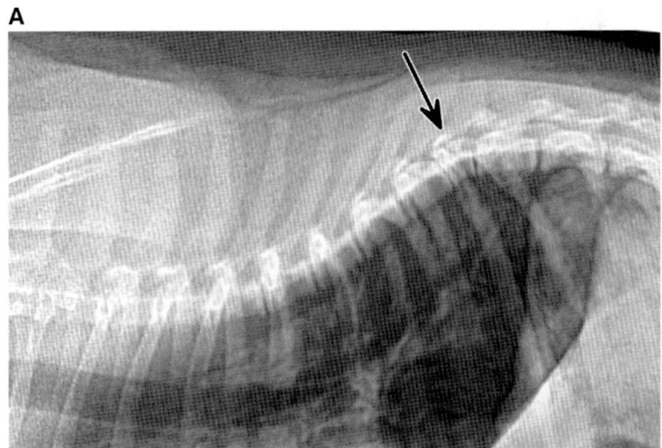

B

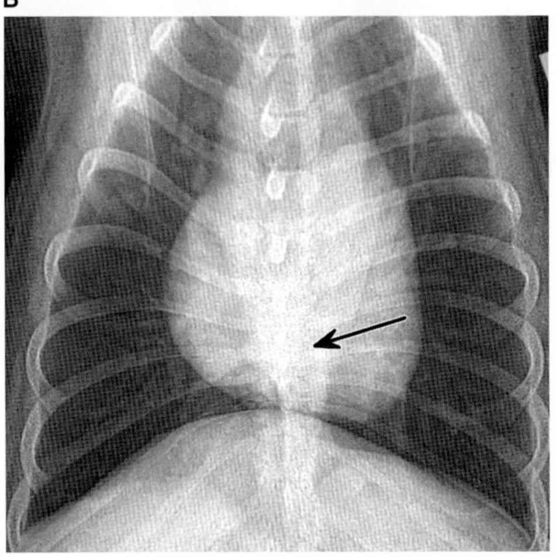

Figure 3.11 Hemivertebra. Lateral view (**A**) and VD view (**B**) of a dog thorax depicting a partially developed, wedge-shaped vertebra in the caudal thoracic spine (black arrow). There is spinal kyphosis and crowding of the proximal ribs. In the VD view, the ribs radiate from the hemivertebra to resemble the spokes in a bicycle wheel.

Rib abnormalities

The ribs are thin and sometimes indistinct in radiographs due to summation with other structures. To make the ribs more conspicuous, try altering your viewing perspective. Inverting the radiograph, either by turning the image upside down or by reversing the black-and-white scale of a digital image, tends to draw more attention to the ribs. Supplemental radiographs also can be helpful. Many rib lesions are easier to see when viewed tangentially (in profile rather than *en face*). Follow-up radiographs often aid in confirming or refuting suspected rib lesions. Keep in mind that in a lateral view, the "up" ribs (furthest from the image receptor) will be larger and less distinct due to magnification distortion.

Congenital rib abnormalities may alter the number or shape of the ribs. Abnormalities may be unilateral or bilateral. Extra ribs occur more often at the first cervical and first lumbar vertebrae. Fewer ribs are seen more often in the caudal thorax. Congenital alterations that affect the shapes of ribs include flaring at the ends, fusion of adjacent ribs, and bipartite development. In chondrodystrophic breeds, notably Bassett Hounds, the distal parts of the ribs normally curve inward at the costochondral junctions (Figure 3.12). Inward curving ribs also can occur in animals with pectus excavatum.

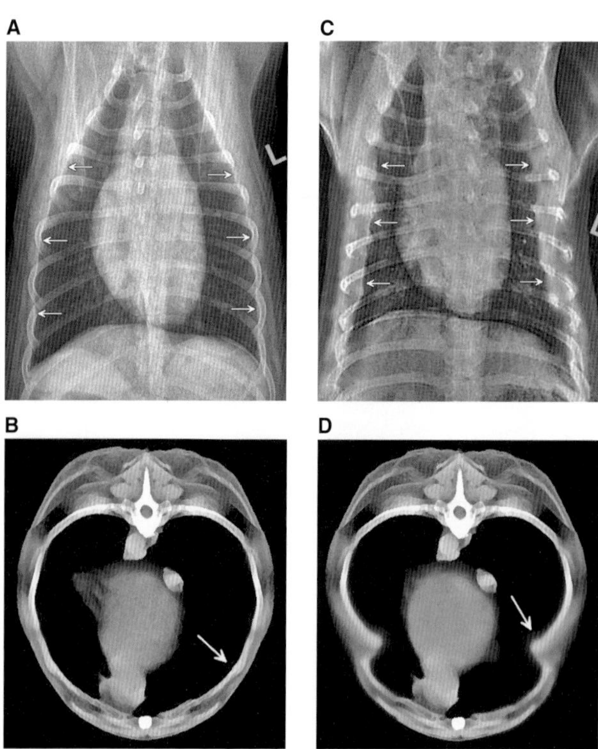

Figure 3.12 Inward curving ribs. VD radiograph (**A**) and CT image (**B**) of a typical dog thorax. The lungs extend to the inner margins of the ribs (arrows). VD view (**C**) and CT image (**D**) of a Bassett Hound thorax. The inward curving ribs (arrow in **D**) create soft tissue opacity along the inner thoracic walls (arrows in **C**) which may be mistaken for pleural fluid.

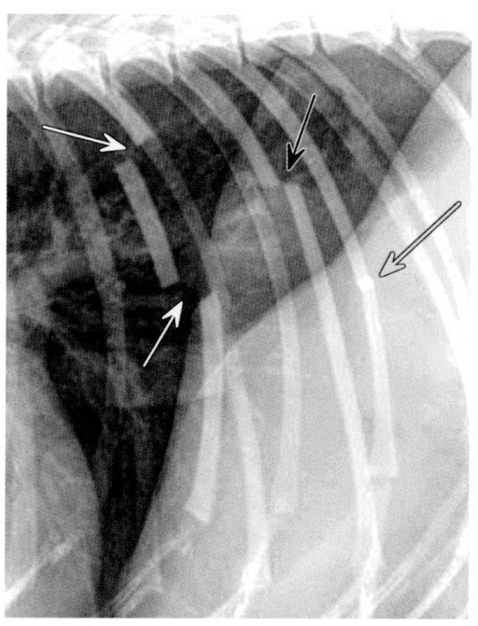

Figure 3.13 R Types of rib fractures. Lateral view of a dog thorax depicting three types of rib fractures, including a cranially displaced segmental rib fracture (white arrows), a caudally displaced transverse rib fracture (black arrow), and a minimally displaced, overriding rib fracture (yellow arrow). In the latter, notice the increased opacity caused by overlap of the fracture ends.

An **acquired absence of one or more ribs** may be due to disease or surgical removal and can occur anywhere along the thorax. Diseases include nutritional, metabolic, neoplastic, and infectious disorders.

Rib fractures typically result from blunt force trauma. Fractures tend to be transverse or oblique and often involve multiple ribs, usually sequentially (Figure 3.13). Other signs of trauma may be concurrent with rib fractures, such as subcutaneous emphysema, pneumothorax, and pulmonary contusions. Minimally displaced rib fractures may be difficult to detect unless the x-ray beam is aligned with the fracture line. Oblique views sometimes are helpful. Follow-up radiographs often reveal osseous remodeling at the fracture site(s). Healing that has progressed without complication produces a localized area of expansile remodeling with smooth, well-defined margins and little or no soft tissue swelling (Figure 3.14). Respiratory motion during healing may lead to larger than expected callus formation. A lot of motion at a fracture site can result in a malunion or non-union rib fracture.

Spontaneous rib fractures have been reported in patients with prolonged dyspnea, severe coughing, or metabolic disease. In these cases, there is no history of trauma. Spontaneous fractures most often occur in the caudal ribs, particularly in older cats with underlying respiratory or renal disease.

Pathologic rib fractures frequently are associated with neoplasia or severe osteomyelitis. Neoplasia is a more

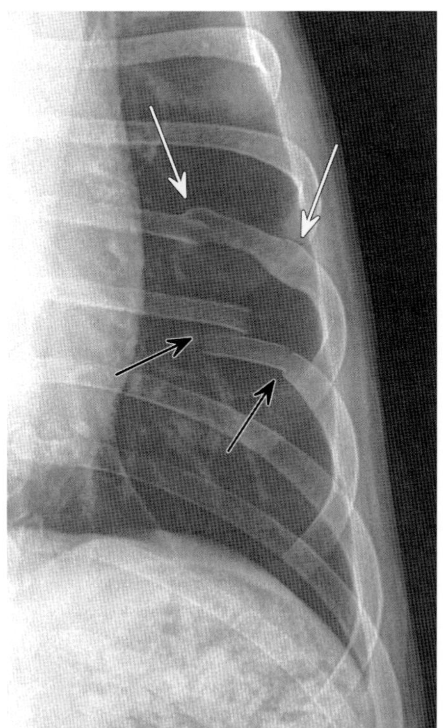

Figure 3.14 Rib fractures. VD view of a dog thorax depicting older, healing rib fractures (white arrows) and a new segmental rib fracture (black arrows). The margins of the healing fractures are smooth and well-defined. The more medial fracture is healing in slight malunion. The more lateral fracture appears as an expansile area in the rib. The ends of the newer, segmental fracture are sharply marginated without evidence of periosteal new bone production.

common cause than osteomyelitis, but the two cannot be differentiated in radiographs. Both can produce a productive or/and lytic bone response (Figure 3.15). Swelling in or near a rib without history or radiographic evidence of trauma should be investigated for neoplasia.

Rib tumors in dogs and cats more often are secondary than primary. Metastatic rib tumors typically are small, slow-growing, and arise in the middle (shaft) of a rib. Slow-growing tumors tend to create expansile areas of osseous remodeling that may be difficult to distinguish from healing fractures. Any solitary rib lesion should be monitored with serial radiographs until proven benign. Primary rib tumors often arise further distally in a rib, near the costochondral junction. They can become quite large and may mineralize. Pleural effusion is absent unless a tumor erodes through the pleura. Primary rib tumors more often are reported in large-breed dogs.

Flail chest is a condition that results from segmental fractures in two or more adjacent ribs (Figure 3.16). The middle fragments become functionally free and move paradoxically with respiration. The fragments are pulled inward during inspiration and pushed outward during expiration (Figure 3.17). The conflicted movement of the chest wall leads to ineffective breathing and can quickly become an emergency, life-threatening situation. In some patients, pain and muscle contractions may limit respiration and initially hide the paradoxical movements.

Abnormal intercostal spaces

Intercostal spaces (ICS) that are significantly wider or narrower than nearby ICS should be investigated. **Abnormal widening** may be due to traumatic swelling, a space-occupying mass,

A

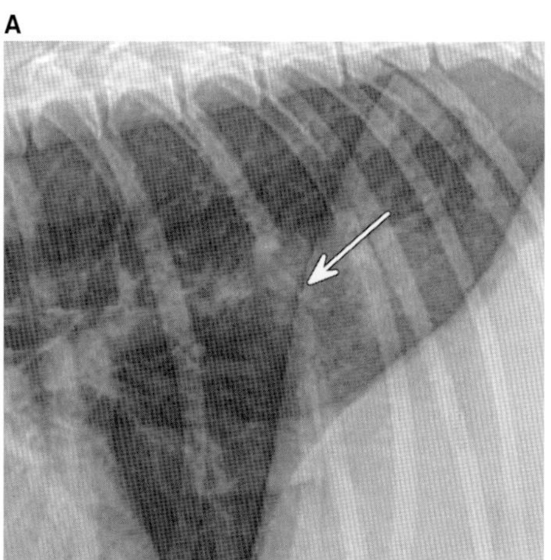

B

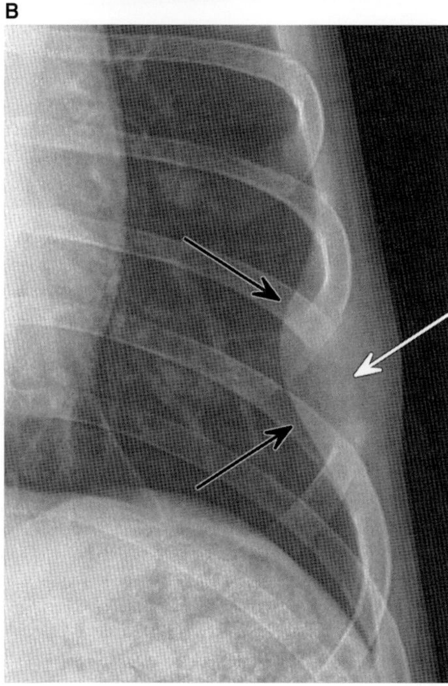

Figure 3.15 Rib tumor. Lateral view (**A**) and VD view (**B**) of a dog thorax depicting localized soft tissue swelling and osteolysis in the left eighth rib (white arrow). No periosteal response is visible. The lesion is easier to see in the VD view because it is tangential to the x-ray beam and there is less superimposition artifact. The soft tissue swelling produces an extra-pleural sign (black arrows). Possible causes for these radiographic findings include tumor and osteomyelitis.

or uneven hyperexpansion of the thorax. Trauma that widens ICS often is accompanied by other signs of injury (e.g., fractured ribs, subcutaneous emphysema). An intercostal mass generally widens one ICS and causes narrowing in the adjacent ICS. Hyperexpansion of the thorax may be due to emphysema or a tension pneumothorax and widens multiple ICS. **Abnormal narrowing** of ICS may be due to muscle contractions, poor lung inflation, or previous thoracotomy. Muscle contractions secondary to pain or struggling cause transient ICS narrowing, which changes in appearance in serial radiographs.

Sternal abnormalities

As mentioned earlier, congenital fusion or malalignment of two or more sternebrae often are incidental findings that may be differentiated from pathology by a lack of soft tissue swelling and an absence of bone remodeling (Figure 3.18). **Sternal dysraphism** is a rare congenital abnormality that causes a "split sternum." The split typically begins in the xyphoid and extends cranially to involve one or more additional sternebrae. The splitting itself is asymptomatic, but sternal dysraphism may be associated with peritoneal-pericardial diaphragmatic hernia.

Pectus excavatum is a congenital dorsal deviation of the sternum. It is also called *funnel chest* or *sunken chest*. The sternum curves inward, which results in dorsoventral narrowing of the thorax and a concave ventrum (Figure 3.19). Part or all of the sternum may be involved. The caudal sternebrae tend to be more severely affected, with the caudal ribs and costal cartilages usually curving inward, too. Moderate to severe pectus excavatum can reduce lung volume and displace the cardiac shadow dorsally and laterally. Cardiac displacement may be mistaken for a mediastinal shift. In a lateral view, the dorsally curving sternebrae may be superimposed on the cardiac silhouette.

A temporary pectus excavatum can result from severe inspiratory efforts that draw a normal sternum inward. This

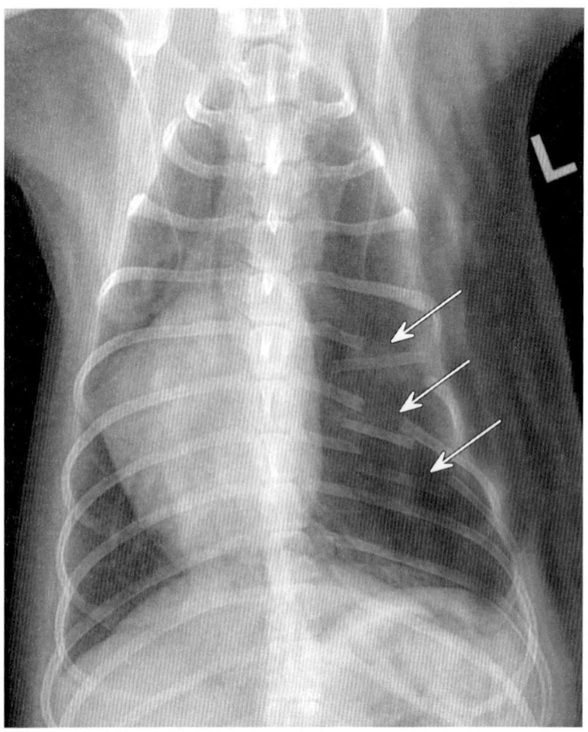

Figure 3.16 Flail chest. VD view of a dog thorax depicting segmental fractures in three adjacent ribs on the left side (white arrows) with soft tissue swelling and subcutaneous emphysema. The mediastinum is shifted to the right due to pneumothorax and higher pressure in the left hemi-thorax than in the right.

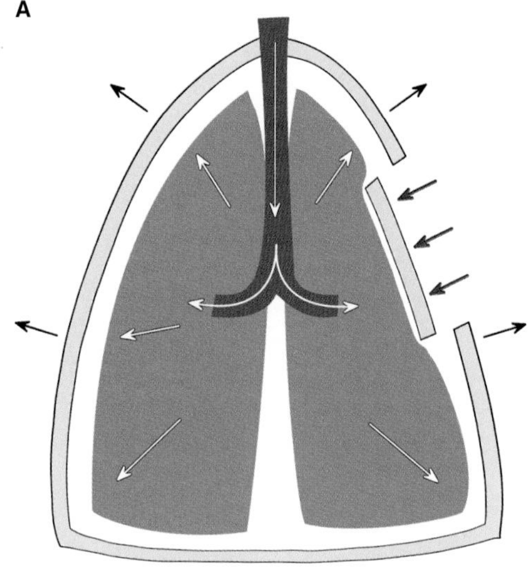

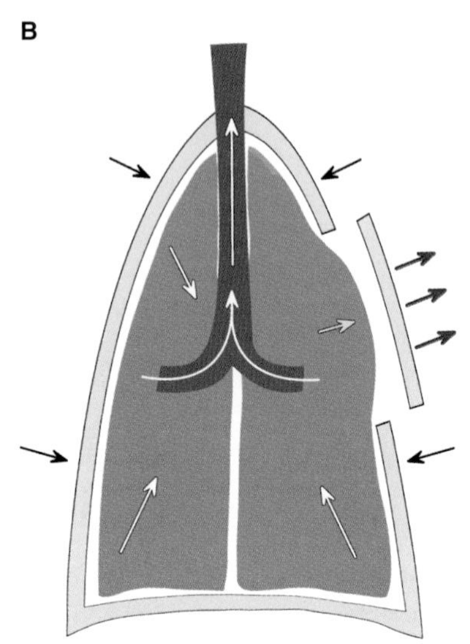

Figure 3.17 Flail chest. These illustrations depict the paradoxical movements of a flail chest. (**A**) During inspiration the thorax expands (black arrows), decreasing the intra-thoracic pressure and allowing the lungs to expand and fill with air (white arrows). The flail section, however, is sucked inward due to the lower intra-thoracic pressure (red arrows). (**B**) During expiration the thorax contracts, increasing the intra-thoracic pressure to expel the air from the lungs. The flail part is pushed outward by the higher intra-thoracic pressure.

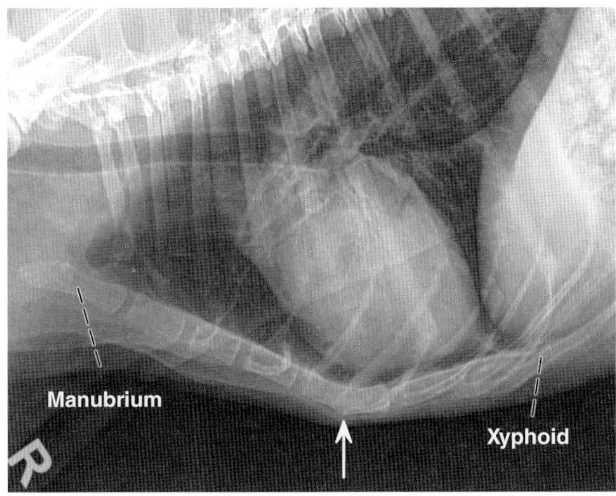

Figure 3.18 Fused sternebrae. Lateral view of a dog thorax depicting congenital fusion and slight misalignment of the fifth and sixth sternebrae (white arrow). No soft tissue swelling nor evidence of degenerative change or active bone remodeling is seen.

is a rare occurrence that is more likely to happen in immature animals with less rigid sternums.

Swimmers syndrome is a congenital abnormality that may appear similar to pectus excavatum. In affected puppies and kittens, the thorax is dorsoventrally flattened and the associated muscles are so weak that the animals are unable to stand. Their movements resemble a paddling or swimming motion.

Pectus carinatum is a congenital ventral deviation of the sternum. It also is called *pigeon chest* or *keel chest*. Typically, the caudal sternum protrudes outward or caudoventrally, resulting in dorsoventral widening of the thorax and a more upright cardiac shadow (Figure 3.20). In a VD/DV view, the thorax may appear laterally narrowed. Rarely, pectus carinatum may result from severe cardiomegaly in an immature animal.

Acquired sternal abnormalities may result from trauma, infection, or neoplasia. These conditions usually are accompanied by soft tissue swelling and frequently include bony abnormalities (Figure 3.21). Traumatic fractures and luxations more often are reported in younger animals, particularly cats and small-breed dogs. Causes include blunt force injuries and bite wounds.

A soft tissue mass on the sternum may represent an abscess, granuloma, hematoma, seroma, or tumor. Sternal masses that protrude inward, toward the thoracic cavity, may produce an extra-pleural sign.

Diaphragm

Normal radiographic anatomy

The diaphragm physically separates the abdominal and thoracic cavities and provides nearly 50% of the force needed for respiration. It consists of a *cupula* and two *crura* (Figure 3.22).

A

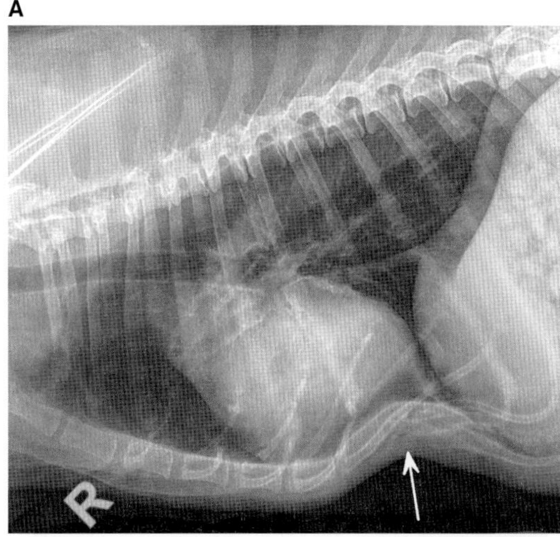

B

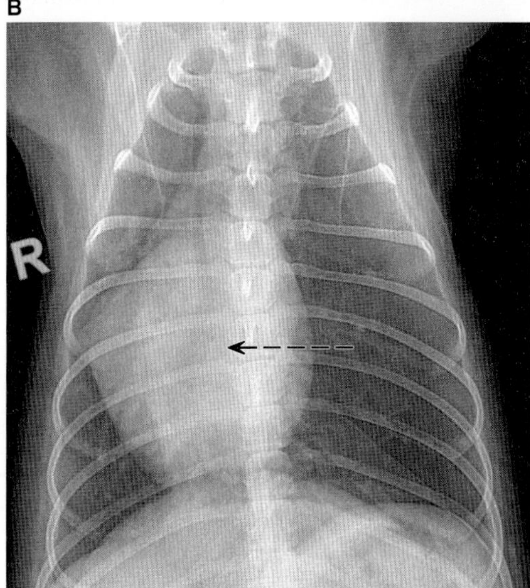

Figure 3.19 Pectus excavatum. Lateral view (**A**) and VD view (**B**) of a dog thorax depicting dorsal deviation of the caudal sternum (white arrow). The caudal thorax is dorsoventrally narrowed. The cardiac shadow is displaced dorsally and to the right by the deformed sternum.

The **cupula** is the convex, dome-shaped part of the diaphragm that bulges centrally and ventrally into the thoracic cavity. It is anchored to the sternum and ribs by fibrous tissue and connected to the spine by the crura.

The **crura** are the two muscular "legs" of the diaphragm (singular *crus*). The word crus is used to describe an anatomical structure that resembles a leg. Crus is the name given to the distal part of a pelvic limb, the part between the stifle and the tarsus. Each diaphragmatic crus extends dorsally and caudally from the cupula to an attachment on the L3-4 lumbar vertebrae. The ventral margins of L3 and L4 frequently are less distinct than the adjacent vertebral bodies, a normal finding that may be mistaken for a periosteal response.

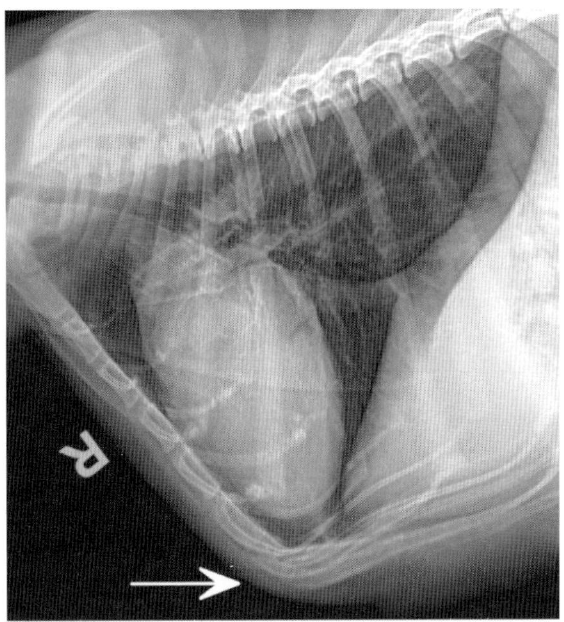

Figure 3.20 Pectus carinatum. Lateral view of a dog thorax depicting ventral protrusion of the caudal sternum (white arrow). The dorsoventral dimension of the thoracic cavity is increased, allowing the cardiac silhouette to be more upright in position.

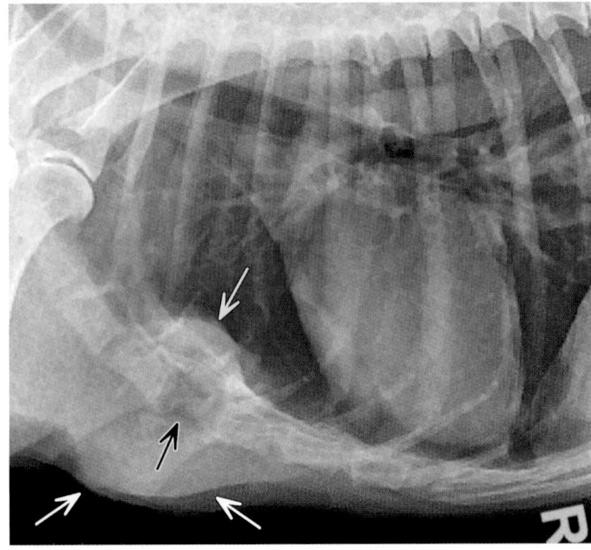

Figure 3.21 Sternal lysis. Lateral view of a dog thorax depicting localized osteolysis in the fourth sternebra (black arrow) with adjacent soft tissue swelling (white arrows). Inward swelling produces an extra-pleural sign (yellow arrow). Possible causes for the radiographic findings include tumor and infection.

There are three natural openings in the diaphragm. Each opening, or hiatus, allows certain structures to normally pass through, but also serves as a potential site for a diaphragmatic hernia. Ventrally and to the right of midline is the **caval hiatus**, through which the caudal vena cava and lymphatic vessels pass. The lymphatics carry fluid in one direction, from the abdominal cavity to the sternal lymph node in the thoracic cavity. Centrally and left of midline is the **esophageal hiatus**, through which the esophagus and vagal nerves pass. Dorsally and near midline is the **aortic hiatus**, through which the aorta, azygos vein, and thoracic duct pass.

The **costophrenic recesses** are the well-defined, wedge-shaped junctions between the diaphragmatic crura and the thoracic wall (Figure 3.22). The appearance of these recesses may be helpful to assess the degree of lung inflation and to detect pleural fluid. Fluid that collects in a costophrenic recess makes that recess appear more rounded, more opaque, and less distinct.

The cranial or "thoracic" margin of the diaphragm tends to be sharply-defined due to the opacity interface with lung air.

A

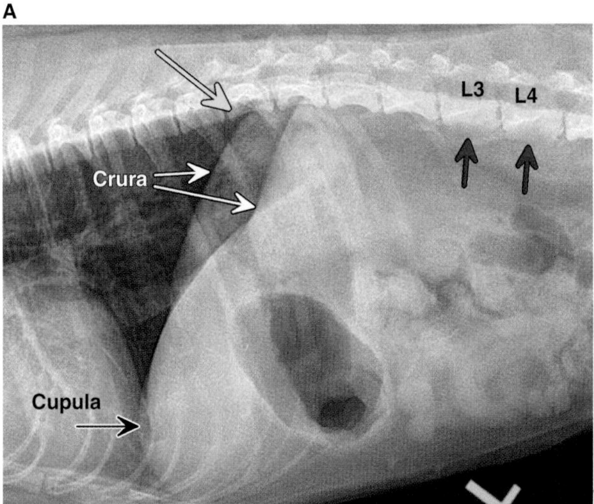

B

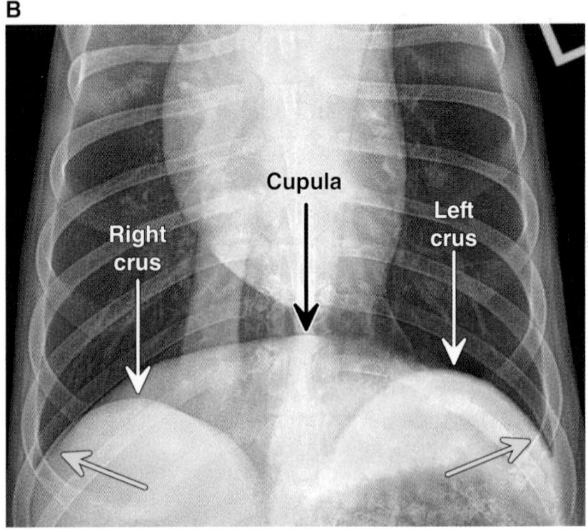

Figure 3.22 Parts of the diaphragm. Lateral view (**A**) and VD view (**B**) of a dog thorax depicting the parts of the diaphragm. The cupula is the central ventral "dome" of the diaphragm. The right and left crura insert on the L3 and L4 vertebrae. The ventral margins of L3 and L4 are less distinct than the adjacent vertebrae (red arrows). The yellow arrows point to the costophrenic recesses, where the diaphragm meets the thoracic wall.

The caudal or "peritoneal" margin often is only partially visible because it blends with the liver and stomach. Ventrally, the caudal margin of the diaphragm may be visible when adjacent to fat in the falciform ligament.

The **position** of the diaphragm is determined by the degree of lung inflation and the forces exerted by the abdominal contents, both of which are affected by patient position and gravity. When the patient is recumbent, the dependent (down) lung partially collapses and the weight of the abdominal viscera push the down side of the diaphragm cranially. The greater the abdominal contents, the greater the push against the diaphragm. In **left lateral** recumbency (left lateral view), the left crus commonly is seen cranial to the right crus. In **right lateral** recumbency, the right crus often is cranial to the left (Figure 3.23). The left crus often can be identified by the nearby gas in the fundus of the stomach (the stomach is located just caudal to the left crus). Note: a full stomach can push the left crus cranial to the right, even with the patient in right lateral recumbency. The right crus can be identified by the caudal vena cava, which emerges from the right side of the diaphragm.

Another difference between right and left lateral views is that the diaphragmatic crura tend to cross or overlap when in left lateral recumbency and they tend to be more parallel in right lateral recumbency (Figure 3.23).

In **dorsal recumbency** (VD view), both crura are dependent (down) and both move cranially. The diaphragm typically appears as three humps in a VD view: right crus, cupula, and left crus. In **ventral recumbency** (DV view), the cupula is down and moves cranially. The diaphragm typically appears as a single hump in a DV view because the cupula obscures both crura (Figure 3.24). In some DV views, the cupula moves so far cranially that it contacts the heart. The dome of the diaphragm may appear indented by the cardiac silhouette and its margin may be indistinct. The effects of patient orientation and gravity on the position of the diaphragm tend to be more evident in large dogs than in cats and small dogs.

A

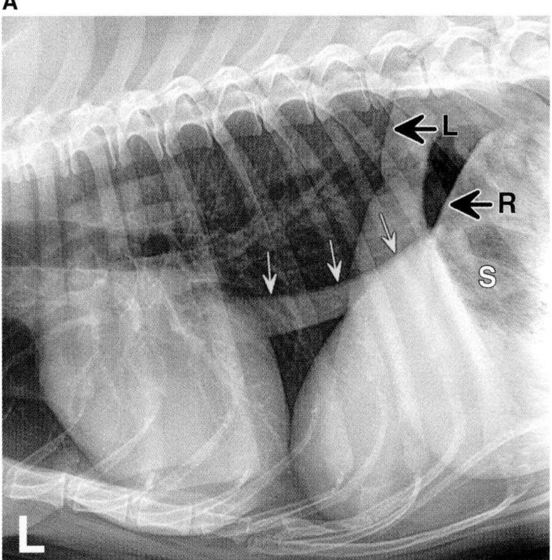

B

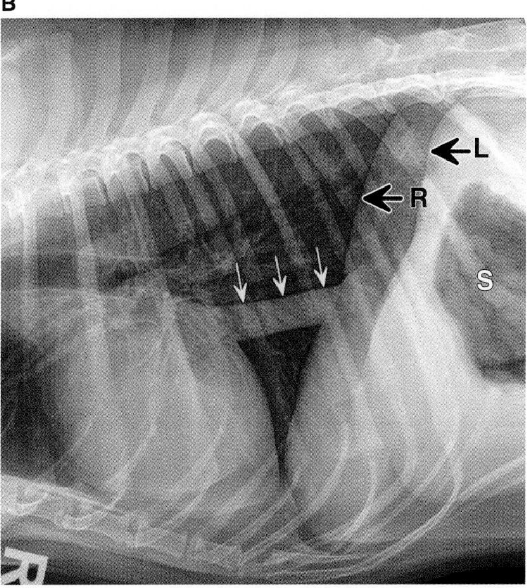

Figure 3.23 Left lateral vs. right lateral. Left lateral view (**A**) and right lateral view (**B**) of the same dog thorax depicting the positions of the left and right crura (L and R). In left lateral recumbency, the left crus (L) is cranial to the right crus (R), and the crura overlap. In right lateral recumbency, the right crus is cranial to the left, and the crura are more parallel. Gas in the stomach (S) is caudal to the left crus. The caudal vena cava (yellow arrows) emerges from the right crus.

Abnormal position of the diaphragm

A diaphragm may not appear as expected due to an error in radiographic technique. Errors that can distort the apparent position of the diaphragm inlcude rotation of the patient and off-centering of the x-ray beam. If the appearance of the diaphragm is not as you expect, first look for a normal cause of the discrepancy before diagnosing disease. When in doubt, repeat the radiographs paying special attention to proper imaging techniques.

Pathologic displacement of part or all of the diaphragm may be due to an increase or decrease in lung volume, abnormal abdominal content, or a defect in the diaphragm.

Non-visualization of the diaphragm may be due to lack of an opacity interface or loss of diaphragmatic integrity. Any soft tissue opacity material between the diaphragm and air-filled lung will obscure the margin of the diaphragm (e.g., pleural fluid, pulmonary disease, mass or fluid in the caudal mediastinum). Loss of diaphragm integrity may be due to a rupture or hernia (discussed on the next page).

Cranial diaphragm displacement most often is due to partial or complete lung collapse. Displacement may be unilateral or bilateral. Unilateral cranial displacement often is accompanied by a mediastinal shift. A physiologic or pathologic increase in the size of the abdominal contents can displace the diaphragm cranially (e.g., full stomach, advanced pregnancy, organomegaly, large tumor, severe effusion).

Defects in the diaphragm that allow cranial displacement include hernias, ruptures, and eventration.

Eventration of the diaphragm produces a cranial bulge, usually involving only part or one side of the diaphragm (Figure 3.25). It most often is due to a congenitally thin and weak diaphragm, but may be caused by an injury to the phrenic nerve. Many patients with diaphragm eventration have no recent history or radiographic evidence of trauma and most are asymptomatic. In very severe cases, breathing can become compromised. The cranially protruding part of the diaphragm typically appears even, well-defined, and relatively unchanged in serial radiographs. Differential diagnoses for an apparent eventration include diaphragmatic hernia, diaphragmatic mass, and a mass in the adjacent lung or caudal mediastinum.

Caudal displacement of the diaphragm may be due to an expanded thoracic cavity or absence of abdominal content. Expansion may be caused by hyperinflated lungs (e.g., emphysema, inspiratory dyspnea), severe pleural effusion, severe pneumothorax, or a large intra-thoracic mass. Absence of abdominal content may be due to emaciation or loss of body wall integrity (e.g., hernia, rupture). Severe caudal displacement of the diaphragm can reveal its **costal attachments**, particularly in a VD/DV view (Figure 3.26). The attachments appear as sharp projections extending cranially from the cupula, sometimes described as "tenting" of the diaphragm.

A

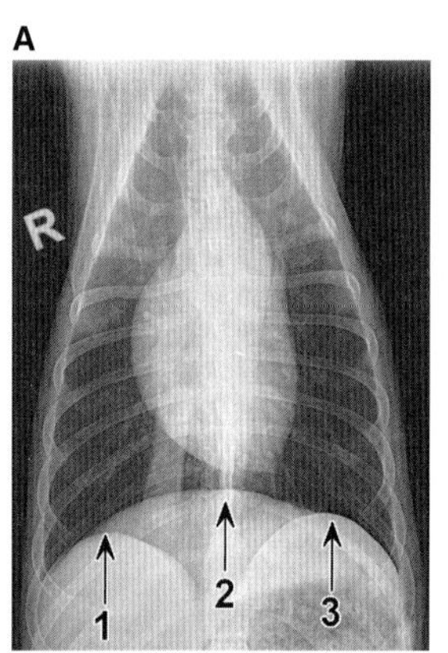

B

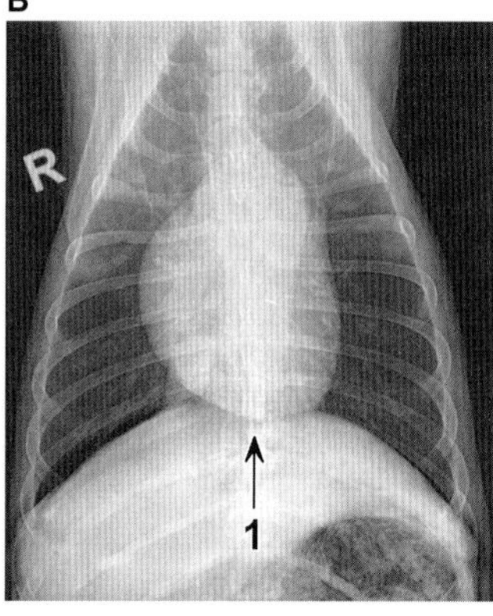

Figure 3.24 VD view vs. DV view. Ventrodorsal view (**A**) and Dorsoventral view (**B**) of a dog thorax. In the VD view, the diaphragm appears as three humps: (1) the right crus, (2) the cupula, and (3) the left crus. In the DV view, the diaphragm appears as one hump: the cupula (arrow). Notice that the cupula and the cardiac silhouette are in the contact in the DV view, indenting the diaphragm.

Diaphragmatic hernia

Protrusion of viscera through a natural opening in the diaphragm is a *hernia* and protrusion through an acquired opening is a *rupture*. Because the two are difficult to differentiate in radiographs, we will use the term "hernia" for both.

Typical **radiographic findings** of a diaphragmatic hernia include a mixed opacity mass in the thoracic cavity and an

A

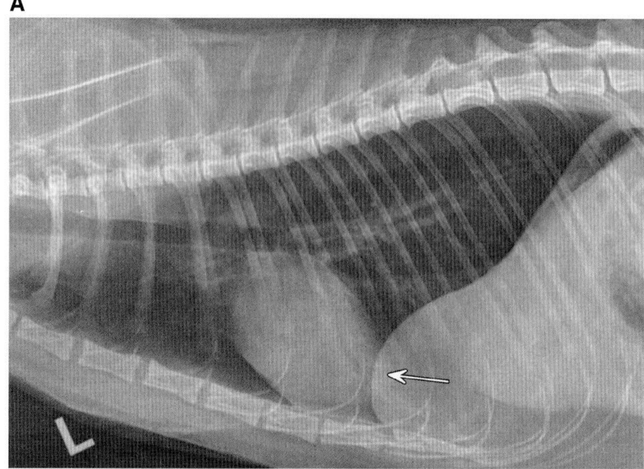

B C

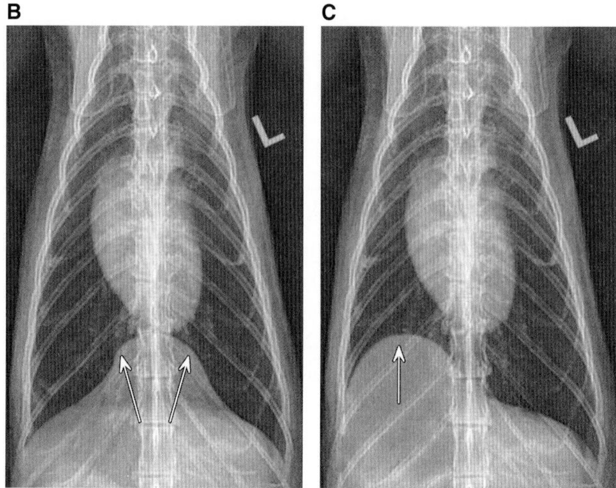

Figure 3.25 Eventration of the diaphragm. Lateral view (**A**) and VD views (**B** and **C**) of a cat thorax depicting a cranial bulge in the ventral part of the diaphragm (white arrows). Any part of the diaphragm may be involved. As depicted in the VD views, the eventration may be centrally located (**B**) or more lateral (**C**).

indistinct or absent diaphragm margin (Figure 3.27). The most commonly displaced structures are the stomach, small intestine, liver, and fat. It may be difficult to identify the displaced viscera unless structures are visibly absent from their normal locations or there is a distinctive shape or pattern associated with the herniated content. Intestines may be recognized as gas or fluid-filled tubes that extend beyond the limits of the abdominal cavity. Visualization of rugal folds helps identify the stomach.

Large protrusions into the thoracic cavity can displace and/or obscure the lungs and the cardiac silhouette. Pleural effusion is a frequent finding with diaphragmatic hernias. Fluid may be unilateral or bilateral and can obscure the displaced viscera and compromise diagnosis. Follow-up radiographs made after thoracocentesis or may improve visualization of the displaced structures and diaphragm margins. Horizontal beam radiography also may be useful (Figure 2.15). The abdominal cavity may appear "empty"

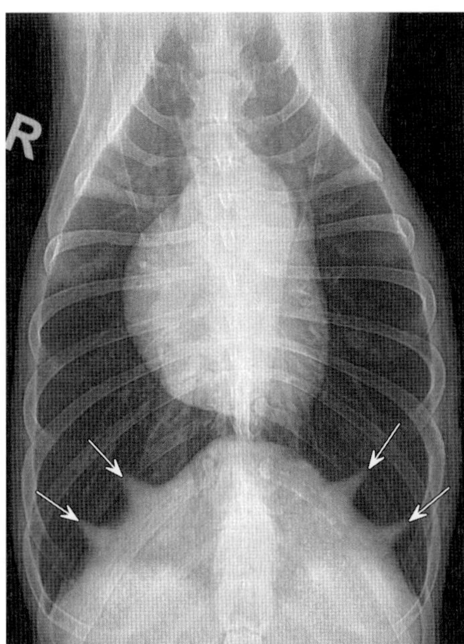

Figure 3.26 Tenting of the diaphragm. VD view of a dog thorax depicting hyperinflated lungs and severe caudal displacement of the diaphragm. The diaphragmatic costal attachments are visible as projections extending from the cupula (white arrows).

due to less viscera. Structures that remain in the abdomen often are cranially displaced or otherwise malpositioned.

Radiographic diagnosis of a diaphragmatic hernia is difficult when the protrusion of viscera is transient or intermittent. Some structures may only be partially displaced. Rarely, a hernia may extend between the soft tissue layers of the thoracic wall instead of into the thoracic cavity. These **paracostal hernias** can present with an extra-thoracic swelling that may be difficult to differentiate from other causes of a thoracic wall mass. The opacity of the hernia mass varies depending on the amount of fat, soft tissue organs, and gas-filled GI structures it contains (Figure 3.28).

A **hiatal hernia** occurs when abdominal contents protrude through a hiatus in the diaphragm. The esophageal hiatus most often is involved and the gastroesophageal junction most often protrudes. Other types of esophageal hiatal hernias include *para-esophageal*, in which part of the stomach is displaced alongside the esophagus without involving the gastroesophageal junction, and *gastroesophageal intussusception*, in which part of the stomach enters the esophagus (see gastroesophageal intussusception). Protrusion through the aortic hiatus is called a *para-aortic* hiatal hernia and protrusion through the vena caval hiatus is a *para-venous* hiatal hernia. Fat or part of the stomach usually is involved in each of these hiatal hernias.

Diagnosis of hiatal hernia frequently is difficult because, in many cases, the abdominal contents are only intermittently displaced, which is called a *sliding* or *dynamic* hiatal hernia. Positioning the patient with the head tilted down may aid in detection.

The classic **radiographic appearance** of a hiatal hernia is an oval or semicircular mass near the left crus of the diaphragm (Figure 3.29). The mass generally is located near midline, between the caudal vena cava and the aorta. The size, shape, and opacity of the mass vary with the type and quantity of displaced viscera. Most hiatal hernias are soft tissue or fat opacity. The intra-abdominal part of the stomach

A

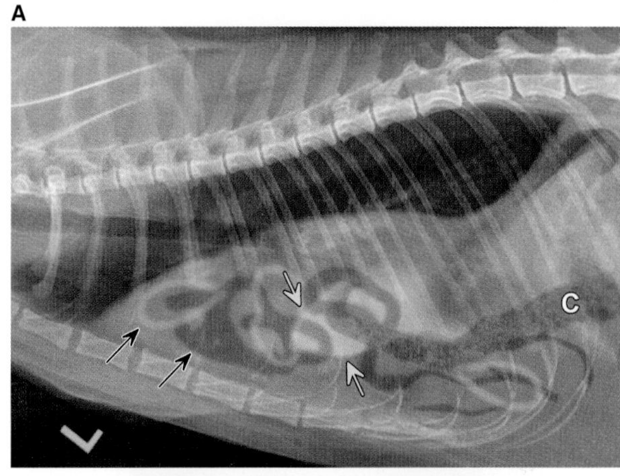

B

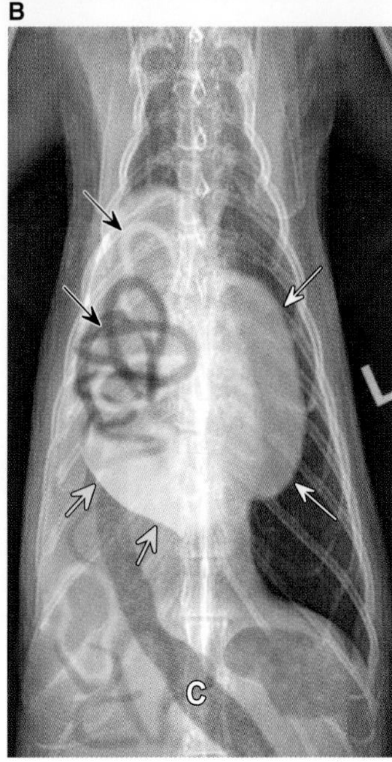

Figure 3.27 Diaphragm hernia. Lateral view (**A**) and VD view (**B**) of a cat thorax depicting a mixed opacity mass in the right hemithorax. Fat opacity is visible, extending from the cranial abdomen into the thoracic cavity mass. Segments of gas-filled and fluid-filled small intestine are visible in the mass (black arrows). Also visible is the well-defined edge of a soft tissue opacity structure (yellow arrows) which may represent displaced liver or spleen. The cardiac silhouette is completely effaced in the lateral view and partially effaced in the VD view. The left border of the cardiac shadow is visible in the VD view (white arrows). The ventral and right lateral margins of the diaphragm are not identified. The colon (**C**) can be followed from the abdomen into the thorax, across the level of the diaphragm.

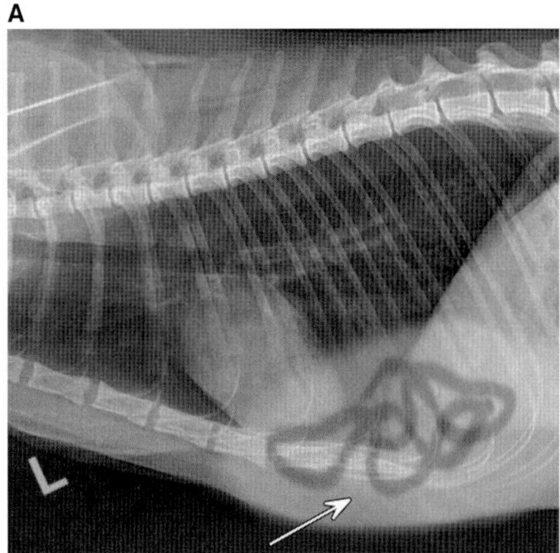

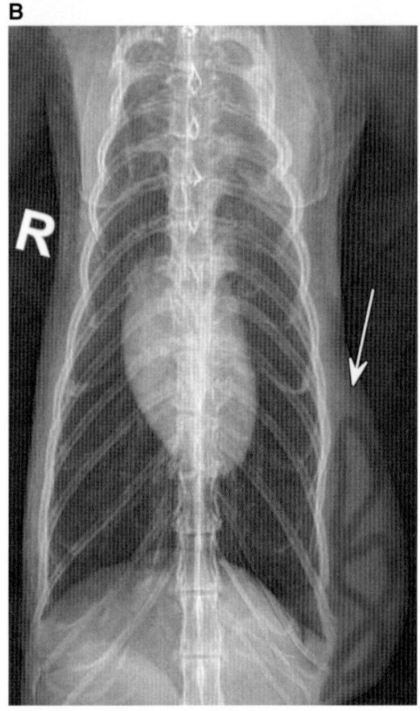

Figure 3.28 Paracostal hernia. Lateral view (**A**) and VD view (**B**) of a cat thorax depicting a swelling along the left lateral body wall (white arrow). The swelling is soft tissue opacity with curvilinear gas-filled segments of small intestine. Notice in the lateral view that the cardiac and diaphragm borders remain visible through the extra-thoracic swelling. This is because the intra-thoracic opacity interface remains.

may be abnormal in shape and the expected gas bubble in the fundus may be absent. The stomach may appear continuous with the hiatal hernia mass if there is only partial gastric displacement. The caudal esophagus may or may not be dilated. A strangulated hernia that traps the stomach can lead to a tension viscerothorax (Figure 3.48).

A **peritoneal-pericardial diaphragmatic hernia** (PPDH) is a congenital condition in which there is an abnormal opening between the peritoneal cavity and the pericardial sac that. The opening allows abdominal viscera to move into the pericardial sac (Figure 3.30). Structures commonly displaced include falciform fat, liver, gall bladder, stomach, and small intestine. The characteristic **radiographic finding** is a large, rounded cardiac silhouette composed of various displaced opacities, such as fat, soft tissues, and gas-filled GI structures. The border of the cardiac silhouette may be irregular or even, but usually it is sharply defined because there is less cardiac motion blur. The cardiac and diaphragm borders frequently merge together without the normal overlap or edge distinction. The dorsal border of a PPDH may be visible in a lateral view as a thin horizontal line between the cardiac silhouette and the diaphragm, located just ventral to the caudal vena cava. This line is seen more often in cats with PPDH than in dogs.

PPDH differs from other diaphragm hernias in that the displaced viscera are confined to the cardiac silhouette. Pleural effusion is uncommon unless secondary right heart failure occurs. If needed, an upper GI study may be useful to identify

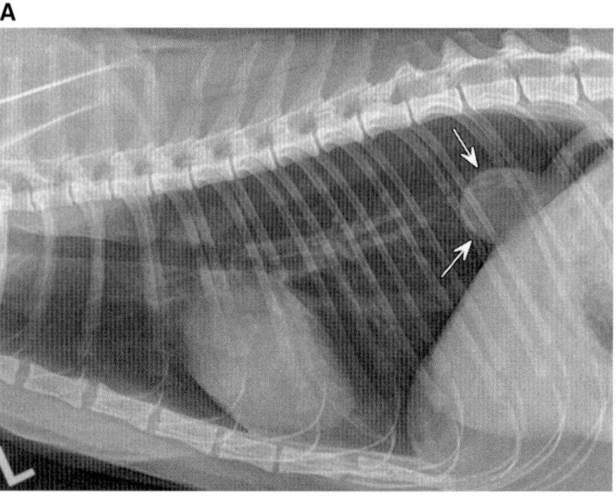

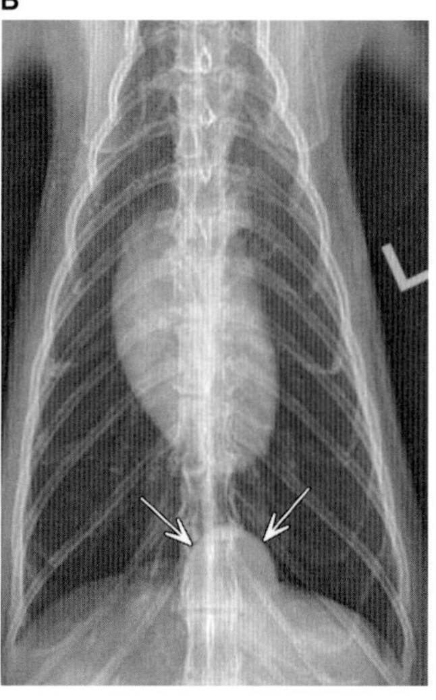

Figure 3.29 Hiatal hernia. Lateral view (**A**) and VD view (**B**) of a cat thorax depicting a soft tissue opacity mass protruding from the dorsal diaphragm near midline and between the aorta and caudal vena cava (white arrows). Pulmonary vessels are visible at the mass because the hernia is located outside the lungs, in the caudal mediastinum.

the contents of the pericardial sac and help differentiate PPDH from pericardial effusion or cardiomegaly.

PPDH is always congenital, never acquired. A sternal deformity such as pectus excavatum or sternal dysraphism may be concurrent with a PPDH. Many affected animals are asymptomatic. When clinical signs are present, they tend to be more GI related in dogs and respiratory related in cats. PPDH most often is reported in long-haired cats and Weimaraner dogs.

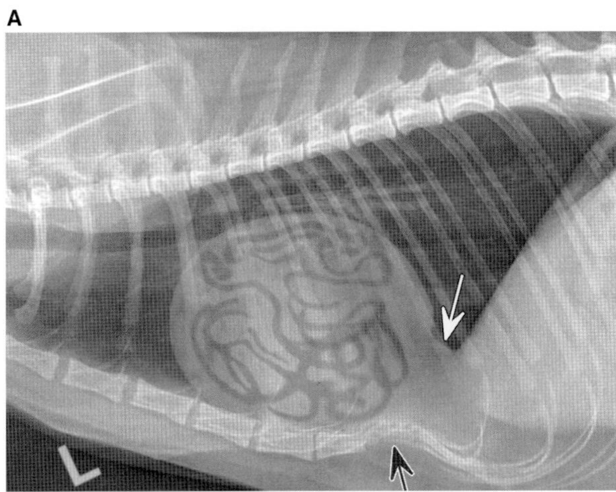

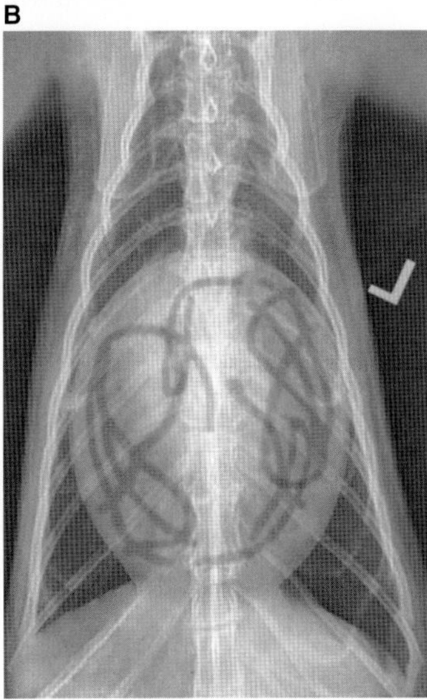

Figure 3.30 Peritoneal-pericardial diaphragmatic hernia. Lateral view (**A**) and VD view (**B**) of a cat thorax depicting a large, rounded cardiac shadow with multiple, curvilinear gas-filled segments of small intestine within the cardiac borders. The caudal cardiac and cranial diaphragmatic margins are not distinguished ventrally. The dorsal border of the PPDH is visible in the lateral view (white arrow). The caudal sternum is mildly deformed due to sternal dysraphism (black arrow).

Diaphragm mass

Masses on the caudal side of the diaphragm usually blend with abdominal structures such as the liver and stomach and therefore are not identified in radiographs. A mass on the cranial side, however, often is outlined against the lung making it visible as a rounded or semi-circular mass. The mass can appear semi-circular because its caudal part is obscurred by the abdominal contents. Possible causes of a diaphragm mass include neoplasia, abscess, granuloma, hernia, and eventration.

Pleura and Pleural Space

Normal radiographic anatomy

The pleura are thin membranes that cover the lungs, line the thoracic cavity, and help form the mediastinum. The **visceral** or *pulmonary* pleura covers the lungs, blood vessels, and bronchi. It does not contain any sensory nerves and receives blood supply from the pulmonary circulation. The **parietal** pleura lines the walls of the thoracic cavity, the mediastinum, and the diaphragm. It contains many sensory nerves and receives blood supply from the systemic circulation. Between the pulmonary and parietal pleura is the *pleural space*.

The **pleural space** is essentially a "potential" space because it normally contains only a capillary thin layer of fluid. The fluid serves to moisten the pleural surfaces and reduce friction. Except for this fluid, the pulmonary and parietal pleura are in virtual contact with each other. The pressure in the pleural space is less than atmospheric pressure, which helps the lungs expand with the chest during inspiration.

Pleural fluid is produced continuously by the parietal pleura and resorbed by the visceral pleura. The turnover is about 75% every hour. Any condition that increases the volume of fluid entering the pleural space or prevents its absorption can increase the volume of pleural fluid. Excess fluid in the pleural space can interfere with lung expansion and convert the potential space into a true cavity. The same is true for gas that accumulates in the pleural space (i.e., pneumothorax).

Pleural fissure lines

Each lung is divided into individual lobes by the pulmonary pleura. The divisions between the lobes are created by inward extensions of the pleura, called **pleural fissures**. Normal pleural fissures rarely are identified in radiographs because the pleura is so thin. The fissures become visible when filled with gas or fluid and when the pleura is thickened.

The locations of the pleural fissures are known (Figures 3.31 and 3.32). When visible in radiographs, they appear as thin, curved, soft tissue opacity lines. Pleural fissure lines that are uniform in thickness with no tapering at either end, generally are caused by pleural thickening (lines that taper suggest pleural fluid as described on the next page). Pleural thickening may result from inflammation, edema, or fibrosis. Pleural fissure lines sometimes are seen in radiographs of older, clinically normal patients. In these patients, pleural thickening likely is a remnant of previous disease that is now inactive. Fissure lines in older animals often are considered to be incidental findings and have been referred to as an "aging change."

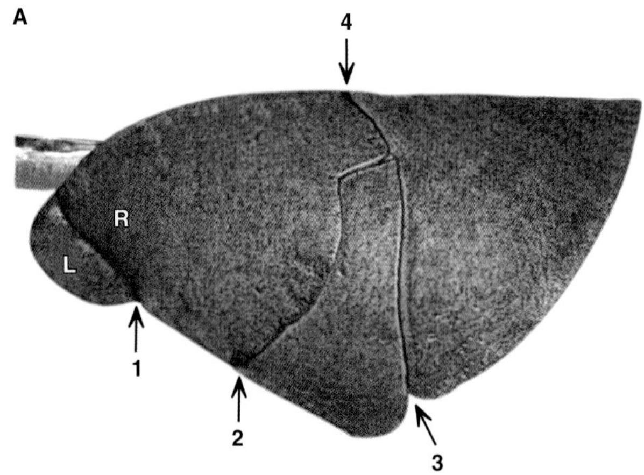

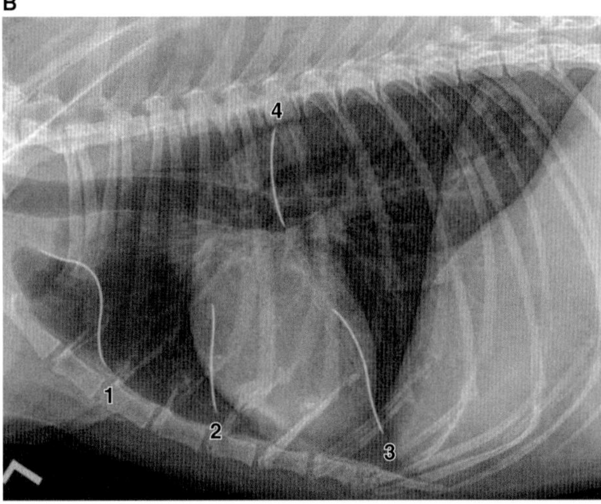

Figure 3.31 Pleural fissure lines. Illustration of a dog lung (**A**) and a lateral radiograph of a dog thorax (**B**) depicting the normal locations of pleural fissures. (**1**) Line produced by the cranioventral mediastinum between the right and left cranial lung lobes. (**2**) Right and left middle pleural fissure lines located between the right cranial and middle lung lobes and between the cranial and caudal sub-segments of the left cranial lung lobe. (**3**) Right and left caudal pleural fissure lines located: between the right middle and caudal lobes and between the left cranial and caudal lobes. (**4**) Right and left dorsal pleural fissure lines located between the right and left cranial and caudal lobes.

Occasionally a normal pleural fissure is visible in a radiograph (Figure 3.33). This occurs when the x-ray beam is perfectly aligned with the fissure (Figure 3.34). Unlike pleural lines caused by disease, normal pleural lines rarely repeat in radiographs because it is unlikely that the x-ray beam will be aligned with the lung fissure every time.

Free fluid or gas in the pleural space is the most common cause of visible pleural fissures. Pleural fluid or gas outlines the lungs and separates the individual lung lobes (Figure 3.35). Separation of the lobes makes the interlobar fissures wider peripherally and narrower centrally. Pleural fluid produces wedge-shaped fissure lines that are more opaque than air-filled. Pleural gas produces wedge-shaped fissure lines that are less opaque than lung (Figure 3.36).

A "reverse pleural fissure line" may be created by fat in the central thorax that extends into a lung fissure. Fat fissure

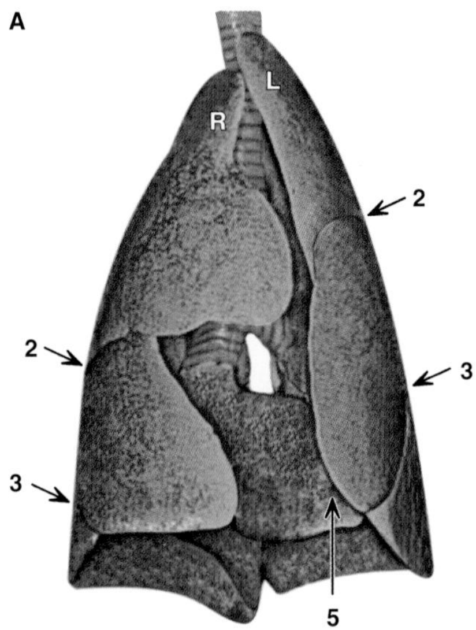

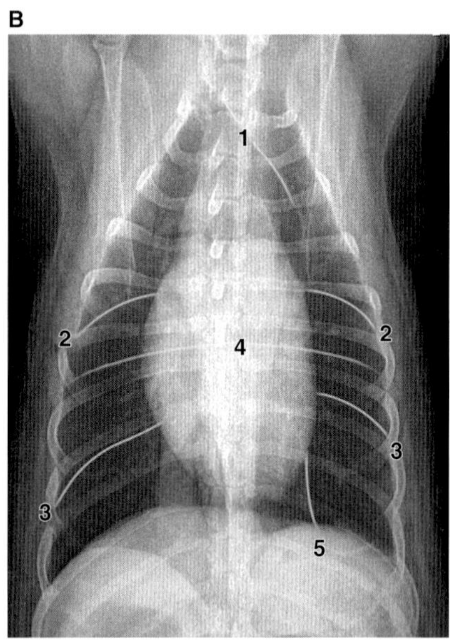

Figure 3.32 Pleural fissure lines. Illustration of a dog lung (**A**) and a lateral radiograph of a dog thorax (**B**) depicting the normal locations of pleural fissures. (**1**) Line created by the cranioventral mediastinum between the right and left cranial lung lobes. (**2**) Right and left middle pleural fissure lines located between the right cranial and middle lung lobes and between the cranial and caudal sub-segments of the left cranial lung lobe. (**3**) Right and left caudal pleural fissure lines located between the right middle and caudal lobes and between the left cranial and caudal lobes. (**4**) Dorsal pleural fissure lines located between the right and left cranial and caudal lobes (not visible in the illustration **A**). (**5**) Line created by the caudoventral mediastinum between the accessory and left caudal lung lobes.

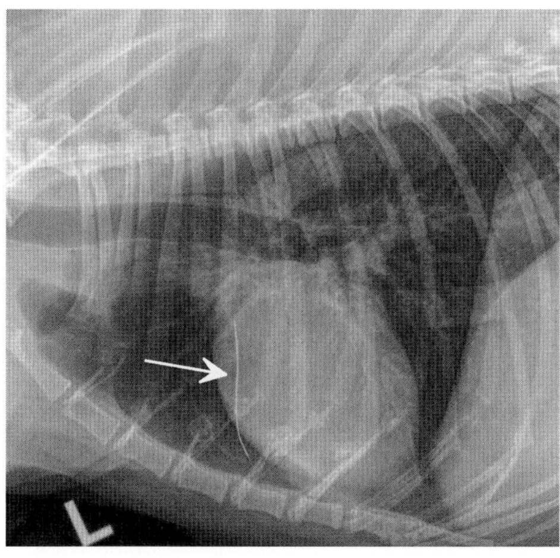

Figure 3.33 Normal pleural fissure line. Lateral view of a dog thorax depicting the appearance of a normal pleural fissure line (white arrow) due to perfect alignment with the x-ray beam.

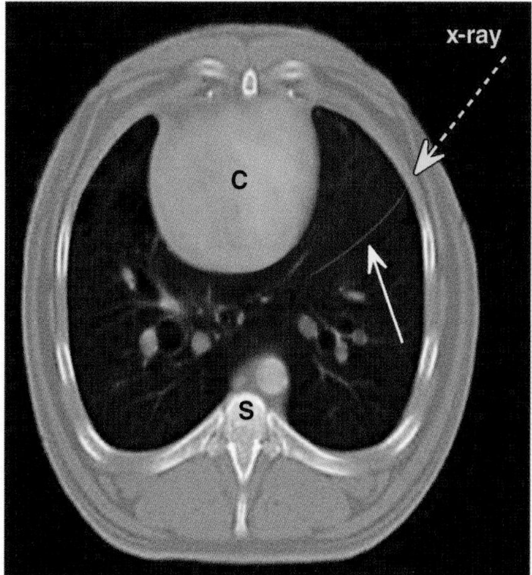

Figure 3.34 Normal pleural fissure line. Cross sectional CT image of a dog thorax depicting the patient in dorsal recumbency with the x-ray beam (yellow arrow) aligned with an interlobar fissure (white arrow). C = cardiac silhouette, S = spine.

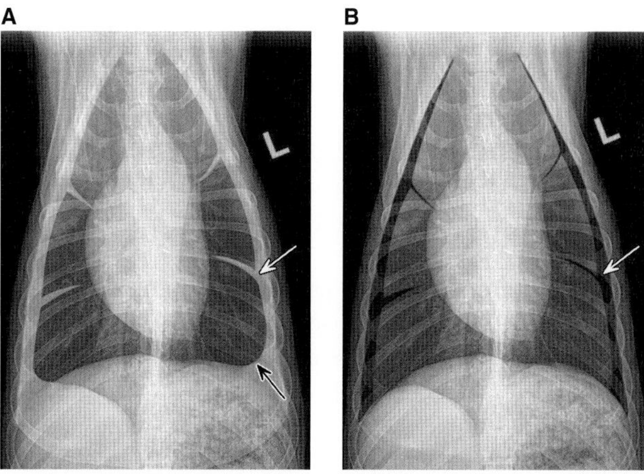

Figure 3.35 Abnormal fluid or gas in the pleural space. VD views of a dog thorax depicting fluid (**A**) and gas (**B**) in the pleural space. Both pleural fluid and pleural gas prevent the lungs from fully expanding. In **A**, the lung lobes are surrounded by fluid (white arrow) which is more opaque than lung tissue. Fluid in the costophrenic recesses makes them more rounded (black arrow). In **B**, the lung lobes are surrounded by gas (white arrow), which is less opaque than lung tissue.

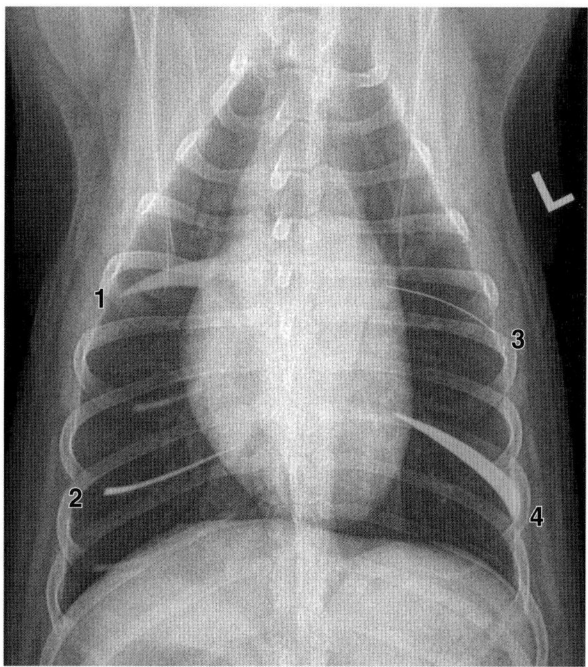

Figure 3.36 Pleural fissure lines. VD view of a dog thorax. (**1**) A reverse fissure line created by fat between the right cranial and middle lung lobes. Notice that the fissure line made by fat is wider centrally and tapers peripherally. (**2**) Mineralized costal cartilage, which may be mistaken for a pleural fissure line. Notice that the cartilage curves in the opposite direction of fissure lines **1**, **3**, and **4**. (**3**) Thin pleural fissure line that is uniform in width, without tapering at either end. This type of fissure line is consistent with pleural thickening or minimal pleural effusion. (**4**) Larger, wedge-shaped pleural fissure line that is wider peripherally and tapers centrally, caused by pleural effusion.

lines are wider centrally and taper peripherally (Figures 3.36 and 3.42). They occur most often between the right cranial and middle lung lobes in overweight dogs.

Pleural fluid

Fluid in the pleural space is called **pleural effusion**. In general, the volume of fluid must exceed 10 ml/kg body weight to be detected in radiographs. This is about 50 ml in a cat or small dog and at least 100 ml in a medium-size dog. As mentioned earlier, pleural effusion may result from excess fluid production, decreased absorption, or both. The type of fluid cannot be determined from radiographs. There are numerous causes of pleural effusion, many of which are associated with disease outside the pleural space (see Differential Diagnoses at the end this chapter).

Fluid in the pleural space usually is freely movable and bilateral in distribution, the latter due to mediastinal fenestrations that are present in most dogs and cats. Unilateral or asymmetric effusion may result from a congenital absence of fenestrations, disease that plugs the existing fenestrations, or fluid so viscous that it cannot pass through the fenestrations. Diseases that can obstruct the fenestrations include severe or chronic inflammation, fibrosis and neoplasia.

The earliest radiographic sign of pleural fluid is **pleural fissure lines**. Fissure lines created by small volumes of pleural fluid may be indistinguishable from pleural thickening. Small volume pleural effusions tend to be easier to see in a VD view than in a DV view. This is because in dorsal recumbency the pleural fluid is more likely to flow with gravity into the interlobar fissures and move laterally away from the mediastinal structures, where it often is easier to see (Figures 3.37 and 3.38). Horizontal beam radiography also may be useful to detect small volumes of pleural fluid (Figure 2.15).

As the volume of pleural fluid increases, the lungs are less able to expand. The lung edges become further separated from the thoracic wall with fluid opacity in between. This finding sometimes is described as "retraction" of the lung lobes. Vascular and bronchial markings do not extend all the way to the ribs. Compared to fully inflated lungs, retracted lungs are more rounded and more opaque. Summation of pleural fluid further increases lung opacity. Pulmonary vessels remain visible in patients with pleural effusion, which is an important finding to help differentiate fluid outside the lungs from fluid inside the lungs (latter may result from pneumonia, pulmonary edema, or hemorrhage). Fluid in the lungs will obscure the vessels because both are soft tissue opacity and there will be no opacity interface.

The central position of the heart within the thoracic cavity is maintained by fully inflated lungs. Less inflated lungs allow the heart to move to one side or the other. Pleural fluid limits lung inflation. When a patient with pleural effusion is placed in lateral recumbency, the heart "falls" toward the dependent side and slides dorsally along the curved thoracic wall (Figure 3.39). In a lateral radiograph, the cardiac shadow will be dorsally separated from the sternum.

Pleural fluid between the heart and sternum often outlines the ventral lung border to create a wavy or "scalloped" appearance (Figure 3.39). Fluid in the costophrenic recesses makes them more rounded and less distinct. Fluid that collects adjacent to the mediastinum often makes it appear widened.

A **large volume of pleural fluid** can lead to very small lungs and widely separated lung lobes. The individual lobes may resemble "leaves on a tree" (Figure 3.40). Large pleural effusions can displace the diaphragm caudally and make it appear flattened and stationary in serial radiographs. Large

A

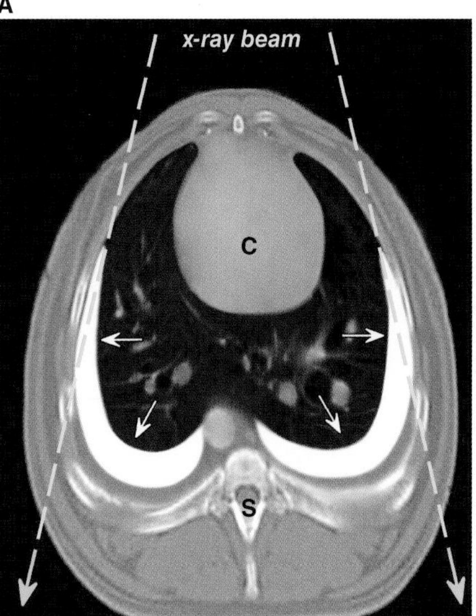

B

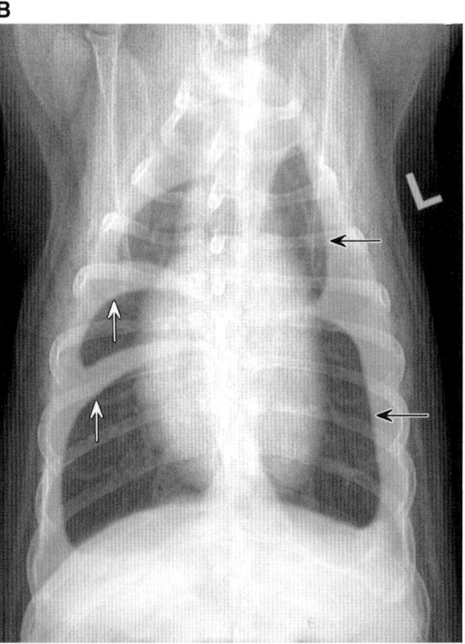

Figure 3.37 Pleural effusion, VD view. **A**. Cross-sectional CT image of a dog thorax depicting the patient in dorsal recumbency. Fluid in the pleural space moves with gravity to the dependent (dorsal) part of the thoracic cavity (white arrows). Because the thorax is wider dorsally than ventrally, fluid moves into the spaces between the lungs and the lateral chest walls. C = cardiac silhouette; S = spine. **B**. VD view of a dog thorax depicting fluid between the lung edges and chest wall (black arrows) and between lung lobes (white arrows). The cardiac shadow is visible because it is adjacent to air-filled lung, as seen in the CT image (**A**).

effusions also expand the thoracic cavity, making the ribs more perpendicular to the spine and the chest more rounded or "barrel-shaped." The overall opacity of the thoracic cavity may be increased to the degree that it resembles an underexposed radiograph; however, underexposure is not the cause if the vertebrae and other extra-thoracic structures

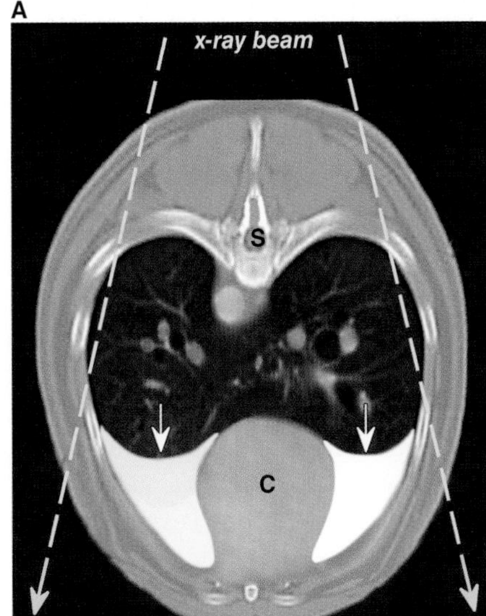

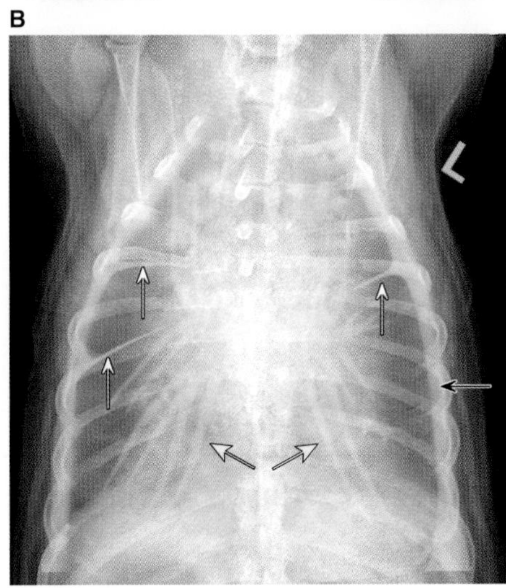

Figure 3.38 Pleural effusion, DV view. **A**. Cross-sectional CT image of a dog thorax depicting the patient in ventral recumbency. Pleural fluid flows with gravity to the dependent (ventral) part of the thoracic cavity where it collects adjacent to the mediastinum and cardiac silhouette (**C**). S = spine. **B**. DV view of a dog thorax depicting a small volume of pleural fluid between the lungs and chest wall (black arrow) and in the interlobar fissures (white arrows). As seen in the CT image (A), most of the fluid collects along the ventral midline where it effaces the cardiac, mediastinal, and diaphragmatic margins. The dorsal lung vessels (yellow arrows) are well-visualized because they are surrounded by well-inflated lung.

are properly exposed. Large volumes of pleural fluid may efface the cardiac and diaphragmatic borders and hide intrathoracic lesions. Follow-up thoracic radiographs made after removing as much fluid as possible may yield additional diagnostic information.

Chronic pleural effusions and inflammatory pleural fluid should be removed with caution because pleural fibrosis may be present. **Pleural fibrosis** reduces lung elasticity, which means the lungs could rupture if they re-expand too quickly. A typical radiographic finding of pleural fibrosis is multiple rounded lung lobes with irregular margins (Figure 3.40).

In patients with **unilateral pleural effusion**, lung not surrounded by fluid tends to be better inflated than the one that is surrounded by fluid. Unilateral effusions may not be evident in a lateral view alone because the edges of the inflated lung typically extend to the thoracic wall. The orthogonal VD/DV view often is needed to confirm the diagnosis.

Variations in body conformation may be mistaken for pleural effusion. As described, the normal inward curvature of

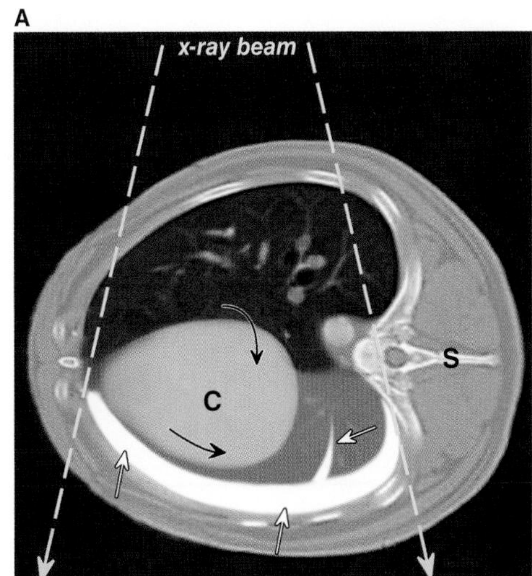

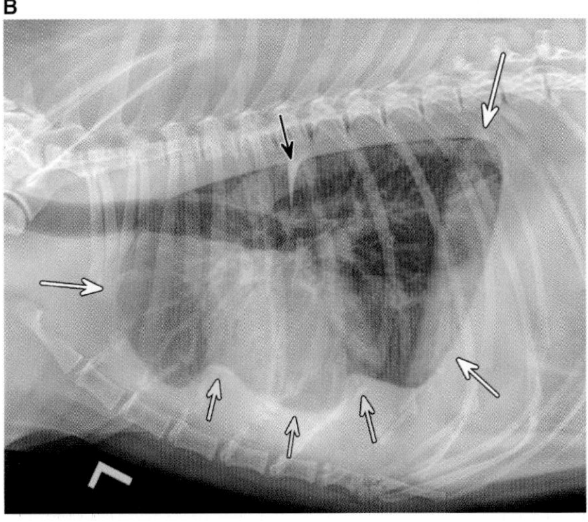

Figure 3.39 Pleural effusion, lateral view. **A**. Cross-sectional CT image of a dog thorax depicting the patient in lateral recumbency. Pleural fluid flows with gravity to collect along the dependent thoracic wall and in an interlobar fissure (white arrows); S = spine, C = cardiac silhouette. The dependent (down) lung is partially collapsed and increased in opacity. The smaller down lung allows the cardiac shadow to "fall" toward the down side and slide dorsally along the curved chest wall (black arrows). **B**. Lateral view of the same dog thorax. Pleural fluid outlines the lung margins (white arrows) and is visible in a dorsal interlobar fissure (black arrow). The ventral lung border appears wavy (yellow arrows).

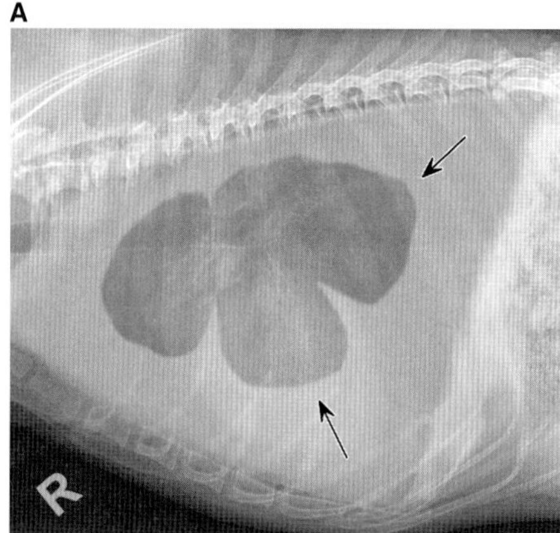

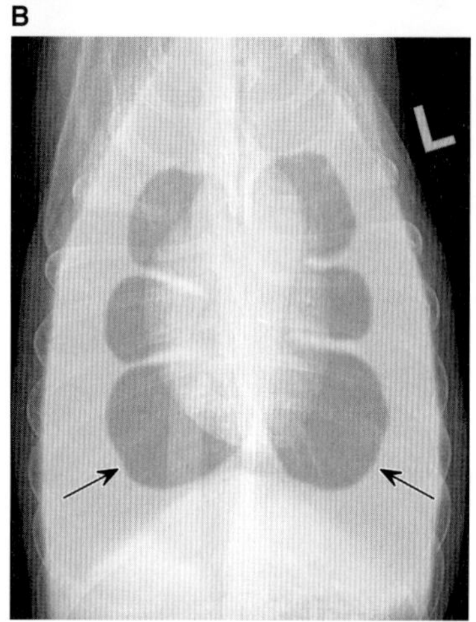

Figure 3.40 Severe pleural effusion with pleural fibrosis. Lateral view (**A**) and VD view (**B**) of a dog thorax depicting a large volume of pleural fluid surrounding lungs that are unable to expand against the fluid (black arrows). Fluid separates the individual lung lobes and outlines their rounded and slightly irregular margins. The appearance of the lungs is concerning for pleural fibrosis. The diaphragm is caudally displaced and flattened by the large effusion.

the ribs in chondrodystrophic breeds can give the false impression of pleural fluid in a VD/DV view (Figure 3.12). Also, the normal hypaxial muscles in cats may resemble rounding of the costophrenic recess in a lateral view (Figure 3.41).

Thin, **mineralized costal cartilages** may be mistaken for pleural fissure lines (Figure 3.36). Cartilages, however, tend to be straighter or curve in the opposite direction than pleural fissure lines. Most costal cartilages can be traced to the end of a rib. Usually, there are multiple mineralized cartilages, most of which are not located in the area of a pleural fissure.

In overweight patients, the thoracic walls are thick and the edges of the lungs may not extend all the way to the ribs (Figure 3.42). In addition, summation of overlying fat increases the overall thoracic opacity and excess mediastinal fat causes widening of the mediastinum. These findings in overweight patients may be mistaken for pleural effusion.

Pleural gas

Free gas in the pleural space is a **pneumothorax**. A pneumothorax may result from a penetrating thoracic wound, a ruptured airway, or a ruptured lung. Free gas in the pleura space increases the pleural pressure, which leads to **lung collapse**. The severity of lung collapse depends on the volume of gas and the pressure in the pleural space.

As with pleural fluid, the earliest radiographic sign of pleural gas is pleural fissure lines. **Gas fissure lines** are more difficult to detect than fluid fissure lines because they produce less contrast with air-filled lung. In most cases, lung collapse is the initial radiographic finding of pneumothorax. The lungs become separated from the chest wall and there is gas opacity in between. The vascular and bronchial markings do not extend to the ribs. The tiny vessels and bronchi in the peripheral lung may not be visible without brightening the radiograph (use a "hotlight" with film radiographs).

Pneumothorax tends to be easier to see in **lateral and DV views**. A DV view may be more diagnostic than a VD view because in ventral recumbency pleural gas rises to the dorsal

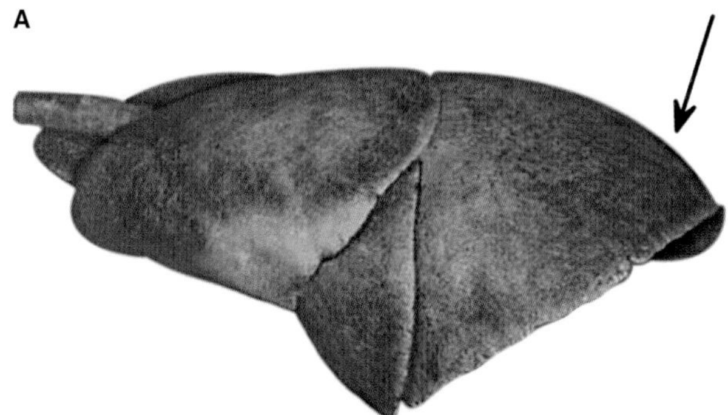

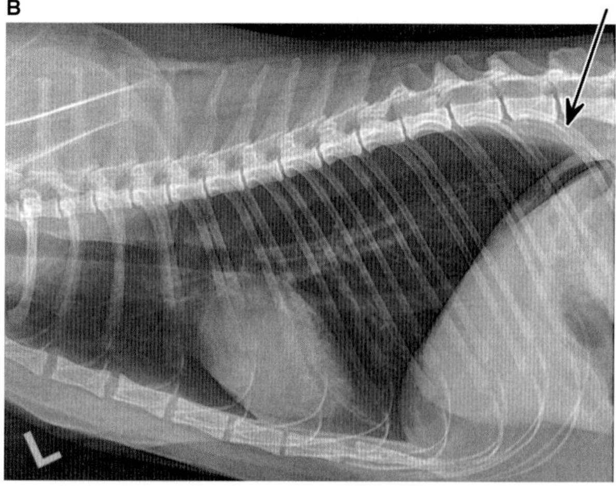

Figure 3.41 Normal cat lung. **A**. Illustration of a normal cat lung specimen. **B**. Lateral radiograph of a cat thorax. The arrows point to the normal curvature of the dorsocaudal lungs due to the hypaxial muscles. In the radiograph, the soft tissue opacity muscle may be mistaken for pleural fluid in the costophrenic recess (arrow).

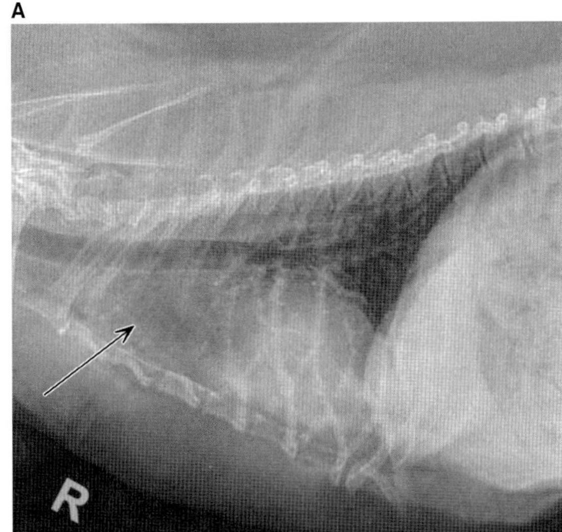

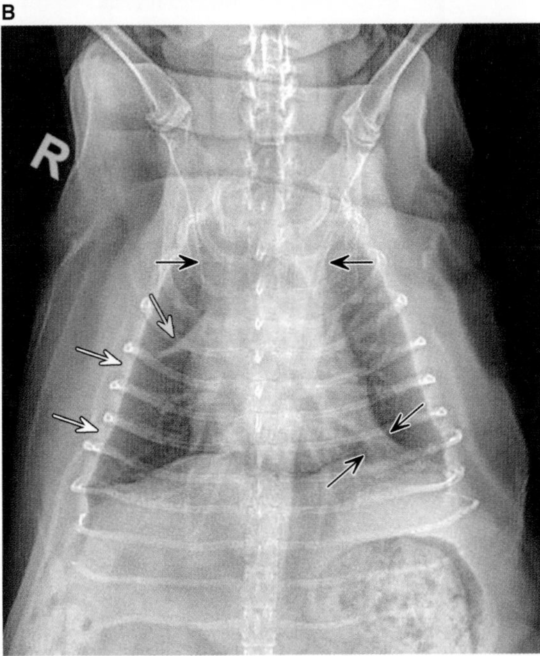

Figure 3.42 Obesity. Lateral view (**A**) and VD view (**B**) of a dog thorax depicting an overweight patient with a large amount of subcutaneous fat and excessive fat deposits in the mediastinum (black arrows indicate the widened cranial and caudal parts of the mediastinum). The lungs do not extend all the way to the ribs (white arrows). Pericardial fat makes the cardiac margins less distinct. Fat extending into the interlobar fissure between the right cranial and middle lung lobes creates a reverse fissure line (yellow arrow).

thorax. The dorsal thorax is wider than the ventral thorax so the gas will be more spread out and less likely to be obscured by the midline structures (Figures 3.43 and 3.44). Horizontal beam radiography may be useful to detect a smaller volume of pleural gas (Figure 2.15).

As the volume of pleural gas increases, the degree of lung collapse increases. Smaller lungs contain less air and are more opaque than inflated lungs. Small lungs also cannot maintain the central position of the heart and other mediastinal structures, which means the **mediastinum can shift** laterally (see mediastinal shift in the next section of this chapter). In a lateral view, a mediastinal shift may

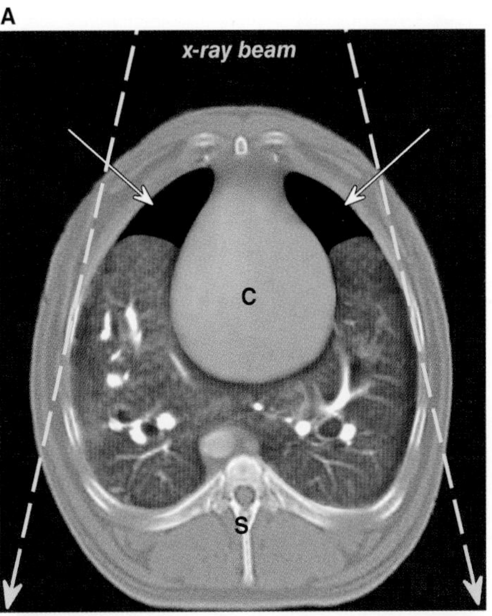

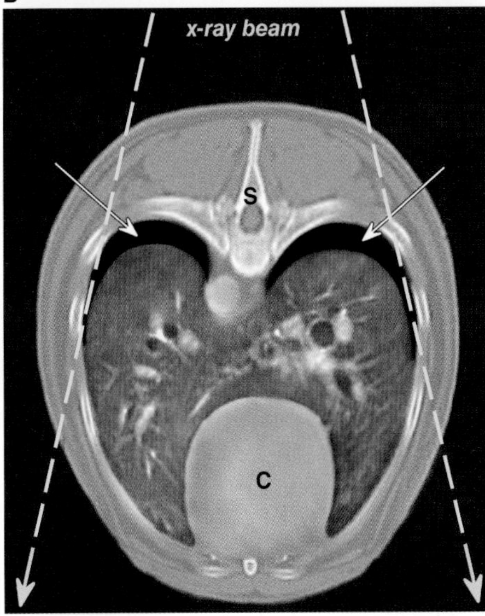

Figure 3.43 Pneumothorax. Two cross-sectional CT images of a dog thorax depicting the patient in dorsal recumbency (**A**) and in ventral recumbency (**B**); S = spine, C = cardiac shadow. Gas always rises. In dorsal recumbency (**A**), gas rises to collect along the narrow ventral midline (white arrows) where it may be obscured in a VD radiograph by the spine, sternum, and mediastinum. In ventral recumbency (**B**), gas rises to the wider dorsal thorax where it can spread between lung and chest wall, making detection easier in a DV view than in a VD view.

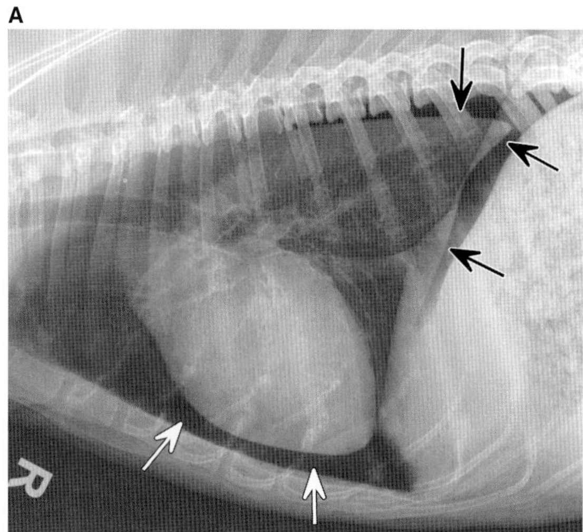

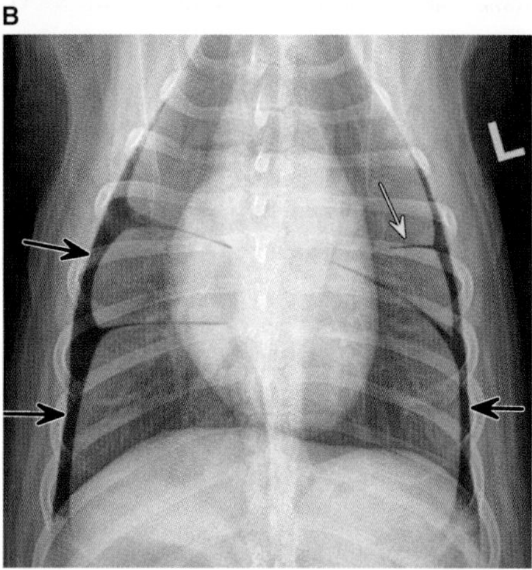

Figure 3.44 Pneumothorax. Lateral view (**A**) and VD view (**B**) of a dog thorax depicting free gas in the pleural space. Pleural gas outlines the lungs, the interlobar fissures, and is visible between the lungs and chest wall (black arrows). The yellow arrow points to gas between the cranial and caudal subsegments of the left cranial lung lobe. In the lateral view, the cardiac shadow is dorsally separated from the sternum with gas in-between (white arrows). Lungs are increased in opacity because they are less inflated.

appear as dorsal displacement of the cardiac silhouette. Dorsal separation of the cardiac shadow from the sternum sometimes is described as "elevation of the heart". The term "elevation", however, is a misnomer. Without the support of an inflated lung, the heart actually falls with gravity toward the dependent thoracic wall and slides dorsally along the normal curvature of the inner chest wall (Figure 3.45).

Free gas in the pleural space increases the opacity interface with the diaphragm, making its cranial margin appear sharper and more distinct. A large volume of pleural gas can caudally displace the diaphragm, making it appear flattened and stationary in serial radiographs.

Severe pneumothorax can reduce the overall opacity in the thoracic cavity to the degree that the thorax appears to

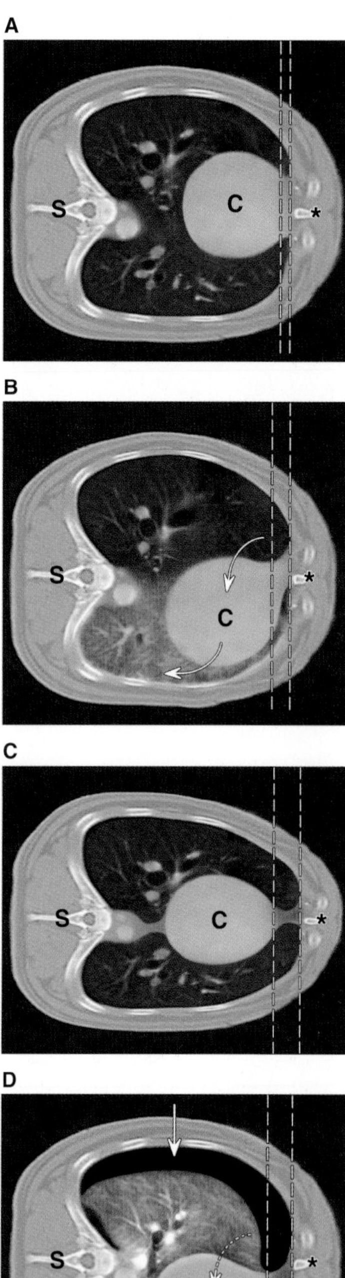

Figure 3.45 Separation of the cardiac shadow from the sternum. Four cross-sectional CT images of a dog thoraces with the patient in lateral recumbency. The dashed yellow lines represent the distance between the cardiac shadow (C) and the sternum (*); S = spine. **A**. Normally inflated lungs support the cardiac shadow in its central position. **B**. Collapse of the dependent lung allows the heart to fall toward the dependent chest wall and slide dorsally along its curved border (arrows). **C**. Deep-chested conformation: the lungs are normally inflated, but the tall narrow thorax leads to greater distance between the cardiac shadow and sternum. **D**. Lung collapse due to pneumothorax (white solid arrow). The heart falls with gravity and slides dorsal to the sternum (white dashed arrows).

be overexposed. However, overexposure is not the cause if the extra-thoracic structures are properly exposed.

Conditions that can **mimic pneumothorax** include emaciation, hyperinflated lungs, hypovolemia, and superimposed skin folds (see Differential Diagnoses). With emaciated patients, there is relatively little tissue overlying the thorax and the lungs tend to be well-inflated, both of which can lead to a thoracic cavity that is less opaque than expected. Hyperinflated lungs also can lead to a less opaque thoracic cavity (e.g., emphysema, manual inflation). Similarly, hypovolemia that results in small cardiovascular structures can diminish overall lung opacity. Hypovolemia also can lead to separation of the cardiac shadow from the sternum. A skin fold superimposed on the thoracic cavity may be mistaken for the edge of a retracted lung (Figure 3.46). The skin fold usually can be traced beyond the limits of the thoracic cavity. Each of these conditions of mimicry is differentiated from pneumothorax by the absence of free gas between the lungs and chest wall.

More common than missing a pneumothorax is an erroneous diagnosis of pneumothorax. This is especially dangerous when the clinician introduces gas into the thorax via chest tap after making an incorrect diagnosis, thus producing a pneumothorax when none existed. A favorite radiographic sign of pneumothorax is "elevation of the heart". Rather than consider it an "elevation", one should more accurately describe it as separation of the cardiac shadow from the sternum. The problem is that there are at least 3 causes for separation of the cardiac shadow from the sternum in addition to pneumothorax. (Figure 3.45). If it is a true pneumothorax, there will be other evidence for that diagnosis in addition to separation of the cardiac shadow.

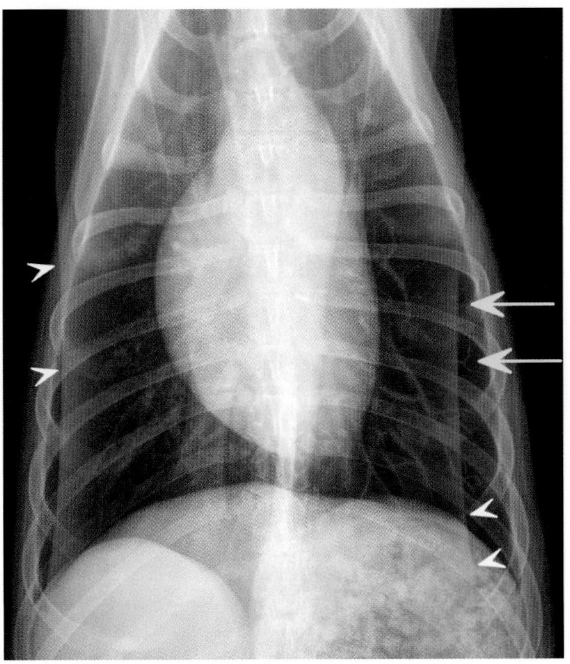

Figure 3.46 Skin folds. VD view of a dog thorax depicting skin folds superimposed on the thoracic cavity (white arrowheads). These may be mistaken for the edges of the lungs, but close inspection reveals the folds can be followed beyond the limits of the thoracic cavity. Also, tiny pulmonary vessels are visible between the skin folds and the ribs (yellow arrows).

Small volumes of pleural gas usually are resorbed within 48 hours, provided that gas does not continue to enter the pleural space.

A **hydropneumothorax** occurs when both fluid and gas are in the pleural space, The most common cause is severe thoracic trauma. Radiographic findings frequently include other signs of damage (e.g., fractured ribs, subcutaneous emphysema). The mixture of fluid and gas opacities in the pleural space can be challenging to interpret. Horizontal beam radiography may be helpful because fluid flows with gravity to the dependent side and gas rises to the "up" side.

A **tension pneumothorax** is present when pleural pressure exceeds atmospheric pressure. Pleural pressure this high can prevent the lungs from expanding, both during inspiration and expiration, which can quickly become an emergency situation. A tension pneumothorax occurs when gas enters the pleural space during inspiration (usually from a ruptured lung) but cannot exit during expiration because the thoracic wall is intact. The lung rupture acts like a one-way valve, allowing gas to continue flowing in but not out. In radiographs, the lungs often are markedly collapsed with very small lobes (Figure 3.47). The lung lobes may be abnormal in shape. Cardiovascular structures usually are small due to hypovolemia and may appear even smaller due to an expanded thoracic cavity. The large volume of pleural gas displaces the diaphragm caudally, sometimes revealing it costal attachments.

A **tension viscerothorax** may develop following herniation and subsequent entrapment of a GI structure within the thoracic cavity. The trapped structure, usually the stomach, can become severely gas-distended to resembles a large, cyst-like mass with rounded, well-defined margins (Figure 3.48). The mediastinum may be displaced to the opposite side. The part of the diaphragm through which the GI structure was displaced may be indistinct, which can help differentiate a viscerothorax from a unilateral pneumothorax. Gas in a pneumothorax outlines the lung, whereas gas in a viscerothorax is confined to the GI structure.

Pleural mass

Masses that originate in the pleura or pleural space usually are accompanied by pleural effusion. Pleural fluid can hide the lesion. A pleural mass may be visible in follow-up radiographs made after removing the pleural fluid or by using horizontal beam radiography to reposition the fluid. Most

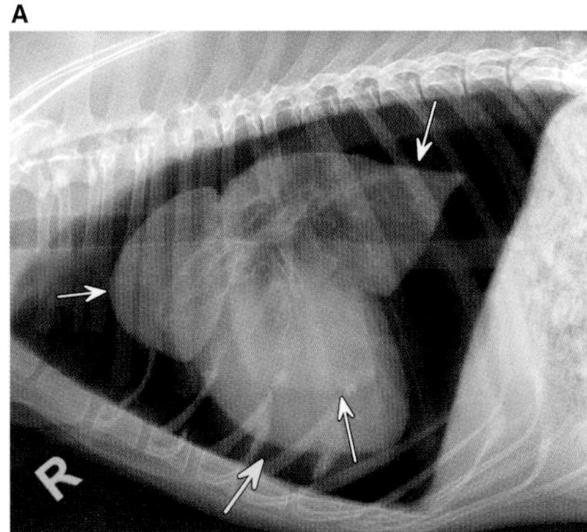

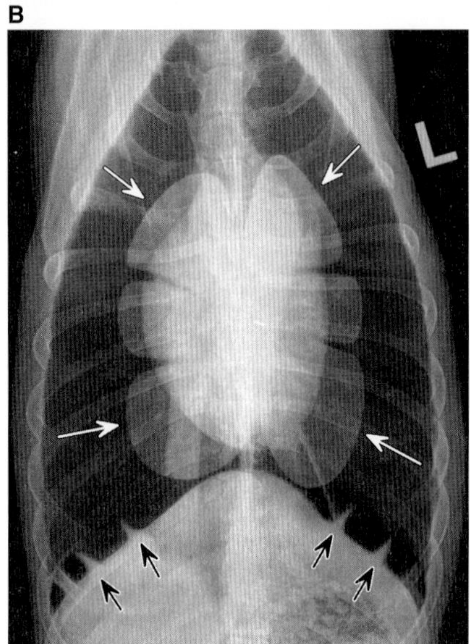

Figure 3.47 Tension pneumothorax. Lateral view (**A**) and VD view (**B**) of a dog thorax depicting an expanded thoracic cavity with severe collapse of all lung lobes (white arrows). The lung edges are widely separated from the chest wall by a large volume of pleural gas. The cardiac shadow is dorsally displaced from the sternum with gas in-between (yellow arrow). The diaphragm is caudally displaced, revealing its costal attachments (black arrows).

pleural masses are difficult to see unless the x-ray beam is tangential to the base of the mass.

Mediastinum

Normal radiographic anatomy

The mediastinum is the central compartment in the thoracic cavity. It is located between the right and left lungs. The mediastinum extends along the midsagittal plane from the thoracic inlet to the diaphragm and from the sternum to the spine. For descriptive purposes, it commonly is divided into *cranial, middle, caudal,* and *dorsal* parts. The **cranial** mediastinum extends from the thoracic inlet to the cranial border of the cardiac shadow. The **middle** mediastinum contains the cardiac shadow. The **caudal** mediastinum extends from the caudal border of the cardiac shadow to the diaphragm. The **dorsal** mediastinum lies dorsal to the level of the trachea.

There are several **openings** in the mediastinum that allow communication with other parts of the body. Fluids, gases, and diseases can easily pass through these openings to enter or exit the mediastinum. Cranially, the mediastinum communicates with the cervical fascia via the thoracic inlet. Caudally, it opens to the retroperitoneal space via the aortic hiatus in the diaphragm. Centrally, it communicates with each lung through the pulmonary root or hilum. The lateral

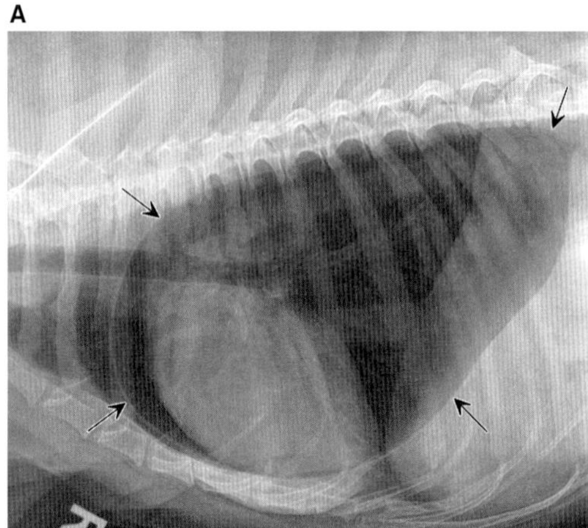

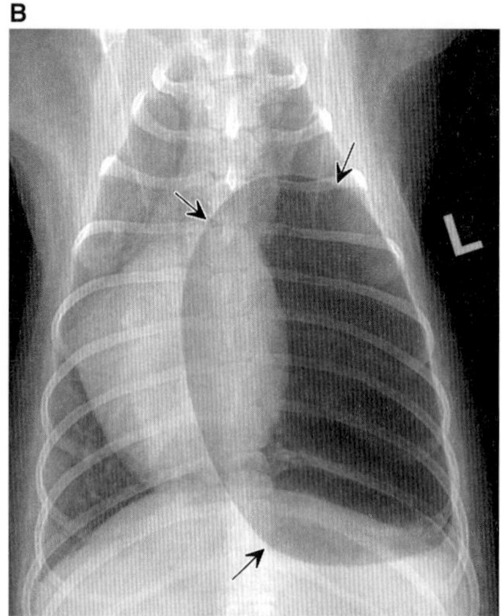

Figure 3.48 Tension viscerothorax. Lateral view (**A**) and VD view (**B**) of a dog thorax depicting a large, gas-distended mass in the left hemithorax (black arrows). The rounded margins are thin and well-defined resembling. The mediastinum is shifted to the right. The normally visible gas bubble in the gastric fundus is not identified. Possible etiologies for the intra-thoracic mass include an incarcerated stomach and a large pulmonary cyst or bulla.

pleural walls that line the mediastinum are delicate and often fenestrated, providing an incomplete barrier between the right and left sides of the thoracic cavity.

Normally visible structures in the mediastinum include the cardiac silhouette, the trachea, the aorta, the caudal vena cava, and in young animals, the thymus (Figure 3.49). The mediastinum is a site for fat deposits, so variable amounts of fat usually are visible, too.

The other mediastinal structures either are too small to be seen or lack the opacity interface to be distinguished in survey radiographs. These include the esophagus, lymph nodes, vessels and nerves (e.g., cranial vena cava, left subclavian artery, brachiocephalic trunk, azygous vein, thoracic duct, phrenic nerves). The normal esophagus may be identified when it contains gas or fluid. In overweight patients, mediastinal structures not normally visible may be identified because excess fat provides the contrast needed to distinguish them. Structures may also be visible in emaciated patients because the absence of fat leads to a thinner mediastinum through which the soft tissue opacity structures may be discernable against air-filled lungs.

The **thymus** often is visible in young dogs and cats. It is located in the ventral part of the cranial mediastinum. In dogs, the thymus may be visible up to about six months of age, rarely up to a year of age. It generally shrinks quickly after the deciduous teeth are lost. The canine thymus tends to be easiest to see in a VD/DV view, appearing as a triangular-shaped, soft tissue opacity structure in the left cranial thorax (Figure 3.50). In cats, the thymus may be visible up to two years of age. It usually is easier to see in a lateral view where it appears as an indistinct soft tissue opacity structure in the cranioventral mediastinum.

Mediastinal lymph nodes may be visible when enlarged or mineralized. Knowledge of their normal locations aids in diagnosis (Figure 3.51). The **cranial mediastinal lymph nodes** are located ventral to the trachea and near the large cranial mediastinal blood vessels. They receive lymphatics from the neck, heart, esophagus, thymus, and thoracic wall. Enlargement of these nodes can widen the cranial mediastinum, increase mediastinal opacity, and displace the trachea dorsally and laterally. Caudal mediastinal lymph nodes frequently are absent in dogs and cats. The **sternal lymph node** is located immediately dorsal to the second or third sternebra. It usually is solitary but may be paired in some dogs. The sternal node receives lymphatics from the abdomen and enlargement generally is due to spread of intra-abdominal disease or lymphoma. **Tracheobronchial** or **hilar lymph nodes** are located near the tracheal bifurcation. They receive lymphatics from the lungs and bronchi. Enlargement produces increased opacity in the hilar region and may lead to a mass effect that displaces the caudal trachea, usually ventrally.

The radiographic appearance of the mediastinum varies with its thickness. In **lateral views**, summation of the cranial mediastinal structures produces a homogenous soft tissue opacity ventral to the trachea (Figure 3.49). The opacity

A

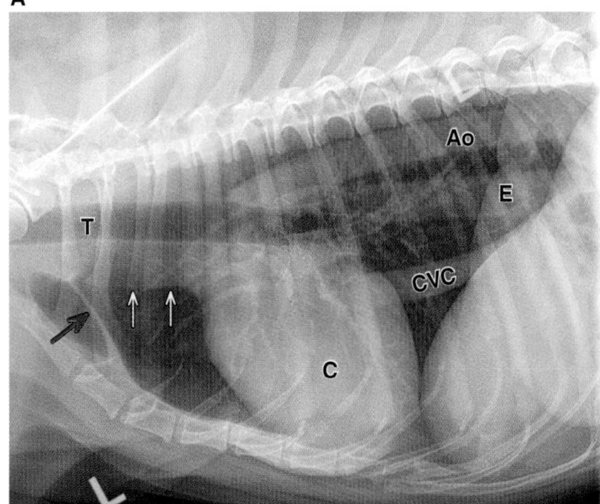

B

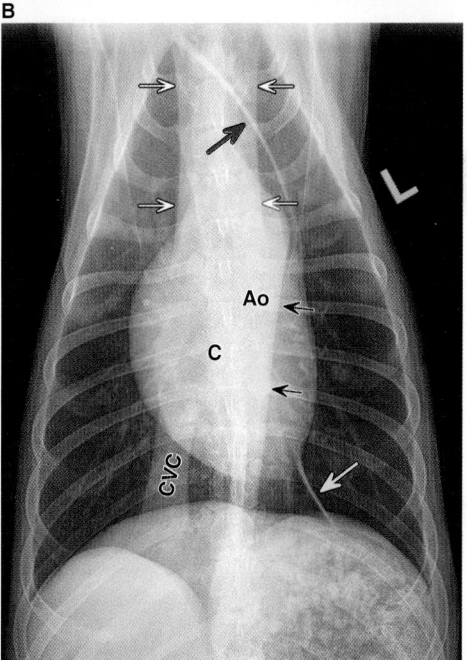

Figure 3.49 Mediastinal structures. Lateral view (**A**) and VD view (**B**) of a dog thorax depicting the normally visible mediastinal structures: trachea (T), cardiac silhouette (C), descending aorta (Ao) and caudal vena cava (CVC). Summation of the cranial mediastinal structures produces soft tissue opacity ventral and lateral to the trachea (white arrows). The ventral mediastinum creates a thin, curved, soft tissue opacity line between the left and right cranial lung lobes (red arrow) and between the accessory and left caudal lung lobes (yellow arrow). In the VD view, the *cranioventral* mediastinum begins at the T1-2 thoracic vertebra and curves caudally toward the left cranial edge of the cardiac shadow. It follows the medial border of the right cranial lung lobe. The right cranial lobe wraps around the heart and extends across midline to the left. The *caudoventral* mediastinum begins at the left caudal edge of the cardiac shadow and curves toward the left diaphragm. It follows the accessory lung lobe, which extends to the left, across the midline. The caudal mediastinum is not identified in a lateral view. In the VD view, only the left border of the aorta usually is visible (black arrows). In a lateral view, fluid in the caudal esophagus (**E**) sometimes produces a soft tissue opacity band between the aorta and caudal vena cava, particularly in a left lateral view.

A

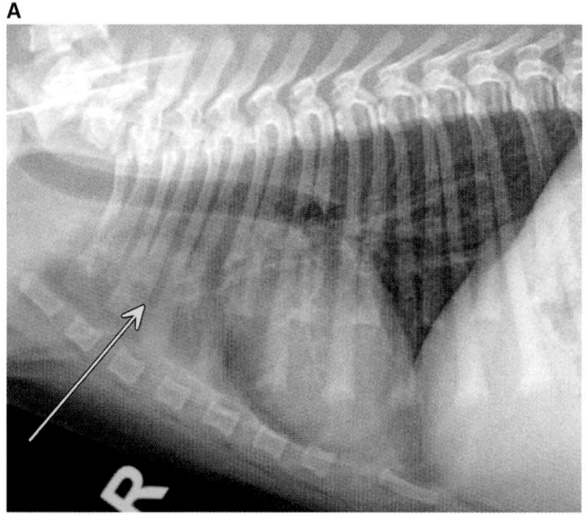

B

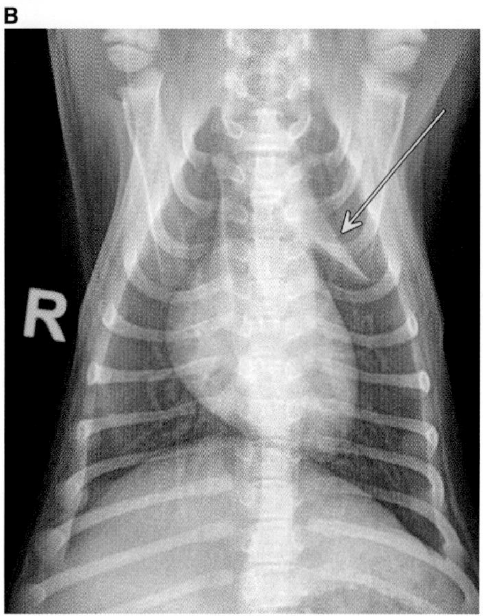

Figure 3.50 Thymus. Lateral view (**A**) and VD view (**B**) of a 5-month-old dog thorax depicting the appearance of the thymus in the cranioventral mediastinum (yellow arrows). In the lateral view, the thymus is less distinct, appearing as an ill-defined soft tissue opacity structure. In the VD view, the thymus appears as a triangular-shaped soft tissue opacity structure, sometimes described as resembling the sail on a sailboat.

quickly fades toward the sternum because there are fewer structures in the ventral part of the cranial mediastinum, and it usually is very thin. The caudal mediastinum also is thin and seldom visualized in a lateral view. In overweight animals, fat deposits often widen the mediastinum (Figure 3.42).

The thin ventral mediastinum frequently produces a curved, soft tissue opacity line that resembles a pleural fissure line (Figures 3.31, 3.32, 3.49). It is visible both cranial and caudal to the cardiac silhouette and varies significantly in width depending on the amount of fat present. It is less evident in chondrodystrophic dog breeds. The **cranioventral** mediastinum conforms to the shapes of the right and left cranial lung lobes. It begins at the thoracic inlet and curves caudally, ventrally and to the left of midline. The **caudoventral** mediastinum conforms to the shapes of the accessory and left caudal lung lobes, curving caudally from the left cardiac border to the middle of the left hemidiaphragm. The caudoventral mediastinum is only visible in the VD/DV view and may be mistaken for the cardiophrenic ligament, which is not visible in radiographs.

Mediastinal shift

The position of the mediastinum is maintained by normal lung inflation. Lungs that are not evenly inflated allow the mediastinum to move or shift toward the smaller lung. Uneven lung inflation also allows the diaphragm on the side with the smaller lung to move cranially.

The most common cause of a mediastinal shift is **lung collapse**. In cases of unilateral collapse, the opposite lung generally is well expanded due to compensatory hyperinflation. Collapse of part of a lung may or may not result in a mediastinal shift; it depends on the degree of compensatory inflation in the unaffected lobes.

Other causes of a mediastinal shift include a large intrathoracic mass and a large volume of unilateral fluid or gas in the pleural space.

In general, the position of the mediastinum is assessed in a VD/DV view based on the position of the cardiac shadow (Figure 3.52). Rotation of the patient during radiography may

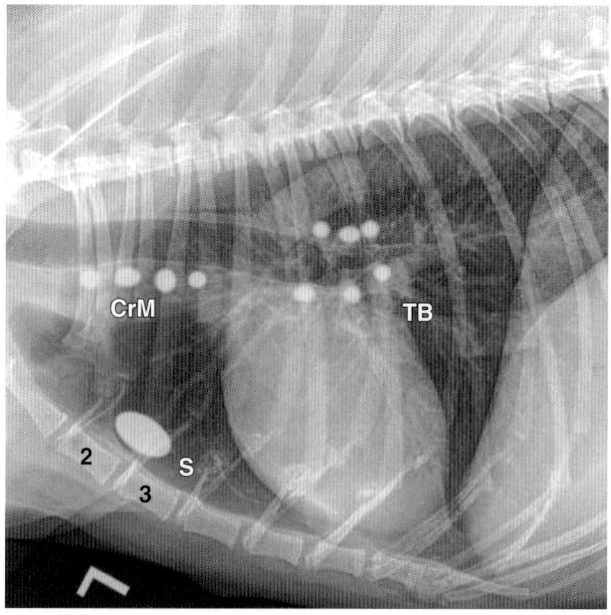

Figure 3.51 Mediastinal lymph nodes. Lateral view of a dog thorax depicting the locations of the mediastinal lymph nodes. The sternal node (S) is dorsal to the second and third sternebrae. The cranial mediastinal nodes (CrM) are ventral to the trachea, near the large cranial mediastinal blood vessels. The tracheobronchial nodes (TB) are in the hilar region, ventral to the esophagus and near the tracheal bifurcation.

be mistaken for a mediastinal shift because **the heart follows the sternum**. It is important to assess patient positioning before diagnosing a mediastinal shift. The spine and sternum should be superimposed and the right and left ribs equal length in a properly positioned VD/DV view. The dorsal spinous processes should be centered on their vertebral bodies.

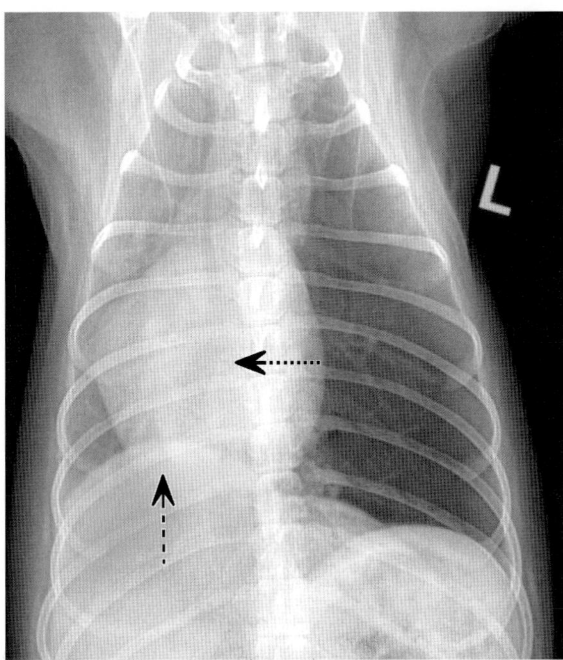

Figure 3.52 Mediastinal shift. VD view of a dog thorax depicting collapse of the right lung. The cardiac shadow is displaced to the right, and the right side of the diaphragm is displaced cranially (black arrows). The right lung is more opaque than the left lung because it contains less air. The left lung is hyperinflated to compensate for right lung collapse. Notice that the patient is not rotated: the spine and sternum are superimposed, the dorsal spinous processes are centered on the vertebral bodies, and the right and left ribs are equal length.

A

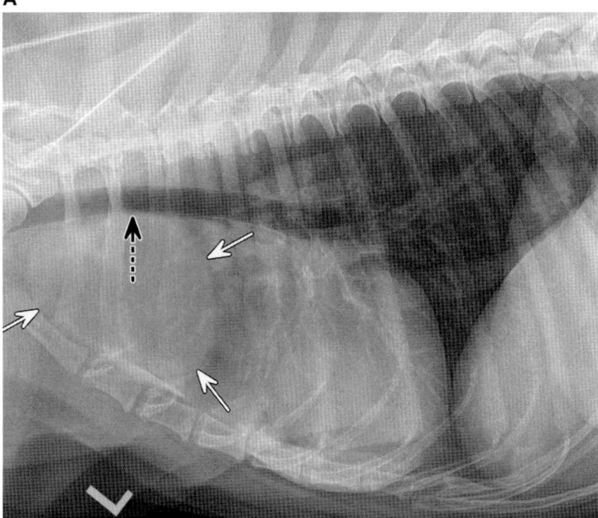

B

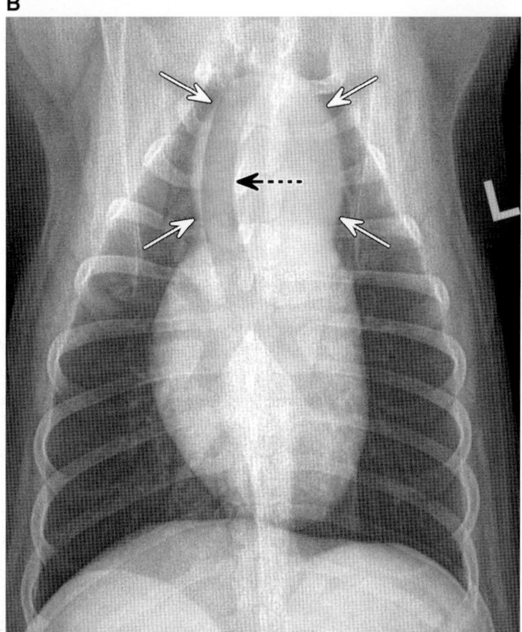

Figure 3.53 Cranial mediastinal mass. Lateral view (**A**) and VD view (**B**) of a dog thorax depicting localized widening of the cranial mediastinum (white arrows). The trachea is displaced dorsally and to the right (black dashed arrows). The margins of the soft tissue opacity mediastinal mass are more distinct in the VD view due to the opacity interface provided by air-filled lung. The cranial cardiac border is partially effaced by the mass.

Abnormal width of the mediastinum

The width of the mediastinum is assessed in a VD/DV view. In dogs, the **normal width** of the cranial mediastinum is about twice the width of a thoracic vertebra. In cats, the cranial mediastinum is about as wide as the spine. A wider than expected mediastinum may be localized due to a mass or it may be diffuse, involving the entire mediastinum. A mediastinal mass may arise in the cranial, dorsal, middle, or caudal part of the mediastinum.

Cranial mediastinal masses that arise ventral to the trachea create increased opacity dorsal to the sternum. When large enough, the mass may displace the trachea dorsally and laterally, usually to the right (Figure 3.53). Very large masses can displace the cardiac shadow caudally and push the tracheal bifurcation caudal to the sixth intercostal space (Figure 3.54). Caudal cardiac displacement usually is accompanied by dorsal cardiac displacement. Possible sites of origin for a cranioventral mediastinal mass include thymus, lymph node, sternum, and ectopic thyroid or parathyroid tissue. A mass may represent a tumor, cyst, abscess, or hematoma (see Differential Diagnoses). A large thymus in a mature dog or cat may be due to neoplasia or sometimes hemorrhage. Thymic tumors can grow to a very large size, particularly thymomas (Figure 3.54). A large sternal lymph node creates a soft tissue opacity mass dorsal to the second or third sternebra (Figure 3.55). Sternal lymphadenomegaly produces an extra-pleural sign, easiest to see in a lateral view. Rarely, a cranial mediastinal mass will involve one or more sternebrae and may cause osteolysis, a periosteal response, or/and adjacent soft tissue swelling.

Cranial mediastinal cysts or *branchial cysts* are congenital, fluid-filled cavities of embryologic origin. They usually are too small to be seen in radiographs of young animals but gradually enlarge over time. Branchial cysts are more common in cats than in dogs and typically produce a well-defined soft tissue opacity mass just cranial to the cardiac shadow (Figure 3.56). An aspirate of the cyst generally yields clear, acellular fluid with low specific gravity.

Conditions that may **mimic a cranial mediastinal mass** include fat deposits and errors in patient positioning. Older, small breed dogs normally store fat in the cranial mediastinum, which may be mistaken for a mass. During positioning for radiography, many patients will tuck their heads and flex

A

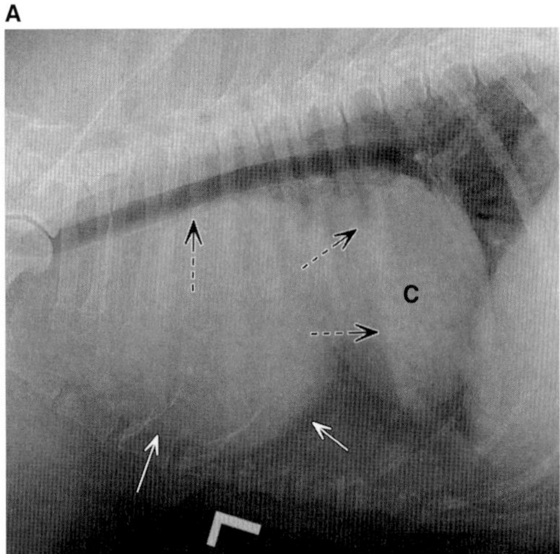

B

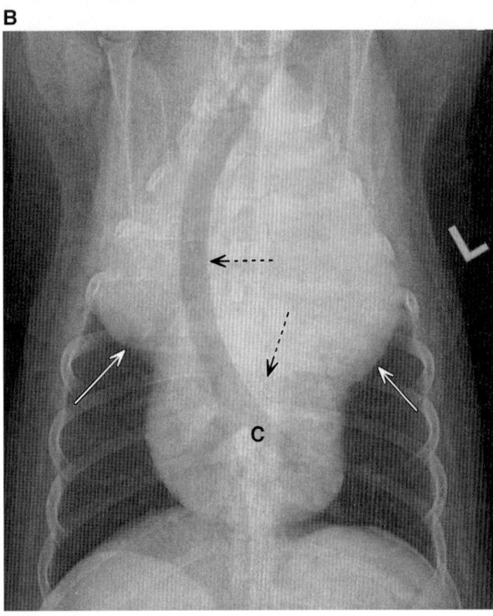

Figure 3.54 Thymoma. Lateral view (**A**) and VD view (**B**) of a dog thorax depicting a large, well-defined, soft tissue opacity mass in the cranial mediastinum (white arrows). The mediastinum is markedly widened, preventing the cranial lung lobes from reaching the thoracic inlet. The mass displaces the trachea dorsally and to the right and displaces the cardiac silhouette (C) caudally and dorsally (black dashed arrows). The cranial cardiac border is partially effaced by the mass.

A

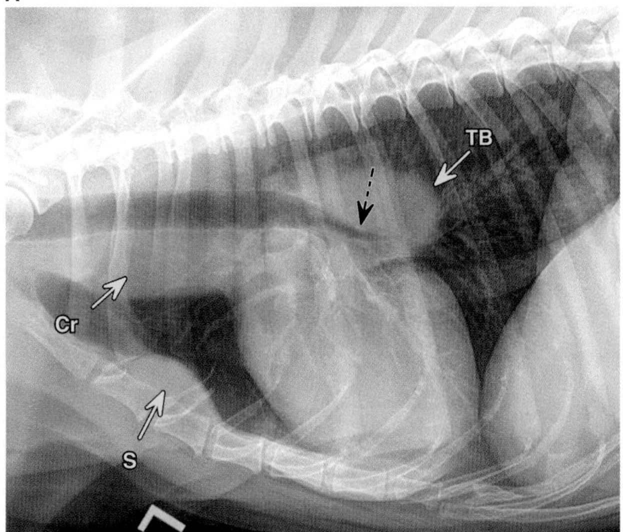

B

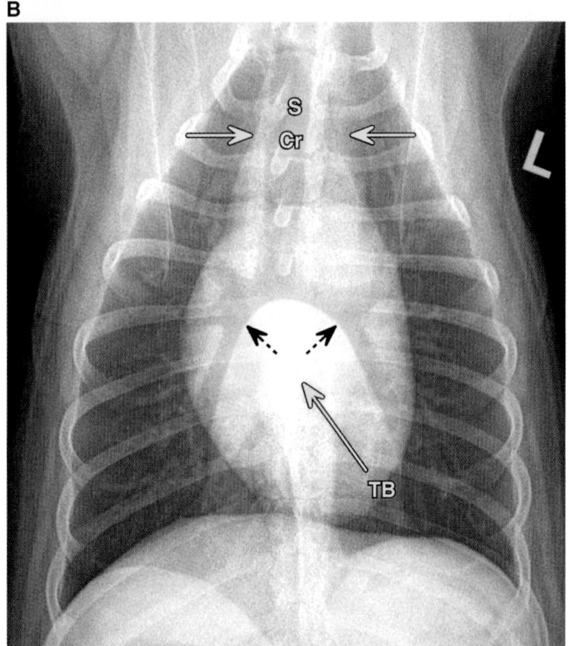

Figure 3.55 Mediastinal lymphadenomegaly. Lateral view (**A**) and VD view (**B**) of a dog thorax depicting enlargement of the sternal (S), cranial mediastinal (Cr), and tracheobronchial (TB) lymph nodes (yellow arrows). TB lymphadenomegaly displaces the caudal trachea ventrally and widens the tracheal bifurcation (black dashed arrows). In the VD view, superimposition of the spine and sternum obscures both the sternal and cranial mediastinal lymph nodes.

A

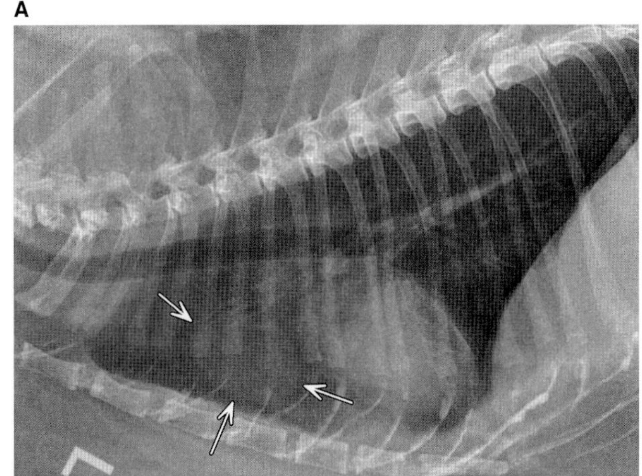

B

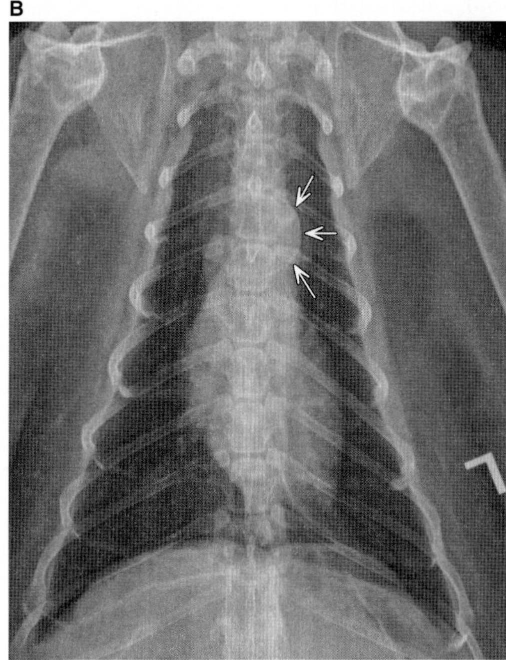

Figure 3.56 Branchial cyst. Lateral view (**A**) and VD view (**B**) of a cat thorax depicting a well-defined, soft tissue opacity mass located immediately cranial to the cardiac shadow (white arrows). In the VD view, only the left border of the mass is visible due to superimposition of the spine and sternum. Notice that the thoracic limbs are pulled caudally in the VD view to eliminate superimposition of the shoulders on the cranial thorax.

their necks which can produce a bend in the trachea that resembles a mass effect (Figure 3.115). Superimposition of the thoracic limb musculature also can mimic a cranial mediastinal mass. When in doubt, repeat the radiograph paying special attention to patient positioning.

Dorsal mediastinal masses occur dorsal to the trachea and most often are associated with the esophagus. Large masses can displace the trachea ventrally and laterally, usually to the right (Figure 3.57). A dilated esophagus can do the same and may be caused by abnormal retention of gas, fluid, food, or a combination of these. The type of esophageal content will affect the opacity of the dorsal mediastinum. An uncommon type of dorsal mediastinal mass is a large vertebral lesion (e.g., paraspinal tumor, severe lordosis, severe spondylosis).

Middle mediastinal masses or **hilar** masses most often represent enlarged tracheobronchial lymph nodes or a heart base tumor. Both of these produce soft tissue opacity along

A

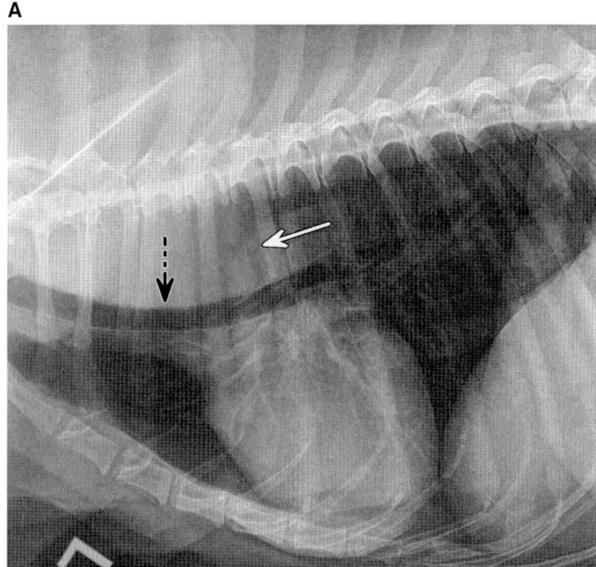

B

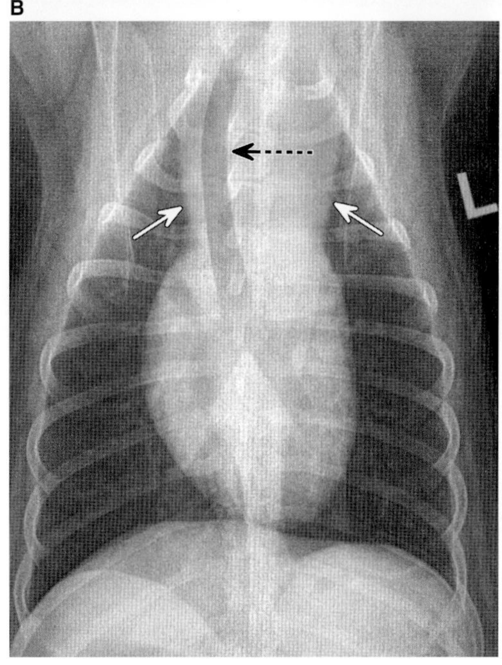

Figure 3.57 Dorsal mediastinal mass. Lateral view (**A**) and VD view (**B**) of a dog thorax depicting increased opacity dorsal to the trachea and widening of the cranial mediastinum (white arrows). The trachea is displaced ventrally and to the right (black dashed arrows). Notice that you cannot determine from the VD view alone whether the mass is located dorsal or ventral to the trachea.

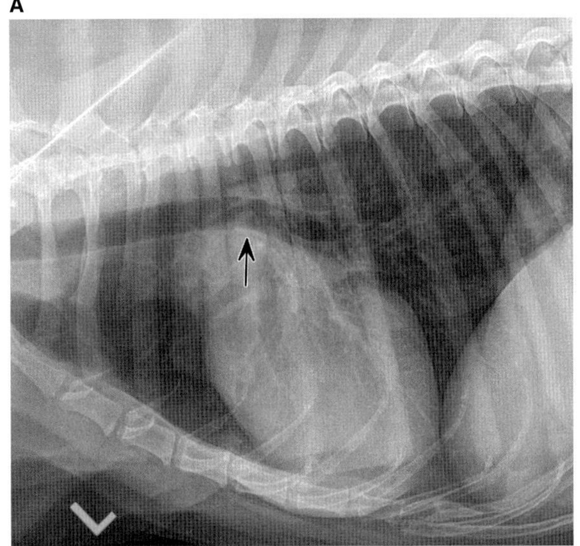

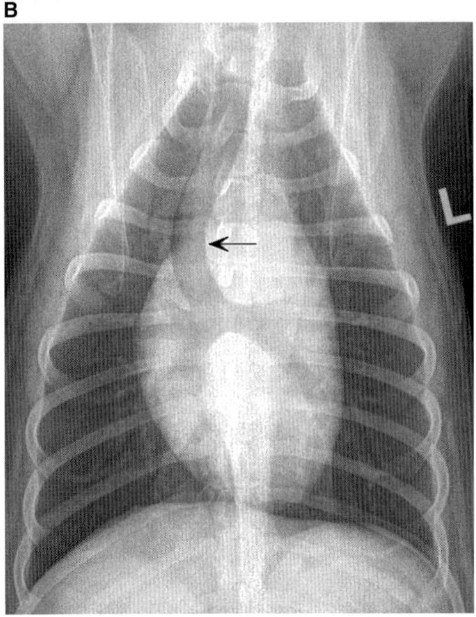

Figure 3.58 Heart base mass. Lateral view (**A**) and VD view (**B**) of a dog thorax depicting soft tissue opacity at the base of the cardiac silhouette and focal dorsal and right lateral displacement of the distal trachea (black arrow).

the distal trachea and both can become large enough to displace and compress the trachea. **Tracheobronchial lymphadenomegaly** occurs at the tracheal bifurcation (Figure 3.55). The enlarged lymph nodes can displace the trachea in any direction, but most often it is ventrally. Dorsal displacement of the trachea most often is due to left atrial dilation. Tracheobronchial lymphadenomegaly may be caused by lymphoma or a mycotic infection. Neoplasms other than lymphoma rarely cause hilar lymph node enlargement. Mineralization in a hilar lymph node typically is a healing response that most often is seen with histoplasmosis.

Heart base masses generally arise cranial to the tracheal bifurcation (Figure 3.58). The margins of a heart base mass often are indistinct due to effacement by pericardial fluid or the adjacent cardiovascular structures. Displacement of the trachea may be the only radiographic finding with a heart base mass. The trachea typically is pushed dorsally and laterally, usually to the right. Heart base tumors frequently are associated with the aorta (e.g., chemodectoma), but may involve the main pulmonary artery or the right atrium (e.g., hemangiosarcoma).

End-on visualization of the **right pulmonary artery** in a lateral view may be mistaken for a hilar mass. This artery, whether normal size or enlarged, can appear as a round, soft tissue opacity "nodule" located ventral to the tracheal bifurcation (Figure 3.99).

Caudal mediastinal masses typically are associated with the esophagus or diaphragm (see Differential Diagnoses). They usually are located on midline or just left of midline (Figure 3.59). Large masses may efface the caudal cardiac and/or cranial diaphragmatic borders. A mass in the accessory lung lobe can be difficult to distinguish from a caudal mediastinal mass.

Diffuse widening of the mediastinum may be due to abundant fat in the mediastinum (i.e., obesity), dilation of the esophagus, or fluid in the mediastinum. Excess mediastinal fat is common and must be differentiated from the other disorders. In overweight animals without mediastinal disease, the width of the cranial mediastinum should not exceed the thickness of the thoracic wall, measured at the same level (Figure 3.42). Dilation of the esophagus is discussed in the next section under "Esophagus". Fluid in the mediastinum may result from a ruptured esophagus, severe inflammation, or hemorrhage (see Differential Diagnoses). Keep in mind that abundant fat or fluid can obscure a mediastinal mass. Conditions that may mimic diffuse widening of the mediastinum include summation with pleural or pulmonary fluid and superimposition of a thoracic mass.

Abnormal opacity in the mediastinum

Orthogonal radiographs are necessary to avoid misinterpreting a structure located outside the mediastinum as something abnormal inside the mediastinum. Summation of dirt, debris, or medication on the skin or hair coat may be mistaken for mineral or metal in the mediastinum. The same is true with summation of a costal cartilage or a mineralized mass in the chest wall. Summation of subcutaneous gas not caused by pneumomediastinum may be mistaken for gas in the mediastinum.

Mineral opacity in the mediastinum may represent esophageal content or dystrophic mineralization (Figure 3.60). Dystrophic mineralization may be associated with a lymph node, a long-standing mass, or a cardiovascular structure. Lymph node mineralization usually is a healing response, most often following a mycotic infection

A

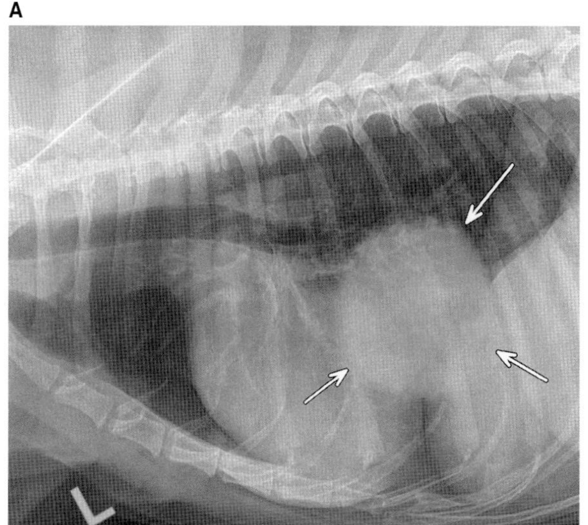

B

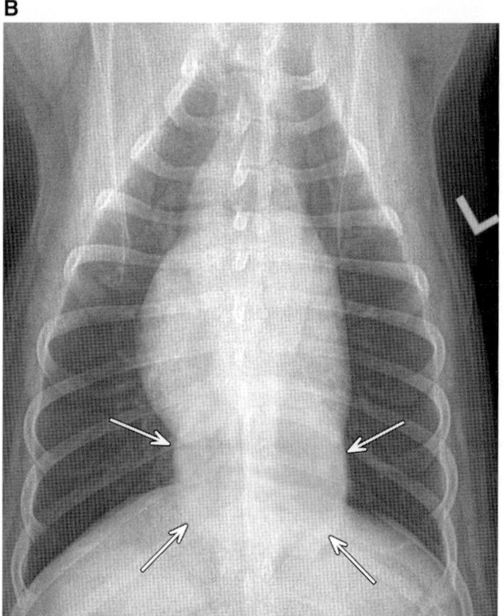

Figure 3.59 Caudal mediastinal mass. Lateral view (**A**) and VD view (**B**) of a dog thorax depicting a soft tissue opacity mass centered between the cardiac silhouette and the diaphragm (white arrows). The mass partially effaces the caudal cardiac and cranial diaphragm borders. The mass may be located in the caudal mediastinum or accessory lung lobe.

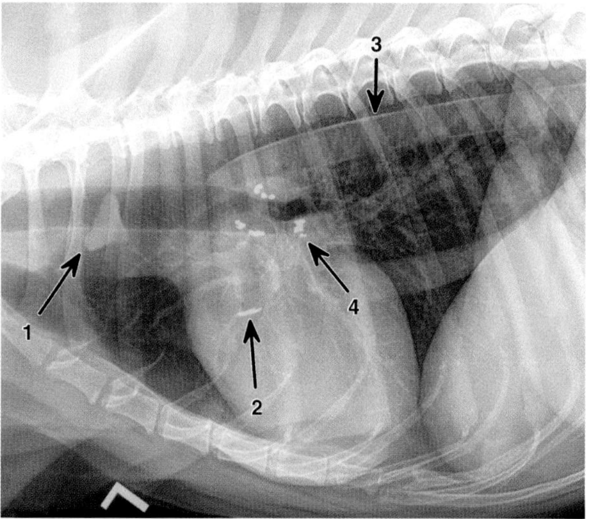

Figure 3.60 Mediastinal mineralization. Lateral view of a dog thorax depicting (1) a mineral opacity foreign object in the esophagus, (2) mineralization of the aortic valve, (3) mineralization in the wall of the descending aorta, and (4) mineralization in the hilar lymph nodes.

(e.g. histoplasmosis). It is rare with neoplasia. A chronic abscess, hematoma, or tumor may mineralize, either focally or diffusely. Cardiovascular mineralization may be incidental or caused by a disease, such as hypercalcemia. Heart valve mineralization usually is small, sharp, and linear. In blood vessels, mineralization tends to be curvilinear and heterogenous, most often in the wall of the aorta or a coronary artery.

Pneumomediastinum means there is free gas in the mediastinum. The gas provides an opacity interface to visualize structures that are not normally seen in survey radiographs. Radiographic signs vary with the amount of gas present. The signs tend to be easier to see in a lateral view where the spine and sternum are not superimposed. Small volumes of mediastinal gas may outline only the outer margin of the trachea and produce subtle, patchy areas of gas opacity (Figure 3.61). Larger volumes of gas may outline the cranial mediastinal blood vessels, the esophagus, and sharpen the margins of the aorta and cardiac silhouette (Figure 3.62). Gas can easily migrate in and out of the mediastinum through the normal openings at the thoracic inlet and aortic hiatus. Through these openings, gas can enter the

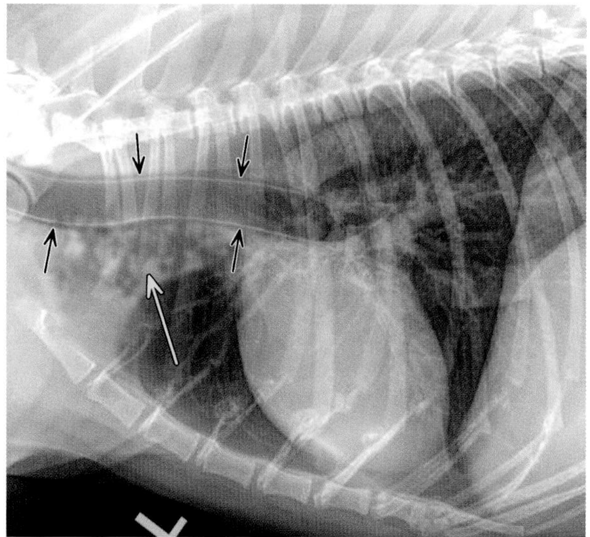

Figure 3.61 Pneumomediastinum. Lateral view of a dog thorax depicting a small volume of free gas in the cranial mediastinum. Gas outlines the outer margin of the trachea (black arrows) and creates a mottled pattern in the tissues ventral to the trachea (yellow arrow).

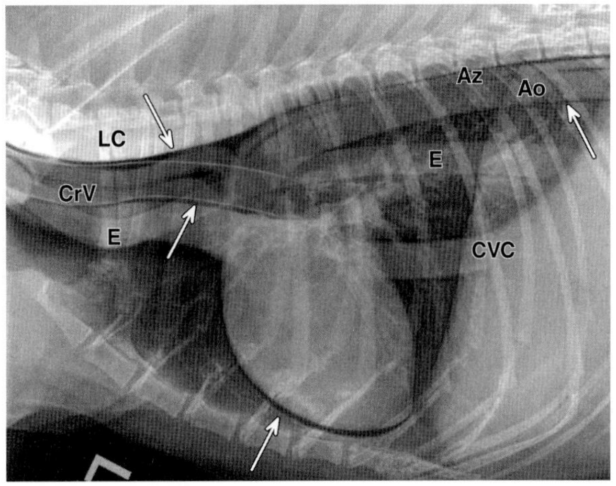

Figure 3.62 Pneumomediastinum. Lateral view of a dog thorax depicting free gas in the mediastinum. Gas outlines structures that are not normally seen, such as the cranial mediastinal blood vessels (CrV), the esophagus (E), and the azygous vein (Az). Gas enhances visualization of the cardiac, aortic (Ao), and longus coli (LC) borders and the outer tracheal margin (white arrows).

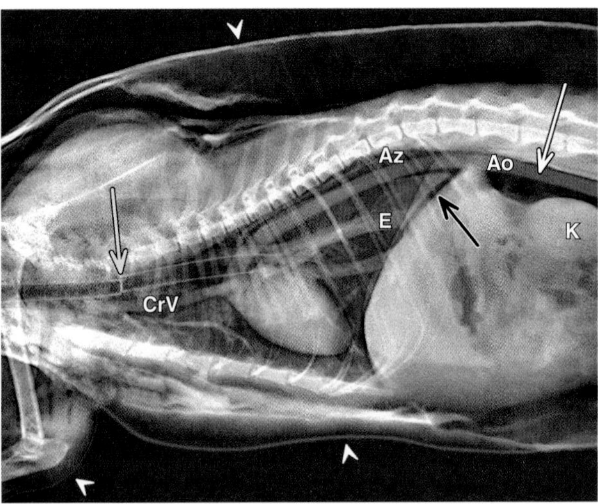

Figure 3.63 Tracheal rupture. Lateral view of a cat thorax depicting marked subcutaneous emphysema (white arrowheads) as well as free gas in the mediastinum, pleural space, and retroperitoneal space. Mediastinal gas sharply outlines the margins of the cardiac silhouette, aorta (Ao), cranial vena cava (CrV), azygous vein (Az), and esophagus (E). Migration of mediastinal gas leads to cervical emphysema, and pneumoretroperitoneum, the latter outlines the borders of the abdominal aorta (Ao) and dorsal kidneys (K) (white arrow). Gas diffusing through the mediastinal pleura causes a pneumothorax (black arrow). In this case, the origin of the free gas is a ruptured trachea. The ends of the torn trachea overlap to create a thin line of increased opacity and a slight discontinuity in the tracheal wall (yellow arrow).

cervical region and retroperitoneal space, respectively. Cervical gas readily spreads into the subcutaneous tissues along the thorax and abdomen (Figure 3.63). Retroperitoneal gas can outline the kidneys, abdominal aorta, and abdominal vena cava. Mediastinal gas also can diffuse through openings in the mediastinal pleura to enter the pleural space. Pneumomediastinum can progress to pneumothorax via the mediastinal fenestrations or a tear in the mediastinum.

A pneumomediastinum may result from a ruptured trachea or ruptured esophagus. It may also be caused by migration of gas from the cervical region or pleural space. Cervical gas may result from a penetrating wound in the neck. Pleural gas may result from a penetrating wound in the thorax or from a tear in a bronchus or lung. Dyspnea is uncommon with pneumomediastinum unless a secondary pneumothorax develops. Iatrogenic causes of pneumomediastinum include faulty intubation, over-distention of a tracheal tube cuff (especially in cats), and faulty venipuncture. An uncomplicated pneumomediastinum often is self-limiting and gas typically is resorbed in 2–10 days. Serial radiographs are useful to monitor the patient's progress and response to therapy.

Conditions that can mimic a pneumomediastinum include both an abundance of mediastinal fat and a lack of mediastinal fat. Abundant fat can separate and outline the mediastinal soft tissues. A lack of fat (e.g., emaciated patient) may allow the mediastinal soft tissues to become more visible against air-filled lungs.

Esophagus

Normal radiographic anatomy

The esophagus is relatively fixed in position at the caudal pharynx and at the diaphragm. The portion in between is freely moveable and quite distensible. The esophagus seldom is identified in survey radiographs because it usually is empty and collapsed. Small volumes of swallowed gas or fluid sometimes are visible, but these tend to be transient and variable in appearance in serial radiographs.

The cervical part of the esophagus runs from the cricopharynx (cranial esophageal sphincter) to the thoracic inlet. It lies dorsal and left lateral to the trachea. At the level of the first and second ribs, there is a slight ventral curvature or **redundancy** in the esophagus (Figure 3.64). The redundancy adds length to the esophagus to allow for movements of the head and neck. During flexion, the ventral curvature is more pronounced and may be mistaken for an esophageal diverticulum, (i.e., a *pseudodiverticulum*). Esophageal redundancy is accentuated in brachycephalic breeds where the length of the esophagus is confined to a shorter body.

The thoracic part of the esophagus extends from the thoracic inlet to the diaphragm. It runs caudally in the median plane, dorsal and left of the trachea, right of the aortic arch, and between the descending aorta and the caudal vena cava. Occasionally, the normal esophagus is visible in a lateral view as a horizontal, soft tissue opacity band between the aorta and caudal vena cava (Figure 3.49). The vagal nerves run alongside

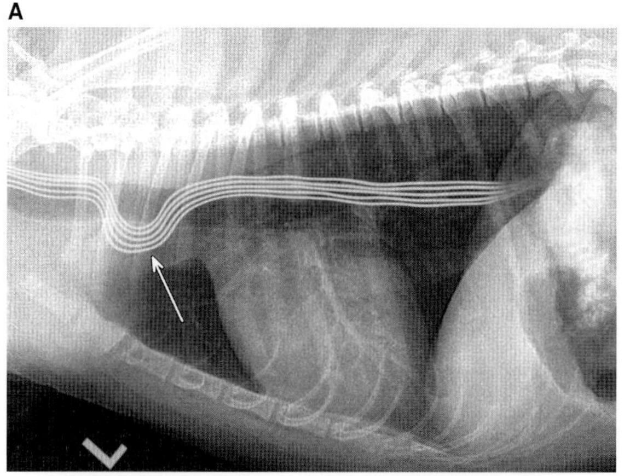

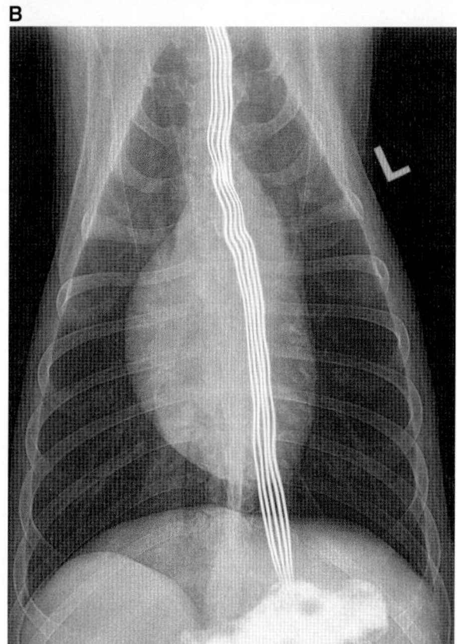

Figure 3.64 Normal canine esophagram. Lateral view (**A**) and VD view (**B**) of a dog thorax depicting a positive contrast esophagram. The longitudinal mucosal folds in the esophagus produce linear filling defects along its entire length. The linear defects are parallel and nearly equal in width. In the lateral view, the normal redundancy in the esophagus is visible near the thoracic inlet (white arrow). Contrast medium is visible in the stomach.

the esophagus and follow it through the diaphragm into the abdominal cavity. The abdominal part of the esophagus runs left of midline from the diaphragm to the cardia of the stomach. The esophagus ends at the gastroesophageal junction.

It is important to make both thoracic and cervical radiographs when examining the esophagus. Abdominal radiographs may be indicated as well because disease in the upper GI tract can affect the esophagus.

Contrast radiography of the esophagus

Complete evaluation of the esophagus often requires an esophagram. The procedure for esophagography, as well as its indications and contraindications, is described in Chapter 2, Contrast Radiography. Esophagrams differ in appearance between dogs and cats. **In dogs**, all of the esophagus contains striated muscle and the mucosal folds are longitudinal (Figure 3.64). The folds produce multiple linear filling defects along the entire length of the esophagus. **In cats**, the cranial 2/3 of the esophagus contains striated muscle and longitudinal mucosal folds, but in the caudal 1/3 there is smooth muscle and the mucosal folds are transverse or oblique in orientation. From about the level of the tracheal bifurcation to the stomach, the feline mucosal folds produce a pattern of filling defects commonly is described as "herringbone" (Figure 3.65).

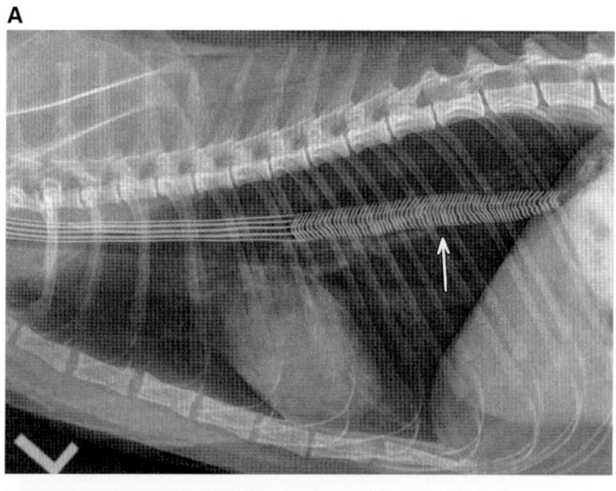

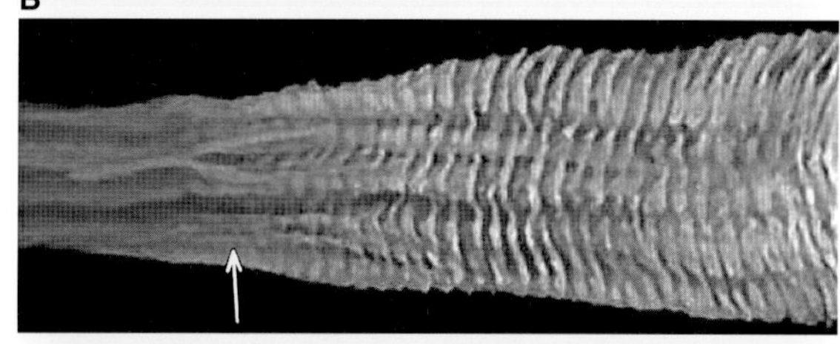

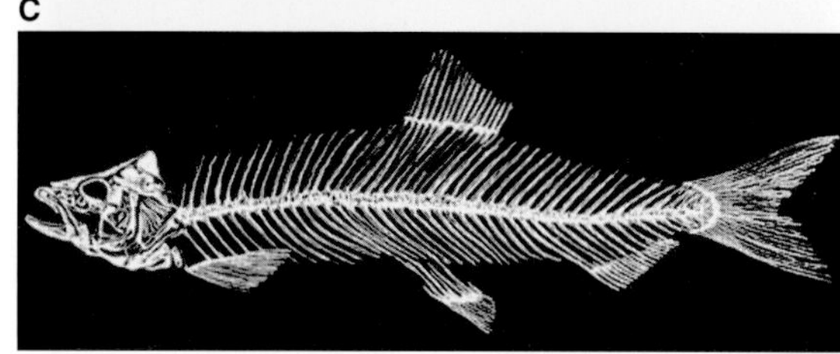

Figure 3.65 Normal feline esophagram. Lateral view (**A**) of a cat thorax depicting a positive contrast esophagram. The mucosal folds in the proximal esophagus are longitudinal and create parallel, linear filling defects, similar to those seen in a dog esophagram. Caudal to the level of the tracheal bifurcation, the mucosal folds are oblique and produce transverse filling defects (arrow). **B**. In this anatomical image of a feline esophagus, you can see the mucosal folds transition from longitudinal to oblique (arrow). The contrast radiographic appearance of the oblique folds has been described as a "herringbone pattern" because it resembles the skeleton of a herring fish (**C**).

In both dogs and cats, contrast medium in the esophagus should be transient and not retained. In some normal dogs, a small amount of contrast may persist for a short period of time near the larynx or thoracic inlet.

Abnormal content or opacity in the esophagus

Persistence of gas, fluid, soft tissue opacity material, or mineral opacity structures in the esophagus needs to be investigated. Abnormal opacity may be localized or diffuse, heterogenous or homogenous. Possible causes of retained gas, fluid, or solid material include physical obstruction, motility disorders, lodged foreign material, and a mass in the esophagus.

Gas in the esophagus may or may not be due to pathology. A small volume of esophageal gas often is incidental and transient. Transient gas commonly is seen between the thoracic inlet and the tracheal bifurcation.

Esophageal gas that is dorsal to the trachea may produce a **tracheal stripe sign**. The tracheal stripe results from the soft tissue opacity wall of the esophagus lying against the soft tissue opacity wall of the trachea with no different opacity between them (Figure 3.66). The two walls blend together to mimic a thickened dorsal tracheal wall.

The tracheal stripe sign may be mistaken for a pneumomediastinum. However, free gas in the mediastinum generally outlines both the dorsal and ventral tracheal walls as well as other mediastinal structures.

Larger volumes of transient esophageal gas sometimes are seen in patients that are sedated, anesthetized, or have swallowed a lot of air (e.g., panting, struggling, coughing, vomiting). Aerophagia usually is accompanied by abundant gas in the GI tract.

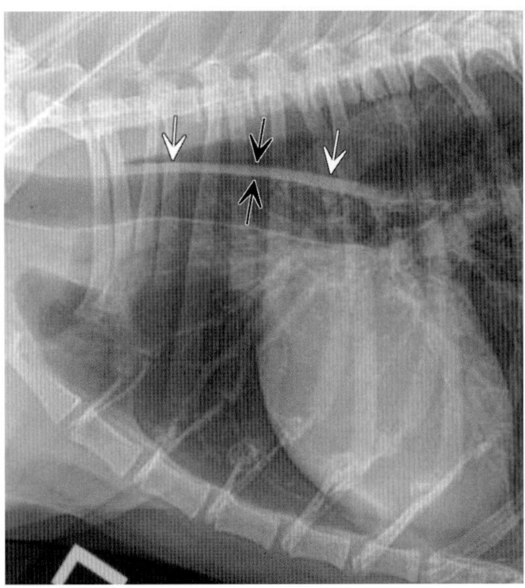

Figure 3.66 Tracheal stripe sign. Lateral view of a dog thorax depicting gas in the esophagus dorsal to the trachea. Gas outlines the ventral mucosal margin of the esophagus (white arrows). The ventral wall of the esophagus blends with the dorsal wall of the trachea to create a soft tissue opacity stripe that may be mistaken for a thickened dorsal tracheal wall (black arrows).

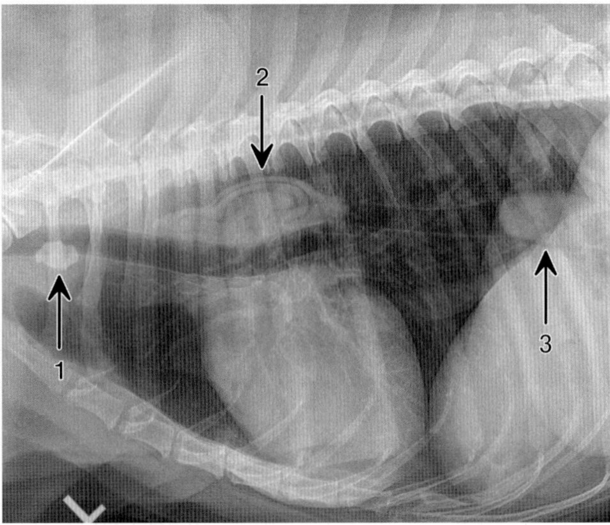

Figure 3.67 Esophageal foreign objects. Lateral view of a dog thorax depicting sites where ingested foreign objects frequently lodge in the esophagus. (**1**) thoracic inlet: an irregular-shaped mineral opacity object is visible here. (**2**) base of the cardiac silhouette: the soft tissue opacity material that is lodged here causes local dilation of the esophagus and ventral displacement of the trachea. (**3**) cranial to the diaphragm: the cranial part of this soft tissue opacity object is partially outlined by gas in the distal esophagus.

Persistent gas in the esophagus may indicate a motility problem. A gas-distended esophagus sometimes is difficult to recognize in radiographs because the esophageal lumen is the same opacity as the lungs (Figure 3.70). In addition, the esophageal walls tend to be thin, faint, and widely separated (Figure 3.71). The walls of a dilated esophagus may be easier to recognize in the caudal thorax where they converge toward the diaphragm. Cranially, the ventral border of the longus coli muscles tends to be more distinct against a gas-distended esophagus.

Foreign materials can lodge in the esophagus of a dog or cat. Common sites include the cranial cervical region, the thoracic inlet, the base of the heart, and just cranial to the diaphragm (Figure 3.67). Metal and mineral opacity objects usually are readily identified in radiographs. Soft tissue opacity materials must be outlined by gas or large enough to be distinguished. Objects that obstruct the esophagus may lead to dilation of the esophagus cranial to the object. The dilated esophagus may fill with gas, fluid, food, or a combination of these. Dilation may not be evident if the patient regurgitated and emptied the esophagus prior to radiography.

Masses associated with the esophagus may be intraluminal, mural, or extraluminal. A large esophageal mass may be difficult to distinguish from a mass in the adjacent lung. Many esophageal masses are soft tissue opacity (e.g., tumor, abscess, granuloma, hematoma). A soft tissue opacity mass in the esophagus often is difficult to detect unless surrounded by gas or a positive contrast medium. In an esophagram, an esophageal mass may appear as a localized thickening of the esophageal wall and/or a filling defect in the esophageal lumen (Figure 3.73). The mucosal margin of the thickened wall may be smooth or irregular, depending on the amount of mucosal damage. Ulcers sometimes are present, appearing as contrast-filled outpouchings that extend away from the esophageal lumen. If the esophagus is obstructed by a mass, contrast fills the dilated lumen cranial to the obstruction.

Spirocercosis is a parasitic infection caused by *Spirocerca lupi*, a nematode with worldwide distribution. It is endemic in warm climates where the incidence can be as high as 85%. After being ingested, the parasites penetrate the gastric mucosa and travel along arteries to the thoracic aorta. They migrate through the aorta and end up in the caudal esophagus where they can produce granulomas along the dorsal esophageal wall. Parasite migration can produce small aneurysms in the wall of the aorta. Spirocera granulomas can grow quite large and may undergo malignant transformation to osteosarcoma. Osteosarcomas can mineralize and they can metastasize to the lungs. Large intra-thoracic granulomas also can cause hypertrophic osteopathy.

The pathognomonic sign of spirocercosis is new bone production along the ventral margins of the thoracic vertebrae (Figure 3.68). New bone occurs in about 25% of affected dogs, most often caudal to the T5 thoracic vertebra. One or more vertebrae may be involved. The border of the new bone may be solid, lamellar, or brush-like and may be well-defined or ill-defined. Diagnosis of spirocercosis is confirmed by endoscopy or finding parasite eggs in the feces.

Abnormal size and margination of the esophagus

An abnormally narrowed or dilated esophagus seldom is detected in survey radiographs unless there is persistent retention of gas, fluid, or food. Usually, an esophagram is needed for diagnosis and to evaluate the mucosal margin.

Abnormal narrowing persists in multiple radiographs and may be focal or regional. Possible causes of a narrowed esophagus include stricture, mural thickening or mass, and external compression, the latter may be the result of a vascular ring anomaly or hiatal hernia (see Differential Diagnoses). Liquid contrast media may be used to evaluate esophageal width and to visualize the mucosal margin. Barium provides the best mucosal coating. An irregular mucosal margin may be due to severe inflammation or neoplasia (Figure 3.69). If the esophageal narrowing does not obstruct the passage of liquids, it may not be evident in a standard esophagram. Mixing the contrast medium with food may aid in diagnosis.

Abnormal dilation of the esophagus commonly is called *megaesophagus*. Although megaesophagus is used as a general

A

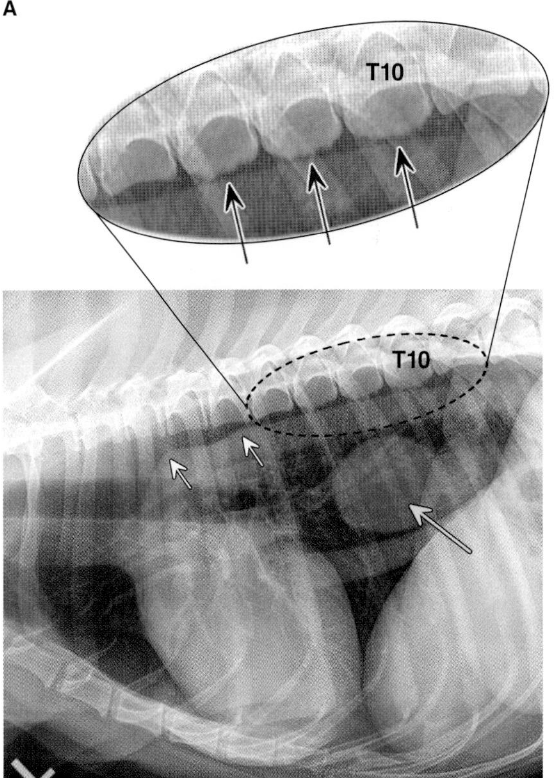

B

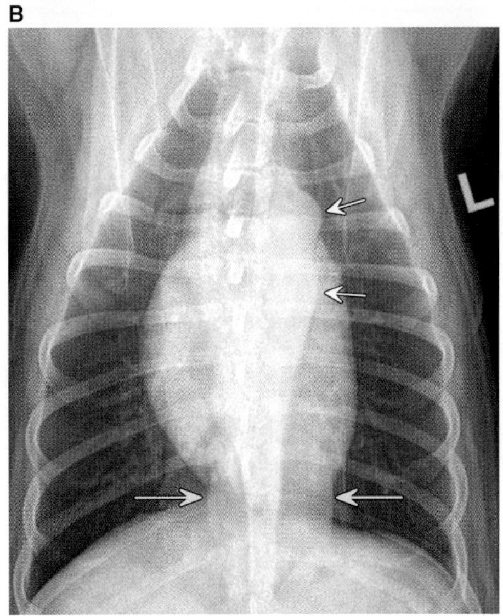

Figure 3.68 Spirocercosis. Lateral view (**A**) and VD view (**B**) of a dog thorax depicting lesions associated with spirocercosis. The pathognomonic finding with spirocercosis is a periosteal response along the caudal thoracic vertebrae. This new bone production is visible in the lateral view along the ventral bodies of T8-10 (black arrows in the ovoid close-up). Compare T8-10 to the normal vertebrae on either side (T7 and T11). In both the lateral and VD views, a soft tissue opacity mass is visible on midline, located between the aorta and caudal vena cava (yellow arrows). This mass is an esophageal granuloma, but a lung mass would have a similar appearance. The two small bulges in the proximal descending aorta (white arrows) are aneurysms caused by the migrating parasites.

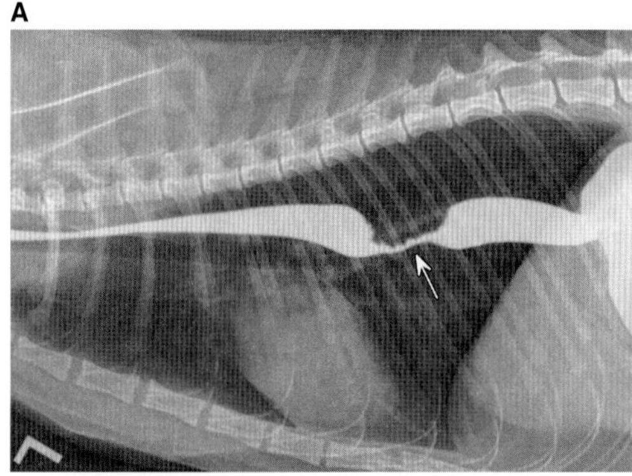

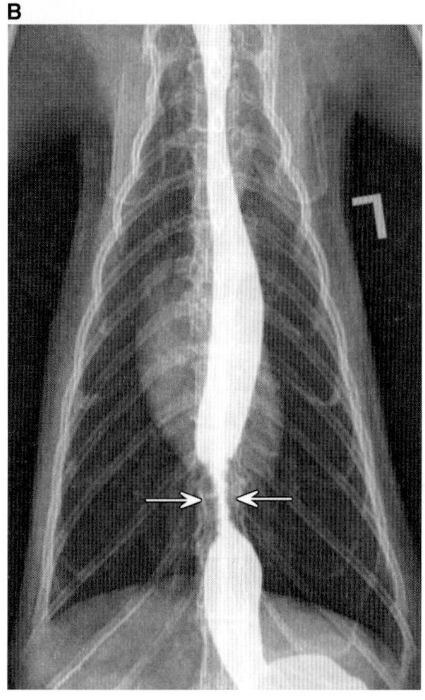

Figure 3.69 Esophageal stricture. Lateral view (**A**) and VD view (**B**) of a cat thorax depicting an esophagram. There is a localized area of persistent narrowing in the caudal esophagus (white arrows). The mucosal margins are irregular, which may be due to severe inflammation or neoplasia.

term to simply describe esophageal dilation, it is also the name given to flaccid dilation of the esophagus due to one of several congenital or acquired causes of weak or absent peristalsis. Congenital megaesophagus is more common in dogs than in cats, particularly in German shepherds. Acquired megaesophagus may result from numerous conditions, including severe or chronic inflammation, neuromuscular disease, immune-mediated disease, chronic obstruction, and others (see Differential Diagnoses). Severe or chronic esophagitis usually is due to gastric reflux and can affect esophageal motility in animals at any age. Neuromuscular and immune-mediated motility disorders often are idiopathic. They tend to occur in older animals (7–15 years of age) and many are incurable. Any cause of acquired megaesophagus may begin as mild or intermittent dilation and progress in severity. Many esophageal obstructions initially present with localized or regional dilation, but any persistent narrowing can progress to general dilation. Certain strong sedatives and anesthetic agents can cause transient esophageal dilation that usually resolves during recovery.

Radiographic diagnosis of esophageal dilation depends on size and content. As mentioned earlier, a large, gas-filled esophagus can easily be missed in survey radiographs because the lumen is the same opacity as the adjacent lungs and the esophageal walls are thin, faint, and widely separated (Figures 3.70 and 3.71). In the lateral view, look for the tracheal stripe sign and a more distinct ventral border to the longus coli muscles. Widening of the mediastinum may or may not be evident with a gas-filled esophagus. A dilated esophagus may displace the trachea ventrally and laterally, usually to the right. The base of the cardiac silhouette may also be displaced ventrally, making the cardiac shadow appear shortened (Figure 3.71). Many patients with a dilated esophagus have concurrent aerophagia and aspiration pneumonia. A gastric outflow problem should always be investigated as a possible etiology of a dilated esophagus.

Performing an esophagram in a patient with megaesophagus carries increased risk of aspiration, but sometimes the procedure is needed to help determine the etiology and full extent of the dilatation. A severely dilated esophagus may require a larger than expected volume of contrast medium for complete opacification. Inadequate dosing can result in an erroneous diagnosis of local esophageal dilation in a patient with general dilation.

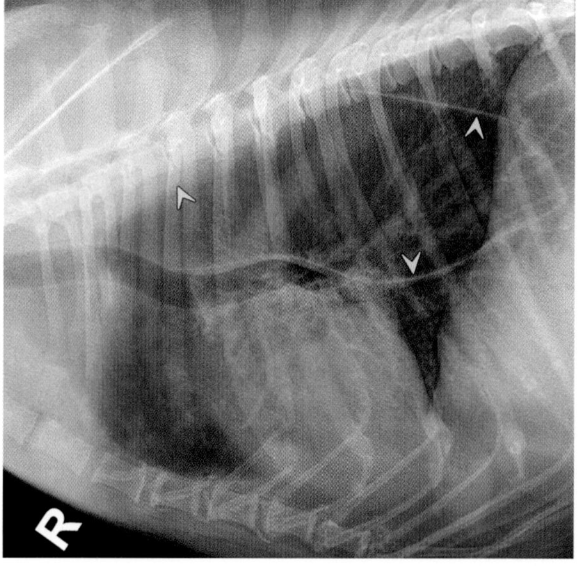

Figure 3.70 Gas-distended esophagus. Lateral view of a dog thorax depicting a largely dilated, gas-filled esophagus. The esophageal walls are thin and widely separated (yellow arrowheads), but converge caudally toward the diaphragm.

A

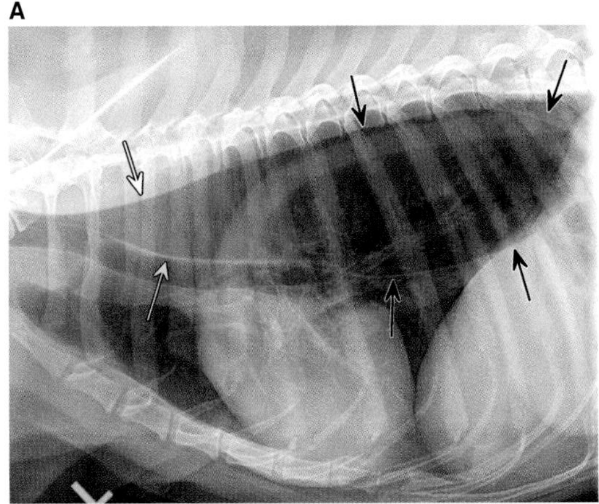

B

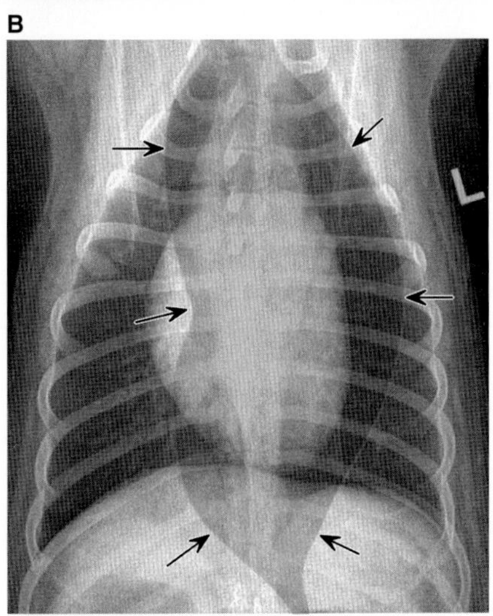

Figure 3.71 Megaesophagus. Lateral view (**A**) and VD view (**B**) of a dog thorax depicting gas-distention of the entire esophagus (arrows). The ventral margin of the longus coli muscles is sharp and distinct against the air-filled esophagus (white arrow). The tracheal stripe sign is visible (yellow arrow). The trachea and cardiac base are displaced ventrally. The cardiac shadow appears shortened due to ventral displacement. In the VD view, the slight indentation along the right lateral border in the middle of the esophagus is a normal finding at the heart base.

Esophagitis

Inflammation of the esophagus may or may not be evident in radiographs. A normal esophagram does not rule out esophagitis. Characteristic radiographic findings include local or regional dilation and variable thickening of the esophageal wall. The mucosal margin may be smooth or irregular. If irregular, rule out neoplasia. Inflammation and neoplasia in the esophagus cannot be reliably differentiated with radiographs. Muscle spasms are common with esophagitis and may be mistaken for an esophageal stricture. Muscle spasms can last longer than normal peristalsis, but they are transient and vary in appearance between radiographs. Strictures persist relatively unchanged. Barium may adhere to damaged mucosa creating a mottled pattern (Figure 3.72).

Mucosal ulcers appear as barium-filled out-pouches that extend away from the esophageal lumen (Figure 3.73).

Esophageal diverticulum

A diverticulum is an abnormal outpouching in the esophageal wall. It may result from a weakness in the wall that allows the mucosa to protrude through (*pulsion diverticulum*) or from an external adhesion that pulls the wall outward (*traction diverticulum*). Esophageal diverticula are reported most often either at the thoracic inlet or just cranial to the diaphragm. They may be visible in survey radiographs when the esophagus contains gas or ingesta. In an esophagram, a diverticulum appears as a contrast-filled bulge that extends

A

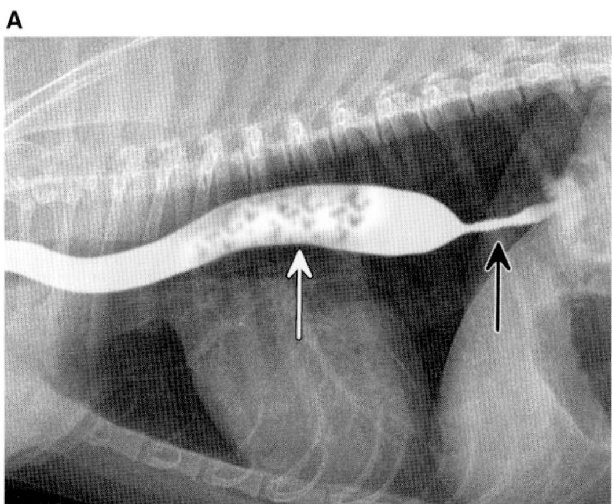

B

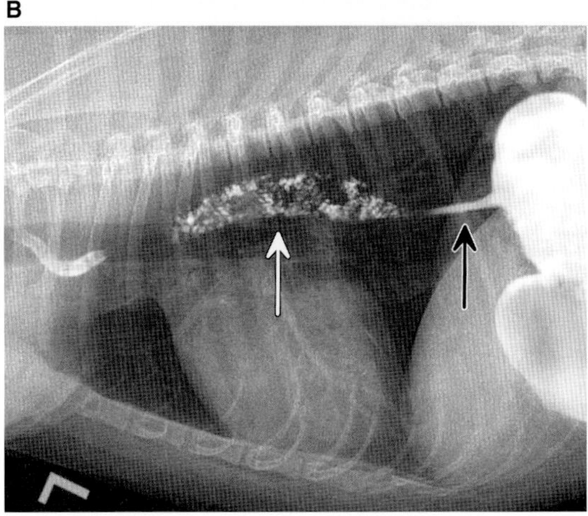

Figure 3.72 Esophageal stricture and inflammation. Two lateral views of a dog thorax depicting a barium esophagram. (**A**) Radiograph made immediately after administering barium reveals filling defects dorsal to the cardiac base (white arrow) and a narrowed area in the distal esophagus (black arrow). (**B**) Radiograph made a few minutes later reveals adherence of barium to damaged esophageal mucosa (white arrow) and persistent narrowing in the distal esophagus (black arrow). Possible etiologies for these lesions include inflammation and neoplasia. Retention of a small amount of barium at the thoracic inlet occurs frequently in normal dogs and its significance in this case is uncertain.

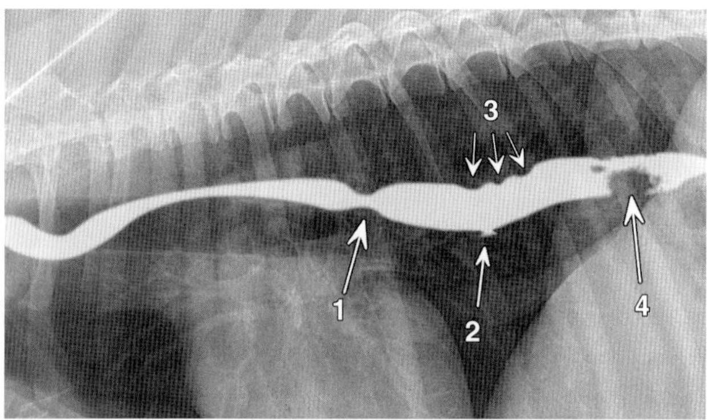

Figure 3.73 Esophageal lesions. Lateral view of a dog thorax depicting a positive contrast esophagram. (**1**) A narrowed area in the esophagus which may be transient (due to peristalsis) or persistent (due to a stricture); a follow up radiograph is needed for diagnosis. (**2**) Esophageal ulcer; a small pocket of barium extends away from the mucosal margin. (**3**) Filling defects along the dorsal esophageal wall; defects are consistent with mural nodules (e.g., granulomas, tumors). (**4**) Irregular-shaped filling defects in the distal esophagus caused by a mural tumor extending into the esophageal lumen.

outward, away from the lumen (Figure 3.74). The lumen may be dilated or it may deviate ventrally or laterally.

As stated earlier, the normal redundancy in the esophagus may be mistaken for a diverticulum at the thoracic inlet, particularly in brachycephalic dogs. To distinguish a true diverticulum from a pseudodiverticulum, repeat the radiograph with the patient's neck extended. There will be little difference in the appearance of a true diverticulum between extension and flexion of the neck, whereas the normal esophageal redundancy will be less apparent with the patient's neck extended.

Gastroesophageal intussusception

Invagination of the stomach into the lumen of the esophagus is rare in dogs and cats. It most often is reported in young dogs, particularly German Shepherds. Many affected animals have preexisting megaesophagus.

Many gastroesophageal intussusceptions occur intermittently which makes them difficult to diagnose with radiographs. The displaced part of the stomach typically creates a well-defined mass in the caudal esophagus (Figure 3.75). The mass may be soft tissue opacity or mixed opacity, the latter due to gas or ingesta in the stomach. Sometimes other viscera is displaced with the stomach (e.g., omentum, spleen, duodenum, pancreas). Often it is difficult to identify the displaced viscera. The stomach may be recognized by its rugal folds or if there is a visible connection between the intra-thoracic mass and the intra-abdominal part of the stomach. The stomach that remains in the abdomen frequently is abnormal in shape or position. Sometimes the area normally occupied by the stomach appears to be empty or contains only small intestine. An incarcerated stomach can become greatly distended with gas and present as an emergency situation (Figure 3.48).

Gastroesophageal intussusception usually leads to caudal esophageal obstruction and cranial esophageal dilation. Dilation may be evident in survey radiographs if there is sufficient gas, fluid, or food in the esophagus. Otherwise an esophagram may be needed for diagnosis. Rarely, contrast medium may enter the stomach during an esophagram to outline the gastric rugae and confirm the diagnosis.

Vascular ring anomaly

Anomalous development of the aorta can lead to constriction of the esophagus at the base of the heart. The most common anomaly is a *persistent right fourth aortic arch*. In this situation, the aorta develops on the right side of the trachea instead of the left side and the esophagus is trapped in a tight ring

A

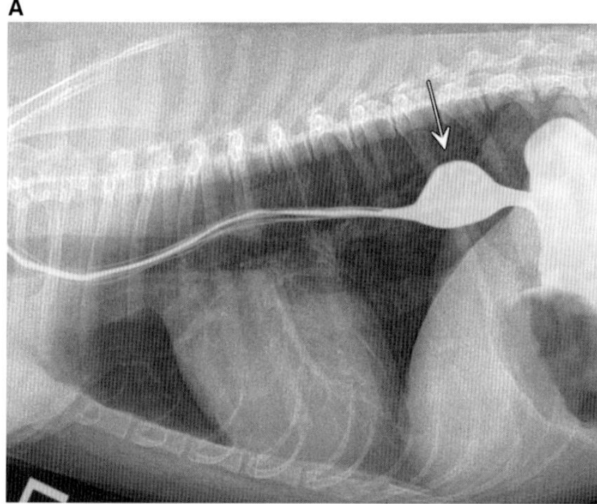

B

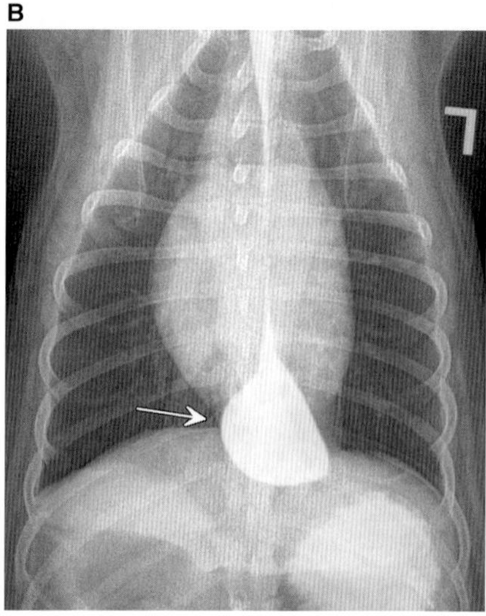

Figure 3.74 Esophageal diverticulum Lateral view (**A**) and VD view (**B**) of a dog thorax depicting a positive contrast esophagram. There is a localized, contrast-filled bulge in the distal esophagus, just cranial to the diaphragm (white arrow).

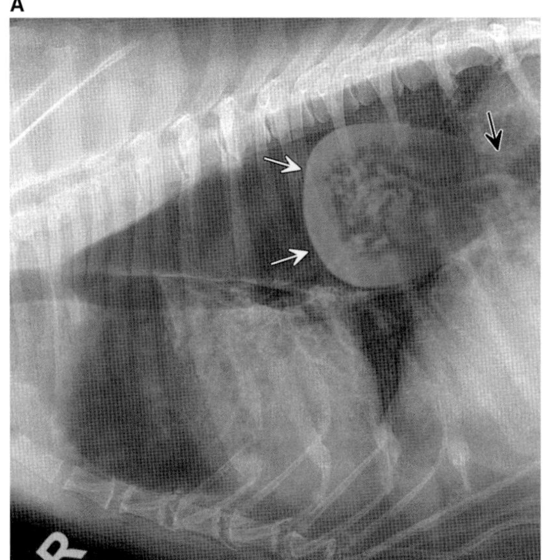

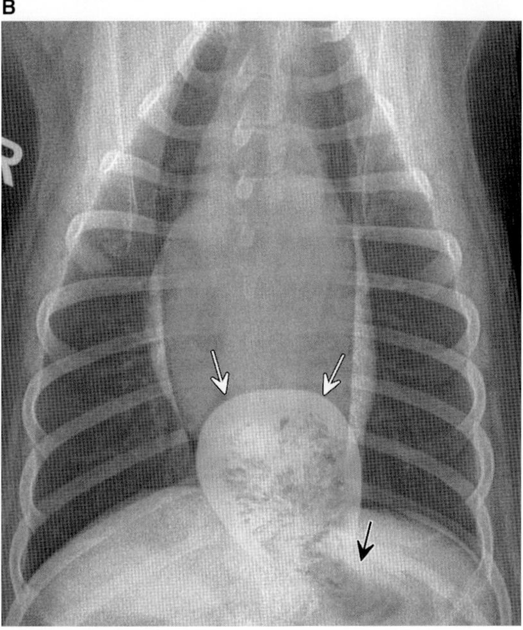

Figure 3.75 Gastroesophageal intussusception. Lateral view (**A**) and VD view (**B**) of a dog thorax depicting part of the stomach extending into the distal esophagus (white arrows). The displaced stomach appears as a mixed opacity mass in the caudodorsal thorax. The mass is continuous with the intra-abdominal part of the stomach (black arrow). The esophagus cranial to the intussusception is dilated with gas. Gas outlines the cranial border of the displaced stomach.

formed by the ligamentum arteriosum and the trachea (Figure 3.76). The result is a functional stenosis that partially or completely obstructs the esophagus. The esophagus proximal to the vascular ring may retain gas, fluid, or food and may be dilated well into the cervical region (Figure 3.77). The esophagus distal to the vascular ring usually is normal size. The dilated proximal esophagus often is large enough to widen the cranial mediastinum and to displace the trachea. Tracheal displacement usually is ventral and to the left (leftward displacement because the anomalous aortic arch usually is on the right).

In an esophagram, the proximal esophagus generally fills with contrast medium and then tapers quickly at the heart base, ending near the fourth intercostal space. Contrast medium may or may not be seen in the distal esophagus, depending on the degree of obstruction.

Heart

Normal radiographic anatomy

What commonly is called the "heart" in a radiograph is actually an image of the pericardial sac and its contents. The contents include pericardial fluid, the origins of major blood vessels, the heart, and blood, all of which are soft tissue opacity and not individually distinguished. Because radiographs reveal only the outer margin of the pericardial sac, the terms **cardiac silhouette** or **cardiac shadow** are more accurate. The word "heart" will be used to describe the actual heart itself. Normal cardiovascular anatomy and circulation are depicted in Figures 3.88 and 3.89.

The **pericardial sac** consists of two layers. The inner *visceral* layer is called the *epicardium* and blends with the surface of the heart. The outer *parietal* layer is tough and fibrous. Between the visceral and parietal layers is a tiny volume of pericardial fluid for lubrication. The pericardiophrenic ligament forms a strong attachment to the diaphragm. It is not visible in radiographs, but the caudal mediastinum sometimes is mistaken for the pericardiophrenic ligament (VD/DV view).

The central **position** of the cardiac silhouette is maintained by normally inflated lungs. In most dogs and cats, the cardiac shadow is located between the T3 and T8 thoracic vertebrae, with its *base* at about the fifth or sixth intercostal space (base refers to the dorsum or "top" of the cardiac shadow). The **cardiac base** is formed by the atria, proximal aorta, main pulmonary artery, and cranial vena cava. Enlargement of any of these can alter the size or shape of the cardiac base. Immediately dorsal to the base lies the tracheal bifurcation and carina. The position of the carina relative to the spine is used to assess cardiac size. The ventrum or "bottom" of the cardiac shadow is called the *apex*. The **cardiac apex** is formed by the interventricular septum.

In a **lateral view**, the cardiac silhouette sits dorsal to the sternum with its long axis tilted cranially about 45° off perpendicular. The **long axis** is the apex-to-base dimension or length of the cardiac shadow. The **short axis** is the width of the cardiac silhouette; the widest dimension perpendicular to the long axis, often at about the level of the caudal vena cava (Figure 3.78). In a lateral view of most healthy dogs and cats, the cardiac base is situated at about 2/3 the height

A

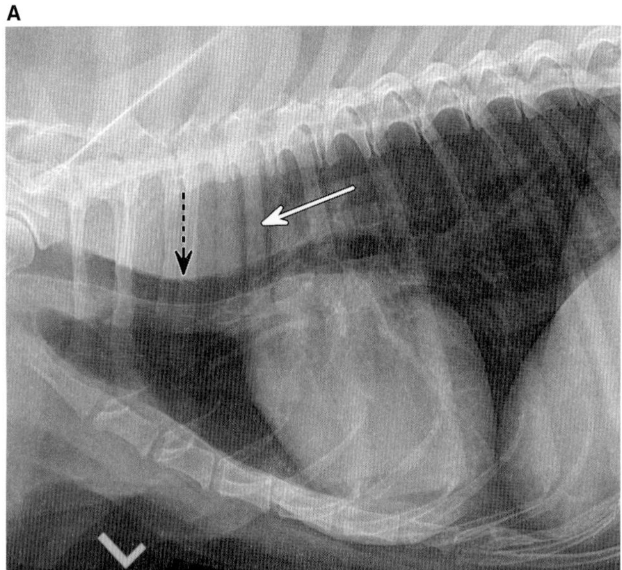

B

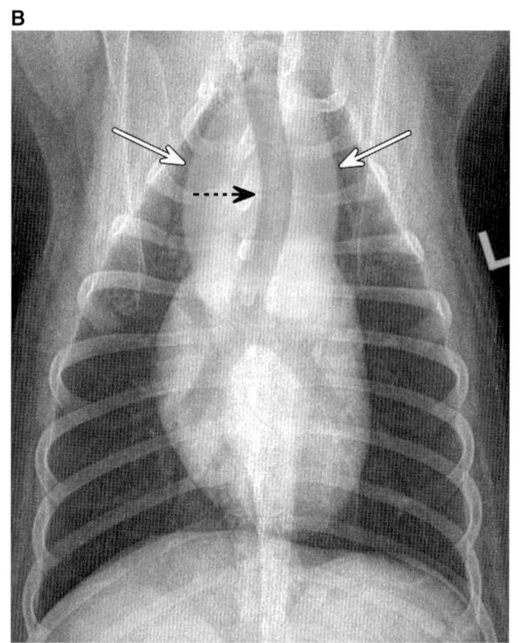

C

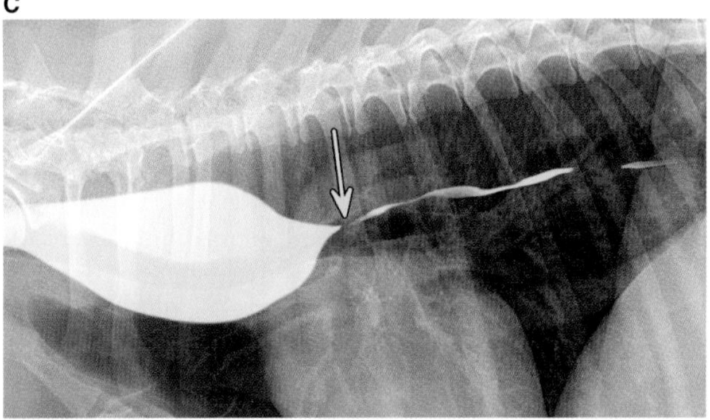

D

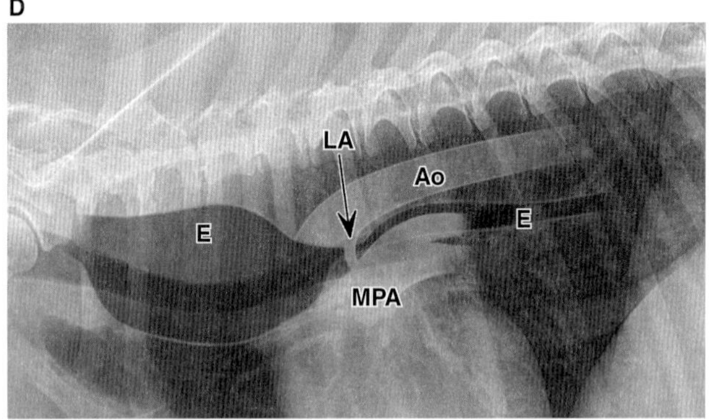

Figure 3.76 Vascular ring anomaly. Lateral view (**A**) and VD view (**B**) of a dog thorax depicting widening of the craniodorsal mediastinum (white arrows). The widening is soft tissue opacity and obscures the ventral margin of the longus coli muscles. The trachea is displaced ventrally and to the left (black dashed arrows). These findings are consistent with a dorsal mediastinal mass, probably involving the esophagus. (**C**) Barium esophagram: the proximal esophagus is dilated with barium and tapers abruptly at the base of the cardiac shadow (yellow arrow). A small amount of barium is visible in the distal esophagus. (**D**) This illustration depicts the anatomy of the persistent right aortic arch: the ligamentum arteriosus (LA), located between the aorta (Ao) and main pulmonary artery (MPA), constricts the esophagus (E) at the base of the heart. The proximal esophagus is distended with gas and the distal esophagus is normal size.

(dorsoventral dimension) of the thoracic cavity (Box 3.1). In most dogs, the cardiac shadow occupies about 2.5–3.5 intercostal spaces. In most cats, it occupies about 2.0–2.5 spaces.

In a **VD/DV view**, the normal position of the cardiac silhouette is on midline with its long axis tilted about 30° off parallel with the spine (Figure 3.78). In most dogs, the width of the cardiac shadow is about 2/3 the width of the thoracic cavity. The cardiac apex generally points left of midline. The canine cardiac silhouette may touch or overlap the diaphragm (Figure 3.79). In most cats, the width of the cardiac shadow is about 1/2 the width of the thoracic. The feline cardiac apex is variable in position (may be right or left of midline) and usually separated from the diaphragm by one or two intercostal spaces of lung (Figure 3.82).

The **shape and apparent size of the cardiac shadow** are related to the shape of the thorax and the size of the thoracic cavity. In dogs with a narrow, deep-chested conformation (e.g., Doberman Pinscher, Irish Setter), the cardiac silhouette is more narrow and upright with relatively little sternal contact and a smaller cardiac-to-thoracic ratio (Figure 3.80). The cardiothoracic ratio is a subjective assessment of the size of the cardiac silhouette in relation to the size of the thoracic cavity. In dogs with a wide, shallow thorax or a "barrel-chested" conformation (e.g., Bulldog, Pug), the cardiac shadow is wider and more rounded with greater sternal contact and a larger cardiothoracic ratio (Figure 3.81). Athletic dogs (e.g., Greyhound) also tend to have a relatively large cardiothoracic ratio (the heart appears relatively large in relation to the size of the thoracic cavity).

In cats, thoracic conformation is more uniform and the size and shape of the cardiac shadow are more consistent among different cat breeds. The feline cardiac silhouette is thinner and more elongated than in dogs with a relatively smaller cardiothoracic ratio (Figure 3.82).

In lateral radiographs of older animals, the cardiac shadow may be tilted further cranially and more parallel with the sternum. This is particularly true in older cats. Also in aged cats, the aortic arch tends to become more vertical and elongated and often bulges to the left (Figure 3.83). In a VD/DV view, the bulge in the proximal aorta cat may be mistaken for a mass in the cranial mediastinum or in the left lung.

Abnormal position of the cardiac silhouette

Recall that the position of the cardiac silhouette is maintained by normally inflated lungs. Uneven lung inflation allows the cardiac shadow to move with gravity, usually toward the smaller lung. Thoracic masses and skeletal deformities also can displace the cardiac shadow.

Cranial cardiac displacement is restricted by the tapering of the thorax. Causes of cranial displacement

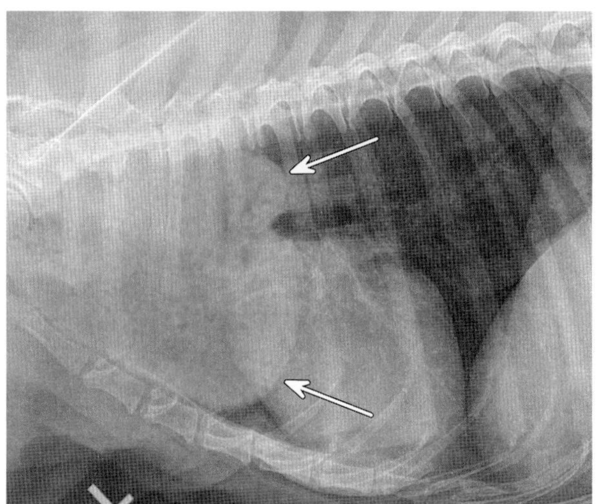

Figure 3.77 Vascular ring anomaly. Lateral view of a dog thorax depicting marked dilation of the proximal esophagus (white arrows) due to constriction near the cardiac base. The dilated esophagus is filled with ingesta that obscures the trachea.

A

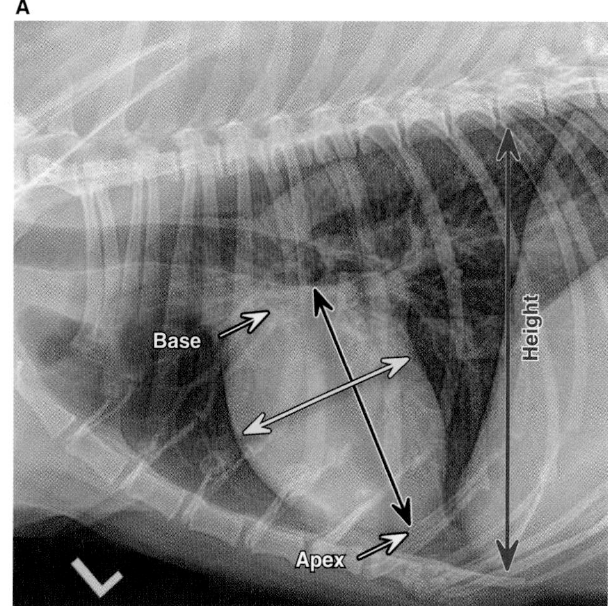

B

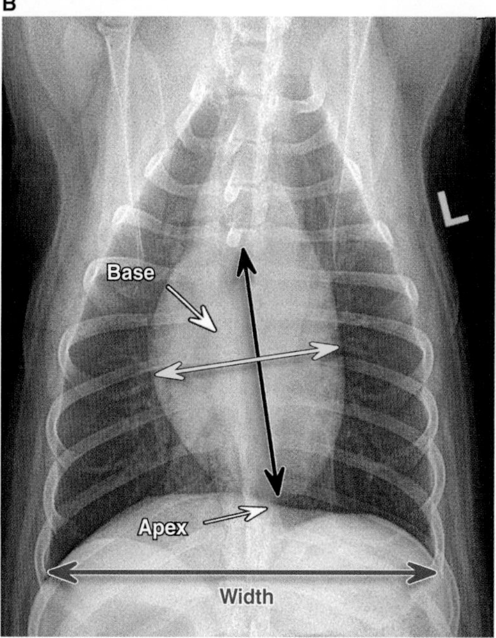

Figure 3.78 The cardiac shadow. Lateral view (**A**) and VD view (**B**) of a dog thorax depicting the cardiac base, apex, long axis (black double headed arrows) and short axis (yellow double headed arrows). In the lateral view, the height of the thoracic cavity is measured from the dorsal border of the last sternebra to the ventral border of the perpendicular vertebra (blue double headed arrow). In the VD view, the width of the thoracic cavity is measured at the widest part of the rib cage (blue arrow).

Box 3.1 Baseline radiographs

Thoracic radiographs made while a patient is healthy can provide a basis to compare the size and shape of the cardiac silhouette in future radiographs of that animal.

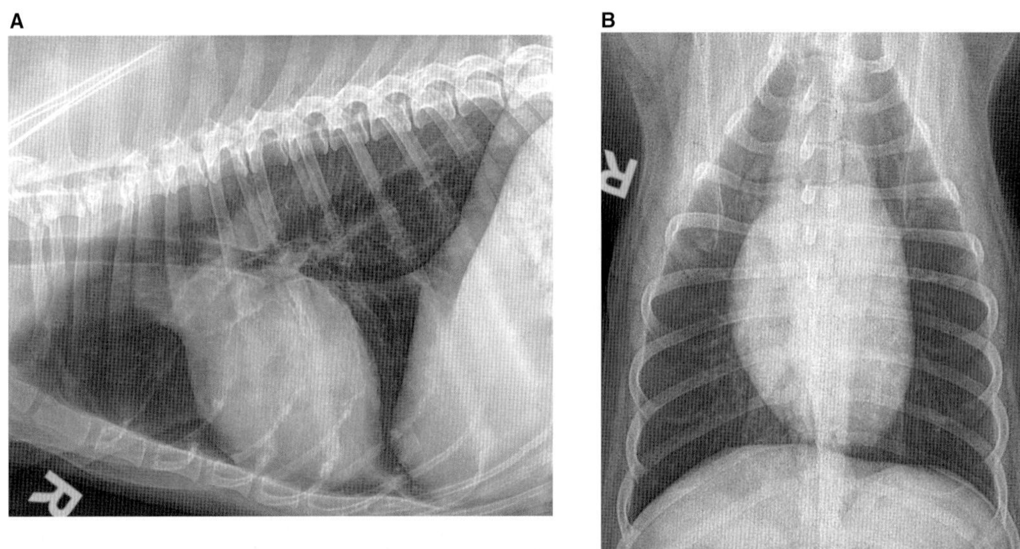

Figure 3.79 Normal canine cardiac silhouette. Lateral view (**A**) and VD view (**B**) of a dog thorax depicting a typical canine cardiac silhouette that is normal in position, size, and shape. Notice in the lateral view the normal slight ventral curvature in the distal trachea. Compare these normal radiographs with the various appearances of the cardiac silhouette depicted in other figures in this chapter.

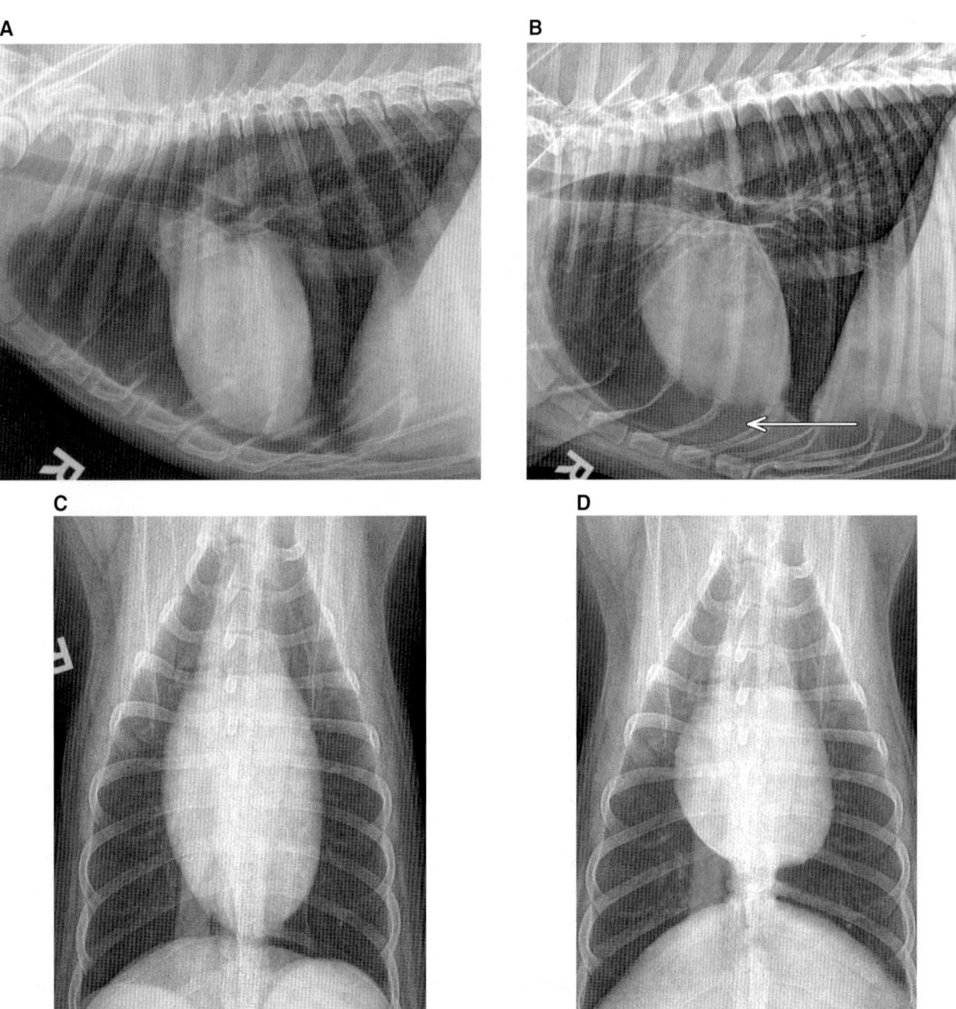

Figure 3.80 Deep-chested conformation. (**A**) Lateral view of a dog thorax depicting the appearance of the cardiac silhouette within a deep, narrow thoracic cavity. Compared to Figure 3.79, the cardiac shadow is more slender and upright with less cardiosternal contact and a smaller cardiothoracic ratio. (**B**) Lateral view of another deep chested dog depicting fat opacity between the cardiac shadow and the sternum (arrow). Separation of the cardiac shadow from the sternum may be a normal finding in a patient with a narrow, deep chest and should not be mistaken for a pneumothorax. (**C**) In a VD view of a deep-chested dog the cardiac shadow appears relatively long and narrow because in dorsal recumbency it is more parallel with the sternum. (**D**) In a DV view of a deep chested dog the cardiac shadow appears relatively small and rounded because in ventral recumbeny it is more perpendicular to the sternum.

A

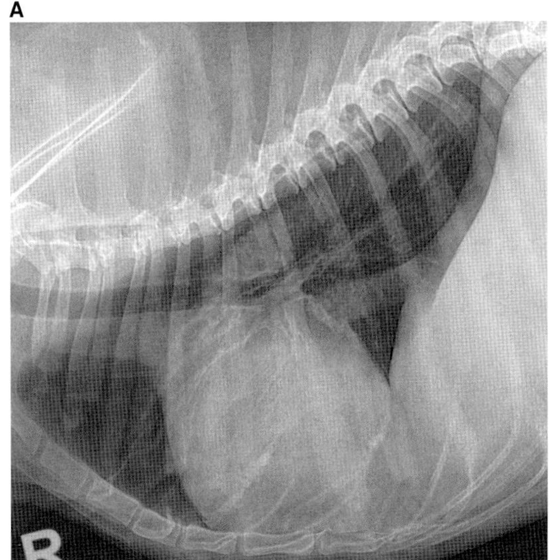

B

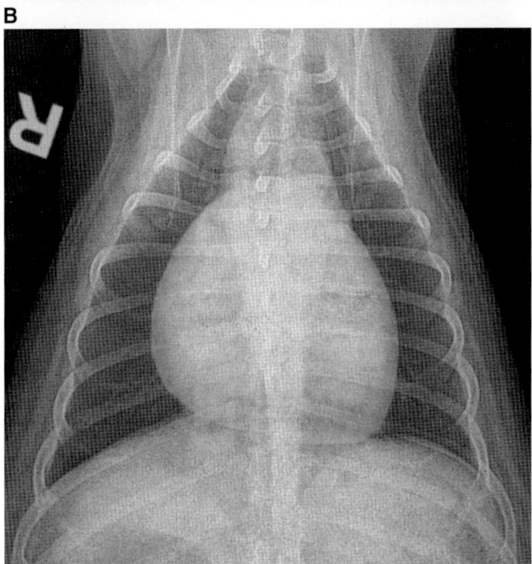

Figure 3.81 Barrel-chest thoracic conformation. Lateral view (**A**) and VD view (**B**) of a dog thorax depicting the appearance of the cardiac silhouette in a wide, shallow thoracic cavity. Compared to Figure 3.79, the cardiac shadow is relatively wider and more rounded with more cardiosternal contact and a larger cardiothoracic ratio. The trachea is closer to the spine, which is expected with this type of body conformation, but may be mistaken for cardiac enlargement.

include abdominal distention and a large mass in the caudal thorax (e.g., diaphragmatic hernia).

Caudal cardiac displacement usually is due to a cranial thoracic mass, typically in the mediastinum or lung. Caudal displacement is recognized when the cardiac base is pushed caudal to the sixth intercostal space. In most cases there is concurrent dorsal cardiac displacement.

Dorsal cardiac displacement is diagnosed in a lateral view. The cardiac shadow is separated from the sternum. Dorsal displacement frequently is accompanied by lateral displacement. The most common cause of dorsal cardiac displacement is lung collapse. Other causes include a large intra-thoracic mass and pectus excavatum. In overweight patients, excess fat between the cardiac shadow and the sternum may give the impression of dorsal displacement. Keep in mind that patients with a narrow, deep thorax may present with a normal separation between the cardiac shadow and the sternum.

A

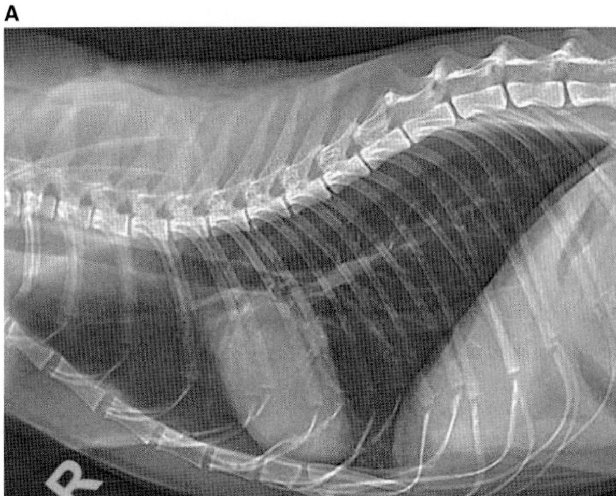

B

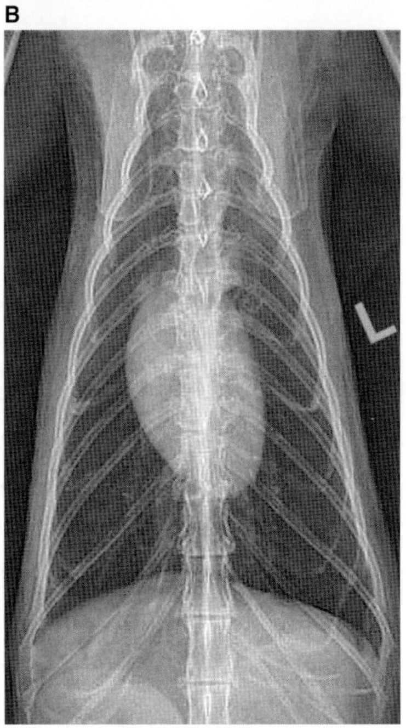

Figure 3.82 Feline cardiac silhouette. Lateral view (**A**) and VD view (**B**) of a cat thorax depicting a cardiac shadow that is normal in position, size, and shape. Compared to dogs, the feline cardiac silhouette is relatively thinner and more tapered at either end. The distal trachea is straight without the distal ventral curvature that is present in some dogs.

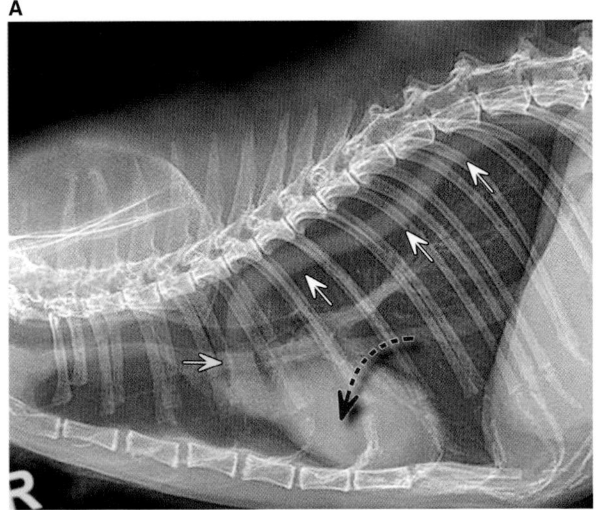

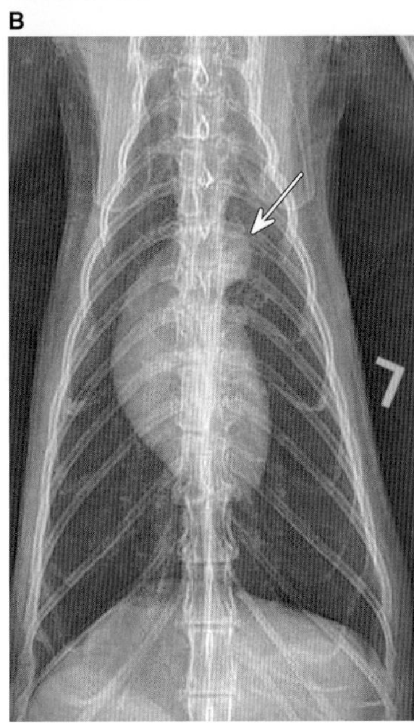

Figure 3.83 Aged feline cardiac silhouette. Lateral view (**A**) and VD view (**B**) of a cat thorax depicting common age-related changes in the cardiovascular structures. Compared to Figure 3.82, the cardiac shadow is more inclined toward the sternum (black dotted arrow), the aortic arch is more vertical (yellow arrow), and the descending aorta is more tortuous (white arrows). In the VD view, the proximal aorta often is visible left of midline (arrow) and may be mistaken for a mass in the cranial mediastinum or lung.

Lateral cardiac displacement is seen in a DV/VD view as a mediastinal shift. The most common cause is lung collapse. Rotation of the patient during radiography may be mistaken for a mediastinal shift. Always evaluate patient positioning before diagnosing cardiac displacement.

Ventral cardiac displacement is restricted by the sternum. Typically only the cardiac base is. The most common cause is a large or dilated esophagus. Ventral displacement may create the appearance of a shortened cardiac silhouette that is more inclined toward the sternum (Figures 3.70 and 3.71).

Abnormal size or shape of the cardiac silhouette

There are subjective and objective methods to evaluate the size of the cardiac shadow. Subjective methods include the cardiac-to-thoracic ratio, the position of the distal trachea, and the number of intercostal spaces occupied by the cardiac shadow. These methods rely greatly on the experience of the reader. An objective method is the vertebral heart score, which may be particularly useful to monitor the progression of heart disease (many acquired heart diseases lead to cardiomegaly about 6–12 months prior to congestive heart failure). Each of these methods is useful and all are discussed further in this section.

Although radiographs are quite useful in determining whether there is cardiac involvement in a disease process, they are a rather insensitive and non-specific means of evaluating the heart. A reader's interpretation of the cardiac silhouette sometimes is influenced by his or her physical examination of the patient and the patient's history. A patient with a heart murmur is more likely to be diagnosed with an enlarged heart.

It is important to realize that severe heart disease can be present without radiographic evidence of abnormal cardiac size or shape. Examples include:

1. Severe cardiac electrical disturbance or arrhythmia.
2. Inflammation of the heart, including endocarditis, pericarditis, myocarditis.
3. Acute rupture of chordae tendinea.
4. Myocardial infarction or neoplasia.
5. Acute cardiac tamponade.
6. Hypertrophic cardiomyopathy with concentric (inward) thickening of the myocardium.
7. Small cardiovascular shunt (e.g., PDA, ASD, VSD).
8. Increased cardiac afterload (e.g., aortic stenosis, pulmonic stenosis, systemic hypertension).

As mentioned earlier, the **cardiothoracic ratio** is a subjective comparison of the size of the cardiac shadow to the size of the thoracic cavity. The ratio can vary significantly among various breeds of dogs and cats due to differences in thoracic conformation. It can also vary in an individual dog or cat depending on the phase of respiration and the phase of the cardiac cycle. The thoracic cavity is larger during inspiration and smaller during expiration. The heart is larger during diastole and smaller during systole. The cardiothoracic ratio also can be influenced by the position of the patient at the time of radiography. In deep-chested dogs the cardiac shadow can appear larger in a VD view than in a DV view due to magnification. Take these factors into consideration when using the cardiothoracic ratio.

Dorsal displacement of the distal trachea is a frequent finding in patients with an enlarged cardiac silhouette. The position of the trachea relative to the thoracic spine is assessed in a lateral view. Dorsal displacement commonly is called "elevation" of the trachea and may occur in conditions other than cardiac disease. For example, the trachea is closer to the spine during expiration and in patients with a wide, shallow thoracic conformation. Over-stretching the patient during radiography also brings the trachea and spine closer together.

The **number of intercostal spaces** (ICS) occupied by the cardiac silhouette in a lateral view has long been used to assess overall cardiac size in dogs and cats. In dogs, the normal range is 2.5–3.5 ICS. Deep-chested dogs are at the lower end of this range (2.5 ICS) and barrel-chested dogs are at the upper end (3.5 ICS). In cats, normal cardiac size is about 2.0–2.5 ICS. Of course, the width of the intercostal spaces can vary between inspiration and expiration. In addition, the ICS may appear narrower when the thorax is off-center in relation to the x-ray beam (due to distortion). Normal and abnormal variations in thoracic conformation also can affect the width of the intercostal spaces (e.g., pectus excavatum).

The **vertebral heart score (VHS)** relates the length and width of the cardiac shadow to the patient's body size. Thoracic vertebrae are used as units of measure. The VHS is also called "vertebral heart size," "vertebral heart scale," and "vertebral heart sum." The method, along with the normal and abnormal values for dogs and cats, is described in Table 3.1 and illustrated in Figure 3.84. Here are a couple of additional tips: (1) When using the VHS in overweight patients, closely inspect the cardiac shadow to find the actual cardiac borders. It is a common error to mistake pericardial fat for the cardiac margin. (2) In patients with severe left atrial dilation, the cardiac base may extend dorsal to the carina. In these patients, the cardiac length is measured from the cardiac apex to the ventral border of the elevated left mainstem bronchus (Figure 3.100).

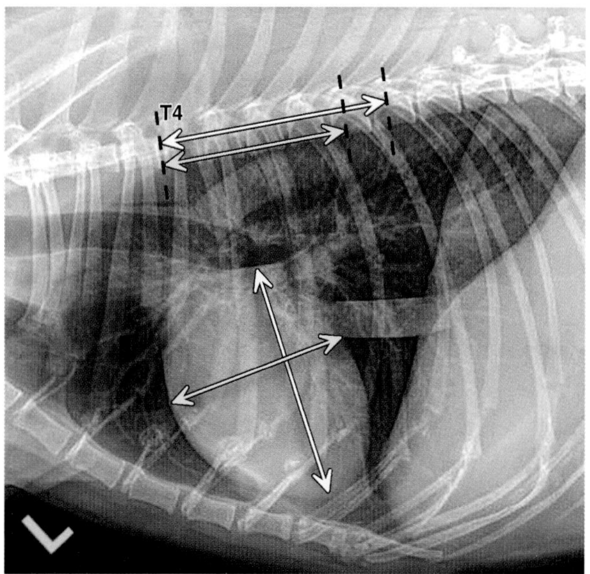

Figure 3.84 Vertebral heart score (VHS). Lateral view of a dog thorax depicting the VHS method to assess the size of the cardiac silhouette. The cardiac length is measured from the ventral border of the distal trachea to the cardiac apex (white double headed arrow). The cardiac width is the widest part of the cardiac shadow, measured perpendicular to the cardiac length at the level of the caudal vena cava (yellow double headed arrow). Both measurements are transposed onto the thoracic spine, each beginning at the cranial edge of the T4 thoracic vertebra. Count the number of vertebrae spanned by each measurement to the nearest 1/10th vertebra. Add the two numbers together to get the VHS. In this example, the cardiac length is 5.4 vertebrae and the cardiac width is 4.3 vertebrae which gives a VHS of 9.7 (5.4+4.3 = 9.7).

Table 3.1 Vertebral heart score (VHS)

1. In a lateral view, measure the length (long axis) and width (short axis) of the cardiac shadow.
2. Transpose both of these measurements onto the thoracic spine, each beginning at the cranial edge of T4.
3. Count the number of thoracic vertebrae spanned by each measurement to the nearest 1/10th of a vertebra.
4. Add the total number of vertebrae along the cardiac length and width to get the vertebral heart score.

	Dog	Cat
Normal range	8.5 – 10.6	6.8 – 8.1
Mild enlargement	11 – 11.9	8.2 – 8.5
Moderate enlargement	12 – 12.9	8.6 – 8.9
Severe enlargement	13 – 14+	9 – 10+

The **vertebral heart width** (VHW) is a variation of the VHS that can be used in cats. It is not used in dogs. The VHW can be useful because cardiac enlargement in cats sometimes is more evident in a DV/VD view than in a lateral view. The VHW method and values are described in Table 3.2 and illustrated in Figure 3.104.

Small cardiac shadow

A smaller than expected cardiac silhouette tends to be a subjective assessment and may or may not be clinically significant. The cardiac shadow may appear relatively small in an expanded thoracic cavity. In cases of true microcardia, the most common cause is hypovolemia. Hypovolemia may result from severe dehydration, massive blood loss, or hypoadrenocorticism (Addison's disease). Hypovolemia not only reduces the size of the cardiac silhouette, it also leads to small pulmonary vessels, a small aorta, and a small caudal vena cava (Figure 3.85). The lungs often are decreased in overall opacity due to less pulmonary blood and compensatory hyperinflation. A small

Table 3.2 Vertebral heart width (cats)

1. In a DV/VD view of a cat thorax, measure the widest part of the cardiac shadow.
2. Transpose this measurement onto the thoracic spine in the lateral view, beginning at the cranial edge of T4.
3. Count the number of vertebral bodies spanned by the measurement, to the nearest 1/10th of a vertebra.

Normal range	2.9 – 4.1
Mild enlargement	4.2 – 4.4
Moderate enlargement	4.5 – 4.9
Severe enlargement	5+

heart may appear cranially displaced because more lung often is visible between the cardiac shadow and the diaphragm. It also may be dorsally separated from the sternum the sternum, which may be misdiagnosed as a mediastinal shift or pneumothorax. Cardiac width tends to decrease more than cardiac length, making the small cardiac silhouette appear narrowed with a more pointed apex.

Causes of microcardia other than hypovolemia include compromised venous return and restrictive pericarditis (see Differential Diagnoses). A reduction in venous return can lead to small intra-thoracic cardiovascular structures similar to hypovolemia. Reduced return can result from severe gastric distention or hepatic cirrhosis.

Pericarditis is uncommon in dogs and cats. Chronic or recurring inflammation can lead to pericardial thickening and fibrosis that prevents the heart from expanding. In these cases, the cardiac margin may be irregular due to uneven pericardial thickening or tiny pericardial nodules (e.g., abscesses, granulomas, pockets of trapped fluid).

In emaciated patients, the cardiac shadow commonly appears small due to loss of pericardial fat, diminished heart muscle mass, and fully inflated lungs.

A

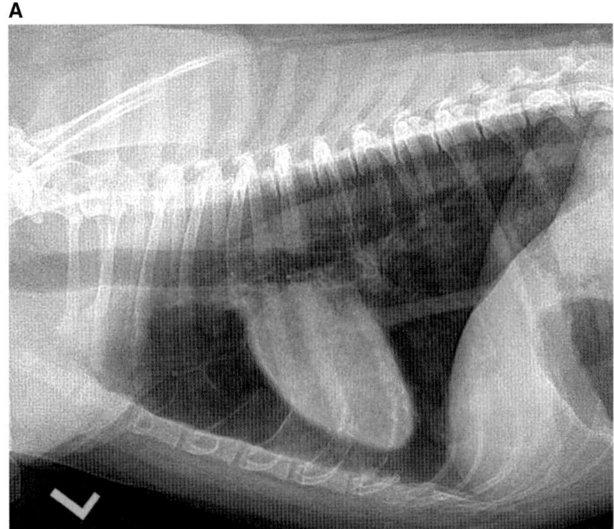

B

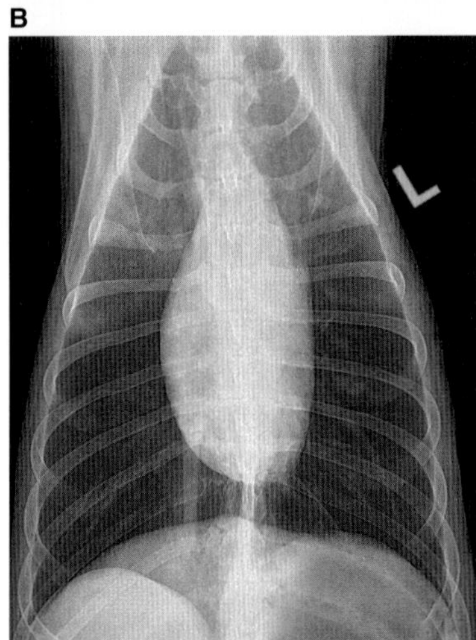

Figure 3.85 Microcardia. Lateral view (**A**) and VD view (**B**) of a dog thorax depicting a small cardiac silhouette. The cardiac shadow is narrowed and dorsal to the sternum. The aorta, caudal vena cava, and pulmonary vessels also are small. The lungs are less opaque due to diminished pulmonary blood flow.

Large cardiac shadow

Overall enlargement of the cardiac silhouette may be due to either abnormal content in the pericardial sac or cardiomegaly (see Differential Diagnoses). Examples of abnormal pericardial content include fluid accumulation, neoplasia, and peritoneal-pericardial diaphragmatic hernia (PPDH). Each of these, and cardiomegaly, are discussed in greater detail on the following pages.

Other causes of a larger than expected cardiac silhouette include patient conformation and errors in radiographic technique. The cardiothoracic ratio is larger in dogs with a wide, shallow chest. The ratio also is larger during expiration. Expiration also reduces the width of the intercostal spaces, allowing the cardiac shadow to span a larger number of ICS. Overstretching the patient during radiography can narrow the thoracic cavity, increasing the cardiothoracic ratio and shortening the distance between the distal trachea and the spine, which may be misdiagnosed as cardiac enlargement. Excess pericardial fat in obese patients may be mistaken for a large cardiac shadow.

Cardiomegaly is used here to describe generalized enlargement of the heart. Both the length and width of the cardiac silhouette are increased (Figure 3.86). The cardiac borders expand outward, becoming more rounded and moving closer to the thoracic walls. The caudal cardiac border may overlap the diaphragm, even during inspiration when the lungs are fully inflated. The distal trachea

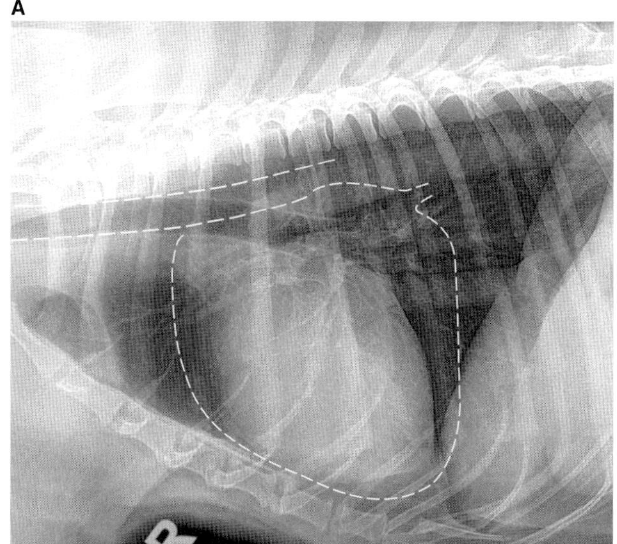

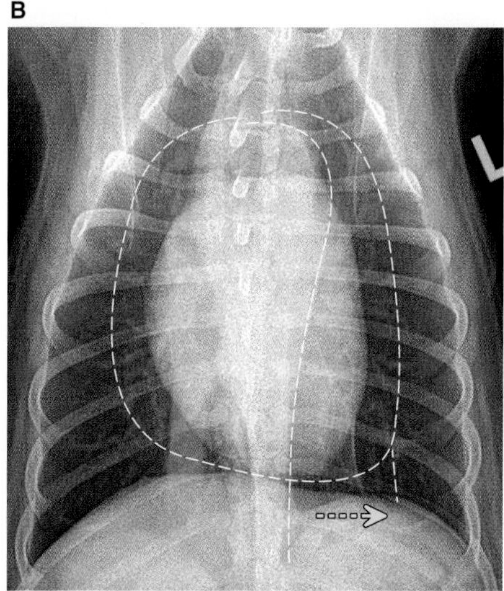

Figure 3.86 Cardiomegaly. Lateral view (**A**) and VD view (**B**) of a dog thorax with a normal cardiac silhouette. The white dashed lines depict the typical appearance of cardiomegaly: the cardiac borders expand, becoming more rounded and moving closer to the thoracic walls. Cardiosternal contact increases and the trachea is dorsally displaced. In the VD view, the cardiac apex and caudal mediastinum are displaced to the left of midline (yellow arrow).

frequently is displaced dorsally. Often there is increased contact between the cardiac shadow and the sternum.

Cardiomegaly may be physiologic or pathologic. Physiologic enlargement is a normal response to increased cardiac demand (i.e., an athletic heart). Pathologic enlargement may be due to congenital heart disease or acquired heart disease (see Differential Diagnoses).

Pericardial effusion refers to excess fluid in the pericardial sac. The fluid may or may not enlarge the cardiac shadow, depending on the amount and rate of accumulation. Effusions that build up slowly over time allow the pericardium to expand and accommodate the excess fluid. Rapid effusions may lead to **cardiac tamponade** before enlarging the cardiac silhouette. Cardiac tamponade occurs when pressure from the pericardial fluid restricts the movement of the heart and causes right heart failure.

Pericardial effusion surrounds the entire heart except at its base. The borders of a cardiac silhouette enlarged by pericardial fluid tend to be very round, even, and sharply-defined (Figure 3.87). The rounded shape has been described as "globoid". The cardiac border is sharply defined because there is

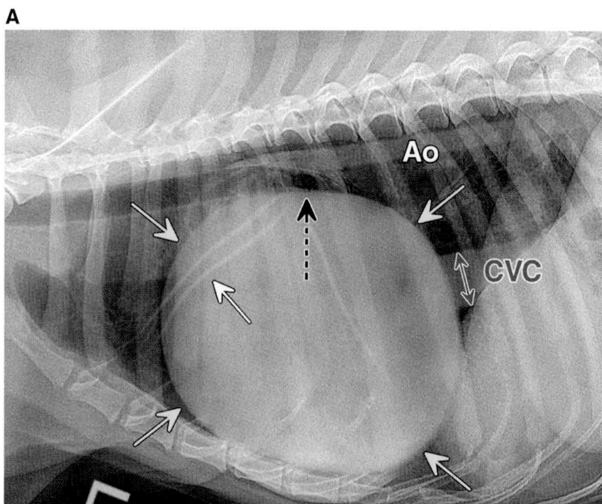

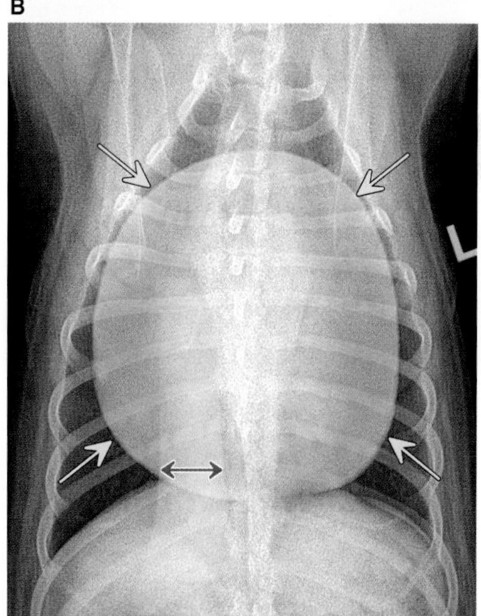

Figure 3.87 Pericardial effusion. Lateral view (**A**) and VD view (**B**) of a dog thorax depicting a very large, rounded cardiac silhouette. The cardiac borders are smooth and even and very well-defined (yellow arrows). The trachea is dorsally displaced (black dashed arrow) but retains its distal ventral curvature. The aorta (Ao) and pulmonary vessels (white arrow superimposed on the cardiac silhouette) are small due to low cardiac output. The caudal vena cava is dilated due to reduced venous return (blue double headed arrow).

less heart motion blur. The caudal trachea usually is dorsally displaced but less severely than with left atrial dilation. In dogs, the trachea may retain its distal ventral curvature with pericardial effusion (Figure 3.87), but the curvature typically is lost with left atrial dilation (Figure 3.92). Pericardial effusion can limit the heart's ability to expand which means it fills with less blood and cardiac output is reduced. Less output leads to a small aorta and small pulmonary vessels. The caudal vena cava in these cases often is dilated because the right heart cannot accept as much blood.

Causes of pericardial effusion include neoplasia, trauma, and infection (see Differential Diagnoses). Pericardial fluid can obscure cardiac masses and hide heart chamber enlargements. Many patients with pericardial effusion exhibit muffled heart sounds and a jugular pulse. Table 3.3 lists some of the radiographic findings that may help distinguish between pericardial effusion and cardiomegaly.

Table 3.3 Pericardial effusion vs. cardiomegaly

	Pericardial effusion	Cardiomegaly
Cardiac shape	Uniformly round, globoid shaped	Rounded, but heart chambers still recognizable
Cardiac margin	Sharply defined due to less heart motion blur	Contours of heart chambers are less distinct, but still recognizable
Left atrium	Usually normal size	Commonly dilated
Heart failure	Right side failure	Usually left side
Pulmonary edema	Absent	Often present
Pleural effusion	May be present	Usually absent
Pulmonary vessels	Normal to small	Veins often are enlarged
Caudal vena cava	Often dilated	Normal size
Aorta	Small	Normal size
Trachea	Mild dorsal elevation; retains caudal ventral curvature	Greater dorsal elevation; Loses caudal ventral curvature

Cardiac neoplasia is uncommon in dogs and cats. Tumors that arise near the heart base tend to be benign and slow-growing whereas intra-cardiac tumors usually are malignant.

The most common heart base tumor is the *chemodectoma* (aortic body tumor). These neoplasms originate from chemoreceptor tissues in the aorta. Examples of intra-cardiac tumors include hemangiosarcoma, fibrosarcoma, rhabdomyosarcoma, and lymphoma. Hemangiosarcoma tends to arise in the right atrium, whereas the other tumors more often occur in the left heart. Lymphoma is more common in cats than in dogs.

Cardiac neoplasms often are accompanied by pericardial effusion, which can hide their visibility. A large tumor at the heart base may be visible as a hilar mass (Figure 3.58). In many cases, tracheal displacement is the only radiographic sign of a heart base tumor. Intra-cardiac tumors are not visible unless large enough to distort the cardiac shadow.

In addition to causing pericardial effusion, heart tumors can induce arrhythmias, obstruct blood flow, and interfere with myocardial contractility and valve function. Most cardiac neoplasms lead to heart failure.

Pneumopericardium refers to free gas in the pericardial sac. It is rare in dogs and cats. Pneumopericardium may result from migration of gas (e.g., recent pericardiocentesis, ruptured alvoeli, pneumomediastinum) or infection with gas-producing bacteria. Gas can migrate along perivascular sheaths into the hilar region and enter the pericardial sac. Pneumopericardium appears as curvilinear pockets of gas between the heart and the pericardium (Figure 3.62). The gas pockets repeat in serial radiographs but they can vary in size and location within the cardiac silhouette.

Heart chamber enlargements

Individual heart chambers enlarge in response to increased volume or increased pressure. Enlargement may be due to dilation or hypertrophy. Dilation increases the size of a heart chamber more than hypertrophy. This is because doubling the size of the lumen makes a bigger difference than doubling the thickness of the walls. Eccentric hypertrophy (outward thickening) enlarges a heart chamber more than concentric hypertrophy (inward thickening).

Heart chamber enlargements occur at specific locations in the cardiac silhouette. The normal heart chambers are illustrated in Figure 3.88 and the normal cardiovascular circulation is illustrated in Figure 3.89. The locations of many cardiac structures can be identified using the long and short axes of the heart (Figure 3.90) or a clock face analogy (Figure 3.91). In general, enlargement of the left heart chambers makes the cardiac shadow longer and taller and enlargement of the right heart chambers makes it wider and more rounded.

Errors in patient positioning may be mistaken for heart chamber enlargement. A patient that is rotated as little as 5-degrees can mimic significant disease. In a VD view, rotation to the right makes the right heart appear larger and the left heart appear smaller. Rotation to the left makes the left heart appear larger and the right heart smaller. Patient rotation also can alter the apparent position of the cardiac silhouette such that it may be mistaken for a mediastinal shift. Remember that "the heart follows the sternum."

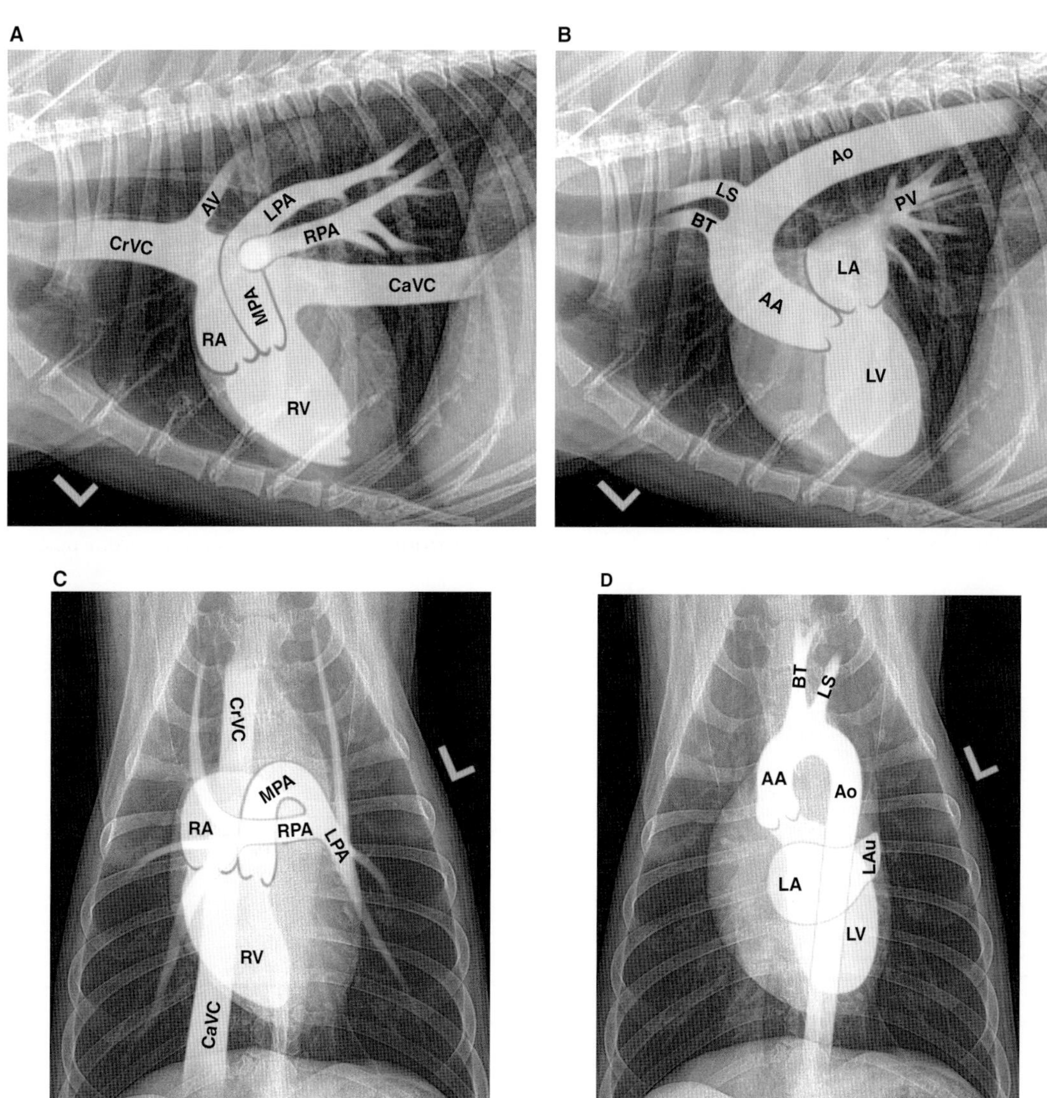

Figure 3.88 Normal anatomy of the heart. Lateral views (**A**, **B**) and VD views (**C**, **D**) of a dog thorax with illustrations that depict the locations and arrangements of structures in the right and left sides of the heart:

AA = ascending aorta
Ao = descending aorta
AV = azygous vein
BT = brachycephalic trunk
CaVC = caudal vena cava
CrVC = cranial vena cava
LA = left atrium
LAu = left auricle
LPA = left pulmonary artery
LS = left subclavian artery
LV = left ventricle
MPA = main pulmonary artery
PV = pulmonary veins
RA = right atrium
RAu = right auricle
RPA = right pulmonary artery
RV = right ventricle

Left atrial dilation

Although there are a number of congenital and acquired causes of left atrial dilation, in adult animals it nearly always is due to mitral valve insufficiency. A dilated left atrium may be directly visible in a radiograph or it may be identified due to displacement of the adjacent structures.

In a **lateral view**, an enlarged left atrium creates soft tissue opacity in the hilar region and dorsal displacement of the distal trachea (Figure 3.92). In dogs, the distal trachea often loses its ventral curvature. Left atrial dilation expands the dorsocaudal cardiac border, making the cardiac shadow taller and wider at the base. Further dilation leads to greater widening at the base and a more triangular shape to the cardiac silhouette (Figure 3.93). Severe dilation can push the caudal cardiac border past vertical, causing it to slope caudally instead of cranially (slope from sternum toward pelvis). Such profound widening can occur in cats with advanced hypertrophic. In these cases, the shape of the cardiac shadow has been compared to that of a "valentine heart" (♥), as shown in Figure 3.109.

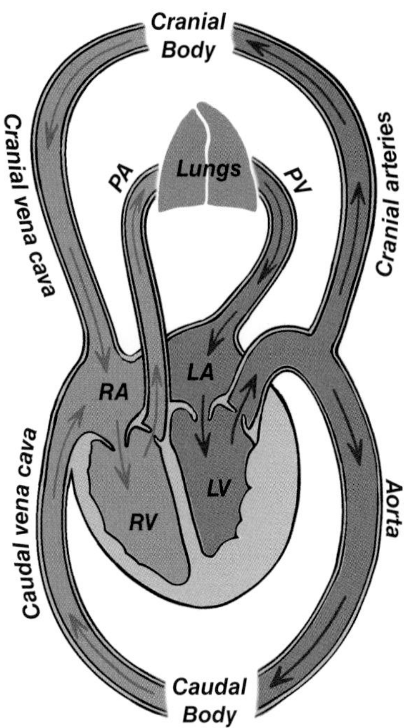

Figure 3.89 Cardiovascular circulation. This illustration summarizes normal cardiovascular blood flow. Blood from the body returns to the heart via the cranial and caudal vena cavae and enters the right atrium (RA). It then passes through the tricuspid valve into the right ventricle (RV). The RV pumps blood past the pulmonary valve into the pulmonary arteries (PA) and to the lungs. Oxygenated blood from the lungs returns to the heart via the pulmonary veins (PV) and enters the left atrium (LA). It then passes through the mitral valve into the left ventricle (LV). The LV pumps blood past the aortic valve into the aorta and to the body. The cranial arteries from the aorta include the brachiocephalic, common carotid, and subclavian.

The left primary bronchus lies dorsal to the left atrium. Atrial dilation can push the left bronchus dorsal to the right bronchus. This is called "splitting of the bronchi" and it occurs more often in dogs than in cats. In dogs, displacement of the bronchus may be accompanied by compression and narrowing. Bronchial compression often leads to coughing.

In cats, the trachea may be dorsally displaced by a dilated left atrium, but splitting of the bronchi and narrowing of the left bronchus are uncommon.

In a **VD/DV view**, the left atrium is not as well visualized. It is centrally located in the cardiac shadow and does not normally contribute to the outer cardiac border. In dogs, the left atrium is situated ventral and just caudal to the tracheal bifurcation. Atrial dilation can displace the right and left primary bronchi laterally and widen the tracheal bifurcation. The left bronchus may be narrowed due to compression. Although the left atrium is the same opacity as the cardiac silhouette, the caudal border of a dilated atrium may be visible due to an opacity interface with the lung (Figure 3.92). As the atrium continues to dilate, its caudal border moves closer to the caudal border of the cardiac shadow, a radiographic finding which has been described as a "double heart border" (Figure 3.93).

In cats, the left atrium is located more cranial and left lateral than in dogs. In a VD/DV view of a cat thorax, left atrial dilation primarily expands the left cranial cardiac border (Figure 3.109). Severe dilation may be accompanied by expansion of the right cranial cardiac. In these cases, the right atrium is laterally displaced, however, sometimes there is concurrent right atrial dilation. As mentioned earlier, in cats with severe left atrial dilation the cardiac shadow may appear triangular or "valentine heart" in shape.

A

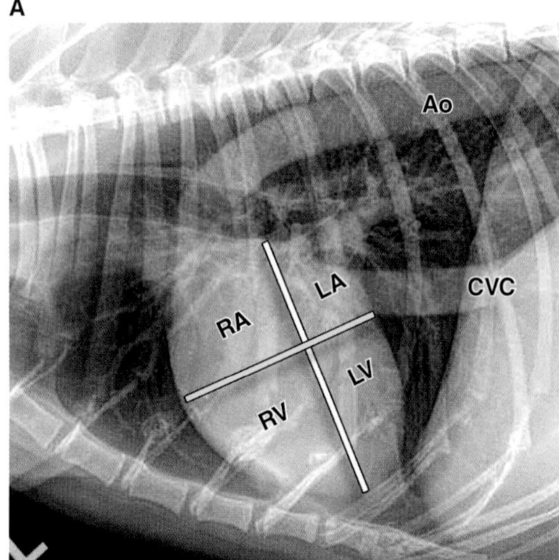

B

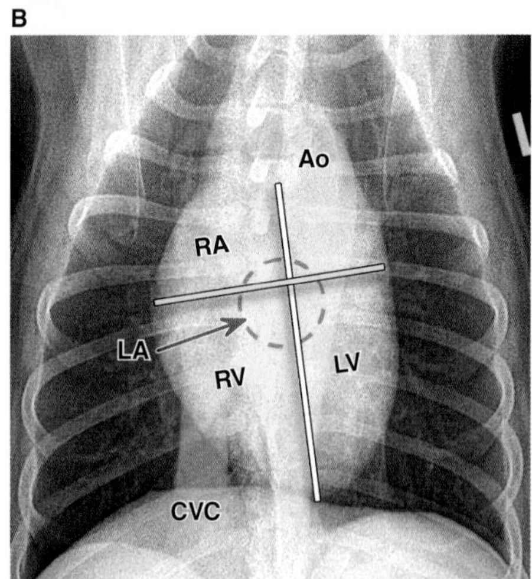

Figure 3.90 Heart chambers. Lateral view (**A**) and VD view (**B**) of a dog thorax depicting the locations of the cardiac chambers based on the cardiac axes. The long axis (white line) divides the heart into right and left sides, normally about a 3:2 ratio. The short axis (yellow line) separates the atria above from the ventricles below. In the VD view, the left atrium (LA) is located in the middle of the cardiac silhouette (arrow and dashed circle). RA = right atrium, RV = right ventricle, LV = left ventricle, Ao = aorta, CVC = caudal vena cava.

A

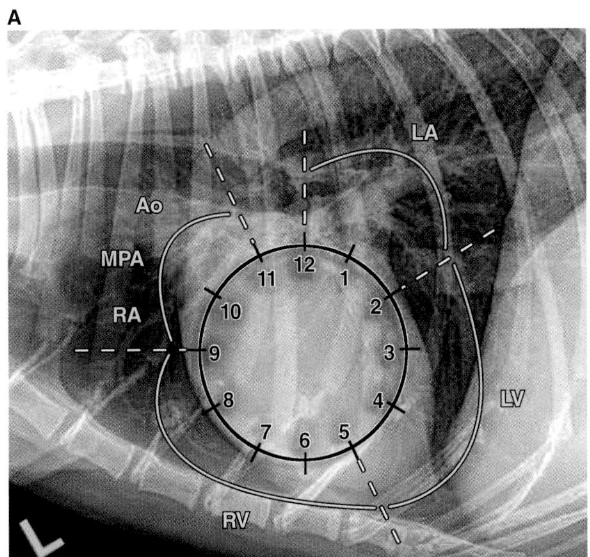

B

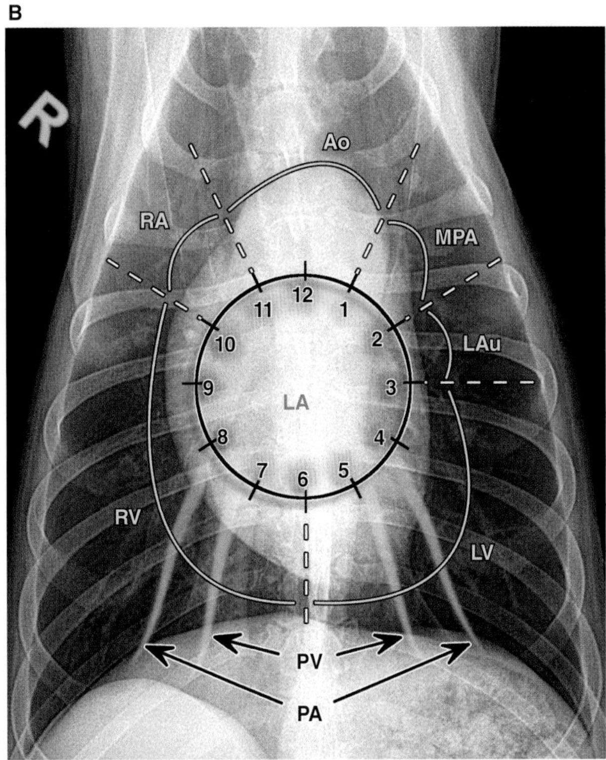

Figure 3.91 Clock face analogy. Lateral view (**A**) and VD view (**B**) of a dog thorax depicting the locations of the cardiac chambers based on a superimposed analog clock face. The clock numbers are used to approximate the borders of individual cardiovascular structures. The curved lines depict the borders of structures when enlarged.

Lateral view:

- Left atrium (**LA**): 12–2 o'clock.
- Left ventricle (**LV**): 2–5 o'clock.
- Right ventricle (**RV**): 5–9 o'clock.
- Right atrium (**RA**), main pulmonary artery (**MPA**), and proximal aorta (**Ao**) are all located at 9–11 o'clock. These structures are difficult to separate in a lateral view; they are better distinguished in a VD/DV view.

VD view:

- Aorta (**Ao**): 11–1 o'clock.
- Main pulmonary artery (**MPA**): 1–2 o'clock.
- Left atrial appendage (**LAA**) or left auricle: 2–3 o'clock.
- Left ventricle (**LV**): 2–6 o'clock.
- Right ventricle (**RV**): 6–11 o'clock.
- Right atrium (**RA**): 9–11 o'clock.
- Left atrium (**LA**) is centrally located and does not contribute to the outer cardiac in a VD/DV view.
- The caudal pulmonary arteries (**PA**) and veins (**PV**) emerge between 7 and 8 o'clock on the right and between 4 and 5 o'clock on the left.

In both dogs and cats, left atrial dilation may lead to dilation or lateral displacement of the **left atrial appendage**. The left atrial appendage (or left auricle) is an ear-like flap attached to the atrium. It is not visible in the lateral view, but in a VD/DV view, dilation or displacement of the left atrial appendage can produce a bulge along the left middle of the cardiac silhouette (Figure 3.93).

Conditions that mimic left atrial dilation include errors in patient positioning and hilar masses. Rotation of the patient during radiography can mimic splitting of the mainstem bronchi in a lateral view and it can accentuate the left heart in a VD/DV view. Hilar masses, such as tracheobronchial lymphadenomegaly, may displace the trachea and create soft tissue opacity in the hilar region, which may be misdiagnosed as atrial dilation.

Left ventricular enlargement

Isolated enlargement of the left ventricle is uncommon. It usually is accompanied by dilation of the left atrium and sometimes by enlargement of other heart chambers as well. Left ventricular enlargement may be due to hypertrophy, dilation, or both. Causes include mitral valve insufficiency, cardiomyopathy, congenital heart disease, and others (see Differential Diagnoses). Enlargement of the left ventricle expands the left lateral and caudal cardiac borders, elongating the cardiac silhouette (Figure 3.94). In dogs, the cardiac apex may be positioned further to the left in a VD/DV view. In cats, the apex is more variable in position and may be left, right, or centered on midline.

Errors in patient positioning can mimic left ventricular enlargement. Rotation of the sternum to the left in a VD

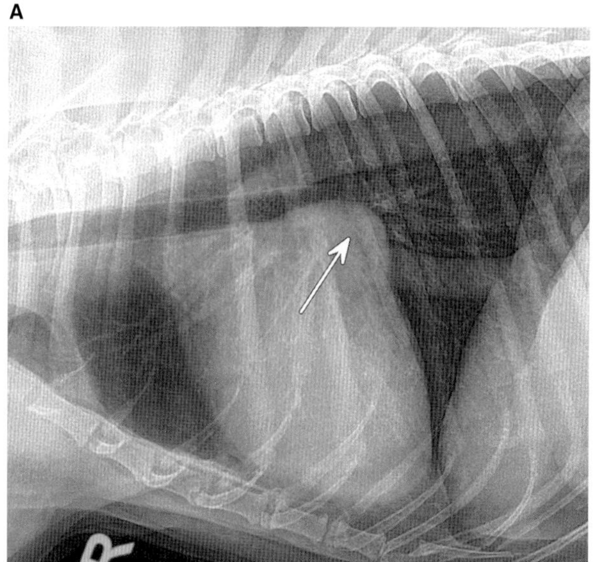

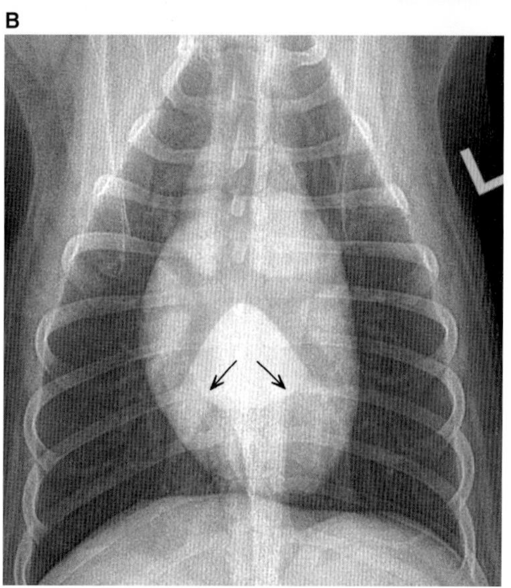

Figure 3.92 Mild left atrial dilation. Lateral view (**A**) and VD view (**B**) of a dog thorax depicting expansion of the dorsocaudal cardiac border (white arrow) and dorsal displacement of the distal trachea. In the VD view, the caudal atrial border is visible (black arrows).

view projects the left cardiac border closer to the left thoracic wall, which may be mistaken for a large left ventricle. Rotation to the right may hide left heart enlargement.

Right atrial dilation

Right atrial enlargement is less common than left atrial enlargement. It frequently is accompanied by right ventricular enlargement, which may obscure the dilated right atrium. Causes include heartworm disease, neoplasia, pulmonic stenosis, and others (see Differential Diagnoses).

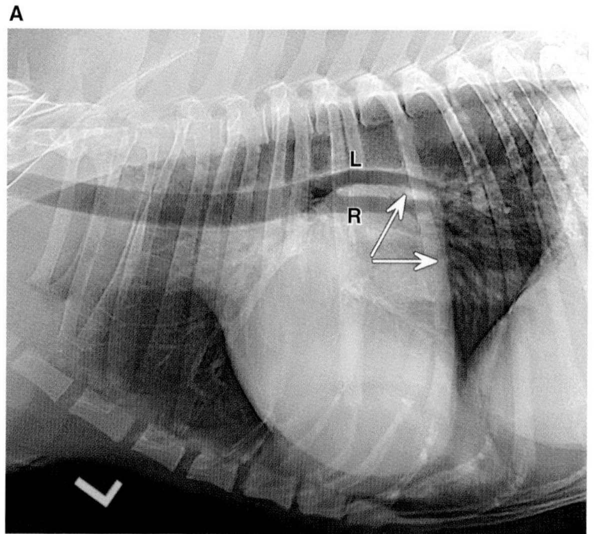

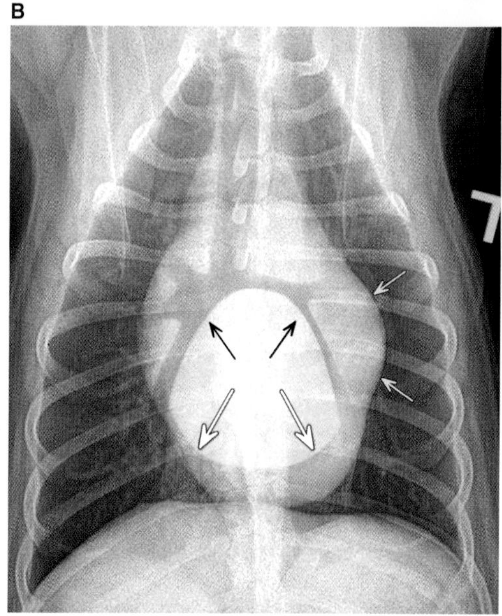

Figure 3.93 Largely dilated left atrium. Lateral view (**A**) and VD view (**B**) of a dog thorax depicting severe left atrial dilation. In the lateral view, the dorsocaudal cardiac border is expanded (white arrows), widening the cardiac base and straightening the caudal cardiac border to make it more vertical. Overall, the cardiac shadow is more triangular in shape, tapering toward the apex. The trachea is dorsally displaced and there is splitting of the primary bronchi with the left bronchus (L) dorsal to the right (R). In the VD view, the tracheal bifurcation is widened and more rounded, resembling an inverted "U" shape rather than an inverted "V" shape (black arrows). The left bronchus is narrowed because it is compressed by the left atrium. The caudal border of the left atrium is pushed toward the caudal cardiac border (white arrows), creating the appearance of a "double cardiac border". The bulge along the left cardiac border (yellow arrows) is the left atrial appendage, which is visible because it is either dilated or laterally displaced.

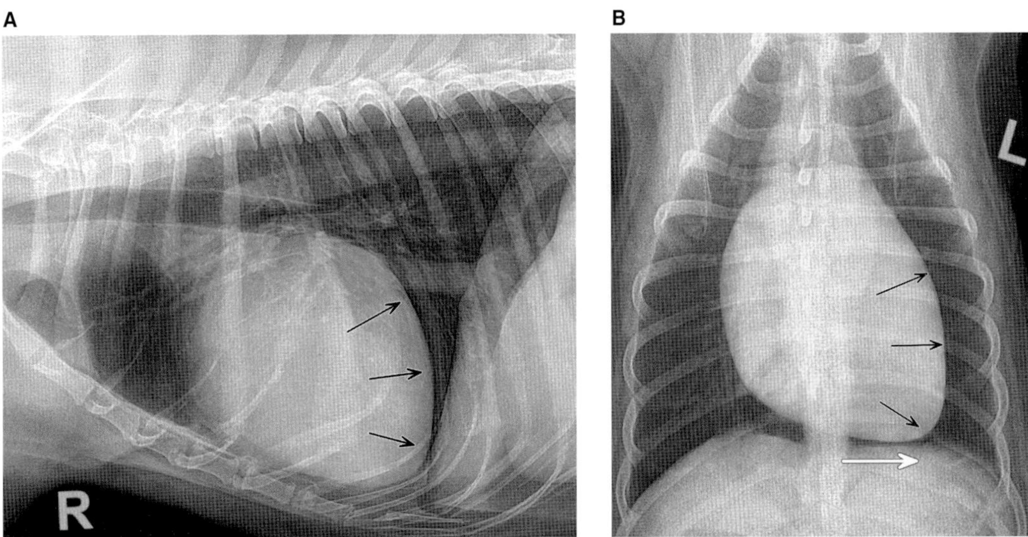

Figure 3.94 Left ventricular enlargement. Lateral view (**A**) and VD view (**B**) of a dog thorax depicting expansion of the caudal and left lateral cardiac borders (black arrows) due to left ventricular enlargement. The cardiac apex is further left of midline (white arrow).

Right atrial dilation expands the right craniodorsal cardiac border, widening the cardiac shadow (Figure 3.95). Severe dilation can extend into the cranial mediastinum and dorsally displace the trachea. The right atrium can become extremely large and even exceed the size of the right ventricle.

Right ventricular enlargement

Dilation or/and hypertrophy of the right ventricle expands the right lateral and ventral cardiac borders, widening the cardiac shadow and increasing its sternal contact. Severe enlargement can distort the cardiac shadow so that it a reverse capital letter D (Figure 3.96). In a lateral view, severe right ventricular enlargement may lead to more focal contact between the cardiac shadow and the sternum and dorsal displacement of the cardiac apex. This degree of ventricular enlargement often is accompanied by dilation of the main pulmonary artery.

Conditions that may be mistaken for right ventricular enlargement include breed conformation and errors in

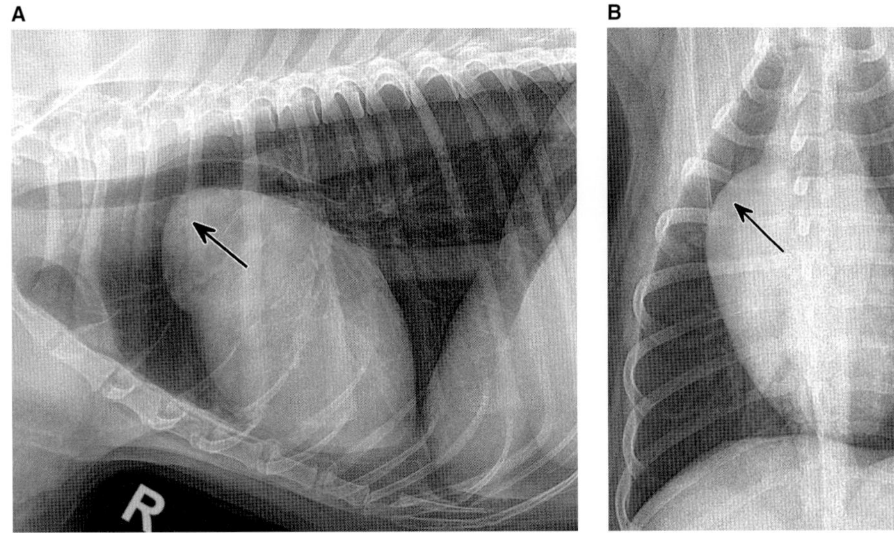

Figure 3.95 Right atrial dilation. Lateral view (**A**) and VD view (**B**) of a dog thorax depicting an outward bulge along the right cranial cardiac border (black arrow). In the lateral view, the right atrium, proximal aorta, and main pulmonary artery all contribute to the cranial cardiac border. Dilation of any of these can expand that part of the cardiac shadow. In the VD view, however, the specific dilated structure often can be identified.

A

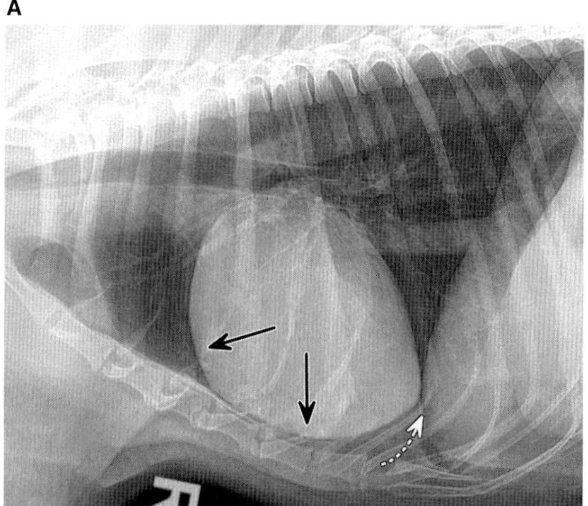

B

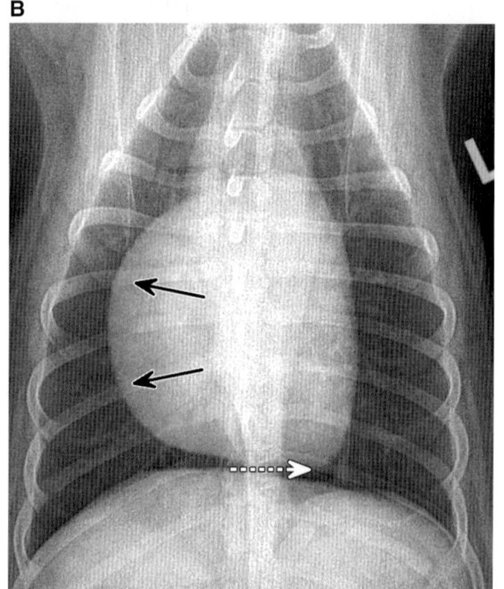

C

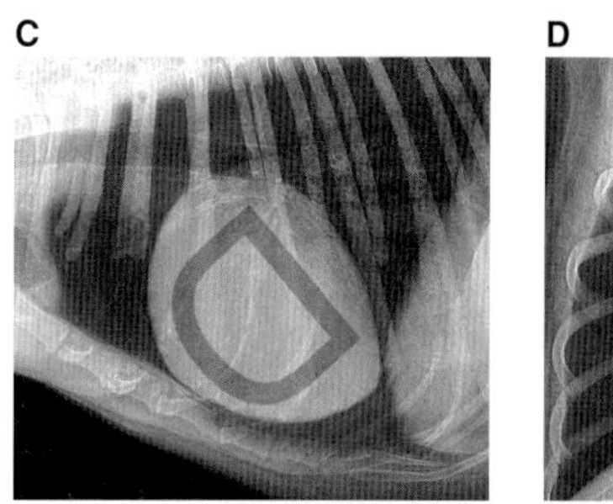

D

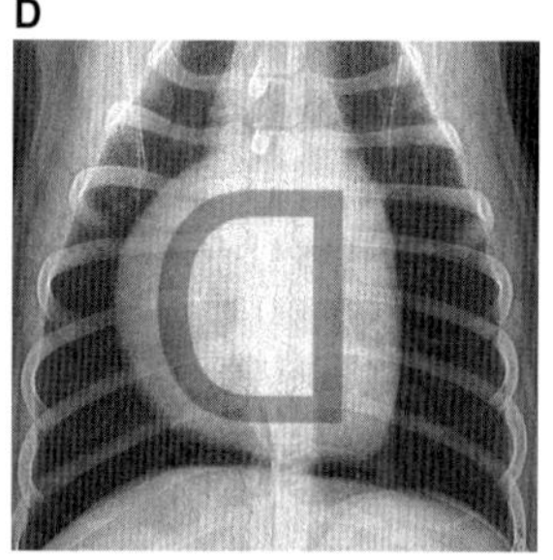

Figure 3.96 Right ventricular enlargement. Lateral view (**A**) and VD view (**B**) of a dog thorax depicting expansion of the ventral and right lateral cardiac borders (black arrows) due to right ventricular enlargement. The cardiac apex is displaced dorsally and to the left (white dotted arrows). Right ventricular enlargement may distort the cardiac silhouette to resemble a reverse capital letter "D", as illustrated in the lateral view (**C**) and the VD view (**D**).

patient positioning. For example, in brachycephalic and chondrodystrophic dogs, the cardiac shadow normally is more rounded and in greater contact with the sternum. In a VD view, rotation of the sternum to the right projects the right cardiac border closer to the right thoracic wall, which can mimic a large right ventricle. Rotation to the left may hide right heart enlargement.

Causes of right ventricular enlargement include heartworm disease, congenital heart disease, and others (see Differential Diagnoses). Right ventricular enlargement tends to alter the size and shape of the cardiac silhouette more than left ventricular enlargement because the walls of the right ventricle are relatively thin.

Aortic arch dilation

The ascending aorta and the aortic arch both contribute to the size and shape of the cardiac silhouette. Dilation of these structures can expand the cranial cardiac border and may widen the cranial mediastinum (Figure 3.97). Causes of dilation include aortic aneurysm and aortic stenosis (see Differential Diagnoses). A mass at the base of the cardiac silhouette may be difficult to distinquish from dilation of the proximal aorta.

In older cats, the aortic arch often is more vertical and may be visible left of midline in a VD/DV. This finding may be mistaken for abnormal enlargement of the proximal aorta or a cranial mediastinal mass (Figure 3.83).

Main pulmonary artery dilation

Dilation of the main pulmonary artery is easiest to see in a VD/DV view. It appears as a focal bulge along the left cranial cardiac border (Figure 3.98). The bulge may not be visible unless quite (this is particularly true in cats). The most common causes of main pulmonary artery dilation are heartworm disease and pulmonic stenosis. In both of these diseases, dilation results from turbulent blood flow distal to a narrowing in the right ventricular outflow tract.

Poor patient positioning can accentuate or diminish the apparent size of the main pulmonary artery. For example, in a VD/DV view, rotation of the sternum to the left may mimic enlargement and rotation to the right may hide it. In older cats, the proximal aorta may be mistaken for a dilated main pulmonary artery (Figure 3.83).

Major vessels

Normal radiographic anatomy

The major vessels (or great vessels) that commonly are visible in thoracic radiographs are the descending aorta, the caudal vena cava, and the right and left primary pulmonary arteries (Figure 3.99). The ascending aorta and the aortic arch are part of the cardiac shadow and are not distinguished in radiographs unless enlarged. The same is true for the cranial vena cava and the main pulmonary artery. These vessels sometimes are visible when surrounded by gas or fat.

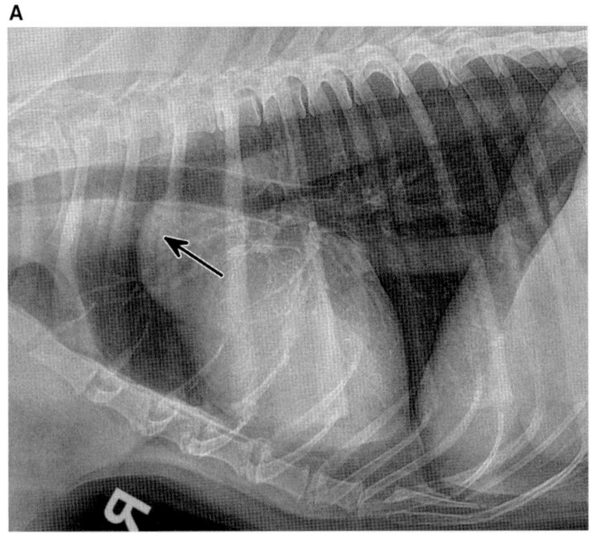

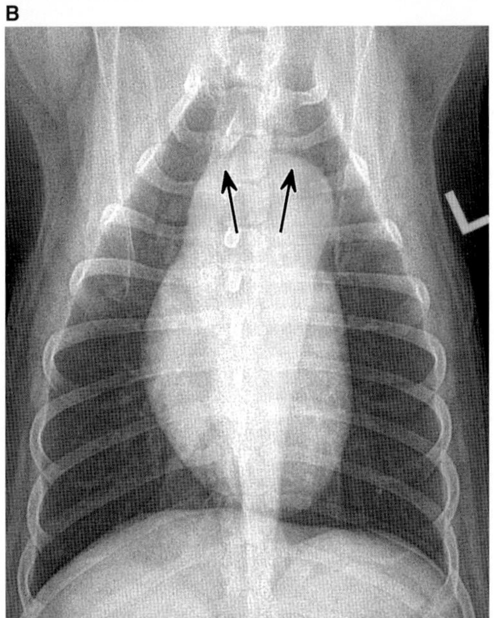

Figure 3.97 Dilation of the aortic arch. Lateral view (**A**) and VD view (**B**) of dog thorax depicting an outward bulge in the cranial cardiac border (black arrows) due to dilation of the aortic arch. In the lateral view, it is difficult to differentiate aortic arch dilation from dilation of either the right atrium or the main pulmonary artery.

The normal **descending aorta** appears as a soft tissue opacity tube curving caudally from the cardiac base to the diaphragm. It is located in the dorsal thorax, ventral to the spine, and slightly left of midline. The abdominal aorta is less distinct but may be visible when surrounded by fat. In a VD/DV view, only the left border of the aorta typically is seen. The right aortic border usually is obscured by superimposition of the spine, sternum, and cardiac silhouette. Sometimes the aorta is easier to follow or trace by beginning at the diaphragm and moving cranially.

The **caudal vena cava** usually is visible between the right crus of the diaphragm and the cardiac shadow. It is centrally located in the lateral view and just to the right of midline in the VD/DV view. The size of the caudal cava is more variable than the size of the aorta. Its diameter changes slightly with the phase of respiration and the stage of the cardiac cycle. In general, the width of the caudal vena cava should not exceed 1.5 times the width of the aorta. Some references suggest the normal width of the caudal cava should not exceed the length of the T5 or T6 thoracic vertebral body.

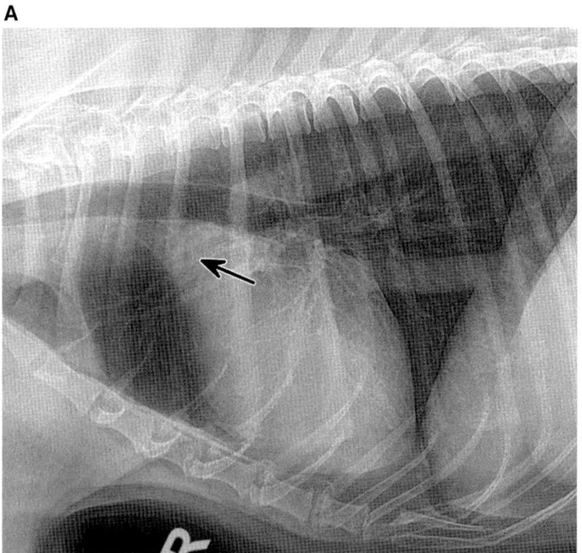

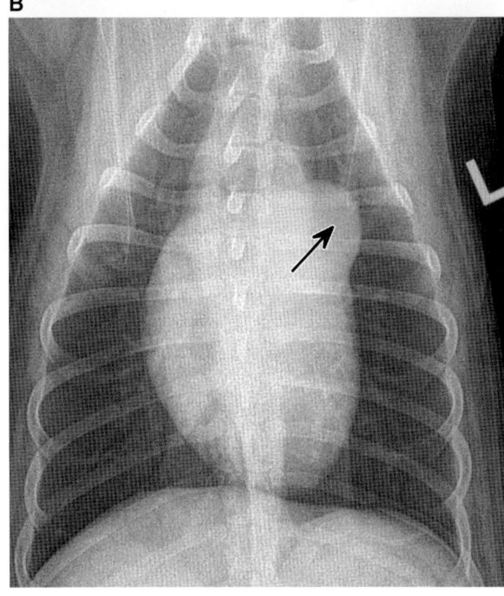

Figure 3.98 Main pulmonary artery enlargment. Lateral view (**A**) and VD view (**B**) of a dog thorax depicting a focal bulge in the left cranial cardiac border (black arrow) due to dilation of the main pulmonary artery. In the lateral view, main pulmonary artery dilation is less evident and difficult to differentiate from dilation of either the right atrium or the proximal aorta.

A

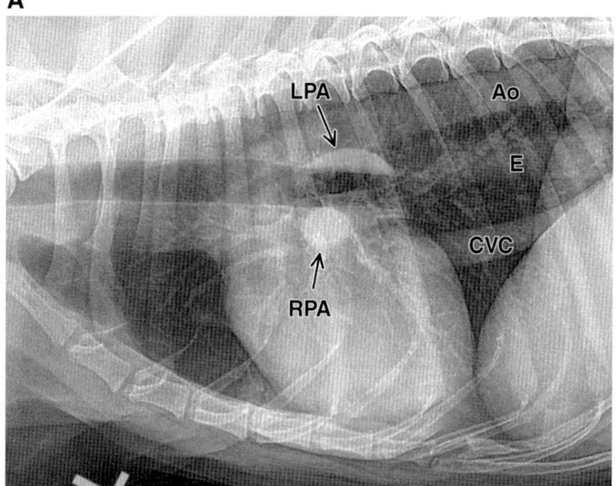

B

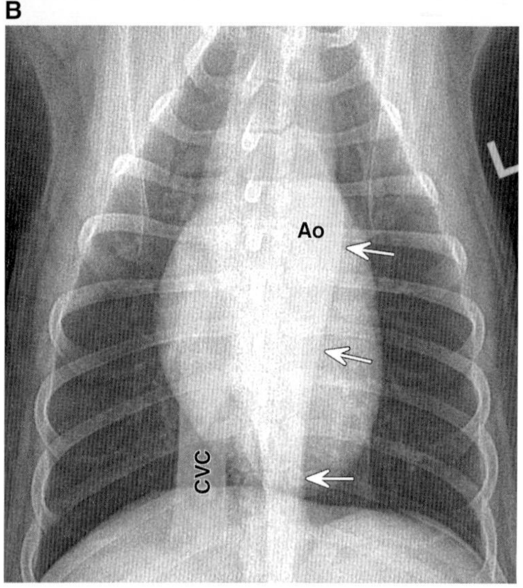

Figure 3.99 Major vessels. Lateral view (**A**) and VD view (**B**) of a dog thorax depicting the major blood vessels commonly seen in thoracic radiographs. Visible are the descending aorta (Ao), caudal vena cava (CVC), and, in the lateral view, the right and left primary pulmonary arteries. In the lateral view, The left pulmonary artery (LPA) often appears as a soft tissue opacity "bulge" dorsal to the tracheal bifurcation. The right pulmonary artery (RPA) often is seen end-on and appears a soft tissue opacity "nodule" ventral to the tracheal bifurcation. The caudal esophagus (E) sometimes is visible in a lateral view as a soft tissue opacity band between the aorta and caudal vena cava. In the VD view, the white arrows point to the left aortic border; the right border is not visible.

The **right and left primary pulmonary arteries** are the initial branches from the main pulmonary artery (MPA). They frequently are visible in a lateral view where they sometimes are mistaken for pathology. This is because the right pulmonary artery branches nearly perpendicular to the MPA and when viewed end-on creates a rounded, soft tissue opacity "nodule" ventral to the tracheal bifurcation (Figure 3.99). The "nodule" may be misdiagnosed as a pulmonary or hilar mass. The left pulmonary artery is the caudal continuation of the MPA. In a lateral view, it curves dorsally over the left mainstem bronchus to produce a soft tissue opacity "bulge" dorsal to the tracheal carina (Figure 3.99). The "bulge" may be mistaken for a hilar mass or left atrial dilation; however, there is no tracheal displacement.

Abnormal major vessels

Smaller than expected blood vessels most often is due to hypovolemia. Hypovolemia also leads to a smaller cardiac shadow. A larger than expected major vessel (dilated vessel) may be due to either increased pressure or increased volume.

Dilation of the **aorta** generally is due to systemic hypertension. High blood pressure can dilate the entire aorta and produce a more wavy or tortuous appearance to the descending aorta. Localized aortic dilation usually represents an aneurysm, which may be caused by a patent ductus arteriosus, spirocercosis, and others (see Differential Diagnoses).

Dilation of the **caudal vena cava** generally is due to increased central venous pressure. Increased venous pressure often results from compromised venous return, which may caused by right heart failure or pulmonary hypertension.

Enlargement of the **pulmonary arteries** most often is due to heartworm disease.

Congenital heart disease

Cardiac abnormalities that are present at birth either **restrict** blood flow or **redirect** it. Restriction is caused by a narrowing or **stenosis** that obstructs the normal flow of blood. Redirection is caused by a **shunt** that allows blood to flow in an abnormal direction.

Radiographic signs of congenital heart disease depend on the severity and duration of the abnormality and the degree of cardiac compensation. Most congenital heart diseases are progressive and will lead to heart failure if left untreated. Radiographs are valuable to monitor the progression of heart disease and the response to therapy.

Cardiovascular stenoses

A stenosis is recognized in radiographs by the dilation that occurs past the narrowed area. The stenosis itself seldom is visible. Narrowing disrupts the normal laminar flow of blow, leading to turbulence downstream from the stenosis (Figure 3.100). Turbulent blood flow exerts outward pressure on the vascular walls, which leads to focal dilation of the vessel. Further downstream, the turbulence diminishes and blood flow returns to normal. Upstream from the stenosis, the blood pressure is elevated because the heart is trying to push a sufficient volume of blood past the narrowed area. The higher blood pressure leads to dilation and/or hypertrophy of the upstream heart chamber.

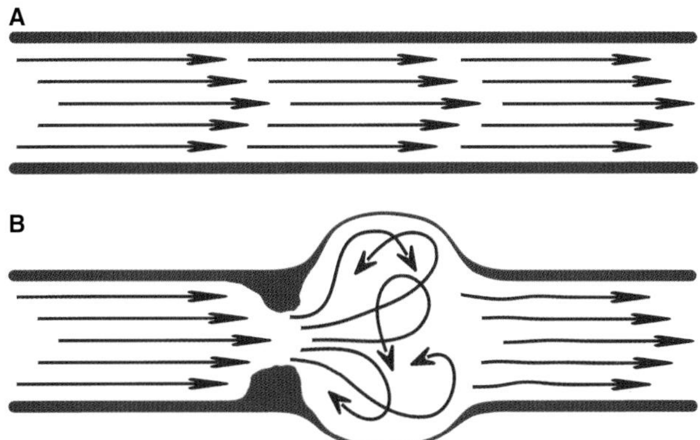

Figure 3.100 Cardiovascular stenosis. **Illustration A** depicts normal *laminar* blood flow. Laminar means the blood is moving downstream in "layers". The layers of blood move together in an even, linear motion that is parallel to the long axis of the blood vessel. Blood in the center of the vessel is moving at a higher velocity than blood at the periphery. **Illustration B** depicts a stenosis. The narrowed area disrupts the laminar flow of blood, causing turbulence past the stenosis. Turbulence exerts outward pressure on the vascular walls that leads to post-stenotic dilatation. Further downstream, past the stenosis and turbulence, blood flow eventually returns to normal laminar flow.

Pulmonic stenosis

Pulmonic stenosis is an abnormal narrowing in the right ventricular outflow tract. It is the most common congenital stenosis in dogs. The narrowing most often occurs at the pulmonary valve (*valvular* stenosis), but it can occur before the valve (*subvalvular* stenosis) or after the valve (*supravalvular* stenosis).

Radiographic signs include focal dilation of the main pulmonary artery and right ventricular enlargement (Figure 3.101). The lung vasculature may be small, especially in the periphery, because the stenosis limits cardiac output. The caudal vena cava may be large due to reduced venous return and increased central venous pressure. In chronic or severe cases, high blood pressure in the right ventricle can lead to tricuspid valve insufficiency and right atrial dilation. Untreated pulmonic stenosis may progress to right heart failure.

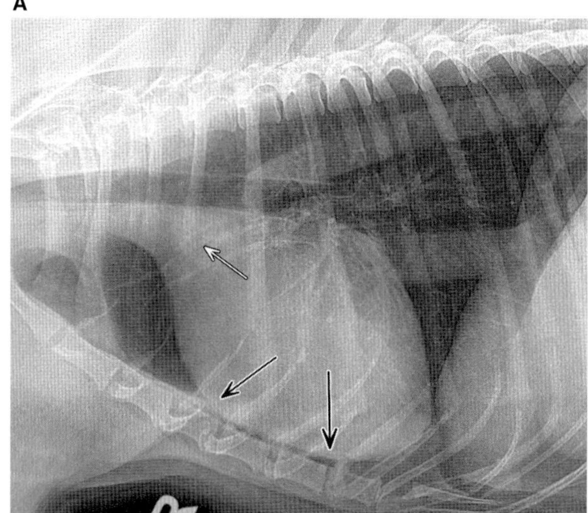

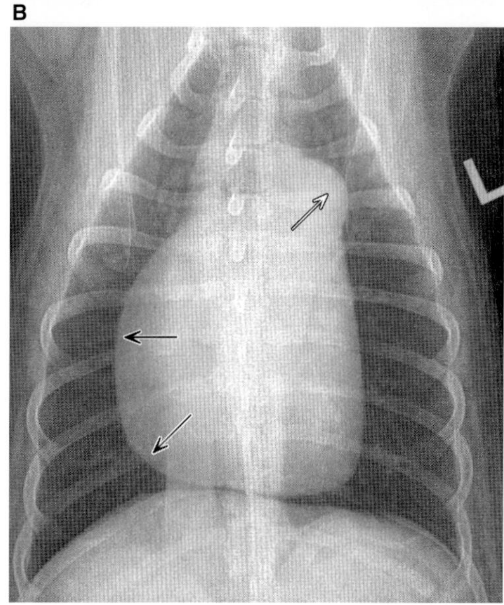

Figure 3.101 Pulmonic stenosis. Lateral view (**A**) and VD view (**B**) of a dog thorax depicting a focal dilation in the main pulmonary artery (white arrow) and right ventricular enlargement (black arrows). The caudal vena cava is enlarged, and the pulmonary blood vessels are small.

Aortic stenosis

Aortic stenosis is an abnormal narrowing in the left ventricular outflow tract. It is the second most common congenital stenosis in dogs. The narrowing most often is caused by nodules or a fibrous band before (below) the aortic valve (*subvalvular* or *subaortic* stenosis). Sometimes the narrowing occurs at the valve (*valvular* stenosis) or after (above) the valve (*supravalvular* stenosis).

Radiographic signs include focal dilation of the ascending aorta and aortic arch and enlargement of the left ventricle (Figure 3.102). The descending aorta and pulmonary vessels usually are normal size. In chronic or severe cases, high pressure in the left ventricle can lead to mitral valve insufficiency and left atrial dilation. Untreated aortic stenosis may progress to left heart failure.

Atrioventricular stenosis

Abnormal narrowing between an atrium and its ventricle is a rare congenital heart defect. It is reported more often in cats than in dogs. The involved right or left atrium may dilate greatly due to elevated pressure within its relatively thin atrial walls. The associated ventricle often is only mildly or moderately enlarged, less than expected with such severe atrial dilation.

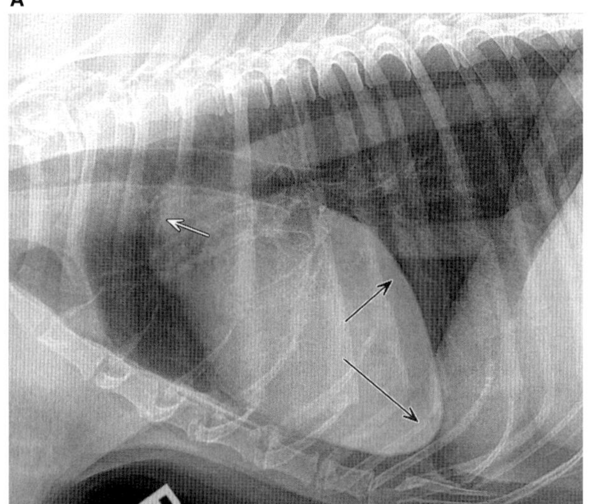

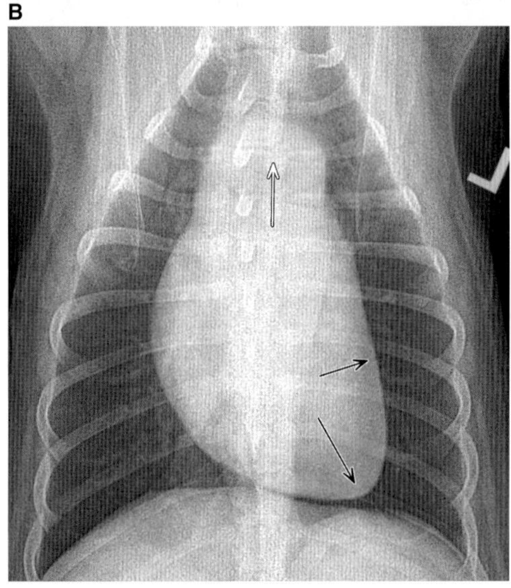

Figure 3.102 Aortic stenosis. Lateral view (**A**) and VD view (**B**) of a dog thorax depicting focal dilation in the aortic arch with widening of the cranial mediastinum (white arrow). The left ventricle is enlarged (black arrows) and the cardiac apex is shifted to the left of midline.

Cardiovascular shunts

Congenital blood shunts result from either the failure of a normal in utero opening to close at birth or a developmental problem that results in an abnormal communication. Shunts may be located between heart chambers (*intra-cardiac*) or between blood vessels (*extra-cardiac*). Patent ductus arteriosus is the most common cardiovascular shunt in dogs and cats. The next most common are ventricular septal defects and atrial septal defects. Each of these is discussed further in this section.

The flow of blood in a cardiovascular shunt is from high pressure to low pressure. Most shunts, therefore, are **left-to-right** because left heart pressure usually is greater than right heart pressure. If right heart pressure exceeds left heart pressure, then a **right-to-left** shunt may develop. A right-to-left shunt can occur when a shunt is combined with stenosis, such as Tetralogy of Fallot. Sometimes a left-to-right shunt will reverse later in life to become a right-to-left shunt due to pulmonary hypertension (see *Eisenmenger's syndrome*).

Left-to-right shunts increase the workload on both the right and left sides of the heart. The left heart works harder because the physiologic receptors that govern output aren't adequately stimulated. The right heart works harder due to the increased pressure and larger volume it receives directly from the left heart without the dampening effect of the lungs.

Patent ductus arteriosus (PDA)

The ductus arteriosus is a normal in utero opening between the main pulmonary artery (MPA) and the aorta. It exists prior to birth so blood can bypass the non-oxygenating fetal lungs. Normally the ductus arteriosus closes within the first few days after birth and becomes the *ligamentum arteriosus*. Failure of the ductus to close results in a left-to-right shunt with blood flowing from the higher pressure aorta into the lower pressure MPA. The redirected blood disrupts laminar flow in both the aorta and the main pulmonary artery MPA (Figure 3.103). Turbulence in each vessel leads to focal dilations in both. In radiographs, the dilatations create the characteristic bulges or "bumps" that help diagnose a PDA (Figure 3.104).

In many patients with a PDA, there are three focal expansions in the cardiac silhouette that are considered

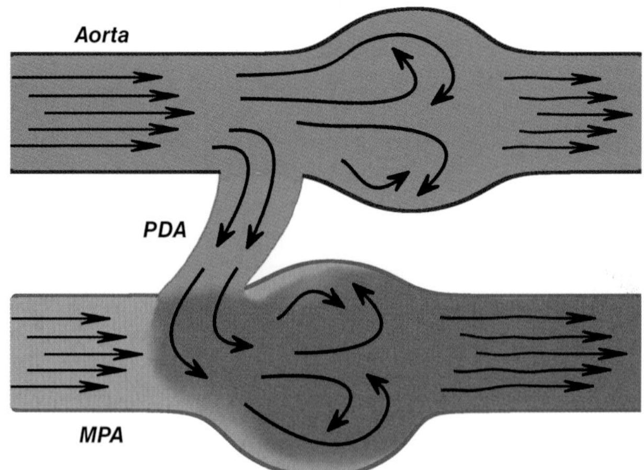

Figure 3.103 Patent ductus arteriosus (PDA). This illustration depicts oxygenated blood (red) from the aorta flowing through a PDA shunt into non-oxygenated blood (blue) in the main pulmonary artery (MPA). Arterial blood from the higher pressure aorta mixing with venous blood in the lower pressure MPA disrupts normal laminar flow in both, leading to turbulence and focal dilation in each vessel (downstream from the shunt). As blood moves past the turbulence, it eventually returns to normal laminar laminar flow.

A

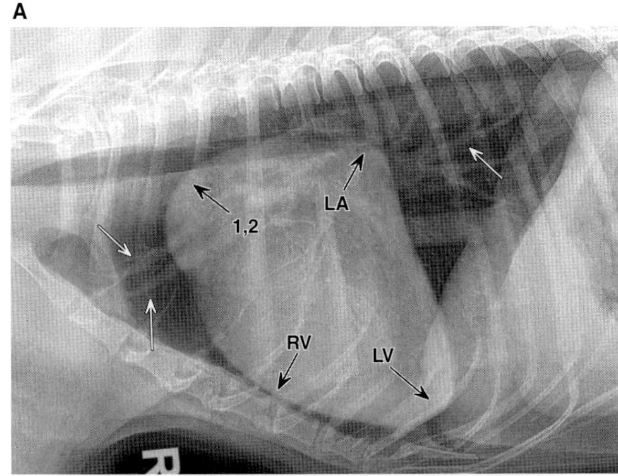

B

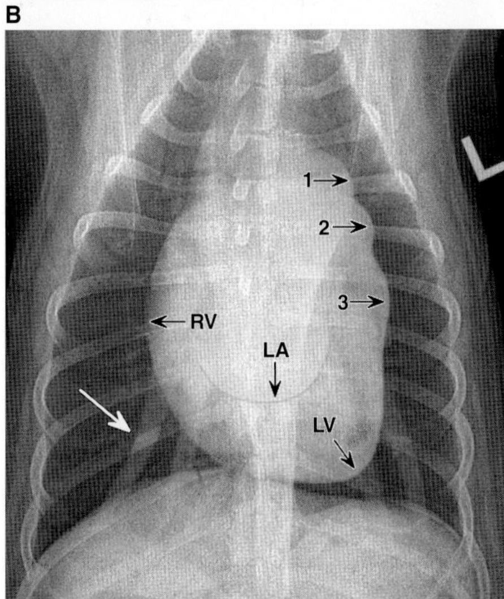

Figure 3.104 Patent ductus arteriosus (PDA). Lateral view (**A**) and VD view (**B**) of a dog thorax depicting the classic radiographic signs of a PDA. The cardiac silhouette is enlarged and abnormal in shape due to left atrial dilation (LA), left ventricular enlargement (LV), right ventricular enlargement (RV) and the three "ductus bumps": (1) focal dilation in the proximal descending aorta; (2) focal dilation in the main pulmonary artery; and (3) bulge created by the left atrial appendage. The aortic bulge (1) typically is seen at about the level of the fourth rib. It may be easier to find by tracing the left border of the aorta from the diaphragm cranially. The main pulmonary artery bulge (2) usually is just caudal to the aortic bulge. Both (1) and (2) are located at the site of the PDA. The left atrial appendage bulge (3) is in the middle of the left cardiac border and only visible in the VD view. The pulmonary vessels are enlarged due to overcirculation (white arrows).

pathognomonic: (1) a bulge in the proximal descending aorta, (2) a bulge in the main pulmonary artery, and (3) a bulge along the left lateral cardiac border created by the left atrial appendage. These three "ductus bumps" are easiest to see in a VD/DV view. They tend to be more apparent in dogs than in cats. Other radiographic signs of a PDA are associated with pulmonary over-circulation (Table 3.4). Blood flow

Table 3.4 Radiographic signs of PDA

1. Focal dilation in the proximal descending aorta.
2. Focal dilation in the main pulmonary artery.
3. Focal bulge caused by the left atrial appendage.
4. Dilation of the left atrium.
5. Enlargement of both the right and left ventricles.
6. Large pulmonary vessels.
7. Increased lung opacity due to hypervascularity and possibly pulmonary edema.

redirected by a PDA increases the volume sent to the lungs. Pulmonary vessels subsequently enlarge and the overall lung opacity increases because there is more blood in the lungs. The pulmonary veins tend to enlarge more than the arteries because their walls are thinner. Thinner walls also are more permeable and high venous blood flow can lead to perivascular leakage and pulmonary edema. Edema further increases lung opacity. Over-circulated lungs also means a larger volume of blood will enter the left atrium. The left atrium can become quite dilated in patients with a PDA, which often leads to dilation or lateral displacement of the left atrial appendage. The left ventricle enlarges to compensate for the larger volume of blood it receives from the left atrium. The right ventricle also enlarges due to increased resistance to output caused by the higher volume and pressure in the main pulmonary artery. The degree of cardiovascular enlargements depends on the magnitude and duration of the shunt.

Atrial septal defect

An abnormal opening between the right and left atria may be due to failure of the *foramen ovale* to close at birth or due to abnormal developmental of the inter-atrial septum. Atrial septal defects typically result in a left-to-right shunt because left heart pressure normally is greater than right heart pressure. Small defects may not produce detectable radiographic signs. Larger defects lead to right atrial dilation and enlargement of the right ventricle, the latter due to the higher pressure and volume of blood coming from the left atrium (Figure 3.105). More blood flow to the right heart leads to over-circulation in the lungs and enlarged pulmonary vasculature. Severe or chronic atrial septal defects may produce a very large and rounded cardiac shadow. Heart disease and can progress to pulmonary hypertension and right heart failure.

Ventricular septal defect

An abnormal opening between the left and right ventricles is due to a deformity in the interventricular septum. The abnormal communication typically leads to a left-to-right shunt between the ventricles. Most interventricular defects

A

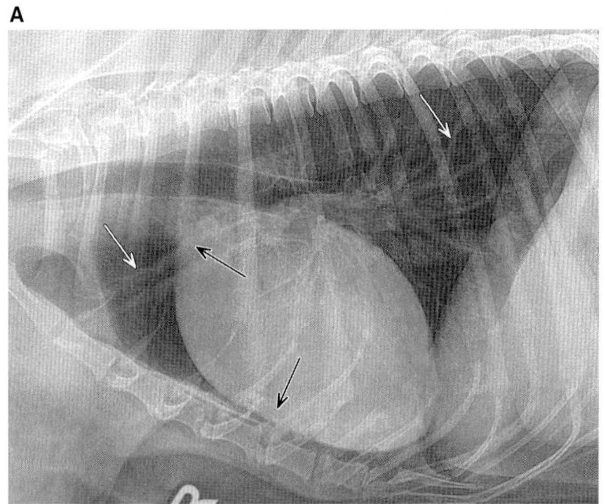

B

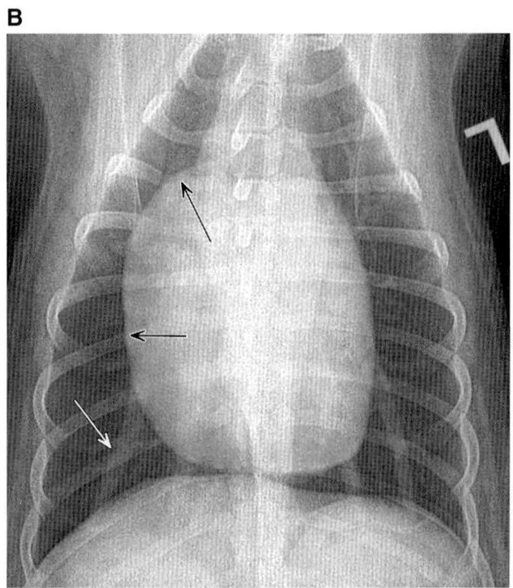

Figure 3.105 Atrial septal defect. Lateral view (**A**) and VD view (**B**) of a dog thorax depicting enlargement of the right atrium and right ventricle (black arrows). The pulmonary vessels are large due to over-circulation (white arrows).

are small and located high in the septum, just below the aortic valve. A large defect in this area may allow much of the shunted blood to flow directly into the pulmonary artery instead of the right ventricle. Such a high septal defect sometimes is called an "overriding aorta." Blood flowing from the left ventricle increases the pressure and volume in the right ventricle and leads to right ventricular enlargement (Figure 3.106). More blood coming from the right heart leads to over-circulation in the lungs and enlargement of the pulmonary vasculature. The left ventricle also enlarges because it must compensate for the volume of blood lost to the right ventricle.

Endocardial cushion defects

The endocardial cushion is the division between the atria and the ventricles. Developmental defects in this area are rare, but they can lead to atrioventricular valve dysfunction and

A

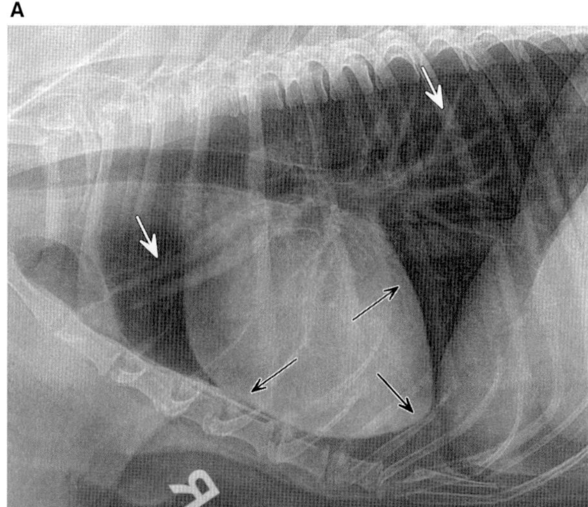

B

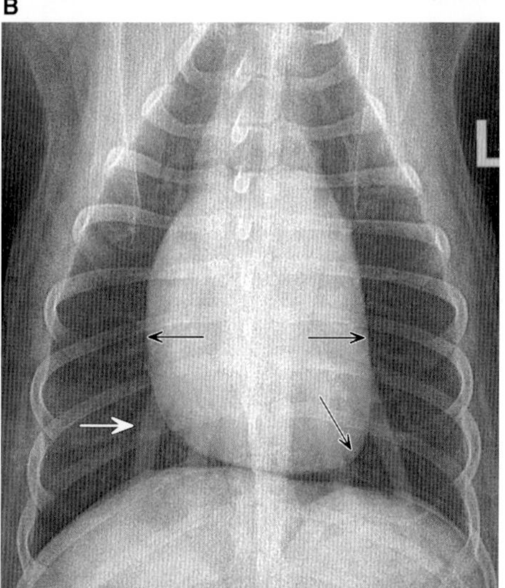

Figure 3.106 Ventricular septal defect. Lateral view (**A**) and VD view (**B**) of a dog thorax depicting biventricular enlargement (black arrows) and enlarged pulmonary vessels (white arrows), the latter due to over-circulation.

intra-cardiac shunts. Partial deformities cause varying degrees of mitral or tricuspid valve insufficiency and enlargement of the left or right heart chambers. Complete defects allow all four heart chambers to communicate, which results in generalized cardiomegaly and rounding of the cardiac silhouette.

Right-to-left cardiovascular shunts

A right-to-left cardiovascular shunt may be congenital or acquired. Acquired shunts are more common than congenital, but both are rare in dogs and cats.

The most common congenital right-to-left shunts are Tetralogy of Fallot and Eisenmenger's complex. **Tetralogy of Fallot** is a ventricular septal defect (VSD) combined with pulmonic stenosis. It generally is described by four characteristics: (1) a high VSD, (2) an overriding aorta, which actually is a high VSD, (3) a pulmonic stenosis, and (4) right ventricular hypertrophy, which is secondary to the pulmonic stenosis. **Eisenmenger's complex** is a VSD with congenital pulmonary hypertension. In both Tetralogy and Eisenmenger's, right ventricular pressure exceeds left ventricular pressure and results in a right-to-left shunt through the VSD. The predominate radiographic finding in both is right ventricular enlargement. The left atrium and left ventricle usually are normal size. Pulmonary vessels may be small due to reduced pulmonary blood flow.

Acquired right-to-left shunts most often are due to **Eisenmenger's syndrome**, which is the reversal of a long-standing left-to-right shunt. The reversal results from chronic over-circulation in the lungs that leads to pulmonary hypertension and increased pressure in the right heart. When right heart pressure exceeds left heart pressure, the left-to-right shunt becomes a right-to-left shunt. Eisenmenger's syndrome has been reported in patients with PDA, VSD, and atrial septal defects.

"Reversal" of a PDA produces a unique clinical finding known as *differential cyanosis*. When a left-to-right PDA reverses to become a right-to-left PDA, blood flows from the main pulmonary artery to the aorta, bypassing the lungs. This means the caudal portions of the body receive poorly oxygenated blood. The cranial parts of the body continue to receive oxygenated blood because they are supplied by branches from the aorta that emerge prior to the PDA. Patients with a reverse PDA typically present with clinical findings of cyanosis in the genitalia and pelvic limbs and normal mucous membranes cranially. In radiographs, some right-to-left shunting PDAs will maintain the appearance of a left-to-right PDA, whereas others will develop right heart enlargement and a more generalized enlargement of the cardiac shadow.

Acquired heart disease

In contrast to congenital heart diseases, acquired cardiac abnormalities are those that develop during an animal's lifetime. Disorders of the heart muscle (cardiomyopathies) are the most common acquired heart diseases in cats and the second most common in dogs. Endocardiosis is the most common in dogs.

Cardiomyopathy

Disorders of the heart muscle generally are classified as either dilated cardiomyopathy or hypertrophic cardiomyopathy. Both frequently progress to systolic and/or diastolic dysfunction and congestive heart failure.

Dilated cardiomyopathy

Dilated cardiomyopathy is characterized by thinning of the myocardium, dilation of the heart chambers, and poor cardiac contractility. It is more common in dogs than in cats, particularly in large and giant breeds (e.g., Doberman Pinscher, Great Dane, Boxer). Dilated cardiomyopathy sometimes is called *congestive cardiomyopathy* because it frequently progresses to congestive heart failure. It has been associated with a taurine deficient diet.

Radiographic signs are those of generalized cardiomegaly, including overall enlargement of the cardiac silhouette and rounding of the cardiac borders (Figures 3.107 and 3.108). Left atrial dilation often predominates. Pulmonary vessels may be small due to diminished cardiac output and the caudal vena cava may be large due to reduced venous return.

Hypertrophic cardiomyopathy

Hypertrophic cardiomyopathy (HCM) is characterized by thickening of the ventricular walls and myocardial stiffness. It is the most common cardiomyopathy in cats, but HCM is

A

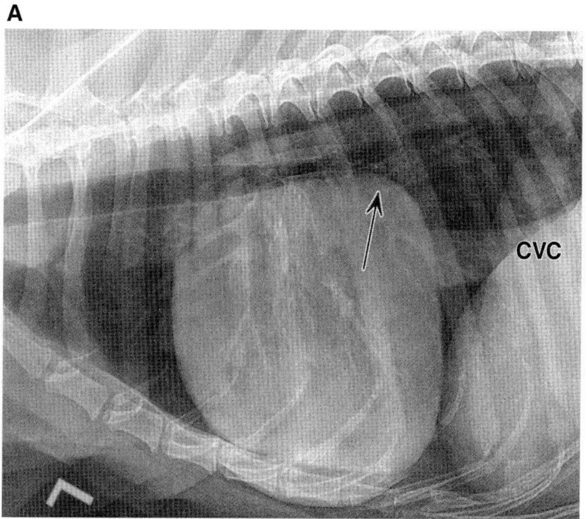

B

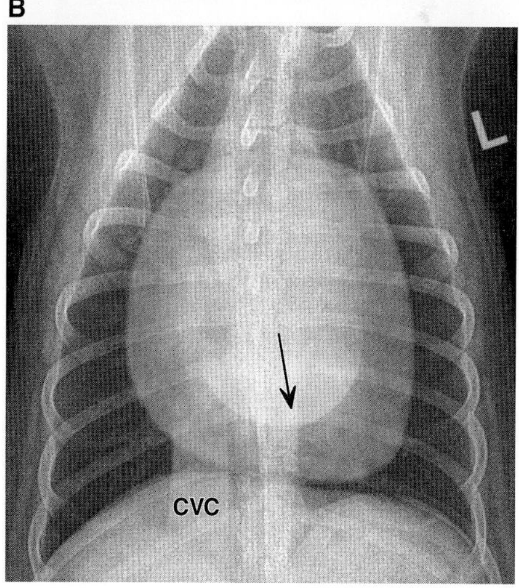

Figure 3.107 Canine dilated cardiomyopathy. Lateral view (**A**) and VD view (**B**) of a dog thorax depicting generalized enlargement of the cardiac silhouette. The cardiac borders are expanded, making them more rounded and moving them closer to the thoracic walls and in greater contact with the sternum. The left atrium is largely dilated (arrow) causing dorsal displacement of the trachea. The pulmonary vessels are small due to lower left heart output and the caudal vena cava (CVC) is large due to lower right heart function.

A

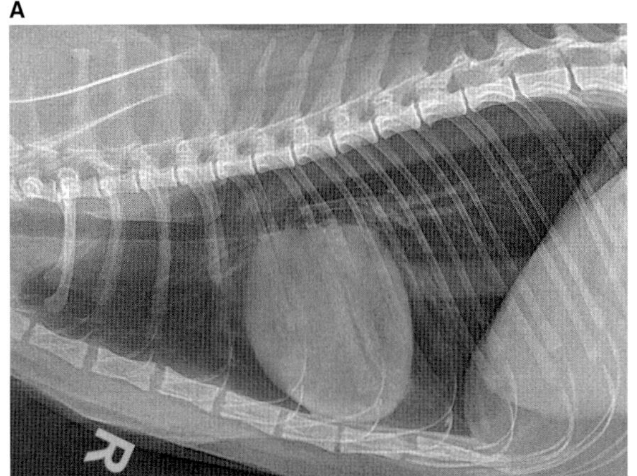

B

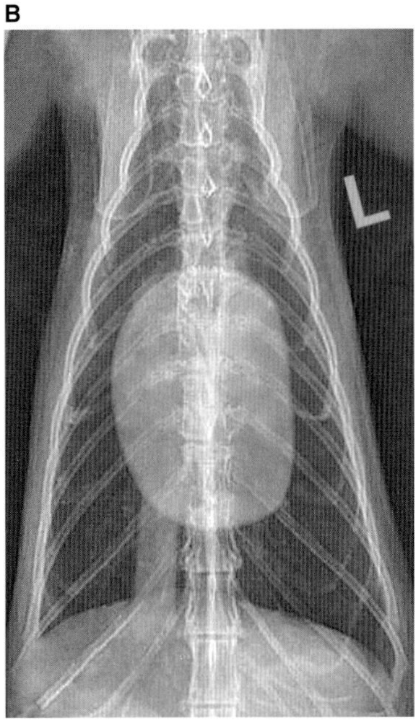

Figure 3.108 Feline dilated cardiomyopathy. Lateral view (**A**) and VD view (**B**) of a cat thorax depicting a longer, wider, and more rounded cardiac silhouette. In cats with dilated cardiomyopathy, the cardiac shadow tends to sit more upright with little sternal contact. The trachea is dorsally displaced and the caudal vena cava is large.

uncommon in dogs. Thickening of the ventricular walls is mostly inward (concentric). Concentric hypertrophy leads to more of a decrease in the size of the lumen than an outward expansion of the heart chamber. This means that radiographic signs of concentric thickening often are less evident than with eccentric hypertrophy or dilation of a heart chamber.

Thickening of the ventricular walls eventually leads to atrial dilation due to the increased pressure in the heart. The left ventricle usually is more severely affected.This means that radiographic signs of concentric thickening often are less evident than with eccentric hypertrophy or dilation of a heart chamber.

Thickening of the ventricular walls eventually leads to atrial dilation due to the increased pressure in the heart. The left ventricle usually is more severely affected.This means that radiographic signs of concentric thickening often are less evident than with eccentric hypertrophy or dilation of a heart chamber.

Thickening of the ventricular walls eventually leads to atrial dilation due to the increased pressure in the heart. The left ventricle usually is more severely affected.

The predominate radiographic finding with HCM is atrial dilation, which may be marked (Figure 3.109). A largely dilated atrium can significantly widen the cardiac base and create a triangular-shaped cardiac silhouette, sometimes described

A

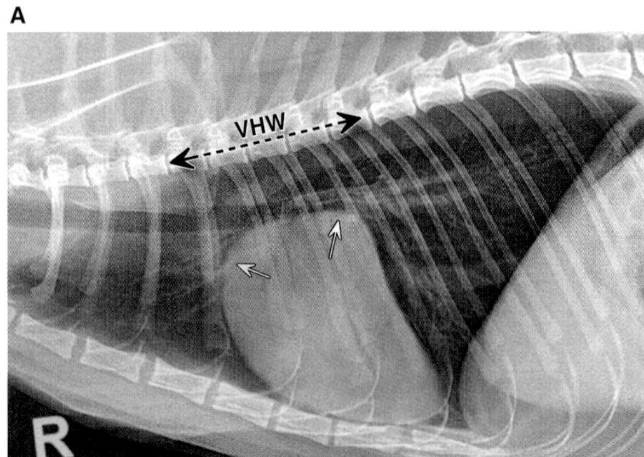

B

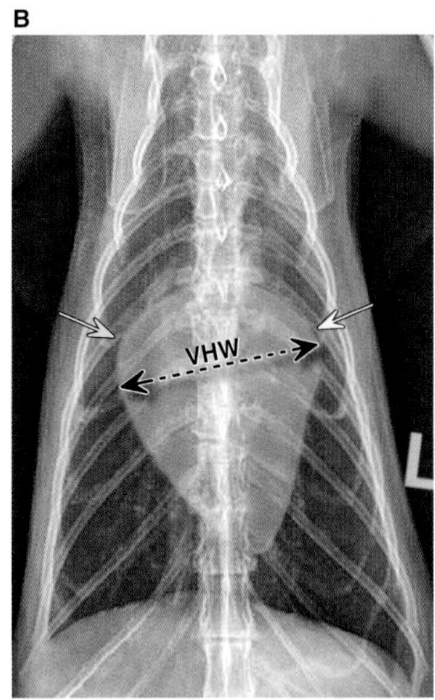

Figure 3.109 Hypertrophic cardiomyopathy. Lateral view (**A**) and VD view (**B**) of a cat thorax depicting an enlarged, triangular-shape cardiac silhouette. The cardiac base is widened due to left atrial dilation (white arrow) and a large or displaced right atrium (yellow arrow). There is increased cardiosternal contact. The vertebral heart width (VHW) is illustrated on these radiographs (Table 3.2). The maximum width of the cardiac shadow (black double headed arrow in the VD view) is transposed to the thoracic spine in the lateral view. Beginning at the cranial edge of T4, count the number of vertebrae spanned by the cardiac width to the nearest 1/10th of a vertebra. In this example, the VHW is 4.8 (normal range is 2.9–4.1).

as a "valentine heart" shape. Both atria may be dilated in cats with HCM or the left atrium may be so dilated that it displaces the right atrium laterally. The ventricles often appear normal in size in radiographs or only mildly enlarged. The cardiac apex may be more pointed due to ventricular hypertrophy.

In cats, HCM may result from hyperthyroidism. Cats with HCM also are at risk for thromboembolic disease. Emboli more often lodge in the distal aortic trifurcation and iliac arteries, but can travel anywhere in the body.

Other cardiomyopathies

Less common myocardial diseases in dogs and cats include arrhythmogenic right ventricular cardiomyopathy, restrictive cardiomyopathy, myocardial inflammation, and endocardial fibroelastosis.

Arrhythmogenic right ventricular cardiomyopathy is characterized by severe ventricular tachycardia. It most often is reported in Boxers. Radiographic signs may resemble dilated cardiomyopathy, but in many cases the cardiac shadow appears normal. The disease is rare in cats and may appear as enlargement of the right ventricle and atrium.

Restrictive cardiomyopathy or unclassified cardiomyopathy, is characterized by stiff ventricular walls with little or no thickening and diastolic dysfunction. It is an uncommon disease that occurs in cats more often than dogs. Radiographic signs are similar to hypertrophic cardiomyopathy.

Myocardial inflammation may result from infection (viral, bacterial, or parasitic) or it may be caused by certain drugs, toxins or a dietary deficiency. Radiographic signs typically are those of congestive heart failure.

Endocardial fibroelastosis is a rare myocardial disease of unknown etiology that causes diffuse thickening of the left atrial and ventricular endocardium. Radiographic signs may resemble those of dilated cardiomyopathy.

Endocardiosis

Endocardiosis is a progressive, non-inflammatory, degenerative disease of the heart valves. It is also known as *myxomatous valve disease*. Degeneration leads to valvular insufficiency, which is the inability of the valve to maintain unidirectional blood flow. Untreated cases of valvular insufficiency can progress to heart failure. Other causes of valvular insufficiency include endocarditis and ruptured chordae tendinea (see Differential Diagnoses).

Radiographic signs depend on the valve affected, the severity and duration of the regurgitant blood flow, and the degree of cardiac compensation. Although the mitral valve is most often involved, endocardiosis can also affect the tricuspid, pulmonary, and aortic valves. These other valves are affected less frequently and usually less severely than the mitral valve.

Mitral valve insufficiency

Endocardiosis of the mitral valve is by far the most common acquired heart disease in dogs. It predominately affects small

A

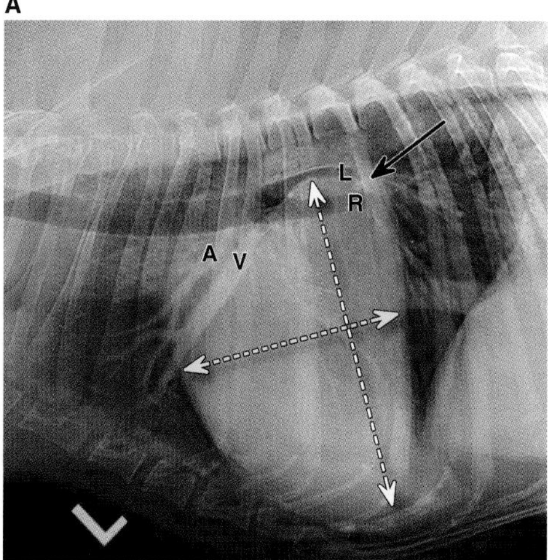

B

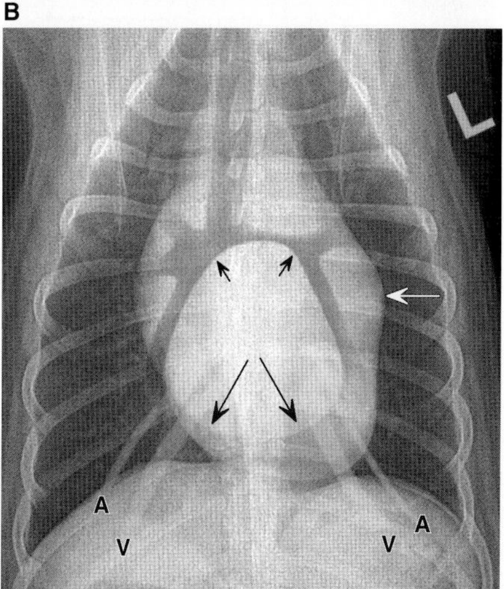

Figure 3.110 Mitral valve insufficiency. Lateral view (**A**) and VD view (**B**) of a dog thorax depicting an enlarged cardiac shadow, increased in both length and width due to left heart enlargement. The cardiac axes are illustrated in the lateral view to depict the measurements used to obtain a vertebral heart score (Figure 3.84). Notice that the long axis (white dashed line) extends from the cardiac apex to the ventral border of the left primary bronchus (L), which in this case is the dorsal cardiac border. Left atrial dilation (black arrows) displaces the trachea dorsally, splits the mainstem bronchi, and widens the tracheal bifurcation. In the lateral view, the left primary bronchus (L) is pushed dorsal to the right (R). The left bronchus is narrowed in both the lateral and VD views due to compression by the dilated left atrium. In the VD view, there is a focal bulge along the left cardiac border caused by dilation or displacement of the left atrial appendage (white arrow). In both views, the pulmonary veins (V) are larger than their paired arteries (A) due to venous congestion and early left heart failure.

breeds that are middle-aged or old, but it can occur in any dog. Mitral valve endocardiosis is rare in cats.

The earliest and most frequent radiographic finding is dilation of the left atrium (Figure 3.110). Dilation is progressive and the left atrium can become quite large. The left atrial appendage may also dilate or it may be laterally displaced. The left ventricle enlarges to compensate for the diminished output caused by regurgitant flow into the left atrium. Mitral valve insufficiency can progress to left heart failure, venous congestion and pulmonary edema.

Rarely, the wall of a severely dilated left atrium can rupture and bleed into the pericardial space, causing a pericardial effusion or cardiac tamponade.

An acute onset of severe mitral valve insufficiency may be caused by a ruptured chordae tendinea. In these cases, there often is insufficient time for the left atrium to dilate before left heart failure occurs. Radiographs may reveal severe pulmonary edema and a relatively normal-appearing cardiac silhouette.

Tricuspid valve insufficiency

Tricuspid valve insufficiency is uncommon in dogs and cats. It most often occurs secondary to another disease, such as chronic mitral valve insufficiency. Regurgitant tricuspid blood flow leads to progressive dilation of the right atrium (Figure 3.111). The right ventricle enlarges to compensate so it can supply sufficient output to the lungs. The pulmonary vessels may be small due to less blood flow and the caudal vena cava may be large due to reduced venous return.

A

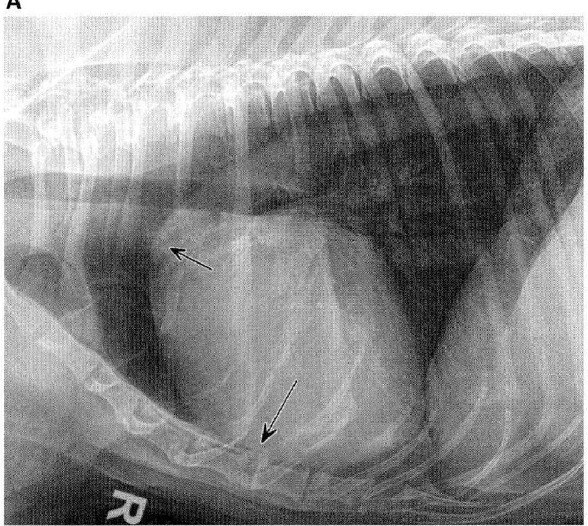

B

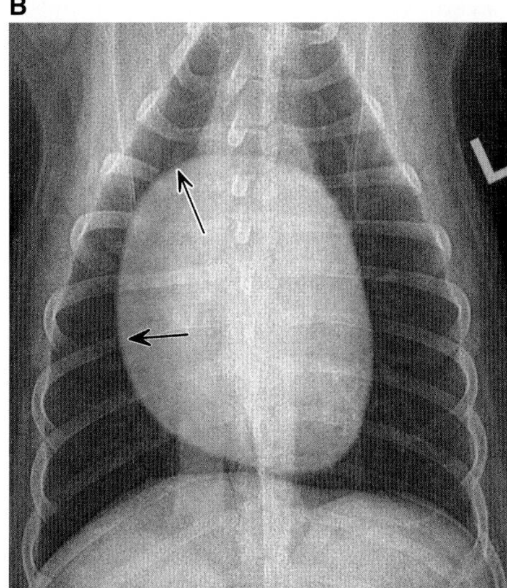

Figure 3.111 Tricuspid valve insufficiency. Lateral view (**A**) and VD view (**B**) of a dog thorax depicting a widened cardiac shadow due to enlargement of the right atrium and right ventricle (black arrows). The ventral, right cranial, and right lateral cardiac borders are expanded, and there is increased cardiosternal contact. The pulmonary vessels are small due to under-circulated lungs.

Heartworm disease

Heartworms are blood-borne parasites that invade the cardiovascular systems of dogs and cats. *Dirofilaria immitis* is the most commonly encountered species. Dirofilaria occur worldwide and are transmitted by mosquitoes. Another species is *Angiostrongylus vasorum*, which is transmitted by slugs or snails in Europe, Canada, South America, and Africa.

Heartworm disease is more common in dogs than in cats. **In dogs**, heartworms cause inflammation in the right heart and in the pulmonary arteries. Inflammation leads to thromboembolism, pulmonary hypertension, and eventual right heart failure. **In cats**, heartworms tend to be fewer, smaller, and shorter-lived than in dogs and disease often is self-limiting. Radiographic and clinical signs of feline heartworm disease frequently resemble those of asthma. In general, the severity of the radiographic findings in both dogs and cats is influenced more by the patient's immune response to the heartworms than the parasite burden itself. The more severe the response, the more severe the signs.

In dogs, the most common radiographic findings are right ventricular enlargement and dilated pulmonary arteries (Figure 3.112). The right ventricle enlarges because the heartworms partially obstruct the outflow tract, which increases the pressure in the ventricle. The outflow obstruction also leads to turbulent blood flow in the main pulmonary artery and local dilation of the artery. In the lungs, the pulmonary arteries dilate due to thromboemboli and vasculitis caused by the heartworms. The veins usually remain normal size. The arteries can become quite large proximal to an embolic obstruction and then taper very quickly distal to the obstruction. The abrupt tapering has been described as "pruned" or "blunted" arteries. The right ventricle and pulmonary arteries will continue to increase in size as long as the infection remains active. Large pulmonary arteries can become tortuous and when viewed end-on may be mistaken for lung masses. Patchy areas of increased lung opacity may develop due to inflammation caused by the thromboemboli or due to an allergic response to the parasites themselves (i.e., eosinophilic pneumonia). Heartworm disease can progress to right heart failure.

A

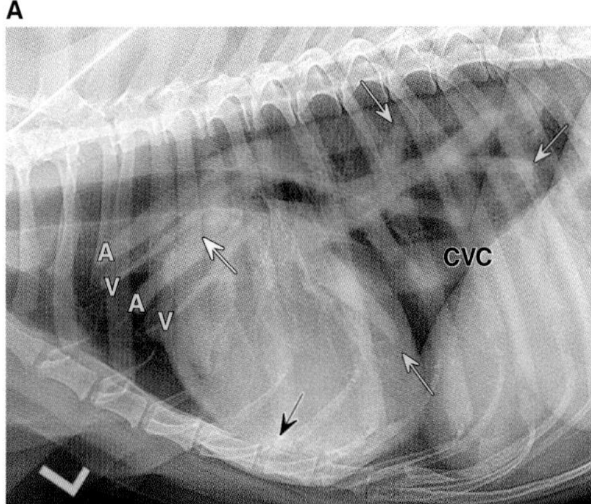

B

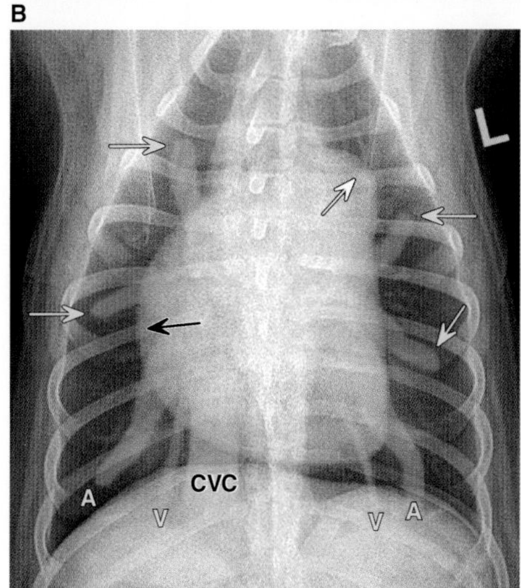

Figure 3.112 Heartworm disease. Lateral view (**A**) and VD view (**B**) of a dog thorax depicting right ventricular enlargement (black arrow) and focal dilation in the main pulmonary artery (white arrow). The pulmonary arteries (A) are larger than the corresponding veins (V). The arteries taper abruptly and appear blunted (yellow arrows). The caudal vena cava (CVC) is large due to increased central venous pressure.

In cats with heartworm infections, radiographic signs of right ventricular and main pulmonary artery enlargement tend to be less evident than in dogs, and enlargement of the lung arteries often is less severe and more dynamic. In cats, the arteries typically enlarge and then reduce in size and then enlarge again as the cat's immune system responds to the parasites. Each time the heartworm larvae transition from one stage in their lifecycle to the next, a new immune response is triggered. The immune response leads not only to artery enlargement, but also to lung inflammation. Inflammation increases lung opacity and frequently resembles feline asthma. Feline heartworm disease rarely progresses to right heart failure.

Heart failure

Heart disease and heart failure are not the same thing. **Disease** refers to any congenital or acquired disorder of the heart. **Failure** occurs when the heart is unable to maintain adequate blood circulation.

Congestive heart failure means blood is backed up in an organ. Radiographic signs of congestive heart failure include lung edema, hepatomegaly, and splenomegaly.

Both heart disease and heart failure commonly enlarge the cardiac silhouette. Heart failure is differentiated from heart disease by an accumulation of fluid in the lungs or in the pleural or peritoneal space.

Left heart failure

Left heart failure occurs when the left ventricle is ineffective in moving blood out of the heart and to the rest of the body. Reduction in left ventricular output causes back up in the left atrium. This results in pulmonary venous congestion and leakage of fluid into the parenchyma of the lungs (see the discussion of pulmonary edema later in this chapter). Fluid in the lungs can lead to increased pressure in the right ventricle, which means left heart failure can progress to right heart failure. Causes of left heart failure include mitral valve insufficiency, cardiomyopathy, and others (see Differential Diagnoses). Radiographic signs of left heart failure (Figure 3.113) include:

1. Pulmonary edema.
2. Pulmonary veins larger than arteries.
3. Left atrial dilation.
4. Enlargement of the left ventricle.

In dogs, **cardiogenic pulmonary edema** typically begins in the hilar region and spreads bilaterally and symmetrically into the central lungs (Figure 3.165). The peripheral lungs usually are spared. A more patchy pattern of lung edema occasionally is seen in dogs, but a patchy pattern is much more common in cats.

In cats, cardiogenic pulmonary edema tends to be more random and asymmetric (Figure 3.166). It generally involves both the central and peripheral lungs. Cats in left heart failure can develop pleural effusion, but effusion is rare in dogs unless left heart failure has progressed to right heart failure.

In both dogs and cats, pulmonary venous congestion leads to enlarged pulmonary veins (the veins are wider than their paired arteries). Venous congestion also can lead to pleural edema and pleural fissure lines.

In most patients with left heart failure, the left heart is visibly enlarged. In some cases, however, the cardiac shadow is normal size. Examples include: patients with sudden or acute left heart failure where is insufficient time for the heart to enlarge before failure occurs (e.g., ruptured chordae tendinae,

A

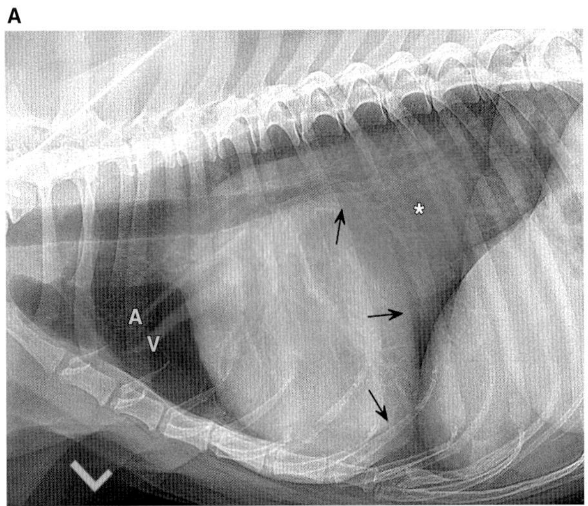

B

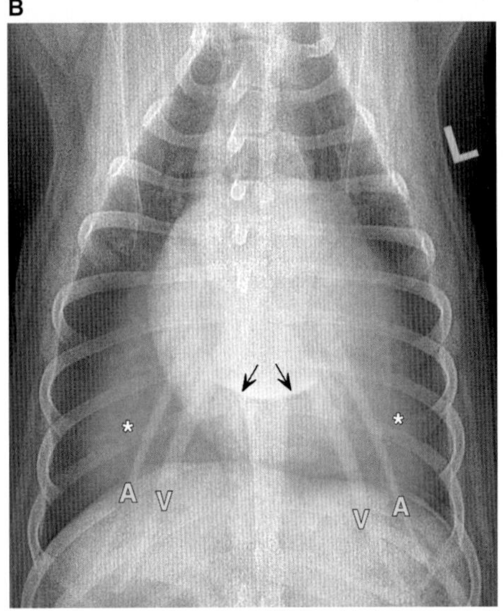

Figure 3.113 Left heart failure. Lateral view (**A**) and VD view (**B**) of a dog thorax depicting a large cardiac silhouette due to left atrial dilation and left ventricular enlargement (black arrows). The trachea is dorsally displaced by the dilated left atrium. The pulmonary veins (V) are larger than their paired arteries (A) due to venous congestion. Lung opacity is bilaterally increased in the hilar and central regions (*) due to cardiogenic pulmonary edema.

A

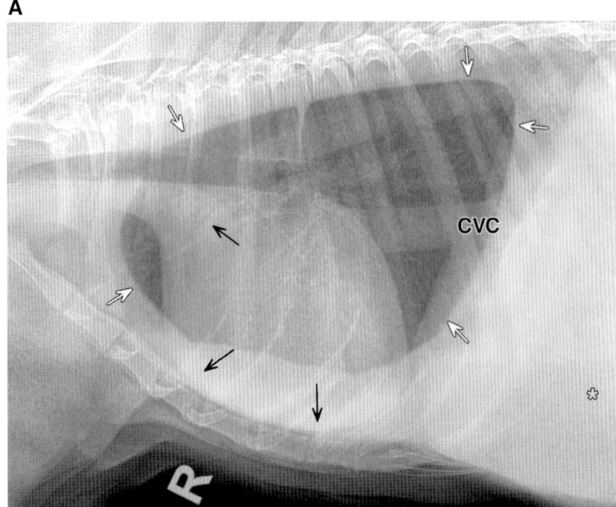

B

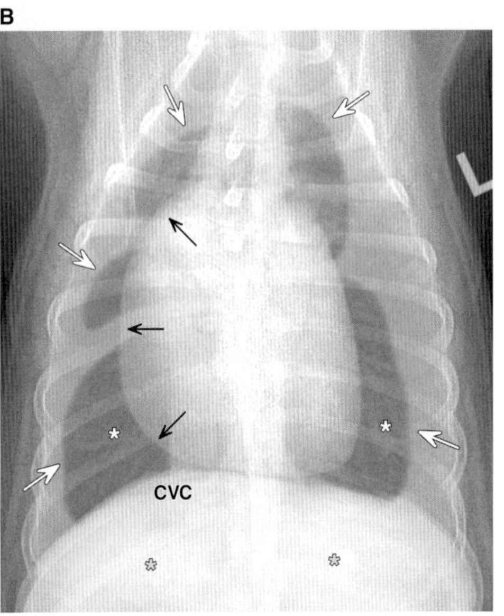

Figure 3.114 Right heart failure. Lateral view (**A**) and VD view (**B**) of a dog thorax depicting pleural effusion. Fluid in the pleural space separates the lungs from the chest wall (white arrows) and causes a diffuse increase in thoracic opacity. The cardiac silhouette is widened due to enlargement of the right atrium and right ventricle (black arrows). The pulmonary vessels are small due to reduced right ventricular output. The caudal vena cava (CVC) is large due to increased central venous pressure. At the periphery of the radiographs, the abdomen is distended, and the serosal margins are indistinct due to peritoneal effusion (*).

severe cardiac arrhythmia, electrocution). Also, an enlarged heart may return to nomal size following diuretic therapy.

Right heart failure

Right heart failure occurs when the right ventricle is ineffective in moving blood out of the heart and into the lungs. Reduced right ventricular output means the right atrium is less able to accept blood returning from the body, which increases systemic venous pressure. Elevated venous pressure can lead to venous congestion and leakage of fluid into the pleural and peritoneal cavities. Venous congestion can cause visible organomegaly, particularly in the liver and spleen. Causes of right heart failure include pericardial effusion, heartworm disease, progression of left heart failure, and others (see Differential Diagnoses). Radiographic signs of right heart failure (Figure 3.114) include:

1. Right heart enlargement.
2. Pleural effusion.
3. Peritoneal effusion.
4. Hepatomegaly and splenomegaly.

In dogs with right heart failure, peritoneal effusion tends to be more severe than pleural effusion. In cats, pleural effusion often is more evident. In both dogs and cats, the pulmonary vessels may be small due to less blood flow to the lungs. The caudal vena cava may be large due to compromised venous return.

Trachea

Normal radiographic anatomy

The trachea extends from the larynx to the base of the cardiac silhouette. It is parallel with the cervical spine and diverges ventrally from the thoracic spine. At the cardiac base, the trachea bifurcates into the right and left primary bronchi. The primary bronchi form a sharp angle at the **carina**. The carina is a ridge of cartilage at the point of branching. The terms "carina" and "tracheal bifurcation" frequently are used interchangeably. The carina is centrally located at about the fifth or sixth intercostal space.

There are approximately 35 C-shaped, cartilaginous rings in the wall of the trachea. The rings help maintain a patent airway. Each ring is open dorsally where its ends are covered by the *trachealis muscle*. The trachealis muscle (also called the **dorsal tracheal membrane**) runs along the entire length of the trachea. In young animals, the tracheal rings are soft tissue opacity and rarely distinguished in radiographs. As the animal ages, the rings commonly mineralize. Mineralization tends to occur sooner in chondrodystrophic breeds.

The inner or mucosal margin of the trachea usually is well visualized in radiographs due to the opacity interface provided by gas in the tracheal lumen. The outer or serosal tracheal margin is less distinct because it is adjacent to soft tissue and fat.

The **size of the trachea** varies normally with the patient's age and breed. The trachea is relatively smaller in immature animals than in adults. It may also be smaller in older, small breed dogs due to loss of rigidity in the tracheal rings. Some dog breeds have a relatively large trachea in relation to body size (e.g., Poodles). Some dog breeds have a relatively small trachea (e.g., English bulldogs). Tracheal size changes slightly between inspiration and expiration, but this tends to be minimally evident in radiographs of normal animals.

In many dogs, but not in cats, the distal trachea often curves slightly ventrally at the cardiac base. This normal ventral curvature may be accentuated or diminished by a mass in the hilar region. The amount of distal curvature in the canine trachea may help differentiate left atrial dilation from tracheobronchial lymphadenomegaly. In general, dilation of the left atrium elevates and straightens the distal trachea, whereas hilar lymphadenomegaly tends to push it ventrally, increasing the amount of curvature. As we indicated earlier, however, there are lymph nodes on all sides of the trachea and sometimes lymphadenomegaly will push the trachea in a different direction.

Abnormal position of the trachea

The trachea is fixed in position at the larynx and at the carina. The middle portion is flexible and easily displaced, especially in the thoracic cavity, where the trachea is least confined. Displacement of the trachea often is due to esophageal or cardiac enlargement. The direction of displacement provides clues to the etiology.

Ventral tracheal displacement most often is caused by a dilated esophagus. **Dorsal** displacement may be due to cardiac enlargement or a ventral mediastinal mass. In obese patients, the trachea may be pushed dorsally and laterally by excess mediastinal fat. **Lateral** tracheal displacement may result from a mediastinal shift, a dilated esophagus, or a large mass in the mediastinum.

Severe skeletal deformities such as pectus excavatum and spinal lordosis can distort the shape of the thorax and alter the position of the trachea.

A normal trachea may appear abnormal in position due to **flexion of the patient's head and neck**. Flexion shortens the distance between the larynx and the heart and causes the trachea in between to curve or bend (Figure 3.115). Keep in mind that many patients will try to tuck their head while being restrained for radiography. If they are allowed to do so, you may see this temporary bend in a radiograph of the trachea.

In brachycephalic and chondrodystrophic breeds, the trachea naturally appears more "curvy" because its length is confined to a shorter body. The curviness of the trachea sometimes is exaggerated during expiration when the heart moves slightly cranially.

Rotation of the patient during radiography can mimic a displaced trachea. Rotation in a VD/DV view projects the trachea to the right or left side which may be mistaken for lateral displacement. Rotation in a lateral view can make the trachea appear closer to the spine and may be mistaken for dorsal displacement and cardiac enlargement. When in doubt regarding the cause of an abnormally positioned trachea, repeat the radiographs while paying particular attention to patient positioning.

Non-visualization of the trachea may be due to tracheal collapse, tracheal rupture, or increased opacity in the mediastinum (e.g., inflammation, hemorrhage, ruptured esophagus). The trachea sometimes is less distinct in obese and heavily muscled patients due to the larger amount of overlying tissue. The same is true with summation of a large, fluid-filled esophagus, a large thoracic mass, or nearby lung disease.

Abnormal size of the trachea

The size of the trachea generally is assessed in a lateral view. The normal **width** (internal diameter) of the cervical trachea should be similar to the width of the larynx. The width of the thoracic trachea normally is about three times the width of the proximal third of the third rib. The **tracheal ratio** compares the width of the trachea to the width of the

A

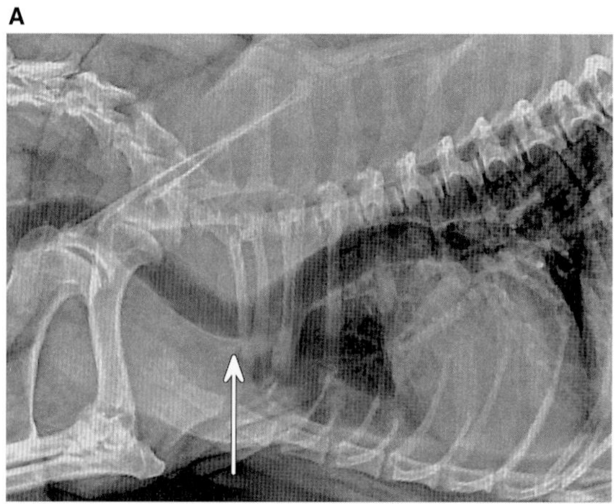

B

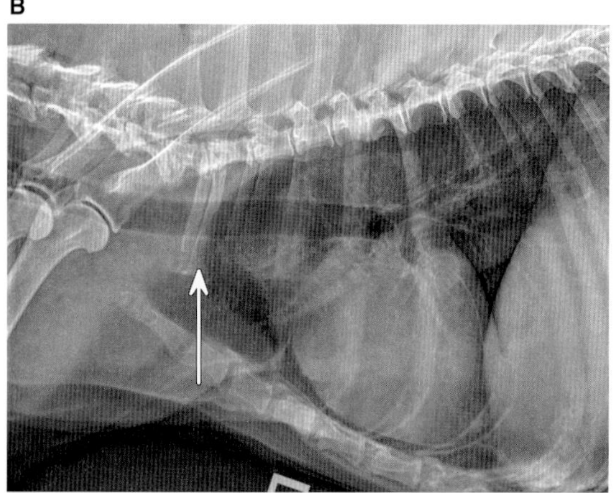

C

D

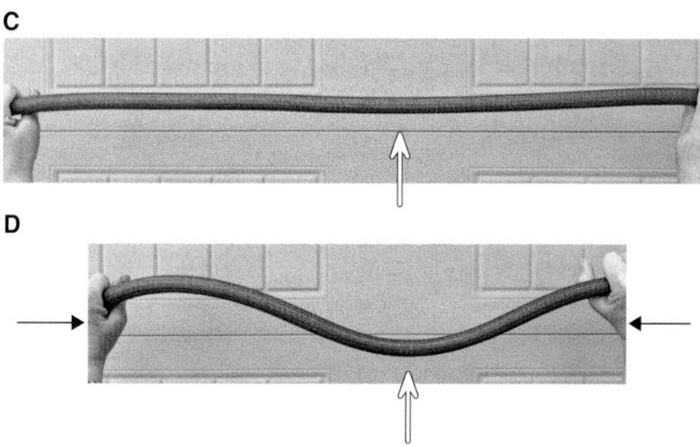

Figure 3.115 Trachea positioning artifact. **A**. Lateral view of a dog thorax with the head and neck flexed. Flexion shortens the distance between the larynx and the hilus, causing a temporary bend in the trachea (arrow). **B**. Lateral view of the same dog with the head and neck extended. There is no bend in the trachea (arrow). **C**. In this picture, a section of flexible garden hose is stretched between two hands. The middle portion is straight (arrow). **D**. In this picture, the same hands are holding the same garden hose, but the hands are moved closer together. Shortening the distance between the ends of the hose causes a bend in the middle (arrow).

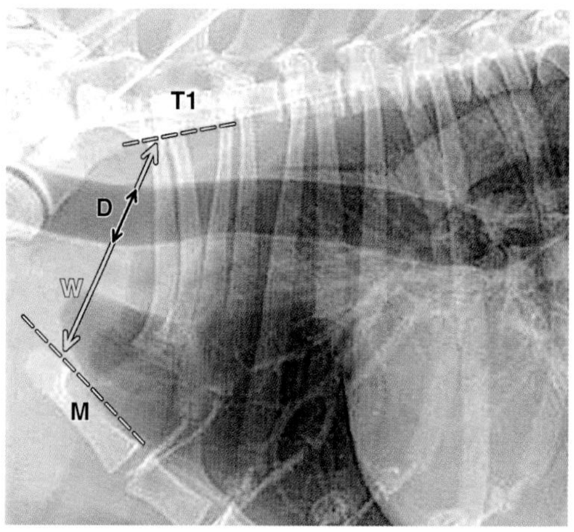

Figure 3.116 Tracheal ratio. Lateral view of a dog thorax depicting the tracheal ratio method for assessing tracheal size. This method compares the internal diameter of the trachea (D) to the width of the thoracic inlet (W). D is measured from mucosa to mucosa. W Thoracic inlet width is measure from the craniodorsal edge of the manubrium (M) to the cranioventral edge of the T1 thoracic vertebra. The Tracheal Ratio (TR) is calculated by dividing D by W (TR = D/W). TR = D/W. Normal TR for most dogs is $\geq$0.20. For brachycephalic dogs it should be $\geq$0.16 and for Bulldogs it should be $\geq$0.12.

thoracic inlet (Figure 3.116). As with all measurement techniques used in radiography, tracheal ratio should be considered a general guideline or "rule of thumb" and not an absolute measurement.

Small or narrowed trachea

Greater than 50% narrowing of the tracheal lumen is abnormal. Narrowing may be localized, segmental, or diffuse. **Static** narrowing repeats unchanged in serial radiographs. **Dynamic** narrowing varies between radiographs and may only be evident during either inspiration or expiration. Causes of a small trachea include stenosis, hypoplasia, tracheal collapse syndrome, and thickening of the tracheal wall. Each of these can partially or completely obstruct airflow (as discussed on the following pages). Clinical signs associated with a small trachea may not manifest unless narrowing is greater than 80%.

Conditions that may mimic a narrowed trachea often are related to positioning artifacts. Over-stretching the patient during radiography can temporarily narrow the tracheal lumen, especially in cats (Figure 3.117). Rotation of the patient in a lateral view may lead to summation of the dorsal tracheal membrane on the tracheal lumen, which may be mistaken for a narrowed lumen or a redundant membrane. Close inspection, however, often reveals the true dorsal margin of the trachea. When in doubt, repeat the radiograph paying particular attention to patient positioning.

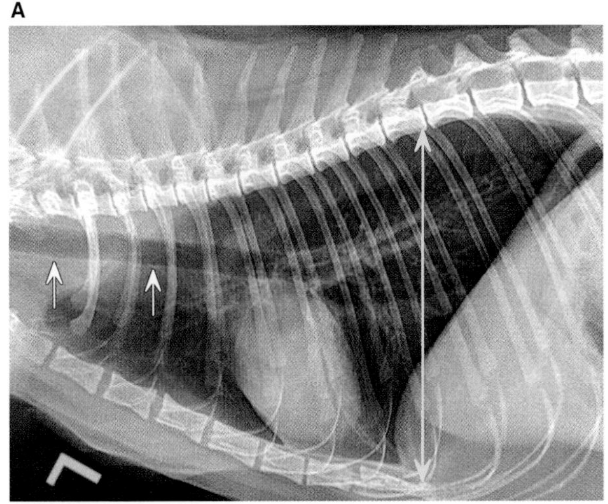

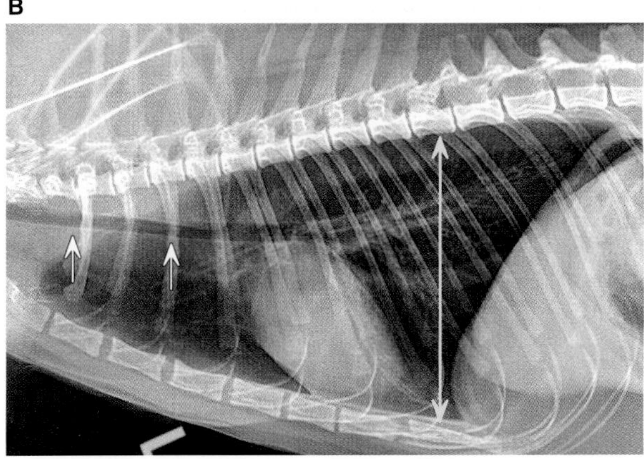

Figure 3.117 Artifactual narrowing of the trachea. Lateral views of a cat thorax depicting the patient in a relaxed position (**A**) and hyperextended due to overstretching (**B**). Notice that overstretching the cat causes significant dorsoventral narrowing of the thoracic cavity (yellow double-headed arrow) and narrowing of the trachea (white arrows).

Sometimes the trachea is oblique to the x-ray beam even in a well-positioned patient. This occurs because the trachea naturally rotates as it courses from the cervical region to the thoracic region (Figure 3.118). Where the trachea is oblique to the x-ray beam, its dorsal membrane may be superimposed on its lumen.

Tracheal stenosis is a static, localized narrowing that can occur anywhere along the trachea (Figure 3.119). A stenosis may be congenital due to a developmental abnormality or it may be acquired secondary to trauma or severe inflammation. External compression can cause a functional stenosis, but this is rare because the trachea is quite rigid and more likely to be displaced than narrowed.

Tracheal hypoplasia is a congenital, static narrowing that usually involves the entire trachea, but can be segmental (Figure 3.120). It most often occurs in brachycephalic and chondrodystrophic dogs due to abnormal development of the tracheal rings. The rings develop as complete or nearly complete circles with little or no dorsal tracheal membrane. In a skyline view (Figure 3.123), a hypoplastic trachea appears very round with a small size lumen. The mainstem bronchi may be as large or larger than the or they too may be hypoplastic. When tracheal hypoplasia is suspected in an immature patient, confirm the diagnosis by making follow-up radiographs as the animal matures. Tracheal growth sometimes is slower in certain individuals and the trachea may eventually grow to normal size.

Tracheal collapse syndrome is a dynamic narrowing that can affect part or all of the trachea. Because it is dynamic,

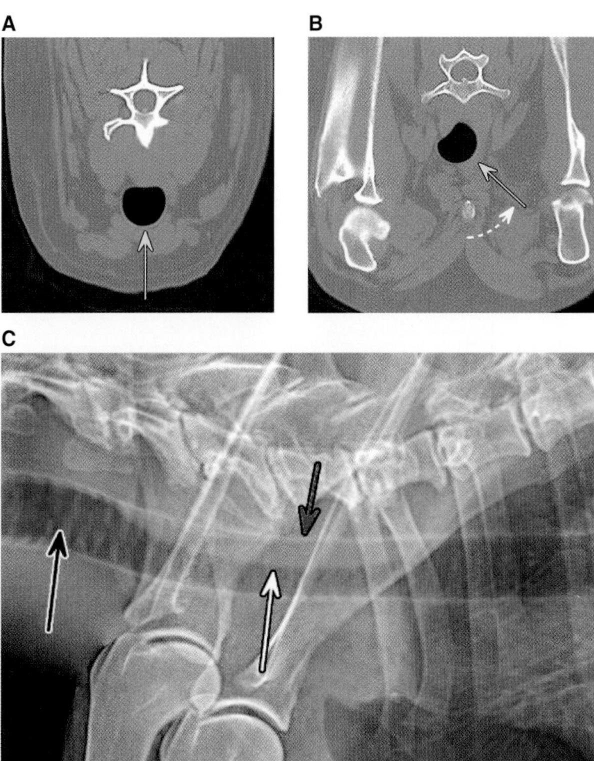

Figure 3.118 False narrowing of the trachea. Cross-sectional CT images of a dog neck depicting the appearance of the trachea in the middle cervical region (**A**) and further caudally, near the thoracic inlet (**B**). The trachea (yellow arrow) naturally rotates in the caudal cervical region (dashed arrow). (**C**) Lateral view of a dog trachea. The dorsal tracheal membrane is visible in the lumen of the caudal cervical trachea (white arrow) because the trachea is rotated here. The dorsal tracheal membrane is not seen in the mid-cervical tracheal lumen (black arrow) because here the trachea is aligned with the x-ray beam. The soft tissue opacity created by the dorsal membrane in the caudal cervical region may be mistaken for the dorsal border of the trachea, leading to a false diagnosis of a narrowed tracheal lumen. Close inspection, however, reveals the true dorsal tracheal border (red arrow). Notice that this artifactual narrowing of the trachea is not caused by superimposition of an adjacent structure, such as the esophagus, longus coli muscles, or mediastinum.

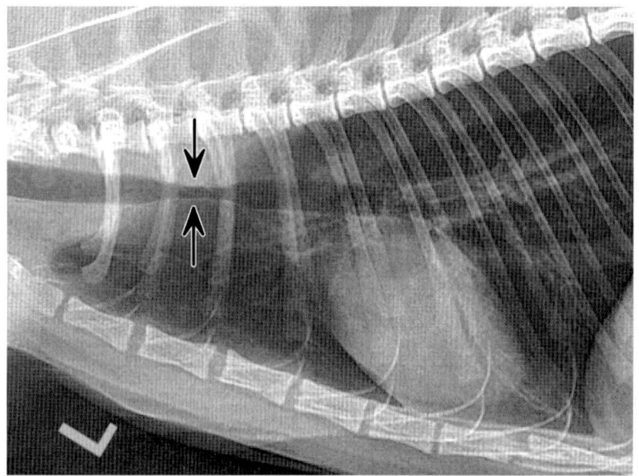

Figure 3.119 Tracheal stenosis. Lateral view of a cat thorax depicting a localized narrowing in the trachea (arrows) due to a stricture.

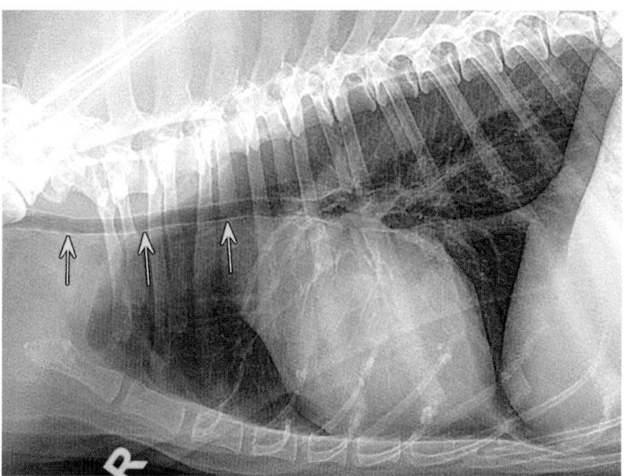

Figure 3.120 Tracheal hypoplasia. Lateral view of a dog thorax depicting uniform narrowing of the tracheal lumen (arrows) due to congenital malformation of the tracheal rings.

collapse may only be intermittently evident in radiographs (Figure 3.121). Diagnosis often requires radiographs made during both inspiration and expiration – and even then the full extent and severity of tracheal collapse may not be apparent.

Tracheal collapse syndrome most often is reported in middle-aged, small breed dogs (Yorkshire terriers are over-represented). It is rare in cats and large breed dogs. The collapse is due to a congenital or acquired weakness in the cartilage. The weakening is progressive and eventually leads to irreversible flattening of the tracheal rings. As mentioned, the bronchi may also be involved. As the rings flatten, the dorsal tracheal membrane stretches, becoming more flaccid and *redundant*. A **redundant dorsal membrane** may be sucked into the tracheal lumen during inspiration and blown outward during expiration.

As mentioned earlier, diagnosis of tracheal collapse syndrome often requires both inspiratory and expiratory radiographs. The cervical trachea is more likely to collapse during inspiration and the thoracic trachea during expiration. Collapse of a weak cervical trachea is caused by the vacuum effect that occurs during inhalation, pulling the tracheal walls inward like sucking air through a straw (Figure 3.122). During expiration, a redundant dorsal membrane in the cervical trachea may "balloon" outward, widening the tracheal lumen. Collapse of a weak thoracic trachea is caused by the increased pressure in the thoracic cavity that occurs during expiration (Figure 3.121). The primary bronchi also may collapse.

In a lateral view, the dorsal border of the trachea may appear indistinct or "doubled" due to superimposition of a

A

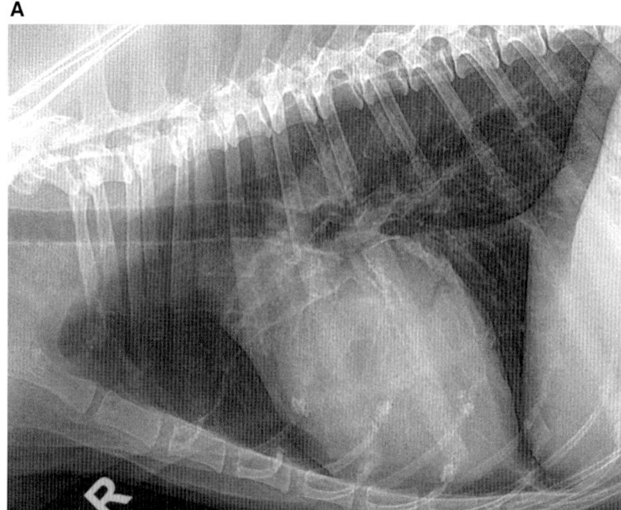

B

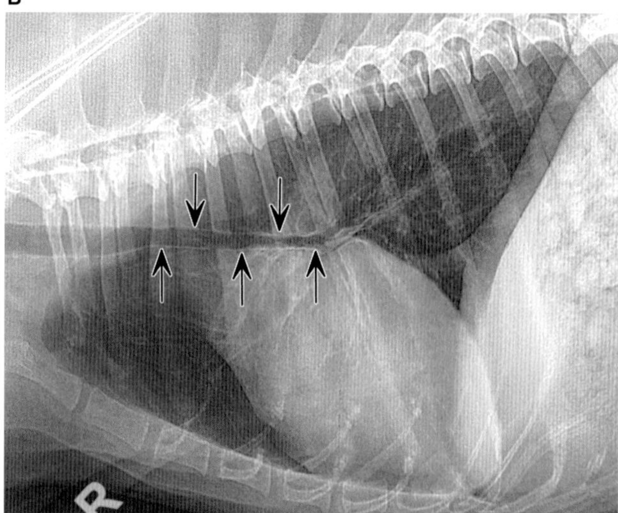

Figure 3.121 Tracheal collapse syndrome. Two lateral views depicting the same dog thorax. **A**. During inspiration, the tracheal lumen is normal size. **B**. During expiration, increased intra-thoracic pressure collapses the distal trachea and primary bronchi (black arrows).

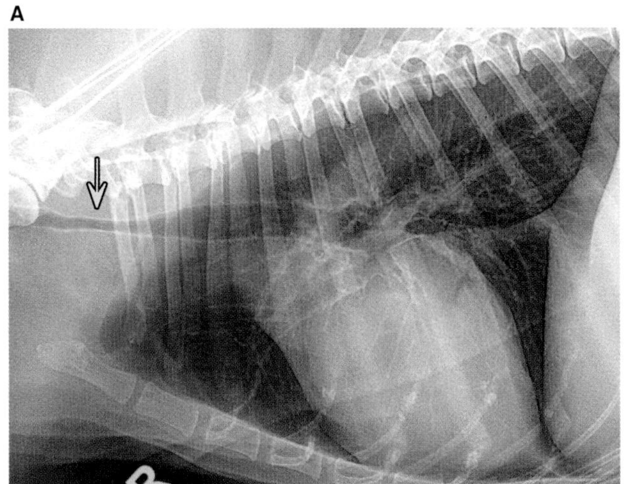

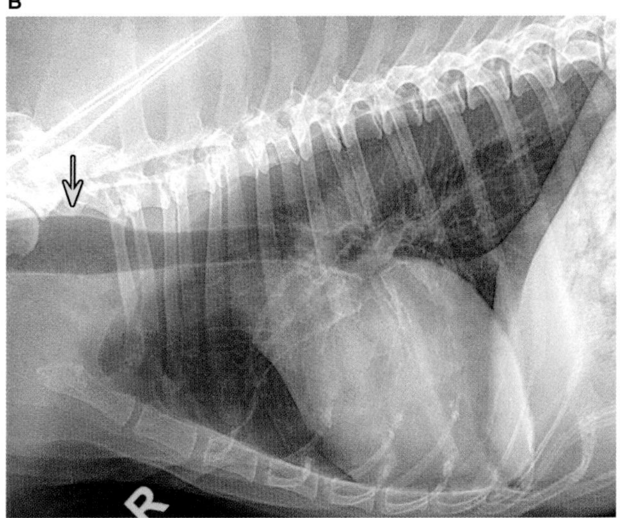

Figure 3.122 Cervical tracheal collapse syndrome. Two lateral views depicting the same dog thorax. **A**. During inspiration, the redundant dorsal tracheal membrane in the caudal cervical region is sucked inward, narrowing the tracheal lumen (arrow). **B**. During expiration, the dorsal membrane balloons outward, widening the tracheal lumen (arrow).

redundant dorsal membrane. The ventral tracheal border usually remains well-defined, but sometimes it too is indistinct or irregular due to inflammation, exudates, or deformed tracheal rings. In a skyline view, a collapsed trachea typically appears crescent-shaped (Figure 3.123).

The characteristic clinical sign of tracheal collapse syndrome is a chronic, non-productive, "honking" cough. The cough increases in severity over time and may be aggravated by conditions such as obesity, pulling against a collar, secondhand smoke, and others. The carina is the most sensitive part of the trachea and anything that pushes on a weakened distal trachea can induce coughing (e.g., left atrial dilation, tracheobronchial lymphadenomegaly, megaesophagus). Secondary complications associated with chronic or

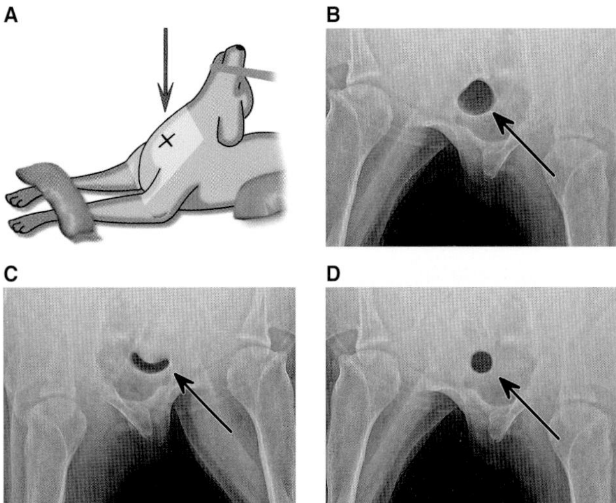

Figure 3.123 Skyline views of the trachea. **A**. This illustration depicts the patient positioning for a "skyline" radiograph of the trachea. **B**. Skyline view depicting a normal trachea (arrow). **C**. Skyline view depicting tracheal collapse with the characteristic crescent-shaped lumen (arrow). **D**. Skyline view depicting a hypoplastic trachea with a small, round lumen (arrow).

severe tracheal collapse syndrome include airway inflammation, aspiration pneumonia, and pulmonary hypertension.

Thickening of the tracheal wall may be diffuse or focal and creates static narrowing of the trachea. Diffuse thickening (Figure 3.124) may be due to edema, inflammation, or hemorrhage. Thickening often results in an indistinct serosal

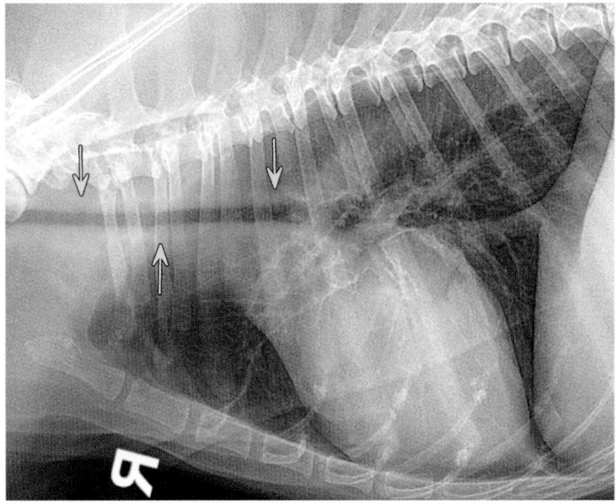

Figure 3.124 Thickened tracheal wall. Lateral view of a dog thorax depicting diffuse thickening of the tracheal wall (arrows) and uniform narrowing of the tracheal lumen. The serosal (outer) borders of the trachea are indistinct, making it difficult to identify the edges of the tracheal wall. The primary radiographic finding is a narrowed tracheal lumen.

margin and sometimes the only radiographic finding is a narrowed tracheal lumen. It may be difficult to differentiate a thickened tracheal wall from stenosis, hypoplasia, or collapse. Focal thickening (Figure 3.125) usually is due to a mass (e.g., tumor, granuloma, polyp, abscess, cyst, hematoma). Soft tissue opacity masses may be visible as they project into the tracheal lumen. Tracheal masses sometimes mineralize. The mucosal margin of the trachea may be even or irregular at the site of a mass.

Large or widened trachea

Generalized enlargement or dilation of the trachea is uncommon and often a subjective assessment. As a normal variant, the trachea is relatively large in some dog breeds. Severe inspiratory dyspnea due to upper airway obstruction may cause tracheal dilation.

Localized or segmental widening of the trachea may be due to ballooning of a redundant dorsal tracheal membrane in a patient with tracheal collapse syndrome (Figure 3.122). This "ballooning" of the trachea tends to be a temporary condition that usually occurs during expiration. A seldom reported cause of focal widening of the trachea is external adhesions that pull on the tracheal wall.

Abnormal opacity associated with the trachea

Growths, foreign objects, and aspirated materials in the tracheal increase its luminal opacity and may obscure its mucosal margin. Growths such as tumors, polyps, granulomas, etc., tend to be well-defined due to the gas opacity interface provided by air in the tracheal lumen. Indistinct margins may be caused by adjacent fluid (e.g., exudates, inflammation). Tracheal growths must be large enough to be detected in radiographs, typically at least 5–10 mm in size. Growths that mineralize may be visible at a smaller size.

Foreign objects in the trachea also must be large enough or opaque enough to be detected in radiographs (Figure 3.126). Mineral and metal opacity objects usually are readily identified. Soft tissue opacity objects frequently are visible because they are surrounded by gas but may be obscured by superimposition of adjacent structures.

Foreign objects may enter the trachea via inhalation or migration. **Inhaled** objects that are small enough to pass through the trachea frequently lodge at the tracheal bifurcation. Smaller inhaled objects may pass into a primary bronchus or beyond. Solid materials tend to enter the right caudal bronchus because it is a straight path from the trachea. Fluids are more likely to flow with gravity into the right middle bronchus due to its anatomy.

Mineralization of the tracheal rings is a common aging change in older dogs and cats. It occurs earlier in large breed and chondrodystrophic dogs. Dystrophic mineralization in other parts of the trachea may result from chronic inflammation or hypercortisolism.

Ruptured trachea

Tracheal rupture most often is caused by external trauma (e.g., penetrating wound, laceration, blunt force). It also can result from foreign objects and invasive or necrotic masses. Iatrogenic causes of tracheal rupture include faulty intubation, overinflation of an endotracheal tube cuff, and a complication from venipuncture.

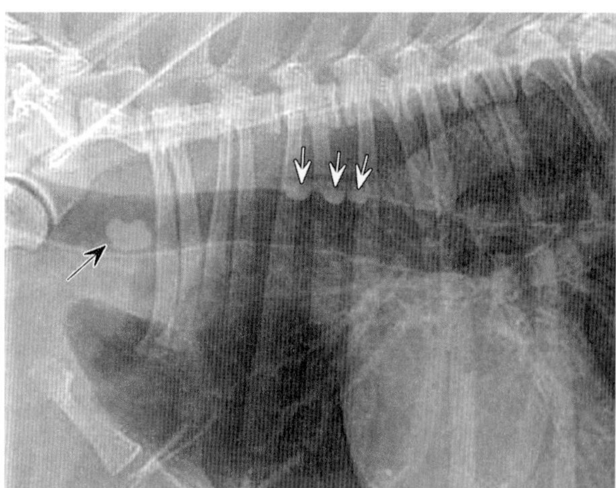

Figure 3.125 Tracheal mass. Lateral view of a dog thorax depicting mural lesions along the trachea. There is an irregular shaped, soft tissue opacity structure near the thoracic inlet (black arrow), which may represent a tumor, polyp, or foreign object. Further distally along the dorsal tracheal wall, there are three soft tissue nodules (white arrows), which are typical in appearance and location for granulomas caused by parasites. Notice that the margins of structures that project into the tracheal lumen are well-defined because they are surrounded by gas.

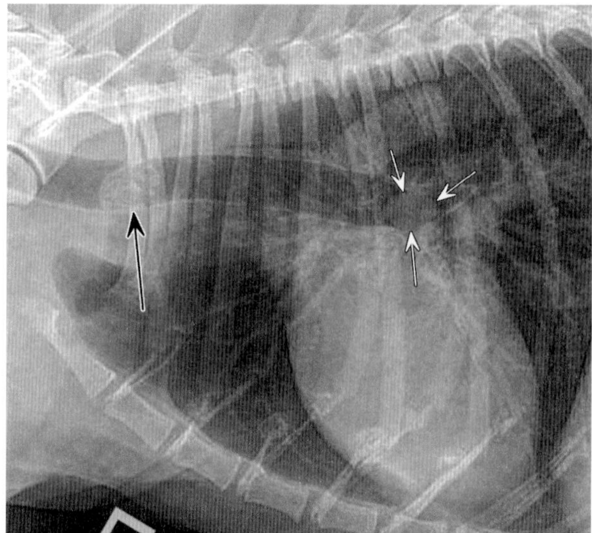

Figure 3.126 Tracheal foreign objects. Lateral view of a dog thorax. Soft tissue opacity objects are depicted in the tracheal lumen, one located near the thoracic inlet (black arrow) and another lodged distally at the tracheal bifurcation (white arrows).

Complete tearing of the trachea is called an avulsion. Tracheal avulsions tend to occur more often in the thoracic cavity. Soft tissue swelling usually accompanies an acute tracheal rupture, but the actual lesion site rarely is identified due to the severe emphysema that commonly follows. Gas leaking from the trachea readily migrates into the cervical fascia, mediastinum, and subcutaneous tissues (Figure 3.63).

Tracheal avulsion more often is reported in cats, usually secondary to blunt force thoracic trauma. In cats that survive the avulsion, healing may result in the formation of a gas-filled sac or "pseudo-airway" that appears in radiographs as an ill-defined area of localized dilation in the trachea.

Lungs

Normal radiographic anatomy

The paired lungs contain over 1000 kilometers of airways, hundreds of millions of air sacs, and receive two separate blood supplies. The pulmonary **parenchyma** is the functional part of the lungs. This is where gas exchange occurs. The parenchyma is composed of numerous air spaces called **alveoli**. Note: the alveoli are not tissue, they are air spaces. The alveoli form groups at the end of each terminal bronchiole. A group of alveoli with their terminal bronchiole is called an **acinus** (pleural **acini**). The diffusion of oxygen and carbon dioxide actually occur at the acini. The pulmonary **interstitium** is the supportive framework of the lungs. It includes connective tissue, capillaries, nerves, lymphatics and it forms the walls of the alveoli.

The two lungs are similar but not identical. They differ in the number of **lung lobes** and in their vascular and bronchial anatomy. The right lung consists of four lobes (cranial, middle, caudal, and accessory). The left lung consists of two lobes (cranial and caudal). The left cranial lung lobe is subdivided into cranial and caudal segments, which are analogous to cranial and middle lung lobes (Figure 3.127).

To help describe radiographic findings, the lungs are divided into three **lung regions**; *hilar, central,* and *peripheral* (Figure 3.128). These regions also aid in distinguishing lobar diseases such as pneumonia from generalized lung diseases such as pulmonary edema.

The hilar region is the innermost part of the lungs. It includes the tracheal bifurcation, primary bronchi, tracheobronchial lymph nodes, and the base of the cardiac silhouette. The central region is the middle part of the lungs. It contains the easily visible pulmonary vessels and bronchi. The peripheral region refers to the outermost parts of the lungs. These areas are mostly air-filled with only tiny vascular and bronchial markings.

The lung vasculature includes *bronchial* and *pulmonary* arterial supplies. The bronchial arteries are part of the systemic circulation and provide oxygenated blood for lung nutrition. They are too small to be seen in radiographs. The **pulmonary arteries** bring deoxygenated blood from the

A

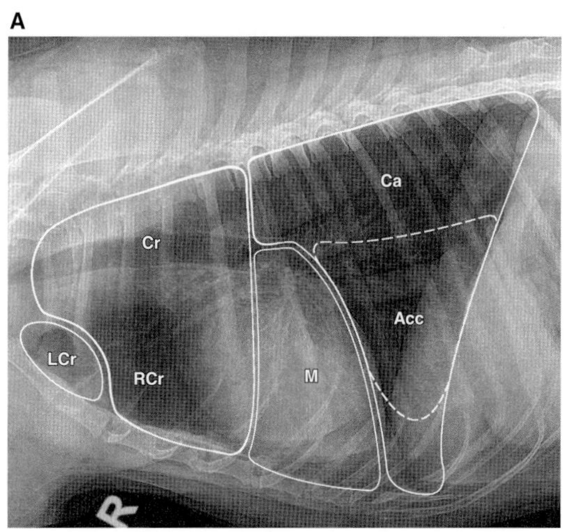

B

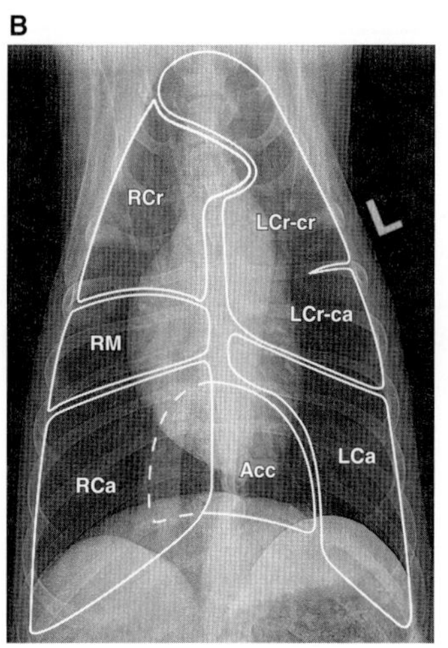

C

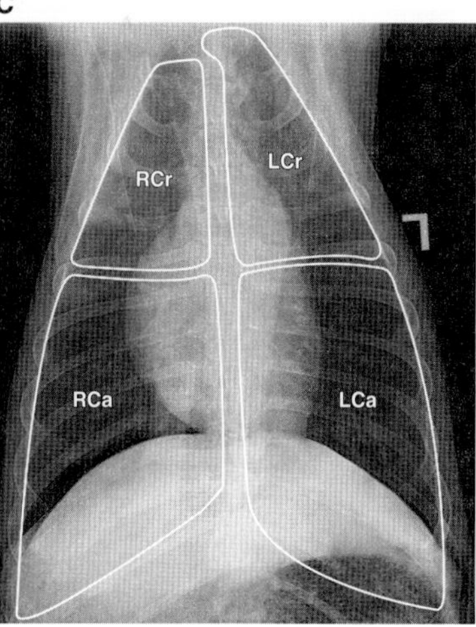

Figure 3.127 Lung lobe borders. Lateral view (**A**), VD view (**B**), and DV view (**C**) of a dog thorax illustrating the edges of the individual lung lobes. The lung lobe edges that are ventral to the trachea are illustrated in the VD view (**B**) and the lung lobe edges that are dorsal to the trachea are shown in the DV view (**C**).

Acc = accessory lobe.
Cr = cranial lung lobes.
Ca = caudal lung lobes.
M = middle lung lobes.
RCa = right caudal lobe.
RCr = right cranial lobe.
RM = right middle lobe.
LCa = left caudal lobe.
LCr = left cranial lobe.
LCr-cr = left cranial lobe, cranial segment,
LCr-ca = left cranial lobe, caudal segment.

A

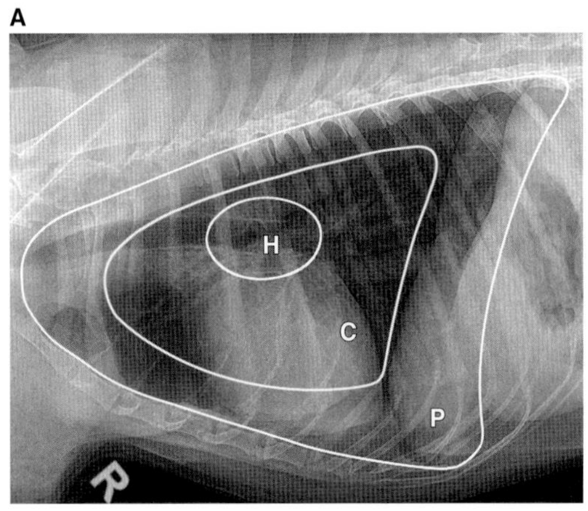

B

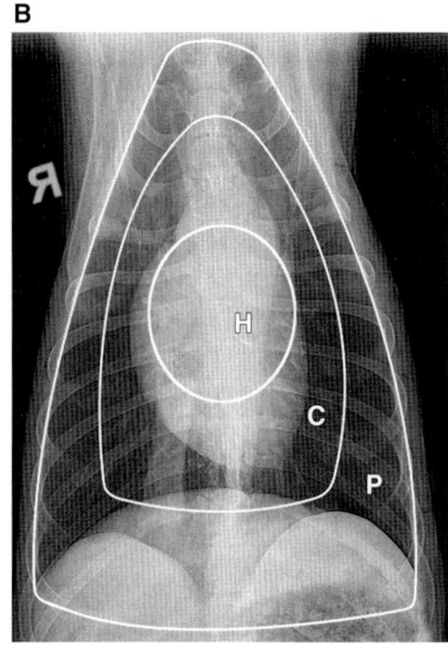

Figure 3.128 Lung regions. Lateral view (**A**) and VD view (**B**) of a dog thorax illustrating the lung regions used to describe radiographic findings.

H = hilar; the innermost lung field.
C = central; the middle lungs where the larger blood vessels and bronchi are visible.
P = peripheral; the outermost lungs that are mostly gas opacity, where tiny vessels and bronchi may be visible.

heart to the lungs for gas exchange. Pulmonary vessels account for nearly 99% of the blood volume in the lungs.

The main pulmonary artery emerges from the right ventricle and divides into the right and left primary pulmonary arteries, which extend into the right and left lungs (Figure 3.129). The lung vessels are largest and most visible near the heart (hilar and central lung regions) and gradually taper into the lung periphery.

Pulmonary arteries and veins travel in pairs. The paired vessels normally are similar in size and course. The arteries are positioned cranial, dorsal, and lateral to the veins (or the veins are caudal, ventral, and medial to the arteries). A helpful memory device: *"veins are ventral and central to arteries."*

The right and left **cranial lobar pulmonary vessels** usually are easier to see in a lateral view than in a VD/DV view, particularly in a left lateral view. This is because the anatomical arrangement of the vessels allows them to be further separated when the patient is in left lateral recumbency as opposed to right lateral recumbency. The right cranial vessels are ventral to the left pair (Figure 3.130). The right cranial artery and vein often are easier to distinguish because fewer mediastinal structures are superimposed. The right and left pulmonary vessels in the other lung lobes are superimposed in lateral views and not as easily distinguished.

The right and left **caudal lobar pulmonary vessels** usually are easier to see in a DV/VD view, particularly in a DV view. They tend to be more distinct in a DV view because in ventral recumbency, the dorsocaudal lungs are better inflated, and the vessels are more perpendicular to the x-ray beam. As a rule of thumb, the normal width of the caudal pulmonary vessels should not exceed the width of the ninth rib, where vessel and rib overlap (Figure 3.131).

Between each pair of pulmonary vessels is a bronchus. The arrangement is **artery-bronchus-vein** or A-B-V, moving from cranial-to-caudal, dorsal-to-ventral, or lateral-to-medial (Figures 3.132 and 3.133).

The **bronchi** form a tree-like structure of branching tubes that serves to conduct gas to and from the lung parenchyma (Figure 3.134). The **primary** or *mainstem* bronchi are the initial branches that come from the trachea and lead into the right and left lungs. The primary bronchi divide into **secondary** bronchi to supply the individual lung lobes. The **tertiary** bronchi currently are considered to be the smallest airways visible in radiographs; however, advances in digital imaging are constantly improving radiographic detail. Bronchial branching ends with the terminal bronchioles that supply the alveoli, which are not visible in radiographs.

The bronchial walls contain cartilage to prevent collapse. The cartilage helps make the bronchi visible in radiographs. When viewed end-on, bronchi appear as circles or **rings**. When viewed in profile, bronchi appear as gradually converging lines, commonly called **tramlines** or sometimes "railroad tracks" (Figures 3.135 and 3.136). Collectively, bronchial rings and tramlines are called **bronchial markings**. As with the pulmonary vessels, the bronchi are largest and easiest to see near the heart (in the hilar and central lung regions) and gradually taper into the peripheral lungs. Many bronchial markings will appear incomplete because the rings or tramlines are not well-aligned with the x-ray beam. Bronchi generally cannot be traced as far into the lung periphery as the vessels. That said, a few peripheral rings and tramlines will be visible in every radiograph because some normal bronchi will be aligned with the x-ray beam. However, a large number of peripheral bronchial markings suggests bronchial disease.

Evaluating the lungs

Most pulmonary diseases lead to increased lung opacity. A few diseases can lead to decreased lung opacity, either due to an increase in pulmonary gas (e.g., destruction of lung tissue) or a decrease in pulmonary soft tissue (e.g., reduced blood flow to the lung).

A

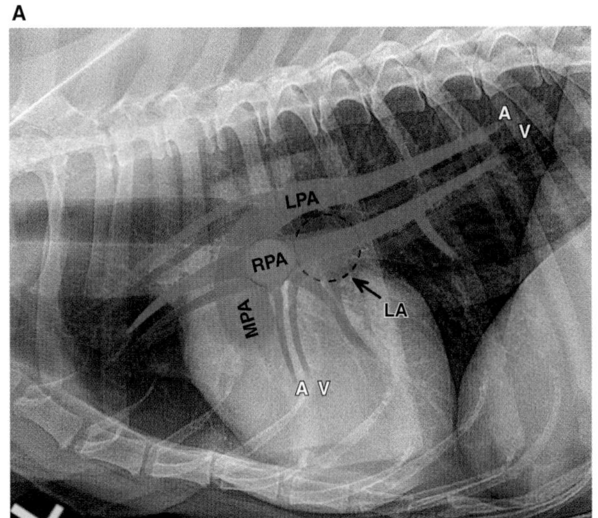

B

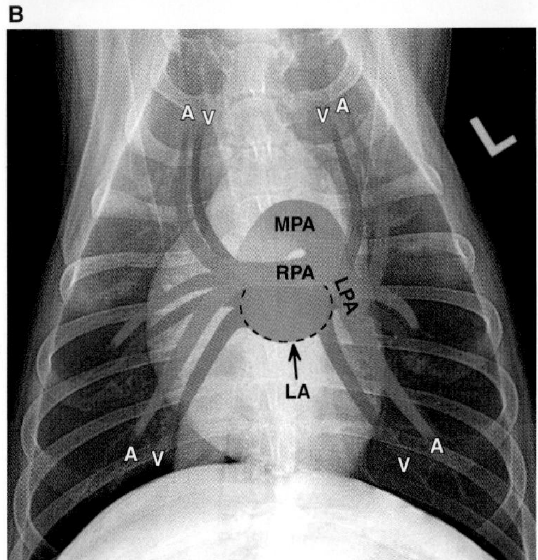

Figure 3.129 Normal pulmonary vasculature. Lateral view (**A**) and DV view (**B**) of a dog thorax illustrating the pulmonary arteries (A, highlighted in blue for deoxygenated blood) and the pulmonary veins (V, highlighted in red for oxygenated blood). In the lateral view, the arteries are cranial and dorsal to their paired veins. In the DV view, the arteries are caudal and lateral to the veins. MPA = main pulmonary artery, LPA = left pulmonary artery, RPA = right pulmonary artery, LA = left atrium.

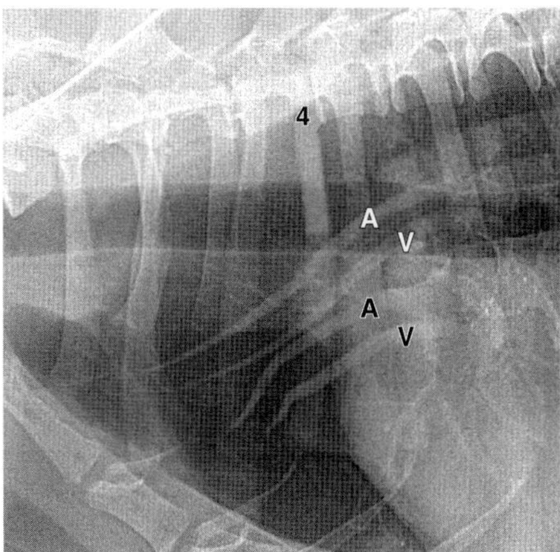

Figure 3.130 Cranial lobar pulmonary vessels. Left lateral view of a dog thorax depicting the normal sizes and positions of the paired cranial lobar pulmonary vessels. The left cranial artery and vein (white A,V) are dorsal to the right cranial artery and vein (black A,V). The width of each vessel should not exceed the width of the narrowest part of the fourth rib (4), measured at the third or fourth intercostal space.

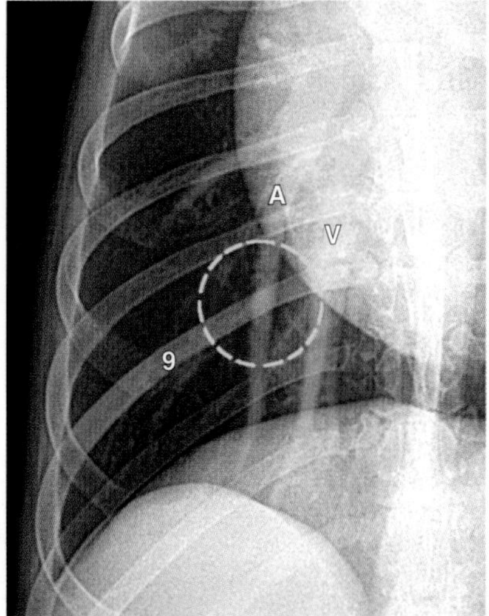

Figure 3.131 Caudal pulmonary vessels. VD view of a dog thorax depicting the appearance of the right caudal pulmonary artery (A) and vein (V). The width of each vessel should not exceed the width of the ninth rib (9), where vessel and rib overlap (dotted circle).

A systematic approach is essential when evaluating the lungs. Otherwise you may miss valuable information. Here's one approach: begin with the pulmonary vessels because they tend to be the first things we see when looking at normal lung radiographs. Blood vessels viewed end-on may resemble nodules, so the next thing to look for are pulmonary nodules. After the blood vessels, the next most likely structures we expect to see are the bronchi. We need to determine whether the number of bronchial markings is abnormally increased. After evaluating the bronchi, we assess the lung parenchyma, looking for regions of abnormal opacity. Finally, we examine the areas outside the lungs for evidence of disease, such as gas or fluid in the pleural space, damage to the thoracic wall, or an abnormal cardiac silhouette. We will discuss each of these in the following pages:

1. Abnormal pulmonary vessels.
2. Nodular lung lesions.
3. Abnormal bronchi.
4. Abnormal lung parenchyma.

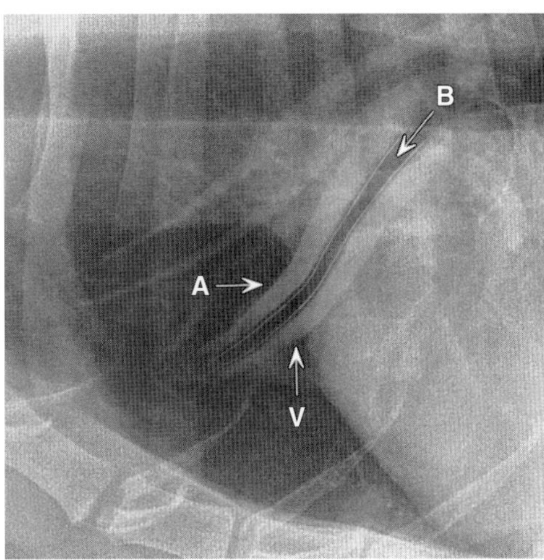

Figure 3.132 Artery-bronchus-vein. Lateral view of a dog thorax depicting the right cranial lobar bronchus (B) between the paired right cranial pulmonary artery (A) and vein (V). Notice the bronchus does not occupy the entire space between the vessels.

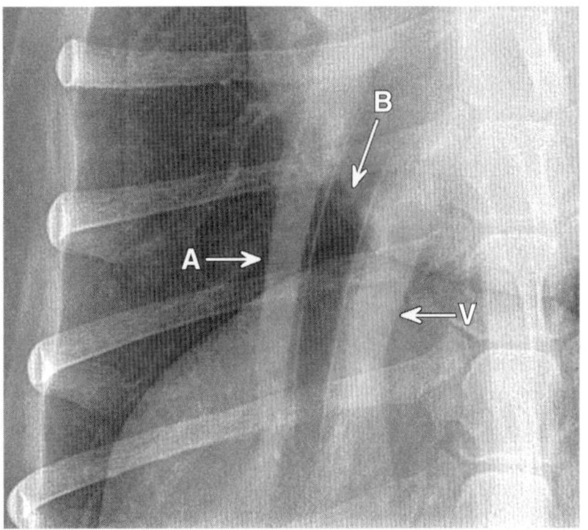

Figure 3.133 Artery-bronchus-vein. VD view of a dog thorax depicting the right caudal lobar bronchus (B) between the paired right caudal pulmonary artery (A) and vein (V). The bronchus does not occupy the entire space between the vessels.

A

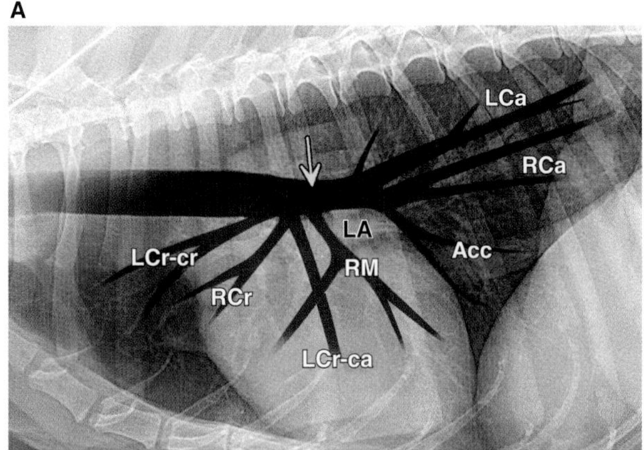

B

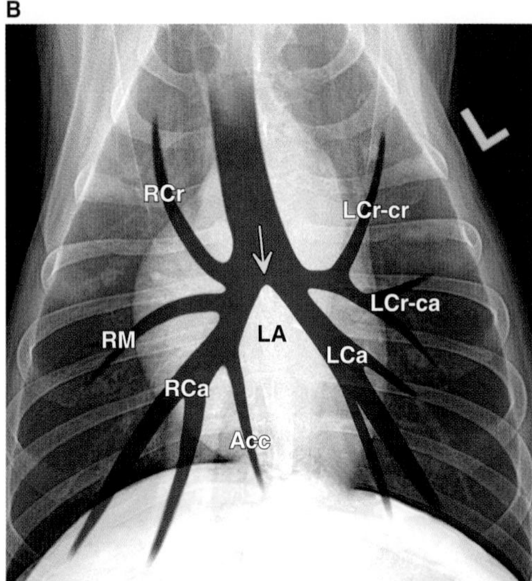

Figure 3.134 Normal bronchi. Lateral view (**A**) and DV view (**B**) of a dog thorax illustrating the bronchial tree. The trachea bifurcates into the right and left primary bronchi at the carina (white arrow). The primary bronchi diverge from the trachea at a sharp angle, about 60°–90°. The left atrium (LA) is located immediately ventral and slightly caudal to the carina. The right primary bronchus branches to supply the right cranial lung lobe (RCr), the right middle lobe (RM), the right caudal lobe (RCa), and the accessory lobe (Acc). The accessory bronchus actually stems from the right caudal bronchus. The left primary bronchus branches to supply the left cranial lobe and the left caudal lobe (LCa). The branch to the left cranial lobe immediately divides to supply the cranial and caudal subsegments of the left cranial lobe (LCr-cr and LCr-ca respectively).

Prior to interpreting your radiographic findings, it is important to evaluate the technical quality of the radiographs and the patient's body habitus. Expiration, underexposure, and obesity all can increase lung opacity and may be misinterpreted as parenchymal disease. Disease outside the lungs, such as pleural effusion, also can cause an apparent increase in lung opacity.

If the lungs are more opaque than normal and it is not due to artifact or extrapulmonary disease, then it is time to describe the lesions. Determine the location of the lung opacification (e.g., ventral, central, dorsal, hilar, cranial, caudal) and its distribution (e.g., focal, lobar, multifocal, diffuse, symmetrical, asymmetrical). It is not important to classify parenchymal disease as an "interstitial pattern" or an "alveolar pattern," both patterns are caused by the same diseases.

Lung patterns have long been used in an attempt to narrow the list of possible causes for abnormal appearing lungs (Box 3.2). We like patterns because they help us with learning and recognition. However, lung diseases rarely fit one specific pattern. Trying to select a pattern that fits the radiographic findings can be confusing and frustrating.

The lungs respond to pathology in only a limited number of ways. Different diseases frequently produce similar

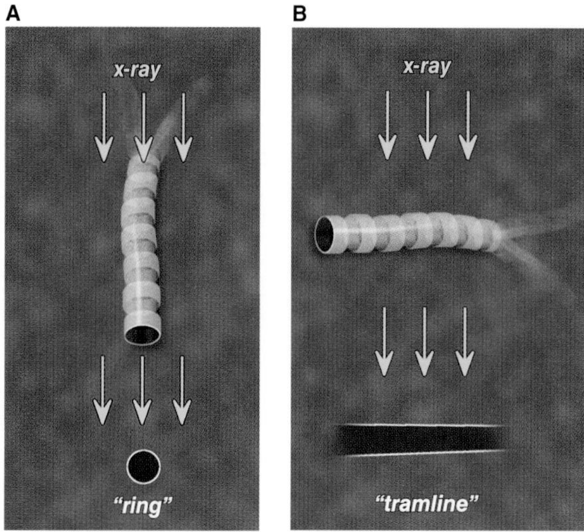

Figure 3.135 Rings and tramlines. **A**. This illustration depicts an isolated bronchus that is aligned with the x-ray beam. The bronchus is viewed end-on and would appear as a "ring" in the radiograph. **B**. Another isolated bronchus, but this one is perpendicular to the x-ray beam. The bronchus is viewed from the side or in profile and would appear as a "tramline" in the radiograph.

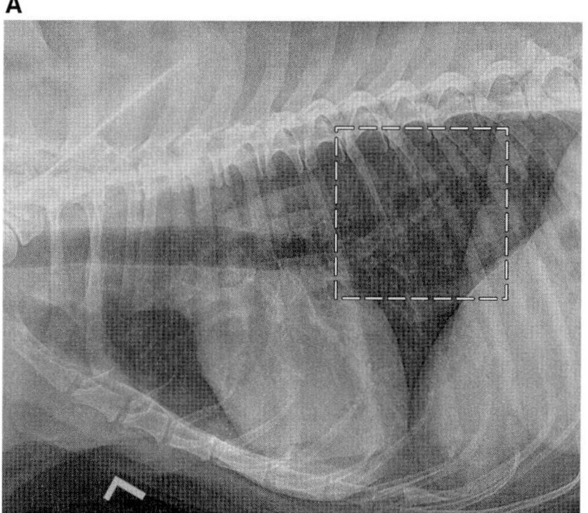

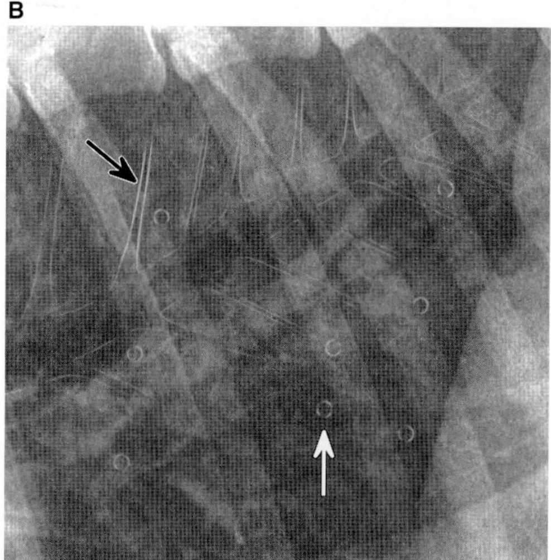

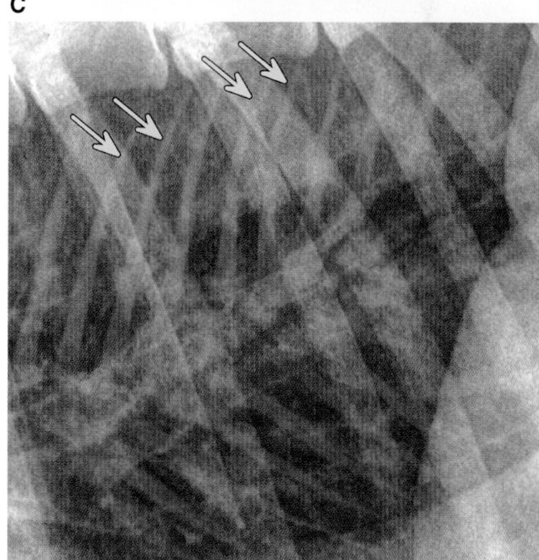

Figure 3.136 Bronchial and vascular markings. **A**. Lateral view of a normal dog thorax depicting the area to be viewed close up (white dashed square). **B**. Close-up view of A with some of the bronchial walls highlighted to produce more visible rings (white arrow) and tramlines (black arrow). **C**. Close-up view of A with the caudal pulmonary blood vessels highlighted (yellow arrows); the vessels may be mistaken for bronchial walls.

radiographic signs. The radiographic appearance of many lung diseases will vary as the disease progresses or regresses, changing from one pattern to another. Remember, a radiograph is a snapshot in time. It represents the appearance of the lungs only at the instant the radiograph was made. A simpler and more straightforward approach to evaluating the lungs is to simply describe the abnormalities you see (Table 3.5). Radiographs are useful to determine whether the lungs are abnormal and which parts are involved (e.g., vessels, bronchi, parenchyma). A definitive diagnosis seldom is made from radiographs. Your radiographic findings, however, often help determine your next diagnostic steps (e.g., airway sampling, lung aspirate, medical therapy with follow-up radiographs). Follow-up radiographs are valuable to monitor the progression of disease and the patient's response to therapy.

Abnormal pulmonary vessels

Radiographic evaluation of the lung vasculature is essentially looking for abnormal vessel size (Figure 3.137). The shapes of the vessels may be considered, but if an artery or vein appears tortuous, it is because it is enlarged. Paired arteries and veins normally are similar in size and about the width of a rib. In a lateral view, the width of the cranial lobar vessels should not exceed the proximal portion of the fourth rib (Figure 3.130). In a VD/DV view, the width of the caudal lobar vessels should not exceed the width of the ninth rib where the vessel and the rib cross (Figure 3.131). Assessing the sizes of the vessels is important in the evaluation of cardiovascular disease.

The pulmonary vasculature responds relatively quickly to changes in volume or pressure. Recent medical treatments such as fluid therapy or diuretic therapy can significantly

Box 3.2 Traditional lung patterns

1. *Alveolar lung pattern*: characterized by soft tissue opacity lungs, border effacement of adjacent soft tissues; lobar sign; air bronchograms; pattern can can change quickly over short periods of time.
2. *Bronchial lung pattern*: characterized by an increase in the number of bronchial markings; abnormal bronchial diameters.
3. *Structured interstitial lung pattern*: discrete nodules or masses in the lungs.
4. *Unstructured interstitial lung pattern*: characterized by increased lung opacity, usually diffuse; vascular and bronchial markings are less distinct, but remain visible ("ground glass appearance").
5. *Vascular lung pattern*: characterized by abnormal size or shape of the pulmonary vessels.

Table 3.5 Describing lung abnormalities

1. Are the lungs increased in opacity?
   a. Rule out artifact (e.g., expiration, obesity).
   b. Determine whether lung volume is lost or maintained.
2. Which parts of the lungs are abnormal?
   a. Vessels
   b. Bronchi.
   c. Parenchyma.
3. What is the distribution of lesions?
   a. Local (confined to a single lung lobe).
   b. Diffuse (two or more lung lobes are involved).
   c. General (all lung lobes are involved).
4. Where are the lesions located?
   a. Hilar region (innermost lung field).
   b. Central region (middle lung field).
   c. Peripheral region (outermost lung field).
   d. Cranial lungs (between thoracic inlet and carina).
   e. Caudal lungs (between carina and diaphragm).
   f. Dorsal lungs (above the trachea).
   g. Ventral lungs (below the trachea).
5. What do the lesions look like?
   a. Solitary, multiple, or numerous.
   b. Unilateral or bilateral.
      - symmetrical or asymmetrical distribution.
   c. Round or irregular in shape.
   d. Distinct or indistinct margins.
   e. Gas, soft tissue, or mineral opacity.
      - homogeneous or heterogeneous in appearance.

alter the sizes of the pulmonary vessels and mask or mimic disease.

Blood vessels normally are well-visualized in air-filled lungs. Indistinct vascular margins often is due to fluid opacity in the adjacent lung, as may occur with inflammation or edema.

Enlargement of both the arteries and veins is caused by higher than normal blood flow in the lungs. Pulmonary

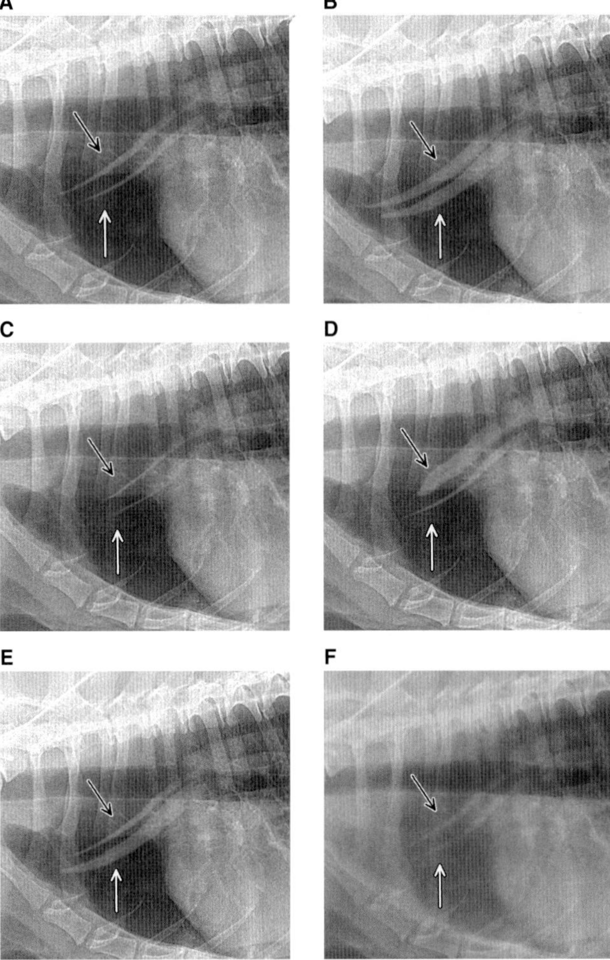

Figure 3.137 Abnormal size of pulmonary vessels. Close-up lateral views of a dog thorax. The cranial lobar artery and vein are highlighted. **A**. Normal paired cranial vessels for comparison: artery (black arrow) and vein (white arrow) are similar in size and course. **B**. Dilation of both the artery and the vein due to over-circulation in the lungs. **C**. Small artery and vein due to hypovolemia. **D**. The artery is larger than the vein due to heartworm disease; the artery tapers abruptly at the site of a thromboembolic obstruction. **E**. The vein is larger than the artery due to venous congestion caused by left heart failure. **F**. The vascular margins are less distinct due to fluid in the adjacent lung (e.g., inflammation, edema).

over-circulation may result from a left-to-right cardiovascular shunt, bilateral heart failure, or iatrogenic fluid overload (see Differential Diagnoses). In over-circulated lungs, the veins may be slightly larger than arteries because venous walls are thinner and more elastic. In radiographs, enlarged pulmonary vessels can be followed further into the lung periphery. Over-perfused lungs contain more fluid and may be increased in overall opacity.

Smaller than expected arteries and veins is due to diminished blood flow to the lungs (under-circulated lungs). The most common cause is hypovolemia. Hypovolemia may result from severe blood loss, shock, dehydration, or hypoadrenocorticism. In addition to small pulmonary arteries and veins, the cardiac shadow, aorta and caudal vena cava are typically small in patients with hypovolemia. In radiographs, small blood vessels cannot be followed as far into the lung periphery. Under-perfused lungs contain less fluid and often are hyperinflated, both of which may decrease overall lung opacity.

Arteries that are larger than veins most often is caused by heartworm disease. The thromboembolic obstructions and endarteritis caused by the heartworms can lead to marked arterial dilation, sometimes to the point that the arteries become tortuous. Arteries can dilate due to pulmonary hypertension alone, but they seldom enlarge enough to be diagnosed in radiographs.

Veins that are larger than arteries most often is due to left heart failure and venous congestion. Pulmonary edema is common in patients with left heart failure and can obscure the vascular margins.

Arteries that are smaller than veins may be caused by reduced output from the right ventricle (e.g., pulmonic stenosis) or severe thromboembolic disease that obstructs numerous arteries.

Nodular lung lesions

Pulmonary nodules are discrete areas of increased opacity. Unlike bronchial, vascular and parenchymal lesions, they are not directly related to any anatomical structure. Nodules can form anywhere in the lungs. The most common pulmonary nodules in dogs and cats are tumors and granulomas. Tumors may be primary or secondary and granulomas typically are caused by either a mycosis or parasites. Other types of lung nodules include abscesses, hematomas, and fluid-filled cysts (see Differential Diagnoses). Acute flooding of the alveoli can produce acinar nodules (Figure 3.160), but these tend to be transient and usually accompanied by alveolar filling in other parts of the lungs.

Pulmonary nodules can be any size. Larger nodules are called masses. The only difference between a nodule and a mass is size. In general, rounded lesions that are less than 3 cm in diameter are called nodules and those larger than 3 cm are called masses. Nodules less than 0.5 cm typically are too small to be seen in radiographs unless mineralized or numerous. Numerous small nodules sometimes are described as "miliary," which is a comparison to millet seeds.

For descriptive purposes, nodules 2–5 mm in size may be considered "small," 5–10 mm in size "medium," and 11–30 mm in size "large" (Figures 3.141 and 3.142). Multiple nodules that are all similar in size suggest an acute arrival to the lungs (a "showering" of the lungs). Multiple, variably sized nodules are more likely to have metastasized over time.

The margin of a lung nodule may be even or irregular, well-defined or ill-defined, depending on its etiology and the condition of the adjacent lung. A distinct margin suggests a slow-growing, long-standing, or healing lesion. An indistinct margin suggests active growth or disease in the adjacent lung (e.g., inflammation, edema, hemorrhage). Tumors are more likely to be well-defined, whereas abscesses and granulomas often are ill-defined. Respiratory motion can make nodule margins appear hazy.

The visibility of a pulmonary nodule depends on its size, opacity, location, and the quality of the radiographs. Orthogonal views are essential to confirm the presence of a lung nodule and to establish its location. The larger and more opaque the nodule, the easier it is to see. Mineralized nodules may be visible when quite small. Soft tissue nodules are more likely to be detected in fully inflated lungs because air-filled lung enhances the gas-to-soft tissue opacity interface.

Patient positioning can significantly influence the degree of lung inflation and therefore the visibility of pulmonary nodules.

In a recumbent patient, the dependent (down) lung partially collapses and there is more blood in the down lung due to the effects of gravity. Because the down lung contains less gas and more fluid, it is more opaque than the up lung. This causes the gas-to-soft tissue opacity interface to be weaker in the down lung than in the up lung. Therefore, a soft tissue structure (e.g., nodule) is more likely to be detected in the up lung than in the down lung (Figures 3.138 and 3.139). Because nodules can form in any part of the lungs, it is important to make both right and left lateral views of the thorax. In addition, to minimize the effects of lung collapse due to gravity, you may want to add both the VD and DV views to your study (Table 3.6).

As you can see, gravity can alter the degree of lung inflation, which can affect the visibility of pulmonary nodules. This is also true for any soft tissue opacity lung lesion, including pneumonia, hemorrhage, atelectasis, and others. Gravity also can alter the degree of inflation within the individual lung lobes (Figure 3.140). The down part of a lung lobe sometimes is partially collapsed and more opaque than the up part. This means that a lesion in the non-dependent portion of a right lung lobe occasionally will be more visible in a right lateral view than in a left lateral view, just the opposite of what we discussed earlier. This is yet another reason to make both lateral views in addition to a VD or/and DV view of the thorax when evaluating the lungs.

Pseudo-nodules are "false nodules" created by superimposition or summation of structures either inside or outside of the lungs. They appear as discrete, rounded, soft tissue or mineral opacity structures that must be differentiated from actual nodules. Most pseudo-nodules are recognized in the orthogonal view.

Perhaps the most common pseudo-nodule is end-on visualization of a pulmonary blood vessel (Figure 3.143). End-on vessels often appear almost mineral opacity, which makes them visible at a very small size (often less than 5 mm). The

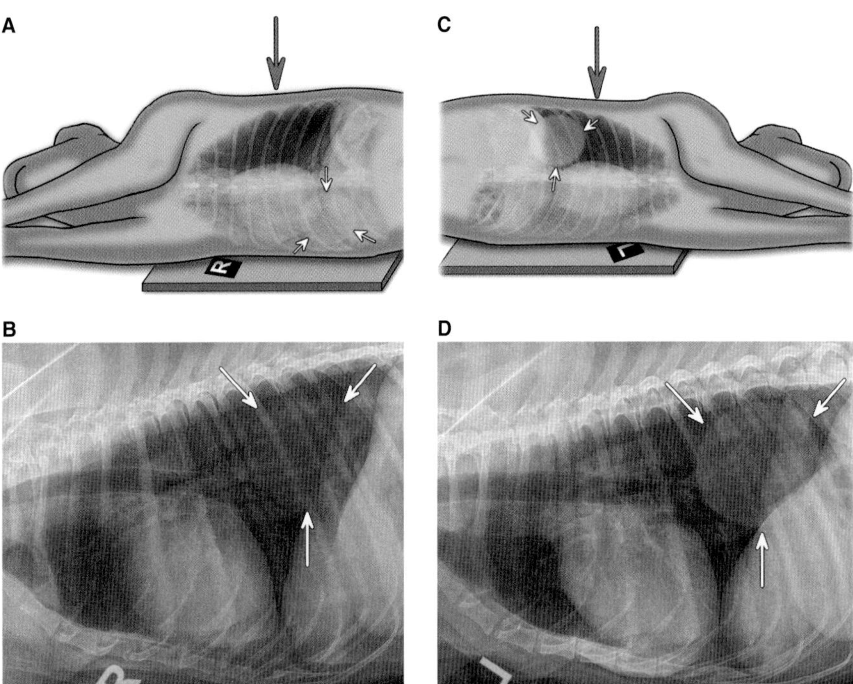

Figure 3.138 Right lateral vs. Left lateral. These illustrations depict a dog in right lateral and left lateral recumbency and the associated radiographs. There is a soft tissue opacity mass in the dorsal part of the dog's right caudal lung lobe (white arrows). **A**. In right lateral recumbency, the right lung is down and partially collapsed. The mass is poorly visualized due to a weak gas-to-soft tissue opacity interface. **B**. Right lateral radiograph: the margins of the mass are not well visualized because there is little alveolar gas adjacent to it. **C**. In left lateral recumbency, the right lung is up and well-inflated. The mass is well-visualized due to a strong gas-to-soft tissue opacity interface. **D**. Left lateral radiograph: the margins of the mass are well visualized because they are surrounded by gas.

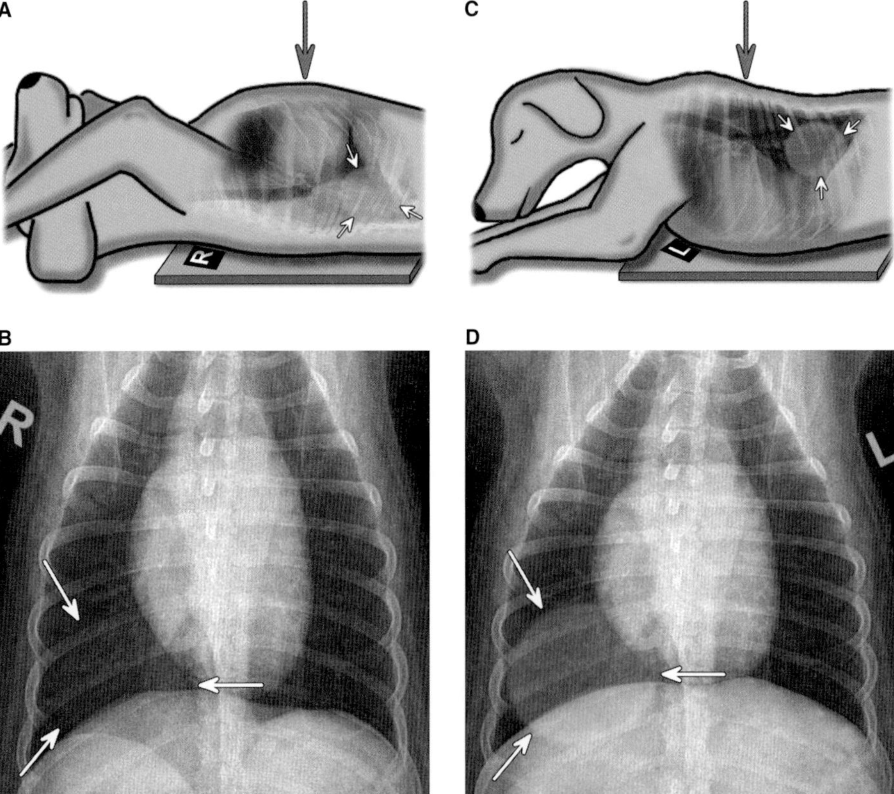

Figure 3.139 VD vs. DV. These illustrations depict the same dog as in Figure 3.138, but now in dorsal and ventral recumbency. The associated radiographs are below each illustration. Again, there is a soft tissue opacity mass in the dog's right caudodorsal lung (white arrows). **A**. In dorsal recumbency, the dorsal part of the lung is down and partially collapsed. The mass is poorly visualized due to the weak gas-to-soft tissue opacity interface. **B**. VD radiograph: the margins of the mass are not well visualized because there is little to no alveolar gas in the adjacent lung. **C**. In ventral recumbency, the dorsal lung is up and well-inflated. The mass is well-visualized due to a strong opacity interface. **D**. DV radiograph: the margins of the mass are well visualized because they are adjacent to air-filled lung.

Table 3.6 Visualization of pulmonary nodules

1. A nodule in the right lung is more likely to be seen in a left lateral view (with the patient lying on its left side, the left lung is down, and the right lung is up).
2. A nodule in the left lung is more likely to be seen in a right lateral view (the patient is lying on its right side with the right lung down and the left lung up).
3. A nodule in the dorsal lungs is more likely to be seen in a DV view (the patient is on its sternum with the ventral lungs down and the dorsal lungs up).
4. A nodule in the ventral lungs is more likely to be seen in a VD view (the patient is on its back with the dorsal lungs down and the ventral lungs up).
5. Variations in aeration within individual lung lobes can result in the opposite effect as described above (see Figure 3.140).

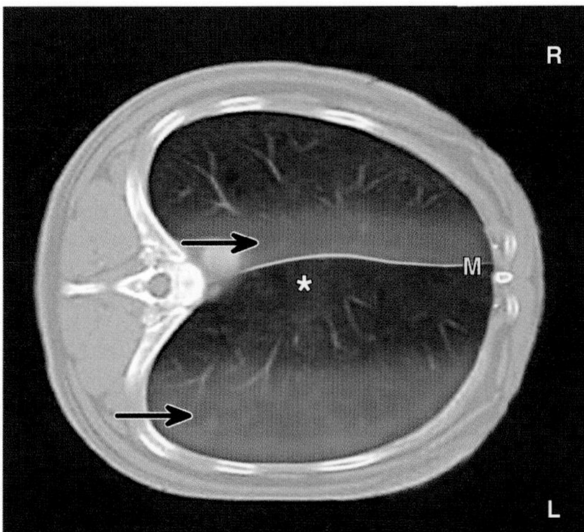

Figure 3.140 Partial lung lobe collapse due to gravity. Cross-sectional CT image of a dog thorax depicting the appearance of the right and left caudal lung lobes with the patient in left lateral recumbency. The mediastinum (M) is highlighted in yellow. The down parts of both caudal lung lobes are more opaque (black arrows) than the up parts because the down parts are less ventilated and more perfused due to gravity. A lesion in the up part of the left lobe (*) may be better visualized in this left lateral view than in a right lateral because that part of the left lung lobe is better inflated. The degree of collapse in different parts of the lungs varies among individual patients and lung conditions. Four view radiographs of the thorax can be very useful.

key differences between end-on pulmonary vessels and actual lung nodules are opacity and size. Most visible lung nodules are soft tissue opacity and larger than 5 mm. End-on vessels may be seen anywhere in the lungs. They usually are continuous with a nearby longitudinal blood vessel of the same size. End-on vessels seldom repeat in serial radiographs because it is unlikely the vessel with be aligned with the x-ray beam every time. Actual lung nodules usually are visible in serial and orthogonal radiographs.

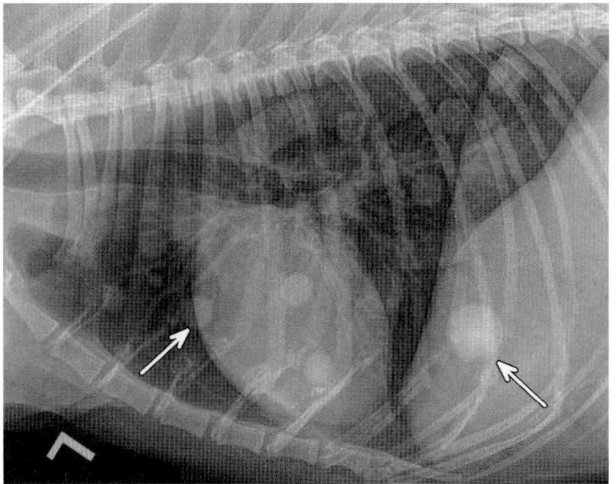

Figure 3.141 Multiple pulmonary nodules. Lateral view of a dog thorax depicting multiple, variable-sized, pulmonary nodules distributed throughout the lungs. The margins of the soft tissue opacity nodules are even and well-defined. Nodules sometimes are more visible when summated with the cardiac silhouette or diaphragm (white arrows).

Pulmonary pseudo-nodules also may be created by superimposition of a nipple, skin growth, costal cartilage, skin parasite, or other focal cutaneous or subcutaneous structure. These types of pseudo-nodules often are identified in orthogonal views. Careful inspection may also reveal that the margins of a cutaneous structure are sharper and more distinct that those of the intra-thoracic structures (Figure 3.144) because the cutaneous structures are adjacent to room air.

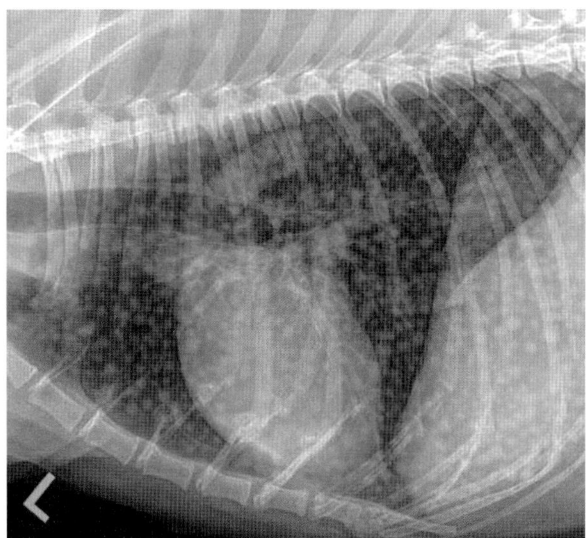

Figure 3.142 Numerous lung nodules. Lateral view of a dog thorax depicting many soft tissue opacity nodules scattered throughout the lungs (sometimes described as a "snowstorm" pattern). Nodules are superimposed on the diaphragm because lung wraps around the diaphragm. Numerous pulmonary nodules may represent metastatic tumors or mycotic granulomas.

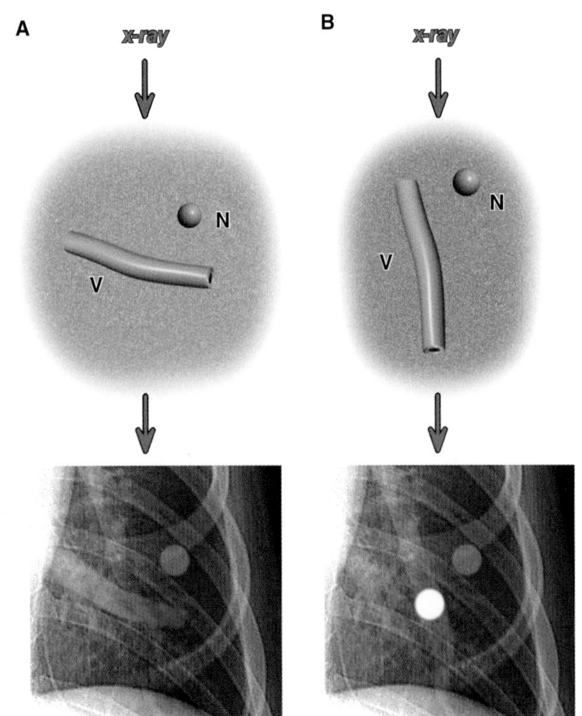

Figure 3.143 End-on vessel. These illustrations depict a vessel (V) and a nearby nodule of similar size (N). **A**. When the vessel is perpendicular to the x-ray beam, it appears as a curvilinear soft tissue opacity structure in the radiograph. The nodule appears as a round soft tissue opacity structure, similar in diameter to the vessel. **B**. When the vessel is aligned (parallel) with the x-ray beam, it is seen end-on and appears as a rounded structure that is nealy mineral opacity due to summation; the x-rays traveled through a larger or longer amount of soft tissue/fluid. The nodule remains the same shape and opacity in both radiographs because it is spherical and the same thickness in all directions.

When in doubt as to the actuality of a suspected lung nodule, carefully palpate the patient's thorax and repeat the radiographs after marking any suspicious cutaneous structures with a small amount of positive contrast medium (Figure 3.145).

Mineral opacity lung nodules in dogs frequently are benign, but in cats they are more likely to be neoplastic. In dogs, multiple, well-defined, mineralized lung nodules often represent **pulmonary osteomas** (Figure 3.146). Pulmonary osteomas usually are less than 3 mm in size, slightly irregular in shape, and scattered in the lungs. They tend to be more numerous in the ventral lung fields. Other names for pulmonary osteomas include *pulmonary osseous metaplasia, heterotopic bone,* and *microlithiasis*. They are more common in certain dog breeds, including Collies, Boxers, and Shetland Sheepdogs.

Similar in appearance to lung osteomas are mineralized granulomas. Mycotic infections such as histoplasmosis can regularly produce granulomas in the lungs. Long-standing and healing granulomas may mineralize. Mineralized lung granulomas differ from pulmonary osteomas in that some of the granulomas usually are larger than 3 mm. Chronic abscesses or tumors in the lungs also may mineralize.

Cavitary lung lesions are pulmonary nodules with gas-filled cavities. Those with thin walls are called **cysts** or **bullae**. Those with thick walls typically represent solid nodules or masses that secondarily developed a gas-filled cavity. A thick-walled cavitary lesion may result from an abscess or tumor that eroded through a bronchus, lost its contents, and filled with gas. Another possibility is an abscess that contains gas-producing bacteria. The cavities in thick-walled lesions often are compartmentalized and irregular in shape (Figure 3.147).

Cysts and bullae appear similar in radiographs and rarely can be differentiated. Both may be congenital or acquired. Very large thin-walled cavitary lesions are more likely to be cysts.

A **bronchogenic cyst** is a rare developmental abnormality that is actually a dilated bronchus. A bronchogenic cyst can become quite large and may compress the adjacent lung and displace the mediastinum (Figure 3.48).

Pulmonary cysts are acquired, usually secondary to an infection (e.g., mycotic, bacterial, parasitic). They can be located anywhere in the lung parenchyma, but they are not part of a bronchus. These cysts also can grow very large.

Bullae are formed when adjacent alveoli merge together (Figure 3.148). A lung bulla may represent a congenital or

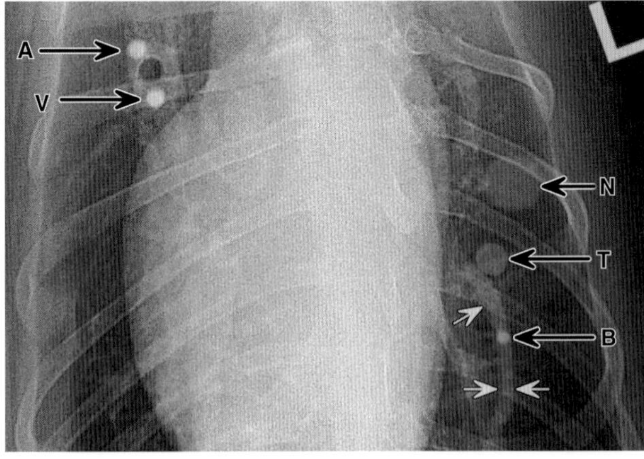

Figure 3.144 Pseudo-nodules. Close up VD-oblique view of a dog thorax depicting various "nodules." The right cranial lobar artery (A) and vein (V) are seen end-on with the bronchus in between. The vessels produce nearly mineral opacity pseudo-nodules and the end-on bronchus appears as a thin, well-defined ring. In the left hemithorax, there is a lung nodule (N), a superimposed skin tumor (T), and an end-on blood vessel (B). The margin of the skin tumor is sharper than the lung nodule because it is extra-thoracic. The end-on vessel is near mineral opacity and continuous with a longitudinal vessel of the same width (white arrows).

A

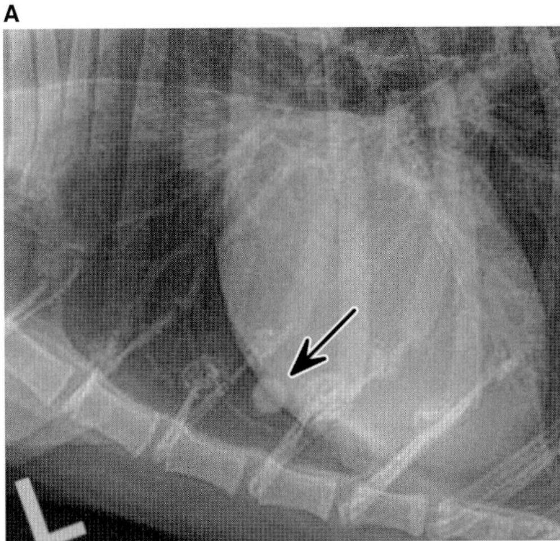

B

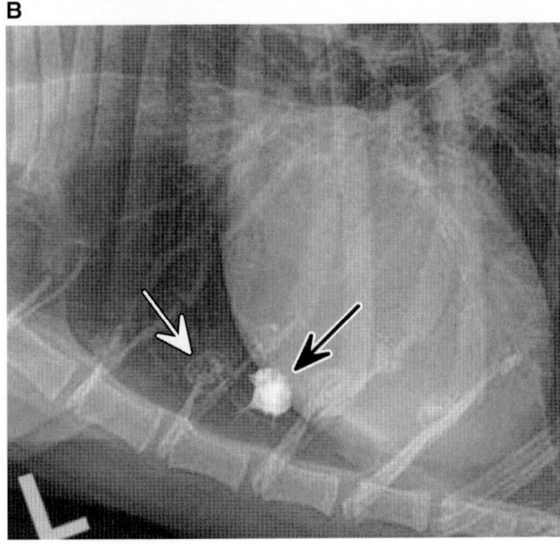

Figure 3.145 Investigating pseudo-nodules. Two close-up lateral views of the same dog thorax. The first radiograph (**A**) depicts a soft tissue opacity nodule at the cranioventral cardiac border (black arrow). In this case, the nodule was suspected to be caused by superimposition of a cutaneous growth. The radiograph was repeated (**B**) after dabbing a small amount of barium on the skin growth. The barium confirms the pseudo-nodule. The white arrow points to mineralized costal cartilage, which also may mimic a pulmonary lesion.

developmental abnormality or it may be acquired, usually secondary to trauma. Bullae may be solitary or multiple, may be located anywhere in the lung, and can vary greatly in size.

Blebs are small bullae that are located under the pleura, usually in the peripheral lungs. They most often are acquired, secondary to trauma, but can be congenital. In patients with a concurrent pneumothorax, blebs may resemble soap bubbles on the surface of the lung.

Pneumatoceles are thin-walled cavitary lesions that develop secondary to trauma (Figure 3.149). Additional signs of trauma often are present at the time of diagnosis, such as fractured ribs, subcutaneous emphysema, and lung contusions. Other names for a pneumatocele include *traumatic cyst* and *traumatic bulla*. Pneumatoceles may be solitary

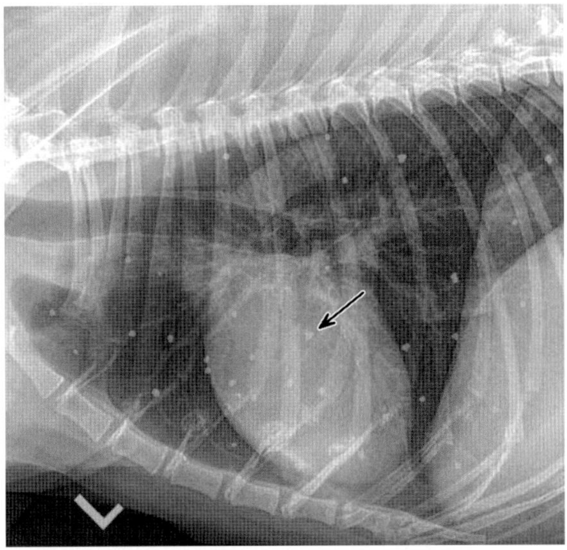

Figure 3.146 Pulmonary osteomas. Lateral view of a dog thorax depicting multiple, well-defined, mineral opacity structures scattered in the lungs (black arrow). The nodules are slightly irregular in shape, less than 3 mm in size, and predominate in the ventral lungs, consistent with pulmonary osteomas. Mineralized granulomas may be similar in appearance.

or multiple. They usually are transient, rarely persisting in serial radiographs. Most pneumatoceles disappear in a few weeks.

The outer margin of a cavitary lung lesion may be well-defined or indistinct, depending on the condition of the adjacent lung. Pulmonary inflammation, hemorrhage, or edema can obscure the margins of a lesion. Expiratory radiographs may enhance visualization of cavitary lesions

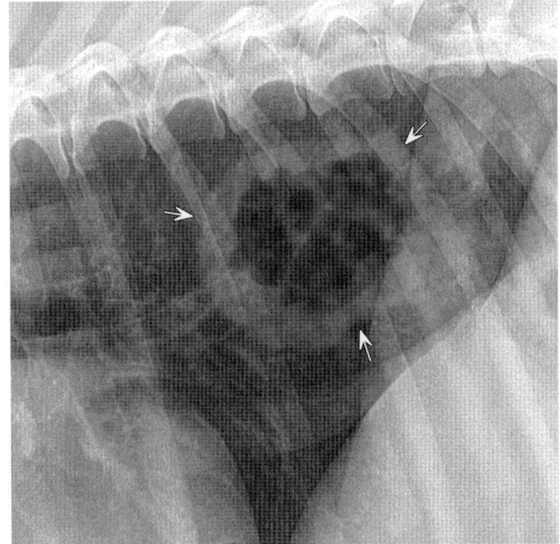

Figure 3.147 Cavitary lung mass. Lateral view of a dog thorax depicting a soft tissue mass with multiple, irregular-shaped, gas-filled cavities in the dorsocaudal lung (white arrows). The thick-walled, cavitary lesion may represent a tumor or long-standing abscess.

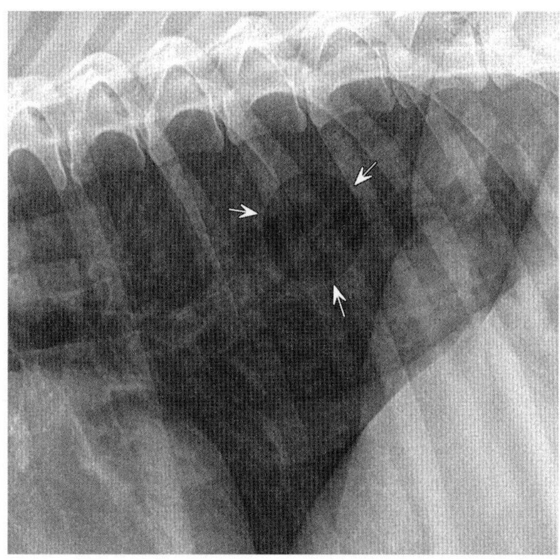

Figure 3.148 Lung bulla. Lateral view of a dog thorax depicting a sharply-defined, thin-walled, gas opacity structure in the dorsocaudal lung (white arrows). The appearance is characteristic of a pulmonary bulla or cyst.

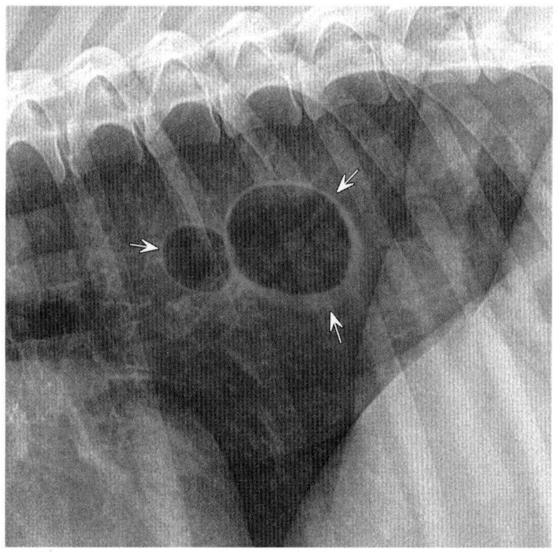

Figure 3.149 Pneumatocele. Lateral view of a dog thorax depicting cavitary lesions with thin to mildly thickened walls (white arrows). The adjacent lung is more opaque due to hemorrhage. Patient history and follow-up radiographs confirm the diagnosis of traumatic lung bullae.

because more opaque lungs provide greater contrast with gas-filled lesions. Some cavitary lesions contain both gas and fluid, appearing as a soft tissue opacity nodule with a less opaque center. Horizontal beam radiography may be useful to reveal a gas:fluid interface in these lesions. Vascular and bronchial markings are not present within a cavitary lesion, but they may be superimposed from the overlying lung. Many cavitary lung lesions remain asymptomatic unless they become infected, rupture, or grow large.

Abnormal bronchi

Bronchial disease usually is recognized in radiographs as an increase in the number of bronchial markings, particularly in the **lung periphery**. Look for more numerous rings and tramlines toward the edges of the lungs, not in the middle of the lungs. The bronchi in the hilar and central lung regions are well-visualized in most thoracic radiographs because they are larger and their walls thicker and more opaque. It is important to not confuse these normal larger bronchi with bronchial disease. Rings are a more reliable finding than tramlines because paired pulmonary vessels may be mistaken for thickened bronchi (Figure 3.136).

Before one can correctly identify an abnormal increase in bronchial markings, it is necessary to know the normal visibility of the bronchi for a particular x-ray system. The high resolution of some digital image receptors allows us to see more of the smaller bronchi than are visible with other imaging systems. Familiarity with radiographs made using a particular receptor and display will help avoid over-diagnosing bronchial disease.

Bronchial markings increase in visibility due to thickening or mineralization of the bronchial walls and due to peribronchial fluid or cells. Thickening and peribronchial diseases are difficult to differentiate in radiographs. With a very high-quality imaging system one may be able to distinguish disease adjacent to a bronchial wall from disease in the lining of the bronchus based on whether the ill-defined thickening is on the inside or outside of the bronchus.

Bronchial wall thickening most often, but not always, is due to inflammation. Airway inflammation may be caused by inhaled irritants, allergies, or an upper respiratory obstruction (see Differential Diagnoses). Bronchial rings that are well-defined suggests a more chronic history of airway inflammation, whereas thick rings with less distinct margins suggest a more acute and severe inflammation or peribronchial disease (Figures 3.150–3.152). Thick, hazy rings commonly are called "donuts."

Peribronchial disease refers to an abnormal accumulation of fluid or cells around the bronchi. The terms *peribronchial infiltrates* and *peribronchial cuffing* are used to describe the increased opacity adjacent to the bronchial walls that makes them appear thicker and less distinct in radiographs.

Peribronchial infiltrates may develop during the early stages of left heart failure. Pulmonary edema surrounding the bronchial walls can increase the number of visible bronchial rings and may be misinterpreted as primary airway disease. In cats especially, it is important to not confuse peribronchial edema due to heart failure with airway inflammation (e.g., asthma). There usually are other radiographic findings that help differentiate the two, including cardiac enlargement and abnormal vasculature.

Peribronchial infiltrates sometimes are mistaken for multiple tiny lung nodules. Close inspection reveals dark centers

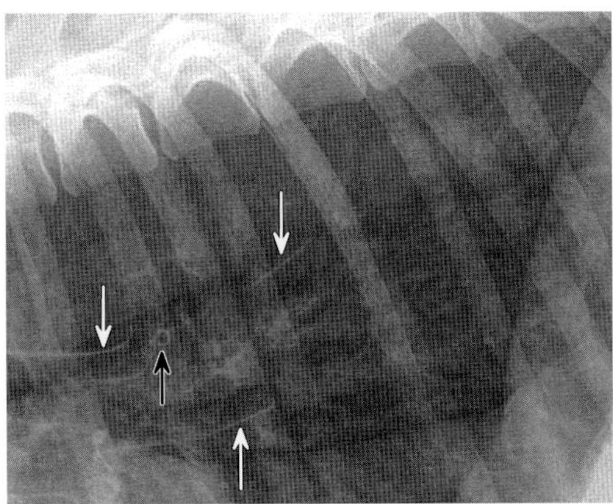

Figure 3.150 Normal bronchial markings. Lateral view of a dog thorax depicting normal lung. The walls of the larger bronchi in the hilar and central lung regions are visible (white arrows). When seen end-on, the bronchi appear as well-defined rings (black arrow).

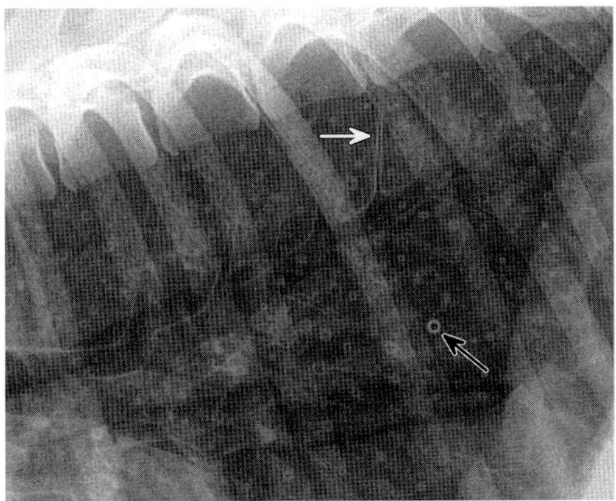

Figure 3.151 Increased bronchial markings. Lateral view of a dog thorax depicting an increase in bronchial markings. Compared to Figure 3.150, there are more visible rings (black arrow) and tramlines (white arrows) due to thickening of the bronchial walls.

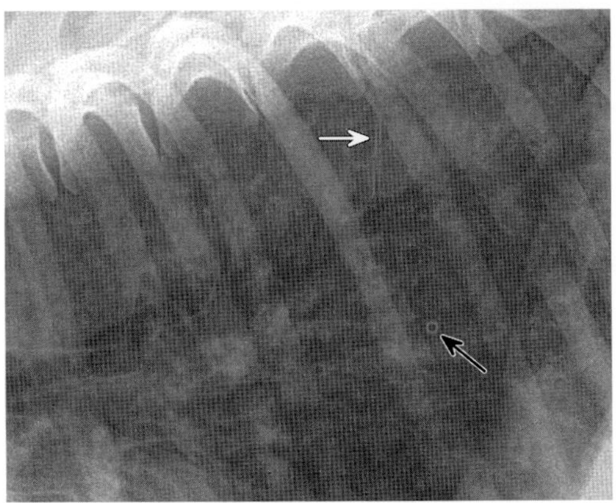

Figure 3.152 Lung inflammation. Lateral view of a dog thorax depicting increased bronchial markings and increased lung opacity (sometimes called a "bronchointerstitial lung pattern"). Compared to Figure 3.151, the bronchial markings are less distinct because there is more fluid in the lungs, the latter due to inflammation.

A

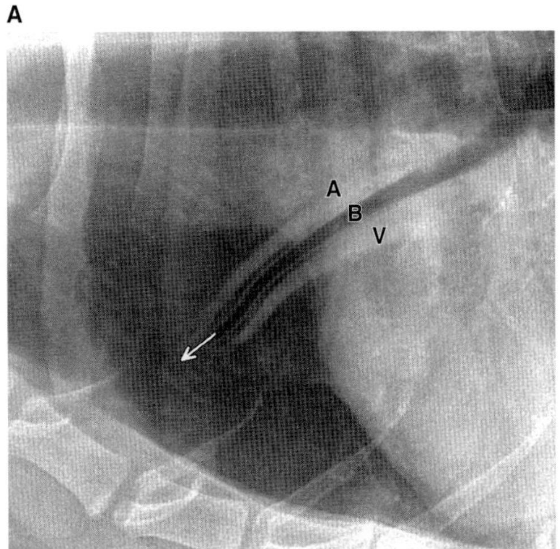

B

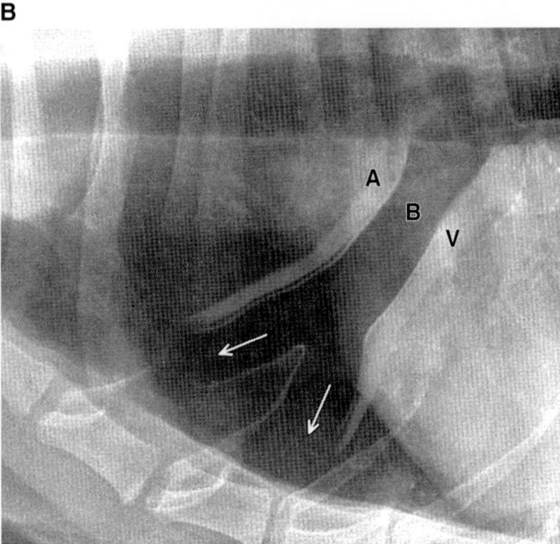

Figure 3.153 Bronchiectasis. Lateral views of a dog thorax. **A**. Normal cranial lobar artery, bronchus, and vein (ABV). The vessels and bronchus taper together into the lung periphery (white arrow). Notice again that the bronchus does not fill the entire space between the vessels. **B**. Bronchiectasis: the bronchus is largely dilated with irregular-shaped walls that do not taper normally (arrows).

in these "nodules" due to gas in the bronchial lumen, confirming that they are, in fact, bronchi.

Chronic or recurrent airway inflammation can lead to an abnormal dilation of the bronchi called **bronchiectasis**. Bronchiectasis appears as widened bronchi with irregular-shaped, non-linear walls that do not taper normally (Figures 3.153 and 3.154). The bronchial dilation usually is irreversible and the function of the mucociliary structures often is impaired, increasing the patient's susceptibility to respiratory infections.

Mineralization of the bronchial walls is a common finding in older dogs and cats, especially chondrodystrophic breeds. It often is considered an "aging change," however, mineralized bronchi most likely are the result of previous airway disease that is now inactive. Bronchial mineralization also may result from an endocrinopathy, such as hypercortisolism (reported more often in dogs than in cats).

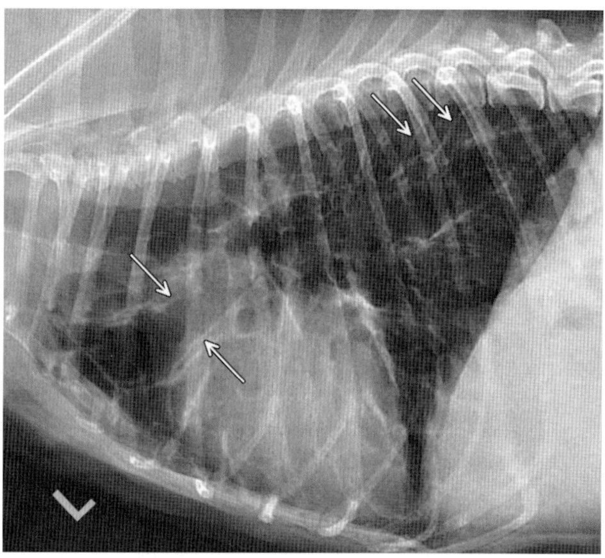

Figure 3.154 Severe bronchiectasis. Lateral view of a dog thorax depicting numerous greatly dilated bronchi (arrows).

Broncholithiasis is mineralized material in a bronchial lumen. It occasionally is reported in cats with chronic lower airway disease, but not in dogs. In cats, broncholithiasis typically appears as multiple, irregular-shaped mineral opacity structures, about 3–6 mm in size, scattered in the lungs.

Abnormal lung parenchyma

The lung parenchyma includes the alveoli and the interstitium. Recall that the alveoli are air spaces, not tissue. Any disorder that causes a loss of alveolar air leads to increased opacity in the lung. Gas in the alveoli may be lost due to either **lung consolidation** or **lung collapse**. Consolidation occurs when there is an influx of fluid or cells into the alveoli and little to no loss of lung volume (Box 3.3). Collapse refers to reduced size of the alveoli and decreased lung volume.

Because there is no "alveolar tissue," virtually all parenchymal disorders that lead to lung opacification begin in the interstitium. In radiographs, however, the accumulations of fluid or cells in the lung interstitium seldom are visible until there is alveolar involvement. The alveolar gas is diminished either due to spillage into the alveolar spaces or because the alveoli cannot expand against the interstitial material. Interstitial fluids and cells can easily pass into and out of the alveolar spaces because the alveolar walls are thin and delicate (the walls are thin to facilitate gas exchange).

Box 3.3 Lung consolidation

The term consolidation is familiar in pathology, but in radiology, it is used to differentiate lung opacification caused by alveolar filling from that caused by alveolar collapse. Consolidation increases lung opacity without loss of lung volume, whereas collapse decreases lung volume.

During the early stages of parenchymal lung disease, filling or/and reduced size of the alveoli appears as a diffuse increase in lung opacity. There is less gas in the alveoli which weakens the gas-to-soft tissue opacity interface. This means that the margins of the adjacent pulmonary vessels, bronchial walls, or cardiac shadow will be less distinct (Figures 3.157–3.159). The soft tissue structures remain visible and can be readily identified, but their edges are more hazy and less-defined adjacent to the more opaque lung.

Continued alveolar filling or further collapse leads to complete loss of alveolar gas and that part of the lung becomes soft tissue opacity. Soft tissue opacity lung adjacent to a soft tissue opacity structure means there is no opacity interface. The margin of the soft tissue structure completely disappears in the radiograph and will not be visible at all.

Commonly, an increase in lung opacity that blurs the soft tissue margins but does not completely obscure them is called an "interstitial lung pattern" or a "ground glass appearance." A ground glass appearance refers to looking at something through an opaque piece of glass such as "bathroom glass". Whatever you're looking at appears fuzzy. An increase in lung opacity that completely obscures the adjacent margins of soft tissue structures is commonly called an "alveolar lung pattern". The lung becomes soft tissue opacity because there is no air in the alveoli.

Attempts to classify lung opacification as either an "interstitial pattern" or an "alveolar pattern" can be confusing because both of these "patterns" typically represent different stages of the same disease processes. If you look at a list of causes for each pattern, you will see the same diseases on both lists. Histopathology of lung specimens has revealed that there is extensive alveolar involvement in many patients with an "interstitial lung pattern" (Figure 3.156). Struggling to classify lung opacification as an alveolar or interstitial "pattern" does not help to differentiate the disease process, only its degree of severity and stage of progression at the time the radiographs were made. What is important is to identify whether or not the lung parenchyma is involved and to determine where the lesions are located (Table 3.7). You can then use these findings along with any other abnormalities you find involving the bronchi, pulmonary vessels, and structures outside the lungs to establish a list of differential diagnoses.

Parenchymal lung disease can be quite dynamic, progressing and regressing over short periods of time. The rate of change provides valuable diagnostic information, which often can be obtained in serial radiographs. For example, with appropriate treatment lung opacification caused by pulmonary edema may improve within hours, whereas opacification due to pneumonia may require days or weeks. Lung opacification that persists longer may represent neoplasia or mycosis.

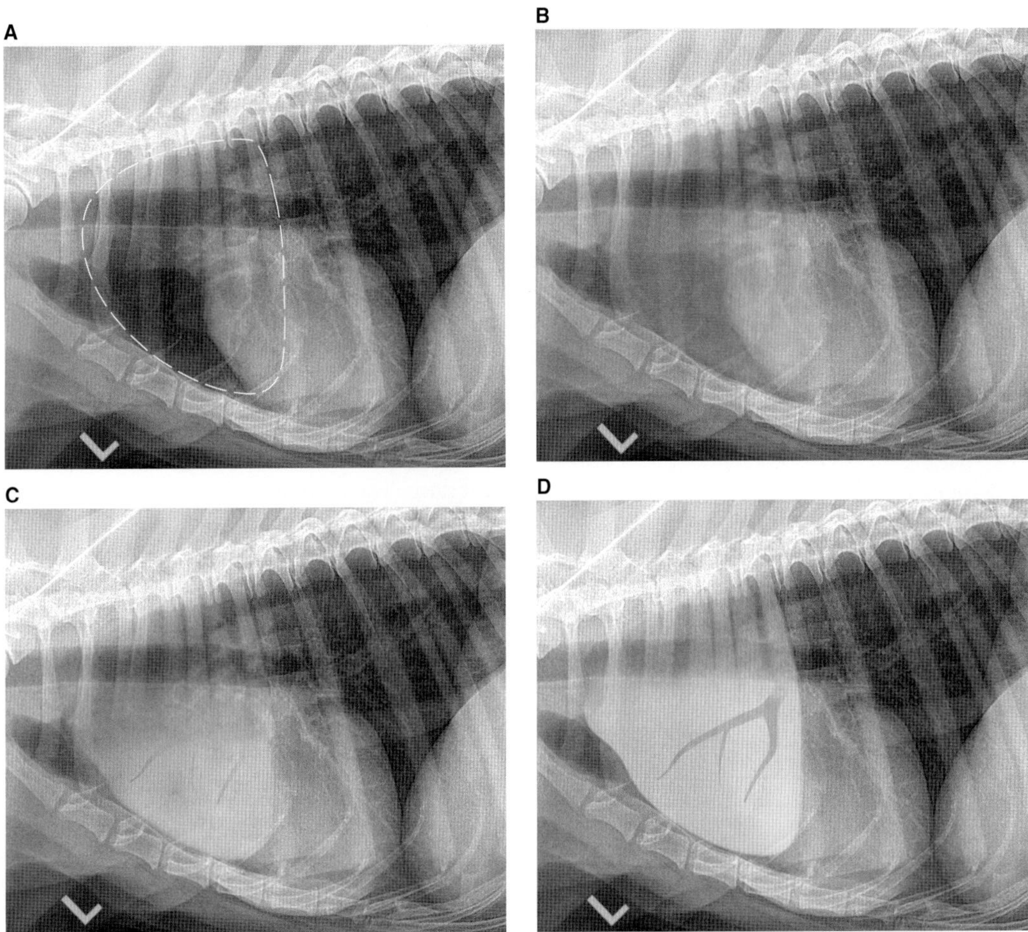

Figure 3.155 Progression of lung parenchyma disease. **A**. Lateral view of a dog thorax depicting the appearance of normal lungs. The right cranial lung lobe is outlined. **B**. During the initial stages of parenchymal lung disease (in this case, pneumonia), there is a diffuse increase in lobar opacity due to an influx of fluid and cells. The cardiovascular margins are less distinct, but they remain visible and readily identified. **C**. Continued alveolar filling leads to more effacement of the cardiac and vascular margins. Notice that the lung lobe is more opaque ventrally than dorsally due to the effects of gravity. There are faint air bronchograms. **D**. Complete filling of the alveoli results in a more uniform lobar opacification and more visible air bronchograms. The vascular and cranial cardiac margins are completely effaced. Note: during the regression or healing of parenchymal lung disease (resolving of the pneumonia), this sequence of radiographic findings will occur in reverse order as cells and fluid leave the alveolar spaces and interstitium.

The alveoli may fill with blood, pus, water, cells, or other materials. Conditions that lead to alveolar filling include cardiovascular disease, lung inflammation, neoplasia and trauma (see Differential Diagnoses). As the alveoli fill with fluid or cells, the borders of any adjacent soft tissue structures become effaced, as described earlier. Any soft tissue opacity margins that were visible because of the gas-to-soft tissue opacity interface will become less distinct or not visible at all due to the loss of alveolar gas (Figure 3.157).

In essence, the loss of alveolar gas "flips" the lung parenchyma from gas opacity to soft tissue opacity. If any gas remains in the bronchi or in small groups of alveoli, it may become sharply visible because there is now a soft tissue-to-gas

Table 3.7 The role of radiography in lung parenchyma disease

1. Confirm lung opacification.
2. Differentiate consolidation from collapse when possible.
3. Help determine the etiology of the lung opacification (e.g., signs of heart failure, signs of trauma).
4. Identify complications such as bacterial pneumonia, abscess formation.
5. Demonstrate accompanying pathology such as pleural effusion, rib fractures.
6. Determine the severity and extent of the disease (e.g., number of lung lobes involved, unilateral or bilateral).

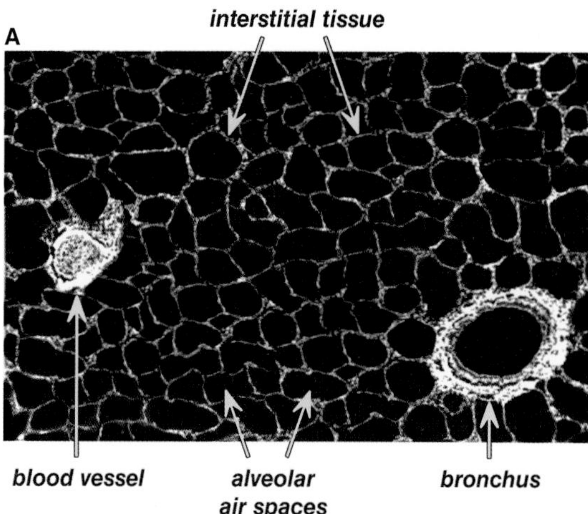

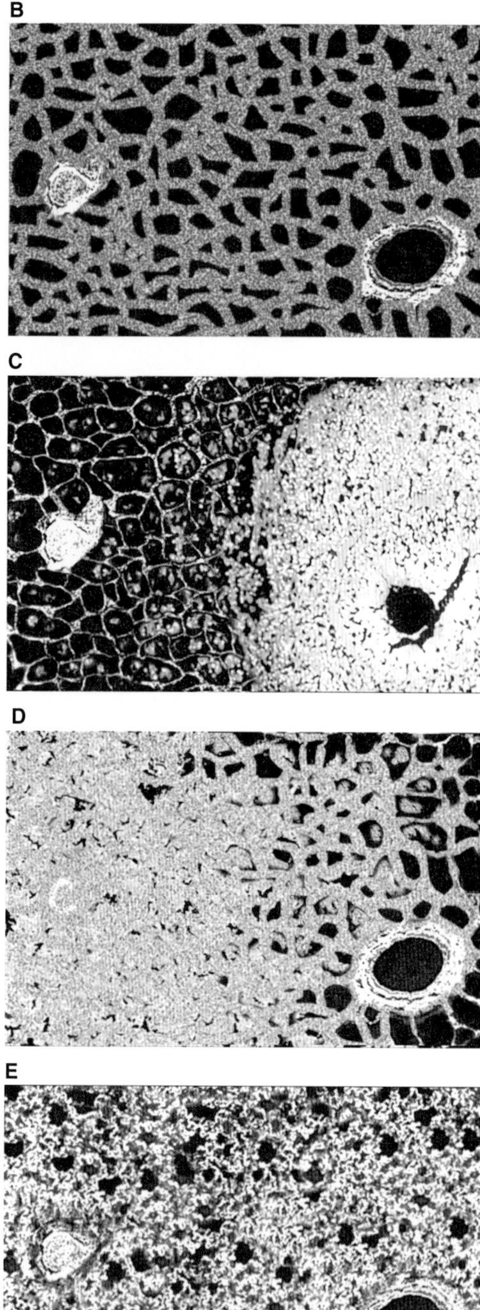

Figure 3.156 Lung parenchyma disease. These illustrations depict the microscopic appearance of lung parenchyma disease. The images are rendered in shades of gray to simulate a radiographic image.

A. Normal lung tissue: depicted are a pulmonary blood vessel, a bronchus, the alveolar air spaces and the interstitial tissue that surrounds the alveoli and forms the alveolar walls.

B. Thickened lung interstitium: the alveolar spaces are smaller than normal due to an infiltration of cells in the alveolar walls and other interstitial tissues. The cellular infiltration increases the amount of soft tissue in the lungs and limits alveolar expansion, both of which increase lung opacity.

C. Peribronchial infiltrates: abnormal cells and fluid fill the alveoli adjacent to the bronchial wall, which may appear in radiographs as thickening of the bronchus. The outer margin of the bronchial wall is obscured by the adjacent alveolar filling, giving the impression of a very thick bronchial wall.

D. Lung hemorrhage: blood cells leaking from the damaged vessel flow into the interstitium and fill the alveoli, both of which increase lung opacity. Blood, or any other fluid that fills the lungs, will obscure the adjacent soft tissue margins.

E. Pulmonary edema: fluid accumulates in the interstitium and alveolar spaces, increasing lung opacity and blurring the soft tissue margins of the vessel and bronchial wall.

opacity interface (Figure 3.158). The bronchi that retain air may be visible as *air bronchograms* (Box 3.4) and the alveoli that retain air may form *air alveolograms*.

Air bronchograms appear as sharply-defined, linear or branching, gas-opacity tubes that are clearly distinct from the soft tissue opacity lung (Figure 3.155). They occur in less than 25% of parenchymal lung diseases that progress to alveolar filling. This is because bronchial gas also is displaced by fluid/cells or it is soon resorbed. Air bronchograms are more likely to occur in consolidated lungs as opposed to collapsed lungs. Note: alveolar filling can occur without air bronchogram formation, but air bronchograms will not occur without alveolar filling.

Air bronchograms sometimes are difficult to detect, especially when they are not well aligned with the x-ray beam. More commonly, air bronchograms are over-diagnosed.

A

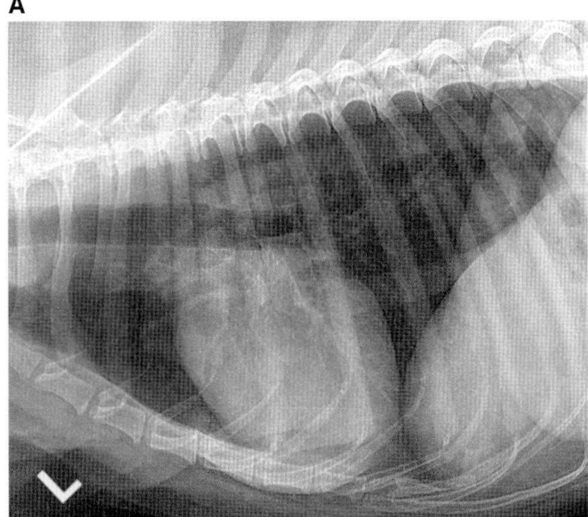

B

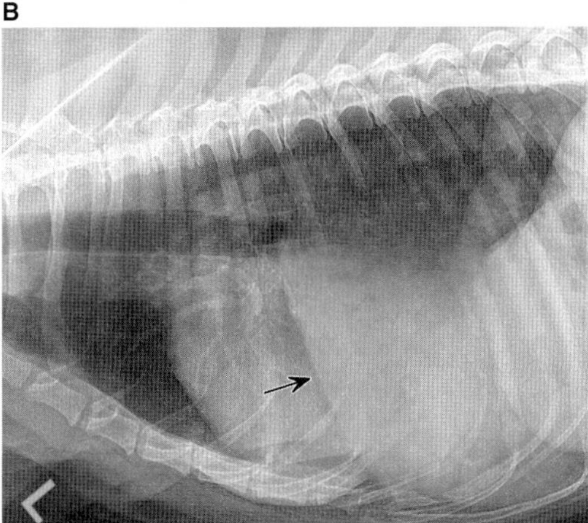

C

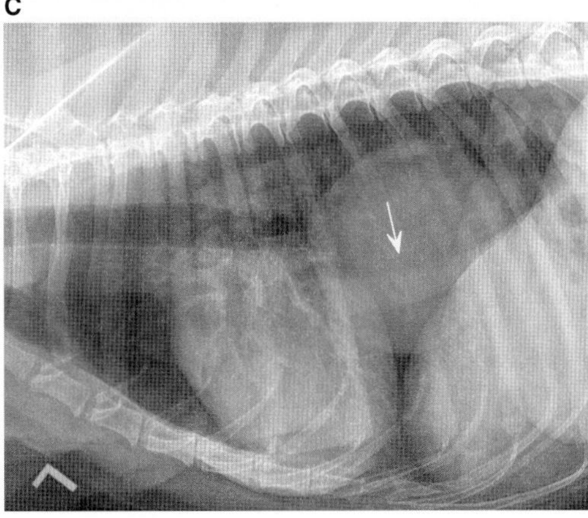

Figure 3.157 Effacement. **A**. Lateral view of a dog thorax depicting normal lungs and well-defined margins associated with the cardiac silhouette, caudal vena cava, and diaphragm. **B**. Lateral view of the same dog as in (A) but depicting alveolar filling in the caudal lung lobes (arrow points to lobar sign). Loss of alveolar gas eliminates the gas-to-soft tissue opacity interface, effacing the caudal cardiac, cranial diaphragmatic, and vena caval margins. **C**. Lateral view of the same dog as in (A) but depicting a soft tissue mass in the caudal lung lobe. The mass does not efface the nearby soft tissue margins because there is some air-filled lung in between. The borders of the mass and the caudal vena cava (arrow) remain visible because there is a gas-to-soft tissue opacity interface.

A frequent error is mistaking a normal bronchus between its paired artery and vein for an air bronchogram (Figures 3.133 and 3.134). Close inspection usually reveals the vascular and bronchial margins, which would be effaced by alveolar filling.

Air alveolograms appear as multiple tiny, rounded areas of gas opacity (Figure 3.159). These are actually pockets of retained gas and not individual alveoli. The alveoli are too small to be seen in radiographs.

Alveolar filling typically begins as patchy, ill-defined areas of increased lung opacity. The alveoli rarely fill in a uniform and contiguous manner (Figures 3.159 and 3.160).

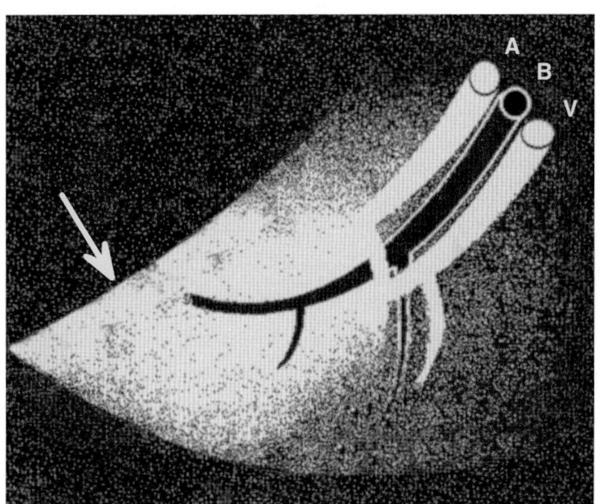

Figure 3.158 Alveolar filling. This illustration depicts an individual lung lobe with its artery (A), bronchus (B), and vein (V). Fluid is filling the alveolar spaces, to a small degree proximally and progressing toward the tip of the lobe where it effaces the margins of the pulmonary vessels and bronchial wall. Gas remaining in the bronchial lumen contrasts sharply with the soft tissue opacity lung parenchyma, forming an air bronchogram. Alveolar filling can extend throughout an entire lung lobe, but spread to other lobes is prevented by the pleura. The sharp pleural edge of the consolidated lung lobe adjacent to air-filled lung produces a lobar sign (arrow).

Box 3.4 History of the "air bronchogram"

The word "-gram" when used as a suffix means "picture" and it commonly is used to describe an image. For example: a *diagram* is an image of a structure; an *electrocardiogram* is an image of the electrical activity in the heart; a *cystogram* is an image of the urinary bladder. An *air bronchogram*, therefore, is an image of a bronchus. Specifically, it is a negative contrast radiographic image of a bronchus. The term air bronchogram was coined by Dr. Ben Felson in the 1950s to help distinguish parenchymal lung disease from disease outside the lungs, such as pleural effusion.

Usually, there is some residual alveolar gas in the early or mild stages of parenchymal disease. Alveolar filling generally occurs in individual lung lobes (called a lobar distribution), but more than one lung lobe may be affected at the same time. The lobar distribution may be symmetrical or asymmetrical. As alveolar filling progresses, the patchy areas spread and coalesce to form a more uniform soft tissue opacity. The spread of alveolar filling is aided by the *alveolar pores*. Alveolar pores link the acini, providing collateral pathways to maintain lung inflation should the proximal airway become obstructed. Unfortunately, the alveolar pores also facilitate the spread of disease.

Unchecked, alveolar filling will continue to spread, eventually displacing all of the gas from the affected lung lobe and resulting in **lobar consolidation**. Further spread is blocked by the pleura. The edge of a consolidated lung lobe next to an air-filled lobe produces a sharp, soft tissue opacity line called the **lobar sign** (Figures 3.157–3.159). The lobar sign confirms alveolar filling and is useful to determine which lung lobes are involved. The affected lobes may be identified by the location of the lung opacification and the effacement of adjacent soft tissues. The lobar sign will not be present if alveolar filling has not progressed to the edge of the lung lobe. A lobar sign sometimes is difficult to see when the lung border is not well-aligned with the x-ray beam.

The most common cause of lung lobe consolidation is pneumonia. Other causes include neoplasia and hemorrhage (see Differential Diagnoses). Acute alveolar filling sometimes produces a mottled pattern of lung opacification that resembles pulmonary nodules (Figure 3.160). This occurs because a rapid influx of fluid can quickly flood the acini to create ill-defined foci of soft tissue opacity (e.g., severe bacterial pneumonia, acute lung hemorrhage). These foci or **acinar nodules** tend to be numerous, ill-defined, and small (about 5–10 mm in size). They often are less discrete toward the lung periphery. Acinar nodules rarely occur without other evidence of alveolar filling.

Rarely, radiographic signs of parenchymal lung disease are confined to the interstitium. Diseases that produce cellular infiltrates and little fluid may result in minimal alveolar filling. Examples include viral pneumonia and septicemia (see Differential Diagnoses). In these cases, increased lung opacity is primarily due to thickening of the interstitial tissues and the inability of the alveoli to expand against the thickened tissues. This degree of lung opacification only blurs the soft tissue margins, it does not completely obscure them (Figure 3.161).

Thickening of interstitial connective tissues may produce faint linear or **reticular markings** in the lungs (Figure 3.162). Reticular markings appear as a "lacey" or "honeycomb" arrangement of thin, faint, soft tissue opacity lines. These fine lines may be confused with tiny blood vessels or bronchi, but they are too small to be visible vessels or bronchi. Reticular markings occur more often in older animals where they probably represent fibrotic remnants from previous disease. They commonly are called an "aging change." Summation of numerous reticular markings can resemble numerous tiny nodules or *reticulonodular* structures (Figure 3.162), but they are too small to be actual nodules. Reticulonodular markings have been reported in patients

A

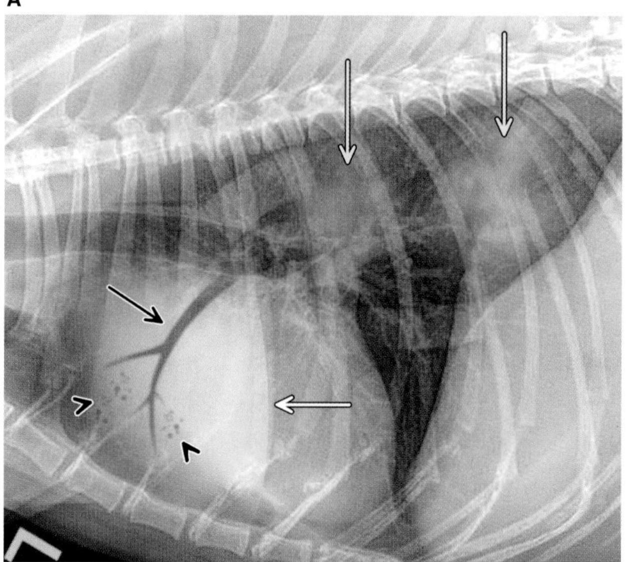

B

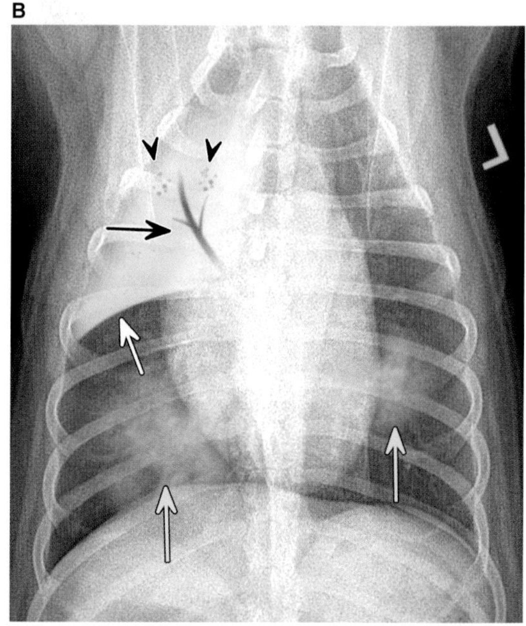

Figure 3.159 Alveolar filling. Lateral view (**A**) and VD view (**B**) of a dog thorax depicting alveolar filling. In the right cranial lung lobe there is homogeneous soft tissue opacity that effaces the right craniolateral cardiac border. The caudal edge of the right cranial lobe is sharply defined against the air-filled right middle lobe, (white arrow points to the lobar sign). Air bronchograms (black arrow) and air alveolograms (black arrowheads) are visible. In the dorsal lung fields, there is patchy alveolar filling appearing as ill-defined, soft tissue opacity areas in both the right and left caudal lung lobes (yellow arrows).

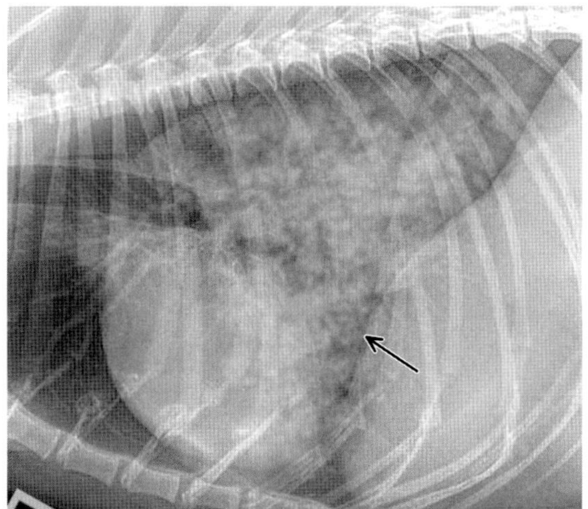

Figure 3.160 Acinar nodules. Lateral view of a dog thorax depicting a mottled pattern of ill-defined soft tissue opacity "nodules" in the caudal lungs (black arrow). The mottled lung opacification is caused by acute alveolar flooding. The appearance of the lungs is likely to change in follow-up radiographs, either becoming more uniform due to continued alveolar filling or decreasing in opacity as fluid leaves the alveolar spaces. Actual pulmonary nodules would persist unchanged in serial radiographs.

with large infiltrates of cells in the lung interstitium (e.g., lymphoma, mycoses, hemangiosarcoma).

Expiratory radiographs and other conditions that prevent the lungs from fully inflating may be mistaken for parenchymal lung disease (Figures 3.3 and 3.163).

Specific lung diseases

1. Lung collapse
2. Pulmonary edema
3. Allergic lung diseases
4. Pulmonary emphysema
5. Pneumonia
6. Lung hemorrhage
7. Lung neoplasia
8. Lung lobe torsion

Lung collapse is not a disease in itself, rather it is a consequence of disease. Pulmonary edema is discussed next because the disease process differs from that of most other lung diseases. Allergic lung diseases, pneumonia, and lung hemorrhage all produce similar radiographic signs and often are difficult to differentiate using radiographs alone. Allergic lung diseases can lead to emphysema or COPD. Pneumonia may be caused by a bacterial, mycotic, viral, or parasitic infection. Lung neoplasia often acts and appears different than the other lung diseases. Lung torsion is a rather unique and uncommon disease process.

Lung collapse

Lung collapse may result from airway obstruction or a condition that prevents the lung from re-expanding, such as fluid or gas in the pleural space or the effects of gravity during prolonged recumbency (see Differential Diagnoses). Lung collapse leads to increased lung opacity and decreased

A

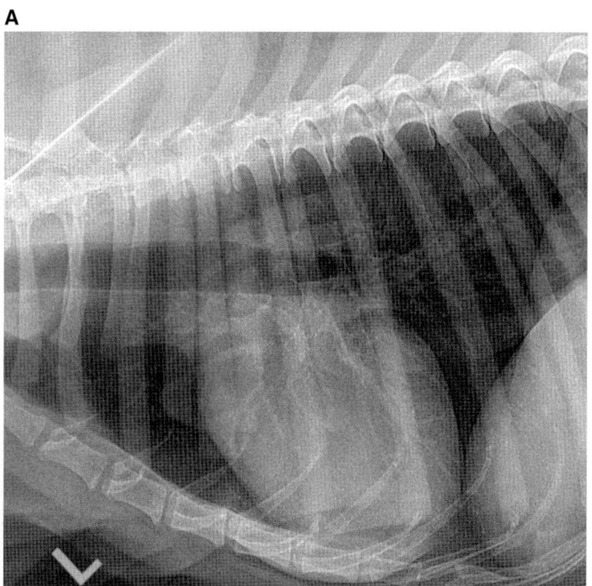

B

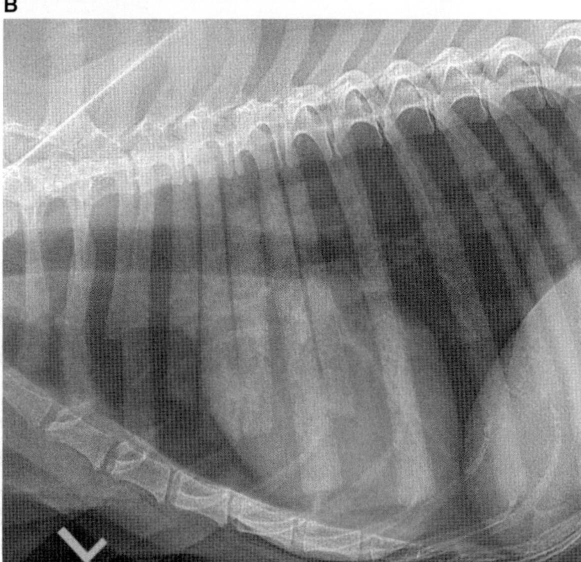

Figure 3.161 Parenchymal lung disease. Two lateral views of a dog thorax. **A**. Normal lungs for comparison. **B**. A diffuse increase in lung opacity. The soft tissue margins are partially effaced. The margins are blurry and less distinct than in (**A**), but the cardiovascular structures, diaphragm, and other soft tissues are easily recognized. This degree of lung opacification has been called "dirty lungs," "ground glass opacity," and "interstitial lung pattern". It is caused by parenchymal lung disease.

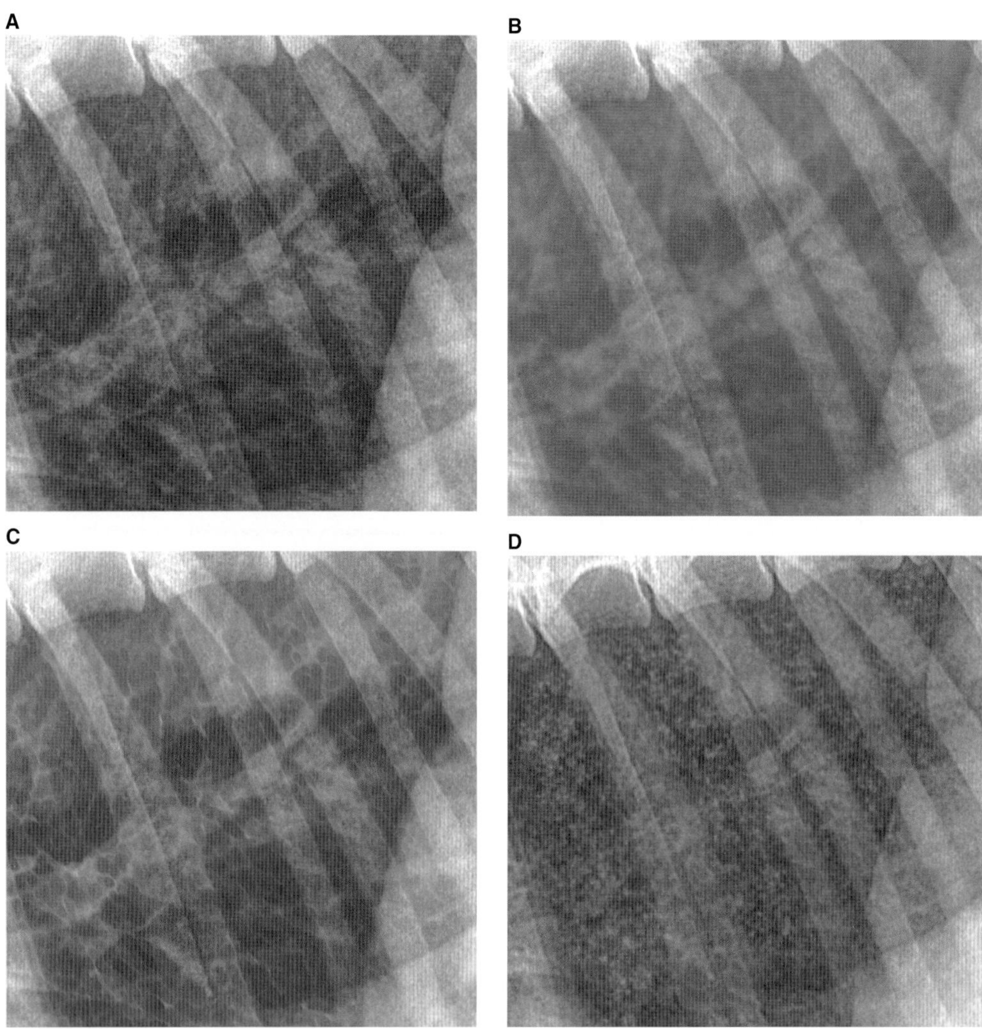

Figure 3.162 Lung interstitial disease. Lateral views of a dog thorax depicting normal and diseased lung. (**A**) Normal lung for comparison. (**B**) Parenchymal lung disease resulting in a diffuse mild increase in lung opacity with less distinct vascular and bronchial markings. (**C**) Reticular lung markings caused by thickening of the interstitial connective tissues; the markings resemble a lacey or honeycomb pattern. (**D**) Summation of interstitial markings creates a reticulonodular appearance in the lungs; however, the numerous tiny "nodules" are too small to be actual nodules and there are too many of them to be bronchi.

lung. Reduced lung volume allows the mediastinum and ipsilateral side of the diaphragm to move toward the smaller lung (Figure 3.164). In lateral recumbency, the cardiac shadow may move dorsally away from the sternum. Compensatory hyperinflation of the unaffected lung lobes sometimes will restore overall lung size and correct the displacement of the intra-thoracic structures. Collapsed lung lobes sometimes are irregular in shape with concave borders.

Lung collapse frequently is called *atelectasis*, which means "incomplete expansion." Some people use both terms interchangeably, while others reserve atelectasis for a lung that never fully expanded and collapse to describe a lung that was expanded, but now is not.

Pulmonary edema

Pulmonary edema is an abnormal accumulation of fluid in the lungs. The fluid usually leaks from the capillaries. The lungs can accommodate up to two times their normal blood volume before edema occurs. When the ability of the lymphatics to maintain adequate drainage is exceeded, fluid leaking from the capillaries builds up in the lung interstitium. Continued leakage spills into the alveoli. If unchecked, pulmonary edema eventually displaces all of the alveolar gas, leading to complete lung consolidation and total effacement of the adjacent soft tissues.

Pulmonary edema is caused by a disorder outside the lungs, such as cardiovascular disease or neurologic disease.

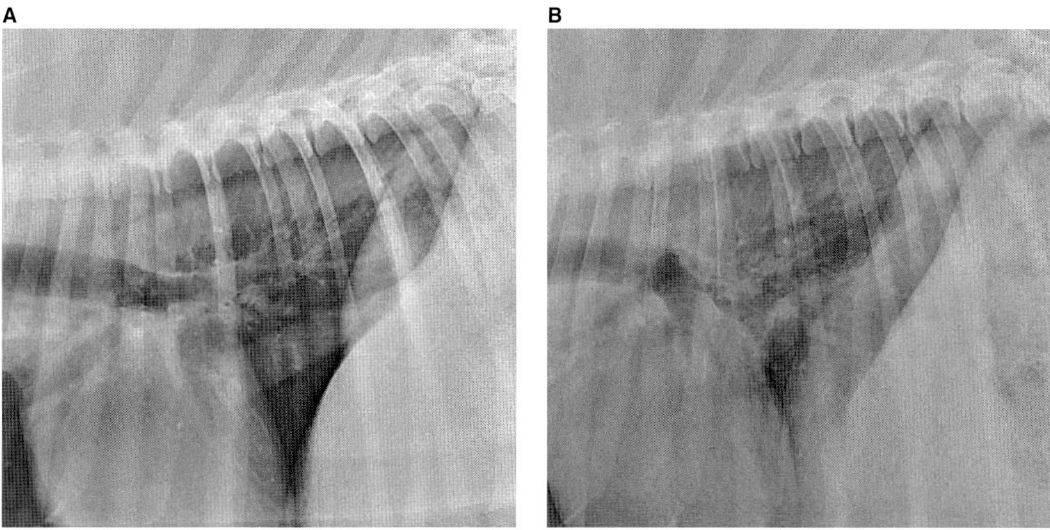

Figure 3.163 Inspiration vs. Expiration. Lateral views of a dog thorax depicting the appearance of the lungs during inspiration (**A**) and expiration (**B**). Expiratory radiographs may be misinterpreted as lung disease because during expiration there is less air in the lungs, reducing the gas-to-soft tissue opacity interface and making the margins of soft tissue structures less distinct. In addition, bronchial and vascular markings are closer together which can make them appear more numerous than actual.

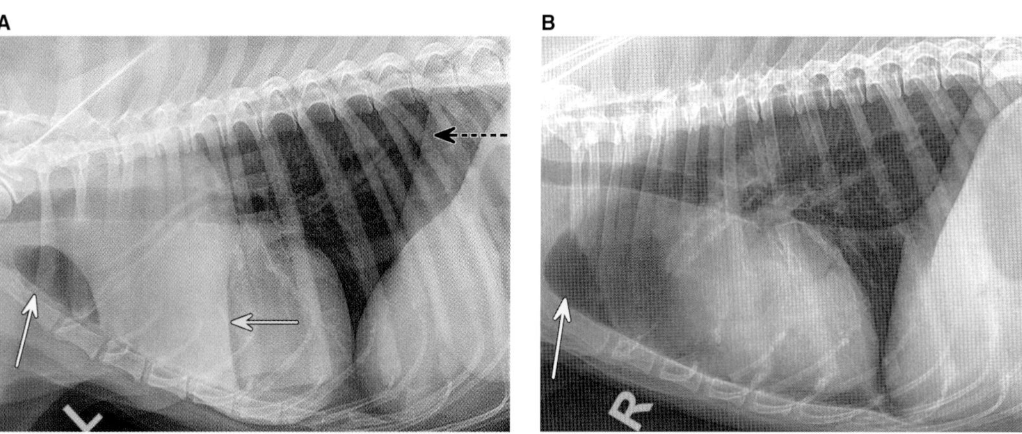

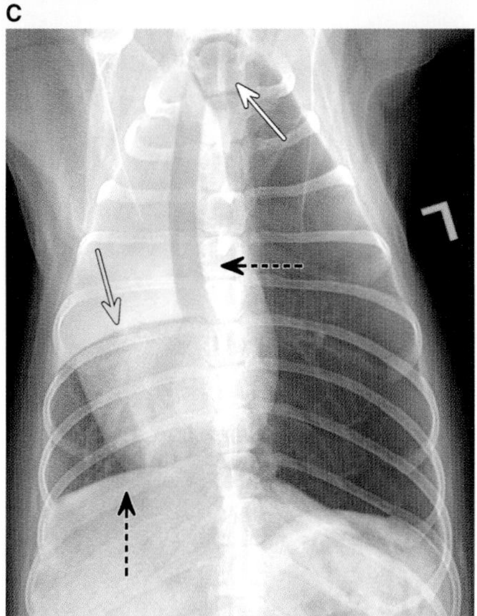

Figure 3.164 Lung lobe collapse. Left lateral view (**A**), right lateral view (**B**), and VD view (**C**) of a dog thorax depicting collapse of the right cranial lung lobe. The collapsed lobe is increased in opacity and its caudal edge creates a lobar sign against the inflated right middle lobe (yellow arrow). The mediastinum, trachea, and cardiac shadow are shifted to the right, and the right side of the diaphragm is cranial to the left (black arrows). The right cranial lobar vessels and the cranial cardiac border are effaced due to loss of gas in the collapsed lobe. The left cranial vessels and cardiac border are well-visualized due to compensatory hyperinflation of the left lung. The white arrow points to the tip of the left cranial lung lobe in each radiograph. Notice the collapsed right lung lobe is better visualized in the left lateral view (A) because it is "up" and adjacent to air-filled lung. It is less evident in the right lateral view but still visible because the right cranial lung lobe extends across midline and wraps around the cranial border of the cardiac shadow.

Because of this, all of the lung lobes tend to be similarly affected. However, variations in anatomy and the effects of gravity can alter the distribution of the fluid.

Pulmonary edema usually is bilateral, but it may appear unilateral in patients that are laterally recumbent. It tends to be more severe in the right caudal lung lobe due to the arrangement of the lymphatics.

In radiographs, early or mild pulmonary edema produces a diffuse, ill-defined increase in lung opacity and less distinct soft tissue margins. Bronchial markings may be more visible due to peribronchial fluid. Interlobar fissure lines sometimes are seen due to concurrent pleural edema. As lung edema and alveolar filling progress, lung opacification increases and the adjacent soft tissue margins become less and less visible until they are completely effaced. Lung volume usually is not reduced with pulmonary edema. Air bronchograms and lobar sign are more likely to occur with pneumonia. The rate of change in lung opacification is valuable to differentiate pulmonary edema from other diseases such as pneumonia.

The most common cause of lung edema is left heart failure. *Cardiogenic* pulmonary edema results from increased capillary venous pressure. *Non-cardiogenic* lung edema may be caused by inflammation or neurologic disease that leads to an increase in capillary permeability.

Cardiogenic pulmonary edema usually is accompanied by cardiovascular enlargement. A dilated left atrium and pulmonary veins larger than their paired arteries are typical findings with left heart failure. These findings may be less evident in patients receiving diuretic therapy. Diuresis can reduce the sizes of the heart and vessels, making them appear normal or even small in radiographs. Diuresis also can lessen pulmonary edema. Cardiovascular enlargement may not be apparent in patients with sudden or acute heart failure because there is insufficient time for enlargement.

In dogs, cardiogenic lung edema typically begins in the hilar region and spreads to the central region (Figure 3.165). It rarely spreads to the peripheral lungs. The distribution of lung edema tends to be bilateral and symmetrical, sometimes described as "butterfly-shaped" in appearance. Occasionally, dogs in left heart failure will present with a patchy and asymmetrical distribution (reported in a few large breed dogs with dilated cardiomyopathy).

In cats, cardiogenic lung edema often is more random, patchy, and asymmetric. The central and peripheral regions tend to be more severely affected (Figure 3.166). Left heart failure due to feline cardiomyopathy may initially produce perivascular and peribronchial edema. Fluid around the bronchi may be misinterpreted as bronchial thickening and the disease misdiagnosed as feline asthma. It is important to thoroughly evaluate the cardiovascular structures. Cats in left heart failure occasionally develop a pleural effusion. Pleural fluid is rare in dogs with left heart failure, unless it has progressed to right heart failure.

A

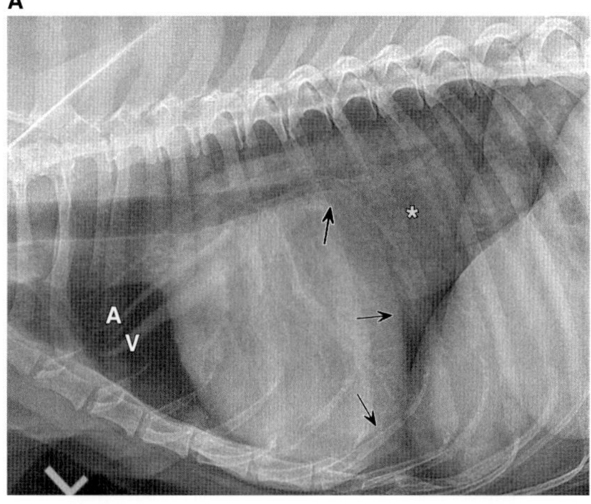

B

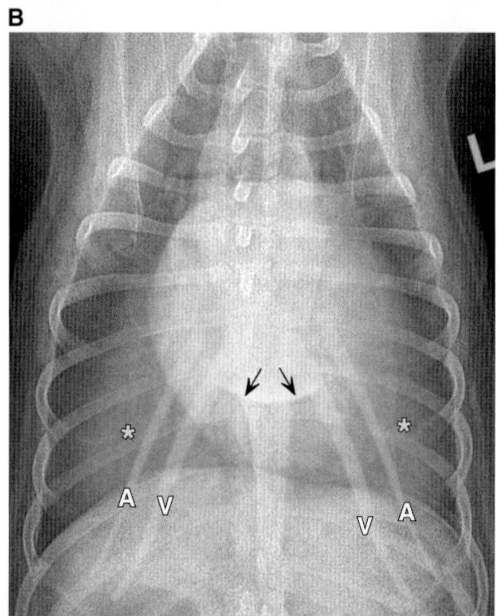

Figure 3.165 Cardiogenic pulmonary edema in a dog. Lateral view (**A**) and DV view (**B**) of a dog thorax depicting left heart failure. There is a bilateral and symmetrical increase in lung opacity in the hilar and central regions (*). The left atrium and left ventricle are enlarged (black arrows). The pulmonary veins (V) are larger than their paired arteries (A).

In both dogs and cats, cardiogenic pulmonary edema is quite labile and its radiographic appearance can change rapidly. With appropriate therapy, lung edema generally resolves within hours rather than days or weeks. Persistent lung opacification and suggests a complication such as pneumonia or acute respiratory distress syndrome. Follow-up radiographs are valuable to monitor the patient's progress and response to treatment.

Non-cardiogenic pulmonary edema results from disease other than left heart failure. It typically begins in the more peripheral lungs and spreads inward (Figure 3.167). The hilar region often is spared. The lung edema usually is bilateral, but not symmetrical, and tends to be more severe in the caudal lung lobes. Causes of non-cardiogenic pulmonary edema include neurologic disease, adverse drug reactions, and

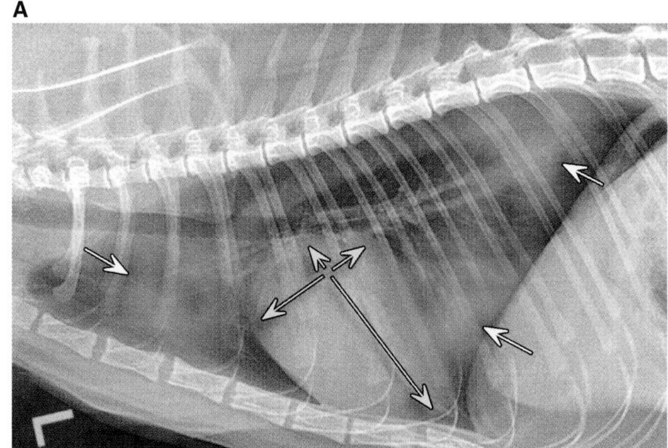

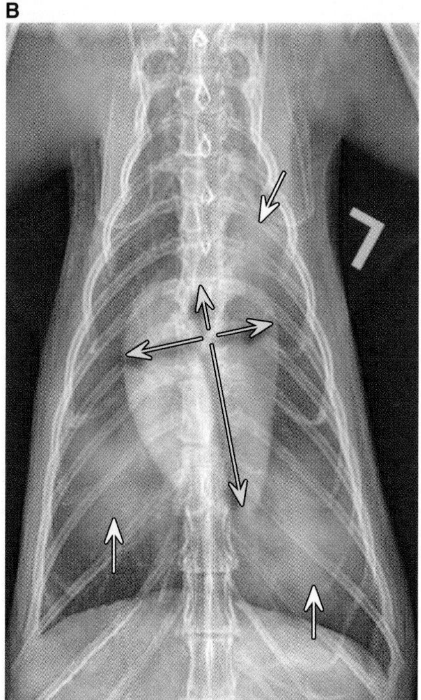

Figure 3.166 Cardiogenic pulmonary edema in a cat. Lateral view (**A**) and VD view (**B**) of a cat thorax depicting increased left heart failure. There is a patchy and asymmetrical increase in lung opacity in the central and peripheral regions (white arrows). The cardiac shadow is enlarged, both in length and at the base (yellow arrows), resulting in a more triangular shape.

severe inflammation (see Differential Diagnoses). With appropriate therapy, non-cardiogenic edema may require a longer period of time to see radiographic improvement than cardiogenic edema (days instead of hours).

Acute respiratory distress syndrome (ARDS) is an emergency situation caused by severe lung inflammation that leads to rapidly progressing pulmonary edema and respiratory failure. Inflammation may be due to infection, trauma, toxins, or inhaled irritants. Clinical signs may mimic those of heart failure but often are unresponsive to supportive care. By the time ARDS is recognized, it frequently is irreversible and fatal. Other names for ARDS include *acute lung injury* (ALI) and *shock lungs*.

In radiographs, the lungs may initially appear normal or hyperinflated. A diffuse increase in lung opacity soon develops due to the severe inflammation and early pulmonary edema. The edema progresses rapidly to produce

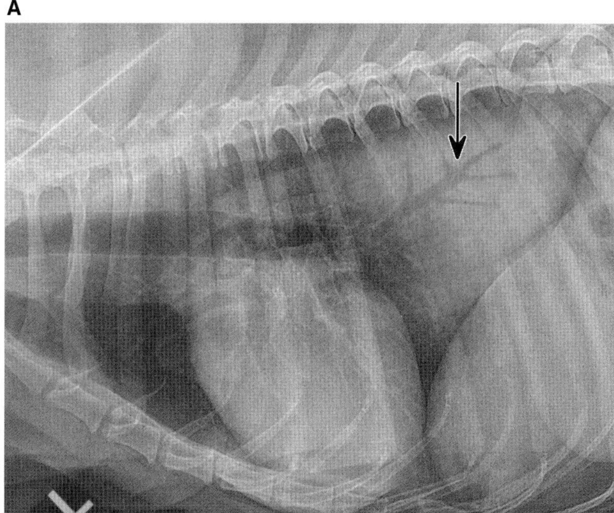

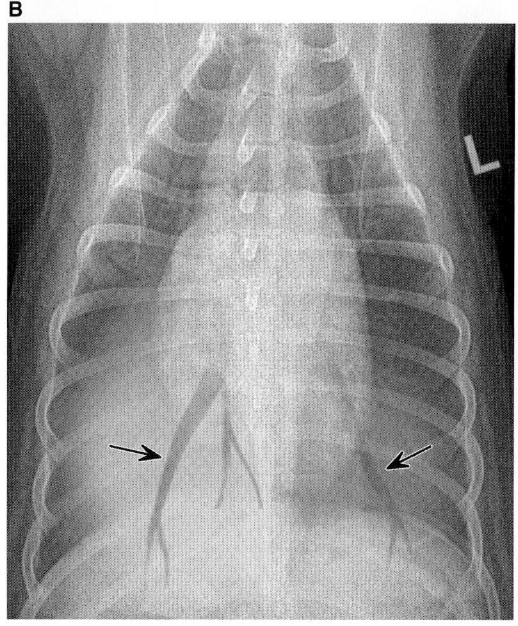

Figure 3.167 Non-cardiogenic pulmonary edema. Lateral view (**A**) and VD view (**B**) of a dog thorax depicting increased opacity in the dorsocaudal lungs. Lung opacification is bilateral and asymmetric, with greater opacity in the right caudal lung lobe. Cardiovascular structures are normal in size and shape. Air bronchograms are visible caudally (black arrows), which is concerning for more severe disease such as acute respiratory distress syndrome.

patchy and then more uniform lung opacification (Figure 3.168). Air bronchograms are common. With lung edema this severe, any remaining air-filled alveoli cannot fully expand and the lungs may appear small, even during inspiration. The trachea may be dilated due to increased inspiratory effort. Cardiovascular structures typically are normal or small in size.

Allergic lung disease

Allergic lung disease is caused by chronic or repeated inflammation in the lower airways. Other names include *asthma, chronic lower airway disease,* and *chronic bronchitis*. Allergic lung disease is more common in cats than in dogs. The etiology seldom is evident in radiographs and usually requires further testing.

Chronic airway inflammation leads to thickened bronchial walls and peribronchial infiltrates. The characteristic radiographic finding is an increase in the number of bronchial markings (Figure 3.169). The bronchial margins may be indistinct due to endobronchial and peribronchial secretions. The secretions can lead to bronchial obstruction and **lung lobe collapse**. Collapse of a lung lobe occurs most often in cats with asthma and usually involves the right middle lung lobe. A collapsed right middle lobe produces a triangular shaped, soft tissue opacity structure adjacent to the cardiac silhouette (Figure 3.170). It may be easier to see the collapsed lobe in a left lateral view with the right lung "up." Lung collapse may or may not be accompanied by a mediastinal shift. Sometimes compensatory hyperinflation of the adjacent lobes prevents a shift.

Progression of allergic lung disease can lead to **air trapping**. The term "air trapping" refers to the retention of gas in part or all of the lungs, even during expiration. An inability to exhale completely can lead to pulmonary emphysema or chronic obstructive pulmonary disease (COPD). Allergic lung disease also can lead to bronchiectasis. In many animals with allergic lung disease, the lungs appear well-inflated or even hyperinflated.

Eosinophilic pneumonia is a type of allergic lung disease that presents with pulmonary nodules. Other names include *eosinophilic pneumonitis, pulmonary infiltrates with eosinophilia* (PIE), and *eosinophilic bronchopneumopathy*. Eosinophilic pneumonia most often is caused by an allergic response to either parasites (e.g., heartworms) or an inhaled allergen. It sometimes is associated with a systemic disease or an adverse reaction to a drug (see Differential Diagnoses). The typical radiographic appearance is a diffuse, patchy, increase in lung opacity with multiple, small nodules widely scattered throughout the lungs (Figure 3.171). The degree of lung opacification and nodule formation varies with the type of allergic response, the amount of antigen, and the duration of exposure. In some dogs, an allergic response to heartworms can lead to **granulomatosis**, a condition in which much larger nodules form in the lungs (up to 2 cm in size) and hilar lymphadenomegaly often develops.

A

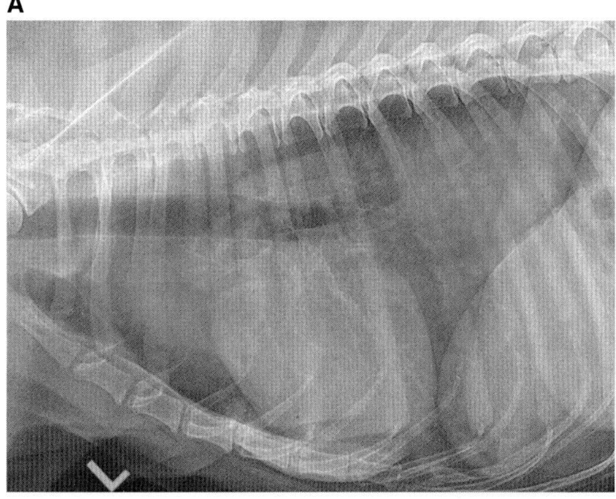

B

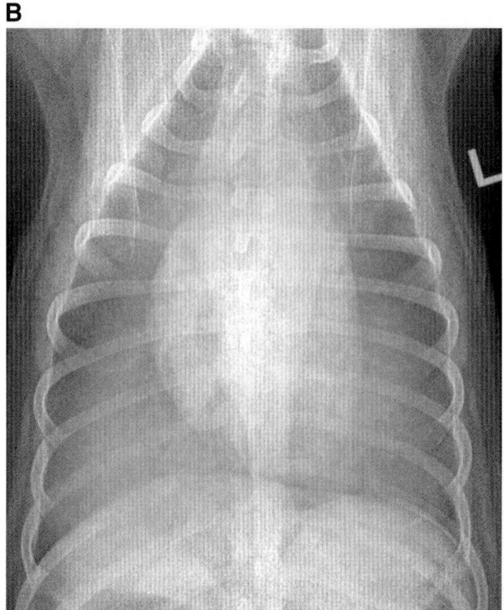

Figure 3.168 Acute respiratory distress syndrome. Lateral view (**A**) and VD view (**B**) of a dog thorax with ARDS. Depicted in the radiographs is a diffuse increase in lung opacity caused by pulmonary edema. The distribution is bilateral and symmetrical, more severe in the central lung region. Cardiovascular structures are partially effaced by the alveolar filling, but appear normal in size and shape. In patients with ARDS, the pulmonary edema fails to respond to therapy.

Pulmonary emphysema

Lung emphysema is an irreversible condition. It is characterized by larger than normal air spaces in the lungs caused by weakened and ruptured alveolar walls. Air cannot be completely exhaled from these areas resulting in "air-trapping" and retention of gas in the lungs. The affected lungs are persistently expanded. Emphysema may be localized or diffuse and may involve a single lung lobe or an entire lung. It may be congenital or acquired, the latter usually secondary to chronic bronchial inflammation.

A

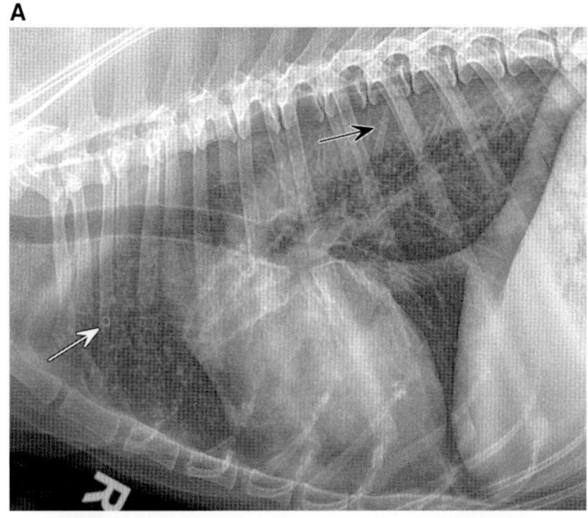

B

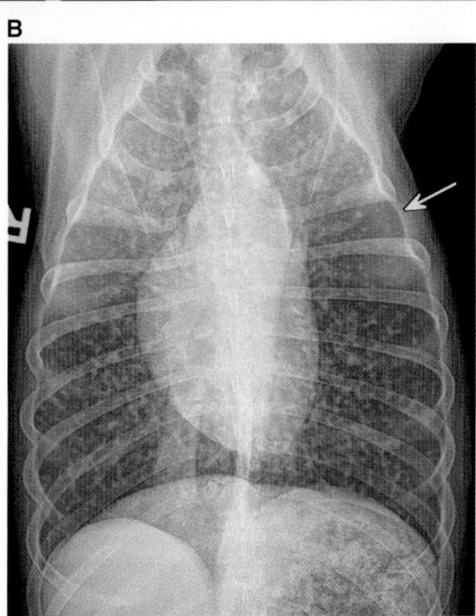

Figure 3.169 Chronic bronchitis. Lateral view (**A**) and VD view (**B**) of a dog thorax depicting hyperinflated lungs and an expanded thoracic cavity. In the VD view, the intercostal muscles bulge slightly outward (yellow arrow) due to repeated episodes of forced expiration. There are numerous bronchial rings (white arrow) and tramlines (black arrow). Many of the rings appear incomplete because not all of the bronchi are well-aligned with the x-ray beam.

In radiographs of emphysematous lungs there is little change in lung size and opacity between inspiration and expiration. The diaphragm may appear stationary in serial radiographs. Pulmonary bullae sometimes are present. Bilateral emphysema can lead to a barrel-chested appearance and a reduced cardiothoracic ratio. Severe, unilateral emphysema may lead to compression of the adjacent lung lobes, a mediastinal shift away from the expanded lung, and caudal displacement of the ipsilateral diaphragm (Figure 3.172). Horizontal beam radiography may be useful for diagnosis because an emphysematous lung may not collapse as would be expected with a normal lung while the patient is in lateral recumbency.

A

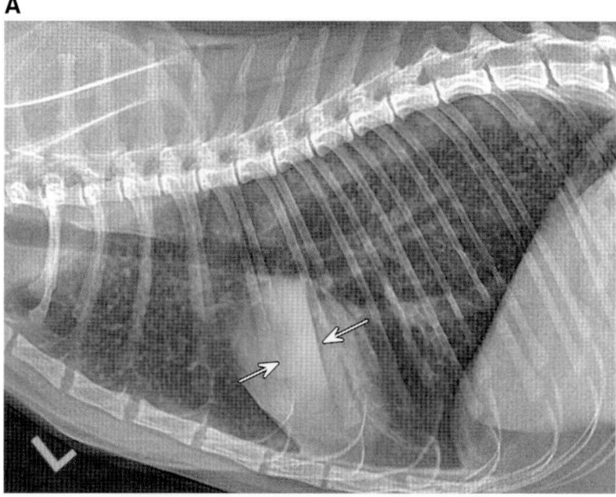

B

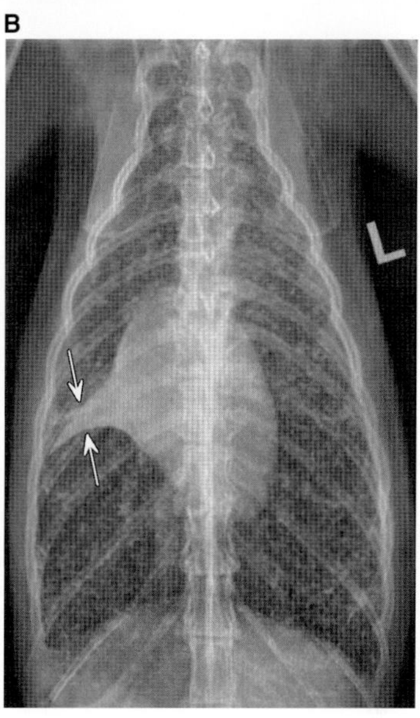

Figure 3.170 Feline asthma. Lateral view (**A**) and VD view (**B**) of a cat thorax depicting numerous bronchial markings within hyperinflated lungs. The thoracic cavity is expanded and the diaphragm is caudally displaced and flattened. The right middle lung lobe is collapsed, creating a triangular-shaped, soft tissue opacity structure that blends with the cardiac silhouette (arrows). In the lateral view, the collapsed lobe is superimposed on the cardiac shadow. It is visible because of the lobar sign created by its caudal border. In the VD view, the collapsed lobe partially effaces the right cardiac border. Compensatory hyperinflation of the right cranial and caudal lung lobes prevents a mediastinal shift to the right.

Pneumonia

Pneumonia generally is defined as lung inflammation. It most often is caused by an infection, either bacterial, viral, mycotic, or parasitic. The infectious agent may enter the lungs via aspiration, inhalation, or hematogenous spread. Pneumonia may be localized to a single lung lobe or it may be diffuse, involving an entire lung or both lungs. Serial radiographs are useful to help determine whether the

A

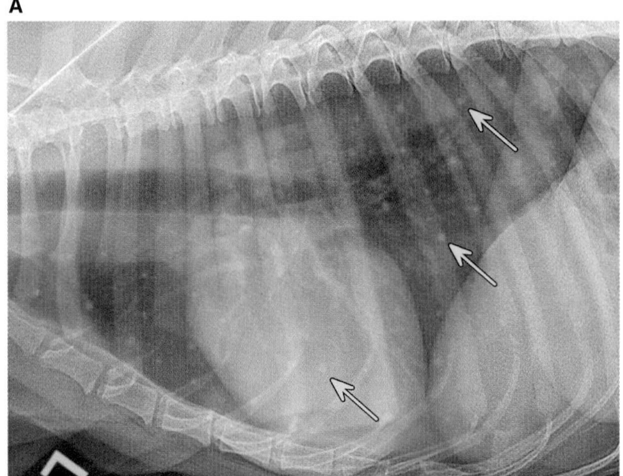

B

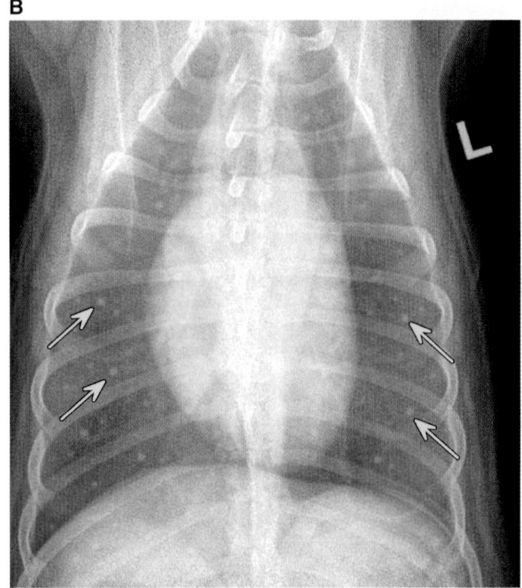

Figure 3.171 Eosinophilic pneumonia. Lateral view (**A**) and VD view (**B**) of a dog thorax depicting increased lung opacity that is diffuse and slightly patchy. There are multiple, small, indistinct nodules widely scattered in the lungs (arrows).

pneumonia is an acute one-time event, a long-standing persistent disease, or a recurring condition.

Radiographic signs of pneumonia primarily are those of alveolar filling and lung consolidation. Bronchial markings do not increase unless there is concurrent airway disease. Lung volume rarely is reduced, which means there is no mediastinal shift. Pneumonia tends to be quite labile and its radiographic appearance can change quickly over a short period of time.

Aspiration pneumonia is caused by inhalation of fluid or particulate matter that leads to lung inflammation and often a secondary bacterial infection. Patients with diseases that affect swallowing are at increased risk (e.g., pharyngeal disorders, megaesophagus). The severity of pneumonia depends on the type and quantity of aspirated material, as well as its distribution and duration in the lungs. Alveolar filling may be radiographically evident in less than 24 hours following aspiration, usually along the bronchial tree. Air bronchograms are common. Cardiovascular structures, intra-thoracic lymph nodes, and the pleural space usually

A

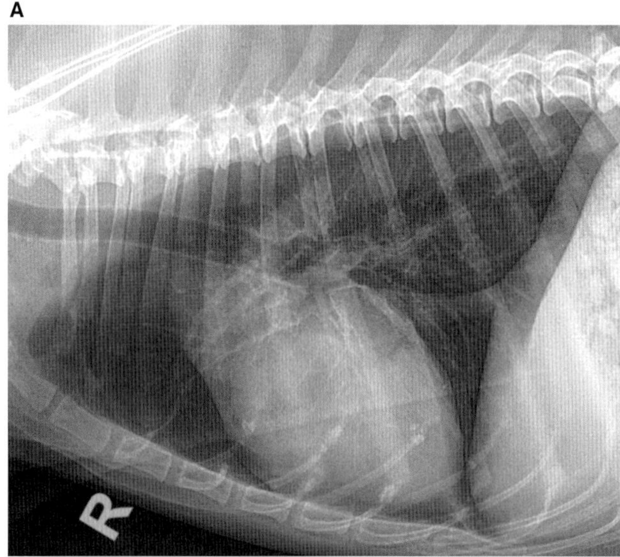

B

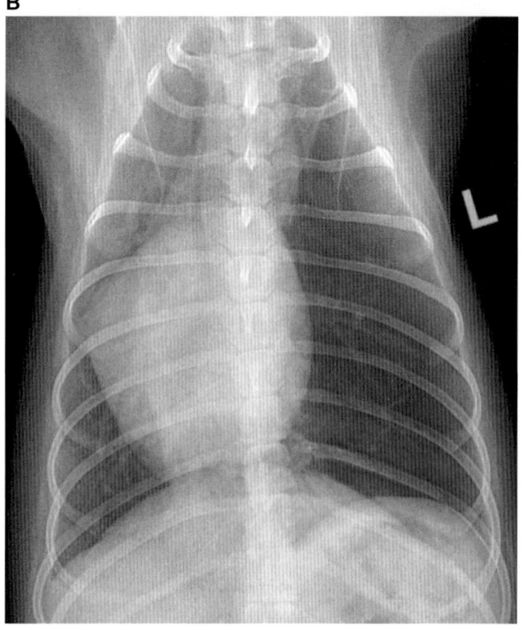

Figure 3.172 Pulmonary emphysema. Lateral view (**A**) and VD view (**B**) of a dog thorax depicting hyperexpansion of the left lung. There is a mediastinal shift to the right. These findings are readily evident in the VD view, but in the lateral view, the only finding is well-inflated lungs.

are normal. Aspiration of very irritating substances, such as gastric contents, can lead to bronchoconstriction, pulmonary edema, and systemic hypotension.

The distribution of aspiration pneumonia is affected by gravity and anatomy. Because of gravity, alveolar filling tends to be more severe in the dependent lungs. Patients that were standing at the time of aspiration are likely to fill the ventral lungs, whereas animals that were laterally recumbent are more likely to fill whichever lung was down at the time. However, many patients that remain standing or sternal are likely to present with pneumonia in the cranioventral lungs at the time of radiography, regardless of their body position at the time of aspiration. This is because fluid flows with gravity from anywhere in the lungs to the dependent parts, whether the pneumonia was caused by aspirated materials or not.

Due to the anatomy of bronchial branching, the right middle lung lobe most often is involved when liquids are aspirated (Figure 3.173). The caudal lung lobes more often are affected by inhaled solid materials. Larger objects can lodge in a caudal lobar bronchus and may obstruct airflow, typically to the dorsal part of the lung lobe. The accessory lung lobe frequently is involved when small objects such as pills are inhaled because it is a straight path from the trachea.

Bacterial pneumonia usually is a secondary complication that follows another lung disease, (e.g., viral infection, mycosis, pulmonary neoplasia, aspiration, trauma). As described with aspiration pneumonia, the dependent lungs tend to be more severely affected. Since most patients are able to remain standing or sternal, lung opacification most often is seen in the ventral lungs. Alveolar filling typically begins in the periphery of the affected lung lobe and spreads inward. More than one lobe may be involved. At the time of diagnosis, most patients with bacterial pneumonia present with lung opacification that completely effaces the vascular margins and the margins of any other adjacent soft tissue structures (Figure 3.174). Air bronchograms and lobar sign are common.

Actinomycosis and ***nocardiosis*** can cause pneumonia in both dogs and cats. The route of infection may be via migrating plant material or from a bite wound or other penetrating injury. Pleural effusion is a frequent finding. Fluid analysis may yield firm, yellowish, sulfur granules. Granulomas may be present in the lungs and can also develop in the skin and abdominal viscera. Abdominal infection can lead to peritoneal effusion, hepatomegaly, and splenomegaly. Nocardiosis can cause hilar and cranial mediastinal lymphadenomegaly in dogs but rarely in cats.

Tuberculosis is a zoonotic disease that can cause pneumonia in both dogs and cats. The typical route of infection in dogs is inhalation, whereas In cats, ingestion is the more common route. Dogs can acquire tuberculosis from an infected person. Lung granulomas are frequent findings in both dogs and cats. They typically begin as small, ill-defined,

A

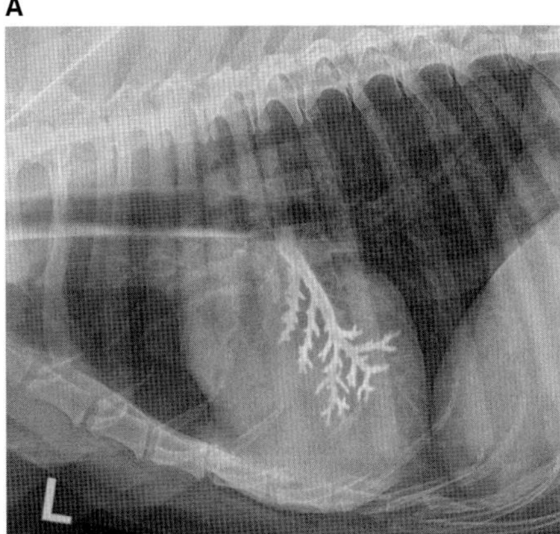

B

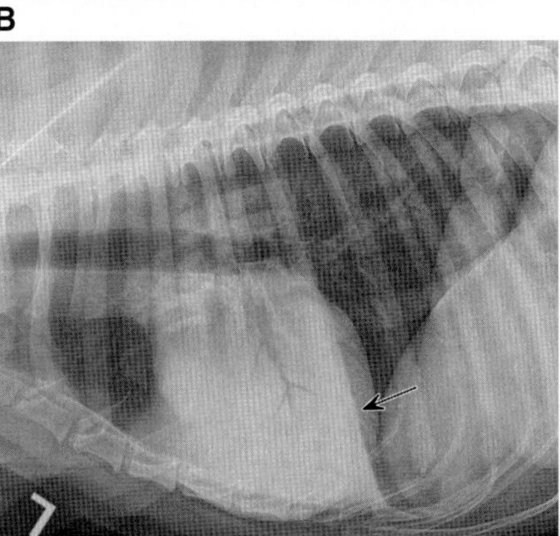

C

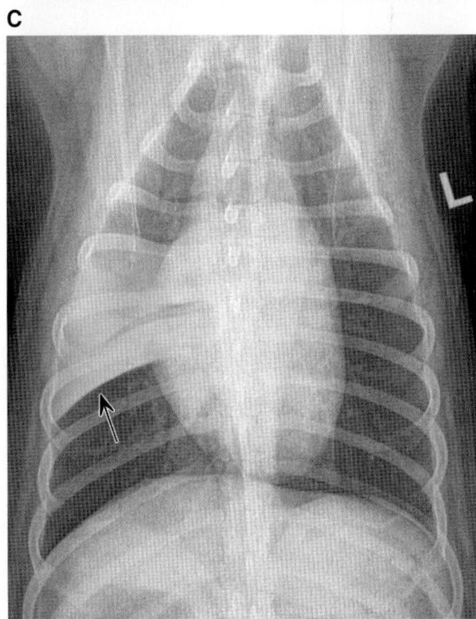

Figure 3.173 Aspiration pneumonia. **A**. Lateral view of a dog thorax depicting aspiration of positive contrast medium. Contrast is visible in the right middle lobar bronchus and also along the ventral trachea. **B**. Lateral view of a dog thorax depicting soft tissue opacity in the right middle lung lobe with lobar sign (arrow) and an air bronchogram extending into the lobe from the tracheal bifurcation. Alveolar filling in this lobe is due to bacterial pneumonia secondary to aspiration. **C**. VD view of same dog thorax depicting alveolar filling in the right middle lung lobe. There is partial effacement of the right cardiac border and a caudal lobar sign (arrow). The air bronchogram is again visible.

A

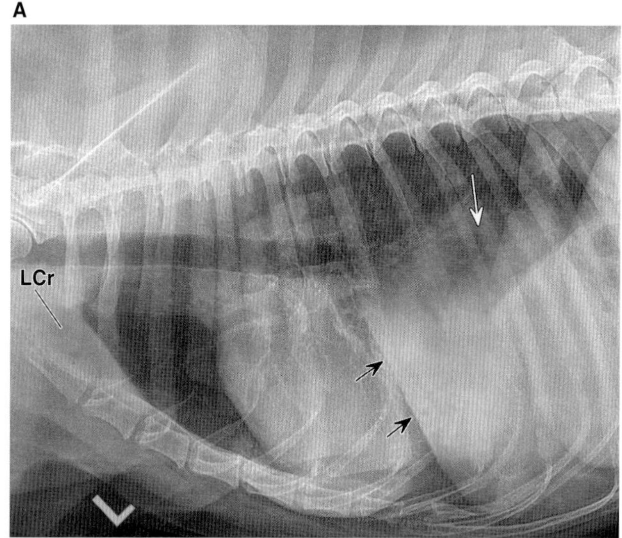

B

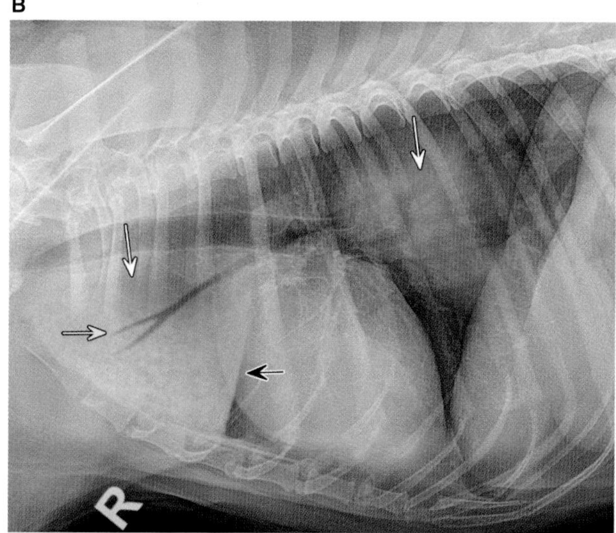

C

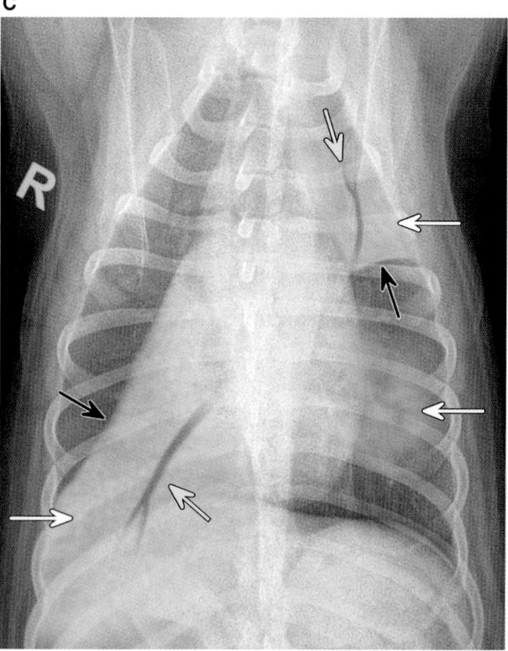

Figure 3.174 Bacterial pneumonia. Left lateral view (**A**), right lateral view (**B**), and VD view (**C**) of a dog thorax depicting multiple areas of increased lung opacity (white arrows). Parenchymal disease is bilateral and lobar in distribution but not symmetrical. The degree of alveolar filling in the right caudal and left cranial lung lobes completely effaces the adjacent soft tissue margins and produces lobar sign (black arrows) and air bronchograms (yellow arrows). Filling is more complete ventrally due to gravity. Alveolar filling in the left caudal lobe is less complete and appears as an ill-defined, "fluffy" area of opacification that remains dorsal at this time. Notice that disease in the left lung is better visualized in the right lateral view and disease in the right lung is more evident in the left lateral view. Recall that the "up" lung is better inflated, which provides a stronger gas-to-soft tissue opacity interface. Notice also that the cranial cardiac border remains visible through the opacified left cranial lung lobe. This is because the inflated right cranial lung lobe wraps around the cardiac silhouette. In the left lateral view, the only evidence of pneumonia in the left cranial lobe is opacification in the cranial tip (LCr) and a lack of visualization of the left cranial lobar vessels; only the right cranial vessels are visible.

soft tissue opacity nodules, but often mineralize and may cavitate. In dogs with tuberculosis, pleural effusion, pleural thickening, and large intra-thoracic lymph nodes are common, but these seldom occur in cats.

Viral pneumonias seldom lead to the influx of fluid and cells that is seen with bacterial infections. Typically there is less alveolar filling and the lower degree of lung opacification tends to be more widely and evenly distributed (Figure 3.161). Soft tissue margins may be blurry, but usually remain visible. Bronchial markings may be more visible due to peribronchial infiltrates. Lungs that are soft tissue opacity and efface the soft tissue margins suggests a secondary complication, such as bacterial pneumonia or pulmonary edema.

Parasitic pneumonia is caused by organisms that reside in the lungs or migrate through the lungs as part of their life cycle. Radiographic signs of parasitic pneumonia generally are non-specific. They include a diffuse increase in lung opacity and sometimes pulmonary nodules are visible (parasite granulomas). Lesions usually are bilateral but not symmetrical. The caudal lung lobes may be more severely affected due to parasite migration through the diaphragm. Parasite granulomas can vary greatly in size and number. They tend to be ill-defined initially, due to active inflammation, but become better defined over time. Diagnosis of parasitic pneumonia generally is confirmed by finding ova or larvae in the feces or in a tracheal aspirate.

Aelurostrongylus is a lung-worm of cats with worldwide distribution. It is prevalent in Europe, the southeast United States, and Australia. Infection most often is reported in young cats, usually hunting animals. The route of infection is via ingestion of an intermediate or transport host. *Aelurostrongylus* typically produces small, peribronchial granulomas (2–6 mm in size). Hilar lymphadenomegaly and pleural effusion may be present.

Eucoleus (*Capillaria*) is a nematode with worldwide distribution that can invade the respiratory tract of both dogs and cats. The route of infection is ingestion, after which the parasites migrate to the lungs. Radiographic signs include a diffuse increase in both lung opacity and bronchial markings.

Paragonimus is a lung fluke that can infect both dogs and cats. It is endemic to North America (mainly east of the Rockies), Africa, and eastern Asia. The route of infection is via ingestion of an intermediate host. Adult parasites migrate through the diaphragm, into the lungs, and invade the lower airways, where they cause inflammation and form cysts. Each fluid-filled cyst contains a developing fluke. At maturity, the fluke opens the cyst, which frequently allows bronchial air to enter the cyst. Cysts that fill with gas are called **pneumatocysts**. Pneumatocysts appear as rounded, thin-walled, cavitary lesions with smooth, well-defined inner margins and irregular, ill-defined outer margins (Figure 3.175). Some pneumatocysts will develop into lung bullae. Pulmonary nodules, pneumatocysts, and bullae may all be present at the same time. Rupture of a bulla or pneumatocyst can lead to a pneumothorax.

Toxoplasmosis is a single-cell parasite with worldwide distribution. It infects cats more often than dogs (because cats are both an intermediate and a definitive host). Radiographic signs are non-specific. Chronic or recurring toxoplasmosis may lead to a diffuse increase in lung opacity and more numerous bronchial markings.

Visceral larva migrans refers to the migration of parasitic nematodes through the lungs and other organs. In dogs and cats, the most common parasites are *Toxascaris* and *Toxocara*, both of which are found worldwide. The parasites migrate from the GI tract through the diaphragm and into the caudal lungs. In the lungs, they cause inflammation and form subpleural granulomas. Unless numerous, the granulomas usually are too small to detect in radiographs (typically 2–5 mm in size).

Pneumocystis carinii are extracellular parasites that normally live in the alveoli of most dog and cat lungs. They are opportunistic and may proliferate in young, immune-suppressed animals. Large numbers of parasites can block the alveolar capillaries, producing a diffuse increase in lung opacity. This is an uncommon disease. It has been reported in Miniature Dachshunds, Cavalier King Charles Spaniels, and Yorkshire Terriers. Pneumocystis pneumonia may be non-responsive to therapy and resemble other antibiotic-resistant diseases such as mycoplasma and mycotic infections.

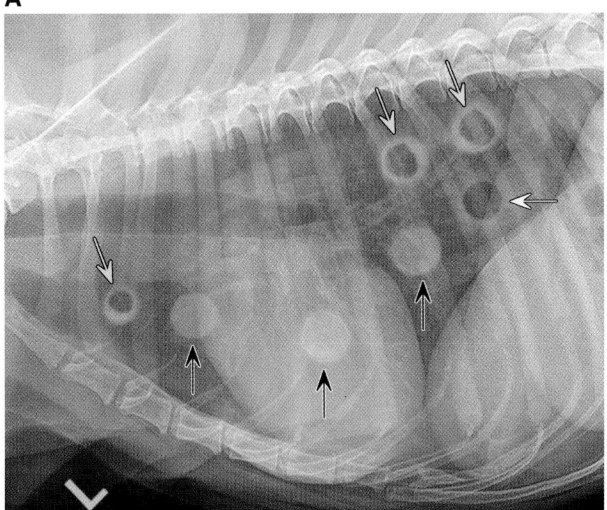

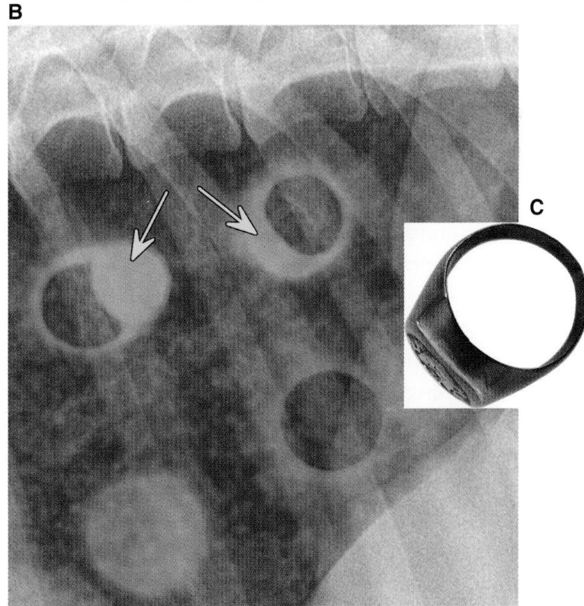

Figure 3.175 Paragonimiasis. (**A**) Lateral view of a dog thorax depicting pulmonary lesions associated with paragonimus infection. There is a diffuse increase in lung opacity that partially effaces the soft tissue structures (soft tissue margins appear hazy but remain visible). The soft tissue opacity nodules (black arrows) are fluid-filled cysts. The cavitary lesions (yellow arrows) are pneumatocysts. The white arrow points to a pneumatocyst that resembles a bulla. (**B**) Close-up of the dorsocaudal lung field in (**A**). The arrows point to adult flukes in the pneumatocysts. A fluke that is outlined by gas has been described as resembling a signet ring (the inset photograph (**C**) is a signet ring). There are reticulonodular markings in the lung caused by thickening of the interstitial connective tissues.

Mycotic pneumonia is more common in endemic areas. Knowledge of the patient's travel history and where fungi are prevalent is valuable for diagnosis. Failure of respiratory disease to respond to appropriate therapy for bacterial pneumonia should raise suspicion for a mycotic infection.

Radiographic signs of mycotic pneumonia often are nonspecific. Signs may resemble allergic lung disease. It is possible that the pulmonary response to a mycotic infection is an allergic response. A diffuse increase in lung opacity is a common finding with mycotic pneumonia, but it rarely effaces the soft tissue margins completely. More severe lung opacification suggests a secondary complication such as bacterial pneumonia. Bronchial markings may be increased and bronchial walls may be mineralization. Bronchial mineralization is more common with *coccidioidomycosis*. Pleural effusion is uncommon, other than with *blastomycosis*. Lung **granulomas** are a frequent finding with mycotic pneumonia (Figure 3.176). They often are multiple, ranging in size from tiny to about 15 mm, but solitary granulomas do occur. Chronic mycoses can lead to numerous granulomas, which has been described as a "snowstorm" of lung nodules (Figure 3.142). As with parasitic granulomas, the margins of actively growing mycotic granulomas may initially be ill-defined due to adjacent inflammation, but often become better defined over time. Granulomas can cavitate or mineralize. Mineralization of small nodules may resemble pulmonary osteomas in dogs. Serial radiographs are valuable to monitor the progress of pneumonia and the response to therapy.

Lymphadenomegaly occurs with some mycotic infections. It is seen more often in dogs than in cats. Hilar lymph node enlargement produces increased opacity near the tracheal bifurcation and may displace or compress the distal trachea. Lymphadenomegaly may help differentiate mycotic pneumonia from pulmonary neoplasia. Other than lymphoma, lung tumors rarely cause enlargement of the intra-thoracic lymph nodes (Figure 3.177).

Aspergillosis pneumonia is uncommon in dogs and cats. *Aspergillus sp.* occur worldwide, and the primary route of infection is inhalation. The fungal spores can lodge in the nasal cavity, paranasal sinuses, or/and lungs. Pulmonary nodules or a solitary lung mass may be present, but lung nodules are less common with aspergillosis than with histoplasmosis or blastomycosis.

Blastomycosis pneumonia is much more common in dogs than in cats. It most often is reported in young adult, large breed, male dogs. *Blastomyces sp.* are endemic in the southeastern and eastern United States, in the mid-Atlantic states, and in parts of Canada. The most common route of infection is inhalation. The tracheobronchial lymph nodes frequently enlarge and sometimes the sternal and cranial mediastinal nodes also enlarge. Multiple pulmonary nodules or a solitary lung mass may be present. Pleural effusion is a frequent finding. Mineralization of the lymph nodes or lung nodules is rare with blastomycosis; it is more common with histoplasmosis.

A

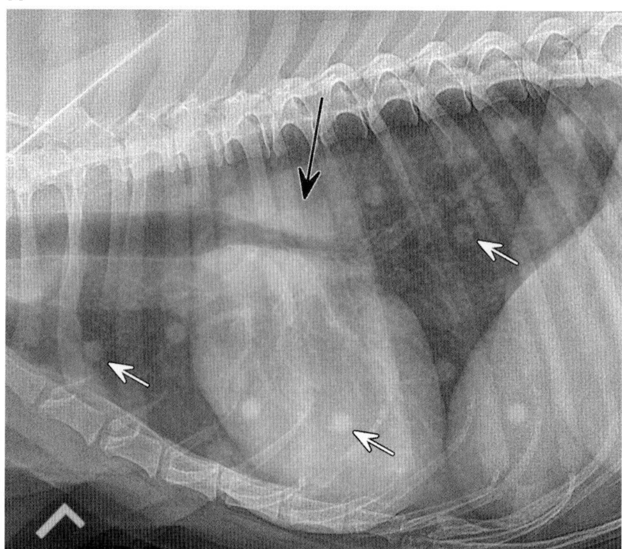

B

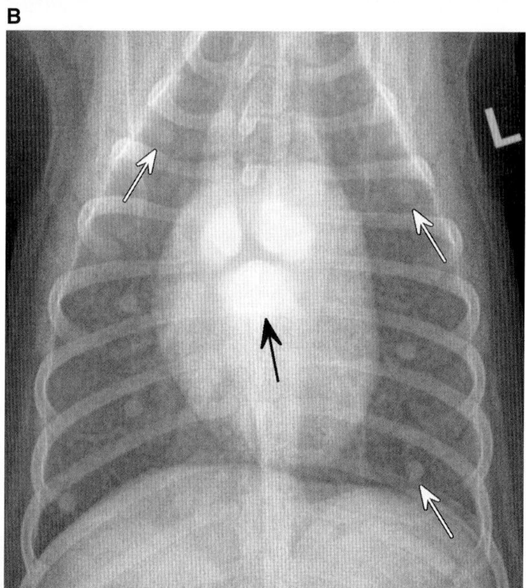

Figure 3.176 Mycotic pneumonia. Lateral view (**A**) and VD view (**B**) of a dog thorax depicting a diffuse increase in lung opacity with multiple small nodules (white arrows). The nodules are fungal granulomas. There is tracheobronchial lymphadenomegaly (black arrows) which increases the opacity in the hilar region. The trachea and primary bronchi are compressed (narrowed) and displaced ventrally by the enlarged lymph nodes.

Coccidioidomycosis pneumonia (*Valley Fever* or *San Joaquin Valley fever*) is more common in dogs than in cats. *Coccidioides* is endemic in the hot, arid regions of North America (southwestern and western United States), Central America, and South America. The typical route of infection is inhalation. Clinical signs may develop shortly after exposure or years later. Pulmonary nodules may be present, but they are less common than with histoplasmosis or

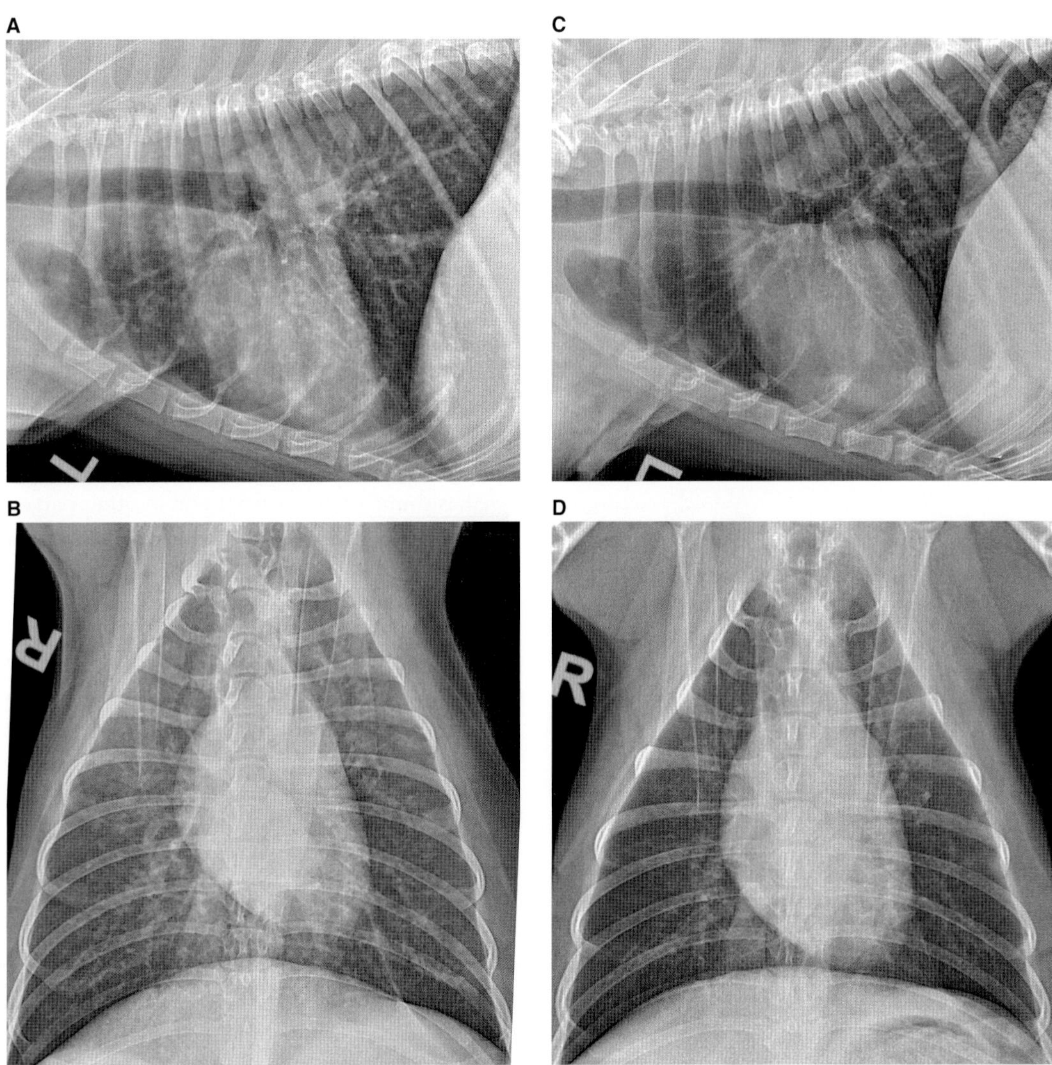

Figure 3.177 Blastomycosis. The initial radiographs of a dog with blastomycosis are on the left and the three-year follow up radiographs are on the right. In the initial lateral view (**A**) and VD view (**B**), there is a diffuse increase in lung opacity with numerous bronchial markings and increased hilar opacity. In the follow-up lateral view (**C**) and VD view (**D**) the lungs are less opaque, there are fewer bronchial markings, cardiovascular margins are more distinct, and hilar opacity is normal.

blastomycosis. Nodules may cavitate. Mediastinal lymph nodes may be mildly enlarged. Mineralization of the bronchial walls is more common with *Coccidioidomycosis* than with the other mycoses.

Cryptococcosis pneumonia is more common in cats than in dogs. Outdoor male cats and Siamese breeds are at increased risk. *Cryptococcus sp.* occur worldwide in temperate climates, especially in areas with excessive bird droppings. Routes of infection include inhalation and via skin lesions. Chronic rhinitis that is unresponsive to antibiotics is a common clinical sign. Rhinitis can progress to facial deformity, nasopharyngeal obstruction, and neurologic signs. Pulmonary nodules or a solitary lung mass may be present. The intra-thoracic lymph nodes sometimes are enlarged.

Histoplasmosis pneumonia is common in both dogs and cats. Young adult dogs are at increased risk. *Histoplasma sp.* are found worldwide in temperate and subtropical regions. The fungus is more prevalent in areas with abundant bird or bat feces. The primary route of infection is inhalation. Tracheobronchial lymphadenomegaly is common and can be severe. Large hilar lymph nodes may displace and/or compress the distal trachea and primary bronchi. Pulmonary nodules are common and frequently mineralize during healing.

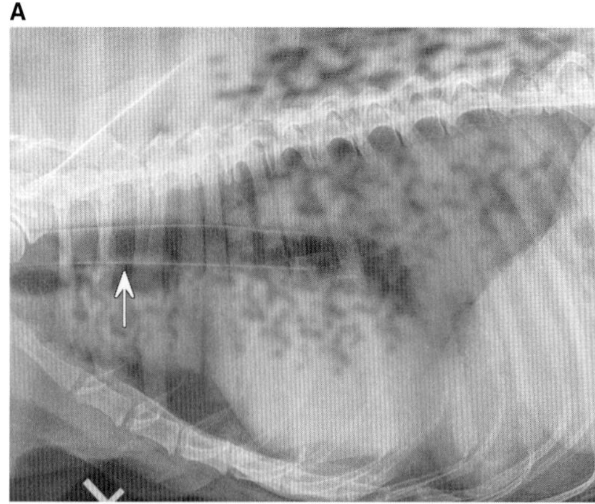

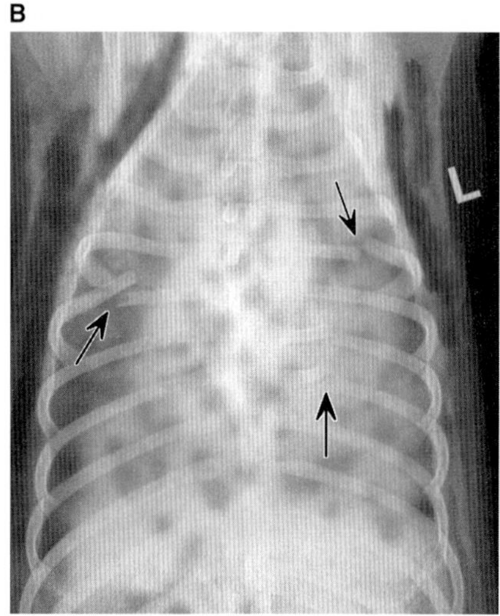

Figure 3.178 Thoracic trauma. Lateral view (**A**) and VD view (**B**) of a dog thorax depicting diffuse, patchy, lung opacification that effaces the cardiovascular and diaphragmatic borders. Subcutaneous emphysema is visible along the dorsal and lateral thorax and is superimposed on the pulmonary and mediastinal structures. In the lateral view, a pneumomediastinum enhances visualization of the outer tracheal margin (white arrow). There are multiple rib fractures, easiest to see in the VD view (black arrows). Radiographic findings and patient history support a diagnosis of pulmonary hemorrhage.

Pulmonary hemorrhage

Bleeding into the lungs may result from trauma, a coagulopathy, or erosion of a blood vessel. **Trauma** is most common and typically results in patchy lung opacification at the site of injury. Bleeding that is severe or unchecked leads to more widespread and uniform alveolar filling and effacement of the adjacent soft tissues (Figure 3.178). Other signs of trauma frequently are present (e.g., fractured ribs, soft tissue swelling, subcutaneous emphysema). Lungs filled with blood do not lose significant volume so there is no mediastinal shift, which may help differentiate a lung bleed from a lung collapse. With appropriate therapy lung contusions often resolve within a few days to a couple of weeks, disappearing in radiographs. Persistence of lung opacification may represent a hematoma or a secondary complication such as pneumonia.

Pulmonary hemorrhage due to a **coagulopathy** typically produces a generalized increase in lung opacity. The degree of opacification depends on the volume of blood in the lungs. Bleeding tends to be more severe in areas with higher blood flow and more numerous capillaries. In most quadrupeds this is in the dorsal lungs. In patients that are able to stand or remain sternal, blood eventually flows with gravity from the dorsal lungs to the ventral lungs. In patients that remain in lateral recumbency, lung opacification may be more unilateral. In addition to bleeding into the lungs, coagulopathies often lead to hemorrhage in the tracheal wall, mediastinum, pleural cavity, and in other parts of the body.

Erosion of a pulmonary blood vessel may be caused by a nearby tumor or abscess, migration of parasites, or thromboembolic disease. Bleeding initially occurs at the site of rupture but can quickly spread if unchecked.

Pulmonary embolism

Pulmonary embolism occurs when a piece of material obstructs an artery in the lung. Most emboli come from a thrombus and therefore the condition commonly is called pulmonary *thromboembolism*. In addition to blood clots, migrating gas bubbles, fat particles, bacteria, and foreign materials can cause a lung embolism. Pulmonary emboli block the flow of blood, but not the flow of air into the lung.

Thoracic radiographs are neither sensitive nor specific for pulmonary embolism, but they are useful to rule out other causes of the patient's clinical signs (e.g., pneumonia, pneumothorax). The lungs can appear normal in radiographs of patients with lung embolism even when the clinical signs are severe. The classic radiographic findings of a pulmonary embolism include (1) dilation of the affected artery proximal to the obstruction, (2) abrupt tapering of the artery distal to the obstruction, and (3) a less opaque area of lung due to diminished blood flow (Figure 3.179). Vascular markings will be small or absent in the area of diminished blood flow. The lack of blood flow eventually progresses to localized pulmonary edema and an ill-defined area of increased lung opacity. In most cases, it is the localized area of lung opacification that is detected in radiographs. Pleural effusion occasionally develops. The cardiac silhouette usually is normal unless the embolic disease is severe or widespread, as may occur with heartworm disease.

Patients with small or only a few pulmonary emboli usually are asymptomatic. Larger or more numerous emboli can be fatal. In most animals, more than 40% of the pulmonary blood supply must be obstructed before clinical signs of respiratory distress develop. Distress due to lung embolism generally responds poorly to oxygen therapy and supportive care.

A

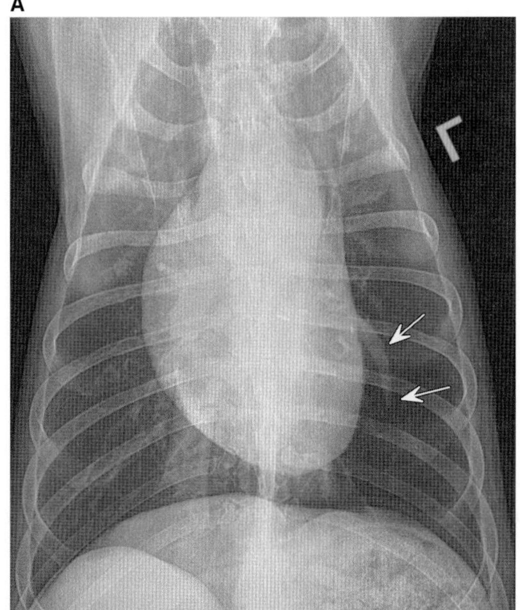

B

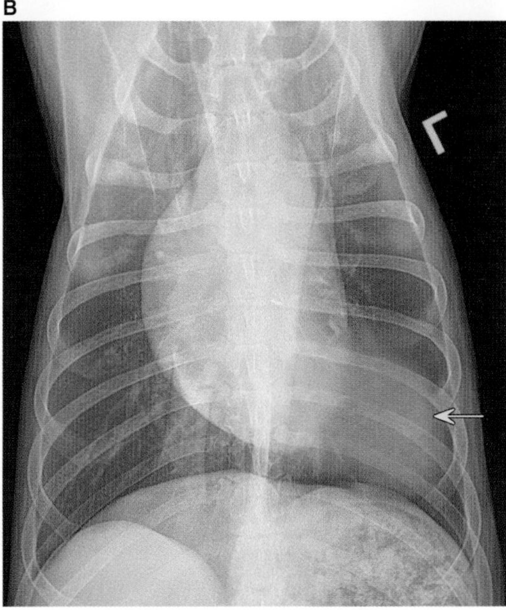

Figure 3.179 Pulmonary embolism. **A**. VD view of a dog thorax depicting the classic signs of pulmonary embolism. A left caudal pulmonary artery is enlarged and tapers abrubtly (white arrows), leading to a less opaque area in the left caudal lung lobe. There are few vascular markings here. **B**. Follow-up VD view of the same dog. There is now a localized, ill-defined area of increased lung opacity caused by pulmonary edema (yellow arrow).

Pulmonary neoplasia

Secondary lung tumors are much more common in dogs and cats than primary lung tumors. Metastatic tumors can form one or more nodules anywhere in the lungs. Nodules that are all similar in size suggests a shower of metastases over a relatively short period of time. Variably sized nodules likely arrived over a more extended time span. Examples of neoplasms that regularly metastasize to the lungs include hemangiosarcoma, osteosarcoma, thyroid carcinoma, and mammary carcinoma. Hemangiosarcoma tends to produce numerous lung nodules, ranging from about 3–10 mm in size.

Tumors that originate in the lungs frequently are malignant and locally invasive. Primary lung tumors can spread to other parts of the lungs, the pleural space, and to extrathoracic sites. Most primary lung tumors produce a solitary, soft tissue opacity mass, usually in the middle of a lung lobe. The mass often is larger than 4 cm in size at the time of diagnosis. The margins of the tumor tend to be uneven and may be indistinct, depending on the condition of the adjacent lung. The alveoli in the adjacent lung can lose gas because they are compressend by the tumor or due to alveolar filling. The alveoli may fill with blood due to tumor erosion through a pulmonary vessel or they may fill with purulent material from a secondary bacterial infection. A primary lung tumor that erodes through a bronchus may become a cavitary lesion. Primary tumors sometimes mineralize. Both cavitation and mineralization are rare with metastatic lung tumors.

Large lung tumors can displace nearby mediastinal structures and may lead to hypertrophic osteopathy. Pleural effusion may or may not be present (more common in cats than in dogs).

Bronchogenic carcinoma is a primary lung tumor in dogs. It tends to form a well-defined and sometimes lobar-shaped mass. It is reported more often in the right caudal lung lobe. In the early stages, as a bronchogenic carcinoma is growing in the bronchial wall, a bulla may develop next to the tumor nodule. **Adenocarcinoma** is a primary lung tumor in cats. It sometimes is associated with metastases to the digits.

Lymphoma in the lungs can present with a variety of radiographic appearances. In cats, it ranges from a generalized, mild increase in lung opacity to complete consolidation of a lung lobe. In dogs, lung lymphoma is more likely to produce multiple discrete pulmonary nodules and thin linear reticular markings. In both dogs and cats, pulmonary lymphoma frequently is accompanied by enlargement of the intra-thoracic lymph nodes and intra-abdominal organomegaly. Lymphadenomegaly is rare with most lung tumors (it is more common with lung mycoses than lung neoplasia).

Lung lobe torsion

Torsion occurs when a lung lobe rotates around its axis, twisting its bronchus, artery, and vein. Rotation obstructs the bronchus and vein, but not the artery. The lung lobe enlarges as it continues to fill with arterial blood. Over time, blood and air leak out of the lobe, reducing its size.

In radiographs, lung lobe torsion generally begins as an ill-defined increase in lobar opacity. As the lung lobe enlarges, its borders bulge outward to become more convex. A greatly swollen lobe can displace the mediastinum.

Because the bronchus is twisted, air cannot flow into the lung lobe and alveolar gas is gradually lost. Blood continues to enter the lobe and is trapped in the parenchyma, increasing the lobar opacity and effacing the lobar vessels and the adjacent soft tissue borders (Figure 3.180). Small pockets of gas may be visible in the opacified lobe due to retained air in groups of alveoli or due to necrosis and infection with gas-producing bacteria. Air bronchograms occasionally are present early, but not later. The lung lobe or its bronchus may appear abnormal in shape or position. Pleural effusion is common and frequently obscures a lung lobe torsion. Additional radiographs made after removing the pleural fluid may be needed for diagnosis.

Blood eventually leaks out of the engorged lung lobe, reducing its size and making its margins more concave. The lobe remains soft tissue opacity because it is not ventilated. Any mediastinal shift that was away from the swollen lobe, now is toward the smaller lobe. Compensatory inflation of the unaffected lung lobes may prevent or correct a shift.

The cause of a lung lobe torsion often is unknown. Many cases are considered idiopathic or labeled spontaneous. Predisposing conditions may include pleural effusion, diaphragmatic hernia, and recent thoracotomy. Note: it often is difficult to determine whether pleural fluid was present prior to a torsion or if it developed after the torsion. Secondary complications to a lung lobe torsion include chylothorax, rotation of a different lung lobe, and bronchial rupture, the latter can lead to a pneumothorax. Patients with lung lobe torsion may present with recurrent pneumonia.

Torsion can affect any lung lobe. In large dogs, the right middle lobe most often is involved. In small dogs (particularly pugs), it is the left cranial lobe. Torsion of the right cranial lobe is uncommon and torsion of the caudal lung lobes is rare.

Differentials for a lung lobe torsion include pneumonia and pulmonary contusion. Pneumonia rarely is accompanied by pleural effusion and frequently improves in follow-up radiographs with proper therapy. Pulmonary contusion may be accompanied by pleural effusion (i.e., hemothorax), but other signs of thoracic trauma frequently are present, such as rib fractures and subcutaneous emphysema.

A

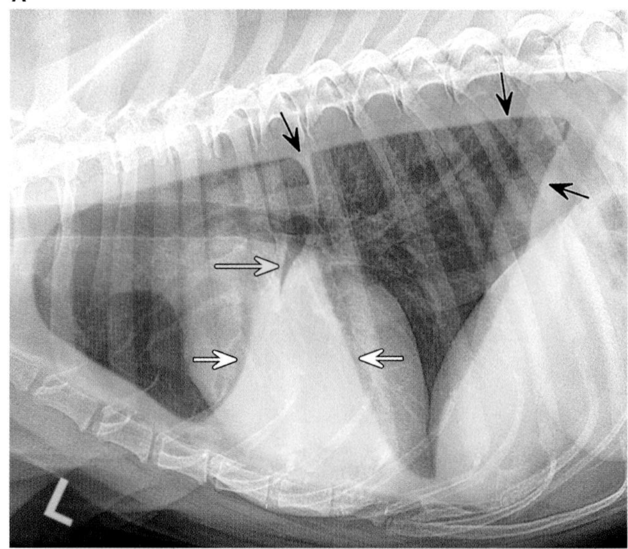

B

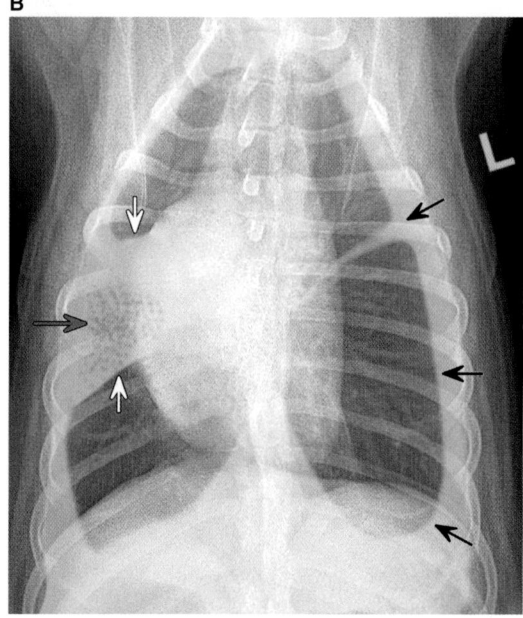

Figure 3.180 Lung lobe torsion. Lateral view (**A**) and VD view (**B**) of a dog thorax depicting a torsion of the right middle lung lobe. There is increased lobar opacity and lobar sign (white arrows). The right cardiac border is partially effaced. Foci of gas are visible in the right middle lobe (blue arrow) due to retained alveolar gas. In the lateral view, the right middle lobar bronchus is cranially displaced, narrowed and blunted (yellow arrow) due to twisting of the bronchus. Pleural fluid is present (black arrows) and there is a pleural fissure line between the cranial and caudal segments of the left cranial lung lobe.

CHAPTER 3

Differential diagnoses for thorax

All areas of each radiograph should be evaluated in a systematic manner. Each anatomic structure must be carefully examined for abnormal position, size, shape, and opacity. Abnormalities caused by trauma frequently are accompanied by other signs of trauma (e.g., fractured ribs, pulmonary contusions, subcutaneous emphysema, free gas or fluid in the pleural space).

Types of masses
- Tumor
- Abscess
- Granuloma
- Hematoma
- Seroma
- Lipoma
- Cyst
- Hernia

Thoracic wall
- Rib abnormalities
- Sternal abnormalities
- Vertebral abnormalities
- Abnormal intercostal spacing
- Abnormal opacity in thoracic wall
- Abnormal thickening of thoracic wall
- Mass in thoracic wall

Diaphragm
- Abnormal position of diaphragm
- Abnormal shape or margin of diaphragm

Pleura and pleural space
- Pleural fissure lines
- Pleural mass
- Pleural effusion
- Pneumothorax

Mediastinum
- Abnormal position of mediastinum / Mediastinal shift
- Abnormal widening of mediastinum
  - Mediastinal mass
- Abnormal opacity in mediastinum
  - Pneumomediastinum

Esophagus
- Abnormal position of esophagus
- Abnormal opacity in esophagus
- Abnormal size of esophagus
  - Megaesophagus

Cardiac silhouette
- Abnormal position of cardiac silhouette
- Abnormal size of cardiovascular structures
  - Small cardiac shadow (microcardia)
  - Enlarged cardiac shadow
    - Cardiomegaly
    - Pericardial effusion
    - Left atrial dilation
    - Left ventricular enlargement
    - Right atrial dilation
    - Right ventricular enlargement
    - Aortic enlargement
    - Caudal vena cava enlargement
    - Main pulmonary artery enlargement
- Right heart failure
- Left heart failure
- Severe cardiac disease without radiographic evidence of cardiac enlargement
- Abnormal opacity in cardiac silhouette

Trachea
- Abnormal position of trachea
- Abnormal opacity of trachea
  - Enhanced visualization of tracheal margins
  - Poor visualization of tracheal margins
- Abnormal size of trachea
  - Narrowed trachea
  - Dilated trachea
- Bronchial obstruction

Lungs
- Increased lung opacity
  - Non-pathologic causes of increased lung opacity
  - Pulmonary edema
  - Pneumonia
  - Lung collapse
  - Pulmonary hemorrhage
  - Pulmonary nodule/mass
  - Mineral opacity in lungs
- Decreased lung opacity
- Abnormal thickening of bronchial walls
- Abnormal size of bronchi
- Abnormal size of pulmonary vessels
- Abnormal opacity in pulmonary vessels

Thoracic wall

1. Pathology associated with the bony thorax usually is accompanied by soft tissue swelling, active bone remodeling, or both.

Rib abnormalities

1. Trauma (e.g., fracture, luxation, healing fracture, bruise/periosteal response).
2. Displacement due to torn intercostal muscle.
3. Infection/inflammation (osteomyelitis).
4. Primary tumor:
   a. Chondrosarcoma (most common).
   b. Osteosarcoma (usually distal rib).

  c. Fibrosarcoma.
  d. Multiple myeloma (multiple areas of decreased opacity).
5. Secondary or metastatic tumor (usually lytic).
6. Cartilaginous exostosis (osteochondroma).
7. Congenital abnormality (e.g., supernumerary or extra ribs, vestigial, flaring at rib ends).

Conditions that may mimic rib abnormalities
1. Poor technique (e.g., overexposed, underexposed).
2. Breed conformation (e.g., chondrodysplasia, brachycephalic).
3. Expanded thorax (e.g., lung hyperinflation, tension pneumothorax).

Sternal abnormalities
1. Congenital condition
  a. Sternal dysraphism.
  b. Fusion of sternebrae (no soft tissue swelling).
  c. Misalignment of sternebrae (no swelling).
2. Sternal spondylosis (older dogs, resembles vertebral spondylosis).
3. Trauma (e.g., fracture, luxation).
4. Osteomyelitis (e.g., puncture wound, foreign object).
5. Neoplasia.
6. Sternal mass:
  a. Hematoma.
  b. Abscess (e.g., bite wound, foreign material).
  c. Granuloma (e.g., chronic inflammation).
  d. Seroma (e.g., trauma, recent surgery).
  e. Tumor (e.g., chondrosarcoma, osteosarcoma, fibrosarcoma).

Vertebral abnormalities
1. Spondylosis deformans.
2. Fracture/luxation.
3. Spondylitis (e.g., *Spirocerca lupi*).
4. Infection/inflammation (e.g., osteomyelitis).
5. Neoplasia.
6. Congenital abnormality (e.g., hemivertebra, transitional vertebra).

Abnormal intercostal spacing
1. Muscle contraction (e.g., pain, struggling).
2. Trauma (e.g., muscle tear, rib fracture).
3. Mass effect (e.g., hematoma, lipoma, tumor).
4. Uneven lung inflation (e.g., pleural disease, intrathoracic mass).
5. Post-thoracotomy.
6. Hyperexpansion of thorax (e.g., emphysema, pneumothorax).
7. Hemivertebrae (result in crowding of proximal ribs).
8. Anomalous curvature of spine or sternum (e.g., scoliosis, pectus excavatum).

Conditions that mimic abnormal intercostal spacing
1. Poor centering of x-ray beam.
2. Breed conformation (e.g., barrel chested).
3. Positioning artifact.

Decreased opacity in thoracic wall
1. Subcutaneous gas:
  a. Penetrating wound (e.g., bite wound, laceration, iatrogenic injection or fluid administration).
  b. Extension of pneumomediastinum.
  c. Infection with gas-forming organism.
2. Subcutaneous fat:
  a. Obesity.
  b. Lipoma; more localized fat opacity.

Increased opacity in thoracic wall
1. Calcinosis cutis (e.g., hypercortisolism).
2. Dystrophic mineralization (e.g., long-standing abscess or granuloma).
3. Neoplastic mineralization (e.g., mammary tumor).
4. Foreign material (e.g., BB, air rifle pellet, bullet fragment, wire fragment, wood, glass, needle).
5. Periosteal response.
6. Microchip.
7. Tattoo.

Conditions that mimic abnormal thoracic wall opacity
1. Poor exposure technique.
2. Dirty or damaged imaging receptor, cassette, or phosphor screen.
3. Superimposition artifact:
  a. Wet or dirty skin or hair coat.
  b. Medication or contrast agent on patient, positioning device, or image receptor.
  c. Cutaneous or subcutaneous nodule (e.g., tumor, cyst, injection site, engorged tick).
  d. Nipples; usually bilateral, ventral, and within one intercostal space of each other.
  e. Skin folds; soft tissue opacity lines extend beyond the borders of the thoracic cavity.
  f. Medical equipment (e.g., ECG leads, IV tubing, bandaging material) or positioning device.
  g. Blanket or stretcher; note the similar pattern in the background beyond the thoracic wall.
  h. Body part of patient or radiographer.

Diffuse thickening of thoracic wall
1. Subcutaneous emphysema:
  a. Extension of pneumomediastinum.
  b. Penetrating wounds (e.g., bite wounds, lacerations).
2. Subcutaneous fat:
  a. Obesity.
  b. Large lipoma; often unilateral.

3. Subcutaneous fluid:
   a. Edema (e.g., lymphatic disease).
   b. Cellulitis (e.g., inflammation, infection).
   c. Hemorrhage (e.g., trauma, coagulopathy).
   d. Iatrogenic fluid therapy.

Mass in thoracic wall

1. Bony lesion (see rib, sternum abnormalities).
2. Soft tissue mass (e.g., tumor, abscess, hematoma, seroma, cyst).
3. Fat opacity mass (e.g., lipoma, dissecting lipoma).
4. Cartilaginous exostosis, osteochondroma.
5. Foreign object.
6. Paracostal hernia.
7. Recent injection/subcutaneous fluid administration.

Conditions that mimic thoracic wall mass

1. Costochondral junctions, particularly when large or mineralized (e.g., chondrodystrophic breeds).
2. Positioning artifact (e.g., patient's skin bunching along one side of its body).
3. Superimposition artifact (e.g., bandaging material, positioning aid); note that the lung is not indented or displaced.

Diaphragm

Abnormal position of diaphragm

1. In general, the position of the diaphragm is determined by the sizes of the lungs and abdominal contents.

Non-visualization of diaphragm

1. Pleural effusion (common cause, pleural fluid eliminates the opacity interface with air-filled lung).
2. Diaphragmatic hernia (common cause).
3. Adjacent lung disease (e.g., pneumonia, mass).
4. Caudal mediastinal/esophageal disease.
5. Extrapleural mass adjacent to diaphragm.

Cranial displacement of diaphragm

1. Poor lung inflation:
   a. Expiratory radiograph.
   b. Obesity.
   c. Pleural adhesions.
   d. Pulmonary fibrosis.
   e. Shallow breathing (e.g., severe pain).
2. Lung collapse (see increased lung opacity):
   a. Recumbent atelectasis.
   b. Airway obstruction.
   c. Pneumothorax, pleural effusion.
3. Diaphragmatic hernia.
4. Abdominal distension:
   a. Severe peritoneal effusion.
   b. Large intra-abdominal mass or organomegaly.
   c. Gastric distention (e.g., bloat, GDV).
   d. Advanced pregnancy.
   e. Severe pneumoperitoneum (e.g., post laparotomy).
5. Phrenic nerve paralysis (e.g., neuropathy, trauma, severe inflammation, myopathy).
6. Eventration of diaphragm.
7. Intra-thoracic adhesions to diaphragm:
   a. Postsurgical complication.
   b. Remnant from previous trauma.
   c. Chronic or severe inflammation.
8. Spinal or sternal deformity:
   a. Pectus excavatum, pectus carinatum.
   b. Severe scoliosis.
9. Absence of a lung:
   a. Prior lobectomy.
   b. Lung agenesis or hypoplasia.

Conditions that mimic cranial displaced diaphragm

1. Caudal centering of the x-ray beam can falsely project the diaphragm cranially.
2. Mass on diaphragm.
3. Adjacent lung disease or pleural effusion.
4. Patient positioning:
   a. In lateral recumbency, the dependent hemidiaphragm moves cranially.
   b. Patient rotation can project one side of the diaphragm cranial to the other.
   c. Contracted thorax due to pain or struggling.

Caudal displacement of diaphragm

1. Hyperinflated or overexpanded lungs:
   a. Deep inspiration (dyspnea, struggling).
   b. Manual ventilation (anesthesia).
   c. Chronic lower airway disease (e.g., asthma).
   d. Pulmonary emphysema.
2. Severe pleural effusion.
3. Severe pneumothorax.
4. Large intra-thoracic mass:
   a. Pulmonary (e.g., lung cyst, emphysema).
   b. Pleural (e.g., herniated viscera).
   c. Mediastinal (e.g., megaesophagus).
5. Empty abdomen; decreased abdominal content due to emaciation or displacement/hernia.
6. Intra-abdominal adhesions to diaphragm.

Abnormal shape or margin of diaphragm

1. Hernia (e.g., hiatal, peritoneal-pericardial, traumatic).
2. Exposed diaphragm attachments due to severe caudal displacement of diaphragm.
3. Eventration of the diaphragm.
4. Adhesions between diaphragm and thoracic or abdominal wall.
5. Mass or nodule(s) on the diaphragm:
   a. Tumors on the diaphragm are uncommon in dogs and cats (rhabdomyosarcoma is reported most often).
   b. Abscess or granuloma due to peritonitis or migrating foreign material.

6. Paralysis of hemidiaphragm.
7. Muscular hypertrophy.

Conditions that mimic abnormal diaphragm margin

1. Summation with adjacent soft tissue mass in lung, pleural space, or caudal mediastinum/ esophagus.
2. Disease in caudal lung, adjacent to diaphragm.
3. Dome of diaphragm deformed by cardiac shadow (particularly during expiration and in a DV view).

Pleura and pleural space

Pleural fissure lines

1. Radiographic signs:
   a. Thin, curvilinear, soft tissue opacity lines at known locations for pleural fissures.
   b. Lines that are wider at the periphery and taper centrally indicate fluid or gas in pleural space.
   c. Fat in a pleural fissure is wider centrally and tapers peripherally ("reverse fissure line"); occurs most often between right cranial and middle lung lobes.
2. Normal pleural fissure; x-ray beam is perfectly aligned with a fissure; seldom repeats between radiographs.
3. Obesity; fat in an interlobar fissure.
4. Older animal; pleural fibrosis from previous disease that is now inactive (e.g., "aging change").
5. Small volume of pleural fluid; pleural fissure lines are earliest finding with pleural effusion.
6. Pleuritis that leads to pleural thickening:
   a. Systemic disease (e.g., septicemia, viral infection).
   b. Intra-thoracic disease (e.g., viral pneumonia, lung parasites, thoracic trauma, mediastinitis).
7. Pleural edema that leads to pleural thickening:
   a. Acute left heart failure.
   b. Sudden or acute thoracic trauma.
8. Pleural scarring and adhesions ("pleural peel") due to chronic or recurring pleural effusion (e.g., pyothorax, chylothorax, hemothorax).

Conditions that mimic pleural lines

1. Superimposed wet or dirty hair coat; often identified in orthogonal views.
2. Mineralized costal cartilage, particularly in cats; cartilage tends to be more linear than a pleural line and often can be followed to the end of a rib; adjacent cartilages tend to be mineralized as well.

Pleural mass

1. Diaphragmatic hernia (common).
2. Tumor:
   a. Primary neoplasia (e.g., mesothelioma).
   b. Secondary neoplasia (e.g., metastatic carcinoma).
3. Abscess, granuloma (e.g., foreign object, parasites, chronic inflammation/infection).
4. Hematoma (e.g., trauma, coagulopathy).
5. Foreign object (e.g., projectile).
6. Trapped fluid (e.g., pleuritis, trauma).

Extra-pleural lesions that mimic pleural mass:

1. Rib mass (e.g., tumor, healing fracture).
2. Osteomyelitis of ribs, sternum, or vertebrae.
3. Thoracic wall mass (e.g., abscess, granuloma, hematoma, tumor, lipoma).
4. Large mediastinal/sternal lymph node.
5. Diaphragm lesion (e.g., eventration, mass).
6. Caudal esophageal mass.

Pleural effusion

1. Radiographic signs:
   a. Pleural fissure lines.
   b. Edges of lungs do not extend to chest wall.
   c. Vascular and bronchial markings do not extend to ribs.
   d. Fluid opacity between lungs and chest wall.
   e. Costophrenic recesses are rounded and indistinct.
   f. Dorsal displacement of cardiac shadow in lateral view.
   g. Increased lung opacity.
   h. Less distinct cardiac and diaphragmatic borders.
2. The type of fluid cannot be determined from radiographs. Fluid analysis helps classify the fluid as transudate or exudate, which provides clues to its etiology:
3. Transudate: Thin and clear fluid with low specific gravity, low protein, low fibrin, and low cell count, that results from pressure filtration without capillary damage. Pleura and thoracic wall often are normal in radiographs; lung borders generally are sharp and well-defined; effusion usually is bilateral and symmetrical. A modified transudate is serous to serosanguinous fluid, which may contain a variety of cell types, often inflammatory, which may eventually lead to an exudate.
   a. Hypoproteinemia is a common cause:
      1) Nephrotic syndrome (glomerulonephritis).
      2) Protein-losing nephropathy.
      3) Protein-losing enteropathy.
      4) Hepatic insufficiency.
   b. Iatrogenic fluid overload.
   c. Right heart failure; pericardial effusion.
   d. Lymphatic obstruction (e.g., lymphoma, fibrosis).
   e. Diaphragmatic hernia.
   f. Pneumonia.
   g. Lung lobe torsion.
   h. Sterile foreign object.
   i. Thromboembolism.
   j. Systemic disease (e.g., pancreatitis).
   k. Idiopathic.
4. Exudate: Fluid is high in protein and cellularity. Pleura may be thickened and fibrotic, which can restrict lung expansion and block mediastinal fenestrations. Pleural effusion may be asymmetric.

a. **Hemothorax**: fluid resembles peripheral blood but may not clot:
   1) Trauma (common cause); other signs of thoracic trauma may be present (e.g., fractured ribs, subcutaneous emphysema).
   2) Erosion through a blood vessel by tumor, abscess, or parasites (e.g., heartworm disease, spirocercosis).
   3) Coagulopathy (e.g., rodenticide poisoning).
   4) Autoimmune disease.
   5) Blood in the pleural space tends to be rapidly resorbed (autotransfusion) unless the pleura is damaged.

b. **Pyothorax** (*empyema*): large number of neutrophils in fluid.
   1) Systemic infection, pneumonia (e.g., bacterial, viral, mycotic, nocardiosis, tuberculosis).
   2) Foreign material, lung abscess.
   3) Autoimmune disease (e.g., systemic lupus erythematosus, rheumatoid arthritis).

c. **Chylothorax**: numerous chylomicrons (fat globules) and lymphocytes in fluid, making it appear milky opaque.
   1) Thoracic duct rupture (common cause) (e.g., trauma, iatrogenic, idiopathic).
   2) Thoracic duct blockage (e.g., thrombosis, fibrosis, congenital malformation).
   3) Lymphangiectasia.
   4) Heart failure (cats).
   5) Cranial vena cava obstruction (e.g., thrombosis).
   6) Lung lobe torsion.
   7) Heartworm disease.
   8) Mycotic infection.
   9) Neoplasia.
   10) Diaphragmatic hernia (especially in cats).

d. *Pseudo-chylous* effusion; fluid is inflammatory, but sterile:
   1) Cats: lymphosarcoma, cardiomyopathy.
   2) Dogs: idiopathic.

e. **Pyogranulomatous effusion**: thick, viscous, straw-colored fluid with high protein, high specific gravity, and relatively few inflammatory cells; fluid may clot.
   1) Feline infectious peritonitis (most common).
   2) Neoplasia (e.g., mesothelioma).

Unilateral or asymmetric pleural effusion:

1. Functionally complete mediastinum; fenestrations are absent or obstructed:
   a. Congenital variation.
   b. Severe or chronic pleural inflammation.
2. Severe pulmonary disease and altered lung compliance.
3. Trapped fluid; there is an unequal distribution of fluid, but the fluid moves with gravity.
4. Encapsulated fluid; fluid does not move with gravity; fluid retains its shape in all radiographs.
5. Loculated fluid; small volume of fluid that is held in a pocket, frequently by adhesions.

Conditions that mimic pleural effusion

1. Underexposed radiograph; extra-thoracic structures are underexposed, too.
2. Normal pleural line due to x-ray beam aligned with the interlobar fissure; seldom repeats in other views.
3. Superimposed costal cartilage or a wet/dirty hair coat that may be mistaken for a pleural line.
4. Inward curvature of ribs in chondrodystrophic breeds (VD/DV view).
5. Normal hypaxial muscles in cats may resemble rounding of the costophrenic recess in a lateral view.
6. Obesity; excessive fat in thoracic wall, along sternum, in mediastinum, and between lung lobes (Note: fat is less opaque than fluid). Lung margins may not extend to the ribs. Lungs may appear more opaque than expected due to incomplete inflation and overlying fat.
7. Thick thoracic wall (e.g., heavy musculature, subcutaneous swelling or fluid). Note that the widening is outside the thoracic cavity and lung borders extend to the inner chest wall.

Pneumothorax

1. Radiographic signs:
   a. Edges of lungs do not extend to chest wall.
   b. Vascular and bronchial markings do not extend to ribs.
   c. Gas opacity between lungs and chest wall and between lung lobes.
   d. Dorsal displacement of cardiac shadow in lateral view.
   e. Overall decreased opacity in thoracic cavity.
2. Perforation of thoracic wall (e.g., trauma).
3. Rupture of lung or airway:
   a. Trauma.
   b. Ruptured lung bulla or cyst (e.g., "spontaneous pneumothorax").
   c. Airway erosion (e.g., paragonimus, tumor, abscess).
4. Extension of pneumomediastinum (e.g., ruptured trachea, ruptured esophagus).
5. Iatrogenic causes of pneumothorax:
   a. Complication of thoracocentesis or lung aspirate.
   b. Recent thoracotomy.
   c. Transthoracic biopsy of liver.
   d. Aggressive CPR.
6. Severe or chronic lung disease that leads to erosion through a bronchus (e.g., abscess, tumor, pneumonia, paragonimus, dirofilariasis).
7. Idiopathic (spontaneous) pneumothorax.

Conditions that mimic pneumothorax

1. Overexposed radiograph.
2. Superimposed axillary skin fold; follow the skin fold to see it extends beyond the thoracic cavity.

3. Cardiac shadow is dorsal to the sternum, but no free gas is in the pleural space and the lungs are not collapsed:
   a. Deep-chested thoracic conformation.
   b. Hypovolemia.
   c. Mediastinal shift.
   d. Recumbent atelectasis with partial collapse of the dependent lung.
   e. Hyperinflated lungs (e.g., manual inflation).
4. Superimposition of adjacent gas:
   a. Subcutaneous emphysema.
   b. Pneumomediastinum.
   c. Gas-filled GI structure in thoracic cavity (e.g., diaphragmatic hernia).
5. Patient was rotated in a DV/VD view, making the peripheral lungs appear less opaque.
6. Emaciated patient with well-inflated lungs and little tissue overlying the thorax.

Mediastinum

Abnormal position of mediastinum

1. Radiographic signs of a mediastinal shift:
   a. The cardiac shadow and other mediastinal structures are displaced to the right or left side.
   b. The ipsilateral hemidiaphragm may be displaced cranially.
2. Unilateral lung collapse (see increased lung opacity):
   a. Airway obstruction.
   b. Recumbent atelectasis.
   c. Inability of one lung to expand:
      1) Unilateral pleural fluid or gas.
      2) Pleural fibrosis.
3. Lung lobe torsion:
   a. Acute torsion: shift is away from the engorged lung lobe.
   b. Chronic torsion: shift is toward the smaller lobe.
4. Absence of a lung:
   a. Lung lobectomy.
   b. Lung agenesis or lung hypoplasia.
5. Large intra-thoracic mass:
   a. Diaphragmatic hernia.
   b. Lipoma; fat opacity.
6. Unilateral increase in lung volume:
   a. Severe emphysema.
   b. Large or multiple pulmonary cysts.
   c. Large lung mass (e.g., tumor).
   d. Unilateral phrenic nerve paralysis; lung on the affected side does not fully inflate because that part of the diaphragm cannot move.
7. Skeletal deformity; shift may be to either side:
   a. Pectus excavatum.
   b. Severe spinal lordosis or scoliosis.
8. Pleural adhesions that pull the mediastinum:
   a. Previous trauma.
   b. Severe or chronic inflammation.
   c. Radiation therapy.

Conditions that mimic mediastinal shift

1. Patient was rotated during positioning for radiography ("the heart follows the sternum").
2. Muscle contractions or splinting of the thorax; shift is away from the contracted side (e.g., pain).
3. Situs inversus; rare congenital condition in which the organs develop in a mirror image to normal.

Abnormal widening of mediastinum

1. Radiographic signs:
   a. Dogs: mediastinum is wider than twice the width of a vertebral body.
   b. Cats: mediastinum is wider than a vertebral body.
   c. Obese animals: mediastinum is wider than the width of a thoracic wall.

Diffuse widening of mediastinum:

1. Obesity is most common cause.
2. Megaesophagus.
3. Fluid in mediastinum (e.g., blood, transudate):
   a. Inflammation (mediastinitis).
   b. Penetrating wound.
   c. Tracheal rupture.
   d. Esophageal rupture.
   e. Infection (e.g., feline infectious peritonitis).
   f. Edema (e.g., congestive heart failure, hypoproteinemia).
   g. Coagulopathy.
   h. Neoplasia.

Conditions that mimic diffuse widening of mediastinum:

1. Summation with pleural fluid.

Mediastinal mass

1. Radiographic signs:
   a. Focal widening and increased opacity in mediastinum.
   b. Trachea may be displaced and compressed.
   c. Cardiac shadow may be displaced or effaced.

Cranioventral mediastinal mass:

1. Normal thymus; dogs less than 1-year-old, cats less than 2-years-old.
2. Tumor (e.g., thymoma, malignant histiocytosis, ectopic thyroid or parathyroid tumor, fibrosarcoma).
3. Lymphadenomegaly:
   a. Sternal lymph node; extra-pleural sign (e.g., lymphoma, spread of intra-abdominal disease).
   b. Cranial mediastinal nodes (e.g., lymphoma).
4. Branchial cyst; particularly in cats.
5. Lipoma; fat opacity mass.
6. Hematoma (e.g., trauma, coagulopathy, neoplasia, spirocercosis).
7. Abscess or granuloma (e.g., foreign object).
8. Esophageal diverticulum.
9. Sternal mass; extra-pleural sign (e.g., tumor, osteomyelitis).

Conditions that mimic a cranial mediastinal mass

1. Flexion of the patient's head and neck during positioning for radiography that causes the trachea to bend dorsally and laterally (usually to the right). Repeat the radiograph without allowing the patient to tuck its head and neck.
2. Superimposition of thoracic limb musculature.
3. Brachycephalic and chondrodystrophic dog breeds with an exaggerated redundancy in the esophagus at the thoracic inlet.
4. Older, small breed dogs with localized fat stores in the cranial mediastinum.
5. Cardiovascular enlargement that extends cranially (e.g., aortic dilation, large right atrium).
6. Summation with adjacent lung disease (e.g., pneumonia, pulmonary mass).
7. Obesity (excess fat in mediastinum).

Craniodorsal mediastinal mass

1. Esophageal dilation:
   a. Megaesophagus.
   b. Vascular ring anomaly.
   c. Foreign material.
   d. Mass (e.g., abscess, granuloma, tumor).
2. Mediastinal mass (e.g., tumor, abscess, granuloma).
3. Vertebral lesion (rare):
   a. Tumor.
   b. Osteomyelitis.
   c. Severe spondylosis.
   d. Spirocercosis.
4. Aortic aneurysm (rare).

Middle (hilar) mediastinal mass

1. Tracheobronchial lymphadenomegaly (e.g., neoplasia, mycotic infection, granulomatosis).
2. Heart base tumor (e.g., chemodectoma); more often is reported in older brachycephalic dogs.
3. Esophageal mass (e.g., foreign object, abscess, granuloma, tumor).

Conditions that mimic a hilar mediastinal mass

1. Cardiovascular enlargement (e.g., left atrium, right atrium, aorta, main pulmonary artery).
2. End-on visualization of right pulmonary artery in a lateral view radiograph.
3. Adjacent lung lesion (e.g., pulmonary mass, localized area of alveolar filling).

Caudal mediastinal mass

1. Esophageal enlargement:
   a. Foreign material.
   b. Mass (e.g., granuloma, tumor, abscess).
   c. Esophageal diverticulum.
   d. Gastroesophageal intussusception.
2. Hiatal hernia.
3. Diaphragm mass (e.g., tumor, abscess, granuloma).
4. Mediastinal mass (e.g., granuloma/abscess caused by migrating foreign object).

Conditions that mimic a caudal mediastinal mass

1. Disease in adjacent lung.
2. Thoracic wall mass.
3. Diaphragmatic hernia.
4. Fluid in esophagus.
5. Eventration of diaphragm.

Abnormal opacity in mediastinum

1. Gas opacity in mediastinum:
   a. Pneumomediastinum (see below).
   b. Gas in esophagus (e.g., megaesophagus).
2. Soft tissue (see mediastinal mass below).
3. Mineral opacity in mediastinum:
   a. Esophageal content (e.g., food, foreign material, bone fragments).
   b. Lymph node mineralization.
   c. Cardiovascular mineralization; linear or heterogenous mineral opacity in cardiac shadow (e.g., aortic valve, coronary artery) or along a vessel wall (e.g., aorta).
      1) Hypercortisolism.
      2) Chronic renal disease.
      3) Hypercalcemia.
      4) Idiopathic.

Conditions that mimic mediastinal mineralization

1. Costal cartilage.
2. Thoracic wall lesion.
3. Debris on skin or hair coat.
4. Lung mineralization (e.g., pulmonary osteomas).

Pneumomediastinum

1. Radiographic signs: free gas outlines outer margins of trachea and other mediastinal structures not normally visible and may migrate into cervical, subcutaneous, retroperitoneal, and pleural areas.
2. Tracheal rupture:
   a. Trauma (e.g., bite wound, laceration).
   b. Faulty intubation or overly distended tracheal cuff, particularly in cats.
   c. Complication of jugular venipuncture, tracheal aspirate, or transtracheal wash.
3. Esophageal rupture:
   a. Trauma, swallowed foreign material.
   b. Long standing tumor, granuloma, abscess.
   c. Complication from endoscopy, intubation.
4. Penetrating wound in neck or oral cavity with gas migrating into mediastinum:
   a. Trauma (e.g., bite wound, laceration).
   b. Recent surgery, tracheostomy.

5. Ruptured lung or bronchus with gas migrating into mediastinum:
    a. Trauma, severe dyspnea.
    b. Ruptured cavitary lesion, "spontaneous" pneumomediastinum.
    c. Lung hyperinflation during anesthesia or resuscitation.
6. Mediastinal infection with gas-producing organism.
7. Migration of retroperitoneal gas.
8. Idiopathic.

Conditions that mimic pneumomediastinum

1. Gas in esophagus (e.g., transient swallowed air, esophageal obstruction, megaesophagus).
2. Superimposed subcutaneous emphysema; orthogonal radiographs aid in localizing gas.
3. Pneumothorax; lung borders and pulmonary vessels do not extend to thoracic wall.
4. Emaciation; reduced mediastinal width against well-inflated lungs enhances visualization of mediastinal structures.
5. Obesity; fat adjacent to mediastinal structures may enhance their visibility; evaluate other fat stores in the patient to determine whether obese; fat is more opaque than gas.

Esophagus

Abnormal position of esophagus

1. Mediastinal shift (e.g., lung collapse).
2. Hernia (e.g., diaphragmatic, hiatal).
3. Adjacent mass.
4. Congenital anomaly (e.g., redundant esophagus).

Conditions that mimic a displaced esophagus

1. Patient was rotated during positioning for radiography (mediastinum follows sternum).

Abnormal opacity in esophagus

1. Radiographic signs: persistent gas, soft tissue, or mineral opacity that repeats in serial radiographs.

Gas in the esophagus

1. Swallowed air; small volumes of transient gas typically are seen near the cranial esophageal sphincter, at the thoracic inlet, and at the heart base. Persistence of gas in multiple radiographs warrants further investigation.
2. Aerophagia due to struggling or excitement; usually there is abundant gas in the GI tract, too.
3. Sedation/anesthesia; certain drugs allow the esophagus to fill with gas; may be mistaken for megaesophagus, but resolves after patient has recovered.
4. Megaesophagus.
5. Obstructed esophagus (e.g., foreign object, stricture).
6. Abnormal esophageal function (e.g., megaesophagus, esophagitis); follow-up radiographs confirm persistence of esophageal gas, often with esophageal dilation.
7. Esophageal diverticulum.

Conditions that mimic gas in the esophagus

1. Superimposition artifact:
    a. Subcutaneous emphysema.
    b. Cavitary lesion in the lung (e.g., bulla).
    c. Pneumothorax.
    d. Pneumomediastinum; however, esophageal disease may be the etiology.
2. Hyperinflated lungs.

Increased opacity in the esophagus

1. Retained fluid or food:
    a. Poor esophageal function (e.g., megaesophagus, esophagitis, gastroesophageal reflux).
    b. Partial or complete obstruction (e.g., vascular ring anomaly; esophageal stricture).
    c. Esophageal diverticulum.
2. Foreign material.
3. Esophageal mass:
    a. Tumor, primary or metastatic.
    b. Abscess (e.g., foreign material, toxin).
    c. Granuloma (e.g., spirocercosis).
    d. Gastroesophageal intussusception.
    e. Hiatal hernia.
4. Swallowed medication (e.g., Pepto-Bismol) or positive contrast agent.

Conditions that mimic increased esophageal opacity

1. Normal caudal esophagus sometimes is visible in a lateral view (particularly the left lateral view).
2. Superimposition artifact; often identified in the orthogonal view:
    a. Wet/dirty haircoat.
    b. Costal cartilage or lesion in bony thorax.
    c. Cutaneous/subcutaneous nodule or mass.
    d. Medical and monitoring equipment.
    e. Nearby pulmonary or mediastinal mass.

Abnormal size of esophagus

1. Radiographic signs: persistent narrowing or dilation that repeats in serial radiographs

Narrowed esophagus:

1. Normal peristalsis; transient muscle contractions produce short-term narrowing, which does not persist in follow-up radiographs.
2. Muscle spasms; more prolonged and frequent muscle contractions but still transient; most often caused by esophagitis.

3. Esophageal stricture:
   a. Chronic or recurrent esophagitis (e.g., gastroesophageal reflux, neoplasia, toxin).
   b. Trauma, passage of severe irritant.
4. External compression of the esophagus:
   a. Vascular ring anomaly.
   b. Mediastinal or hilar lymphadenomegaly.
   c. Heart base mass.
   d. Hiatal hernia.
   e. Mass in adjacent lung or mediastinum.
5. Esophageal mass (e.g., tumor, abscess, granuloma).

Dilated esophagus:
1. Certain drugs (e.g., anesthesia, heavy sedation).
2. Aerophagia (e.g., severe dyspnea, upper airway obstruction).
3. Sedation/anesthesia; may lead to transient esophageal dilation.
4. Congenital **megaesophagus**: a sometimes manageable but often incurable condition; clinical signs of regurgitation develop at time of weaning:
   a. Genetics (hereditary in Miniature Schnauzer and Wirehair Fox Terrier).
   b. Familial predisposition (Irish Setter, Chinese Shar-Pei, Great Dane, Newfoundland).
   c. Canine glycogen storage disease (Lapland dogs).
   d. Mucopolysaccharoidosis (Siamese cat).
   e. Congenital myopathy (Labrador Retriever).
   f. Canine giant axonal neuropathy (German Shepherd Dog).
5. Acquired **megaesophagus**: numerous causes are implicated, including inflammatory, neurologic, metabolic, and immune mediated diseases:
   a. Esophagitis; chronic or recurring inflammation.
      1) Gastroesophageal reflux.
      2) Ingested irritants.
      3) Sliding hiatal hernia.
   b. Severe lung disease adjacent to esophagus; uncommon cause of short term esophageal dilation.
   c. Caudal esophageal obstruction:
      1) Foreign material.
      2) Esophageal mass.
      3) Esophageal stricture.
      4) Hiatal hernia.
      5) Large mass in adjacent lung or mediastinum.
      6) Achalasia at gastroesophageal junction.
   d. Gastric outflow problem:
      1) Gastric dilatation and volvulus or GDV.
      2) Gastric foreign material.
      3) Pyloric canal dysfunction.
   e. Neurologic, degenerative, or immune-mediated disease:
      1) Myasthenia gravis.
      2) Central nervous system trauma, meningitis.
      3) Autonomic nervous system disease.
      4) Polyneuritis, polymyositis, polymyopathy.
      5) Systemic lupus erythematosus.
      6) Dermatomyositis.
      7) Muscular dystrophy.
   f. Systemic disease:
      1) Hypoadrenocorticism.
      2) Diabetes mellitus.
      3) Hypothyroidism (questionable).
      4) Hyperinsulinism (insulinoma).
      5) Uremia.
      6) Electrolyte disturbances.
      7) Inflammation/infection (e.g., canine distemper).
      8) Neosporosis; especially in puppies.
      9) Thiamine deficiency.
   g. Toxins:
      1) Heavy metal (e.g., lead, zinc, thallium).
      2) Organophosphates.
      3) Chlorinated hydrocarbons.
      4) Herbicides.
      5) Botulism.
      6) Snake venom (e.g., Australian tiger snake).
      7) Tetanus.
   h. Idiopathic.

Cardiac silhouette

Abnormal position of cardiac silhouette

1. *Caudal displacement of cardiac shadow*; caudal to the sixth intercostal space:
   a. Cranial mediastinal mass.
2. *Cranial displacement of the cardiac shadow*; tapering of the thorax limits cranial movement:
   a. Abdominal distention; diaphragm bulges cranially.
   b. Collapse of cranial lung lobes.
   c. Diaphragmatic hernia.
3. *Ventral displacement of the cardiac shadow*; usually only the cardiac base is displaced because the sternum restricts ventral movement:
   a. Dilated esophagus is most common cause.
   b. Large mediastinal mass dorsal to the heart.
   c. Severe spinal lordosis; also causes left or right lateral displacement of the cardiac shadow.
4. *Dorsal displacement of the cardiac shadow*; recognized in a lateral view as separation from the sternum:
   a. Pneumothorax.
   b. Mediastinal shift (e.g., lung collapse).
   c. Cranioventral mediastinal mass; cardiac shadow is also displaced caudally.
   d. Large volume of pleural fluid.
   e. Obesity; displacement is due to pericardial or mediastinal fat.
   f. Deep-chested patient conformation.
   g. Pectus excavatum.

5. *Lateral displacement of the cardiac shadow*; recognized in a VD/DV view:
   a. Mediastinal shift (e.g., lung collapse, pneumothorax, pleural effusion, large thoracic mass).
   b. Cardiomegaly.
   c. Pectus excavatum.
   d. Severe spinal lordosis.
   e. Situs inversus; rare congenital anomaly in which the viscera develop in a mirror image to normal. Make sure the radiographs are correctly labeled right vs. left (consider repeating the study).

Conditions that mimic cardiac displacement

1. Patient was rotated during positioning for radiography ("the heart follows the sternum").

Abnormal size of cardiovascular structures

1. Hypovolemia is the most common cause of a smaller than expected cardiac shadow and smaller than expected blood vessels and may be caused by:
   a. Shock.
   b. Severe dehydration.
   c. Hypocorticosism (Addison's disease).
   d. Severe anemia or blood loss.

Small cardiac shadow (microcardia)

1. Hypovolemia.
2. Compromised venous return (e.g., GDV, vena cava thrombus, hepatic cirrhosis).
3. Pneumothorax, especially tension pneumothorax.
4. Some forms of cardiomyopathy in cats.
5. Constrictive or restrictive pericarditis:
   a. Bacterial infection (e.g., nocardiosis, tuberculosis).
   b. Mycotic infection (e.g., coccidiomycosis, actinomycosis).
   c. Foreign material (e.g., bullet or other projectile, migrating grass awn).
   d. Neoplasia (e.g., chemodectoma, mesothelioma).
   e. Sequela to hemorrhagic pericardial effusion.
6. Emaciation/cachexia; loss of pericardial fat, diminished heart muscle mass.
7. Atrophic myopathy (rare).

Conditions that mimic small cardiac shadow

1. Deep-chested patient conformation.
2. Hyperinflated lungs, reducing the cardiac-to-thoracic ratio (e.g., deep inspiration, asthma, manual ventilation during anesthesia).
3. Displacement of heart (e.g., megaesophagus, mediastinal shift).

Small aorta

1. Hypovolemia.
2. Proximal aortic stricture leading to reduced size of descending aorta.
3. Severe heart disease resulting in low cardiac output.

Small caudal vena cava

1. Hypovolemia.
2. Tension pneumothorax.
3. Positive pressure ventilation during anesthesia.

Enlarged cardiac shadow

1. Cardiomegaly (see below); the borders of individual cardiac structures often are still discerned.
2. Pericardial effusion (see below); evenly rounded, smooth, and sharply-defined cardiac margin.
3. Peritoneopericardial hernia (PPDH); typically a heterogeneous appearance to the cardiac shadow; PPDH is a congenital condition, never acquired.

Cardiomegaly

1. Athletic heart; a non-pathologic large cardiac shadow seen in certain breeds (e.g., Greyhound) and in animals undergoing physical conditioning.
2. Primary cardiomyopathy; etiology is unknown:
   a. Dilated cardiomyopathy.
   b. Hypertrophic cardiomyopathy.
   c. Restrictive cardiomyopathy.
   d. Unclassified or arrhythmogenic cardiomyopathy.
3. Secondary cardiomyopathy; etiology is known; cardiac changes may predominately be dilation (**D**) or hypertrophy (**H**):
   a. Genetic predisposition.
   b. Endocardiosis and valvular insufficiency.
   c. Congenital heart defects, especially blood shunts.
   d. Systemic hypertension (H).
   e. Arrhythmia; tachycardia or bradycardia, (D).
   f. Metabolic/endocrine disease:
      1) Diabetes mellitus (D).
      2) Hyperthyroidism (H).
      3) Hypothyroidism (D).
      4) Uremia (D).
      5) Acromegaly (H).
      6) Pheochromocytoma (H).
   g. Electrolyte imbalance.
   h. Infiltrative cardiac disease:
      1) Mucopolysaccharidosis (D).
      2) Neoplasia (lymphoma).
      3) Amyloidosis.
   i. Nutritional deficiency (D):
      1) Taurine deficiency (D).
      2) L-carnitine deficiency (D).
      3) Vitamin E or selenium deficiency (D).
   j. Hypoproteinemia (D).
   k. Myocarditis (D):
      1) Lyme disease (borreliosis).
      2) Bartonellosis (cat scratch fever).
      3) Bacterial (usually secondary to immune deficiency).
      4) Mycotic (e.g., aspergillosis).
      5) Viral (e.g., parvovirus, distemper, herpes).

6) Protozoal (e.g., toxoplasmosis, trypanosomiasis).
7) Inflammation without infection (D)

l. Trauma (e.g., blunt force to thorax) (D).
m. Heat stroke (D).
n. Electrocution (D).
o. Drugs (e.g., doxorubicin, catecholamines).
p. Toxins (e.g., heavy metals).

4. Sedation/anesthesia; drugs that induce bradycardia may result in the cardiac shadow appearing larger than expected in radiographs; cardiac size returns to normal after patient is recovered.
5. Sick sinus syndrome; bradycardia leads to radiographic enlargement of cardiac shadow.
6. Iatrogenic fluid overload (hypervolemia).
7. Cardiac inflammation/infection; myocarditis:
   a. Viral (e.g., parvovirus, distemper).
   b. Bacterial (e.g., Streptococcus, brucellosis).
   c. Fungal (e.g., histoplasmosis, Cryptococcosis).
   d. Parasitic (e.g., Bartonellosis, Trypanosomiasis).
   e. Protozoal (e.g., Lyme disease).
8. Infiltrative cardiac disease (e.g., lymphoma, amyloidosis, lipidosis, mucopolysaccharidosis).
9. Ischemic myocardial disease.
10. Systemic hypertension (e.g., chronic renal disease).
11. Metabolic disease:
    a. Hyperthyroidism; more often in older cats.
    b. Hypercorticism.
    c. Diabetes mellitus.
    d. Acromegaly; more often in cats.
12. Chronic anemia.
13. Nutritional deficiency (e.g., L-carnitine, taurine).
14. Immune-mediated disease (e.g., rheumatoid).
15. Toxicity (e.g., doxorubicin, heavy metals, lead, mercury).
16. Neuromuscular disease.

Conditions that mimic a large cardiac shadow

1. Expiratory radiograph; the cardiac-to-thoracic ratio is increased.
2. Obesity with excessive pericardial fat; close inspection often reveals the soft tissue opacity cardiac margin surrounded by fat opacity.
3. Pericardial effusion.
4. Peritoneopericardial diaphragmatic hernia.

Pericardial effusion; more often reported in male dogs over six years of age and larger than 20 kg. Affected animals may exhibit jugular pulse and muffled heart sounds. Etiology may not be present at time of diagnosis.

1. Radiographic signs:
   a. Large, round cardiac silhouette
   b. Sharp margins due to less cardiac motion blur
2. Transudative pericardial effusion:
   a. Congestive right heart failure.
   b. Hypoproteinemia.
   c. Peritoneopericardial diaphragmatic hernia.
   d. Uremia.
   e. Toxemia
   f. Trauma.
   g. Obstructed lymph or blood flow (e.g., neoplasia).
   h. Idiopathic; usually benign.
3. Hemorrhagic pericardial effusion:
   a. Neoplasia; more common in dogs than in cats.
      1) Right atrial or auricular hemangiosarcoma.
      2) Heart base tumor (e.g., chemodectoma).
      3) Mesothelioma.
      4) Lymphoma; more common in cats.
   b. Rupture of a severely dilated left atrium.
   c. Pericardial trauma (e.g., gunshot wound)
   d. Iatrogenic complication from pericardiocentesis.
   e. Coagulopathy (e.g., rodenticide, DIC).
   f. Idiopathic.
4. Exudative pericardial effusion:
   a. Infection (e.g., bacterial, mycotic, actinomycosis, coccidiomycosis, tuberculosis).
   b. Feline infectious peritonitis (FIP).
   c. Sterile foreign object.
   d. Steatitis.
   e. Idiopathic.
5. Pericardial mass
   a. Neoplasia (e.g., mesothelioma, chemodectoma).
   b. Abscess.
   c. Granuloma.
   d. Cyst (congenital or acquired).

Conditions that mimic a heart base tumor

1. Left atrial dilation.
2. Severely dilated pulmonary arteries (e.g., heartworm disease).
3. Hilar lymphadenomegaly; heart base mass usually is cranial to tracheal carina.
4. Esophageal mass or diverticulum.
5. Other mediastinal mass.
6. Adjacent pulmonary mass or alveolar filling.

Left atrial dilation

1. Radiographic signs:
   a. Expansion of dorsocaudal cardiac border.
   b. Increased opacity in hilar region.
   c. Dorsal displacement of distal trachea.
   d. Splitting of mainstem bronchi.
   e. Widening of tracheal bifurcation.
   f. Widening of cardiac base, leading to a more triangular-shaped cardiac shadow
2. Mitral valve insufficiency:
   a. Endocardiosis is most common etiology; particularly older, small breed dogs.
   b. Endocarditis (e.g., bacterial infection).

   c. Ruptured chordae tendinea or papillary muscle.
   d. Congenital mitral valve dysplasia/stenosis.
3. Cardiomyopathy (e.g., dilated, hypertrophic, restrictive, arrhythmogenic).
4. Hyperthyroidism in cats.
5. Systemic hypertension.
6. Patent ductus arteriosus.

Conditions that mimic left atrial enlargement

1. Patient was rotated during position for the lateral view to resemble splitting of the mainstem bronchi.
2. Heart base mass; usually cranial to left atrium.
3. Hilar mass/lymphadenomegaly; tends to push the distal trachea ventrally.
4. Nearby pulmonary mass; the trachea is not displaced.

Left ventricular enlargement

1. Radiographic signs: expansion of left and caudal cardiac borders, elongating the cardiac silhouette.
2. Mitral valve insufficiency.
3. Cardiomyopathy.
4. Hyperthyroidism in cats.
5. Congenital heart disease (e.g., patent ductus arteriosus, aortic stenosis).
6. Hypervolemia (e.g., fluid overload).
7. Aortic insufficiency.
8. Chronic anemia.
9. Peripheral arteriovenous fistula.
10. Chronic renal disease.
11. Systemic hypertension.
12. Coarctation of the aorta (rare).
13. Myocarditis.
14. Neoplasia.
15. Aneurysm.

Conditions that mimic left ventricular enlargement

1. Patient rotated to the left in a DV/VD radiograph (the heart follows the sternum).
2. Obesity with excess pericardial fat.
3. Pericardial effusion.
4. Right ventricular enlargement causing left lateral displacement of the cardiac apex in a VD/DV view.

Right atrial enlargement

1. Radiographic signs: expansion of right cranial cardiac border.
2. Tricuspid valve insufficiency:
   a. Sequela to chronic mitral valve insufficiency is most common etiology.
   b. Tricuspid valve endocardiosis.
   c. Endocarditis; less common in tricuspid valve than mitral and aortic valves.
   d. Sequela to right ventricular dilation/failure.
   e. Ruptured chordae tendinea.
   f. Congenital tricuspid valve dysplasia/stenosis.
3. Cardiomyopathy.
4. Right-atrial hemangiosarcoma.
5. Cor pulmonale (e.g., dirofilariasis).
6. Congenital heart disease:
   a. Pulmonic stenosis.
   b. Tetralogy of Fallot.
   c. Atrial septal defect (left-to-right shunt).
7. Arteriovenous fistula.

Conditions that mimic right atrial enlargement

1. Summation of nearby pulmonary mass, consolidated lung lobe, or cranial mediastinal mass.
2. Severely dilated main pulmonary artery or aortic arch.

Right ventricular enlargement

1. Radiographic signs: expansion of right and ventral cardiac borders leading to a reverse-D shaped cardiac silhouette.
2. Tricuspid insufficiency.
3. Myocardial disease:
   a. Dilated cardiomyopathy.
   b. Arrhythmogenic right ventricular cardiomyopathy (Boxers).
4. Sequela to left heart disease (e.g., chronic mitral valve insufficiency).
5. Cor pulmonale or "pulmonary heart disease"; right ventricular enlargement is secondary to lung disease, e.g., pulmonary hypertension. Causes include:
   a. Heartworm disease.
   b. Chronic obstructive pulmonary disease (COPD).
   c. Pulmonary thromboembolism.
   d. Obesity hypoventilation or "Pickwickian" syndrome; obesity reduces lung capacity leading to increased cardiac workload; term originates from an overweight Charles Dickens character who suffered respiratory difficulties.
   e. Brachycephalic dogs with chronic airway obstruction.
6. Congenital heart disease:
   a. Pulmonic stenosis.
   b. Left-to-right intracardiac shunt:
   c. Patent ductus arteriosus.
   d. Ventricular septal defect.
   e. Atrial septal defect.
   f. Tetralogy of Fallot.
7. Pulmonary valve insufficiency.
8. Myocarditis.
9. Neoplasia.
10. Arteriovenous fistula.
11. High altitude disease.
12. Thoracic deformity (e.g., pectus excavatum).
13. Aneurysm.

Conditions that mimic right ventricular enlargement

1. Sternum rotated to right on DV/VD radiograph (heart follows sternum).
2. Expiratory radiograph (increased cardiac sternal contact and dorsal positioning of trachea).
3. Obesity (pericardial fat may mimic cardiomegaly).

Aortic enlargement

1. Radiographic signs: expansion of cranial cardiac border.
2. Aortic stenosis; narrowed left ventricular outflow tract leads to post-stenotic turbulence and dilation.
3. Coarctation of the aorta; rare congenital narrowing in the aorta itself which leads to distal dilation.
4. Aneurysm; aortic dilation due to a weak or thin aortic wall (e.g., spirocercosis, idiopathic).
5. Patent ductus arteriosus (PDA).
6. Congenital hypothyroidism.
7. Systemic hypertension.
8. Vascular ring anomaly, persistent right aortic arch.

Conditions that mimic aortic enlargement

1. Brachycephalic dogs; aorta may normally appear relatively large in these breeds.
2. Aging change; loss of elasticity in the aortic wall results in a more visible aortic arch.
3. Dilated right atrium.
4. Heart base mass.
5. Cranial mediastinal mass.

Caudal vena cava enlargement

1. Radiographic signs: caudal vena cava is wider than 1.5 × aorta or wider than length of T5 or T6.
2. Reduced venous return to right heart:
   a. Right heart insufficiency or failure.
   b. Mass in right ventricle, right atrium, or caudal vena cava (e.g., tumor, thrombus).
   c. Proximal stenosis of caudal vena cava.

Main pulmonary artery (MPA) enlargement

1. Radiographic signs: expansion of cranial cardiac border.
2. Heartworm disease.
3. Pulmonic stenosis.
4. Patent ductus arteriosus.
5. Large atrial or ventricular septal defect resulting in a large left-to-right blood shunt.
6. Pulmonary hypertension.
7. Pulmonary arterial stenosis (rare).
8. Idiopathic; MPA is enlarged, but right ventricle is normal size.

Conditions that mimic MPA enlargement

1. Patient was rotated during positioning for radiography, projecting the MPA laterally.
2. Summation of nearby pulmonary or mediastinal mass; often resolved in orthogonal view.
3. In a lateral view, a large MPA may be indistinguishable from enlargement of the aorta or right atrium, or a heart base mass; the orthogonal view often provides clarification.

Right heart failure

1. Radiographic signs:
   a. Enlargement of the right atrium and ventricle.
   b. Pleural effusion.
   c. Peritoneal effusion.
   d. Hepatosplenomegaly due to venous congestion.
2. Clinical signs include labored breathing, exercise intolerance, and abdominal distention.
3. Sequela to left heart failure.
4. Pericardial disease (e.g., effusion, inflammation).
5. Heartworm disease.
6. Pulmonary hypertension, cor pulmonale.
7. Tricuspid valve insufficiency (see right atrial enlargement).
8. Cardiomyopathy.
9. Severe left-to-right intracardiac shunting of blood.
10. Pulmonary thromboembolism.
11. Pulmonic stenosis.
12. Severe cardiac electrical disturbance.
13. Arteriovenous fistula.
14. Myocarditis/myocardial infarction.
15. Endocardial fibroelastosis.

Left heart failure

1. Radiographic signs:
   a. Pulmonary edema
      1) Dogs: central and symmetrical distribution, "butterfly" pattern.
      2) Cats: patchy, asymmetrical distribution, may be accompanied by pleural effusion
   b. Pulmonary veins larger than arteries.
   c. Enlargement of left atrium and left ventricle.
2. Clinical signs of left heart failure include cough, dyspnea, tachypnea, and syncope. Cough mainly is due to lung edema and tends to be more severe at night. A patient with left heart enlargement and a cough is not necessarily in left heart failure. A largely dilated left atrium can compress the left mainstem bronchus and induce a cough, which is not in itself a sign of heart failure.
3. Mitral valve insufficiency (see left atrial dilation).
4. Cardiomyopathy (see cardiomegaly).
5. Hyperthyroidism in cats.
6. Systemic hypertension.
7. Congenital heart disease:
   a. Patent ductus arteriosus.
   b. Aortic stenosis.

c. Ventricular septal defect.
d. Mitral valve dysplasia.
e. Atrial septal defect.

8. Myocardial disease (e.g., inflammation, ischemia, neoplasia).
9. Severe cardiac electrical disturbance.
10. Aortic valve insufficiency.
11. Increased cardiac demand (e.g., overexertion, anemia, pregnancy).

Severe cardiac disease without radiographic evidence of cardiac enlargement

1. Cardiac electrical disturbance (e.g., arrhythmias, tachycardia).
2. Myocardial infarction, inflammation, or infection.
3. Myocarditis/endocarditis:
   a. Bacterial infection (most common).
   b. Viral infection (e.g., distemper, hepatitis, parvovirus).
   c. Toxoplasmosis.
   d. Leptospirosis.
   e. Pneumonia.
   f. Immune-mediated disease (e.g., rheumatoid arthritis).
   g. Parasitic infection (rare).
   h. Rickettsial infection (rare).
4. Endocardial or pericardial inflammation.
5. Concentric hypertrophy without dilation:
   a. Severe aortic stenosis.
   b. Severe pulmonic stenosis.
6. Hypertrophic cardiomyopathy.
7. Constrictive pericarditis.
8. Neoplasia of myocardium: Myocardial tumors:
   a. Primary neoplasms:
      1) Hemangiosarcoma (most common):
      2) Fibrosarcoma.
      3) Lymphoma (more often reported in cats).
      4) Myxosarcoma.
      5) Chondrosarcoma.
   b. Metastatic tumors (usually involve left heart):
      1) Adenocarcinoma (from lung or mammary gland).
      2) Melanoma (can extend to heart).
   c. Benign cardiac tumors (uncommon):
      1) Fibroma.
      2) Myxoma.
      3) Rhabdomyoma.
   d. Heart base tumors:
      1) Chemodectoma (aortic body tumor) is most common, and most often is reported in older brachycephalic dogs (e.g., Bulldog, Boxer, Boston Terrier).
      2) Lymphoma.
      3) Ectopic thyroid carcinoma.
      4) Ectopic parathyroid carcinoma.
9. Electrolyte disturbances.
10. Cardiac trauma.

Abnormal opacity in the cardiac silhouette

1. Radiographic signs: gas, fat, or mineral opacity within the cardiac shadow; may be focal, multifocal, or diffuse.
2. Gas opacity:
   a. Peritoneopericardial hernia with gas in displaced GI structures.
   b. Pneumopericardium:
      1) Recent pericardiocentesis.
      2) Infection with gas-producing organism.
      3) Thoracic trauma; migration of gas from ruptured alveoli or pneumomediastinum.
   c. Gas embolism; gas in a heart chamber tends to persistently outline part or all of the chamber.
3. Fat opacity:
   a. Obesity.
   b. Peritoneopericardial hernia with displaced falciform or omental fat.
   c. Lipoma.
4. Mineral opacity:
   a. Mineralized heart valve or coronary vessel.
   b. Long-standing inflammation or mass (e.g., granuloma, abscess, hematoma).
   c. Hyperparathyroidism.
   d. Hypercortisolism.
   e. Hypervitaminosis D.
   f. Neoplasia (e.g., lymphoma).
   g. Idiopathic.
5. **Aortic** mineralization:
   a. Lymphoma.
   b. Renal failure.
   c. Primary or secondary hyperparathyroidism.
   d. Arteriosclerosis.
   e. Hypercorticism (Cushing's syndrome).
   f. Parasites (e.g., Spirocerca lupi).
   g. Hypervitaminosis D.
   h. Inflammation.
   i. Idiopathic.
6. Metal opacity:
   a. Foreign object (e.g., metal projectile, migrating intravascular catheter fragment).
   b. Pacemaker lead.

Conditions that mimic altered cardiac opacity

1. Superimposition artifacts (e.g., skin folds, dirty hair coat, costal cartilages, lung lesions, others); often recognized in orthogonal views.

Trachea

Abnormal position of trachea

Cervical trachea displaced ventrally and/or laterally

1. Soft tissue mass in cervical region:
   a. Tumor; thyroid carcinoma is most common.
   b. Retropharyngeal lymphadenomegaly.

c. Abscess/granuloma (e.g., foreign object).
d. Hematoma (e.g., trauma).
2. Esophageal dilation.
3. Vertebral mass (e.g., osteochondroma).

Thoracic trachea displaced ventrally
1. Esophageal dilation is most common cause.
   a. Vascular ring anomaly.
   b. Megaesophagus.
   c. Esophageal mass (e.g., foreign object, tumor).
2. Tracheobronchial lymphadenomegaly.
3. Aortic dilation (e.g., aneurysm).
4. Dorsal mediastinal mass.
5. Large vertebral mass or severe spondylosis.

Thoracic trachea displaced to the right
1. Megaesophagus.
2. Mediastinal shift (see mediastinum).
3. Cranial mediastinal mass (e.g., lymphadenopathy, tumor).
4. Heart base tumor.
5. Pulmonary mass.

Thoracic trachea displaced to the left
1. Mediastinal shift (see mediastinum).
2. Vascular ring anomaly.

Thoracic trachea displaced dorsally
1. Enlarged cardiac shadow (see page).
2. Cranial mediastinal mass (e.g., enlarged lymph node(s), tumor, cyst).
3. Heart base tumor.
4. Pectus excavatum.

Conditions that mimic abnormal tracheal position
1. Flexion of the head and neck.
2. Patient was rotated during positioning.
3. Expiratory phase of respiration; the heart and lungs move cranially, accentuating tracheal curvature.
4. Obesity; excess mediastinal fat.
5. Normal anatomic variation (e.g., Bulldog, Yorkshire Terrier).

Abnormal opacity in trachea
1. Radiographic signs: soft tissue, mineral, or metal opacity in tracheal lumen.
2. Aspirated foreign object or contrast medium.
3. Endotracheal mass:
   a. Granuloma (e.g., spirocercosis, difficult intubation, tracheostomy).
   b. Abscess (e.g., foreign material).
   c. Polyp.
   d. Tumor (e.g., chondroma, osteoma, carcinoma, sarcoma, lymphoma).
4. Dystrophic mineralization (e.g., hypercortisolism, chronic inflammation).

Conditions that mimic increased tracheal opacity
1. Mineralized tracheal is a normal aging change and it can occur relatively early in chondrodystrophic and large-breed dogs.
2. Underexposed radiograph.
3. Superimposition artifact (e.g., esophageal content, cutaneous mass, pulmonary mass).

Enhanced visualization of tracheal margins
1. Pneumomediastinum; dorsal and ventral margins of trachea are outlined by gas; visualization of other mediastinal margins also is enhanced.
2. Megaesophagus; dorsal margin of trachea is outlined by gas (i.e., tracheal stripe sign); dorsal tracheal wall may appear thickened due to blending with ventral esophageal wall.
3. Emaciation; tracheal margins appear more distinct against inflated lungs due to thinner, less opaque thorax and mediastinum.

Poor visualization of tracheal margins
1. Underexposed radiograph.
2. Obese or heavily muscled patient; superimposition of large amount of overlying tissue may obscure the tracheal margins.
3. Tracheal collapse syndrome; redundant dorsal tracheal membrane blurs the dorsal tracheal margin.
4. Thickened tracheal wall (e.g., inflammation, edema, hemorrhage).
5. Narrowed tracheal lumen (e.g., stenosis, hypoplasia).
6. Increased endotracheal opacity (e.g., exudates, nodules/masses, aspirated material).
7. Mediastinal fluid (e.g., inflammation, hemorrhage).
8. Tracheal rupture or avulsion:
   a. External trauma (e.g., bite wound, blunt force)
   b. Foreign object.
   c. Faulty intubation or overinflated tube cuff.
   d. Complication of venipuncture, endoscopy, or transtracheal wash.
9. Tracheobronchitis:
   a. Infection:
      1) Viral (e.g., distemper, parainfluenza, adenovirus, herpesvirus, calicivirus).
      2) Feline infectious peritonitis.
      3) Bacterial (e.g., Bordetella).
      4) Mycotic.
      5) Parasitic (e.g., larva migrans, aeleurostrongylus, dirofilariasis).
      6) Toxoplasmosis.
   b. Allergies/asthma.

c. Inhaled irritants (e.g., smoke, dust, hot or irritating gases, foreign material, gastric contents).
d. Tracheal collapse syndrome.
e. Compression of bronchi by enlarged heart or hilar lymph nodes.
f. Primary ciliary dyskinesis.
g. Tracheal hypoplasia.
h. Idiopathic.

10. Superimposition artifact; (e.g., large esophagus, cutaneous or subcutaneous mass, adjacent lung disease).

Abnormal size of trachea

1. Radiographic signs:
   a. Greater than 50% narrowing is abnormal.
   b. Tracheal ratio less than 0.20 in average dog, or less than 0.16 in brachycephalic breed, or less than 0.10 in bulldogs.

Narrowed trachea

1. Hyperextension of the head and neck; avoid overstretching the patient during positioning for radiography.
2. Immature patient; trachea is relatively narrower in young animals than in adults.
3. Aged, small breed dog: trachea is narrower due to weakened cartilage rings.
4. Tracheal collapse syndrome.
5. Tracheal stenosis or stricture; usually a focal or localized narrowing.
6. Tracheal hypoplasia; usually a diffuse or generalized narrowing.
7. Thickened tracheal wall:
   a. Inflammation (i.e., tracheitis).
   b. Edema (e.g., allergic response).
   c. Hemorrhage (e.g., trauma, coagulopathy).
8. Endotracheal mass or foreign material.
9. Tracheal compression caused by a large esophagus, mediastinal or hilar mass.
10. Aging change due to loss of tracheal ring rigidity (especially in small dog breeds).

Conditions that mimic a narrowed trachea

1. When the trachea is oblique to the x-ray beam, the dorsal membrane may be superimposed on the lumen; close inspection reveals the true dorsal border of the trachea and normal size lumen.

Dilated trachea

1. Tracheal collapse syndrome; outward "ballooning" of redundant dorsal tracheal membrane.
2. Severe inspiratory distress due to upper respiratory obstruction:
   a. Laryngeal edema.
   b. Laryngeal paralysis.
   c. Aspirated foreign object.
   d. Mass (e.g., tumor, abscess, granuloma, hematoma).
3. Adhesions pulling on the trachea.
4. Breed variation; the trachea may appear relatively large in some dogs (e.g., Poodles).

Bronchial obstruction

1. Inhaled foreign object (e.g., marble, pebble).
2. Excess endobronchial mucous (e.g., asthma).
3. Endobronchial tumor (e.g., lymphoma, bronchogenic carcinoma).
4. Endobronchial granuloma (e.g., parasites).
5. Endobronchial abscess (e.g., migrating plant awn).
6. Lung lobe torsion.

Lungs

Increased lung opacity

1. Pulmonary edema (see below).
2. Pneumonia (see below).
3. Lung collapse (see below).
4. Pulmonary hemorrhage (see below).
5. Neoplasia (e.g., lymphoma, hemangiosarcoma).
6. Hypervascular lungs (e.g., large left-to-right shunt).
7. Pulmonary fibrosis:
   a. Previous lung disease that is now inactive (e.g., "aging change," "old dog lungs").
   b. Chronic inflammation (e.g., inhaled irritants).
   c. Systemic/metabolic disease; chronic condition:
      1) Hypercortisolism.
      2) Pancreatitis.
      3) Uremia.
   d. Toxins (e.g., herbicide paraquat).
8. Inability of lungs to expand:
   a. Pleural effusion or pneumothorax.
   b. Pleural fibrosis; chronic or repeated pleuritis.
   c. Abdominal distention:
      1) Ascites.
      2) Large mass or organomegaly.
9. Pulmonary nodule/mass (see below).
10. Chronic lung lobe torsion.
11. Lung infarct, pulmonary thromboembolism:
    a. Heartworm disease is most common etiology, <u>both</u> before and after therapy.
    b. Recent trauma or surgery.
    c. Prolonged immobilization.
    d. Neoplasia (e.g., lymphoma, metastatic disease).
    e. Heart disease (e.g., cardiomyopathy, valvular regurgitation, endocarditis).
    f. Disseminated intravascular coagulation (DIC).
    g. Systemic disease:
       1) Chronic renal disease.
       2) Hypercortisolism.
       3) Diabetes mellitus.

4) Hyperlipidemia.
5) Pancreatitis.
6) Fever of unknown origin.
7) Immune-mediated disease.

Conditions that mimic increased lung opacity

1. Summation of pleural fluid.
2. Superimposition of nearby disease:
   a. Mediastinal mass, thymus, lymph node.
   b. Esophageal content.
   c. Rib lesion (e.g., healing fracture, tumor).
   d. Cutaneous/subcutaneous nodule, growth, cyst, parasite (e.g., engorged tick).

Non-pathologic causes of increased lung opacity

1. Poor radiographic technique (e.g., underexposure, underdeveloped film radiograph); the extra-thoracic structures are affected, too.
2. Motion unsharpness (e.g., panting, struggling).
3. Thick tissue overlying the thorax (e.g., obesity, heavy musculature, subcutaneous fluid or lipoma).
4. Lateral view; lungs tend to appear more opaque in lateral recumbency than in a VD/DV views due to atelectasis of the dependent lung. Do not rely on lateral views alone to diagnose lung disease. Any suspected increase in lung opacity must be confirmed in the VD/DV view.
5. Poorly inflated lungs:
   a. Expiratory radiograph.
   b. Obesity.
   c. Sedation/anesthesia.
   d. Recumbent atelectasis.
   e. Abdominal distention (e.g., pregnancy).
   f. Shallow breathing (e.g., severe pain).
6. Immature lungs; the water content in juvenile lungs is higher than in adults.
7. Superimposition artifact:
   a. Wet or dirty hair coat.
   b. Medication or contrast agent on hair or skin.
   c. Bandaging material, blanket, stretcher.
   d. Medical equipment (e.g., IV tubing, ECG leads).
   e. Patient's forelegs.
   f. Esophageal content.
8. Pseudo-nodules:
   a. End-on visualization of a pulmonary vessel.
   b. End-on visualization of the right pulmonary artery in a lateral view; appears as a pseudo-nodule located ventral to distal trachea.
   c. Costochondral cartilage.
   d. Nipple, skin growth.
   e. Site of an injection or fluid administration.
9. Many superimposition artifacts are recognized in orthogonal views.

Pulmonary edema

1. Cardiogenic lung edema/left heart failure:
   a. With enlargement of cardiac shadow:
      1) Chronic mitral valve insufficiency.
      2) Cardiomyopathy.
      3) Severe left-to-right blood shunt.
   b. Without enlargement of cardiac shadow:
      1) Ruptured chordae tendinea.
      2) Cardiac trauma.
      3) Severe cardiac arrhythmia.
      4) Some forms of cardiomyopathy.
      5) Myocardial depressant, either endogenous or exogenous.
2. Non-cardiogenic lung edema:
   a. Neurologic disease; lung edema tends to be most severe in the peripheral lungs, sparing the hilar region, and frequently clears within 24–48 hours after resolution of the neurologic condition:
      1) Seizure; post-ictal response.
      2) Head trauma.
      3) Electrocution.
      4) Brain tumor.
      5) Encephalitis.
   b. Upper airway obstruction, severe inspiratory distress:
      1) Foreign object in trachea.
      2) Laryngeal swelling or paralysis.
      3) Tracheal collapse syndrome.
      4) Brachycephalic syndrome.
      5) Strangulation.
   c. Drowning or near-drowning; lung edema may develop hours later.
   d. Infection (e.g., viral, mycoplasma, leptospirosis, toxoplasmosis, babesia).
   e. Inhaled or aspirated irritant (e.g., noxious gas, smoke, gastric contents); can rapidly progress (within 24 hours) to a severe pulmonary edema, predominately in the caudal and peripheral lungs.
   f. Iatrogenic causes of lung edema:
      1) Fluid therapy volume overload; resembles left heart failure; cardiac shadow usually is enlarged; hematocrit and plasma protein concentration are decreased.
      2) Post-cardiac arrest and resuscitation.
      3) Adverse reaction:
      4) Drugs (e.g., theophylline, sulfonamide, iodinated contrast agent).
      5) Oxygen therapy.
      6) Blood transfusion.
      7) Re-expansion lung edema; caused by rapid withdrawal of pleural fluid or pleural gas (e.g., pleural effusion, pneumothorax, post-operative repair of diaphragmatic hernia).
      8) Radiation therapy (i.e., radiation pneumonitis).

g. Systemic disease (e.g., pancreatitis, uremia).
h. Toxin; blood borne toxins can cause a diffuse, bilateral and symmetrical lung edema:
   1) Snake or spider venom.
   2) Alpha-naphthyl thiourea (ANTU).
   3) Herbicides (e.g., Paraquat).
i. Pulmonary thromboemboli:
   1) Fat emboli secondary to extensive fractures.
j. ARDS (acute respiratory distress syndrome); initially causes a diffuse, patchy increase in lung opacity that rapidly progresses to more uniform alveolar flooding, often with air bronchograms.
k. Shock, DIC (disseminated intravascular coagulation).
l. Pulmonary hypertension:
   1) Heartworm disease.
   2) Pulmonary thromboemboli.
   3) High altitude disease.
m. Interstitial neoplasia that obstructs flow of blood or lymph (e.g., lymphoma).

3. Unilateral pulmonary edema:
   a. Prolonged lateral recumbency (hypostasis).
   b. Unilateral blunt force thoracic trauma.
   c. Disease in one lung (e.g., thromboembolism, obstructed flow of blood or lymph).
   d. Unilateral emphysema; edema develops in the contralateral lung.

Pneumonia

1. Bacterial pneumonia; either primary infection or secondary complication to:
   a. Chronic tracheobronchitis.
   b. Aspiration/inhalation (e.g., food, gastric contents, medication, foreign material, contrast medium):
      1) Megaesophagus.
      2) Dysphagia.
      3) Force feeding.
      4) Aspirated mineral oil can lead to formation of lung granulomas, predominately in the central lung region (i.e., "lipid pneumonia").
   c. Secondary to another type of lung infection:
      1) Fungal, mycotic.
      2) Parasitic (e.g., rickettsia, babesia, toxoplasmosis).
      3) Mycoplasma.
      4) Bordatella, kennel cough
   d. Lung neoplasia.
   e. Bronchiectasis.
   f. Ciliary dyskinesia.
   g. Immunosuppression (e.g., chemotherapy, drugs, stress, malnutrition).
2. Viral pneumonia:
   a. Dogs: influenza, distemper, adenovirus, parainfluenza.
   b. Cats: feline immunodeficiency virus (FIV), calicivirus, herpes virus.
3. Mycotic pneumonia; especially in endemic areas.
4. Allergic or adverse response (e.g., eosinophilic pneumonia, eosinophilic bronchopneumopathy):
   a. Parasites:
      1) Heartworm.
      2) Paragonimus.
      3) Toxoplasmosis.
      4) Visceral larval migrans.
   b. Inhaled allergen.
   c. Drug reaction (e.g., contrast medium).
   d. Idiopathic; inciting agent is not identified.
5. Systemic disease:
   a. Septicemia.
   b. Hypercortisolism.
   c. Pancreatitis.
   d. Uremia.
   e. Immune mediated disease.

Lung collapse

1. Recumbent atelectasis:
   a. Sedation/anesthesia.
   b. Debilitating illness.
2. Airway obstruction:
   a. Faulty placement of endotracheal tube.
   b. Endobronchial exudates (e.g., feline asthma).
   c. Inhaled foreign object.
   d. Endobronchial mass (e.g., tumor, granuloma, polyp).
3. Lung is unable to expand:
   a. Severe pleural effusion.
   b. Pneumothorax, tension pneumothorax.
   c. Large thoracic wall mass.
   d. Pleural fibrosis (e.g., chronic pleuritis).
   e. Traumatic lung damage.
4. Lung lobe torsion; usually with pleural effusion.
5. Pulmonary thromboembolic disease, loss of blood supply to lung.
6. Loss of pulmonary surfactant:
   a. Congenital condition, incomplete expansion of lung lobe(s) at birth.
   b. Severe or chronic infection.
   c. Inhalation of a toxic substance.
   d. Pancreatitis.

Pulmonary hemorrhage

1. Radiographic signs: bleeding settles with gravity into dependent lungs; bleeding due to acute trauma initially is located near the site of damage; most hemorrhage resolves in a few days with appropriate therapy, persistence suggests hematoma.
2. Trauma (e.g., lung contusions).
3. Coagulopathy (e.g., rodenticide, poisoning, thrombocytopenia).
4. Eroded blood vessel (e.g., tumor, abscess, severe thromboembolism, parasites, leptospirosis).
5. Exercise induced hemorrhage.

Pulmonary nodule or mass

1. Lung tumor, primary or metastatic:
   a. Bronchogenic carcinoma is most common primary lung tumor in dogs; frequently arises in the right caudal lung lobe as solitary mass.
   b. Adenocarcinoma is most common primary lung tumor in cats; may be associated with metastases to digit(s).
2. Lung abscess:
   a. Chronic bacterial pneumonia.
   b. Inhaled or migrating foreign object (e.g., grass awn).
   c. Neoplasia.
   d. Trauma (e.g., hematoma, pneumatocele).
   e. Parasitic infection (e.g., paragonimus).
   f. Bronchiectasis.
   g. Emboli (e.g., dirofilaria, bacterial, fungal).
   h. Systemic infection.
3. Lung granuloma:
   a. Migrating grass awn; especially in outdoor and working dogs.
   b. Inhaled foreign material (e.g., mineral oil).
   c. Mycotic infection (e.g., histoplasmosis).
   d. Bacterial infection (e.g., mycobacterium).
   e. Eosinophilic pneumonia.
   f. Tuberculosis.
   g. Parasitic infection (e.g., heartworm, toxoplasmosis, paragonimus).
   h. Chronic or recurrent allergic reaction.
4. Lung hematoma (e.g., trauma).
5. Fluid-filled pulmonary cyst (e.g., pneumatocele).
6. Acute alveolar flooding that appears as acinar nodules; "nodules" are transient and seldom repeat in follow-up radiographs due to continued filling of alveoli or resolution of lung disease (e.g., severe pneumonia, rapid pulmonary edema).
7. Smooth-bordered, well-defined lung nodules:
   a. Tumor, primary or metastatic.
   b. Long-standing abscess or granuloma.
   c. Fluid-filled cyst/bulla.
8. Lung nodules with indistinct borders:
   a. Disease in adjacent lung (e.g., inflammation, hemorrhage, edema).
   b. Actively growing granuloma or abscess.

Conditions that mimic a lung nodule

1. End-on visualization of a pulmonary blood vessel.
2. Superimposed costal cartilage.
3. Superimposed extra-thoracic structure (e.g., nipple, skin growth, engorged tick).
4. Very large pulmonary vessels may be mistaken for nodules (e.g., heartworm disease, left-to-right shunt and overcirculated lungs).

Multiple small pulmonary nodules (2–5 mm in size)

1. Pulmonary fibrosis (older animals; often a remnant from previous disease).
2. Granulomas; may mineralize during healing (e.g., mycosis, parasites, tuberculosis, foreign material).
3. Metastatic neoplasia.
4. Eosinophilic bronchopneumopathy (allergic response).

Multiple medium size pulmonary nodules (5–10 mm)

1. Neoplasia (e.g., metastatic tumors, lymphoma).
2. Acute pulmonary edema; ill-defined acinar nodules.
3. Hematomas (e.g., trauma, coagulopathy).
4. Abscess; Granuloma; latter may mineralize (e.g., mycosis, parasites, tuberculosis, foreign material).

Multiple large pulmonary nodules (11–30 mm in size)

1. Metastatic neoplasia.
2. Abscessation (e.g., systemic infection).
3. Granulomas (e.g., mycotic infection).

Numerous nodules ("snowstorm pattern")

1. Metastatic neoplasia.
2. Mycotic infection.
3. Pulmonary lymphoma.
4. Eosinophilic pneumonia/bronchopneumopathy.

Multiple pulmonary masses (larger than 3 cm)

1. Primary or metastatic neoplasia.
2. Abscesses; systemic infection.
3. Multiple, fluid-filled cysts.
4. Hematomas (e.g., trauma).

Mineralized pulmonary nodule or mass

1. Pulmonary osseous metaplasia (heterotopic bone); incidental mineral opacities in dogs, measure less than 3 mm in size; predominately in ventral lung fields.
2. Dystrophic mineralization:
   a. Chronic or healing granuloma.
   b. Tumor (especially in cats).
   c. Chronic inflammation.
3. Inhaled foreign object.
4. Broncholithiasis.

Pseudo-nodules

1. End-on visualization of pulmonary blood vessel.
2. Right pulmonary artery ventral to the distal tracheal.
3. Costochondral cartilage.
4. Rib remodeling (e.g., fracture, tumor, infection).
5. Esophageal content (e.g., food, foreign material).
6. Superimposed extra-thoracic structure; many of these are recognized in orthogonal views:
   a. Nipple, skin nodule, or cyst.
   b. Cutaneous parasite (e.g., engorged tick).

c. Dirt, debris, or medication on skin or hair coat.
d. Local swelling in thoracic wall (e.g., injection site).

Mineral opacity in lungs

1. Pulmonary osteomas.
2. Healing granulomas (e.g., histoplasmosis).
3. Chronic inflammation/infection (e.g., abscess).
4. Neoplasia; primary or metastatic tumor.
5. Metabolic disease; diffuse mineralization:
   a. Hypercortisolism.
   b. Hyperparathyroidism.
   c. Chronic uremia.
   d. Hypervitaminosis D, especially in cats.
6. Alveolar microlithiasis ("pumice lung").
7. Broncholithiasis.
8. Mineralization of peribronchial mucus glands (cats).
9. Inhaled material (e.g., barium sulfate).

Decreased lung opacity

1. Hypovascular lungs:
   a. Hypovolemia (e.g., shock, severe dehydration).
   b. Low cardiac output (e.g., pulmonic stenosis).
2. Air trapping; inability to exhale completely:
   a. Chronic obstructive pulmonary disease.
   b. Emphysema.
3. Lung hyperinflation, overexpansion:
   a. Severe dyspnea, upper airway obstruction.
   b. Compensatory hyperinflation:
      1) Lung lobe collapse.
      2) Lung lobectomy.
      3) Lung agenesis or hypoplasia.
4. Focal decrease in lung opacity:
   a. Cavitary lesion; bulla, bleb, cyst, pneumatocele.
   b. Cavitary mass (e.g., tumor, granuloma, abscess).
   c. Dilated bronchus, bronchiectasis.
   d. Pulmonary thromboembolism.
   e. Emphysema.

<u>Conditions that mimic decreased lung opacity</u>

1. Overexposed radiograph.
2. Oblique positioning of the patient may mimic unilateral reduced lung opacity.
3. Emaciation; less tissue overlying the thorax and lungs usually are well-inflated.
4. Lung hyperinflation (e.g., deep breath, manual ventilation).
5. Summation of gas:
   a. Pneumothorax.
   b. Pneumomediastinum.
   c. Megaesophagus.
   d. Gas-filled viscera displaced into thoracic cavity.
6. Mach lines; a summation artifact created by the curvilinear lines of vessels, bronchi, ribs, or costal cartilages that creates the illusion of decreased opacity.

Abnormal thickening of bronchi

1. Radiographic signs:
   a. Increased bronchial markings in <u>peripheral</u> lungs.
   b. Rings are a more reliable finding than tramlines.
2. Allergy/asthma; common, particularly in cats.
3. Tracheobronchitis; inflammation may be present without visible radiographic signs.
4. Inhaled irritants (e.g., secondhand smoke).
5. Infection (e.g., bacterial, viral, parasitic).
6. Chronic upper airway obstruction:
   a. Laryngeal paralysis.
   b. Tracheal collapse syndrome.
   c. Tracheal hypoplasia.
   d. Tracheal stenosis.
   e. Mass in tracheal or bronchial lumen:
      1) Aspirated foreign material.
      2) Tumor, polyp, granuloma, abscess.
   f. Bronchial compression (e.g., mass, cardiac enlargement).
7. Peribronchial cuffing:
   a. Early pulmonary edema.
   b. Bronchopneumonia.
   c. Lymphatic disease.
   d. Eosinophilic pneumonia.

Chronic lower airway disease

1. Causes of chronic inflammation include:
   a. Allergy (eosinophilic inflammation).
   b. Infection (neutrophilic inflammation).
   c. Upper airway obstruction (e.g., tracheal collapse syndrome, pharyngeal disease).
2. Most often reported in small-breed dogs and cats, but can affect any size or breed of dog.
3. Dogs typically present with dry, harsh, non-productive cough, wheezing, exercise intolerance, labored expiration; cough tends to be worse at night and after excitement and often ends with gagging.
4. Cats commonly exhibit panting, gagging, episodes of wheezing and labored expiration.

<u>Conditions that mimic thickened bronchi</u>

1. Misinterpreting the larger bronchi in the hilar and central lung regions as abnormal.
2. Older dogs, especially chondrodystrophic breeds (but not older cats); bronchial walls may be increased in opacity in older dogs, but they remain thin and appear as well-defined rings as opposed to thicker, less distinct donuts that occur due to pathology.
3. Mistaking the paired blood vessels adjacent to a bronchus for thickened bronchial walls. Close inspection often reveals the actual vascular and bronchial borders. Keep in mind that a bronchus does not always fill the entire space between the artery and vein. Also, the wall of a bronchus is uniform in thickness and does not taper.

Vessels, however, do taper toward the lung periphery. In most cases, an increase in bronchial rings is a more reliable finding than looking for an increase in tramlines because of the tendency to mistake paired vessels for thickened bronchi.

4. High-quality digital radiographs can enhance the visualization of bronchial walls, which may be misinterpreted as a bronchial lung pattern. Familiarity with the imaging system can help avoid this error in interpretation.
5. Peribronchial disease due to pulmonary edema (e.g., left heart failure).
6. Numerous thickened bronchi may be mistaken for tiny pulmonary nodules. Nodules with black dots in the center are bronchi.

Abnormal size of bronchi

1. Bronchiectasis:
   a. Chronic infection/inflammation.
   b. Mucociliary disease.

Abnormal size of pulmonary vessels

1. Radiographic signs:
   a. Lateral view: cranial lobar vessels larger than proximal part of fourth rib.
   b. VD/DV view: caudal lobar vessels larger than ninth rib where vessel and rib cross.

Small arteries and veins

1. Hypovolemia (e.g., shock, severe blood loss, severe dehydration, Addison's disease).
2. Low right ventricular output (e.g., pulmonic stenosis, cardiac tamponade, cardiomyopathy).
3. Right-to-left blood shunt (e.g., Tetralogy of Fallot).
4. Hyperinflated lungs; vessels appear small.

Large arteries and veins

1. Large left-to-right blood shunt:
   a. Patent ductus arteriosus.
   b. Ventricular septal defect.
   c. Atrial septal defect.
2. Iatrogenic fluid overload.
3. Bilateral heart failure.
4. Some forms of feline cardiomyopathy.
5. Systemic hypertension (e.g., hyperthyroidism).
6. Pulmonary congestion (precedes pneumonia).
7. Chronic anemia.
8. Peripheral arteriovenous malformation.
9. Upper airway obstruction.

Arteries larger than veins

1. Heartworm disease is most common etiology.
2. Other causes of pulmonary thromboemboli (e.g., recent trauma, renal disease, septicemia, pancreatitis, hypercortisolism).
3. Large left-to-right shunt (e.g., septal defect).
4. Pulmonary hypertension (e.g., chronic lung disease).

Veins larger than arteries

1. Left heart failure (see left heart failure above).
2. Left atrial obstruction (e.g., neoplasia, thrombus).
3. Right-to-left shunt (e.g., tetralogy of Fallot).

Arteries smaller than veins

1. Pulmonic stenosis.
2. Severe thromboembolic disease that affects many arteries.

Abnormal opacity in pulmonary vessels

1. Gas opacity in pulmonary vessels:
   a. Gas embolism (e.g., pneumocystogram, emphysematous cystitis, venipuncture).
2. Mineral opacity in pulmonary vessels:
   a. Hypercortisolism.
   b. Chronic renal failure.
   c. Hypertension (cats).
   d. Toxins (e.g., cholecalciferol poisoning).
   e. Hypercalcemia.

4 Abdomen

Radiography of the Dog and Cat: Guide to Making and Interpreting Radiographs, Second Edition. M.C. Muhlbauer and S.K. Kneller.

Companion website: www.wiley.com/go/muhlbauer/dog

Introduction to abdominal radiography

Evaluation of abdominal radiographs begins and ends with a systematic approach. We evaluate the quality of the radiographs first and then proceed with an orderly examination of the anatomy (Tables 2.7 and 2.9). When evaluating anatomy, most of us look at a structure's position first, followed by its size, shape, and opacity. We initially look for each organ or body part in an expected location.

All of the abdominal viscera are soft tissue opacity. The individual organs are distinguished because peritoneal and omental fat provide the **opacity interfaces** needed to visualize their serosal margins (Figure 4.1). When intra-abdominal fat is absent or obscured by fluid, serosal margins are less distinct or may not be visible at all. In emaciated animals, there often is insufficient fat to provide an opacity interface. Fluid in the abdominal cavity may result from inflammation or effusion. Because fluid is the same opacity as the soft tissue structures, the serosal margins become less distinct. Visceral crowding also can obscure serosal margins because fat may not visible between the borders of the contiguous soft tissue structures.

An opacity interface also is needed to see mucosal margins. Unless the mucosa is outlined by gas or a positive contrast medium it cannot be accurately evaluated. This is because any adjacent fluid or soft tissue material will blend with the mucosa. The thickness of visceral walls seldom can be reliably assessed with survey radiographs.

In addition to radiography, other non-invasive imaging modalities are available to examine the abdominal viscera. Ultrasonography, computed tomography, magnetic resonance imaging, and nuclear medicine imaging are increasingly utilized in veterinary medicine and may provide diagnostic information not available from radiography. This book is specific to radiography, but keep in mind that these other diagnostic tools may be available.

At the end of this chapter are extensive lists of differential diagnoses for the numerous radiographic findings being discussed.

Procedure for making abdominal radiographs

Patients should be encouraged to urinate and defecate prior to radiography. An empty colon and a small urinary bladder can lessen visceral crowding and reduce summation artifacts.

For elective radiographs, the GI tract should be empty. Many abdominal radiographs are rendered non-diagnostic due to the presence of ingesta. A 12-hour fast allows the stomach to empty and an 18- to 24-hour fast allows the intestines to empty. Patients should have free access to water during fasting.

When practical, drugs that affect GI motility should be discontinued 24–48 hours prior to abdominal radiography, including sedatives and anesthetic agents that slow GI peristalsis (e.g., xylazine).

Cleansing enemas may be needed to empty the large intestine. Either a mixture of water and mild soap or a saline solution are acceptable enemas and should be administered 2–4 hours prior to radiography. Enema solutions that are below body temperature may help stimulate the expulsion of gas from the colon. Enemas are contraindicated in patients with acute abdominal pain, active vomiting, or a palpable abnormality in the abdomen. Enemas are not recommended prior to initial radiographs in patients being evaluated for GI disease. This is because an enema can alter the pattern of gas and fluid in the intestinal tract, which may mask or mimic pathology. Phosphate enemas are not recommended because they can be toxic, especially in cats and small dogs.

Clean and dry the patient's hair coat and skin as needed prior to radiography. Move any monitoring equipment, such as ECG leads, out of the field-of-view (FOV). Note any cutaneous or subcutaneous growths that may create superimposition artifacts.

For accurate technical settings, measure the thickness of the abdomen at its widest part, which typically is over the liver at the level of the xyphoid or 12th rib.

Center the x-ray beam in the middle of the abdomen, midway between the diaphragm and the pelvic inlet. This helps minimize distortion at either end of the abdomen. Landmarks for centering include the level of the umbilicus or just caudal to the last rib.

Collimate the FOV to include the entire abdomen from the diaphragm to the pelvic inlet. The landmark for the diaphragm is about the T8 thoracic vertebra and the landmark for the pelvic inlet is the greater trochanters of the femurs. Collimation should include the spine dorsally and the body walls laterally and ventrally (Figures 4.2 and 4.3)

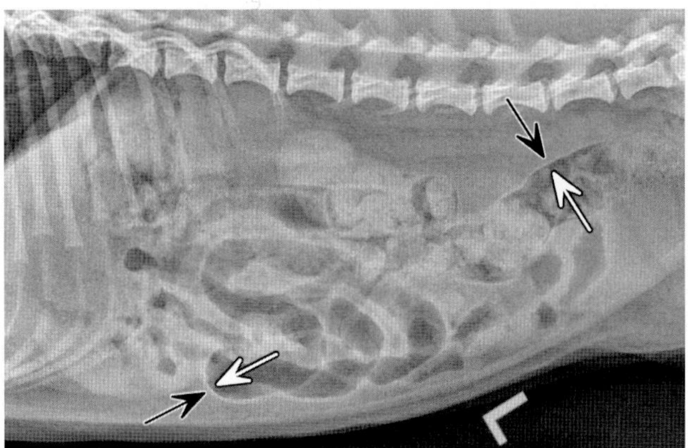

Figure 4.1 Opacity interfaces. Lateral view of a dog abdomen depicting serosal and mucosal margins. The serosal margins (black arrows) are visible because of adjacent fat. The mucosal margins (white arrows) are visible because of adjacent gas.

A

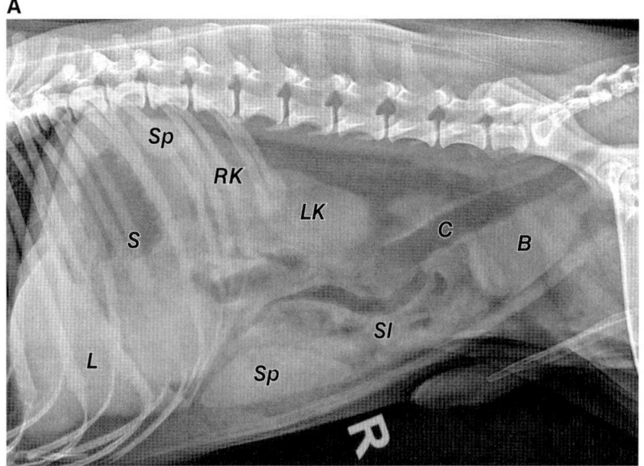

B

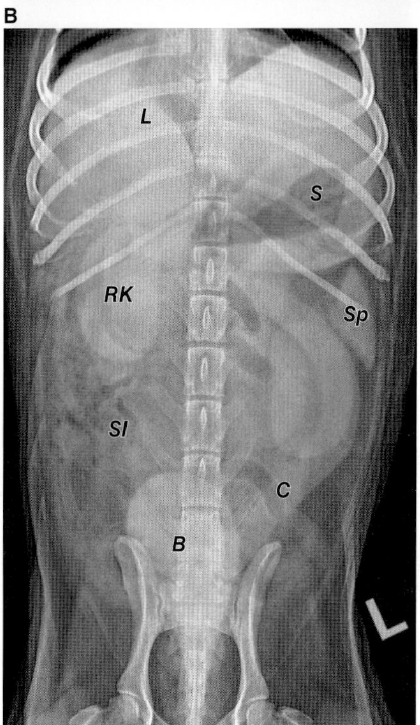

Figure 4.2 Normal canine abdomen. Lateral view (**A**) and VD view (**B**) of a dog abdomen depicting radiographs that are properly positioned, centered, collimated, and exposed. L = liver, S = stomach, RK = right kidney, LK = left kidney, Sp = spleen, SI = small intestine, C = colon, B = urinary bladder.

The pelvic limbs should be moved caudally to eliminate superimposition. **Avoid overstretching** the patient as this will distort the shape of the abdomen and increase visceral crowding, especially in cats and small dogs. Align the spine and sternum in the same anatomical plane.

Use body markers to indicate **R**ight or **L**eft and whether horizontal beam radiography was performed.

Make the exposure at the end of expiration to minimize motion artifact as most patients pause breathing momentarily at the end of expiration. Expiration also allows the

A

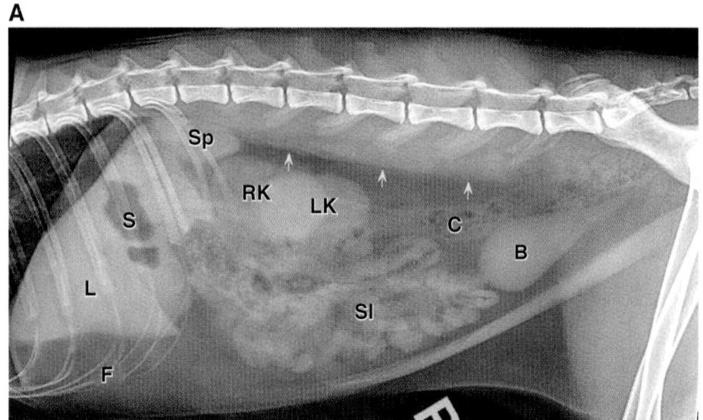

B

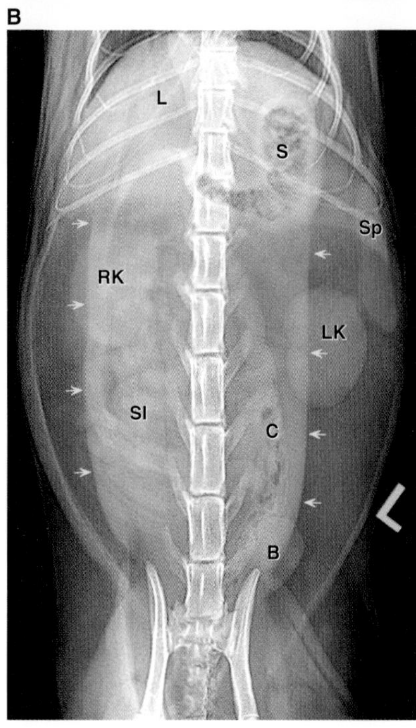

Figure 4.3 Normal feline abdomen. Lateral view (**A**) and VD view (**B**) of a cat depicting a normal abdomen. L = liver, F = falciform fat, S = stomach, RK = right kidney, LK = left kidney, Sp = spleen, SI = small intestine, C = colon, B = urinary bladder. The yellow arrows point to the borders of the hypaxial muscles, which tend to be relatively larger and more visible in cats than in dogs.

diaphragm to move cranially, which expands the abdominal cavity and lessens visceral crowding.

Standard views of the abdomen

Orthogonal radiographs are needed for complete evaluation of the abdomen. Standard radiographs for most abdominal studies include either a right or left lateral view (Figure 2.16) and a VD view (Figure 2.17). The DV view is not routinely made because serosal margins are less distinct due to visceral crowding.

The **right lateral view** is useful to move stomach gas into the fundus and to move stomach fluid into the pylorus (Figure 4.4). The radiographic appearance of fluid and gas in the stomach depends on the volume of each. In a right lateral view, the kidneys tend to be further separated than in a left lateral view and the margins of the liver and spleen may be easier to identify. The **left lateral view** allows stomach gas to rise into the pylorus and stomach fluid to flow into the fundus. This is helpful when differentiating a fluid-filled pylorus from a cranioventral abdominal mass.

The **VD view** is useful to move stomach gas into the body of the stomach and to move stomach fluid into the fundus and pylorus (Figure 4.5). The **DV view** allows stomach gas to rise into the fundus and pylorus and stomach fluid to flow into the body of the stomach. It usually is easier to position

A

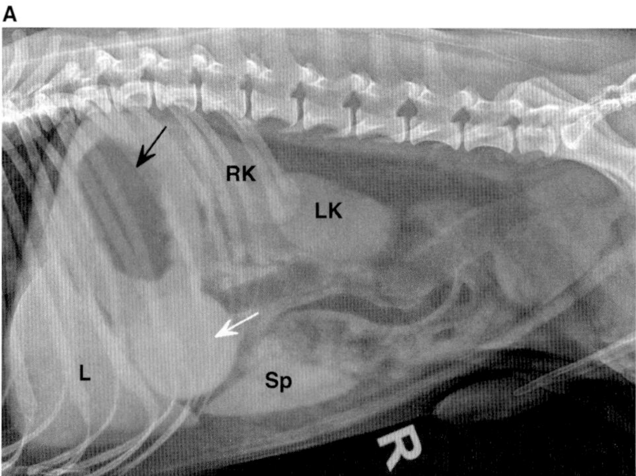

B

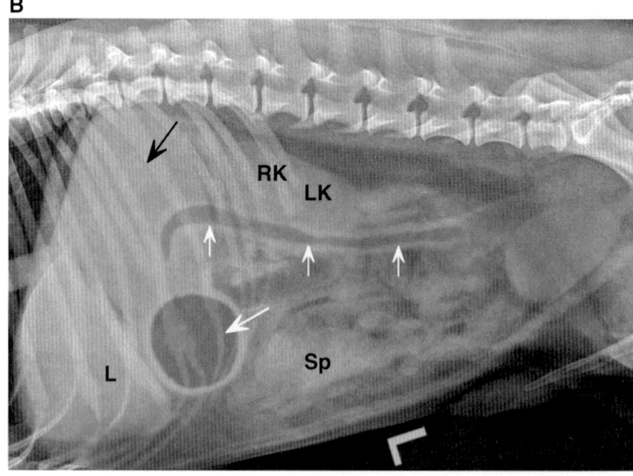

Figure 4.4 Right lateral vs. left lateral. Right lateral view (**A**) and left lateral view (**B**) of a dog abdomen depicting the differences between the two views. In right lateral recumbency, fluid in the stomach flows into the pylorus (white arrow) and gas rises to the fundus (black arrow). In left lateral recumbency, fluid flows into the fundus and gas rises to the pylorus and duodenum (white arrows). The margins of the liver (L) and spleen (Sp) sometimes are better visualized in a right lateral view than in a left lateral. The right and left kidneys (RK and LK) tend to be further separated in a right lateral view.

A

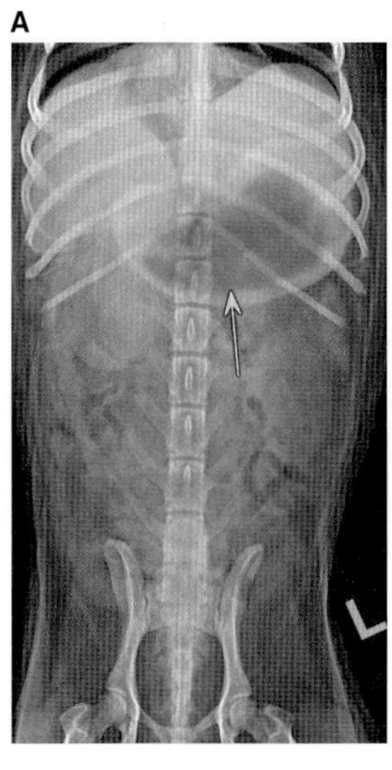

B

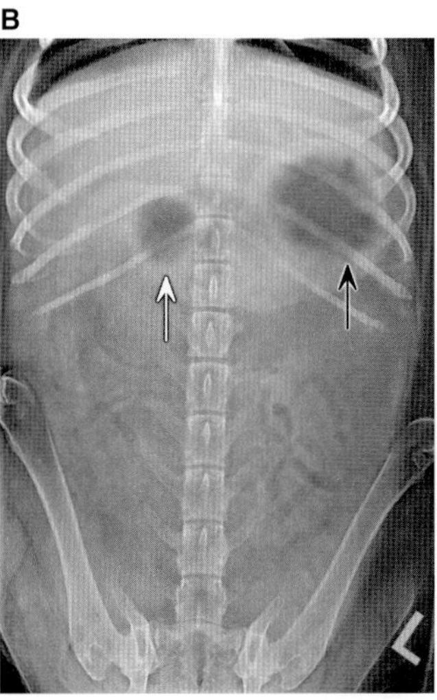

Figure 4.5 VD vs. DV. VD view (**A**) and DV view (**B**) of the same dog abdomen depicting some of the differences between the two views. In dorsal recumbency, there are three humps to the diaphragm and gastric gas rises into the body of the stomach (yellow arrow). In ventral recumbency, there is one hump to the diaphragm and gastric gas rises to the fundus (black arrow) and pylorus (white arrow). The serosal margins are less distinct in a DV view than a VD due to visceral crowding.

a patient straight for a VD view than a DV view (Figure 2.18), however, some patients will not tolerate being in dorsal recumbency. When neither a VD nor DV view is possible, make both the right lateral and the left lateral views. Making both right and left lateral views can alter the positions of the moveable viscera and change the distribution of fluid and gas in the hollow organs, which may reveal lesions that were not initially evident.

Supplemental views of the abdomen

Supplemental views sometimes are needed to confirm or further evaluate a suspected lesion. For example, when the stomach or colon is not recognized in initial radiographs, gas may be added to help identify them. To add gas to the stomach, a small volume of carbonated beverage may be given per os or air administered through a gastric tube. To identify the colon, a small volume of room air can be infused per rectum.

Flexed VD view ("frog-legged view") flexing the pelvic limbs with the patient in dorsal recumbency may be preferred to an extended VD view to eliminate superimposition of the inguinal skin folds and to lessen visceral crowding (Figure 4.6).

Oblique views are used to eliminate superimposition of overlying structures. For example, rotating the patient 10° or 20° from a true VD or lateral view may reduce summation of the spine or intestines on an area of interest (Figure 2.12). The oblique view can be further modified by collimating the field of view to a specific area and centering the x-ray beam on that area to make a tangential view.

Tangential views are used to better visualize a peripheral lesion, such as a mass in an abdominal wall. The patient is rotated or the x-ray tube is angled so the x-ray beam strikes the lesion in profile rather than en face (Figure 2.13). The FOV should be collimated to the size of the lesion to lessen scatter radiation and sharpen radiographic detail.

Horizontal beam radiography takes advantage of gravity to reposition fluid, gas, and viscera. It may be used to detect small volumes of free fluid or gas in the abdominal cavity or to better visualize an intra-abdominal mass that was obscured by viscera or fluid in the initial radiographs. Fluid flows to the dependent (down) part of the abdomen and gas rises to the uppermost part. The patient may be standing, held vertically, or positioned in lateral, dorsal or ventral recumbency, depending on the purpose of the view (Figure 2.15). The image receptor is placed alongside the patient, and the x-ray beam is directed across the table (horizontally) to make a VD or lateral view. The source-to-image distance should be the same as for vertical radiography (typically 100 cm or 40 inches) and you should follow the same guidelines for centering the x-ray beam and collimation.

Abdominal compression is a useful technique to displace overlying viscera away from an area of interest (Figure 2.19). For example, the abdomen may be gently compressed using a low opacity paddle (e.g., a plastic or wooden spoon) to push the intestines away from the urinary

A

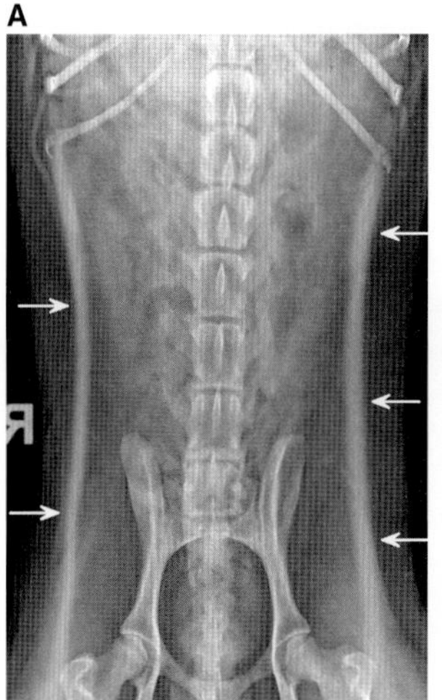

B

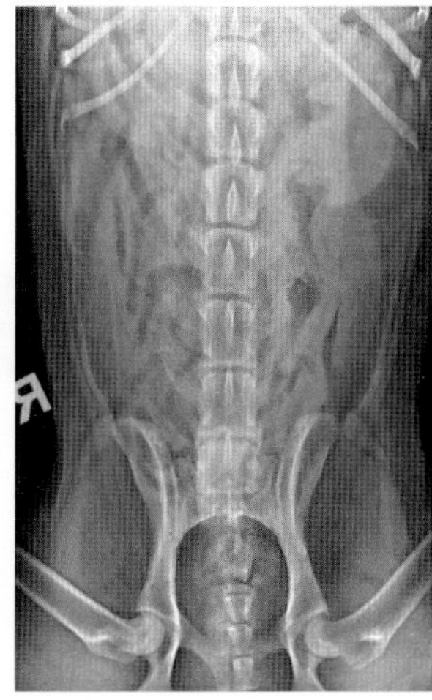

Figure 4.6 Inguinal skin folds. An extended VD view (**A**) and a flexed VD view (**B**) of the same dog abdomen depicting the appearance of skin folds and visceral crowding. With the pelvic limbs extended, the inguinal skin is stretched to create superimposition artifacts (white arrows). Extension also narrows the abdomen, which can crowd the organs and make serosal margins less distinct. The flexion or "frog-leg" view allows the abdomen to expand and may improve the visualization of serosal margins.

bladder, the uterus, a kidney, or a mass. The x-ray exposure is decreased to compensate for the reduced abdominal thickness; typically, the exposure time is reduced by half. Compression radiography is contraindicated in patients with a tense or painful abdomen, peritoneal effusion, or a mass that is at risk for rupture.

The urethral view is used to better visualize the urethra in male dogs by moving the pelvic limbs cranially while the patient is in lateral recumbency (Figure 2.20).

Patient factors

The patient's age, body type, body condition, and position at the time of radiography can affect the appearance of the abdominal structures. Some of the more frequently encountered factors are described below.

Immature animals

1. Liver and kidneys are relatively larger than in adults.
2. Serosal margins are less distinct due to a weaker opacity interface (Figure 4.7). The abdomen of a juvenile (less than six months old) typically contain less fat than in an adult. In addition, juvenile fat is mostly *brown fat*. The brown fat in immature animals is more opaque than adult fat due to its higher water content. To confirm the patient is immature, look for open growth plates.

Aged animals

1. Liver may normally extend caudal to the costal arch.
2. Spleen may be smaller than expected due to atrophy.
3. Abdomen may appear distended due to weak muscles.
4. Mineralized adrenal glands occasionally are visible in older cats as an incidental finding.

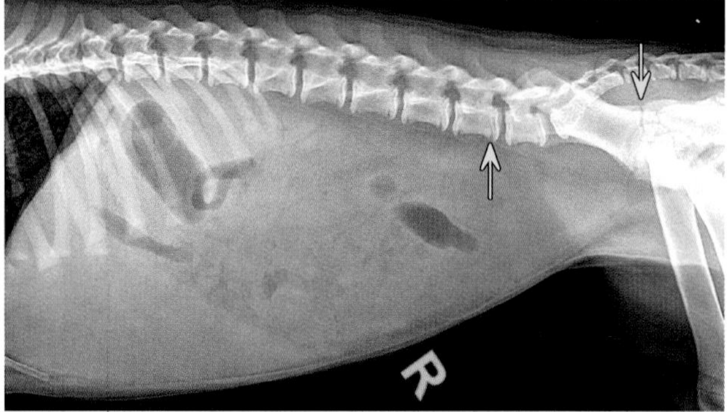

Figure 4.7 Immature abdomen. Lateral view of a 2-month-old puppy abdomen depicting indistinct serosal margins. Immature fat is more opaque than adult, which weakens the opacity interface with soft tissues. The patient's young age is evident from the open growth plates in the vertebrae and pelvis (yellow arrows), the relatively large size of the liver, and the incomplete mineralization of the costal arch.

Obese animals

1. Abdomen commonly appears distended.
2. Large amounts of intra-abdominal fat may displace viscera from their expected locations.
3. Small intestine may be crowded into the central abdomen. It often is displaced toward the right side in obese cats and ventrally in obese dogs.
4. Excessive fat in cats and small dogs can outline the serosal margins and may improve visualization of abdominal viscera. In large dogs, however, obesity increases scatter radiation which degrades radiographic contrast and detail.

Emaciated animals

1. Ventral abdomen may appear tucked or concave.
2. Serosal margins are less distinct due to loss of intra-abdominal fat. Examine other parts of the patient to help confirm emaciation (e.g., lack of subcutaneous fat).

Effects of positioning

1. Spleen tends to be less visible in a left lateral view.
2. Liver sometimes appears larger in a right lateral view than in a left lateral.
3. Spleen and liver are more likely to be in contact with each other in a right lateral view which may result in a mistaken diagnosis of hepatomegaly.
4. Kidneys tend to overlap more in a left lateral view and to be further separated in a right lateral view.
5. Pulling the pelvic limbs caudally can cause visceral crowding in the abdomen and may produce superimposed skin folds in a VD view. Position the pelvic limbs away from the area of interest, but in a neutral position or flexed in a VD view (e.g., frog-leg view).
6. Four views of the abdomen (right lateral, left lateral, VD, and DV) allows gravity to redistribute fluid and gas, which may aid in recognizing lesions, particularly when investigating GI disease.

Abdominal cavity

Normal radiographic anatomy

The borders of the abdominal cavity include the diaphragm cranially, the sublumbar muscles dorsally, the pelvic inlet caudally, and muscular walls laterally and ventrally. The sublumbar muscles are also called hypaxial muscles or psoas muscles.

Parietal peritoneum lines the diaphragm and muscular walls. **Visceral peritoneum** covers most of the abdominal organs and forms the mesentery. Between the parietal and visceral peritoneum is the peritoneal space (Figure 4.8).

The **peritoneal space** is considered a "potential space" because it contains only a small volume of fluid. It is not visible in radiographs. The peritoneal space surrounds the abdominal organs that are covered by the visceral perito-

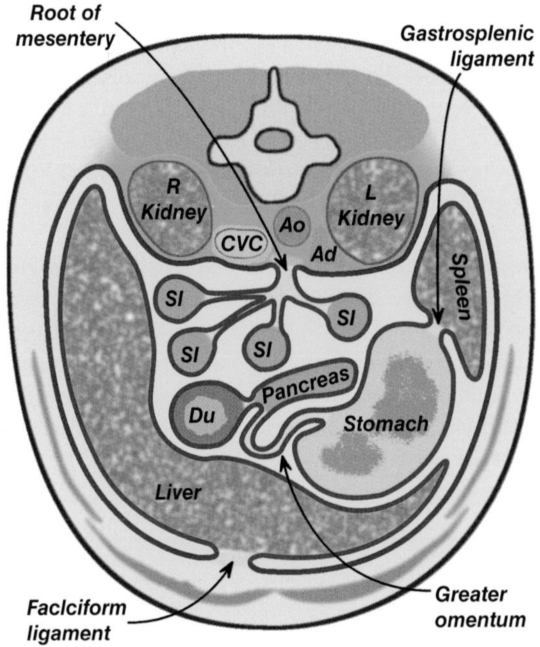

Figure 4.8 Peritoneum. This illustration depicts a cross-sectional view of the abdomen. The peritoneal space is enlarged and colored yellow for demonstration purposes. It normally contains only a small amount of fluid for lubrication. *Parietal* peritoneum is shown in red and *visceral* peritoneum in blue. The kidneys are located in the retroperitoneal space (colored green). Only the ventral borders of the kidneys are covered by peritoneum. Folds of peritoneum form the falciform and gastrosplenic ligaments and the root of the mesentery. SI = small intestine, Du = duodenum, CVC = caudal vena cava, Ao = aorta, Ad = adrenal gland.

neum. The organs that usually are visible in survey radiographs include the liver, spleen, stomach, intestines, and urinary bladder. Peritoneal structures not generally seen include the gall bladder, pancreas, ovaries, uterus, lymph nodes, and blood vessels. The kidneys are located in the retroperitoneal space.

The **retroperitoneal space** is the area dorsal to the peritoneal space and ventral to the sublumbar muscles. It extends from the diaphragm to the pelvis. The retroperitoneal space communicates cranially with the mediastinum (via the aortic hiatus) and caudally with the pelvic canal. In addition to the kidneys, structures in the retroperitoneal space include the adrenal glands, ureters, aorta, caudal vena cava, cisterna chyli, and lymph nodes. The kidneys usually are visible in survey radiographs and the aorta sometimes is identified. The other retroperitoneal structures rarely are distinguished unless enlarged or mineralized. A notable exception are the paired *deep circumflex iliac arteries* which branch from the caudal aorta at nearly a 90° angle. In a lateral view, one or both of these vessels often is seen end-on to appear as a focal mineral opacity structure ventral to the caudal lumbar spine, sometimes mistaken for a ureteral calculus (Figure 4.9). This finding is similar to seeing an end-on pulmonary vessel and mistaking it for a mineralized lung nodule (Figures 3.145 and 3.146). Rarely will more than one of these vessels be visible in radiographs.

There is no direct communication between the peritoneal space and the retroperitoneal space. Disease in one compartment rarely involves the other. Fat, however, is stored in both compartments. Fat deposits tend to be largest in the falciform ligament, omentum, mesentery, and caudal retroperitoneal space. The radiographic appearance of peritoneal and retroperitoneal fat normally is similar in opacity and homogeneity. Large fat deposits may be mistaken for a mass or fluid, particularly in overweight cats (Figure 4.10). However, most masses and all biological fluids are soft tissue opacity and should not be mistaken for fat.

Normal **intra-abdominal lymph nodes** are not visible in survey radiographs. The *visceral* nodes are located in the peritoneal space and the *parietal* nodes are in the retroperitoneal space. The visceral nodes receive lymphatics from the cranial abdomen and drain into the cisterna chyli. The parietal or sublumbar nodes receive lymphatics from the spine, adrenal glands, kidneys, pelvic canal, and pelvic limbs and also drain into the cisterna chyli. The cranial mesenteric nodes are the largest visceral lymph nodes. They are located near the root of the mesentery. The medial iliac nodes are the largest sublumbar nodes and they are located ventral to the L5–7 vertebrae. There is considerable variation in the number and location of the sublumbar lymph nodes among dogs and cats. Sometimes these nodes are absent.

Abnormal size of the abdomen

A small or contracted abdomen may be due to loss of body fat or displacement of the abdominal viscera, the latter resulting from a hernia or rupture of the diaphragm or body

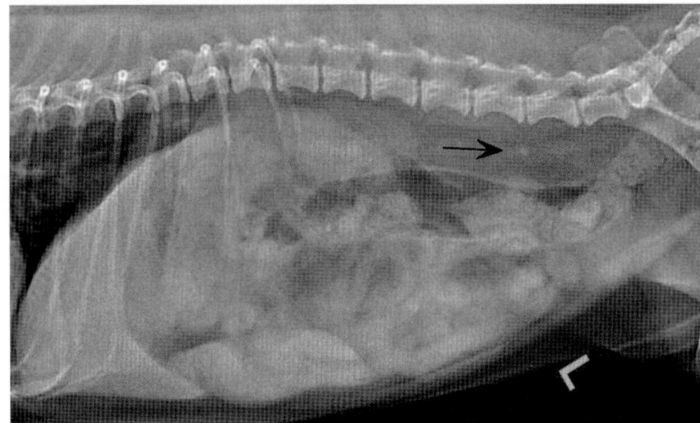

Figure 4.9 Deep circumflex iliac artery. Lateral view of a dog abdomen depicting end-on visualization of a deep circumflex iliac artery (arrow), which may be mistaken for a ureteral calculus.

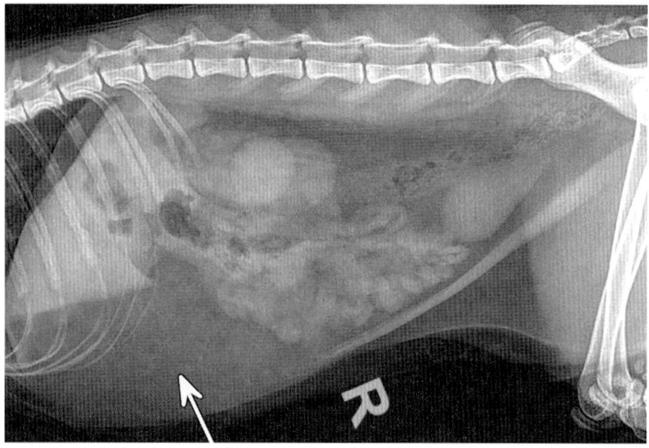

Figure 4.10 Falciform fat. Lateral view of a cat abdomen depicting a large amount of fat in the falciform ligament (arrow). Falciform fat may be mistaken for a mass or peritoneal effusion, but this is fat opacity, not soft tissue, and the falciform is a common site for fat deposition.

wall. In emaciated patients, the abdomen may appear "tucked up" with a concave ventral border (Figure 4.11). The serosal margins often are indistinct because there is insufficient intra-abdominal fat to create a visible opacity interface. Both the peritoneal and retroperitoneal spaces tend to be small.

Abdominal distention may involve the peritoneal space, the retroperitoneal space, or both. Disease in one space usually does not involve the other, which means the other space generally appears normal in radiographs. Conditions that can enlarge both spaces include excess fat in overweight animals and hemorrhage, the latter when caused by coagulopathy or severe trauma. Leakage of urine can also enlarge one or both spaces.

An abdomen may appear distended due to weakening of the supporting ligaments and muscles. Weakening may be associated with old age or Cushing's Syndrome (hypercortisolism). The abdomen may appear to sag or to be pendulous, but serosal margins remain distinct, unless there is concurrent intra-abdominal fluid or inflammation.

Abnormal abdominal wall

Thickening (widening) of a body wall may be localized or diffuse. A thickened wall may or may not be accompanied by altered opacity. Localized thickening typically is due to a mass.

A thickened abdominal wall that contains gas opacity may result from a penetrating wound, herniation of a gas-filled structure, or migration of emphysema. Penetrating wounds (e.g., bite wounds, injections, surgery) generally produce a multifocal gas pattern, whereas a herniated bowel segment tends to be localized and confined. Migration of emphysema typically originates in the thorax (e.g., pneumomediastinum) and can become quite diffuse (Figure 3.63).

Fat opacity in a diffusely thickened abdominal wall may be due to obesity or a dissecting lipoma. Obesity is bilateral, whereas lipomas tend to be unilateral. Localized fat opacity may represent an isolated lipoma or a hernia containing omental or falciform fat. Fat in the body wall may displace and outline muscle layers, providing an opacity interface with the soft tissue opacity of the muscles.

A thickened abdominal wall that is soft tissue opacity may be due to subcutaneous fluid, a mass, or displaced viscera. Soft tissue opacity swelling may obscure fascial planes and muscle layers.

Mineral or metal opacity in the abdominal wall usually is readily identified and may represent dystrophic mineralization or a foreign object. Superimposition artifacts can mimic abnormal opacity.

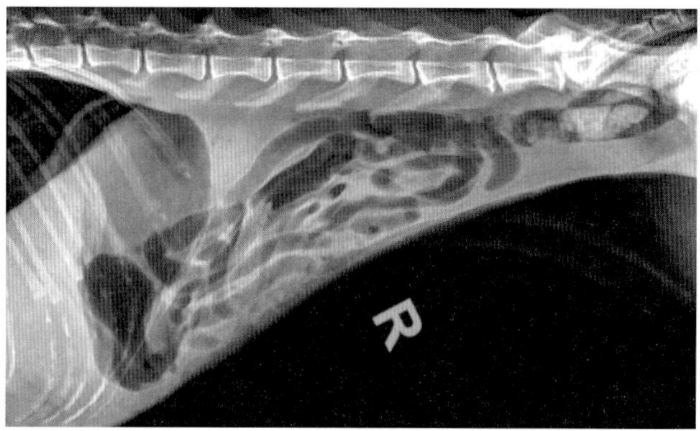

Figure 4.11 Emaciation. Lateral view of a dog abdomen depicting little intra-abdominal fat. The ventral abdomen is concave and tucked-up. The serosal margins are indistinct because there is insufficient fat for an opacity interface. Notice the lack of subcutaneous fat.

Abdominal hernia or rupture

A *hernia* is a protrusion through a natural opening; the peritoneum remains intact. A *rupture* is an acquired loss of body wall integrity; the peritoneum is damaged. The two rarely are distinguished in radiographs. The term hernia, therefore, commonly is used as a catch-all phrase to describe the displacement of abdominal viscera outside the abdominal cavity.

Displaced viscera create variable degrees of extra-abdominal swelling. Swelling caused by a hernia may be difficult to distinguish from swelling caused by a tumor, cyst, or other mass. The opacity of the swollen area may provide clues to its contents.

Fatty tissues tend to enter a hernia first (e.g., omentum, mesentery, falciform ligament). The most commonly displaced soft tissue structures are the intestines, stomach, liver, spleen, urinary bladder, and uterus. The identity of a displaced organ may be determined by recognizing its shape or its pattern or by noticing that it is absent from its normal location. GI structures often can be identified by their intraluminal gas. Displaced intestines commonly create curvilinear gas opacity tubes that extend beyond the limits of the abdominal cavity. A strangulated or incarcerated GI structure can dilate greatly to produce a very large cyst-like mass (Figure 3.48).

The abdominal cavity may appear "empty" when a significant amount of viscera is displaced. The serosal margins of the remaining organs usually are well-visualized unless surrounded by fluid or there is insufficient body fat.

Abdominal hernias vary in etiology and location (Figure 4.12). **Diaphragmatic** hernias, including traumatic, hiatal, and peritoneopericardial, are discussed in Chapter 3: Thorax. An **umbilical**, **inguinal**, or **scrotal** hernia may be congenital or acquired and may appear as either a soft tissue, fat, gas, or mixed opacity swelling in its respective area. **Perineal** hernias result from a weakened or ruptured pelvic floor and most often occur in older, intact males. They typically produce a swelling under the tail and may displace the rectum. Contents in a perineal hernia may include fluid, fat, urinary bladder, prostate gland, uterus, or/and intestine. **Intra-abdominal** hernias occur when an organ protrudes through a tear in the mesentery. These may be visible in radiographs as a static bowel segment or dilated bowel if the segment becomes incarcerated (i.e., mesenteric hernia).

Abnormal opacity in the abdominal cavity

Abdominal radiographs that are less opaque than expected may be due to poor radiographic technique, excess intra-abdominal fat, or free gas in the peritoneal or retroperitoneal space (see differential diagnoses). Excess fat is due to obesity or a large intra-abdominal lipoma (Figure 4.13). Free gas may result from a penetrating wound, ruptured GI structure, recent laparotomy, or infection with gas-producing bacteria.

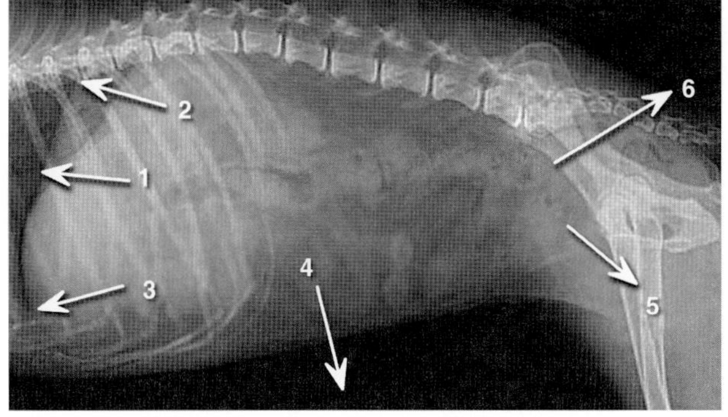

Figure 4.12 Abdominal hernias. Lateral view of a dog abdomen depicting common sites of abdominal hernias: (**1**) diaphragm hiatus; (**2**) dorsal diaphragm; (**3**) ventral diaphragm; (**4**) umbilicus; (**5**) inguinal region; (**6**) perineal region.

A

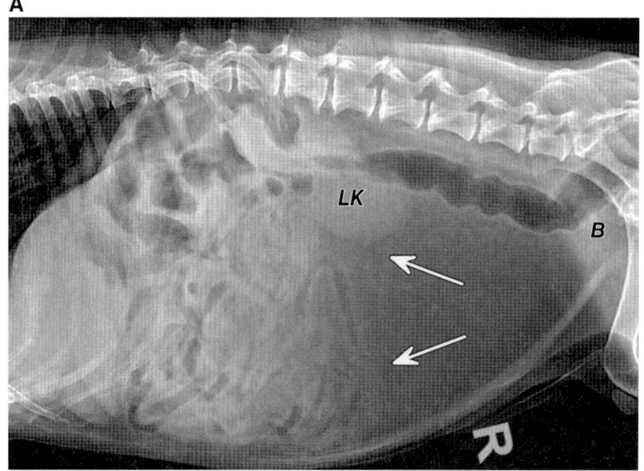

B

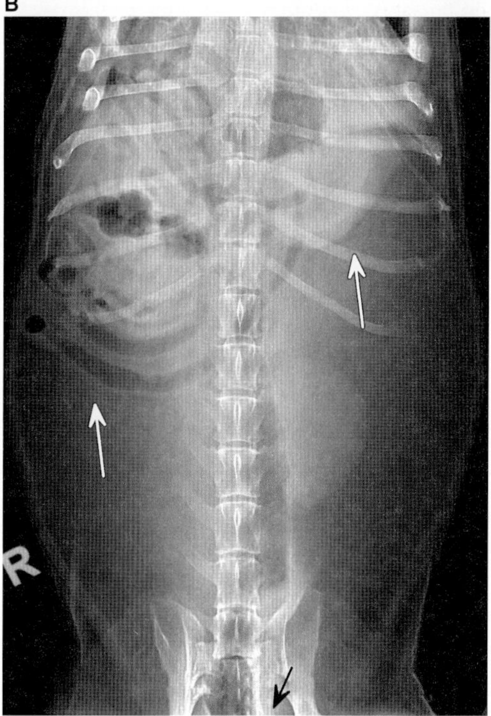

Figure 4.13 Intra-abdominal lipoma. Lateral view (**A**) and VD view (**B**) of a dog abdomen depicting a large lipoma in the caudal abdomen. The lipoma displaces the small intestine cranially, the colon dorsally (arrows), and the urinary bladder (B) caudally. The soft tissue opacity left kidney (LK) is visible through the fat opacity lipoma.

Abdominal structures or areas that appear more opaque than expected in radiographs may be due to poor radiographic technique, increased intra-abdominal fluid, or visceral crowding (see differential diagnoses). Increased fluid and visceral crowding both lead to less distinct serosal margins. Fluid may result from inflammation or effusion. The type of fluid cannot be determined from radiographs because all biological fluids are soft tissue opacity.

Gas in the abdominal cavity

Gas is common in the GI tracts of dogs and cats. The volume of gas can vary greatly between patients and may or may not be clinically significant. Abnormal GI gas usually is accompanied by dilation or a persistently abnormal pattern.

Gas within the wall or parenchyma of an organ (*pneumatosis*) is abnormal. Pneumatosis has been reported in the stomach, intestines, spleen, liver, uterus, gall bladder, and urinary bladder. It most often is caused by a gas-producing bacterial infection (e.g., E. coli, pseudomonas), particularly in animals with diabetes mellitus. Pneumatosis also can result from damage to the mucosa and leakage of gas into the wall of the organ.

Pneumoperitoneum is free gas in the peritoneal space. The etiology of pneumoperitoneum may not be evident from radiographs alone. Patient history and results of physical examination often provide valuable diagnostic information.

Penetrating wounds frequently are accompanied by subcutaneous emphysema. Note: superimposition of subcutaneous gas can mask or mimic a pneumoperitoneum. Post-operative gas generally is resorbed within a week, but gas can persist in the peritoneal space for as long as three to four weeks. In patients with pneumoperitoneum caused by a ruptured stomach or bowel segment, the damaged organ may be abnormally distended.

Small volumes of peritoneal gas appear as irregular-shaped bubbles or pockets of gas. Bubbles usually are unevenly distributed and frequently become trapped among the segments of small intestine. They appear as sharply-marginated pockets of gas that are more linear or triangular in shape than the normal rounded, flowing intestinal gas pattern (Figure 4.14).

Peritoneal gas rises to the highest part of the abdomen. Larger volumes of gas tend to collect between the diaphragm and the liver (Figure 4.14). Gas adjacent to the diaphragm, liver and stomach enhance their visualization due to the gas:soft tissue opacity interface. As gas continues to fill the peritoneal space, more and more serosal margins may become more distinct. However, pneumoperitoneum often is accompanied by peritoneal inflammation or effusion, which may obscure serosal margins.

A large volume of free gas in the peritoneal cavity can cause an overall decrease in abdominal opacity which may be mistaken for an overexposed radiograph. Examine the extra-abdominal structures to determine whether the exposure was correct.

Peritoneal gas tends to be freely moveable. Its distribution is affected by gravity and the position of the patient at the time of radiography. Small volumes of free gas may be easier to detect with horizontal beam views (Figure 2.15). In lateral recumbency, gas rises to the uppermost part of the peritoneal space and tends to collect under the ribs (Figure 4.15). Left lateral recumbency is preferred over right lateral recumbency because the gas that normally is present in the gastric fundus and colon may be mistaken for peritoneal gas. In dorsal recumbency, free gas is likely to collect between the ventral body wall and the liver (Figure 4.16). Keep in mind that it takes some time for peritoneal gas to redistribute, so allow the patient to remain recumbent for about 5–10 minutes prior to making the radiograph. For patients in distress, a standing lateral view may be preferred, in which case free gas rises dorsally to collect in the sublumbar region.

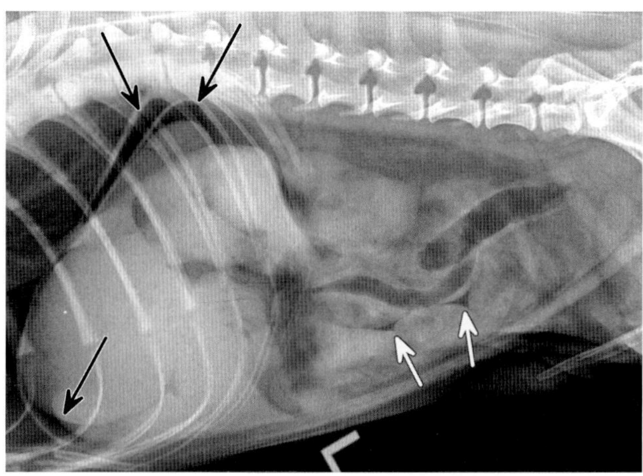

Figure 4.14 Pneumoperitoneum. Left lateral view of a dog abdomen depicting free gas in the peritoneal cavity. Pockets of gas accumulate between the diaphragm and liver (black arrows) and form triangular-shaped bubbles among the segments of small intestine (white arrows).

Pneumoretroperitoneum is free gas in the retroperitoneal space. The margins of the kidneys, aorta, and sublumbar muscles often become more visible due to the gas outlining their margins (Figure 3.63). Causes of a pneumoretroperitoneum include a penetrating wound, migration of gas from a pneumomediastinum, and infection with gas-producing bacteria.

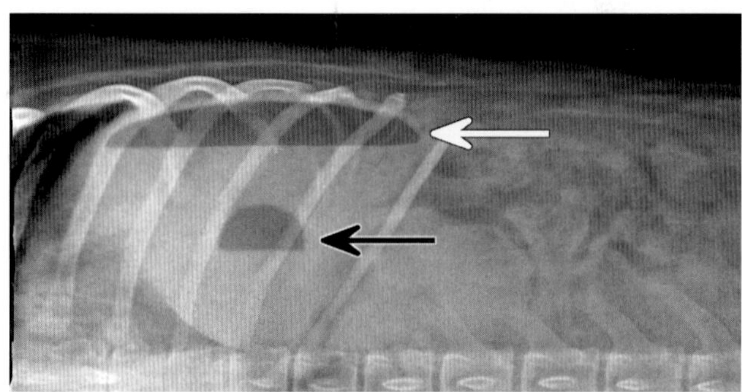

Figure 4.15 Horizontal beam view. VD view of a dog abdomen made with the patient in left lateral recumbency and the x-ray beam directed horizontally (across the table). Free gas rises to the uppermost part of the peritoneal space and is depicted under the ribs (white arrow). A normal gas:fluid line is depicted in the gastric pylorus (black arrow).

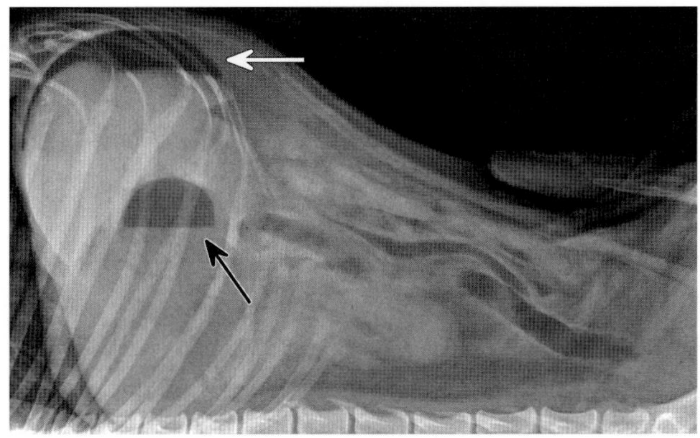

Figure 4.16 Horizontal beam radiography. Lateral view of a dog abdomen made with the patient in dorsal recumbency and the x-ray beam directed horizontally (across the table). Free gas rises to the uppermost part of the peritoneal space and is depicted between the ventral body wall and the liver (white arrow). A normal gas:fluid line is depicted in the stomach (black arrow).

Fluid in the abdominal cavity

An increase in intra-abdominal fluid may result from inflammation or effusion. The type of fluid cannot be determined from radiographs.

Peritoneal inflammation (peritonitis) creates more fluid due to increased blood flow and capillary leakage. The inflammation may be localized or diffuse. Serosal margins in the inflamed area appear hazy and indistinct due to fluid effacement. Peritonitis can progress to effusion and complete loss of visualization of serosal margins. Effusion may or may not cause abdominal distention. The retroperitoneal space is normal as long as the inflammation is confined to the peritoneal space.

Peritonitis can alter peristalsis in the nearby intestines and cause stasis in one or more bowel segments. A static bowel segment is called a *sentinel loop*. Sentinel loops are segments of intestine that persist relatively unchanged in size, shape, content, and position in serial radiographs. Often it is this static gas pattern that is first detected in patients with peritonitis. Pancreatitis is a common cause of localized peritonitis. It may lead to sentinel loops in the duodenum and transverse colon (Figures 4.17 and 4.48).

Peritoneal effusion (or ascites) is free fluid in the peritoneal space. There are numerous possible etiologies (see differential diagnoses). Small volumes of fluid may be visible as streaks of soft tissue opacity mixed with intra-abdominal fat. The fat provides the opacity interface to see the free fluid as thin, faint, curvy or "wispy" lines (Figure 4.18). "Fluid-streaking of fat" tends to be easiest to see at the periphery of the abdominal cavity, where there are fewer superimposed structures. Sometimes a wet hair coat can mimic fluid-streaking of fat, but wet hair extends beyond the limits of the abdominal cavity.

Larger volumes of peritoneal fluid lead to an overall increase in peritoneal opacity and greater effacement of serosal margins (Figure 4.19). The radiograph may appear underexposed. Examine the retroperitoneal space and the skeletal structures to determine whether the exposure was correct. In patients with peritoneal effusion, the small intestine often is suspended in the fluid and evenly distributed (unless displaced by a mass). Gas-filled bowel loops rise to the top of the fluid and commonly collect in the mid-abdomen. Severe peritoneal effusion can distend the abdomen and push the diaphragm cranially. In these cases the diaphragm may appear stationary in serial radiographs.

The retroperitoneal space remains normal as long as fluid is confined to the peritoneal space. The kidneys frequently are visible through the peritoneal effusion because they are surrounded by retroperitoneal fat.

Retroperitoneal fluid typically is due to leakage of urine or blood, but can be caused by inflammation (see differential diagnoses). Fluid partially or completely obscures the margins of the kidneys and sublumbar muscles. Large volumes of fluid may distend the retroperitoneal space and displace the colon and small intestine ventrally (Figure 4.20). Peritoneal serosal margins remain distinct as long as the disease is confined to the retroperitoneal space.

Mineral opacity in the abdominal cavity

Mineral opacity material is a frequent finding in the GI tracts of dogs and cats and may or may not be clinically significant. It may be associated with food, bones, or foreign objects.

Focal mineral opacity structures outside the GI tract may represent calculi or dystrophic mineralization. These are seen more often in the hepatobiliary and urinary tracts.

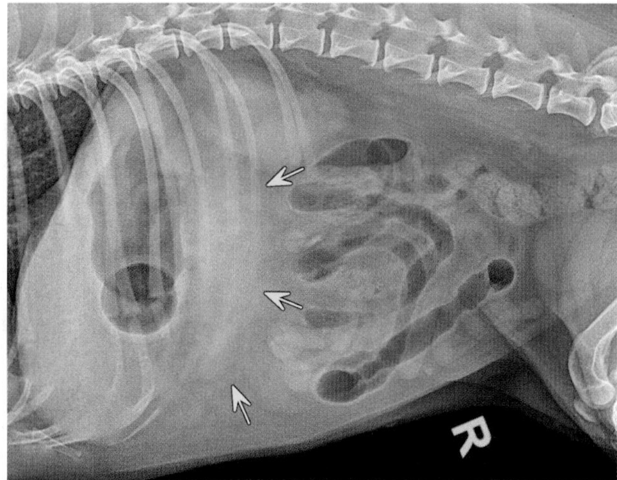

Figure 4.17 Localized peritonitis. Lateral view of a dog abdomen depicting an area of hazy, indistinct serosal margins in the cranial abdomen (arrows). The margins are not well-visualized due to regional inflammation caused by pancreatitis. The more caudal peritoneal serosal margins and the retroperitoneal margins remain distinct.

A

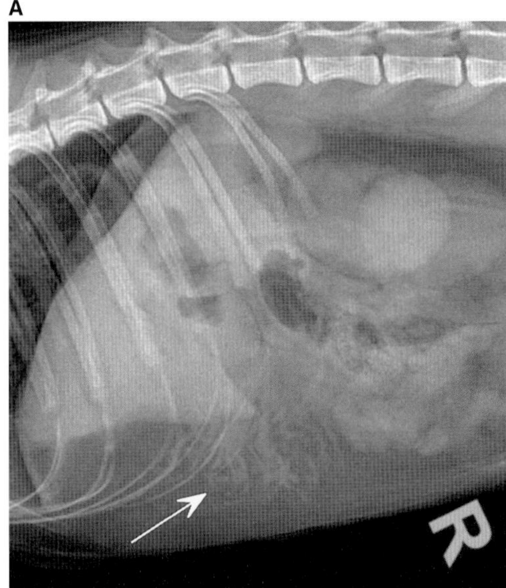

B

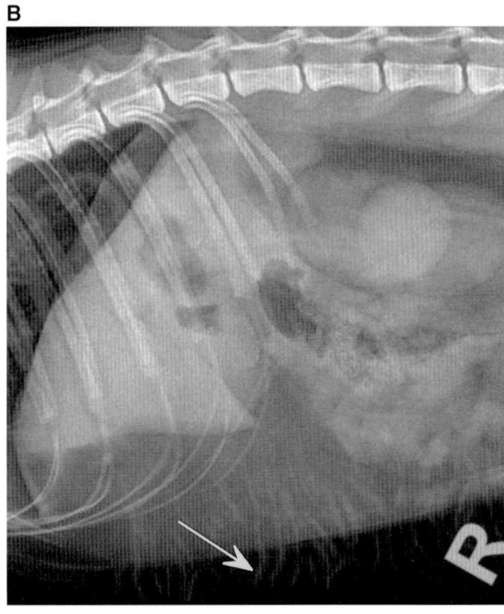

Figure 4.18 Fluid-streaking of fat. **A**. Lateral view of a cat abdomen depicting a small volume of peritoneal fluid. The fluid is interspersed with the fat to create wispy, curvilinear, soft tissue opacity streaks (arrow). **B**. Lateral view of a cat abdomen depicting a wet hair coat. The superimposed wet hair creates a similar pattern to (A), but the wet hair extends beyond the limits of the abdominal cavity (arrow). Peritoneal effusion is confined to peritoneal space.

Some focal areas of mineral opacity appear to be free in the peritoneal cavity. These sometimes are **Bates bodies**, which appear as discrete, round, or oval-shaped structures with smooth borders and less opaque centers (Figure 4.21). Bates bodies can vary in size and may be fixed in position or freely moveable, changing location in serial radiographs. They generally are considered incidental findings, possibly representing nodules of fat necrosis from a previous episode of pancreatitis or peritonitis. They are reported most often in older cats.

Vascular mineralization is uncommon in dogs and cats. It typically appears linear and heterogenous (Figure 4.22) and may be associated with atherosclerosis or hypercalcemia. Mineralization usually involves the arteries (e.g., aorta, iliac, celiac, mesenteric).

Metal opacity in the abdominal cavity may represent a foreign object (e.g., projectile, ingested foreign object), surgical implant (e.g., sutures, vascular band), or contrast medium.

A

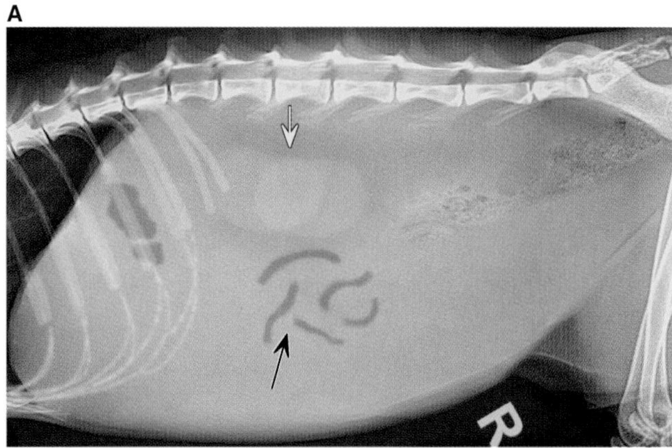

B

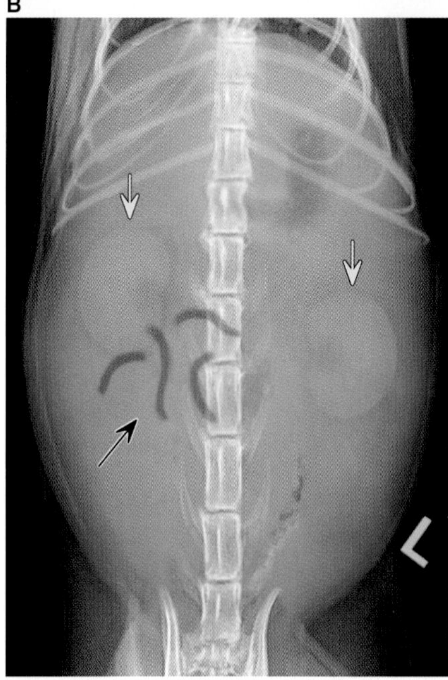

Figure 4.19 Peritoneal effusion. Lateral view (**A**) and VD view (**B**) of a cat abdomen depicting a distended abdomen due to peritoneal fluid. The fluid completely effaces the borders of the peritoneal structures (liver, spleen, intestines, urinary bladder are not identified), but the borders of the kidneys remain visible because they are retroperitoneal (yellow arrows). A few gas-filled segments of small intestine are depicted in the mid-abdomen (black arrows).

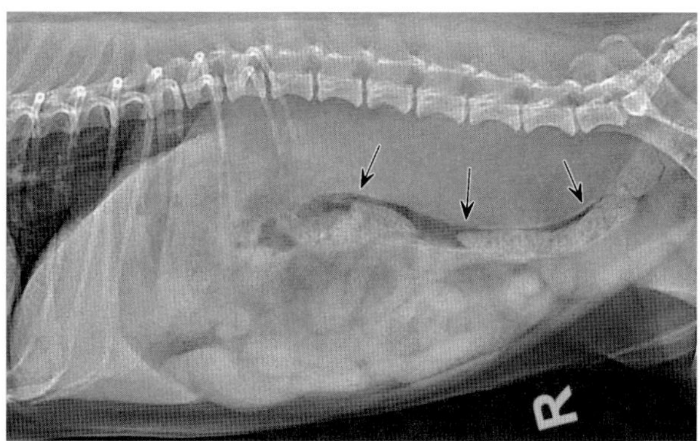

Figure 4.20 Retroperitoneal effusion. Lateral view of a dog abdomen depicting swelling in the retroperitoneal space due to fluid accumulation. The type of fluid cannot be determined from radiographs. The margins of the kidneys and sublumbar muscles are obscured. The descending colon and small intestine are displaced ventrally (arrows).

A

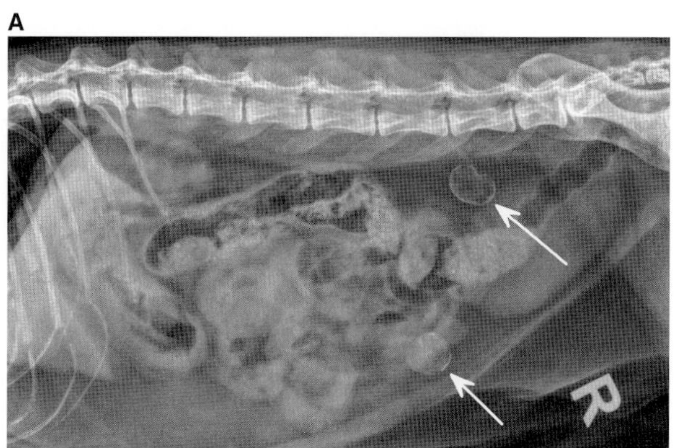

B

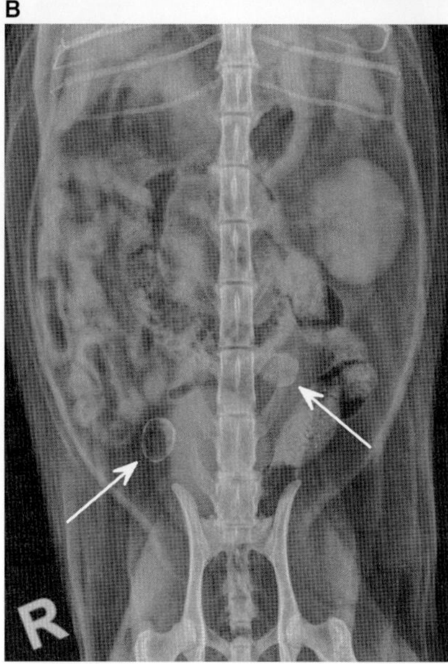

Figure 4.21 Bates bodies (nodular fat necrosis). Lateral view (**A**) and VD view (**B**) of a cat abdomen depicting two mineral opacity nodules in the abdomen (arrows). The margins of the nodules are smooth and well-defined and the centers are less opaque.

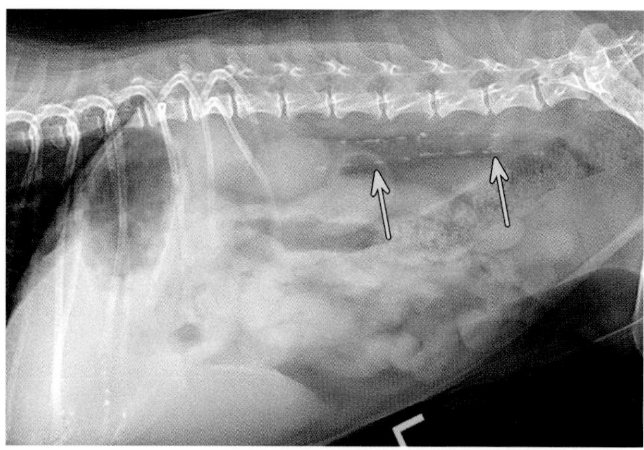

Figure 4.22 Vascular mineralization. Lateral view of a dog abdomen depicting mineral opacity foci in the retroperitoneal space consistent with mineralization in the wall of the abdominal aorta (arrows). May be mistaken for ureteral calculi.

Intra-abdominal mass

A mass in the abdominal cavity must be large enough or sufficiently different in opacity to be distinguished in radiographs. Soft tissue opacity masses generally need to be at least twice the width of the small intestine to be recognized. Larger masses may be identified by the displacement of the nearby structures, which is called a **mass effect**.

A mass effect may be caused by any large, space-occupying structure, including organomegaly, tumors, abscesses, cysts, granulomas, hematomas, and lipomas. Organomegaly may be physiologic or pathologic. Examples of physiologic organomegaly include a full urinary bladder, postprandial stomach, pregnancy, and compensatory renal hypertrophy (latter occurs when the other kidney is absent or not functional). Pathologic organomegaly is discussed with each specific organ later in this chapter.

Clues to the origin of an abdominal mass come from its location and the direction of displacement of the adjacent viscera (Figure 4.23).

Most masses are soft tissue opacity (Figure 4.24), but longstanding and necrotic masses can mineralize or cavitate, the latter sometimes filling with gas. Some neoplastic masses are bone-forming.

The margins of a mass may be well-defined or indistinct, depending on the opacity interface. Indistinct margins may result from visceral crowding or adjacent fluid, the latter due to inflammation, hemorrhage, or effusion. When a large volume of intra-abdominal fluid is present the radiographs should be repeated after removing as much fluid as possible to better visualize the visceral margins.

Lymphadenomegaly may be caused by neoplasia, infection, or inflammation and can produce a visible intra-abdominal mass. Groups of enlarged visceral lymph nodes sometimes blend together to produce an ill-defined, soft tissue opacity mass in the peritoneal space (Figure 4.25).

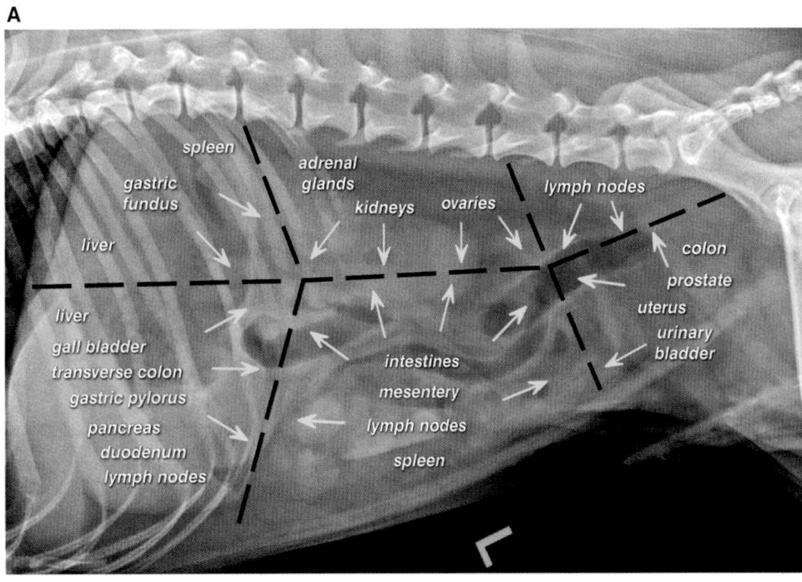

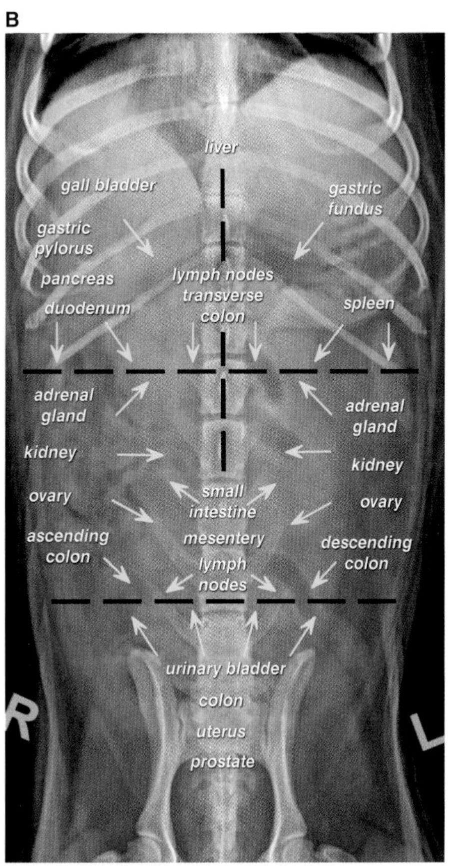

Figure 4.23 Mass effect. Lateral view (**A**) and VD view (**B**) of a dog abdomen depicting the possible sites of origin for an intra-abdominal mass based on its location and the direction of displacement of the adjacent structures (yellow arrows).

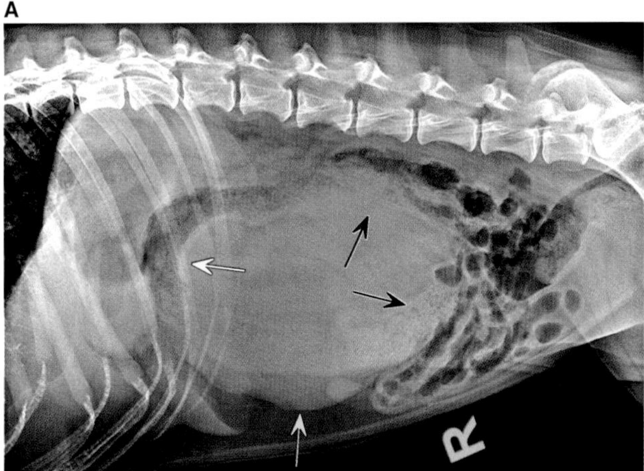

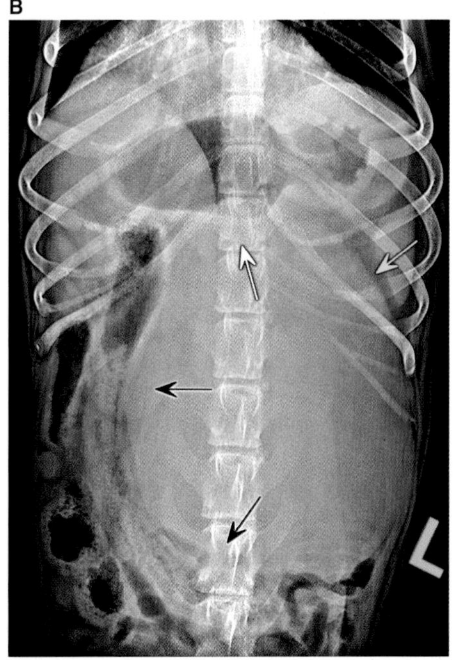

Figure 4.24 Intra-abdominal mass. Lateral view (**A**) and VD view (**B**) of a dog abdomen depicting a soft tissue opacity mass in the mid-abdomen. The mass displaces the intestines dorsally, caudally, and to the right (black arrows). The transverse colon and stomach are displaced cranially (white arrows). The edges of the mass are well-defined by intra-abdominal fat (yellow arrows). Possible origins for this mass include spleen, mesentery, intestine, left kidney. This was a tumor in the left kidney.

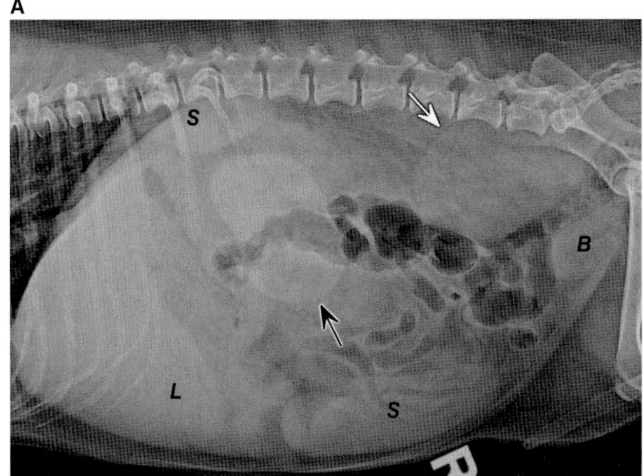

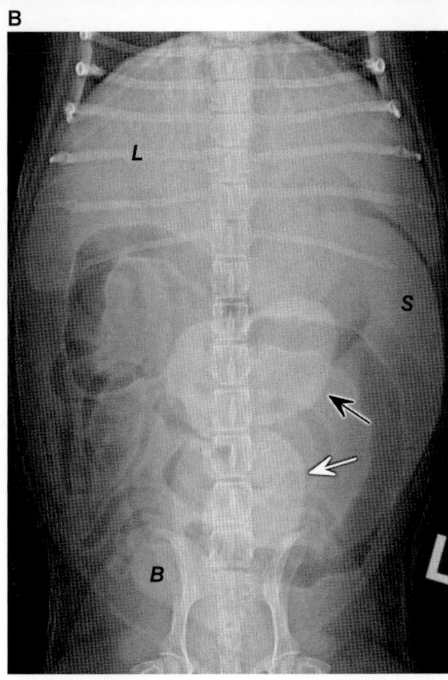

Figure 4.25 Abdominal lymph node enlargement. Lateral view (**A**) and VD view (**B**) of a dog abdomen depicting organomegaly and lymphadenomegaly due to lymphoma. The liver (L) and spleen (S) are enlarged with rounded margins. The mesenteric lymph nodes (black arrow) and sublumbar lymph nodes (white arrow) are enlarged. B = urinary bladder.

Sublumbar lymphadenomegaly most often involves the medial iliac lymph nodes. It typically appears as a retroperitoneal mass ventral to the caudal lumbar spine.

Enlargement of the sublumbar lymph nodes may be accompanied by a periosteal response along the caudal lumbar vertebrae. Periosteal new bone sometimes involves the pelvic bones and proximal femurs but most often develops along the middle ventral borders of the L5-7 vertebral bodies (Figure 4.26). This new bone production differs from spondylosis deformans. Spondylosis tends to be better-defined and forms at the ends of the vertebral bodies, not in the middle.

Liver

Normal radiographic anatomy

The liver is located in the cranial abdomen. It is connected by ligaments to the diaphragm, caudal vena cava, stomach, duodenum, and right kidney. The *falciform* ligament attaches the liver to the ventral body wall and serves as a storage reservoir for fat.

The liver consists of six lobes: right lateral, left lateral, right medial, left medial, caudate, and quadrate (Figure 4.27). The **gall bladder** lies between the quadrate lobe and the right medial lobe. It is not visible in radiographs unless enlarged, emphysematous, mineralized, or filled with contrast medium. The right kidney lies in the renal fossa of the caudate liver lobe. Because the kidney and the liver are the same opacity, the cranial pole of the right kidney may not be visible unless surrounded by fat or gas.

Liver in the lateral view

The triangular-shaped liver is located between the diaphragm and the ventral body wall (Figures 4.2 and 4.3). Its margins normally are even and well-defined. The cranial border of the liver blends with the caudal border of the diaphragm (Both are soft tissue opacity with no other opacity between them). The dorsal liver border is formed by the caudate lobe, but it is not well visualized because it blends with the adjacent soft tissues. The caudal border of the liver is adjacent to the stomach and also poorly visualized. The ventral liver border usually is visible because it is adjacent to falciform fat.

The caudoventral border of the liver forms an acute angle at about the level of the costal arch. The **costal arch** is the curved line formed by the caudal costal cartilages

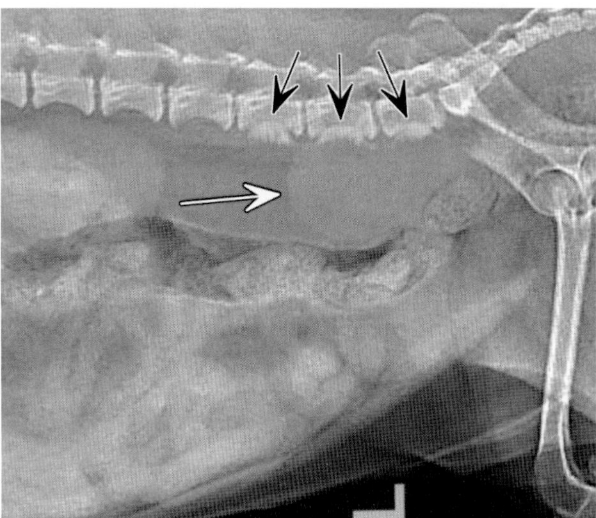

Figure 4.26 Periosteal response. Lateral view of a dog abdomen depicting medial iliac lymphadenomegaly (white arrow) and a periosteal response along the caudal lumbar vertebrae (black arrows).

A

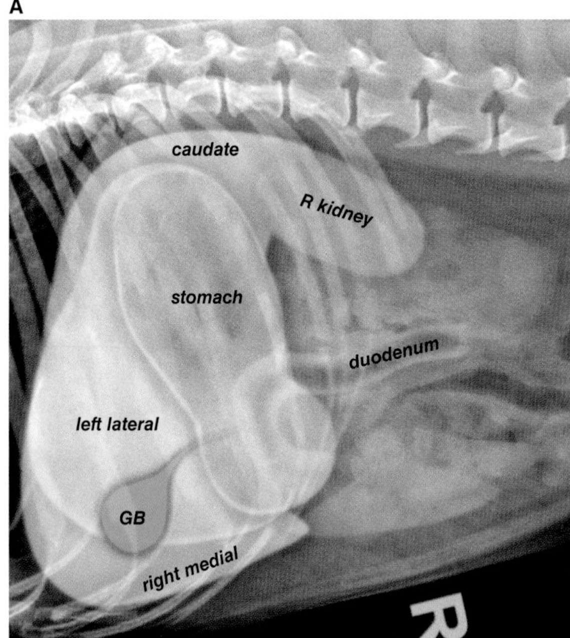

B

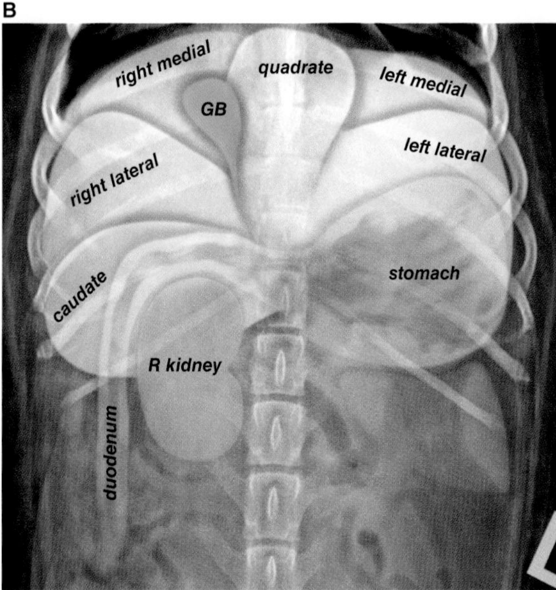

Figure 4.27 Liver anatomy. Lateral view (**A**) and VD view (**B**) of a dog abdomen illustrating the individual liver lobes, gall bladder (GB), stomach, and right kidney. In the lateral view, the left lateral and right medial liver lobes form the caudoventral edge of the liver.

(Figure 4.28). The caudoventral edge of the liver is a frequently used landmark to evaluate liver size. When the edge extends caudal to the costal arch, the liver commonly is considered to be enlarged. However, this interpretation of liver size is based on palpation of the liver in a clinical setting. It is important to realize that palpable findings do not always correlate with radiographic findings. The costal arch is typically mineral opacity. It is located cranial to the palpable arch because muscle, skin, and subcutaneous tissue are between the true arch and the fingers during palpation. In radiographs, of normal dogs and cats, the caudoventral edge of the liver frequently extends caudal to the visible costal arch. This is usually evident during inspiration and in right lateral recumbency. The liver may also extend further caudal than expected in animals with weak supporting ligaments (e.g., old age, endocrinopathy). Do not rely on the position of the

A

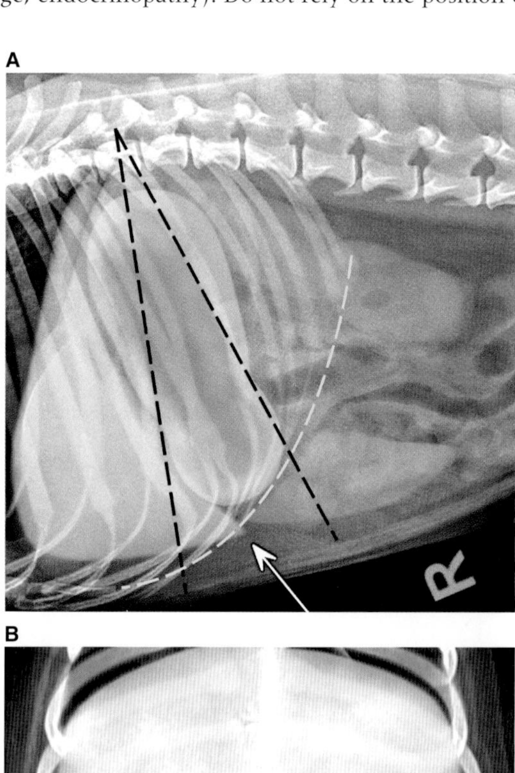

B

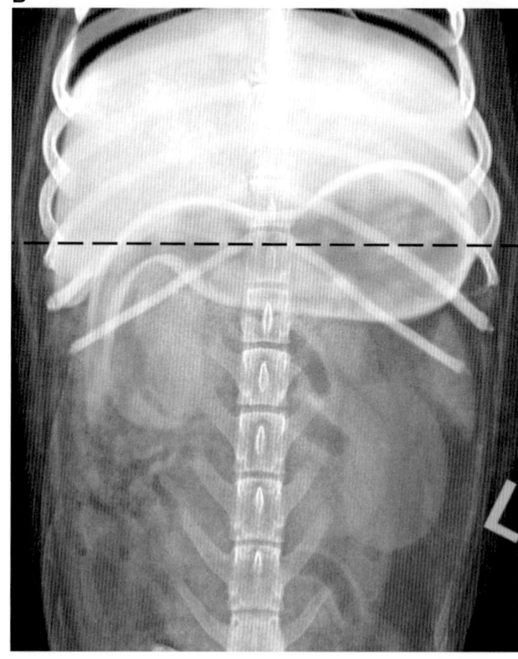

Figure 4.28 Liver size. Lateral view (**A**) and VD view (**B**) of a dog cranial abdomen with the liver and stomach highlighted. In the lateral view, the caudoventral edge of the liver (white arrow) extends to about the level of the costal arch (yellow dotted line). The normal gastric axis (black dashed lines) is angled somewhere between perpendicular to the spine and parallel with the ribs. In general, if the pylorus is more cranial than perpendicular to the spine, the liver is considered small. If the pylorus is further caudal than parallel to the ribs, the liver is considered enlarged. In the VD view, the normal gastric axis is about perpendicular to the spine.

caudoventral edge of the liver to diagnose hepatomegaly. **The key radiographic finding with hepatomegaly is rounding of the liver margins**.

Liver size is also assessed in a lateral view by evaluating the position of the gastric axis. The **gastric axis** is an imaginary line drawn between the fundus and pylorus of the stomach (Figure 4.28). In a lateral view, the normal gastric axis is somewhere between perpendicular to the spine and parallel with the ribs, depending on the patient's body conformation and the size of the stomach. The gastric axis tends to be more perpendicular to the spine in deep-chested dogs (e.g., Afghan Hound, Collie) and in patients with a full stomach. It often is more parallel with the ribs in shallow-chested breeds (e.g., Bulldog, Pug) and in patients with an empty stomach.

The gall bladder in a lateral view is located in the cranioventral part of the liver. Mineral or gas opacity in this area may be associated with the gall bladder. However, artifacts created by superimposition of the ribs, costal cartilages, and the caudal lung lobes must be differentiated from a hepatobiliary lesion.

A large gall bladder can create a convex, soft tissue opacity bulge along the ventral border of the liver, particularly in cats (Figure 4.29).

Liver in the VD/DV view

The liver occupies the space between the diaphragm and the stomach. In dogs, the liver is relatively symmetrical in shape, occupying at least two intercostal spaces on both the right and left sides. The gastric axis tends to be nearly perpendicular to the spine (Figure 4.28), but it is less reliable for assessing liver size in a VD/DV view than in a lateral view.

In cats, there usually is more liver on the right side than on the left. In both dogs and cats, the gall bladder is located right of midline in the cranial part of the liver.

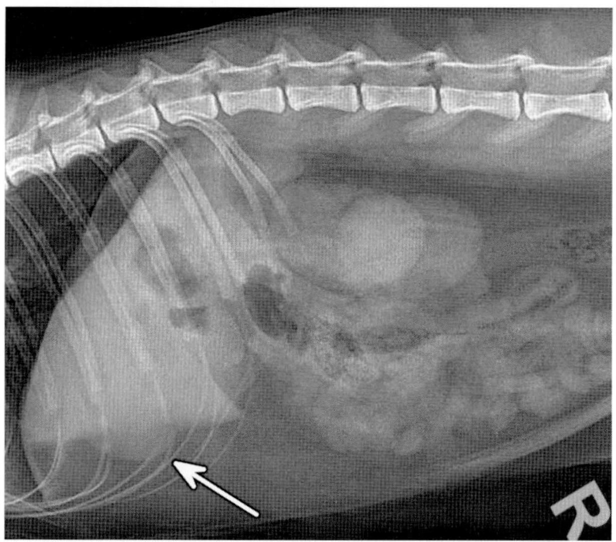

Figure 4.29 Large gall bladder. Lateral view of a cat abdomen depicting a soft tissue opacity bulge along the ventral border of the liver due to a large gall bladder (arrow).

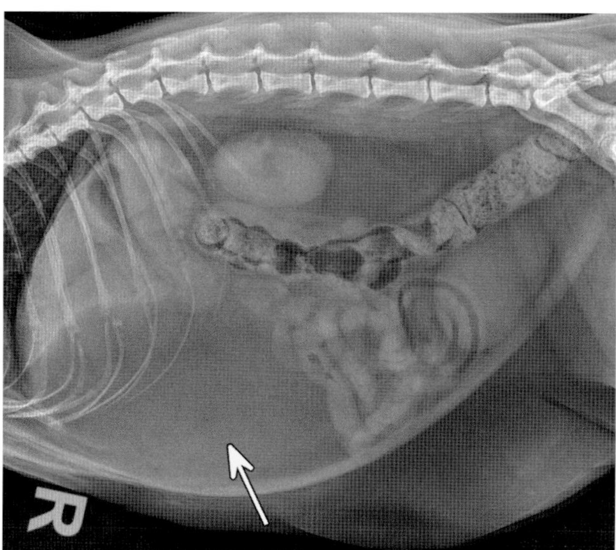

Figure 4.30 Falciform fat. Lateral view of a cat abdomen depicting a large amount of fat in the falciform ligament (arrow). The liver appears to be displaced dorsally (or perhaps the body wall is ventrally displaced).

Abnormal liver position

The liver normally lies within the costal arch. Its position can vary somewhat depending on the patient's body conformation and phase of respiration. Again, the liver tends to be positioned further cranially in deep-chested patients and more caudal in patients with a wide, shallow thorax. Displacement of the liver may be due to a mass effect or loss of abdominal integrity.

Cranial displacement of the liver most often results from a hernia or rupture of the diaphragm. This is because the cranial position of the liver is limited by an intact diaphragm. A large intra-abdominal mass can push both the liver and diaphragm cranially (e.g., distended stomach, advanced pregnancy, severe splenomegaly).

Caudal displacement usually is due to an expanded thoracic cavity (e.g., severe pleural effusion, severe pneumothorax). Weakening of the supportive ligaments along the ventral body wall can lead to a pendulous abdomen that allows the liver to move caudally. Ligaments frequently weaken and stretch in older animals and in patients with hypercortisolism.

Lateral or **ventral displacement** of the liver usually is due to loss of body wall integrity, which may result from trauma or a congenital abnormality.

Dorsal displacement is caused by a ventral mass effect. In patients with a large amount of falciform fat, the liver may appear to be dorsally displaced (Figure 4.30).

Abnormal liver size

As mentioned earlier, liver size is assessed by the shape and position of its caudoventral edge and the position of the gastric axis. Describing a liver as small often is a subjective assessment. Enlargement of the liver is recognized by the rounding of the hepatic margins, caudal extension of the liver edge and caudal displacement of the stomach. Unless the change is severe, the diagnosis of a small liver or a large liver can be difficult from radiographs. The causes and radiographic signs of each are discussed in more detail on the following pages.

Small liver (microhepatia)

In general, a liver that occupies fewer than 2 intercostal spaces is considered small (Figure 4.31). In a lateral view, the caudoventral edge of the liver does not extend to the costal arch. The gastric pylorus may be located cranial to the fundus, making the gastric axis slope from caudodorsal-to-cranioventral.

A

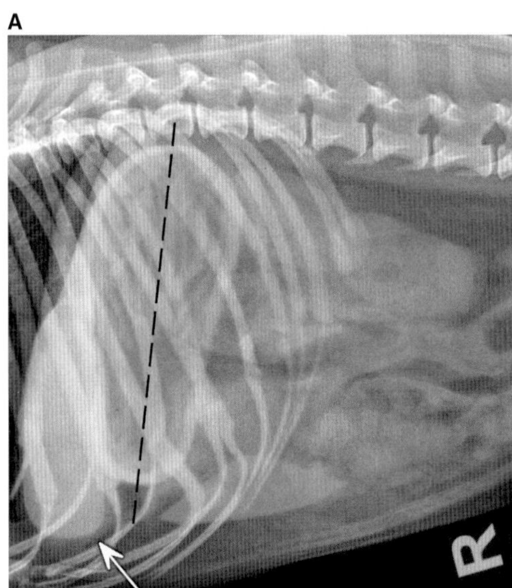

B

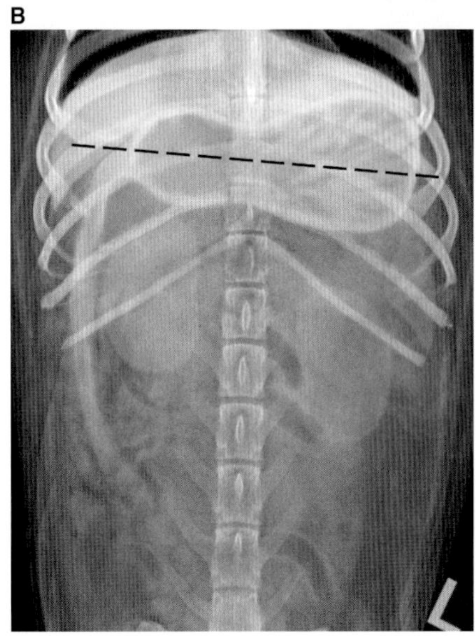

Figure 4.31 Microhepatia. Lateral view (**A**) and VD view (**B**) of a dog abdomen depicting a small liver. There are fewer than two intercostal spaces between the stomach and the diaphragm. The caudoventral edge of the liver (white arrow) does not extend to the costal arch. In the lateral view, the gastric axis slopes from caudodorsal-to-cranioventral (black dotted line).

A

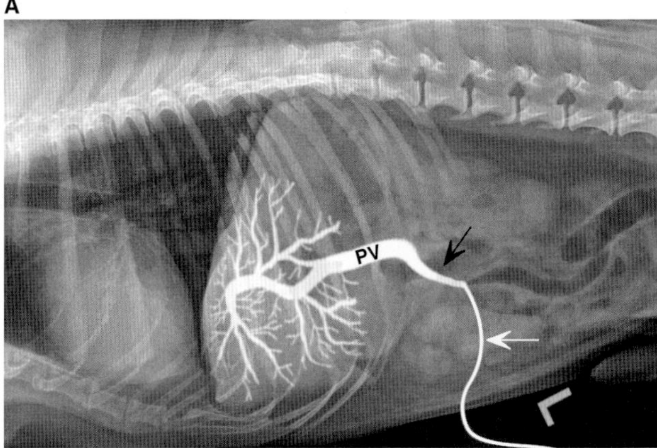

B

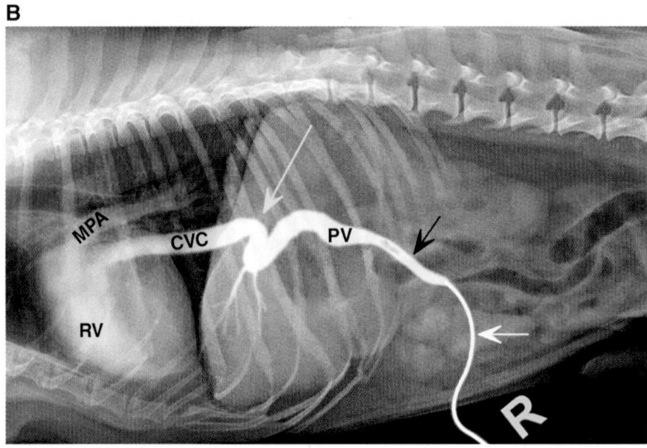

Figure 4.32 Portosystemic vascular shunt. Lateral views of a dog abdomen depicting venous portograms. **A.** Normal study: contrast medium is infused via a catheter (white arrow) that was surgically placed in a jejunal vein (black arrow). Contrast medium flows through the jejunal vein and into the portal vein (PV), which leads to opacification of multiple intra-hepatic branches. **B.** Portosystemic shunt: contrast medium flows from the portal vein directly into the caudal vena cava (CVC). The intra-hepatic shunt (yellow arrow) allows most of the contrast medium to bypass the intra-hepatic branches and enter the right ventricle (RV) and main pulmonary artery (MPA).

The most common causes of microhepatia are a portosystemic vascular shunt and hepatic cirrhosis.

A **portosystemic vascular shunt** is an abnormal communication between the portal vein and the systemic circulation. The shunt may be congenital or acquired, partial or complete, intra-hepatic or extra-hepatic. In all of these, blood from the portal system is allowed to bypass the liver. In radiographs, the liver is small, but the hepatic margins usually remain even and well-defined. The kidneys may be large to compensate for the underperforming liver.

Hepatic cirrhosis is scarring and fibrosis of the liver due to chronic inflammation. In radiographs, the liver is small with irregular margins, the latter due to nodular regeneration. Hepatic cirrhosis frequently progresses to liver failure and peritoneal effusion.

Radiographic diagnosis of microhepatia is easier when the entire liver is small and less obvious when only a portion of the liver is affected. Venous portography can be used to investigate a suspected portosystemic shunt (Figure 4.32). Hepatic vessels will be poorly opacified if there is severe shunting of blood. The procedure for venous portography, as well as its indications and contraindications, is described in the Contrast Radiography section of Chapter 2.

Large liver (hepatomegaly)

Hepatomegaly may involve part or all of the liver. Partial liver enlargement usually is due to a mass. Generalized enlargement may be due to endocrinopathy, venous congestion, inflammation, or neoplasia (see differential diagnoses).

In a lateral radiograph of a patient with generalized hepatomegaly, the caudoventral edge of the liver is rounded and extends a significant distance caudal to the costal arch (Figures 4.33 and 4.34). The stomach is displaced caudally

A

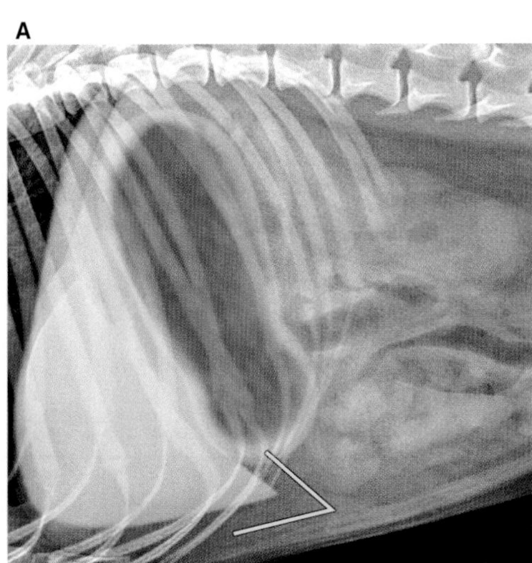

B

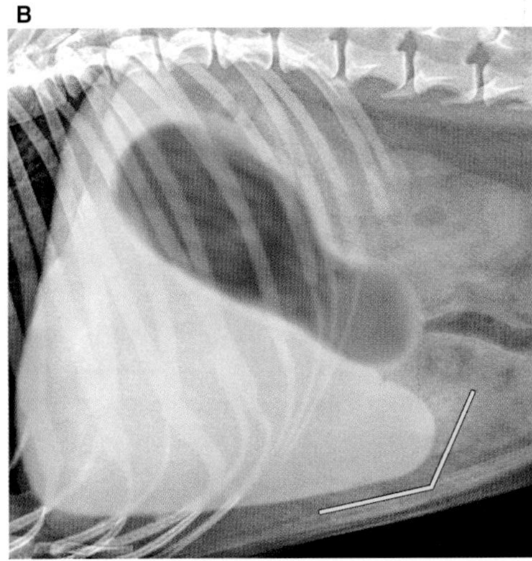

Figure 4.33 Rounding of liver margins. Lateral views of a dog abdomen depicting a normal size liver (**A**) and an enlarged liver (**B**). The caudoventral edge of the normal liver forms an acute angle (less than 90°) near the costal arch. Hepatomegaly causes rounding of the caudoventral edge and extends the edge caudal to the costal arch.

A

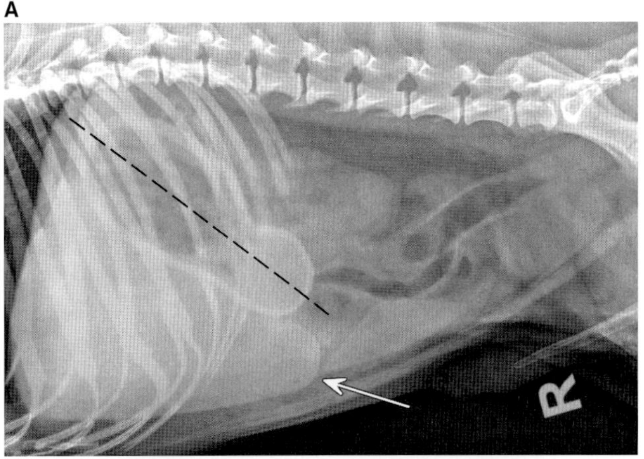

B

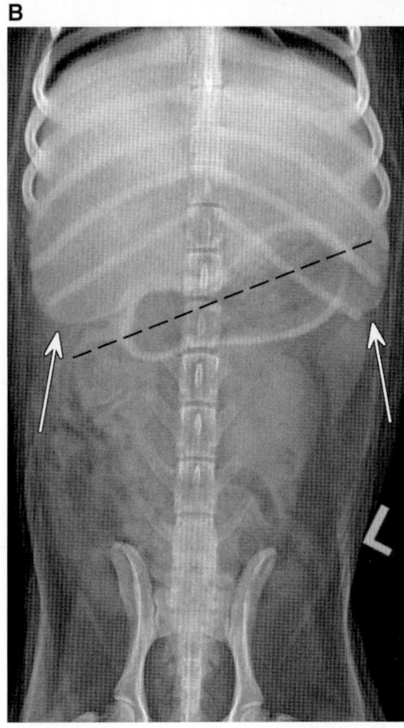

Figure 4.34 Hepatomegaly. Lateral view (**A**) and VD view (**B**) of a dog abdomen depicting generalized liver enlargement. The borders of the liver are rounded (arrows). In the lateral view, the caudal edge of the liver extends significantly caudal to the costal arch. The stomach is displaced caudally and dorsally. The gastric pylorus is caudal to the fundus, altering the slope of the gastric axis (black dotted line).

and dorsally, producing a more craniodorsal-to-caudoventral slope to the gastric axis. The severity of stomach displacement depends on the degree of liver enlargement. Severe hepatomegaly can also push the proximal duodenum, right kidney, and transverse colon further caudally and may limit movement of the diaphragm.

Generalized hepatomegaly often is accompanied by a distended abdomen, either due to the large size of the liver, a weak body wall, enlargement of other viscera, or peritoneal effusion. Venous congestion and infiltrative diseases such as lymphoma frequently lead to enlargement of multiple organs and varying amounts of peritoneal effusion.

Liver mass

Masses growing in or on the liver generally lead to asymmetric hepatomegaly and an abnormal liver shape. The adjacent viscera may be unevenly displaced, depending on the size and location of the mass (Figure 4.35). A left liver mass can displace the gastric fundus caudally and medially, sometimes pushing the fundus caudal to the pylorus. The head of the spleen and the intestines may be pushed caudally. Right liver enlargement can displace the gastric pylorus, proximal duodenum, and right kidney caudally and medially.

A

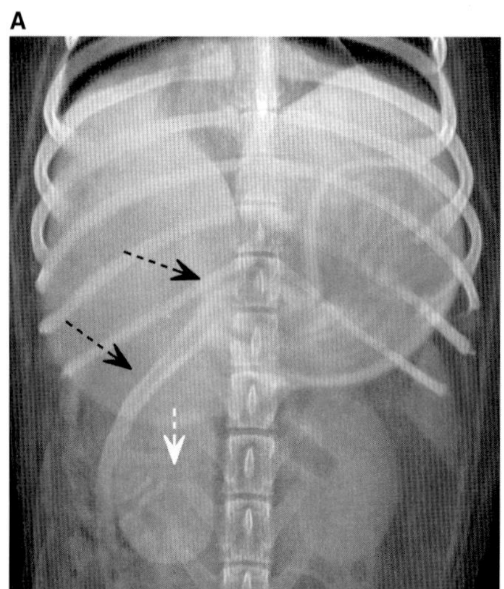

B

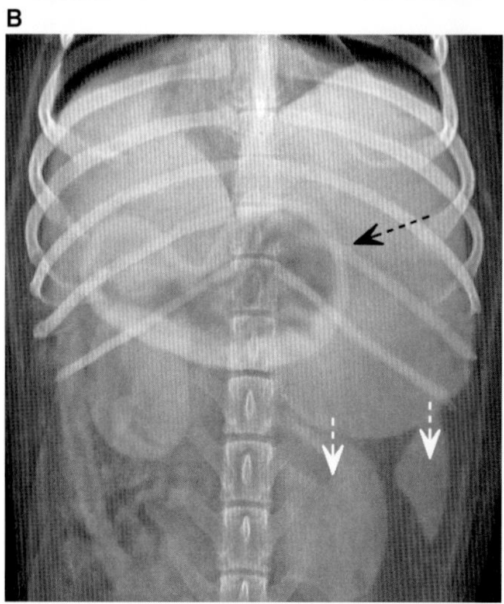

Figure 4.35 Liver mass. Two VD views of a dog abdomen depicting asymmetric liver enlargement. Where the liver is enlarged, its margin is rounded. **A**. A mass in the right side of the liver displaces the gastric pylorus and duodenum caudally and to the left (black dotted arrows). The duodenum is highlighted for demonstration purposes. The right kidney is displaced caudally (white dotted arrow). **B**. Left liver enlargement displaces the gastric fundus to the right and caudally (black dotted arrow) and pushes the spleen and left kidney caudally (white arrows).

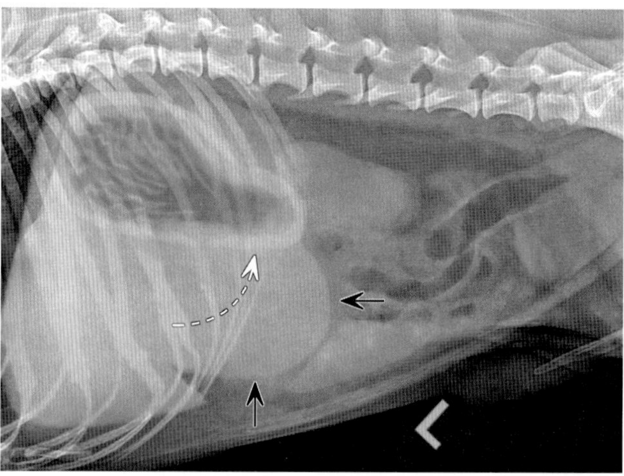

Figure 4.36 Central liver mass. Lateral view of a dog abdomen depicting a soft tissue opacity mass in the cranioventral abdomen (black arrows). The mass displaces the gastric pylorus caudally and dorsally (white dotted arrow) and pushes the intestines caudally. A mass in this area may be associated with the liver, stomach, spleen, or pancreas.

A centrally located liver mass may displace the gastric pylorus caudally and dorsally (Figure 4.36). A central hepatic mass can extend caudal to the stomach, particularly if it is pedunculated, and may appear separate from the liver. In these cases, the liver mass may be misdiagnosed as part of the spleen or other nearby structure.

In addition to mistaking a hepatic mass for part of the spleen, the spleen may be mistaken for part of the liver. In a lateral view the tail of the spleen sometimes blends with the caudoventral edge of the liver, mimicking a large liver. In these cases the opposite lateral view often allows the liver and spleen to be distinguished as separate structures.

A large gall bladder may produce an intra-hepatic mass effect. As mentioned earlier, gall bladder distention may produce a swelling or bulge along the ventral liver border in a lateral view (Figure 4.29).

Abnormal liver opacity

The normal liver is uniform soft tissue opacity. Mineral or gas opacity in the liver is abnormal and frequently involves the biliary system. Occasionally, dystrophic mineralization or a gas-producing bacterial infection occurs in a long-standing hepatic tumor or abscess, or in an area of liver necrosis (e.g., liver lobe torsion). Gas also can enter the liver parenchyma from the GI tract via the portal system, which may occur due to a necrotic stomach (e.g., gastric dilatation and volvulus). Abnormal opacity in the liver parenchyma typically appears as an irregular or mottled pattern localized in part of the liver.

Abnormal opacity in the gall bladder is seen in the right cranioventral part of the liver. An **emphysematous gall bladder** most often is associated with diabetes mellitus. Gas initially forms in the bladder wall and eventually fills the lumen to produce multiple tiny bubbles that conform to the shape of the gall bladder (Figure 4.37). Emphysema can extend into the bile ducts to create a tree-like pattern of gas opacity, similar in appearance to air bronchograms in consolidated lungs.

Mineral opacity in the gall bladder or bile ducts may represent cholelithiasis or dystrophic mineralization. **Choleliths** (gallstones) can vary greatly in size, number, and opacity (Figure 4.38). They may or may not be clinically significant.

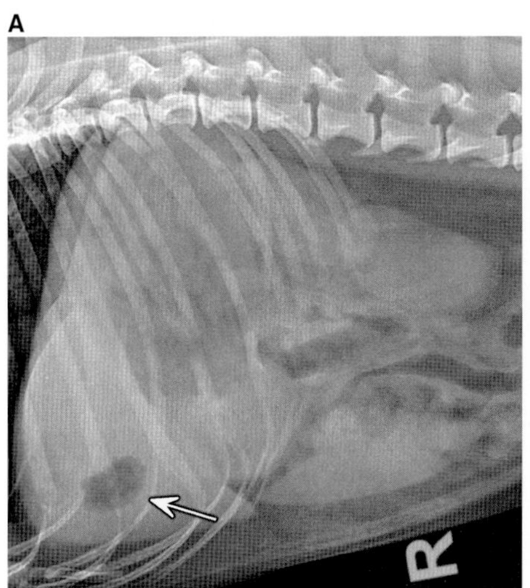

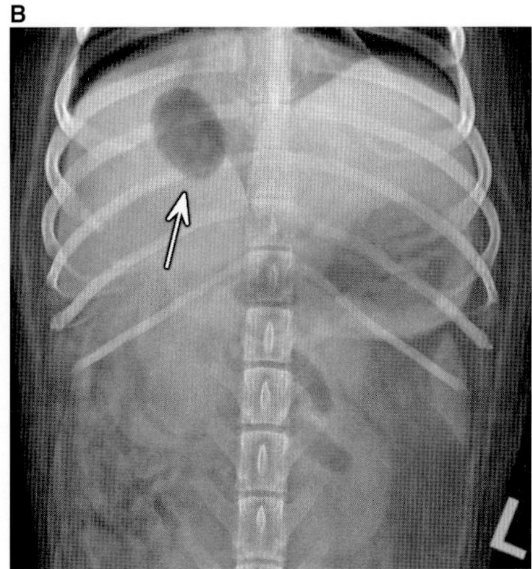

Figure 4.37 Emphysematous gall bladder. Lateral view (**A**) and VD view (**B**) of a dog abdomen depicting localized gas opacity in the right cranioventral part of the liver (arrow). The gas is in the shape and location of the gall bladder.

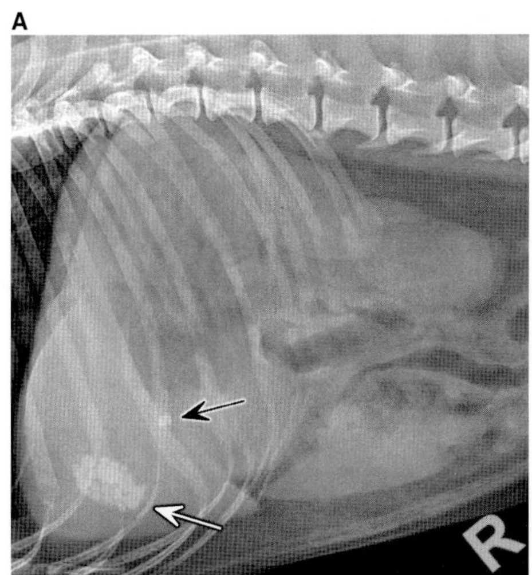

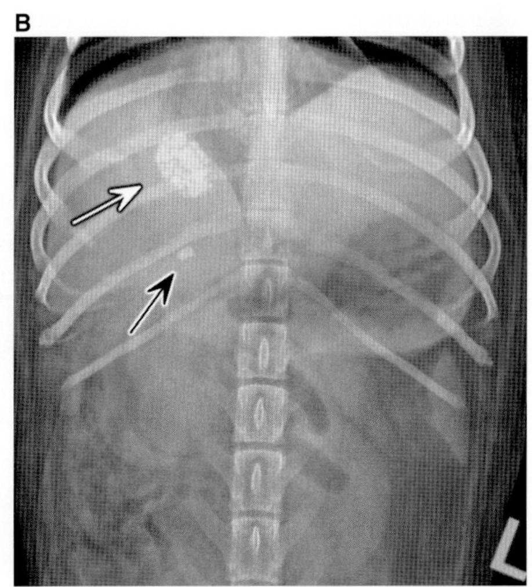

Figure 4.38 Cholelithiasis. Lateral view (**A**) and VD view (**B**) of a dog abdomen depicting multiple, small, mineral opacity structures in the shape and location of the gall bladder (white arrow). There also is a focal mineral opacity located between the gall bladder and the duodenum, consistent with a choledocolith (black arrow).

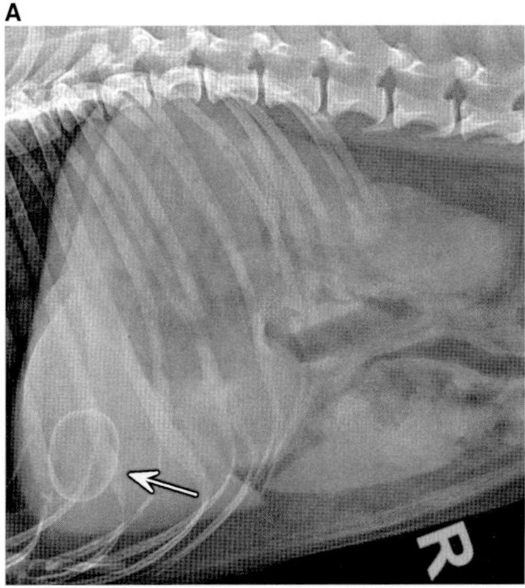

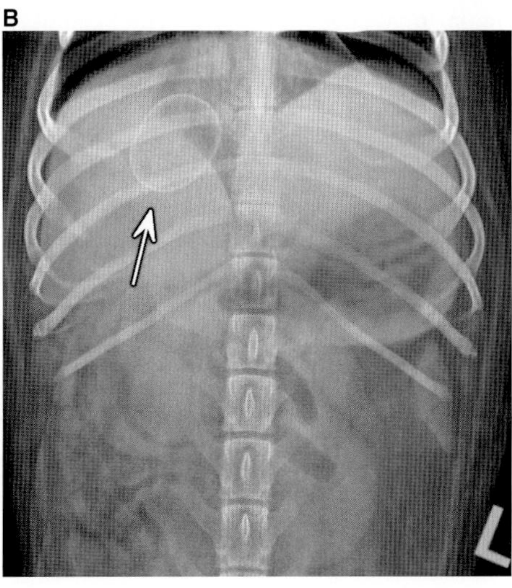

Figure 4.39 Mineralization of the gall bladder wall. Lateral view (**A**) and VD view (**B**) of a dog abdomen depicting a thin, shell-like, mineral opacity structure in the area of the gall bladder (arrow); sometimes called a "porcelain" gall bladder.

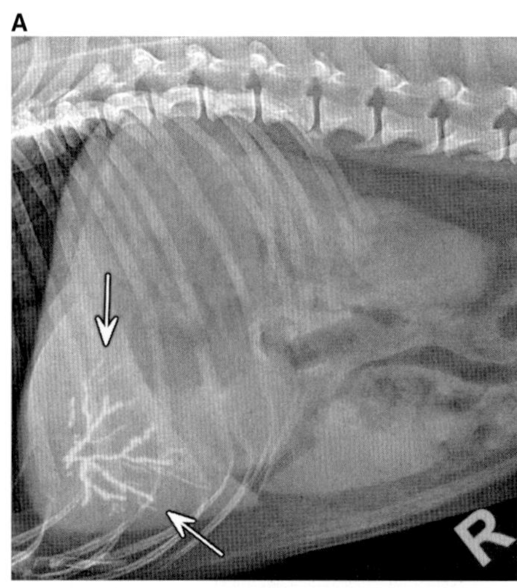

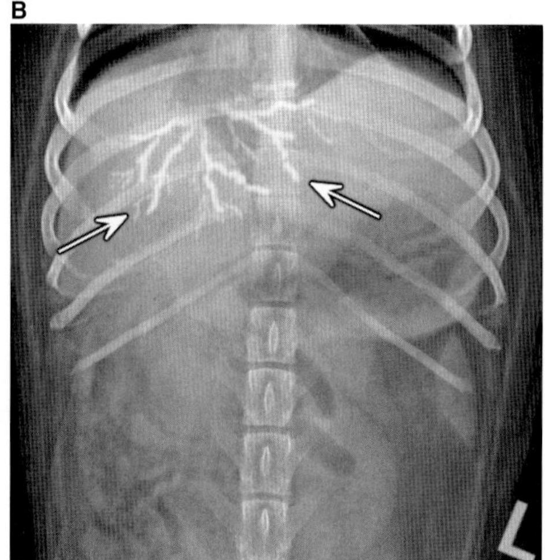

Figure 4.40 Bile duct mineralization. Lateral view (**A**) and VD view (**B**) of a dog abdomen depicting a branching pattern of heterogeneous mineral opacity structures in the liver (arrows), typical of biliary mineralization.

Not all gallstones are mineral opacity. When in the common bile duct, mineral opacity calculi are called *choledocoliths* and may be visible between the gall bladder and the duodenum (Figure 4.38). **Mineralization** of the gall bladder wall typically appears as a thin, well-defined, shell-like structure (Figure 4.39). Mineralization in the bile ducts appears as a linear or branching pattern in either an isolated part of the liver or scattered throughout the liver (Figure 4.40).

Spleen

Normal radiographic anatomy

The spleen is a relatively flat and elongated organ with even, well-defined margins. The edges of the spleen form acute angles (less than 90°). Because it is thin, the spleen often is difficult to identify in radiographs except where it overlaps or "folds" on itself. In these areas the spleen is essentially doubled in thickness and opacity. The two layers of spleen summate to create a triangular or wedge-shaped appearance (Figure 4.41). Seeing a splenic triangle in a radiograph does not mean you have identified the entire spleen; rather, you have found the starting point to begin examining the spleen.

For descriptive purposes, the spleen is divided into three parts; *head*, *body*, and *tail*. The head is the proximal part of the spleen that is anchored to the fundus of the stomach by the *gastrosplenic ligament*. The body of the spleen is the middle part. The tail of the spleen is the distal part. Both the body and tail of the spleen are freely moveable. In dogs, the body and tail can vary considerably in size and position. In cats, they are more constant and proportionately smaller than in dogs.

Spleen in a lateral view

The head of the spleen is located in the craniodorsal abdomen. Overlap of the head and body of the spleen creates a soft tissue opacity triangle between the fundus of the stomach and the kidneys (Figure 4.41). This triangle commonly is called the "head of the spleen," but it represents only a portion of the proximal spleen. The triangle sometimes is difficult to identify in a lateral view because it blends with the adjacent soft tissues. In cats and overweight dogs the triangle may be more distinct because it is surrounded by fat.

The body and tail of the spleen can extend anywhere from the liver to the urinary bladder. Overlap of body and tail often creates a soft tissue opacity triangle in the ventral abdomen, particularly in a right lateral view. The distal spleen is easiest to see when it is positioned near the ventral body wall, which is common in dogs but rare in cats. In many cats, the normal spleen is not identified in a lateral view.

Spleen in a VD/DV view

The head of the spleen is located in the left cranial abdomen. Again, overlap with the body of the spleen produces the familiar soft tissue opacity triangle near the left body wall, located just caudal to the gastric fundus and cranial to the left kidney (Figure 4.41). As we discussed with the lateral view, this triangular-shaped overlap is not the "head of the spleen"; rather, it is a starting point from which to begin evaluating the spleen.

The distal spleen can extend either caudally along the left body wall or toward the mid-abdomen. Its margin tends to be difficult to trace in a VD/DV view because the other viscera are superimposed. With careful inspection, however, the entire spleen often can be identified.

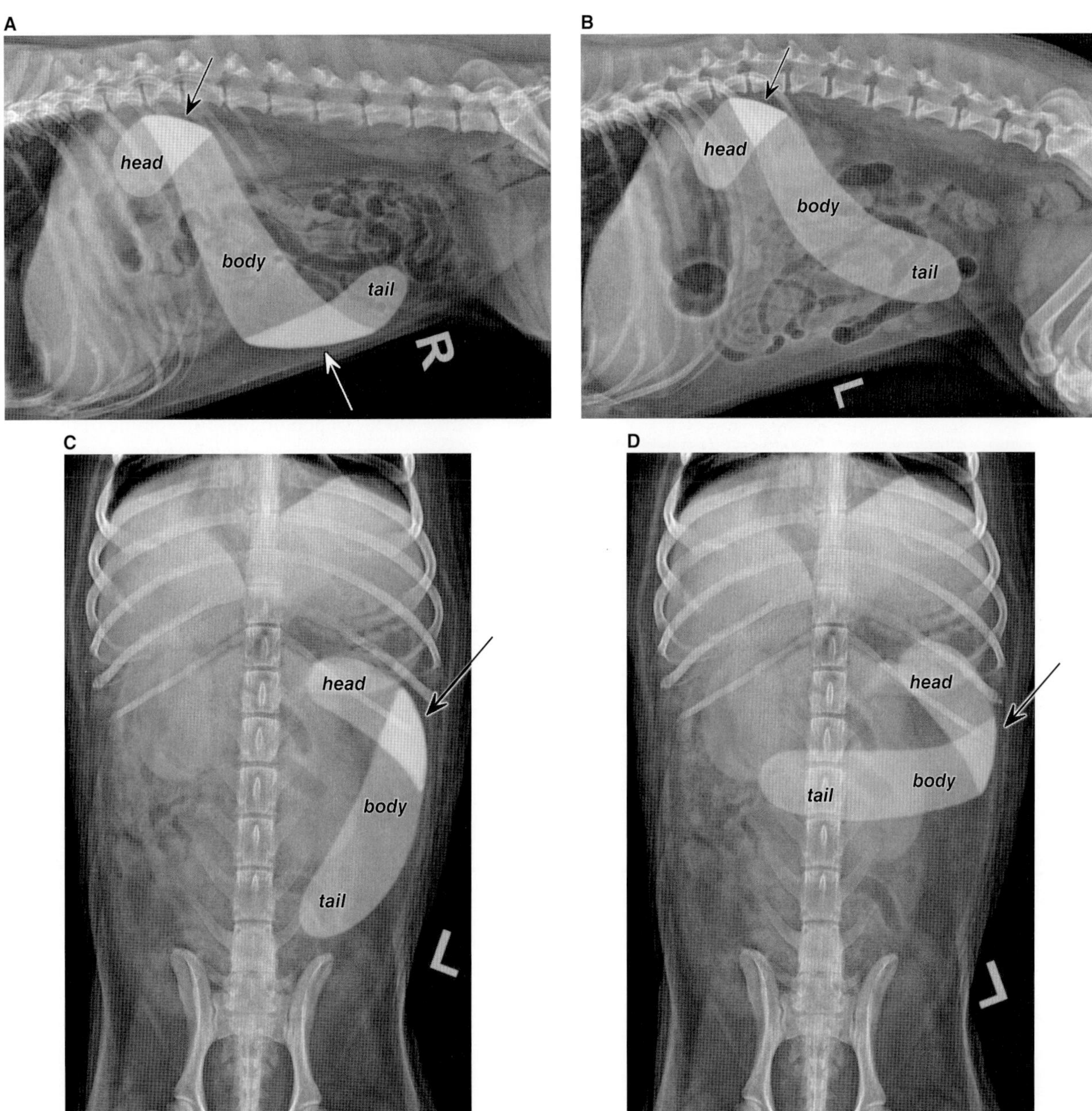

Figure 4.41 Normal spleen. Right lateral view (**A**), left lateral view (**B**), and VD views (**C** and **D**) of a dog abdomen illustrating some of the normal positions of the spleen. Overlap of the head and body of the spleen produces a wedge-shaped soft tissue opacity structure in the left craniodorsal abdomen (black arrow). Overlap of the body and tail can create a similar wedge shape in the ventral abdomen (white arrow).

Abnormal spleen position

Non-visualization of the spleen may be due its absence (e.g., prior splenectomy) or because it is obscured. The spleen may be obscured because it is small and blends with other soft tissue structures or because there is no opacity interface (e.g., visceral crowding, loss of body fat, adjacent fluid accumulation).

Displacement of the spleen can occur in a variety of directions. The body and tail of the spleen are quite mobile and readily displaced by nearby structures or loss of body wall integrity. The position of the head of the spleen is largely determined by the size and orientation of the stomach because the two are connected by the gastrosplenic ligament. In a deep-chested dog with an empty stomach, the proximal spleen may lie near the diaphragm. Gastric dilatation with volvulus or a splenic torsion can displace the proximal spleen so that it is absent from its expected position in the craniodorsal abdomen.

Abnormal spleen size and shape

Unless it is very large, describing the size of the spleen tends to be a subjective assessment. Splenomegaly frequently is over-diagnosed, especially when a long portion of the spleen is visible or the tail of the spleen extends further caudally than expected. The normal spleen is relatively large in certain dog breeds (e.g., German Shepherd, Greyhound). The key radiographic finding with **splenomegaly**, as with hepatomegaly, is rounding of the margins (Figure 4.42).

Splenic enlargement may be generalized or localized. There are numerous causes of generalized splenomegaly (see differential diagnoses). A large spleen may displace the intestines dorsally, caudally, and either to the right or left side. Irregular or uneven splenic borders suggest multiple nodules or masses in the spleen.

A

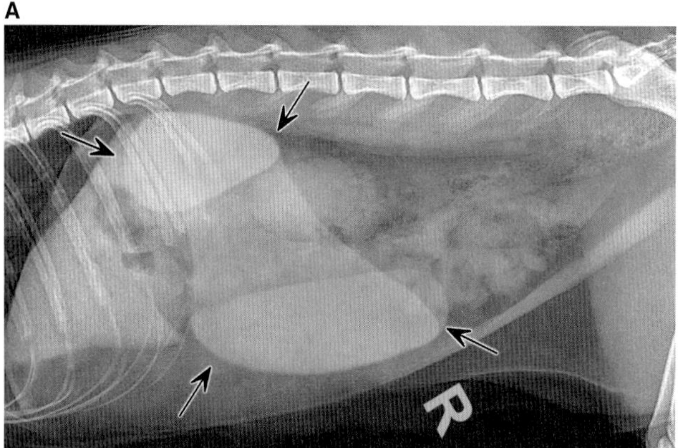

B

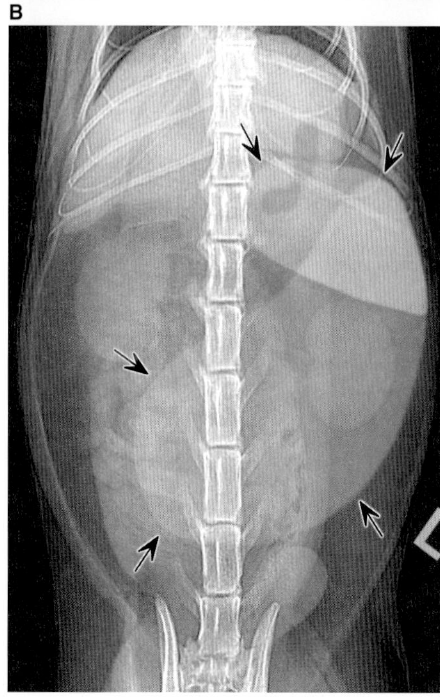

Figure 4.42 Splenomegaly. Lateral view (**A**) and VD view (**B**) of a cat abdomen depicting generalized enlargement of the spleen (arrows). The margins of the spleen are rounded. The small intestine is displaced caudally and to the right.

Localized splenomegaly is due to a **splenic mass**. A mass in the proximal spleen typically produces increased opacity in the left craniodorsal abdomen and causes rounding of the splenic triangle. Larger masses can deform or medially displace the gastric fundus and push the left kidney caudally. Masses in the body and tail of the spleen are much more variable in position. They are seen most often in the ventral mid-abdomen (Figure 4.43).

Peritoneal effusion is a frequent finding with both benign and malignant causes of splenic enlargement. The type of fluid cannot be determined from radiographs, but often it is non-clotting blood. Depending on the volume of fluid, peritoneal serosal margins may be obscured. Repeating the radiographs after removing as much fluid as possible may yield additional diagnostic information.

It often is difficult to determine from radiographs whether a mass in the area of the spleen actually involves the spleen. Masses in the left craniodorsal abdomen, for example, may originate in the left kidney or adrenal gland. Masses in the mid-abdomen may originate from the mesentery, lymph node, or intestine.

A **smaller than expected spleen** may be due to hypovolemia or atrophy, the latter reported most often in aged animals. The feline spleen tends to be proportionately smaller than the canine spleen, but not always. It has been suggested that a feline spleen that is visible in a lateral radiograph must be enlarged; however, just because it is visible does not necessarily mean that the spleen is abnormally large.

Splenic torsion

Rotation of the spleen around its mesenteric axis often is associated with gastric dilatation and volvulus, but may occur independently. Splenic torsion is a rare but potentially life-threatening condition, most often reported in large, deep-chested dogs. Rotation restricts splenic blood flow leading to venous congestion, ischemia, and moderate to severe splenomegaly. The classic radiographic finding is a caudally and medially displaced spleen with a reverse C-shaped appearance (Figure 4.44). This finding, however, may not be apparent unless the spleen is significantly enlarged. In most cases of splenic torsion, the proximal spleen is absent from its expected position in the left craniodorsal abdomen. Pockets of gas sometimes are visible in a rotated spleen due to secondary infection with gas-producing bacteria (Figure 4.45).

Abnormal spleen opacity

The normal spleen is homogenous soft tissue opacity. Gas or mineral opacity in the spleen is abnormal and may be focal or multifocal. Gas in the spleen (splenic emphysema) is rare, most often associated with splenic torsion and a secondary gas-producing bacterial infection (Figure 4.45). **Splenic emphysema** typically appears as a patchy, mottled, or "foamy" gas pattern. Gas in a splenic blood vessel may produce an "air vasculogram," similar in appearance to an air bronchogram in consolidated lungs.

Mineralization in the spleen usually is dystrophic and may result from chronic inflammation or infection. Neoplastic mineralization can occur (e.g., extra-skeletal osteosarcoma).

A

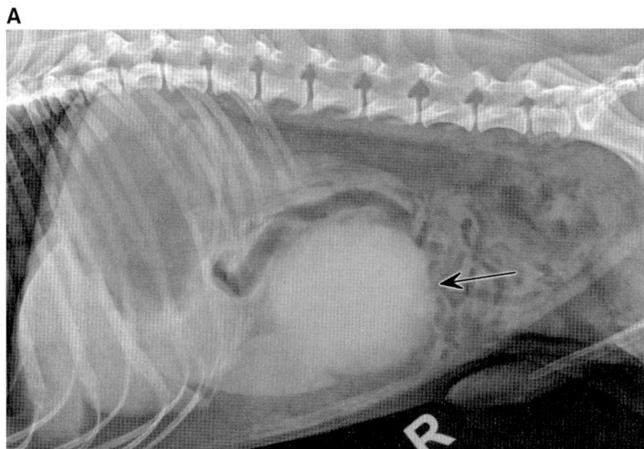

B

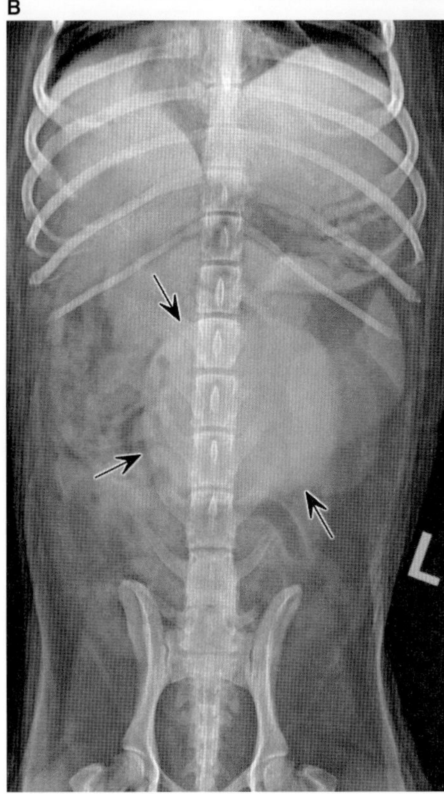

Figure 4.43 Splenic mass. Lateral view (**A**) and VD view (**B**) of a dog abdomen depicting a rounded, soft tissue opacity mass in the ventral mid-abdomen (arrows). The adjacent bowel is displaced caudally, dorsally, and to the right. The mass may originate from spleen, mesentery, lymph node, or intestine.

A

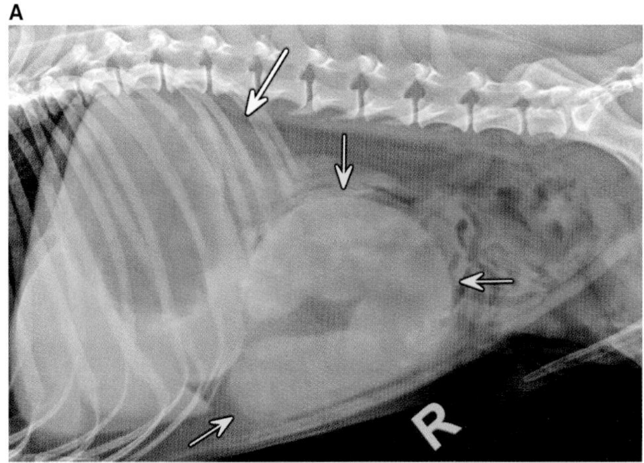

B

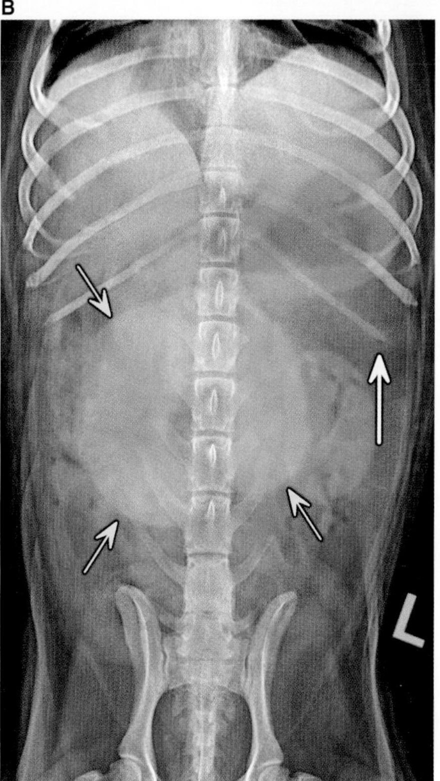

Figures 4.44 Splenic torsion. Lateral view (**A**) and VD view (**B**) of a dog abdomen depicting an enlarged spleen that is displaced medially and caudally (yellow arrows). The shape of the spleen resembles a reverse capital letter C. The splenic triangle is absent from its normal location in the left craniodorsal abdomen (white arrow).

Pancreas

Normal radiographic anatomy

The pancreas is divided into three parts; *right limb, left limb,* and *body*. The body is the part between the two limbs and it is located in the right cranial abdomen near the gastroduodenal angle (Figure 4.46). The gastroduodenal angle

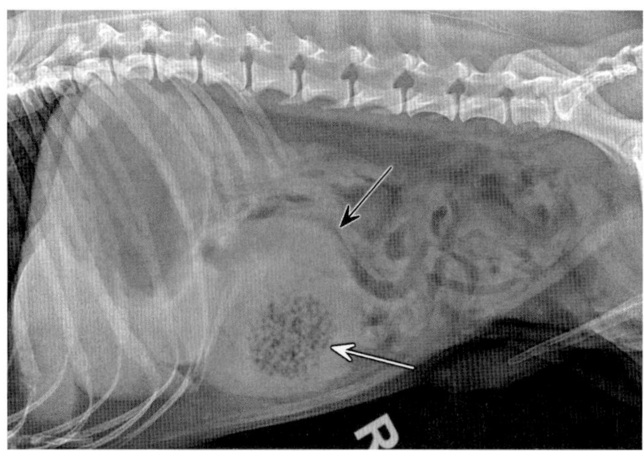

Figure 4.45 Splenic emphysema. Lateral view of a dog abdomen depicting a soft tissue opacity mass in the cranioventral abdomen (black arrow) with multiple foci of gas opacity (white arrow). Gas most likely is due to gas-producing bacteria. The mass may represent a splenic torsion or an abscess associated with the spleen, liver, pancreas, intestine, or mesentery.

refers to the junction between the stomach and the duodenum.

The right limb of the pancreas extends caudally from the body of the pancreas to about the level of the L3-4 vertebrae. It is positioned between the descending duodenum and the ascending colon. The left pancreatic limb extends transversely from the body, across midline, and toward the left kidney. It is positioned between the greater curvature of the stomach and the transverse colon.

The normal pancreas seldom is seen in radiographs due to its small size and similar opacity to the adjacent tissues. When surrounded by fat, the left pancreatic limb may be visible in a VD/DV view, particularly in cats (Figure 4.47). In these cases it appears as a thin, linear, soft tissue opacity structure within a triangle formed by the stomach, spleen, and left kidney.

Pancreatic disease

Diseases of the pancreas may or may not be evident in radiographs. Characteristic findings of pancreatic disease include increased opacity, indistinct serosal margins, and a mass effect in the area of the pancreas (Figure 4.48). These findings may be present near the gastroduodenal angle or along the descending duodenum or caudal to the stomach. Note: when examining these areas, use caution when interpreting subtle increases in opacity and mildly indistinct margins. In a VD view of many patients there is less fat and more visceral crowding in the right cranial abdomen than in the left cranial abdomen.

A mass effect in the area of the pancreas may be caused by pancreatic swelling or a pancreatic mass (e.g., tumor, cyst, abscess). Both pancreatitis and pancreatic neoplasia produce similar radiographic signs and cannot reliably be differentiated.

In a VD view, a pancreatic mass effect may displace the duodenum to the right and widen the gastroduodenal angle. The transverse colon may be displaced caudally, resulting in increased distance from the stomach. In a lateral view, the duodenum may be displaced either ventrally or dorsally.

A

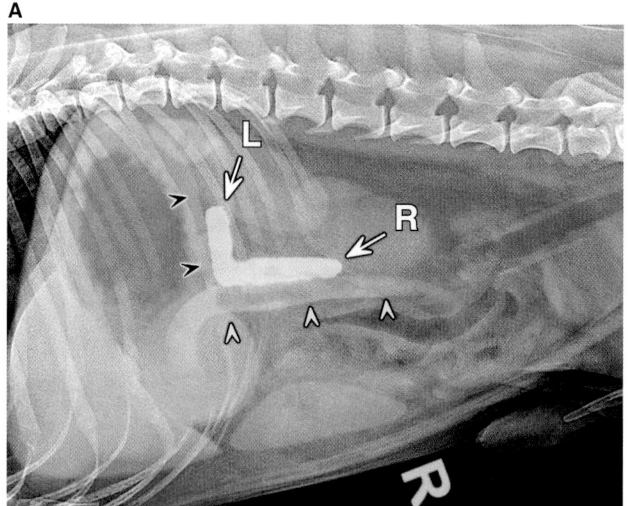

B

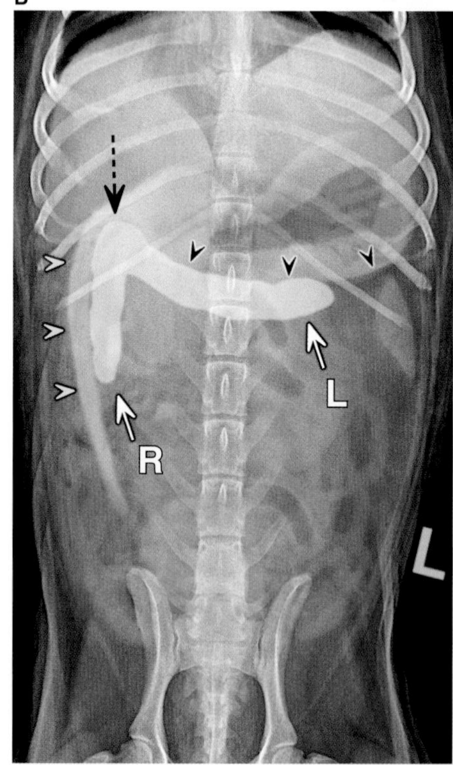

Figure 4.46 Pancreas. Lateral view (**A**) and VD view (**B**) of a dog abdomen with the area of the pancreas highlighted. The body of the pancreas lies in the gastroduodenal angle (black dotted arrow). The right pancreatic limb (R) lies adjacent to the descending duodenum (yellow arrowheads). The left pancreatic limb (L) lies adjacent to the greater curvature of the stomach (black arrowheads).

Pancreatic diseases can cause a regional peritonitis that diminishes peristalsis in the nearby intestines. Regional inflammation near the descending duodenum or transverse colon may lead to a localized functional ileus known as a sentinel loop. A **sentinel loop** is a static segment of bowel, often recognized in radiographs by its static gas pattern that remains relatively unchanged in serial radiographs. The segment appears similar in size, shape, and content between images. Sentinel loops do not only occur with pancreatitis; any site of peritoneal inflammation can lead to a functional ileus.

Pancreatic disease can progress to a more diffuse peritonitis and peritoneal effusion, further obscuring serosal margins. Pancreatic adenocarcinoma can metastasize throughout the peritoneal space to produce a diffuse, mottled, hazy pattern (i.e., carcinomatosis).

Severe pancreatic disease may cause a gastric outflow problem and persistent distention of the stomach. It can also lead to hepatitis and hepatic lipidosis. Pancreatic mineralization is rare but may result from chronic inflammation or fat necrosis.

Normal radiographs do not rule out pancreatic disease. Follow-up radiographs or other imaging modalities may be needed in patients that do not respond to appropriate therapy.

Signs of pancreatic disease sometimes are evident in an Upper GI study. Radiographic signs may include a duodenal sentinel loop, delayed gastric emptying, delayed transit through the intestines, or thickening of the duodenal or gastric wall.

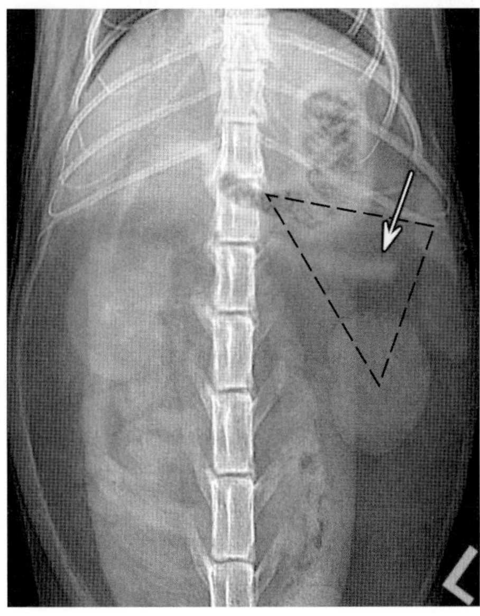

Figure 4.47 Normal pancreas. VD view of a cat abdomen depicting the left limb of the pancreas (arrow). The left limb is visible within the triangle formed by the stomach, spleen, and left kidney because it is surrounded by fat.

A

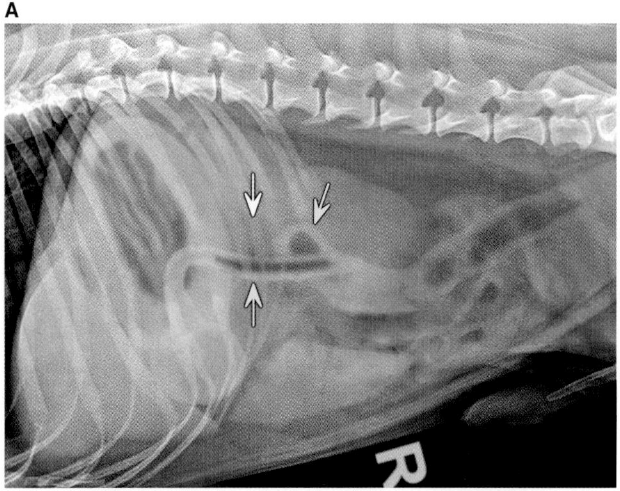

B

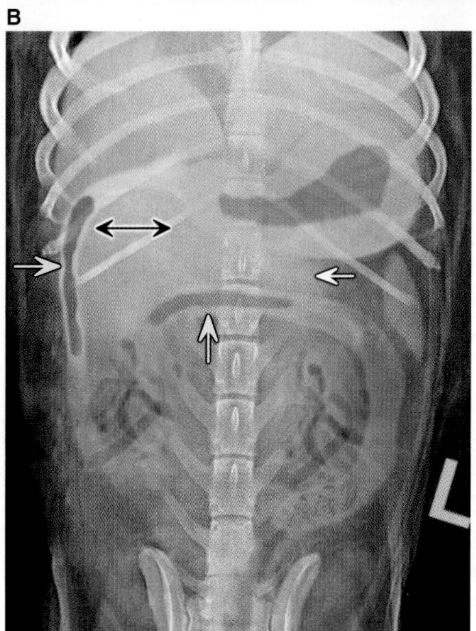

Figure 4.48 Pancreatic disease. Lateral view (**A**) and VD view (**B**) of a dog abdomen depicting increased opacity and indistinct serosal margins in the area of the pancreas. The gastroduodenal angle is widened (black double-headed arrow); there is soft tissue swelling between the greater curvature of the stomach and the transverse colon (white arrow), and there are static gas patterns (sentinel loops) in the descending duodenum and transverse colon (yellow arrows).

Gastrointestinal tract

The GI tract includes the stomach, small intestine, and large intestine. The esophagus is part of the alimentary tract and is discussed in Chapter 3: Thorax.

Normal GI structures are continuously in motion. A radiograph depicts their appearance only at a single instant in time. Multiple views, serial radiographs, and contrast radiography may be needed to detect or confirm lesions. Many GI diseases present with similar signs and any particular disorder can vary significantly in its radiographic appearance. Most GI findings are not pathognomonic for any specific condition. Some diseases of the GI tract rarely produce detectable radiographic abnormalities (e.g., parasitic diseases, dietary problems, GI inflammation).

Radiography generally is a readily available diagnostic imaging modality and can provide information about the GI tract relatively rapidly. Other modalities, however, may be needed for a more definitive diagnosis, including endoscopy, ultrasonography, and computed tomography.

Stomach

Normal radiographic anatomy

The stomach is located caudal to the diaphragm and liver. Its caudal border is convex and called the *greater curvature*. Its cranial border is concave and called the *lesser curvature* (Figure 4.49). For descriptive purposes, the stomach is divided into four parts: *cardia, fundus, body,* and *pylorus*.

The **cardia** is the small area of the stomach that joins the esophagus. It is not radiographically distinct from the fundus.

The **fundus** is the dome-shaped pouch that comprises the dorsal and left lateral portions of the stomach. It stores undigested food and gas.

The **body** of the stomach is the large distensible part located between the fundus and the pylorus.

The **pylorus** forms the distal third of the stomach. It consists of the *pyloric antrum* (the area before the gastric outlet), the *pyloric canal* (the passage that connects the stomach to the duodenum), and the *pyloric sphincter* (a thick muscular ring that helps regulate outflow from the stomach). In most adult dogs, the pylorus is positioned ventral to the fundus and to the right of midline. In cats, puppies, and barrel-chested dogs, the pylorus tends to be closer to midline. The closer the pylorus is to midline, the more U-shaped or J-shaped the stomach appears in a VD/DV view (Figure 4.50).

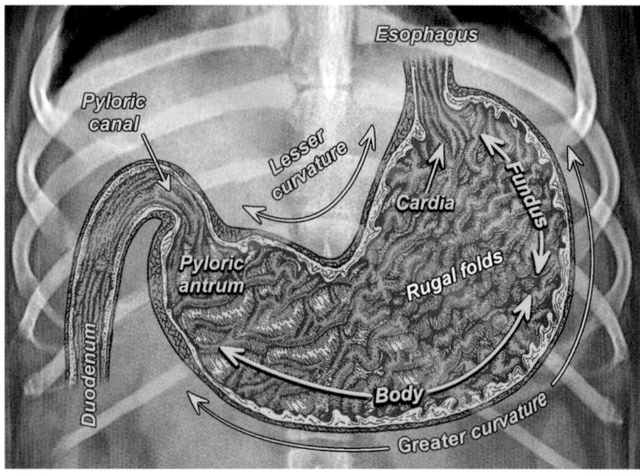

Figure 4.49 Anatomy of the stomach. VD view of a dog abdomen illustrating the parts of the stomach and the rugal folds.

A

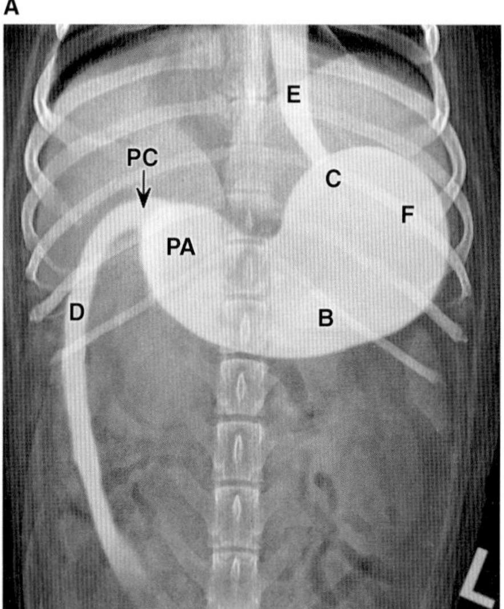

B

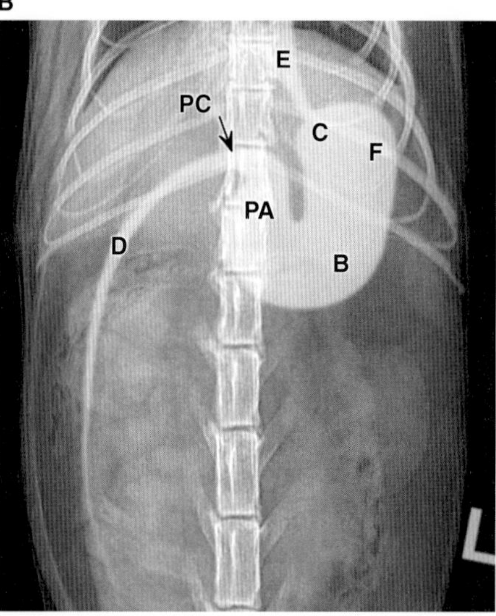

Figure 4.50 Normal stomach. VD views of a dog abdomen (**A**) and a cat abdomen (**B**) with the stomach highlighted to show the relative positions of the esophagus (E), cardia (C), fundus (F), body (B), pyloric antrum (PA), pyloric canal (PC), and duodenum (D).

The size, shape, position, and opacity of the stomach can vary significantly depending on its contents. An empty stomach generally lies within the costal arch, rarely extending caudal to the last pair of ribs. As the stomach fills, the fundus and body expand and the greater curvature becomes more convex. Filling increases the length and diameter of the pylorus and moves it further to the right. In a lateral view, a full stomach may touch the ventral body wall and extend caudally to the level of the umbilicus.

The stomach is able to expand because the gastric mucosa is formed into folds called *rugae*. The **rugal folds** generally are larger and more numerous in dogs than in cats and often more visible in the fundic region (Figure 4.49). Rugal folds can vary significantly in appearance and their radiographic interpretation requires experience and excellent visualization of the gastric mucosa. In general, each fold should be similar in height and width (thickness) to the width of the spaces between folds.

The mucosal margin of the stomach rarely is identified with certainty in survey radiographs, because fluid and most ingesta are the same opacity as the mucosa, contrast radiography is usually needed. Prior to performing gastrography, however, always make **four view survey radiographs of the stomach**: right lateral, left lateral, VD, and DV. In many cases, these four views will redistribute gas and fluid in the stomach lumen and will help clarify questionable findings. Four views are also important during gastrography to allow different parts of the stomach to fill with contrast medium. This is particularly useful when searching for mural lesions and identifying the different parts of the stomach.

In some animals, especially overweight cats, a submucosal layer of fat may be visible in the stomach wall. Submucosal fat appears as a thin line of fat opacity that follows the curvature of the stomach (Figure 4.51). The fat layer may be mistaken for gas in the stomach wall.

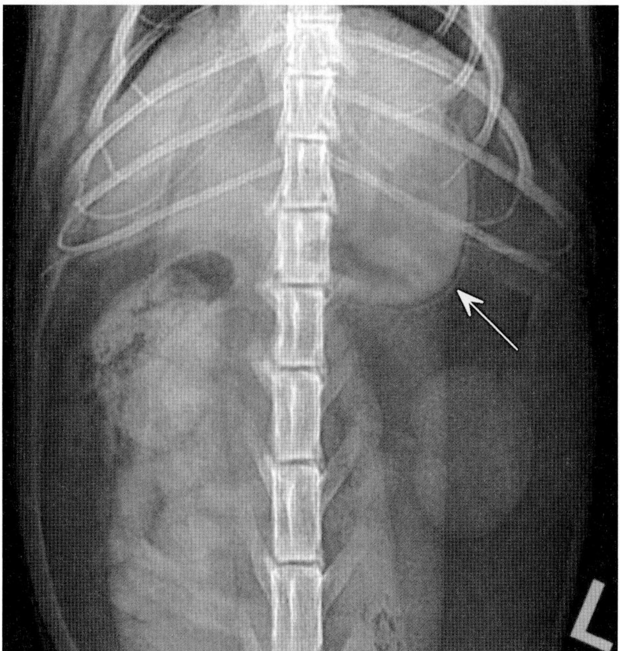

Figure 4.51 Gastric submucosal fat. VD view of a cat abdomen depicting a thin line of submucosal gastric fat (arrow).

Gas and fluid in the stomach

In most patients, the stomach contains some gas or food, making its identification relatively simple. The distribution of material in the stomach varies with its volume and the position of the patient at the time of radiography. Gas generally rises to the highest parts of the stomach and fluid flows with gravity into the dependent parts. Deliberately changing the position of the patient is useful to redistribute gas, fluid, and contrast media in the stomach. In situations where there is only a small volume of material in the stomach, the patient should be rotated a full 180° for a few seconds and then back to the position desired to ensure the gas or fluid moves to a different part of the stomach.

Figures 4.52–4.55 illustrate the distribution of fluid and gas in the stomach based on the position of the patient. Each figure includes both a radiograph and a cross-sectional CT image to help describe the appearance of the stomach in right lateral, left lateral, dorsal and ventral recumbencies. Table 4.1 summarizes the distribution of gas and fluid in different parts of the stomach.

Abnormal stomach position

The normal position of the stomach is influenced by the volume of its contents as well as the patient's body conformation and the phase of respiration. For example, in deep-chested dogs the stomach tends to be more cranial in position than in barrel-chested dogs. The stomach naturally moves caudally during inspiration and cranially during expiration.

Abnormal position of the stomach may be due to a nearby mass effect or a hernia (see differential diagnoses). The cardia is the least mobile part of the stomach because it is relatively fixed in position by its attachment to the esophagus.

Abnormal stomach size

A largely distended stomach may be physiologic or pathologic. Follow-up radiographs sometimes are needed to distinguish the two. Recent ingestion of a large amount of food or water can lead to marked gastric distention (Figure 4.56). Ingestion of a large amount of foreign material can produce a similar appearance (Figure 4.57). Because normal and abnormal gastric contents can appear similar in radiographs, a follow up study often is useful. A stomach that can empty normally will naturally be smaller in follow-up radiographs, provided the patient does not eat, drink, or vomit between studies.

Disorders that prevent normal gastric emptying may be physical or functional, congenital or acquired, acute or chronic, partial or complete. Physical obstructions can result from foreign material, thickening of the stomach wall, or gastric malpositioning. Functional outflow problems usually are due to pyloric disease. The degree of gastric distention depends on the severity and duration of the disorder and the patient's ability to vomit.

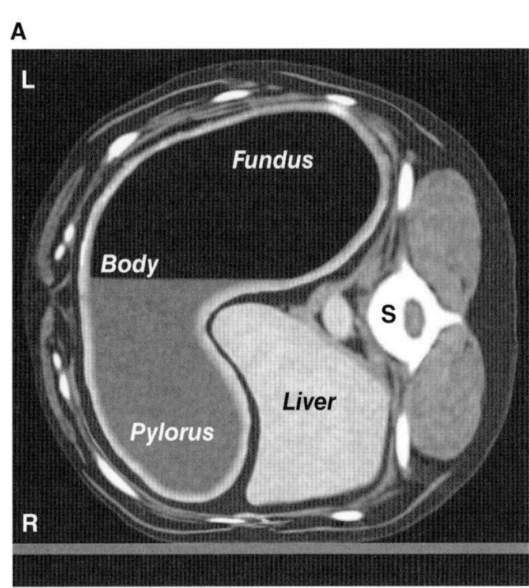

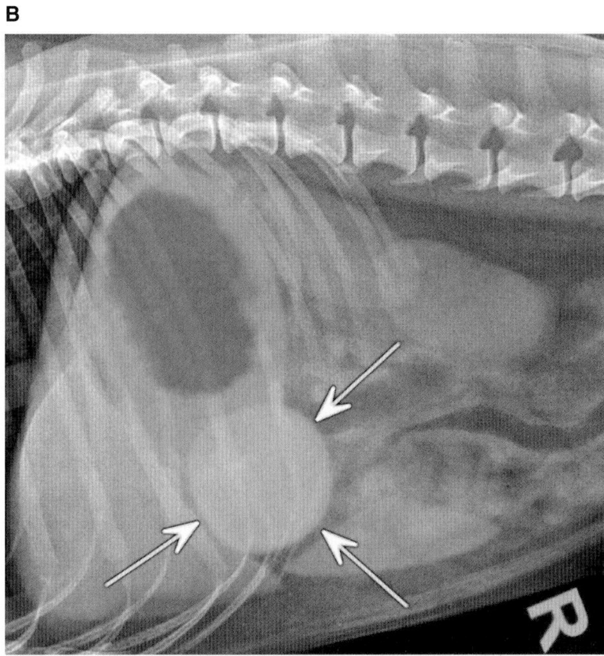

Figure 4.52 Stomach in right lateral view. CT image (**A**) and lateral radiograph (**B**) depicting a dog in right lateral recumbency. S = spine. Fluid flows into the dependent pylorus and gas rises into the fundus. In the radiograph, a fluid-filled pylorus may appear as a discrete, round, soft tissue opacity mass in a right lateral view (arrows), which may be mistaken for pathology. As shown in Figure 4.53, the left lateral view allows gas to enter the pylorus, confirming its identity.

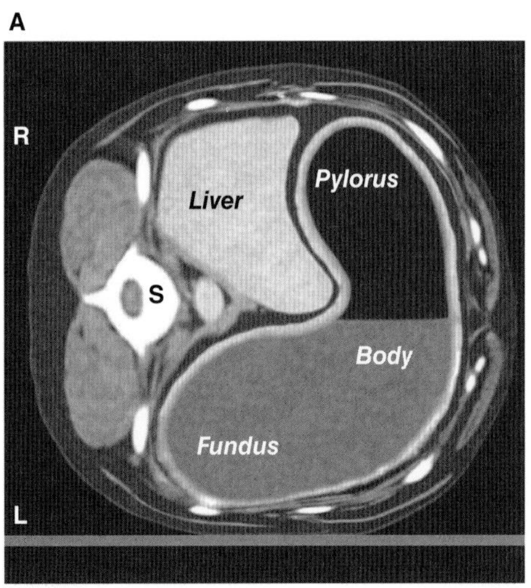

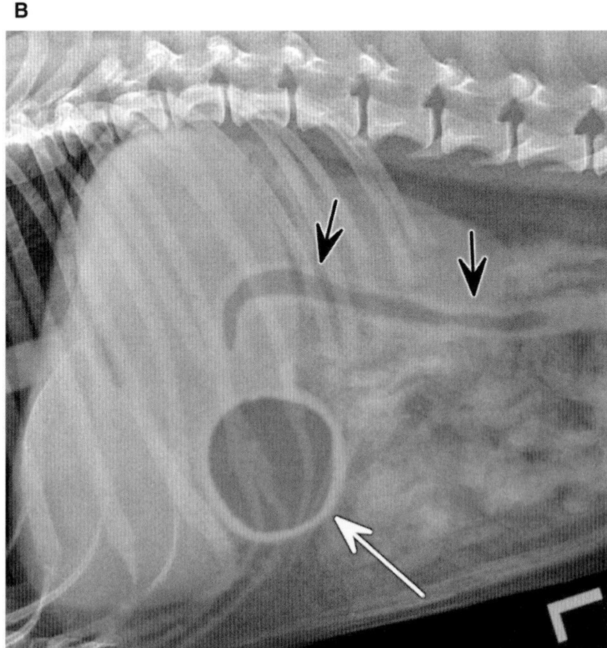

Figure 4.53 Stomach in left lateral view. CT image (**A**) and lateral radiograph (**B**) depicting a dog in left lateral recumbency. S = spine. Fluid flows into the dependent fundus and gas rises into the pylorus. Gas is more likely to enter the duodenum while in left lateral recumbency (black arrows) The body of the stomach may contain fluid or gas, depending on the volume of each.

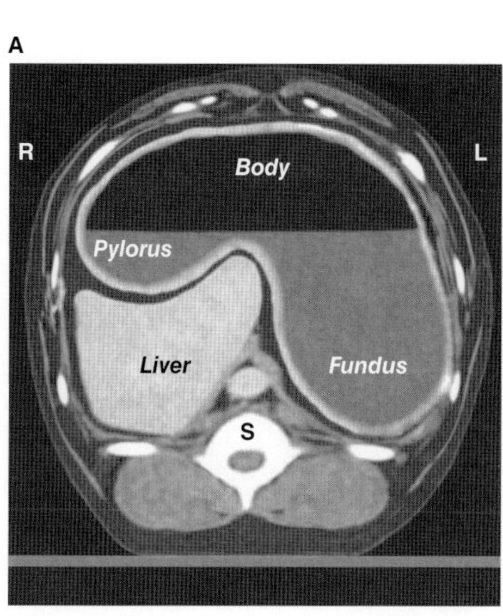

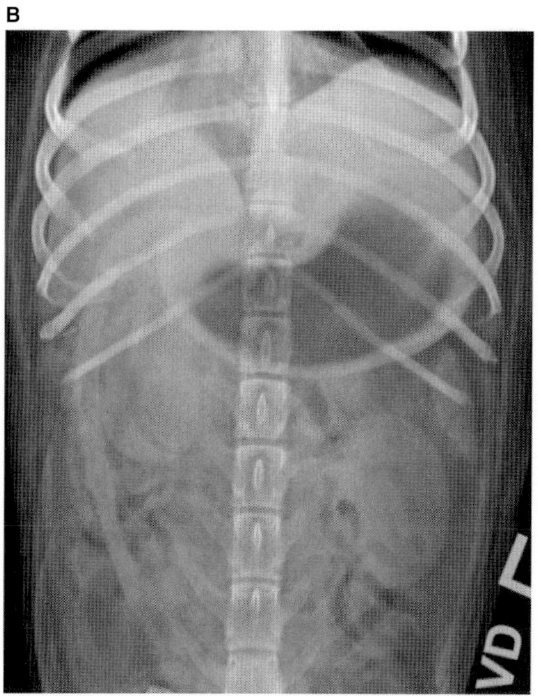

Figure 4.54 Stomach in VD view. CT image (**A**) and lateral radiograph (**B**) depicting a dog in dorsal recumbency. S = spine. Fluid flows into the dependent fundus and gas rises into the body. The pylorus may contain fluid or gas, depending on the volume of each.

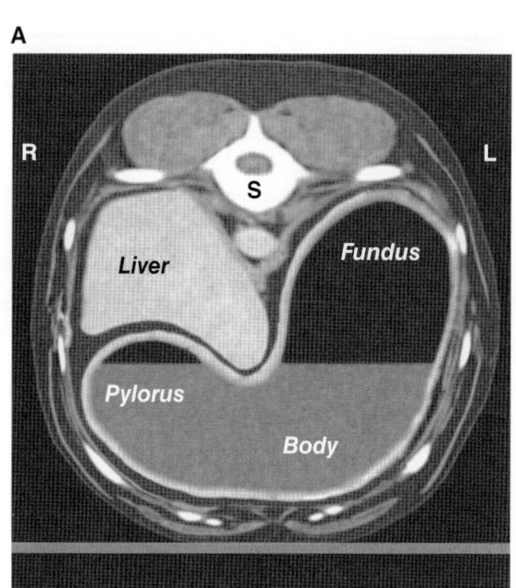

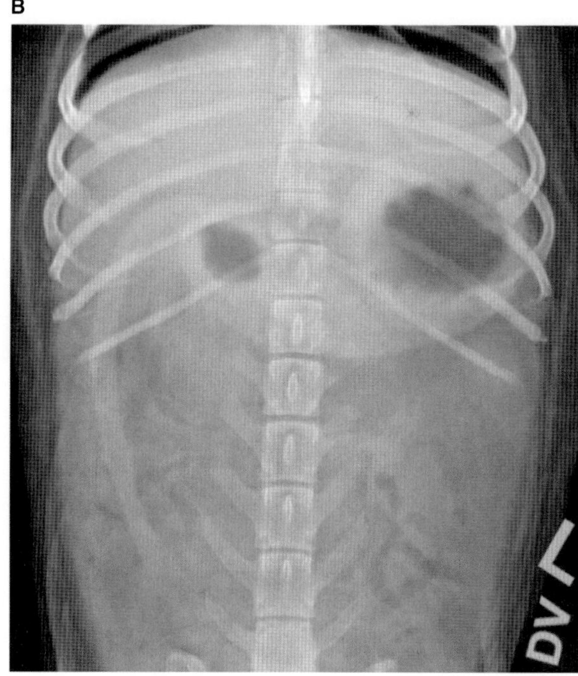

Figure 4.55 Stomach in DV view. CT image (**A**) and lateral radiograph (**B**) depicting a dog in ventral recumbency. S = spine. Fluid flows into the dependent body of the stomach and may fill the pylorus, depending on volume. Gas rises into the fundus and may partially fill the pylorus.

Table 4.1 Typical distribution of gas and fluid in the stomach

Patient position	Fundus	Body	Pylorus
Right lateral	Gas	Gas	Fluid
Left lateral	Fluid	Fluid	Gas
Dorsal (VD view)	Fluid	Gas	Gas/Fluid
Ventral (DV view)	Gas	Fluid	Gas

A

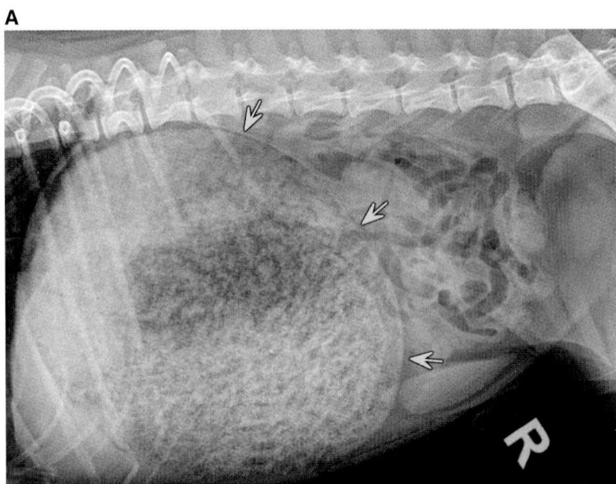

B

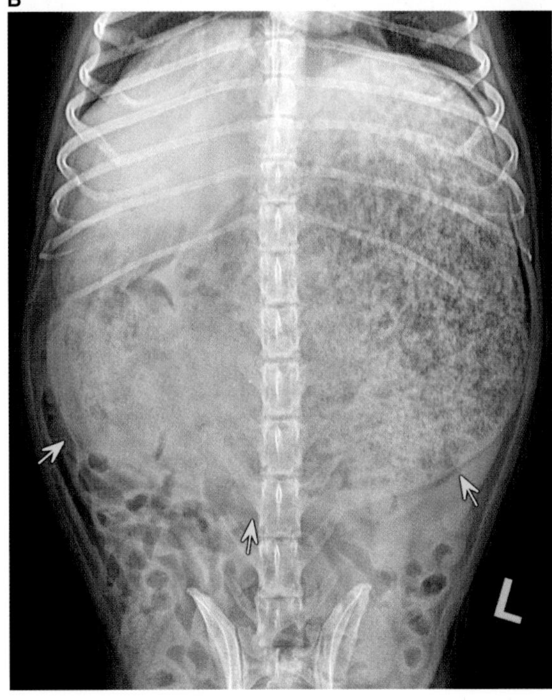

Figure 4.56 Gastric distention due to overeating. Lateral view (**A**) and VD view (**B**) of a dog abdomen depicting a stomach greatly distended with heterogeneous material (arrows). In this case, the material is ingested food, which was confirmed by seeing a smaller stomach and feces in the colon in follow-up radiographs.

A

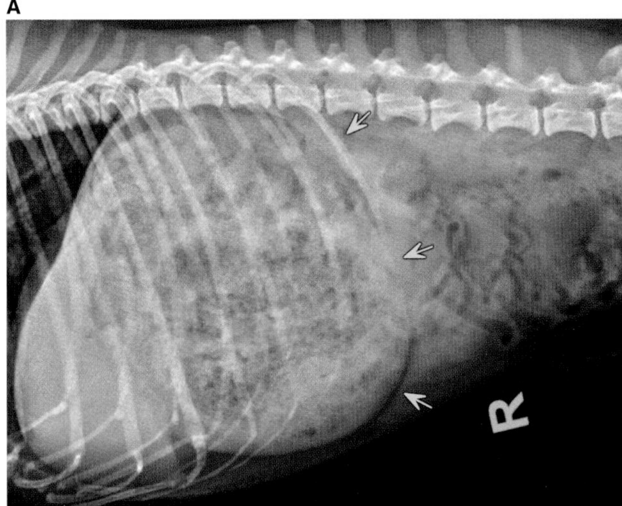

B

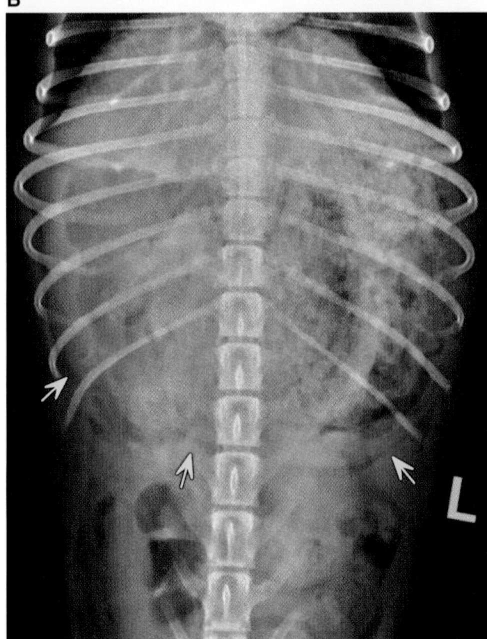

Figure 4.57 Gastric distention due to foreign material. Lateral view (**A**) and VD view (**B**) of a dog abdomen depicting a stomach greatly distended with heterogenous material (arrows). In this case, the material ingested is polyurethane, which is an adhesive agent that expands and hardens when in water (e.g., "Gorilla glue"). Follow-up radiographs documented a lack of emptying.

A stomach that is largely distended has been described as both *dilated* and *dilatated*. The terms often are used interchangeably. Specifically, dilation refers to the passive act of enlarging whereas dilatation describes the state of abnormal enlargement. Dilatation is dilation beyond normal dimensions. Gastric dilatation sometimes is called *gastric bloat*.

A largely distended stomach creates a mass effect in the cranial abdomen. The intestines, spleen, and sometimes the kidneys often are displaced caudally. An extremely distended, mostly fluid-filled stomach may be difficult to recognize in radiographs because it is homogenous in opacity and its margins extend much further caudally than expected (Figure 4.58). A gas pocket floating on top of the gastric fluid may be mistaken for the actual size of the stomach if the fluid-filled portion is not identified.

In patients with a chronic gastric outflow problem, multiple, tiny, mineral opacity objects may be visible in the dependent portion of the stomach (Figure 4.58). This finding is called the **gravel sign**. The gravel sign can occur anywhere in the GI tract. It results from the sand-like sedimentation of heavier particles in an area of chronic obstruction. In the stomach, the gravel sign often is easiest to see in a lateral view and typically in the pylorus.

A

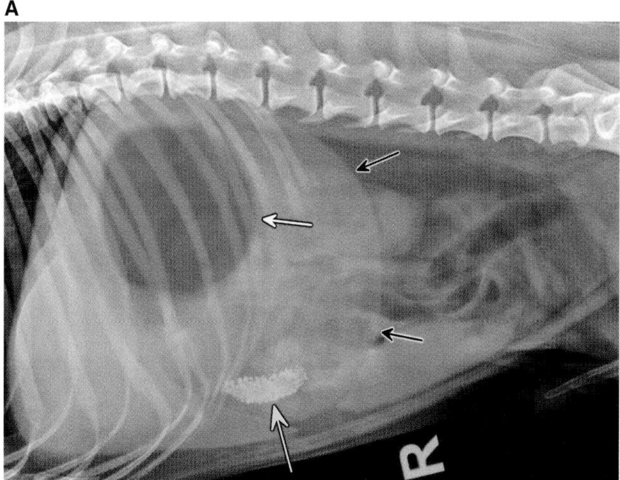

B

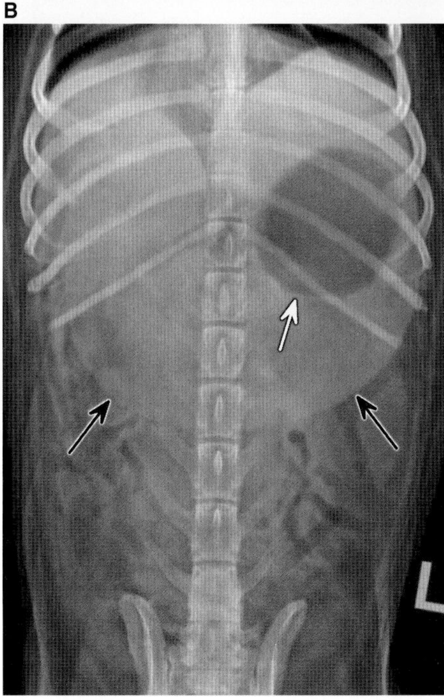

Figure 4.58 Chronic gastric outflow obstruction. Lateral view (**A**) and VD view (**B**) of a dog abdomen depicting a greatly distended, mostly fluid-filled stomach. A gas bubble in the fundus (white arrow) may be mistaken for the entire size of the stomach if the fluid-filled caudal part is not identified (black arrows). In the lateral view, the **gravel sign** is visible in the pyloric region (yellow arrow).

Gastric dilatation and volvulus (GDV)

GDV can occur when the stomach rotates around its axis. It is more common in large, deep-chested dogs, but can occur in any breed of dog and at any age. It is rare in cats but has been reported in a cat with a diaphragmatic hernia. Patients with GDV frequently present as an emergency, in a life-threatening situation. Patients in severe distress must be stabilized prior to imaging.

During gastric volvulus, the pylorus rotates from its normal position in the ventral, right side of the abdomen to the dorsal, left side (Figures 4.59 and 4.60). Volvulus also twists the esophagus at the cardia of the stomach. The duodenum follows the pylorus and moves dorsally and to the left, often wrapping around the esophagus. GDV results in an inability to eructate and an obstructed pyloric outflow.

The radiographic appearance of GDV is summarized in Table 4.2. Note: radiographic findings depend on the stomach contents, the degree of gastric distention, and the extent of rotation. **The key to diagnosis of GDV is to locate the pylorus** (Figures 4.60 – 4.63). Locating the pylorus is essential to differentiate GDV from gastric dilatation only. A displaced pylorus is easiest to identify when it contains gas. Because the pylorus typically rotates dorsally and to the left, the right lateral and DV views tend to be the most diagnostic. Remember, the dependent (down) parts of the stomach fill with fluid (and ingesta) while the non-dependent (up) parts fill with gas. In right lateral and ventral recumbencies, a pylorus that is displaced to the left and dorsally will be "up" and more likely to fill with gas.

The classic appearance of GDV in the right lateral view is commonly called *compartmentalization* of the stomach (Figures 4.60 and 4.61). Compartmentalization appears as a gas-filled pylorus positioned craniodorsal to a gas-and-fluid-filled fundus, and with a band of soft tissue opacity between them. Compartmentalization is considered by many to be pathognomonic for GDV but, like most radiographic signs, it is not 100% diagnostic.

If the pylorus cannot be identified from right lateral and DV views, make all four views of the stomach (right lateral, left lateral, DV, and VD). If identification remains equivocal and the condition of the patient warrants further diagnostics instead of surgery, a gastrogram may be helpful.

Gastric volvulus usually leads to splenic displacement due to the gastrosplenic attachment. The spleen typically is displaced to the right, caudally and ventrally as the stomach rotates. The splenic triangle will be absent from its normal position in the left craniodorsal abdomen. The displaced

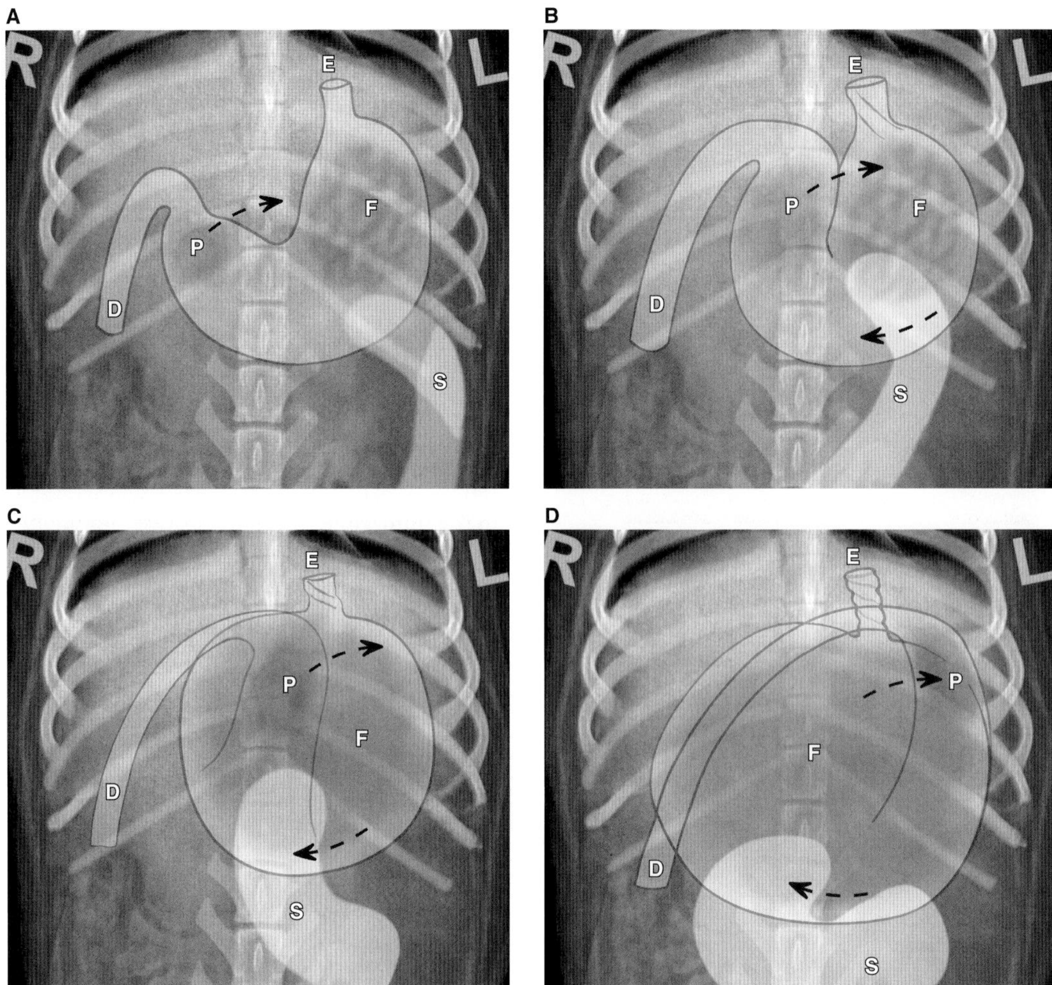

Figure 4.59 Gastric volvulus and dilatation (GDV). DV views of a dog cranial abdomen illustrating the stages of stomach rotation in a patient with GDV. **A**. The pylorus (P) moves to the left, pulling the duodenum (D) with it. **B**. As the pylorus and duodenum move to the left, the fundus moves to the right, pulling the spleen (S) with it. Rotation of the stomach causes a twist in the distal esophagus (E) at the cardia of the stomach. **C**. Continued rotation causes a more severe twisting at the distal esophagus, preventing eructation. The stomach dilates. The displaced spleen enlarges due to venous congestion. **D**. The pylorus ends up in the left cranial abdomen with the duodenum wrapped around the esophagus. The stomach is largely distended. The spleen is absent from its normal location in the left cranial abdomen.

spleen may enlarge due to venous congestion. A splenic torsion sometimes is concurrent with GDV. If the displaced spleen does not enlarge, it may be difficult to identify.

GDV may be accompanied by a **reflex ileus**. In these cases, the small intestine is extensively gas-filled due to weak peristalsis. The bowel is not abnormally distended, but the gas pattern may appear static and unchanged in serial radiographs. Reflex ileus usually resolves following successful treatment of GDV.

Gastric dilatation often leads to compression of the caudal vena cava and restriction of the venous return to the heart. The caudal vena cava and the cardiac shadow may be small. GDV also leads to esophageal dilation, usually with gas, due to gastroesophageal obstruction.

Pneumoperitoneum in patients with GDV can occur due to stomach rupture or recent trocharization of the stomach. Gas occasionally is seen in the liver or gastric wall due to stomach necrosis and migration of gas through the portal system.

Importantly, lack of severe gastric distention does not rule out GDV. It just makes diagnosis more difficult. Sometimes the stomach will de-rotate after the patient is sedated or during positioning for radiography. Remember, four-view radiographs of the stomach often are useful to locate the pylorus, which again, is key to diagnosis of GDV. A difficult-to-diagnose form of GDV occurs when the stomach rotates a full 360°. In these cases, the pylorus and fundus reoccupy their normal positions.

A

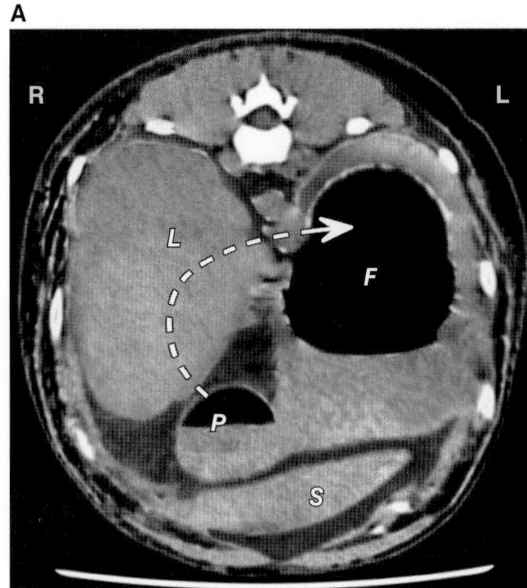

B

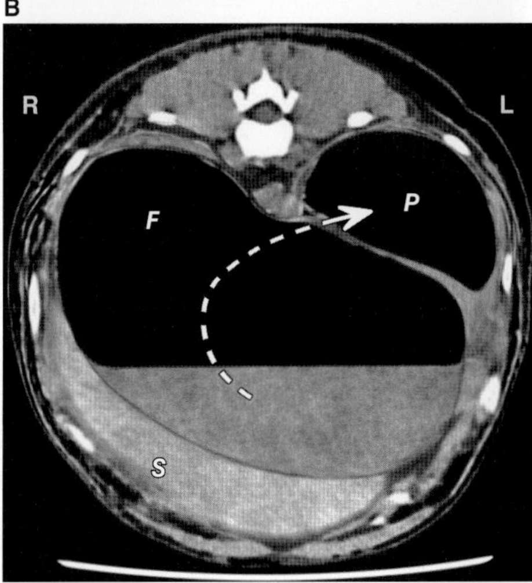

Figure 4.60 Gastric dilatation and volvulus (GDV). **A**. Cross-sectional CT image of a dog abdomen depicting the normal appearance of the gastric fundus (F), the pylorus (P), the spleen (S), and the liver (L). The dashed white arrow indicates the movement of the pylorus during gastric volvulus. **B**. CT image depicting the same area in a dog with GDV. The pylorus is displaced dorsally and to the left and the fundus is displaced to the right. Both are dilated with mostly gas.

Abnormal stomach content and opacity

Foreign materials are common in the stomachs of dogs and cats. Many are recognized by their opacity or distinct shape or pattern (Figures 4.64 and 4.65).

Mineral and metal opacity objects tend to be easily identified and may or may not be clinically significant. Keep in mind that some types of ingested metal can cause poisoning. Oral medications containing bismuth or kaolin may appear mineral or metal opacity in radiographs. Medications gradually dissolve and become smaller over time. Positive contrast medium may be retained in the stomach longer than expected when adhered to foreign material or to damaged mucosa. Re-ingestion of contrast medium (i.e., coprophagia) can produce unexpected mineral/metal opacity in the stomach.

Table 4.2 Radiographic findings with GDV

1. Pylorus is abnormally positioned, usually dorsally and to the left.
2. Compartmentalization of the stomach.
3. Abnormally positioned spleen with variable splenomegaly.
4. Reflex ileus in small intestine.
5. Dilated esophagus.
6. Small caudal vena cava and small cardiac silhouette.

Soft tissue opacity objects in the stomach may be identified when outlined by gas or a positive contrast agent (Figure 4.66). This is also true for soft tissue opacity masses in the stomach (e.g., tumor, abscess, granuloma, others).

Although uncommon in dogs and cats, a mass can develop in any part of stomach. Large masses may partially or completely obstruct gastric outflow. They sometimes distort the shape of the stomach. Note: a stomach that appears abnormal in shape is relevant only if it persists in serial radiographs. Infiltrative masses can alter gastric motility, making that part of the stomach wall appear stiff or fixed in position between radiographs.

Thickening of the gastric wall may be localized or diffuse and generally is caused by either inflammation or infiltrative disease. Fluid in the stomach may be mistaken for wall thickening in survey radiographs (Figure 4.67). Thinning or atrophy of the stomach wall is rare but may follow chronic inflammation. A gastrogram usually is needed to accurately identify the mucosal margin and to evaluate the stomach wall thickness and position.

Gastritis is difficult to diagnose with radiographs because the signs are non-specific. The stomach may be persistently larger than expected in serial radiographs and gastric contents may empty more slowly. Food retained more than 12 hours is abnormal. In some cases, gastritis makes the stomach empty more rapidly. Gastrography may reveal a stomach that is less distensible than expected and an irregular or nodular mucosal margin. Mucosal ulcers may be present, but ulcers are difficult to see in radiographs unless they are large.

Gas or mineral opacity in the stomach wall is abnormal. Gastric pneumatosis can result from deep mucosal ulcers, stomach wall necrosis or perforation of the stomach wall. Mineralization in the wall may be due to chronic inflammation, neoplasia, metabolic disease, or toxicosis (see differential diagnoses).

Gastrography

The procedure for gastrography, as well as its indications, contraindications, and normal transit times, can be found in

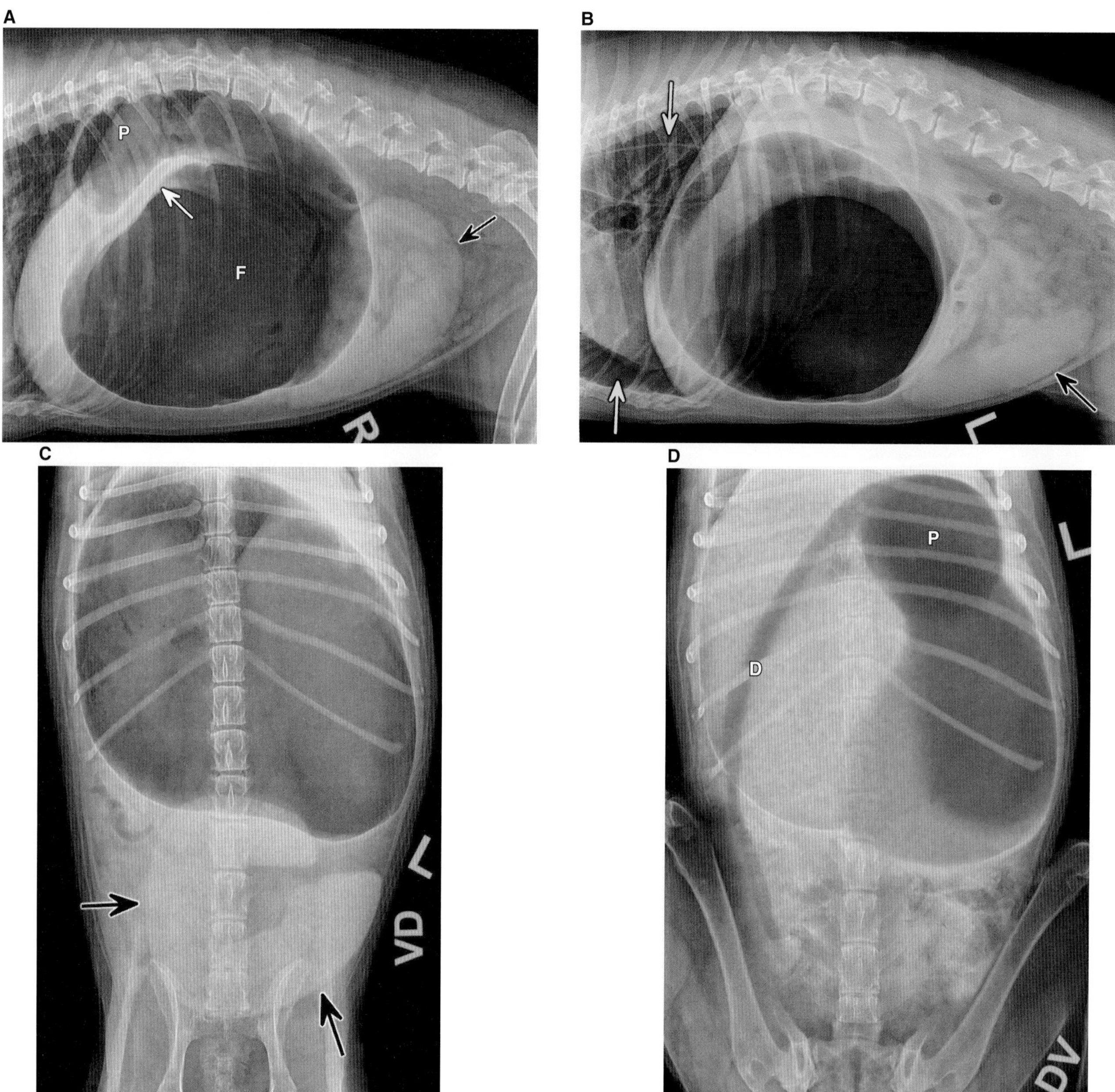

Figure 4.61 Gastric dilatation and volvulus (GDV). The classic appearance of GDV is depicted in these right lateral (**A**), left lateral (**B**), VD (**C**), and DV (**D**) views of a dog abdomen. The stomach is greatly distended with gas and fluid. In the right lateral view (**A**), the pylorus (P) is displaced dorsally and it is cranial to the fundus (F). There is a soft tissue opacity fold between them (white arrow). This finding is commonly called "compartmentalization of the stomach", but it is not as evident in the other views. The spleen is displaced caudally and to the right (black arrows). It is mildly enlarged with rounded margins. The cardiac silhouette appears small (as seen at the periphery of the left lateral view, **B**) and the caudal esophagus is dilated with gas (yellow arrows). The pylorus is not readily identified in either the left lateral or the VD view because it is not filled with gas. In the DV view, gas is visible in the pylorus and duodenum (D), which aids in their identification.

the contrast radiography section of Chapter 2. Before performing a gastrogram, make the four survey radiographs of the stomach (right lateral, left lateral, VD and DV). As mentioned earlier, many questionable radiographic findings can be resolved by simply redistributing gas and fluid in the stomach. If findings remain inconclusive, a negative or positive contrast gastrogram may be useful. With a gastrogram, we are usually looking for filling defects and assessing gastric emptying.

Filling defects are areas that should contain contrast medium but persistently do not. They may be caused by a thickened or otherwise abnormal stomach wall, foreign

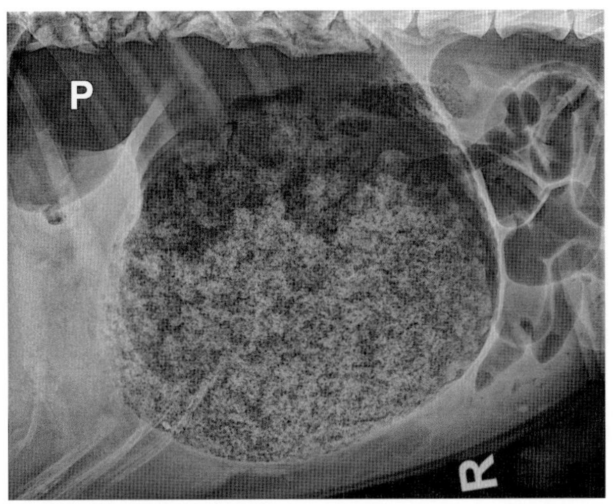

Figure 4.62 GDV with ingesta. Lateral view of a dog abdomen depicting a compartmentalized stomach that is greatly distended with gas and heterogeneous soft tissue opacity material. The gas-filled pylorus (P) is craniodorsal to the food-filled fundus.

material, or retained ingesta. Food in the stomach cannot reliably be distinguished from pathology, which is why it is so important to properly prepare the patient prior to gastrography.

In a normal gastrogram, the mucosal margin is relatively even and well-defined. The rugal folds may be visible as regularly spaced, curvilinear, filling defects (Figure 4.68). A thickened, interrupted, or distorted pattern of folds may be due to inflammation or infiltrative disease (Figure 4.69). Note: there is considerable variation in the appearance of the rugal folds and interpretation relies on experience.

Normal stomach contractions produce transient filling defects in a gastrogram. Filling defects due to peristalsis appears as even indentations along the outline of the stomach and vary in appearance between radiographs (Figure 4.70). Filling defects caused by lesions in the stomach wall persist relatively unchanged in serial radiographs. One of the keys to differentiating peristalsis from pathology is repeatability.

Filling defects caused by gastric wall thickening may be localized, regional, or diffuse. The mucosal margin along the

A

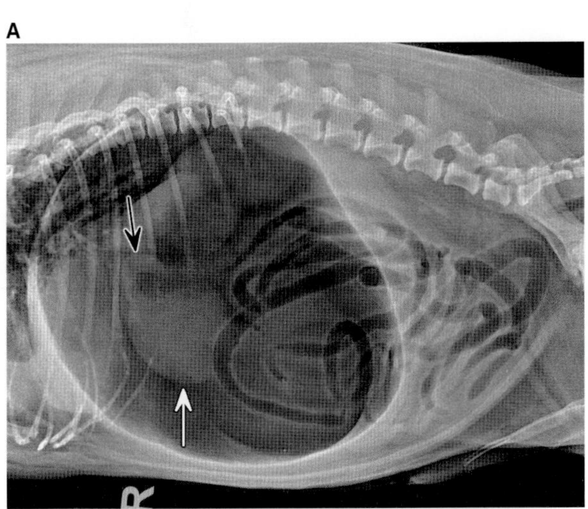

B

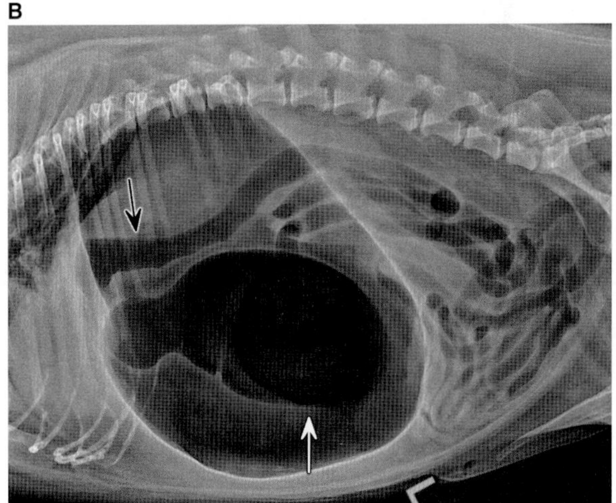

C

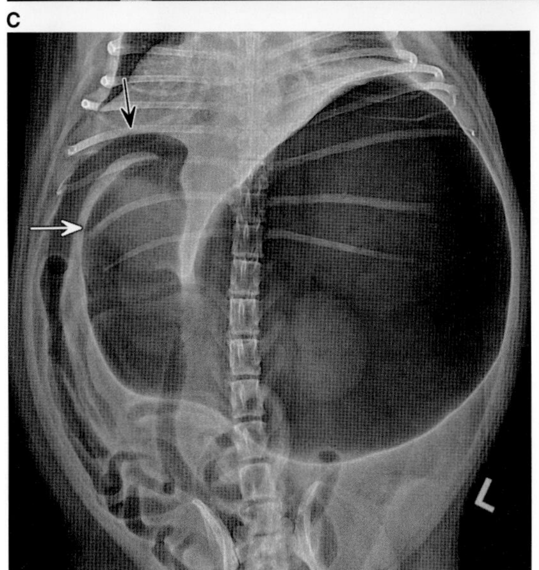

Figure 4.63 Gastric dilatation without volvulus. Three views of a dog abdomen depicting a stomach greatly distended with mostly gas but normal in orientation. **A**. In the right lateral view, fluid flows into the pylorus (white arrow) and duodenum (black arrow). The body and fundus of the stomach are largely distended with gas. **B**. In the left lateral view, gas rises to fill the pylorus (white arrow) and duodenum (black arrow), making them easier to identify. The body and fundus remain largely distended. **C**. In the VD view, gas rises to fill the pylorus (white arrows) and duodenum (black arrows), visible in their normal positions.

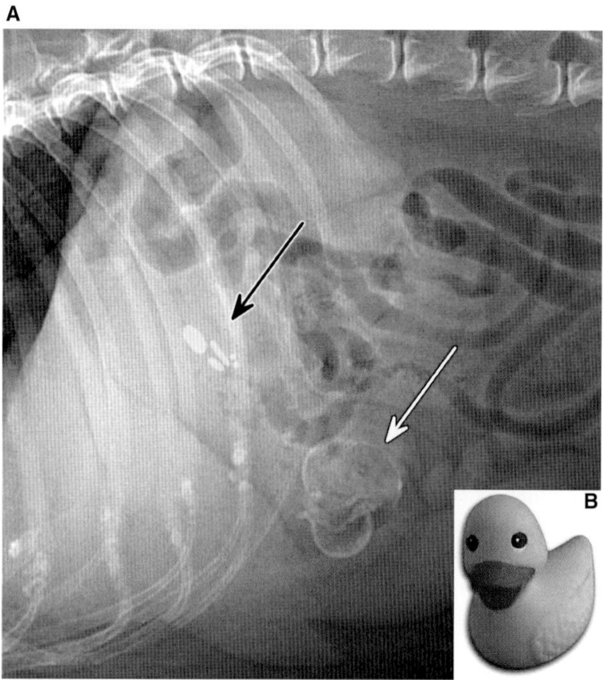

Figure 4.64 Gastric foreign objects. **A**. Lateral view of a dog abdomen depicting mineral opacity foreign objects in the stomach. The ovoid objects in the body of the stomach (black arrow) are pieces of Pepto-Bismol tablets. The object in the pylorus (white arrow) is an upside down rubber ducky toy (as shown in the inset photo **B**).

affected area may or may not differ in appearance from the adjacent, unaffected mucosa. Mucosal ulcers may result from severe, chronic, or repeated episodes of disease. Large ulcers appear as persistent, contrast-filled outpouchings that extend away from the gastric lumen (Figure 4.71). When viewed *en face*, a large ulcer may resemble a bullseye target because the thickened mucosa surrounding the ulcer creates a ring-shaped filling defect around the contrast-filled center.

Filling defects caused by freely moveable material in the stomach can change location between radiographs and sometimes are only visible when the patient is in a certain position. Small objects can be obscured by positive contrast medium, but may become visible as the stomach empties. The same is true for materials that are widely disbursed in the stomach, such as fabric or cloth. Such items may be identified only after the majority of the contrast medium has exited the stomach, leaving a small amount of contrast adhered to the material.

The **rate of gastric empty** can be assessed with gastrography by making serial radiographs at specific times. Both the time required for the stomach to begin emptying and the time required for it to empty completely can be evaluated. Each of these, however, is influenced by many factors, including:

1. Psychogenic and Pharmacologic effects.
2. The amount of ingesta retained in the stomach.
3. The volume of contrast medium in the stomach.
4. Pathology.

Psychogenic factors can slow or accelerate gastric emptying (e.g., fear, pain, rage). When stress is the suspected cause of delayed emptying, allow the patient to calm down for 15 to 30 minutes and then repeat the radiographs.

Drugs such as atropine, narcotics, sedatives, and others can slow gastric peristalsis. Whenever practical, drugs that alter GI motility should be discontinued 24 to 48 hours prior

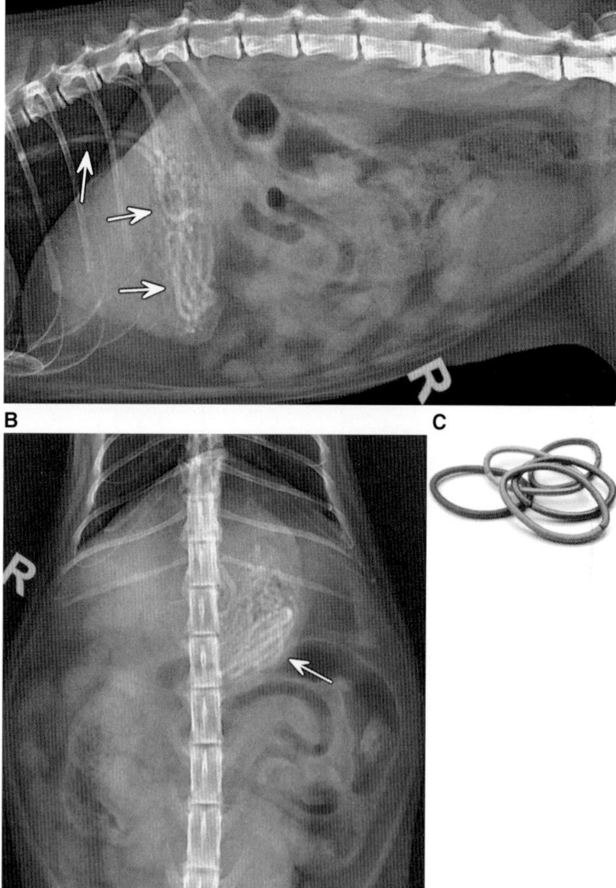

Figure 4.65 Gastric foreign material. Lateral view (**A**) and VD view (**B**) of a cat abdomen. Multiple, curvilinear, mineral opacity objects are visible in the stomach and caudal esophagus (white arrows). These are ingested hair ties, examples of which are shown in the inset photo (**C**).

CHAPTER 4

to gastrography. It is important to know the patient's medication history when interpreting a gastrogram.

If the stomach is not completely emptied of solid material prior to beginning gastrography, gastric emptying may be delayed. Proper patient preparation is important. Always evaluate the gastric contents in survey radiographs and keep this in mind when interpreting the gastrogram.

Liquids tend to remain in the stomach until there is a sufficient volume to stimulate emptying. An insufficient volume of contrast medium can significantly delay gastric emptying. Causes of inadequate contrast medium in the stomach include defecient dosing and patient vomiting. It is

A

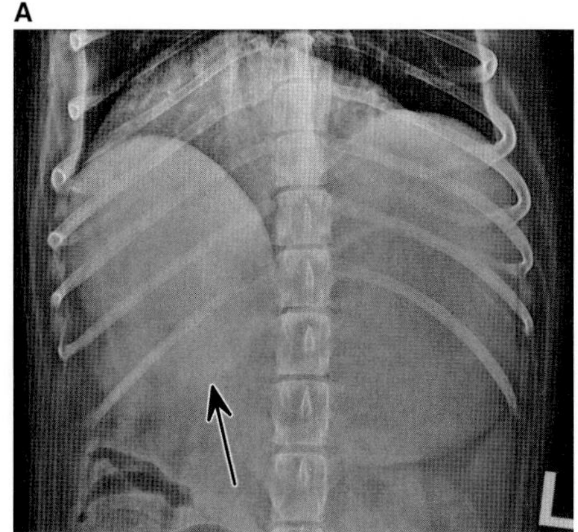

B

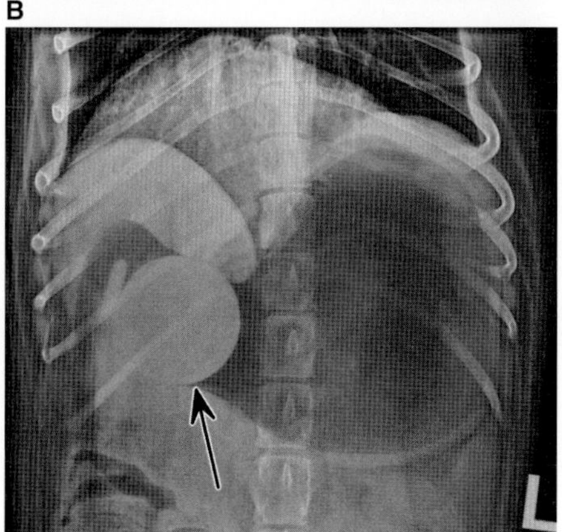

C

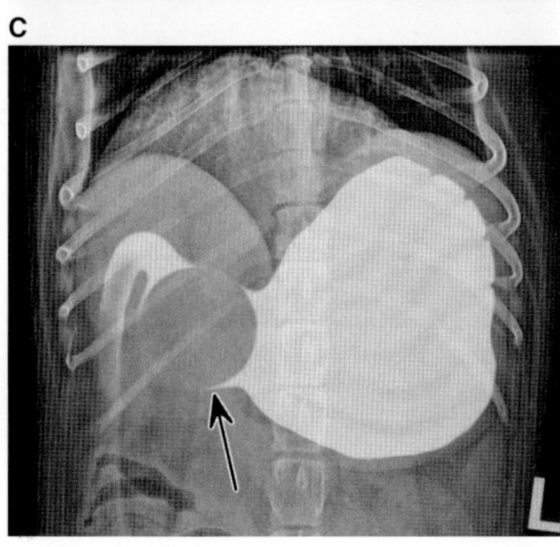

Figure 4.66 Gastric foreign object. VD views of a dog abdomen depicting a round, soft tissue opacity object in the pyloric antrum (arrow). **A**. Survey radiograph: the object is not well seen because it is surrounded by fluid, which is the same opacity as the object. **B**. Negative contrast gastrogram: adding gas to the stomach provides an opacity interface to reveal the outline of the object. **C**. Postitive contrast gastrogram: adding barium to the stomach also provides an opacity interface to identify the object.

A

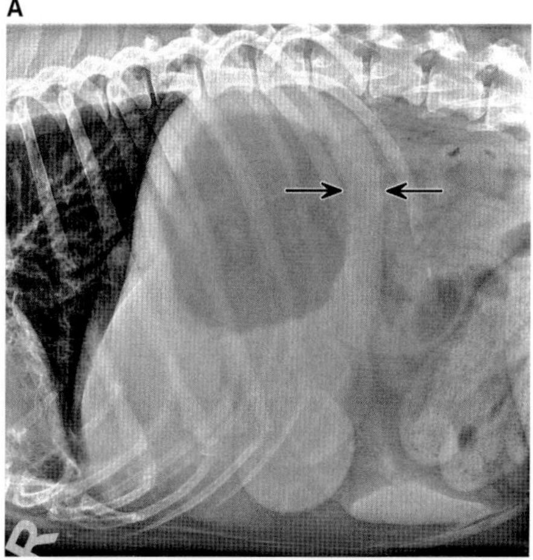

B

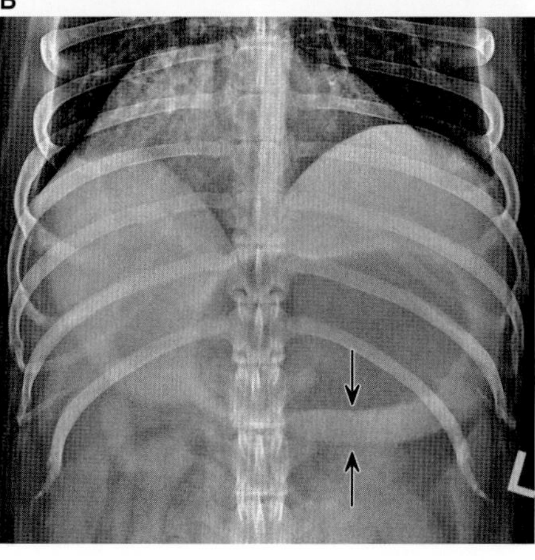

Figure 4.67 Fluid in stomach. Lateral view (**A**) and VD view (**B**) of a dog abdomen depicting a stomach moderately distended with fluid and gas. The mucosal margin cannot be identified with certainty in these images. Fluid blending with the gastric mucosa may be mistaken for a thickened stomach wall (black arrows).

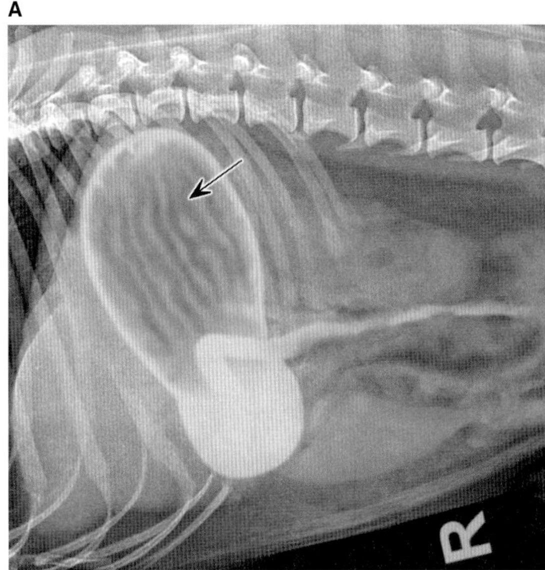

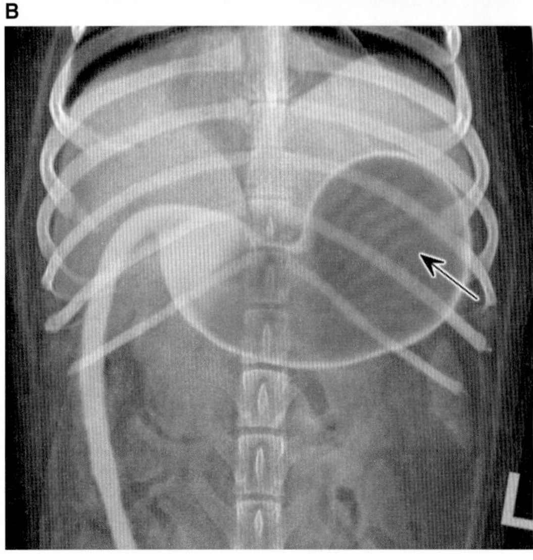

Figure 4.68 Gastric rugae. Lateral view (**A**) and VD view (**B**) of a dog abdomen depicting a positive contrast gastrogram. The rugal folds create curvilinear filling defects (darker areas in the contrast medium); easier to see in the fundic region (black arrows).

important to assess the degree of gastric filling in the initial radiographs and to be aware of any patient vomiting when assessing the rate of gastric emptying.

Rapid gastric emptying generally is a subjective assessment and its clinical significance often is uncertain. It is a notable radiographic finding but not diagnostic of any specific condition. Delayed gastric emptying longer than 4 hours is of significant concern.

Pathologic causes of delayed gastric emptying may be physical or functional (as described with abnormal stomach size). In patients with a partial obstruction to gastric outflow, a liquid contrast medium may move past the obstruction, making the diagnosis more difficult. In these cases, mixing the contrast medium with food often demonstrates the outflow problem. Solid materials are less likely to move past an incomplete obstruction than liquids.

Many gastric outflow problems involve the pylorus. Normal pyloric contractions must be differentiated from pathology. Normal pyloric peristalsis creates a transient, circumferential narrowing of the pyloric canal. This normal narrowing often is absent in a subsequent radiograph (Figure 4.72). Persistent narrowing that is unchanged in serial radiographs indicates pathology (Figure 4.73). Sometimes the pyloric antrum will bulge around a narrowed pyloric canal due to continued contractions from the body of the stomach (Figure 4.74).

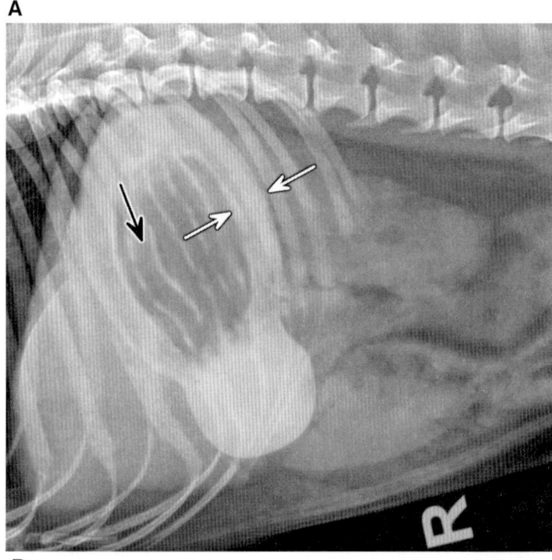

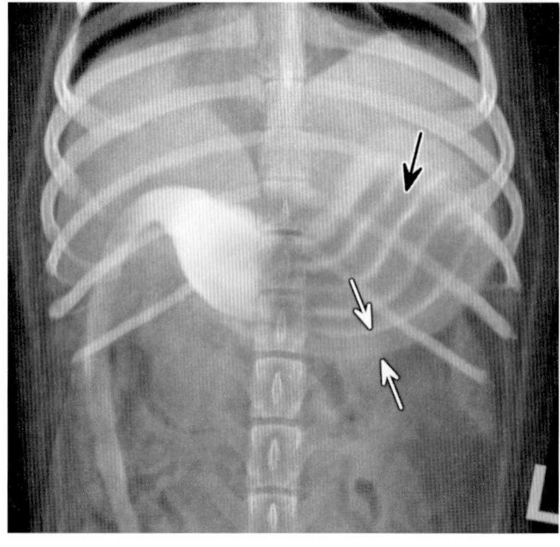

Figure 4.69 Thickened stomach wall. Lateral view (**A**) and VD view (**B**) of a dog abdomen depicting a positive contrast gastrogram. Most of the contrast medium has exited the stomach. A small volume fills the spaces between the rugal folds and outlines the mucosal margin. The gastric wall is thickened (white arrows), and the rugal folds are widened (black arrows).

A

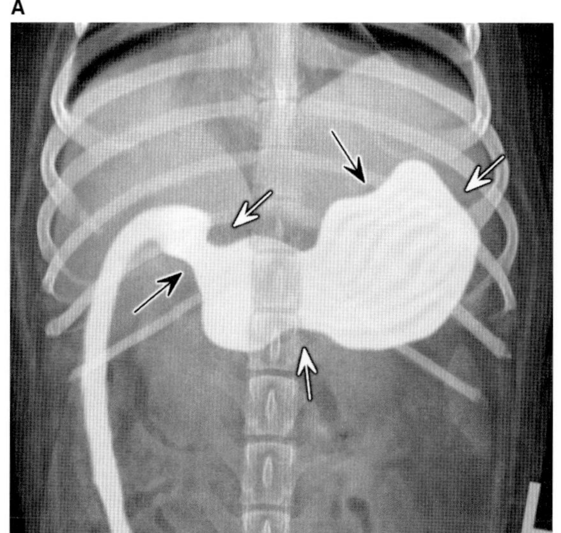

B

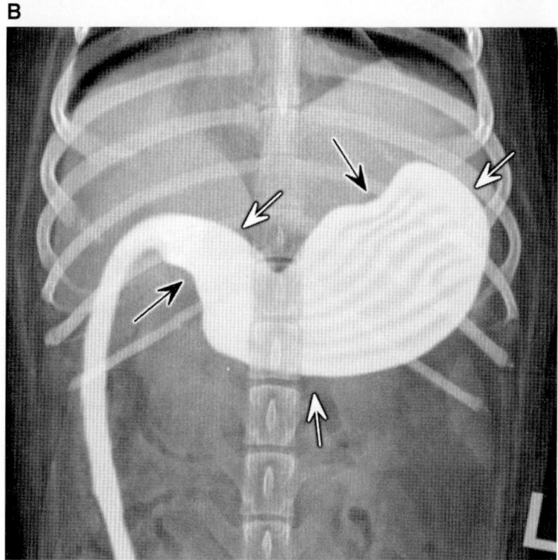

Figure 4.70 Filling defects. Two VD views of a dog abdomen depicting a gastrogram. The two radiographs were made a short time apart. In radiograph **A**, there are multiple filling defects along the outline of the stomach, some caused by peristalsis (white arrows) and others caused by gastric wall thickening (black arrows). In radiograph **B**, the indentations caused by peristalsis (white arrows) do not repeat, whereas those caused by wall thickening (black arrows) persist relatively unchanged. The thickened wall appears stiff and fixed in position.

Small intestine

Normal radiographic anatomy

The small intestine occupies the areas in the mid-abdomen that do not contain fat or other viscera. The normal small bowel appears as a collection of continuously flowing and overlapping tubular segments with even serosal margins. All parts of the small intestine should be similar in size, with no segment larger than twice the diameter of any other segment. The small intestine is divided into three sections: *duodenum, jejunum,* and *ileum*.

The **duodenum** begins at the gastric pylorus, extends a short distance cranially, and then curves caudally. The descending duodenum runs along the right body wall to about the level of the ilial wings where it curves to the left and then cranial as the ascending duodenum. The ascending duodenum runs cranially to join the jejunum just caudal to the stomach. The duodenum is slightly larger in diameter and more constant in position than the other parts of the small intestine.

Along the descending duodenum are pockets of lymphoid tissue called *Peyer's patches*. The mucosa is thin over these patches and when the duodenum is filled with gas or a positive contrast medium they appear as focal out-pouches (Figures 4.75 and 4.88). The out-pouches resemble mucosal ulcers and commonly are called *pseudoulcers*. They are seen most often in young dogs.

In cats, normal peristalsis along the descending duodenum frequently produces a series of segmental or circular contractions, commonly called the *string-of-pearls* sign. The string-of-pearls is easiest to see in an upper GI study (Figure 4.90) and should not be mistaken for linear foreign material.

The **jejunum** begins in the mid-abdomen, just caudal to the stomach, and represents the majority of the small intestine. It is freely moveable and readily displaced. The jejunum ends at the ileum, which is also located in the mid-abdomen.

The **ileum** is the shortest, most distal part of the small intestine. It connects the jejunum to the ascending colon.

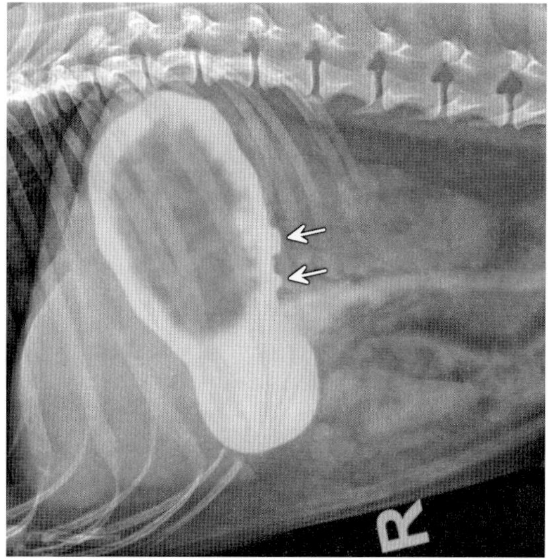

Figure 4.71 Gastric ulcers. Lateral view of a dog abdomen depicting a gastrogram with mucosal ulcers along the greater curvature (white arrows). The ulcers appear as focal, contrast-filled outpouchings that persist in serial radiographs.

A

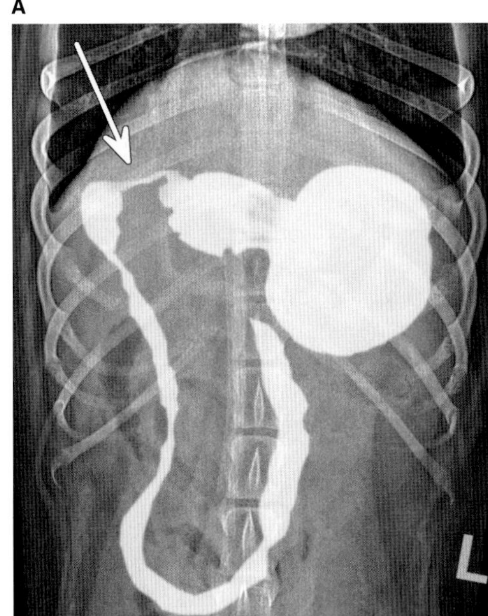

B

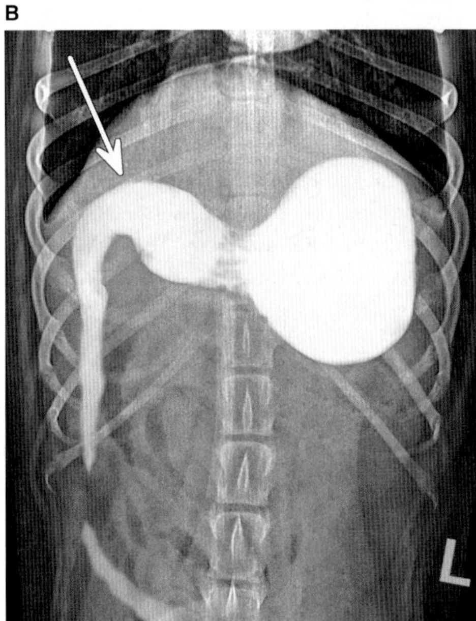

Figure 4.72 Pyloric contraction. Two VD views of the same dog abdomen depicting a gastrogram. **A**. The pyloric canal is narrowed (white arrow) which may be due to normal peristalsis or pathology. **B**. In this second radiograph, made a short time later, the narrowing is not evident because it was caused by a peristaltic contraction.

Other than location, there are no distinguishing radiographic features between the ileum and the jejunum.

Abnormal position of the small intestine

The majority of the small intestine is quite mobile. Its normal distribution is influenced by the patient's body conformation, the amount of intra-abdominal fat, and the sizes of the adjacent viscera. For example, in deep-chested dogs the intestines may be adjacent to the diaphragm. In thin animals the small bowel can extend from the liver to the pelvic inlet. In overweight animals, intra-abdominal fat limits the space available for the small intestine and the bowel is confined to

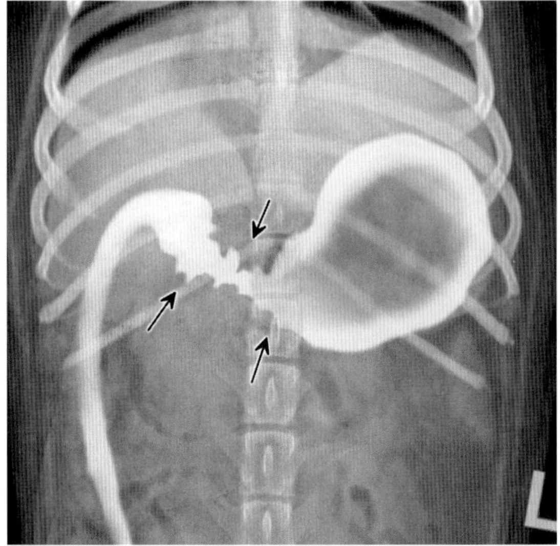

Figure 4.73 Stomach mural lesions. VD view of a dog abdomen depicting a gastrogram with multiple irregular-shaped filling defects in the distal body and pyloric regions (black arrows). The lesions are visible along both the lesser and greater curvatures due to an annular neoplasm invading the stomach wall.

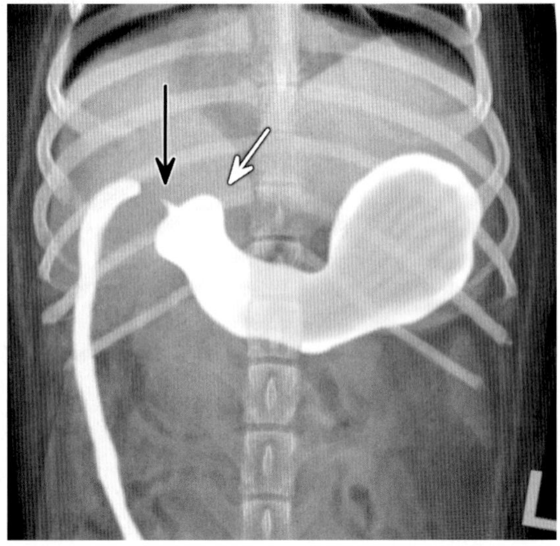

Figure 4.74 Pyloric outflow obstruction. VD view of a dog abdomen depicting a gastrogram with marked narrowing of the pyloric canal (black arrow). Peristalsis pushing against the narrowing causes the stomach wall to bulge outward (white arrow) creating a pointed or "beak-like" appearance near the pyloric canal.

a smaller area (Figure 4.76). Crowding of the small bowel in obese patients may be mistaken for intestinal plication (Figure 4.95). The normal stomach, colon, urinary bladder, and uterus can vary significantly in size and affect the position of the small bowel. Pathologic displacement of the small intestine may be due to a mass effect or loss of abdominal (see differential diagnoses).

Abnormal size of the small intestine

The width of the small intestine is measured from serosa to serosa. An abnormal increase in bowel width may be due to either dilation of the bowel lumen or thickening of the bowel wall.

A

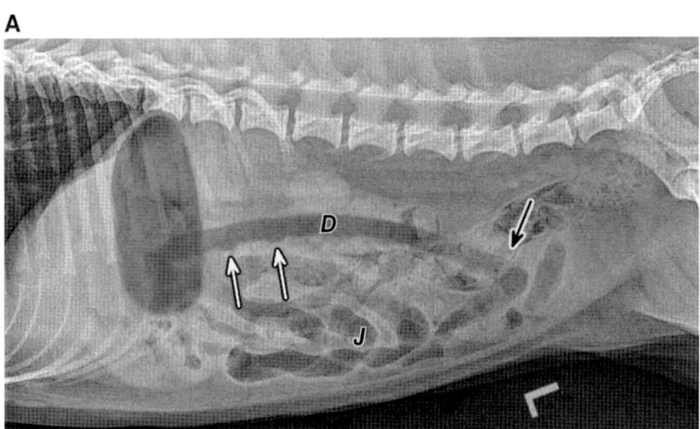

B

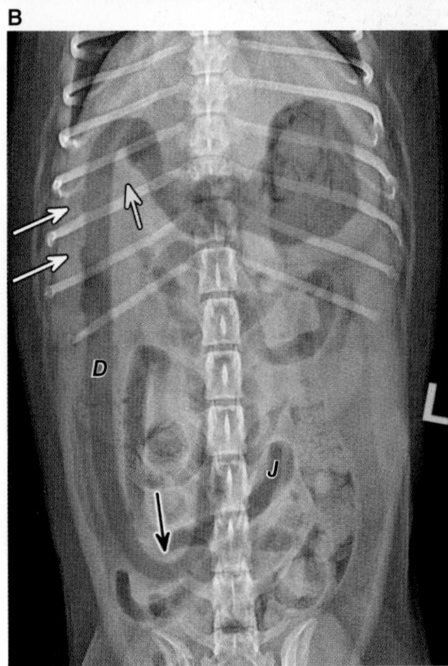

Figure 4.75 Normal small intestine. Lateral view (**A**) and VD view (**B**) of a dog abdomen depicting gas in the stomach, duodenum (*D*) and jejunum (*J*). The cranial duodenal flexure is part of the gastroduodenal angle (yellow arrow). Peyer's patches are visible along the descending duodenum (white arrows), appearing as square-shaped out-pouches that extend away from the lumen. At the caudal duodenal flexure (black arrow), the duodenum curves to the left and then cranially.

A

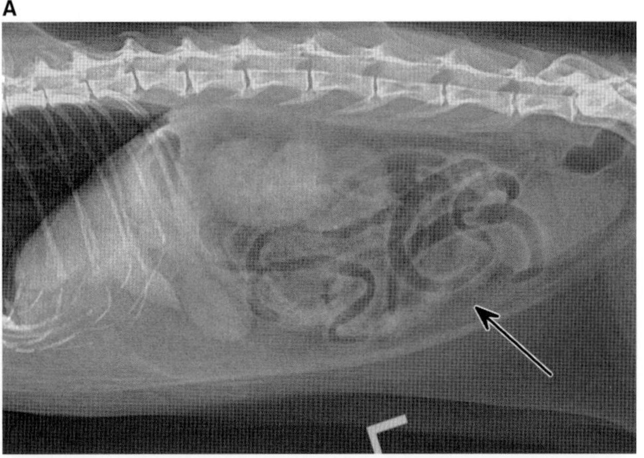

B

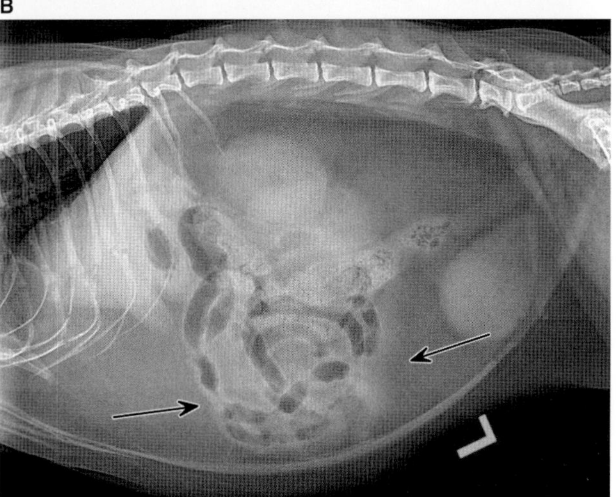

C

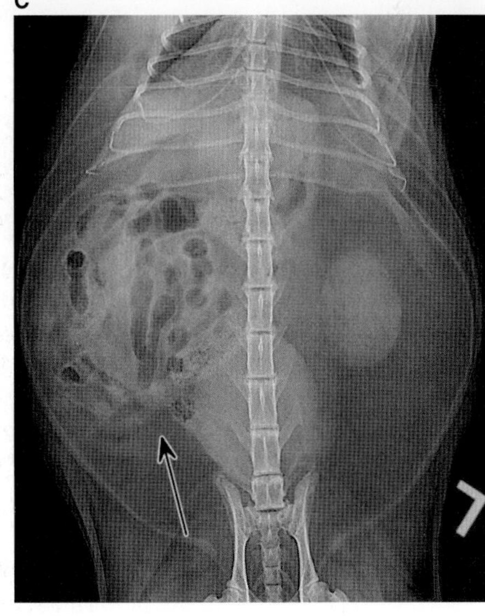

Figure 4.76 Normal distribution of the small intestine. **A**. Lateral view of a cat abdomen depicting even distribution of the small intestine (arrow). **B**. Lateral view of an overweight cat abdomen depicting crowding of the small intestine due to excess intra-abdominal fat (arrows). **C**. VD view of the same cat as in B; the small bowel is confined to the right abdomen by the excess fat (arrow).

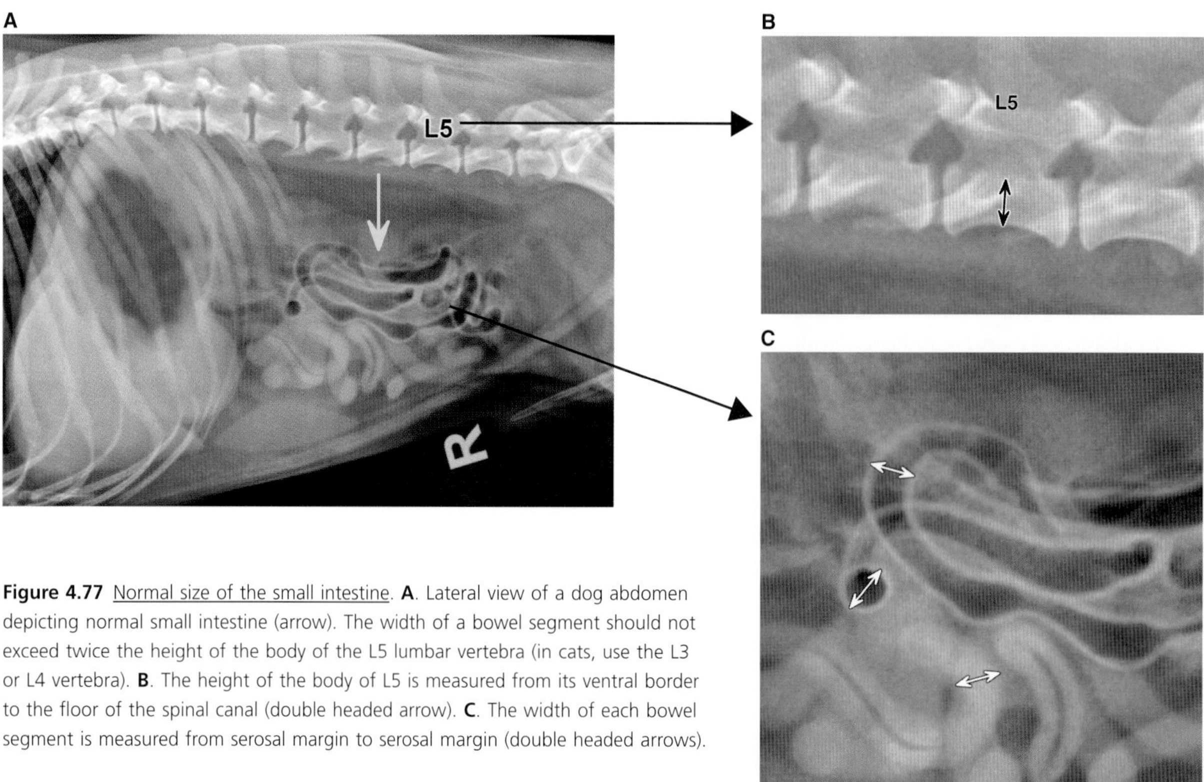

Figure 4.77 Normal size of the small intestine. **A**. Lateral view of a dog abdomen depicting normal small intestine (arrow). The width of a bowel segment should not exceed twice the height of the body of the L5 lumbar vertebra (in cats, use the L3 or L4 vertebra). **B**. The height of the body of L5 is measured from its ventral border to the floor of the spinal canal (double headed arrow). **C**. The width of each bowel segment is measured from serosal margin to serosal margin (double headed arrows).

One method to evaluate the size (diameter, width) of the small intestine is to compare bowel width to the height of a middle lumbar vertebral body (Figure 4.77). Bowel width that exceeds twice the height of the vertebral body may be considered abnormally distended. As with most radiography "rules of thumb", this is a guideline and not an absolute rule. In most cats, normal small bowel width should not exceed 12 mm.

Abnormal dilation of the small intestine is due to ileus. **Ileus** is a motility disorder that leads to bowel stasis, a condition in which the intestinal contents do not progress normally through the intestinal tract. Ileus may be caused by a physical blockage or a functional problem. Physical blockages are called *obstructive, mechanical,* or *dynamic* ileus. Functional problems are due to abnormal peristalsis and are called *functional, paralytic,* or *adynamic* ileus. Some authors use the word "obstruction" to describe a physical blockage and "ileus" to describe a motility disorder (due to something other than a blockage). Obstructive and functional ileus are difficult to distinguish in survey radiographs. Serial imaging often is helpful to monitor the sizes of the bowel segments and to determine whether or not there is aboral movement of intestinal contents. Persistence of abnormal appearing bowel over a 24 to 48 hour period is indicative of ileus.

Bowel wall thickness seldom can be accurately assessed in survey radiographs because the mucosal margin rarely is reliably identified. Fluid in the bowel lumen is the same opacity as the mucosa and the two blend together. Fluid adjacent to the mucosa can be mistaken for a thickened bowel wall (Figure 4.78). To accurately evaluate intestinal wall thickness, the bowel lumen must be filled with gas or a positive contrast medium. When abnormal

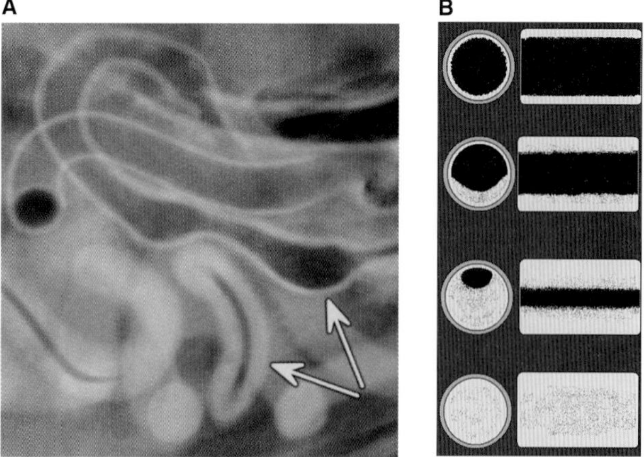

Figure 4.78 Bowel wall thickness. **A**. Same lateral view as in Figure 4.77. The bowel wall thickness appears to differ between segments of small intestine (arrows). This is an artifact caused by fluid in the bowel lumen. **B**. Illustration depicting cross-sectional and longitudinal views of a small bowel segment containing different volumes of fluid and gas. Fluid blends with the mucosal margin to create the appearance of a thickened bowel wall. (Special thanks to Dr. Tim O'Brien for the illustration.)

A

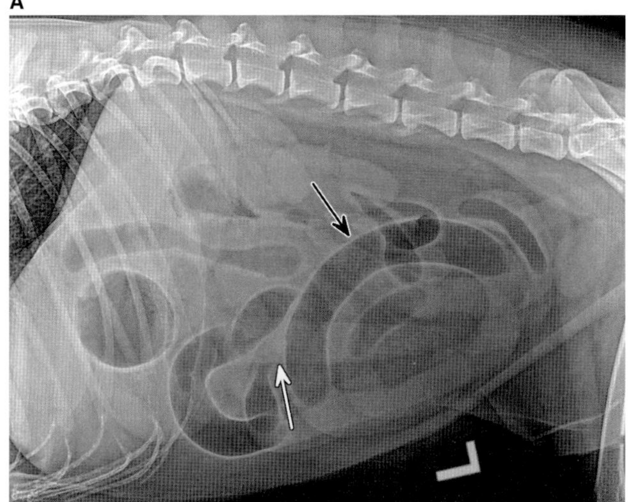

B

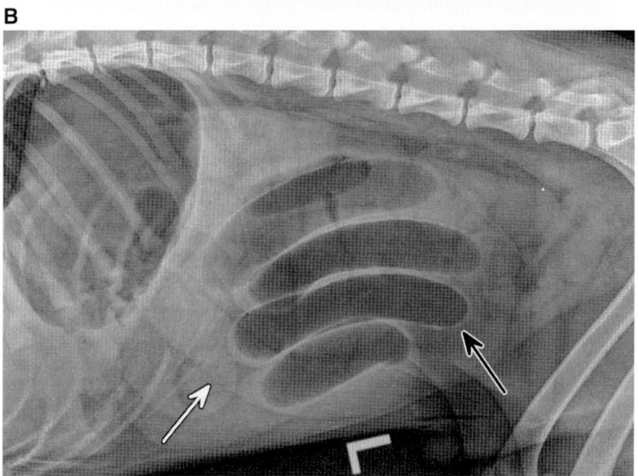

Figure 4.79 Obstructive ileus. **A**. Lateral view of a dog abdomen depicting abnormally dilated small intestine. Bowel segments are both gas-filled (black arrow) and fluid-filled (white arrow). **B**. Lateral view depicting stacking or layering of both gas-filled bowel segments (black arrow) and fluid-filled segments (white arrow). The fluid-filled bowel segments are less obvious.

bowel wall thickening is present, it most often is due to inflammation (enteritis) or infiltrative disease. The two cannot be differentiated in radiographs.

Obstructive ileus

Physical blockage of the small intestine usually leads to dilation of the bowel proximal to the obstruction. The dilated bowel may be filled with fluid, gas, food, or a combination of these. Bowel segments distal to the obstruction often are normal size. Fluid-distended intestines tend to be less obvious in radiographs than gas-distended bowel. It is important to carefully examine the soft tissue opacity intestinal segments for abnormal size (Figure 4.79).

The degree of small bowel dilation depends on the location, duration, and completeness of the obstruction. Proximal obstructions (closer to the stomach) may result in little or no abnormal bowel distention because gas and fluid can move back into the stomach and be vomited. Sometimes a proximal obstruction will result in medial displacement of the descending duodenum. Chronic proximal obstructions can lead to gastric atony and persistent distention of the stomach.

More distal obstructions (in the jejunum) generally produce uneven bowel distention. Intestinal widths can vary greatly. Bowel segments proximal to the obstruction usually are significantly larger than those distal to it. In some cases, the degree of small bowel dilation makes it difficult to distinguish small intestine from colon in survey radiographs. In these cases, the colon may be identified after infusing a small volume of contrast medium via the rectum.

The gravel sign (Figure 4.58) sometimes is present near the site of a small bowel obstruction, particularly in patients with chronic, incomplete blockages.

Small intestine that continues to distend may become layered or stacked. This is because the dilated bowel segments must execute tight, hairpin turns to fit within the limited space of the abdominal cavity (Figure 4.79). Bowel distention this severe usually requires immediate surgical intervention.

Horizontal beam radiography (Figure 2.15) sometimes is used to detect gas-capped fluid lines in static bowel segments (Figure 4.80). It has been suggested that gas:fluid lines at variable levels is more likely to indicate obstructive ileus,

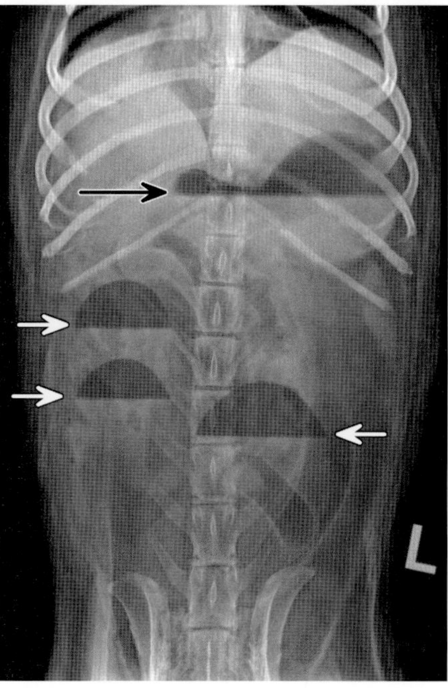

Figure 4.80 Horizontal beam radiograph. VD view of a dog abdomen made with the patient held erect and the x-ray beam directed horizontally. Gas-capped fluid levels are depicted in several abnormally distended segments of small intestine (white arrows). A normal gas:fluid level is depicted in the stomach (black arrow).

whereas lines at the same level are more likely to represent functional ileus.

Functional ileus

Abnormal bowel function due to uncoordinated, weak, or absent peristalsis can lead to intestinal stasis and dilatation, i.e., a functional ileus. Unlike obstructive ileus, the bowel lumen remains patent; there is no physical blockage. The causes of functional ileus are numerous, including inflammation, trauma, electrolyte imbalances, pharmaceutical responses, vascular compromise, neuromuscular disease, and others (see differential diagnoses).

Functional ileus typically appears as mostly gas-distended intestines that are all similar in size (Figure 4.81). There is no layering or stacking and bowel distention tends to be less severe than with obstructive ileus. Untreated functional ileus, however, can progress to more severe bowel dilation that may eventually resemble an obstructive pattern.

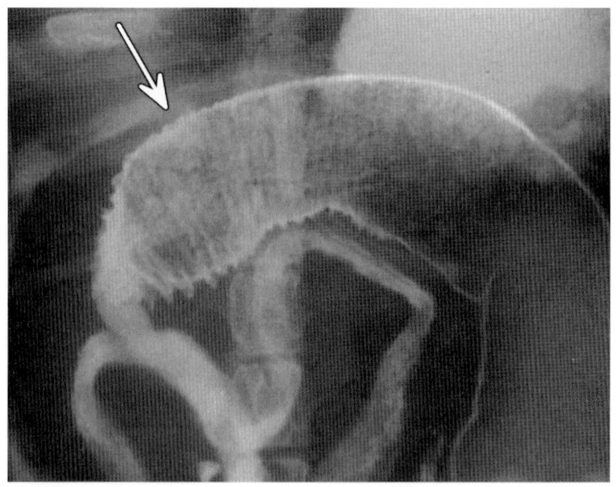

Figure 4.82 Intestinal ischemia. VD view of a dog abdomen depicting a dilated segment of small intestine with irregular margins that appear corrugated (white arrow).

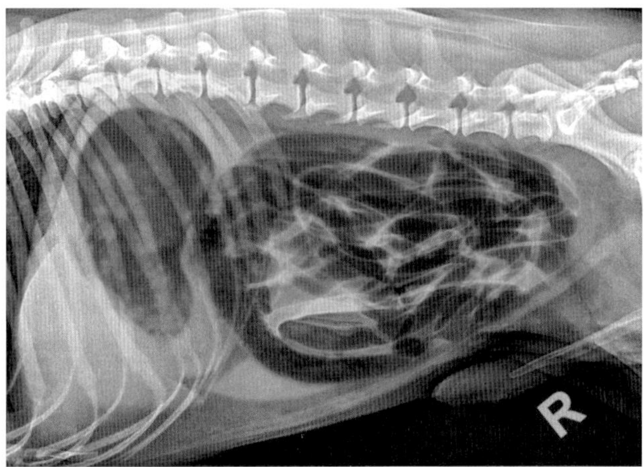

Figure 4.81 Functional ileus. Lateral view of a dog abdomen depicting uniform dilation of the small intestine. The gas-distended bowel segments are evenly distributed and similar in size.

Functional ileus can affect part or all of the small intestine. Pancreatitis is a common cause of localized functional ileus. As described earlier, a key radiographic finding of localized ileus is the sentinel loop, which again is an intestinal segment that remains relatively unchanged in serial radiographs.

The intestinal serosal margins in patients with funcitonal ileus sometimes are irreguar or indistinct (Figure 4.82), especially in cases of severe inflammation, ischemia, or infiltrative disease. Neoplasia can create multiple, persistent indentations in the bowel wall that resemble a corrugated pattern or "thumb prints" (Figure 4.91). Rarely, severe inflammation or infiltrative disease can lead to loss of mucosal integrity and gas in the bowel wall (i.e., *intestinal pneumatosis*, as shown in Figure 4.83).

A

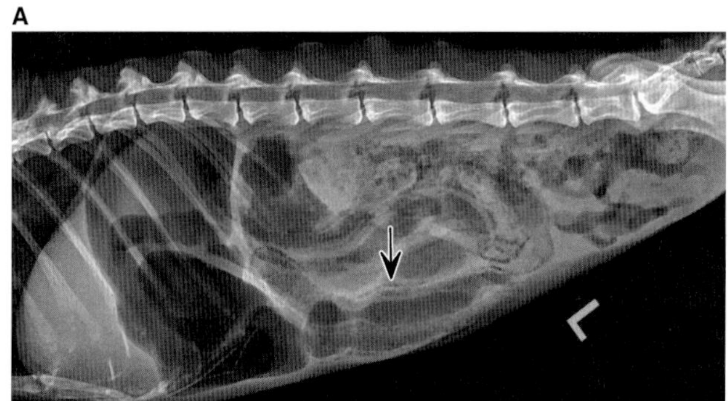

B

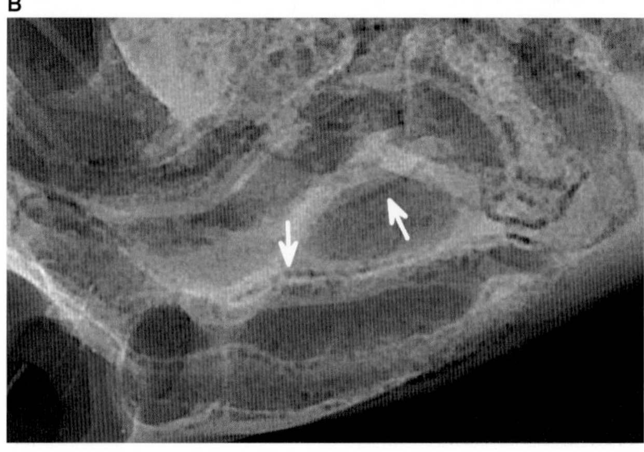

Figure 4.83 Intestinal pneumatosis. **A**. Lateral view of a cat abdomen depicting a functional ileus with gas in the small bowel wall (arrow). **B**. Cropped and enlarged part of radiograph A. Gas in the bowel wall (arrows) is due to mucosal damage caused by severe enteritis. due to severe enteritis and damage to the mucosa.

Mesenteric volvulus

Mesenteric volvulus occurs when the small intestine rotates around the root of the mesentery. Rotation restricts blood flow to the small bowel resulting in a functional ileus. In the initial radiographs, the small intestine often is uniformly distended with gas and fluid. However, dilation progresses rapidly and in radiographs made as soon as 1–2 hours later the sizes of the small bowel segments may have increased dramatically. Peritoneal effusion usually is present and also progressive. Mesenteric volvulus may be accompanied by torsion of other organs. Pneumoperitoneum may be present due to bowel rupture. Patients with mesenteric volvulus frequently present as an emergency and in a life-threatening situation.

Enteritis

Small bowel inflammation rarely produces diagnostic radiographic findings. The bowel wall may be thickened and the small intestine may contain more fluid or gas than expected. Fluid-filled bowel is often seen in patients with diarrhea; however, it is difficult to distinguish thickening of the bowel wall from fluid in the bowel lumen with survey radiographs. Gas-filled bowel may be more significant in cats than in dogs because cats tend to swallow less air than dogs. Enteritis sometimes creates the appearance of turgid bowel segments with increased tonus, but this is a subjective assessment that is based on experience.

Abnormal opacity or content in the small intestine

The small intestine usually contains some fluid and gas, but rarely a significant amount of ingesta. Bowel gas tends to be more plentiful in dogs than in cats. A larger than expected volume of gas may or may not be clinically significant. Panting animals can swallow large volumes of air. Unless the bowel is abnormally distended, intestinal gas may be incidental. Even extreme amounts of air swallowing will not dilate a normal intestine. Other causes of extensive gas in the small intestine (other than aerophagia) include a recent enema, enteritis, and early ileus.

A persistently irregular intestinal gas pattern, one that does not resemble normal physiology or biology, is concerning for pathology (e.g., foreign material, mural lesion). Gas in the bowel wall is uncommon, but can result from damage to the mucosa (e.g., passage of sharp materials, severe enteritis, infiltrative bowel disease).

Foreign materials in the small intestine sometimes are recognized by their opacity, pattern, or when they are outlined by gas or positive contrast medium. Mineral and metal opacity materials usually are readily identified in survey radiographs. Some foods and medications contain mineral opacity materials. Bone fragments are a frequent finding in the GI tracts of dogs and cats. Pay attention to gastric contents since they usually pass into the small intestine. Metal opacity material generally is either a foreign object or a contrast medium. Mineral and metal opacity structures located outside the intestines may be mistaken for abnormal content (e.g., calculi, dystrophic mineralization, surgical implants).

Some soft tissue opacity materials in the small intestine produce a characteristic pattern. Corn cob pieces, for example, appear as regularly repeating pockets of gas (Figure 4.84). Cloth or fabric may appear as a mottled, linear, or streaked gas pattern, particularly when the material is not saturated with fluids (Figures 4.85 and 4.86). Occasionally a soft tissue opacity object is identified because it is outlined by intestinal gas (Figure 4.87).

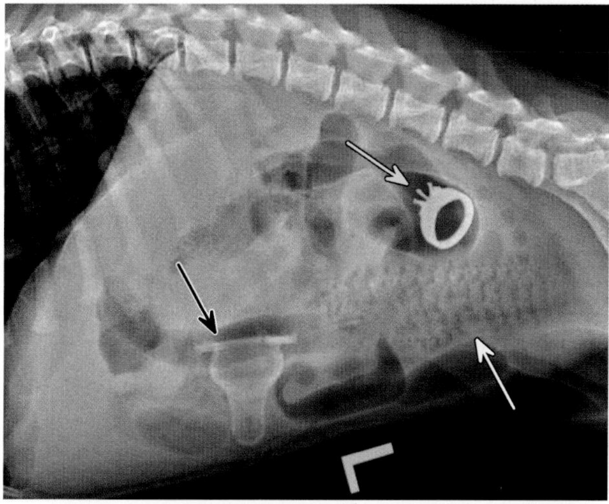

Figure 4.84 Foreign objects in the small intestine. Lateral view of a dog abdomen depicting various ingested foreign objects, including a pacifier nipple (black arrow), diamond ring (yellow arrow), and a large piece of corn cob (white arrow).

Upper GI study

The procedure for an upper GI study, as well as its indications and contraindications, can be found in the contrast radiography section of Chapter 2. Prior to performing an upper GI study in a patient with suspected ileus, both the clinician and the owner must consider the stress to the patient, the amount of time required, and the expense of the contrast study compared to an exploratory laparotomy.

A normal upper GI study is depicted in Figure 4.88. The small intestine is even and flowing with no sharp turns and no segment larger than twice the diameter of any other segment. Normal bowel peristalsis produces transient narrowing which varies between radiographs. The mucosal margin may appear slightly hazy, irregular, or spiculated, particularly in younger animals, due to the numerous tiny villi or *fimbria* that project into the bowel lumen (Figure 4.89).

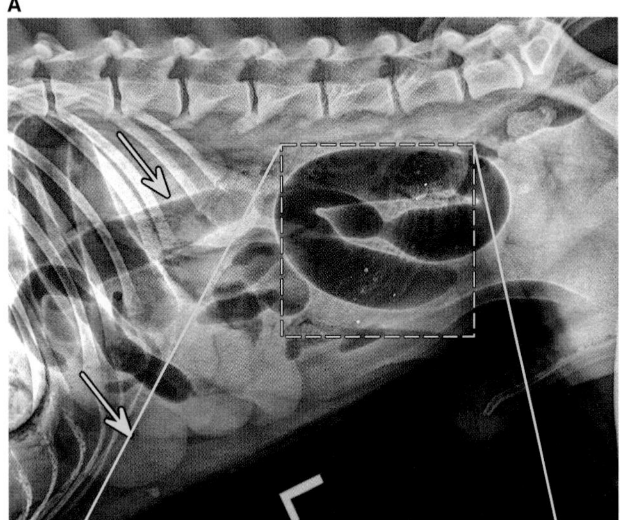

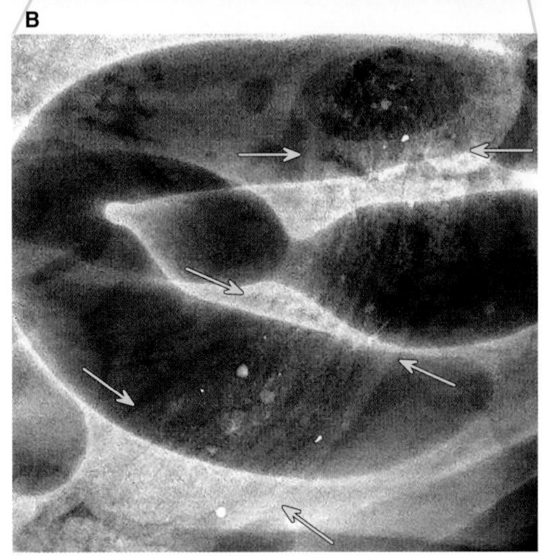

Figure 4.85 Fabric foreign material. **A**. Lateral view of a dog abdomen depicting dilation of the small intestine due to obstructive ileus (arrows). **B**. Cropped and enlarged section of the radiograph depicting the striated pattern of gas and soft tissue opacities that is characteristic of ingested cloth material (arrows).

Filling defects in an upper GI study may be caused by material in the bowel lumen, thickening of the bowel wall, or external compression (e.g. stricture, adjacent mass effect). Defects caused by ingesta in the bowel lumen often are difficult to differentiate from pathology. Thickening of the bowel wall may be localized or diffuse, unilateral or bilateral. Mural masses typically produce focal, unilateral filling defects with even margins that gradually taper on either end. If the mucosa is ulcerated or otherwise damaged, the margin may be more irregular. At the site of a mass the bowel lumen may unilaterally narrow or the lumen may appear to deviate to the opposite side. Circumferential or annular thickening of the bowel wall tends to produce narrowing from both sides, sometimes with a very irregular or corrugated mucosal border (Figure 4.91).

Barium suspensions sometimes break apart in the intestinal tract, creating a mottled or "cobblestone" pattern called **flocculation** (Figure 4.92). Flocculation tends to occur in areas of severe inflammation or excess mucous production. A pattern that resembles flocculation can occur when barium mixes with ingesta or due to a very irregular or ulcerated mucosal margin. Larger mucosal ulcers will persist in multiple radiographs as out-pouches of barium that extend away from the bowel lumen.

An upper GI study provides some information about **small intestinal transit time** (the amount of time required for the contrast medium to pass through the small intestine). A transit time that is shorter than expected (contrast medium passes more quickly through the bowel) generally is due to hyperperistalsis. More frequent intestinal contractions most often occur in bowel that is inflamed or irritated. A longer than expected transit time (passage of contrast medium is delayed) usually is due to reduced or ineffective peristalsis, (i.e., ileus).

In patients with obstructive ileus, contrast medium typically fills the dilated bowel segments proximal to the blockage. Filling may not occur when the flow of contrast is impeded by trapped gas, fluid, or ingesta. Distal to the blockage, contrast medium may or may not be visible, depending on the degree of obstruction. In patients with functional ileus the affected bowel segments tend to fill more slowly and less completely.

Linear foreign material

Ingested string-like materials (e.g., thread, carpet fiber, dental floss) can lead to an obstructive ileus when the proximal end of the string is fixed in position and the distal portion extends into the small intestine. Typically, the proximal end is wrapped around the base of the tongue or anchored in the stomach. Normal peristalsis causes the bowel to "climb up" the distal portion of the linear material and bunch together. The obstruction caused by linear foreign material usually is partial and seldom is the bowel abnormally dilated. A complete obstruction, however, can occur. Continued peristalsis creates a sawing action against the string-like material, which gradually erodes the bowel wall. Perforation of the bowel generally results in peritonitis and pneumoperitoneum.

In radiographs, the bowel segments that contain linear material appear bunched together in a plicated or pleated pattern that may resemble a "scrunchie" hair tie (Figure 4.94). Generally, there is little to no visible content in the plicated bowel other than a few small, irregular-shaped pockets of gas. The gas pockets tend to be crescent-shaped or comma-shaped and more peripheral in the bowel than the rounded and centrally located gas bubbles seen in normal intestine. The serosal

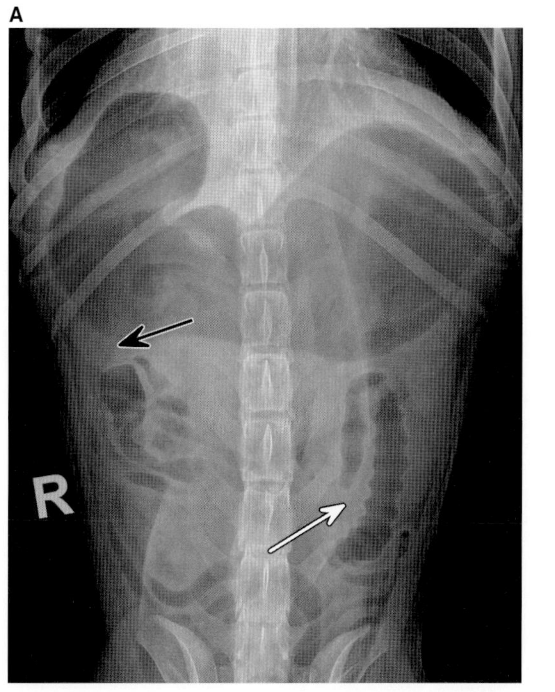

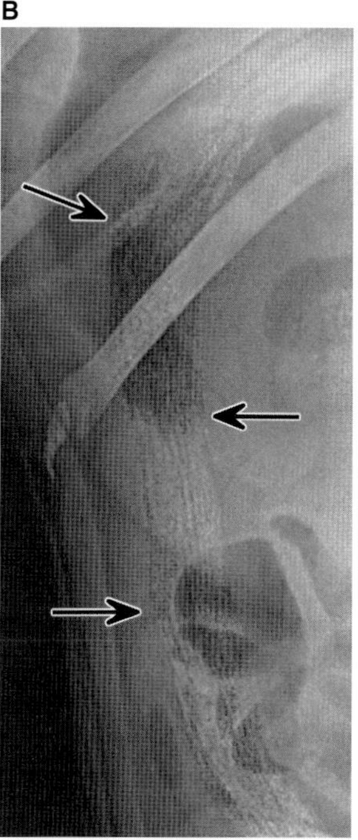

Figure 4.86 Fabric foreign material. **A**. VD view of a dog abdomen depicting the characteristic striated pattern of ingested cloth material in the descending duodenum (black arrow). The stomach is moderately distended with mostly gas. **B**. Cropped and enlarged section of the radiograph depicting a more detailed image of the striated pattern (arrows). In **A**, there is a gas-filled, hyperperistaltic segment of small intestine in the left caudal abdomen (white arrow). Follow-up radiographs would be helpful to differentiate normal peristalsis from pathology in this segment.

margins of the plicated bowel often are indistinct due to visceral crowding or adjacent fluid (e.g., peritonitis, peritoneal effusion). An upper GI study aids in making the diagnosis when the intestinal margins are not well-visualized in survey radiographs (Figures 4.95–4.97).

In obese patients, crowding of the small intestine may be mistaken for plication. Although the excess intra-abdominal fat confines the bowel to a smaller area, the serosal margins and luminal gas patterns remain even and flowing without tight turns.

In an upper GI study of many cats, the normal pattern of segmental contractions along the descending duodenum may be mistaken for intestinal plication (Figure 4.90). In some cats, a normal mucosal fold in the duodenum creates a linear filling defect (known as the *"pseudo-string sign"*), but there is no scrunching of the bowel.

Intussusception

An intussusception occurs when one segment of small intestine slides or "telescopes" into the lumen of an adjacent segment (Figure 4.98). The result is partial or complete bowel obstruction and compromised blood supply to the affected bowel. An intussusception can occur anywhere in the GI tract, but most often in the jejunum.

It is difficult to distinguish an intussusception from other causes of obstructive ileus with survey radiographs alone. Sometimes the curved margin of the inner bowel segment is outlined by a pocket of gas, appearing as a smooth-bordered soft tissue opacity structure within a distended bowel segment. In many cases, contrast radiography is needed to make the diagnosis.

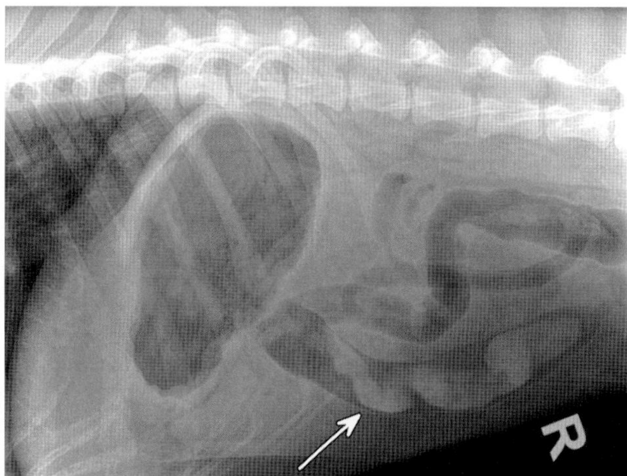

Figure 4.87 Small bowel foreign material. Lateral view of a dog abdomen depicting a soft tissue opacity object in the descending duodenum (arrow points to a sock). It is unusual to see soft tissue opacity materials this well outlined by intestinal gas.

In an upper GI study of a patient with complete obstruction, the contrast medium ends abruptly at the intussusception. With a partial obstruction, a thin line of contrast medium may be visible in the narrow lumen of the intussusceptum. If an ileocolic intussusception is suspected, a barium enema is more likely to demonstrate the lesion than an upper GI study (Figure 4.112). An ileocolic intussusception can prevent gas from entering the cecum and ascending colon.

Large intestine

Normal radiographic anatomy

The large intestine includes the *cecum, colon,* and *rectum.* These parts of the large intestine usually can be identified in survey radiographs based on their location, size, and shape (Figure 4.99).

A

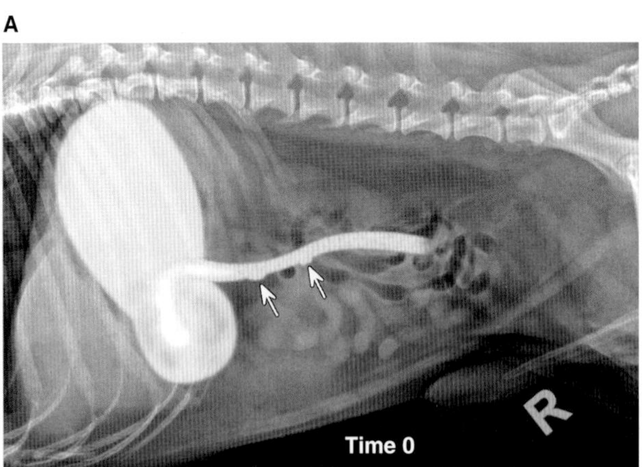

Time 0: barium is visible in the stomach and duodenum. Pseudoulcers along the descending duodenum produce barium filled out pouches (arrows).

B

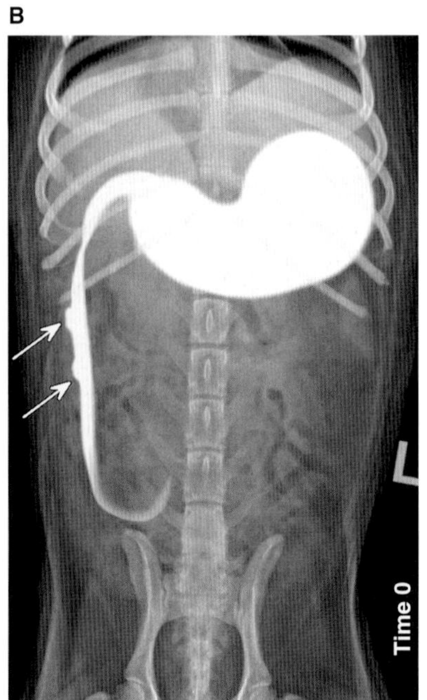

C

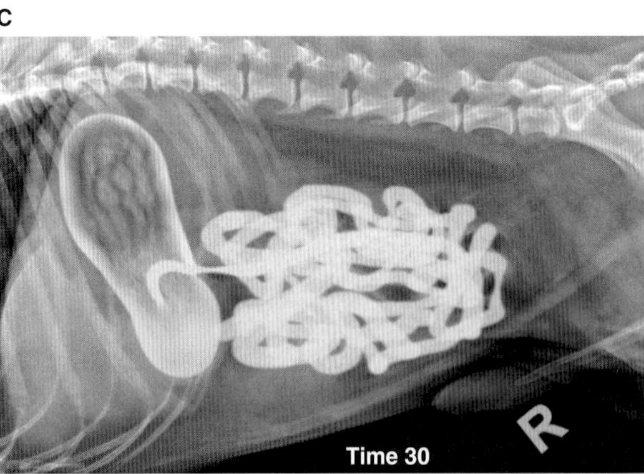

Time 30: barium is visible throughout most of the jejunum and there is less barium in the stomach.

D

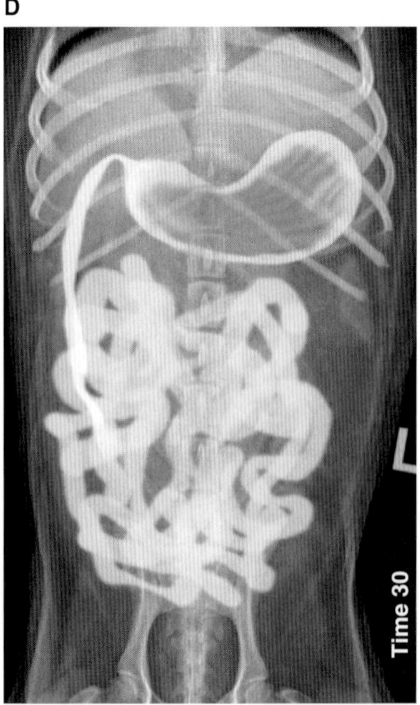

Figure 4.88 Normal upper GI study. Lateral and VD views of a dog abdomen depicting the passage of barium through a normal GI tract. Radiographs **A** and **B** were made immediately after dosing (Time 0) and radiographs **C** and **D** were made 30 minutes later (Time 30), as indicated by the labels in each radiograph.

E

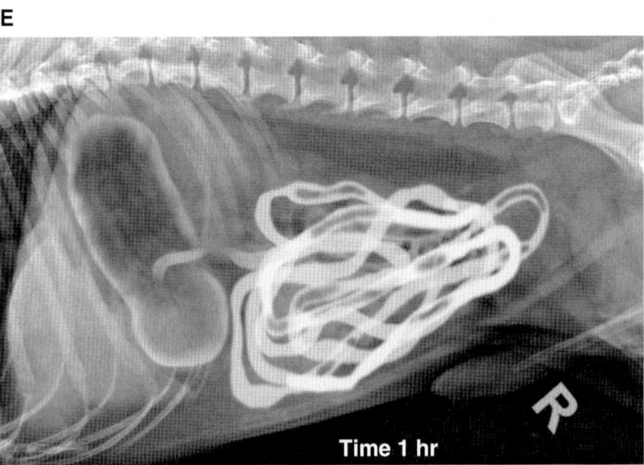

F

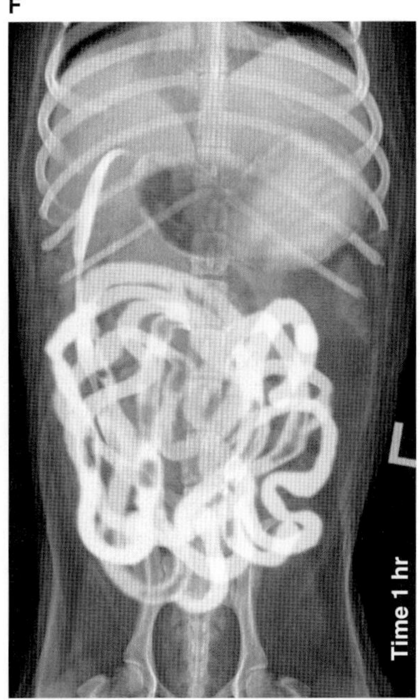

Time 1 hour: the stomach is mostly empty of barium. The majority of the small bowel is opacified, but barium has not yet reached the colon.

G

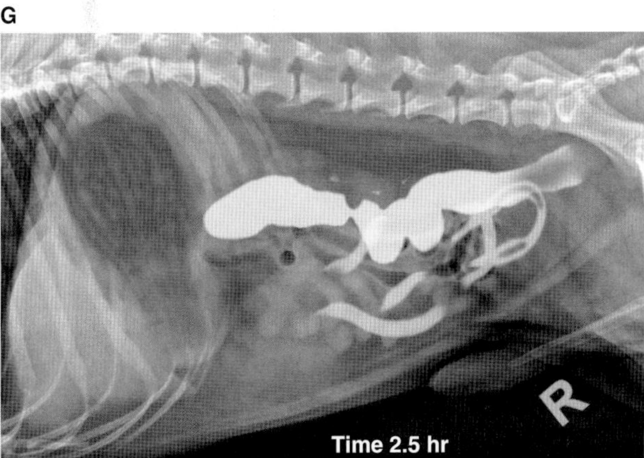

H

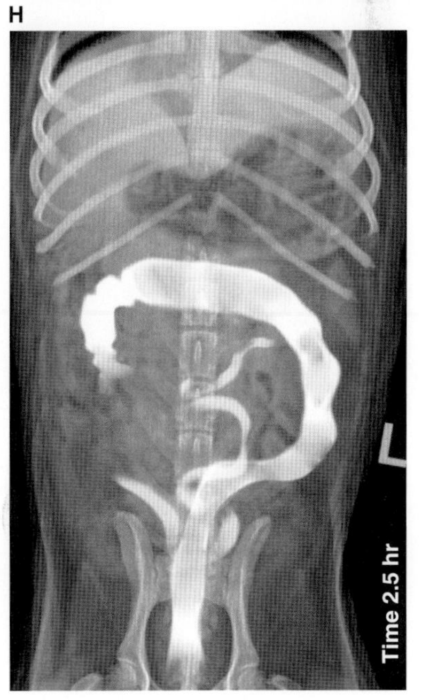

Time 2.5 hours: barium is visible in the colon. The stomach is virtually empty and a small amount of barium remains in the small intestine.

Figure 4.88 (cont.) Normal upper GI study. Lateral and VD views of a dog abdomen depicting the continued passage of barium through a normal GI tract. Radiographs **E** and **F** were made 60 minutes after dosing (Time 1 hr) and radiographs **G** and **H** were made 90 minutes later (Time 2.5 hr), as indicated by the labels in each radiograph.

The **cecum** is a diverticulum of the proximal colon. It is located right of midline in the mid-to-cranial abdomen. The radiographic appearance of the cecum differs between dogs and cats. The canine cecum is compartmentalized and frequently contains gas, appearing as a C-shaped or corkscrew-shaped structure that is joined to the ascending colon via the cecocolic junction. The feline cecum seldom is identified in radiographs. It is a simple comma-shaped extension of the ascending colon without divisions and without a defined cecocolic junction. The cecum in cats rarely contains enough gas or ingesta to be distinguished (Figure 4.100).

The colon usually contains some gas and/or feces, making it identifiable in survey radiographs. It is difficult to reliably assess colon wall thickness, however, because feces tends to be the same opacity as the mucosa. The colon is

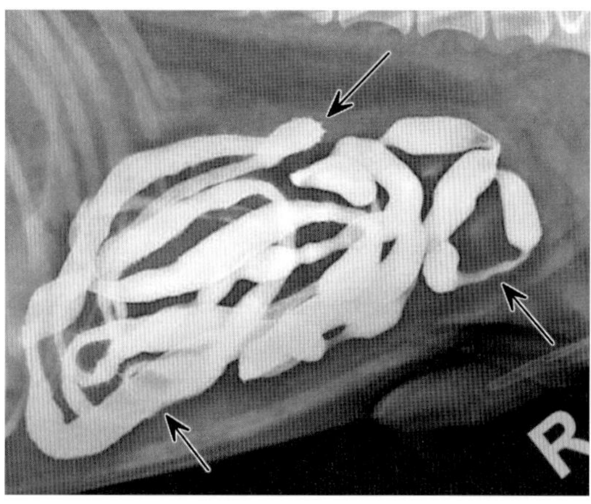

Figure 4.89 Fimbria. Lateral view of a dog abdomen depicting a normal upper GI study. Intestinal villi project into the bowel lumen to create tiny, spiculated filling defects along the mucosal margin (black arrows).

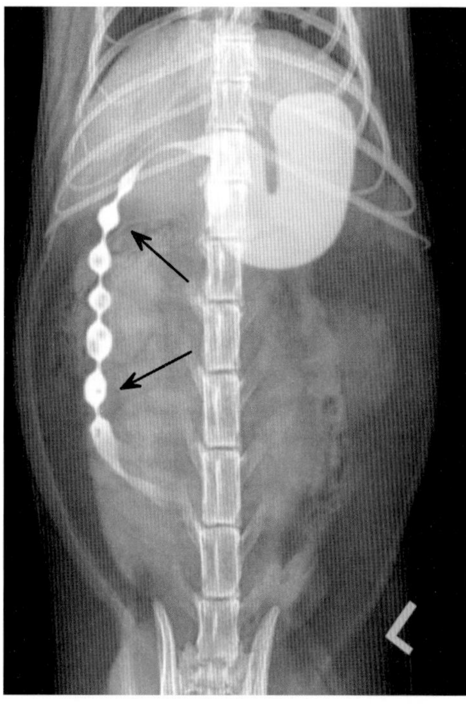

Figure 4.90 String of pearls. VD view of a cat abdomen depicting a normal upper GI study. The circular pattern of segmental peristalsis along the descending duodenum (arrows) is common in cats and known as the *string of pearls* sign.

divided into *ascending, transverse,* and *descending* parts. Together these parts are shaped like a "shepherd's crook" or a "question mark."

The short **ascending colon** runs cranially from the cecum to the transverse colon. It is located right of midline and medial to the descending duodenum. The ileum joins the ascending colon at the ileocolic junction.

The **transverse colon** runs across midline from the ascending colon to the descending colon. It is located caudal to the greater curvature of the stomach. The pancreas lies between the transverse colon and the stomach.

The **descending colon** runs caudally from the transverse colon to the rectum. It generally is positioned left of midline but, because it is more mobile than the other parts of the colon, it may be located on midline or right of midline. In some cats and dogs, the descending colon is excessively long or **redundant**. This is a normal variation that allows even greater mobility (Figure 4.101).

The **rectum** begins at the pelvic inlet and runs caudally from the distal colon to the anal canal. It is located on

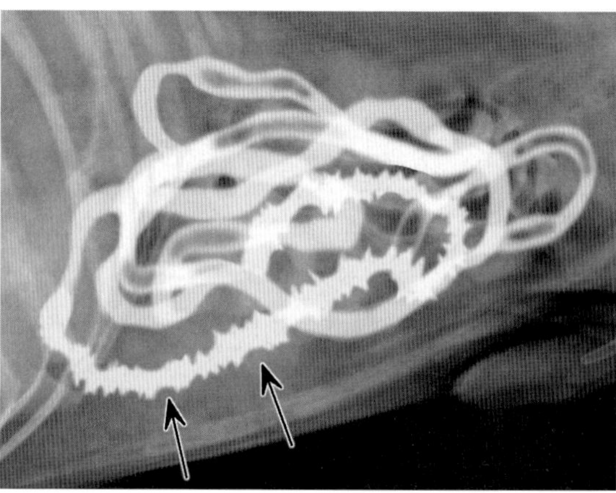

Figure 4.91 Corrugated bowel. Lateral view of a dog abdomen depicting an abnormal upper GI study. The mucosal border along a segment of jejunum is markedly irregular with numerous indentations that resemble "thumb imprints" (black arrows). This finding is typical of an annular, infiltrative disease (e.g., neoplasia, mycosis).

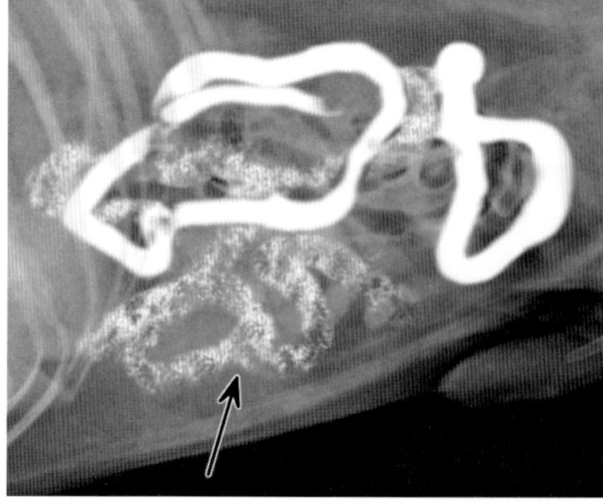

Figure 4.92 Flocculation. Lateral view of a dog abdomen depicting a barium upper GI study. There is a mottled or speckled pattern in the jejunum (black arrow) caused by flocculation of the barium mixture.

CHAPTER 4

A

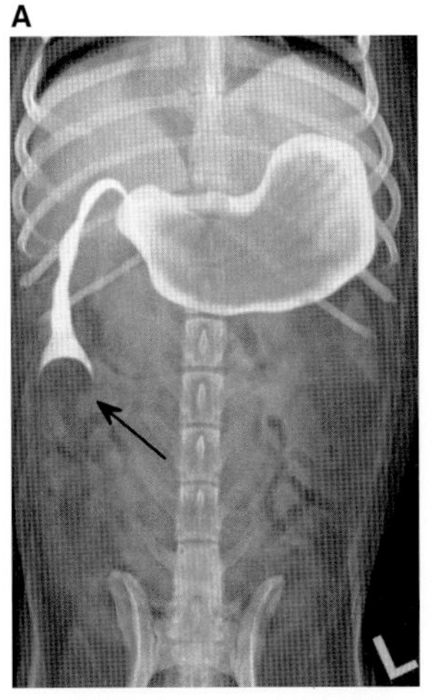

B

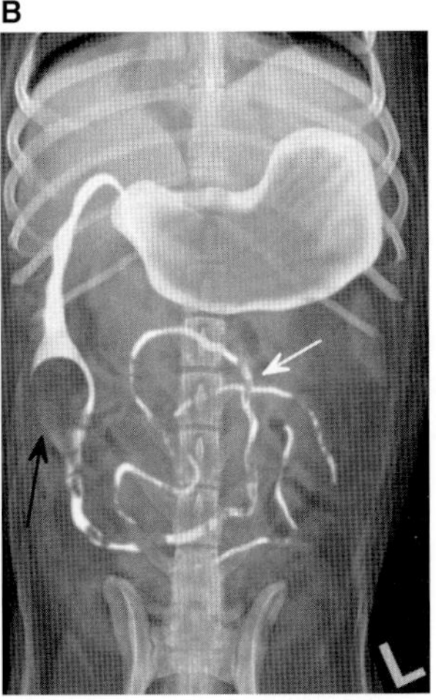

Figure 4.93 Complete vs. partial intestinal obstruction. **A**. VD view of a dog upper GI study depicting a complete blockage in the descending duodenum. The blockage prevents barium from passing into the more distal small intestine. The rounded proximal edge of the obstructing object is outlined by barium (may be a rubber ball, fruit pit, etc.). **B**. VD view of an upper GI study depicting an incomplete blockage in the proximal duodenum (black arrow). Some of the barium is able to pass into the jejunum (white arrow). The transit time, however, most likely is delayed.

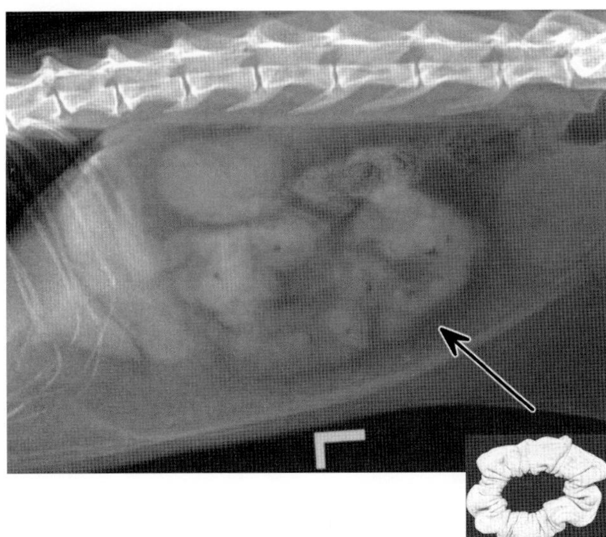

Figure 4.94 Linear foreign material. Lateral view of a cat abdomen depicting plication of the small intesine (arrow). The bowel is "scrunched" together, resembling a "scrunchie" hair tie (inset photo). Notice the tiny, crescent-shaped gas bubbles in the plicated bowel. The bubbles do not resemble a normal intestinal gas pattern.

midline in the pelvic canal, between the pubis and the sacrum. The rectum may be displaced or compressed by enlargement of nearby structures, such as the prostate gland, cervix, vagina, and regional lymph nodes.

Abnormal position or shape of large intestine

The large intestine is easily displaced in a variety of directions by physiologic or pathologic enlargement of nearby structures or due to loss of abdominal integrity (see differential diagnoses).

Non-visualization of the colon may be because it is empty or because other structures are superimposed. Compression radiography is a simple technique that can be used to displace overlying structures and improve visualization of the colon (Figure 2.19). A colon that contains only fluid may blend with adjacent soft tissues and can be difficult to identify unless it is surrounded by fat. When the colon is not recognized in survey radiographs, a small volume of gas or

A

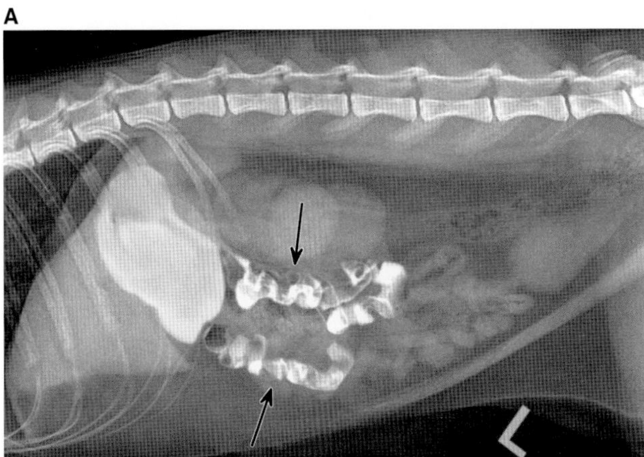

B

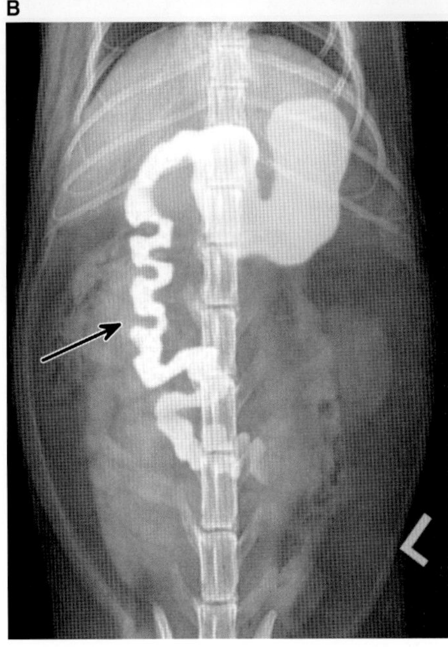

Figure 4.95 Linear Foreign material. Lateral view (**A**) and VD view (**B**) of cat abdomen depicting an upper GI study. The descending duodenum is tortuous with multiple back-and-forth tight turns, i.e., plication (arrow).

A

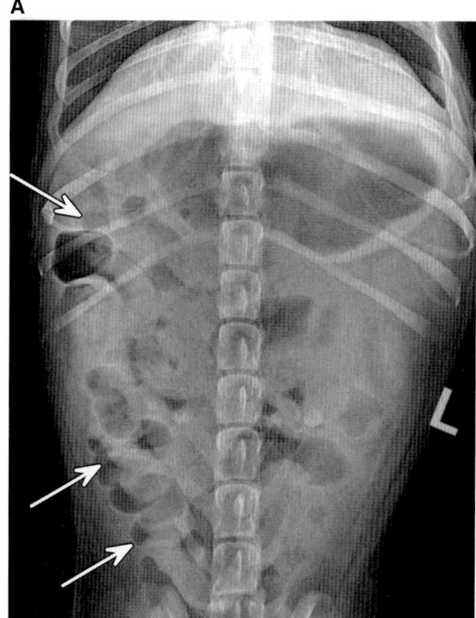

B

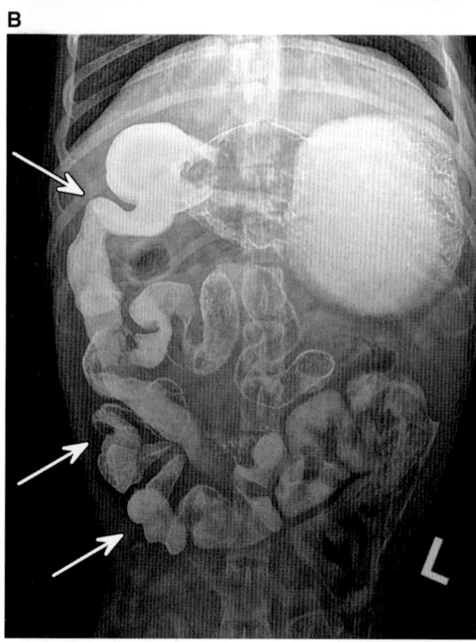

Figure 4.96 Linear foreign material. **A**. Survey radiograph VD view of a dog abdomen depicting an irregular intestinal gas pattern (arrows). **B**. Upper GI VD view of the same dog depicting tight, tortuous turns and bunching in the duodenum and jejunum (arrows).

positive contrast medium can be infused per rectum and the radiographs repeated (Figure 4.102).

Abnormal size of large intestine

The diameter (width) of the colon naturally varies with the volume of its contents and normal peristalsis. It has been reported that a colon width that exceeds three times the width of the small intestine or two times the length of the L7 lumbar vertebra is abnormally distended (note: L7 sometimes is congenitally shortened). Abnormal narrowing or dilation of the colon will persist in serial radiographs, whereas physiologic variations are temporary.

Physiologic narrowing of the colon may be due to a spasm. **Colon spasms** are transient, but tend to persist longer than peristaltic contractions and may produce significant narrowing (Figure 4.105). They can result from severe inflammation or mechanical irritation (e.g., rectal palpation, inserting a catheter, performing an enema, infusing a cold liquid). Patient sedation or anesthesia usually prevents spasms.

A

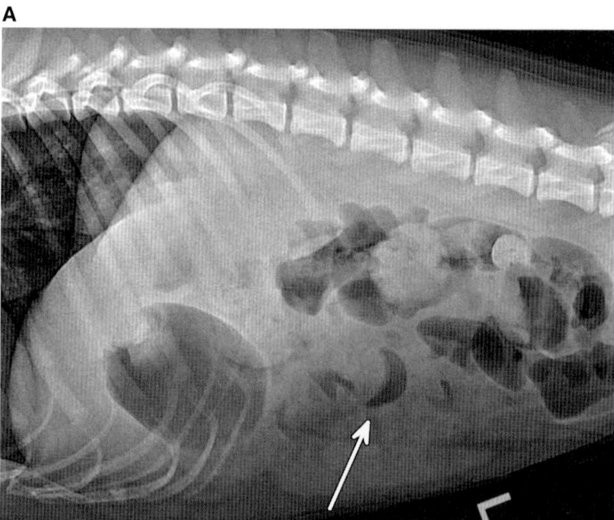

B

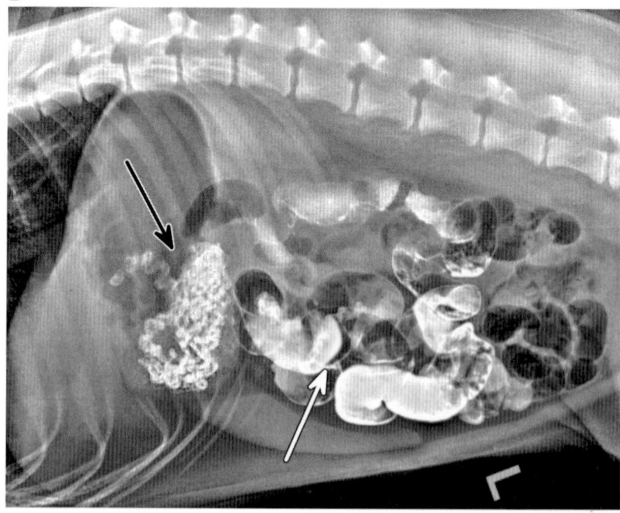

Figure 4.97 Linear foreign material. **A**. Survey lateral view of a dog abdomen depicting indistinct intestinal serosal margins and an atypical crescent-shaped pocket of gas (arrow). **B**. Lateral view of the same dog during an upper GI study. The crescent gas pocket is again visible (white arrow) along with bunching of the small intestine. Some curvilinear material is present in the stomach (black arrow). The material is carpet fibers that are anchored in the stomach and extend into the small intestine. The carpet fibers were masked when the stomach was filled with barium, but are now visible because most of the barium has exited the stomach (some barium remains adhered to the fibers).

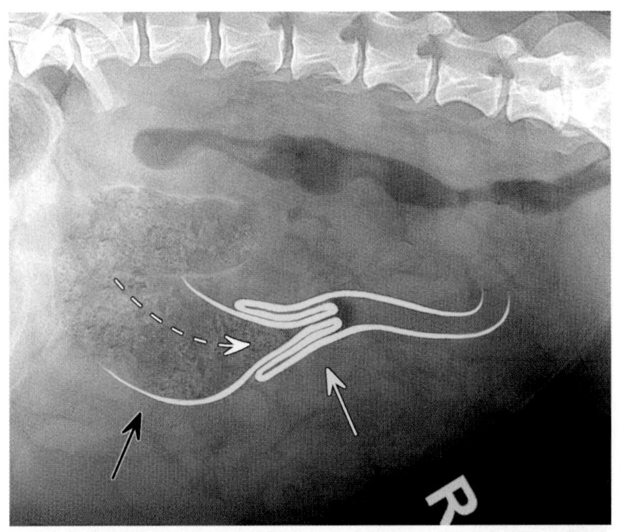

Figure 4.98 Intussusception. Lateral view of a dog abdomen depicting a segment of jejunum (black arrow) sliding into the lumen of a distal jejunal segment (yellow arrow). The bowel walls are highlighted for illustration purposes. The proximal segment is distended with ingesta due to narrowing and obstruction at the intussusception.

Pathologic narrowing of the colon may be due to a stricture, a thickened wall, a mural mass, foreign material, or external compression. The lesion site may not be evident in survey radiographs. Colonography can help locate and define the size of the lesion and the degree of mural involvement. Chronic or repeated episodes of severe colitis can lead to regional or diffuse thickening of the colon wall as well as an irregular mucosal margin and shortening of the colon (Figures 4.106, 4.107, 4.109). In patients with severe colitis, parts of the colon may become atonic, in which case they appear similar in size, shape, and content in serial radiographs. Infiltrative diseases of the colon (e.g., neoplasia, mycosis) and chronic colitis may produce similar radiographic findings. In both cases, the sublumbar lymph nodes sometimes enlarge.

Dilation of the colon generally is evident in survey radiographs. Dilation may result from a physical obstruction or a functional problem caused by ineffective peristalsis. The colon may be distended with gas, fluid, feces, or a combination of these. Feces that is more opaque than expected may be due to constipation or obstipation (Figures 4.103 and 4.104). The increase in fecal opacity results from continued absorbtion of water. Opaque feces also may result from ingested bone materials or a recent upper GI study.

Physical obstructions in the colon may be caused by abnormal narrowing of the lumen, material blocking the lumen, or pathology in the pelvic canal (e.g., fracture, mass). Greater than 50% narrowing of the pelvic canal frequently leads to constipation or obstipation.

Functional problems that lead to colon dilation are labeled megacolon. **Megacolon** is dilation in the absence of a physical obstruction. It is caused by decreased motility in the large intestine, which can result from a number of conditions (see differential diagnoses). In patients with megacolon, the rectum may be normal. In radiographs of these patients, the distended colon typically tapers abruptly at the rectum.

Determining the cause of constipation or a dilated colon often is not possible with radiographs alone. Follow-up radiographs may provide some diagnostic information. After the initial radiographs, empty the colon and repeat the study in a few days or weeks, depending on the patient's condition. If constipation quickly recurs, then causes for megacolon should be investigated.

Colon torsion or volvulus

Rotation of the colon around its long (mesenteric) axis leads to mechanical obstruction and ischemia. It occurs more

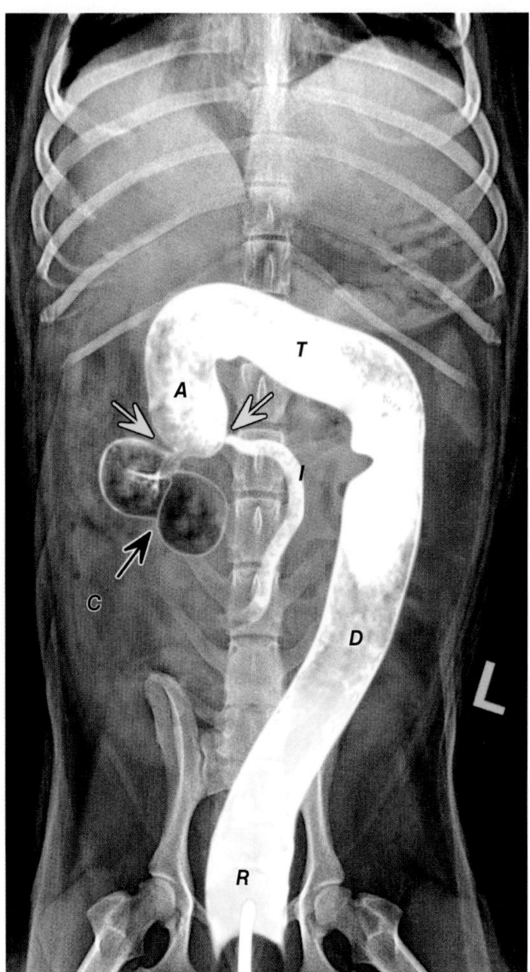

Figure 4.99 Normal canine large intestine. VD view of a dog abdomen depicting a barium enema. **C** = cecum (black arrow), **I** = ileum, **A** = ascending colon, **T** = transverse colon, **D** = descending colon, **R** = rectum. The yellow arrows point to the cecocolic and ileocolic junctions.

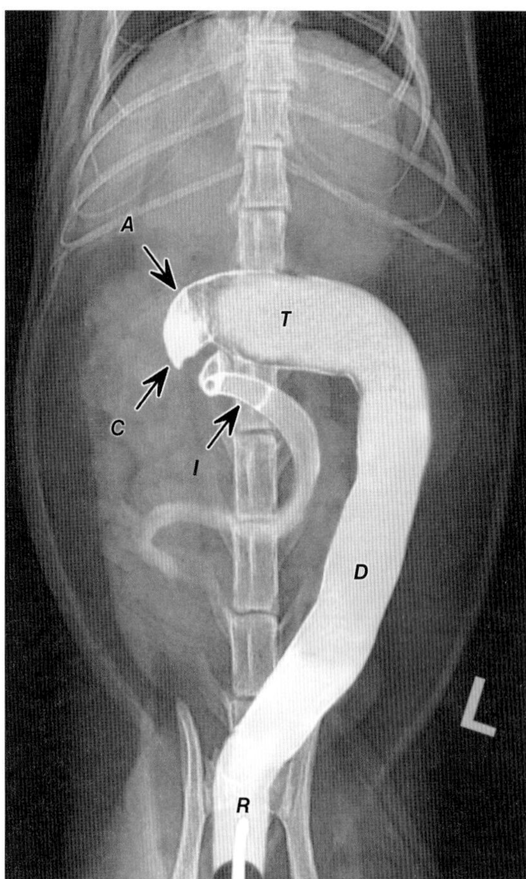

Figure 4.100 Normal feline large intestine. VD view of a cat abdomen depicting a barium enema. **C** = cecum, **I** = ileum, **A** = ascending colon, **T** = transverse colon, **D** = descending colon, **R** = rectum.

often in large breed dogs and frequently is associated with GDV. Rotation typically displaces the descending colon to the right and ventrally and the cecum to the left and dorsally. Rotation also twists the descending colon, which can cause an obstruction that leads to the dilation of the proximal colon and an empty distal colon and an empty rectum (Figure 4.108). The small intestine generally is normal or only mildly distended with mostly gas. Variable amounts of peritoneal effusion often are present.

Abnormal content or opacity in large intestine

Normal feces in the colon often appears heterogeneous with a somewhat granular pattern of gas and soft tissue opacities. Homogenous soft tissue opacity in the colon (without the tiny, evenly dispersed, gas bubbles commonly seen in fecal material) suggests fluid in the colon (e.g., enema, diarrhea). Persistence of a localized soft tissue opacity structure in the colon may represent a mass or foreign material. Mineral or metal opacity objects in the colon usually are readily identified.

Colonography

The procedure for colonography, as well as its indications and contraindications, is described in the contrast radiography section of Chapter 2. When filled with positive contrast medium, a normal colon appears relatively uniform in width with an even mucosal margin. The normal colon wall is relatively thin. Filling defects may be caused by retained

A

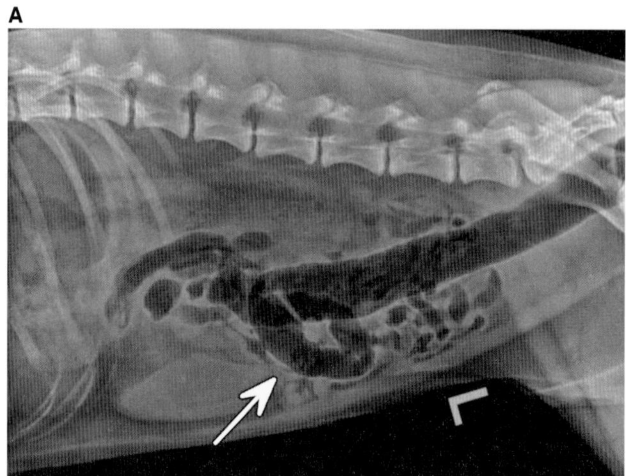

B

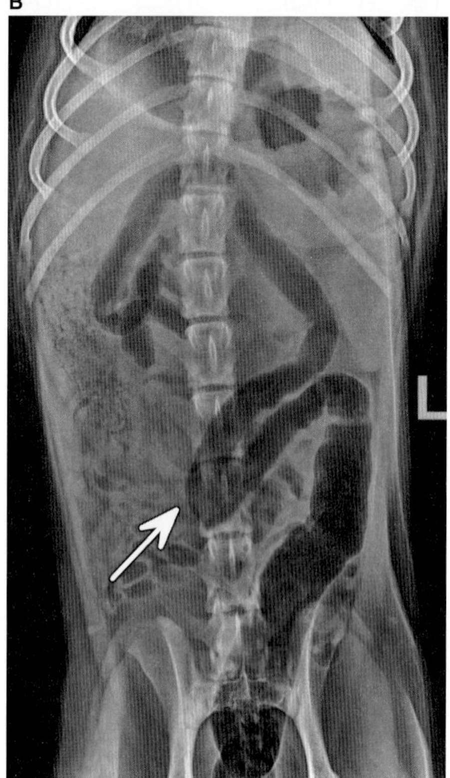

Figure 4.101 Redundant colon. Lateral view (**A**) and VD view (**B**) of a dog abdomen depicting a pneumocolon in a patient with a redundant colon. The excessive length of the descending colon is a normal variant that results in extra bowel loops (arrow).

A

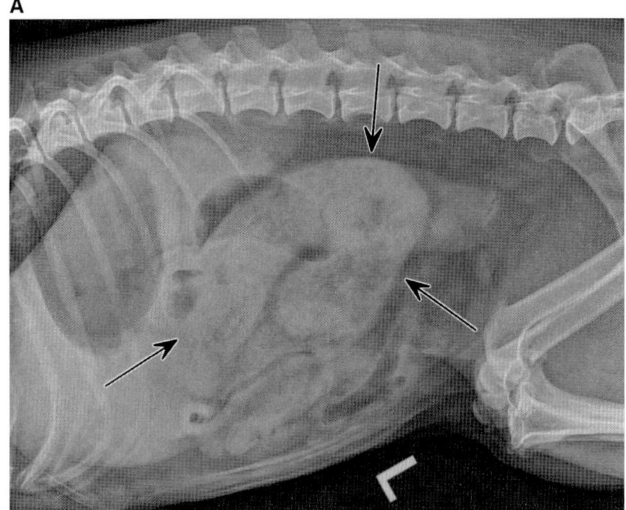

B

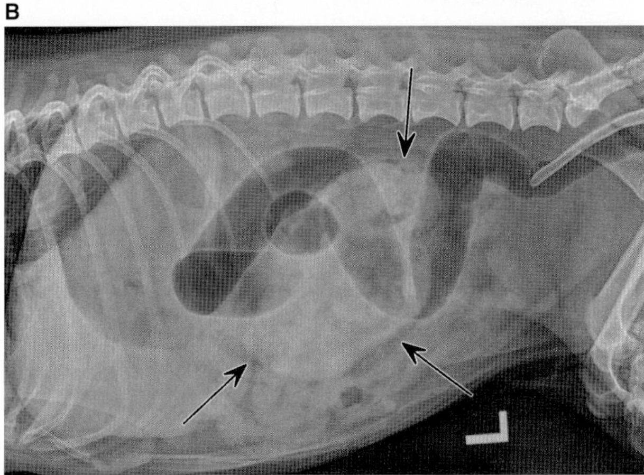

Figure 4.102 Pneumocolon. **A**. Survey lateral radiograph of a dog abdomen. It is uncertain whether the large tubular structure (arrows) is a filled colon or distended (obstructed) small bowel. **B**. Lateral view of the same dog depicting a pneumocolon. Identification of the colon confirms that the large tubular structure seen in A (arrows) is dilated small intestine. A metal catheter is visible in the rectum.

feces, foreign material, thickening of the bowel wall, or mural masses (see differential diagnoses). Feces sometimes is adhered to the mucosa and may be difficult to differentiate from pathology.

Thickening of the colon wall or an irregular mucosal margin may result from chronic inflammation or infiltrative disease (e.g., neoplasia, mycosis). Contrast medium can cling to the colon wall at sites of damaged mucosa or where there is excess mucous production, creating a mottled, heterogeneous pattern. Contrast medium that extends beyond the mucosal margin may indicate an ulcer, diverticulum, or perforation.

Tumors in the colon wall typically produce variably thickened areas with irregular margins. The colon wall may appear "stiff" or "rigid" in serial radiographs. Mural masses can thicken only one side of the colon wall to create an irregular-shaped filling defect and unilateral narrowing or deviation of the colon lumen. Annular tumors often create circumferential thickening and more uniform narrowing of the lumen.

A

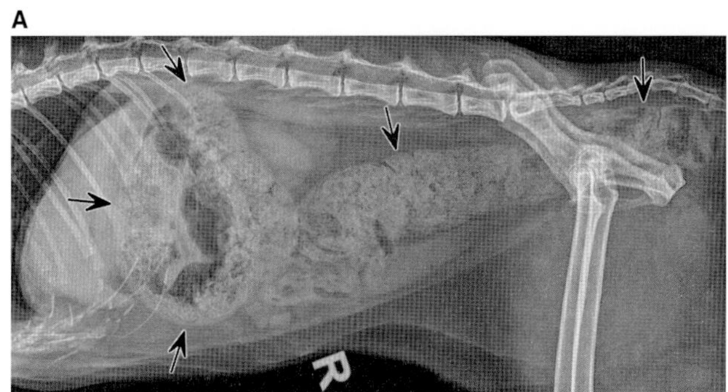

B

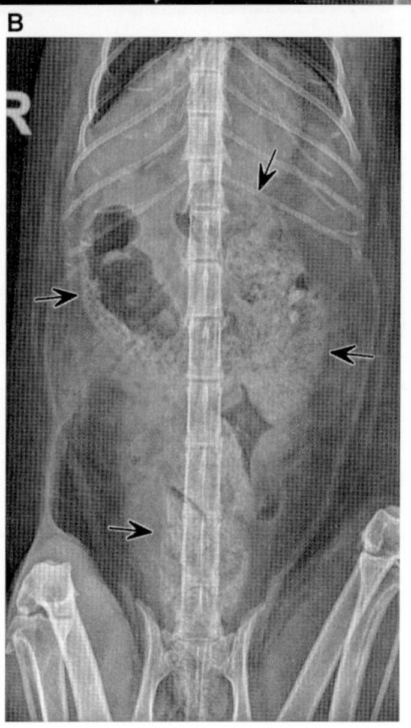

Figure 4.103 Constipation. Lateral view (**A**) and VD view (**B**) of a cat abdomen depicting a large amount of fecal material in the colon and rectum (arrows).

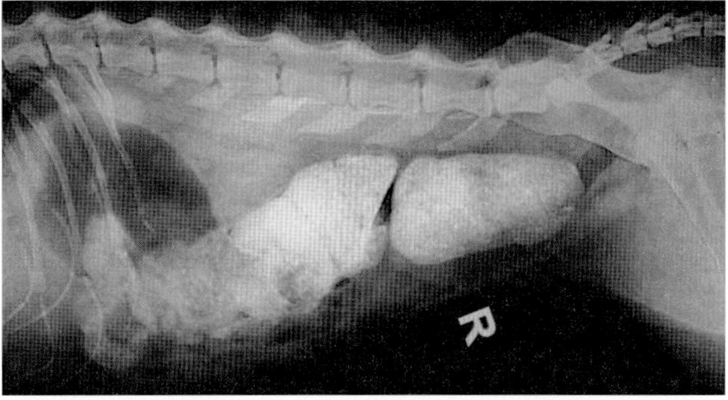

Figure 4.104 Obstipation. Lateral view of a cat abdomen depicting mineral opacity fecal material in the colon.

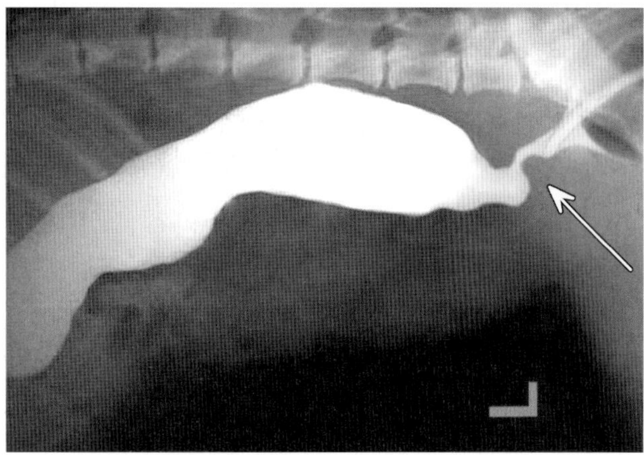

Figure 4.105 Colon spasm. Lateral view of a dog abdomen depicting a barium enema. There is irregular narrowing in the distal colon due a spasm (arrow) probably caused by irritation from the catheter in the rectum.

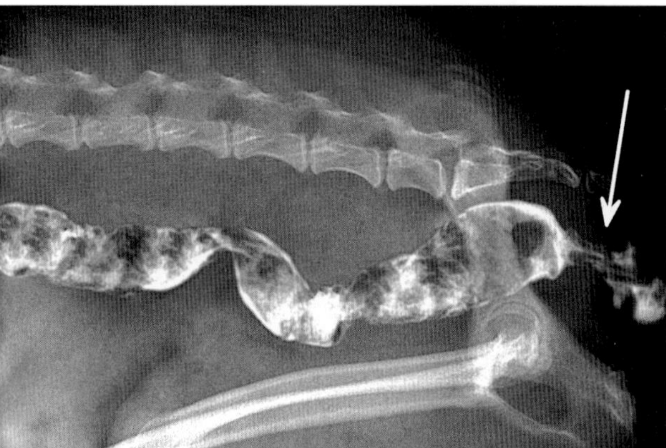

Figure 4.106 Rectal stricture. Lateral view of a cat abdomen depicting a barium enema. The irregular narrowing in the rectum (arrow) may be due to neoplasia or fibrosis. The filling defects in the descending colon are caused by retained feces that could not be removed. The contrast study helps identify the length of the lesion, which could not be determined by palpation alone.

These lesions sometimes resemble an "apple core" or "napkin ring" in appearance. Annular lesions tend to occur in the terminal colon, often due to adenocarcinoma (Figure 4.109). Lymphoma generally presents with multiple filling defects along the colon wall that protrude into the bowel lumen.

Colitis

Inflammation in the colon can lead to variable thickening of the colon wall and an irregular mucosal margin, depending on the severity and duration of colitis. As mentioned earlier, contrast medium may cling to the wall in areas of damaged mucosa or extend beyond the lumen due to ulceration or perforation. Severe colitis can lead to shortening of the colon (Figure 4.109) and granulomatous thickening of the colon wall (Figure 4.110).

Cecal inversion

Cecal inversion is a type of intussusception in which the cecum prolapses into the ascending colon to cause a partial or complete obstruction. It is uncommon in dogs and cats, most often associated with hypermotility, which may be due to parasitism or another cause of inflammation. Cecal inversion can occur at any age but is reported more often in young animals. In radiographs, the cecum is absent from its normal location. A soft tissue opacity mass or filling defect may be visible in the ascending colon (Figures 4.111 and 4.112). A prolapsed cecum may progress further into the colon, pulled by normal peristalsis. It may enter the descending colon.

A

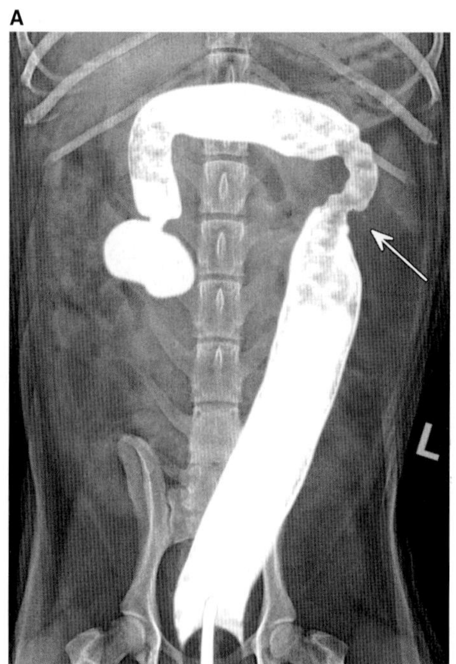

B

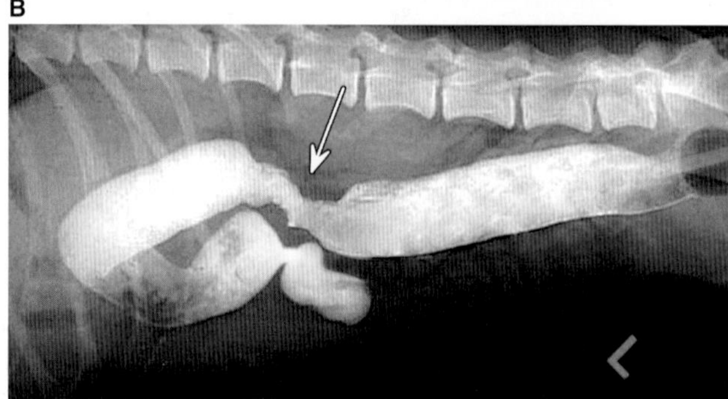

Figure 4.107 Colon narrowing. VD view (**A**) and lateral view (**B**) of a dog abdomen depicting a barium enema. There is an irregular area of persistent narrowing in the proximal descending colon (arrow) which may be due to a stricture or an annular tumor.

A

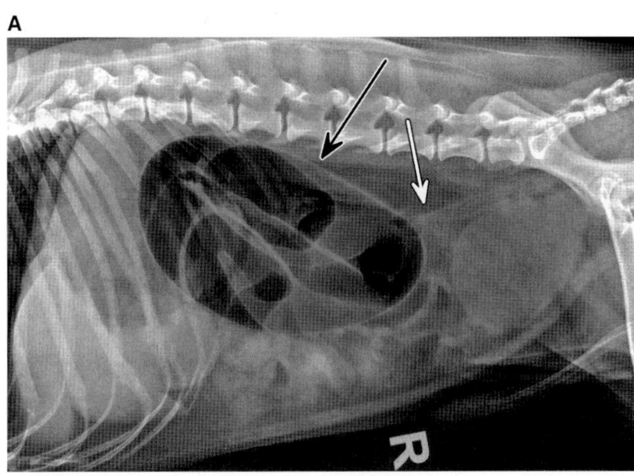

B

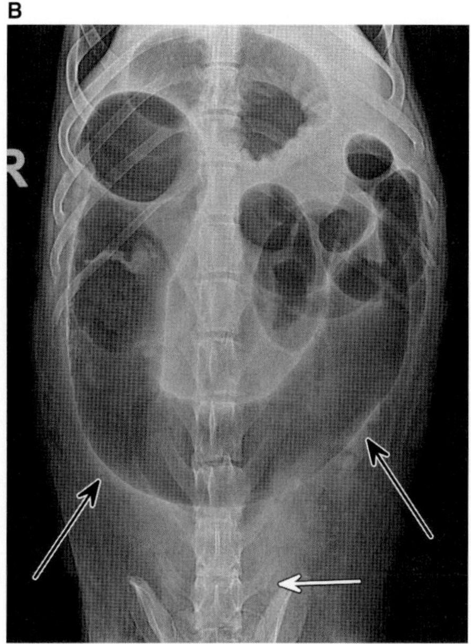

Figure 4.108 Colon torsion. Lateral view (**A**) and VD view (**B**) of a dog abdomen depicting extreme gas distention of the proximal colon (black arrows) and an empty distal colon and rectum (white arrow). It is difficult to determine from these radiographs whether it is small intestine or large intestine that is abnormally dilated. Depending on the patient's condition, this degree of bowel distention probably warrants surgery.

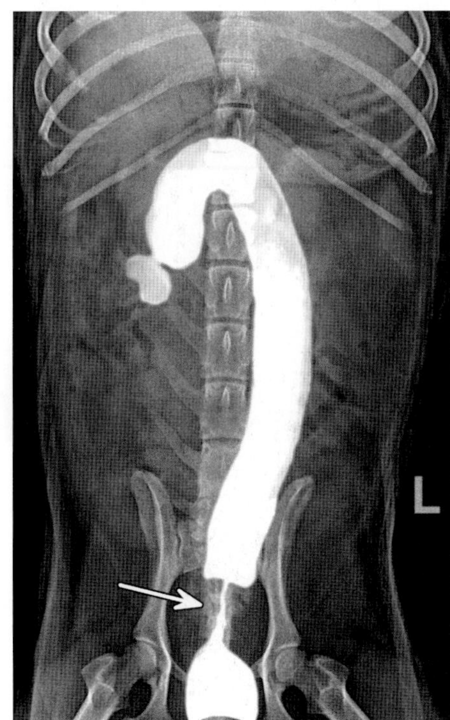

Figure 4.109 Colorectal stricture and short colon. VD view of a dog abdomen depicting a barium enema. The distal colon is markedly narrowed due to an annular tumor (arrow). The constriction resembles an "apple core" with only a thin line of barium in the lumen. The transverse and descending parts of the colon are shortened due to chronic inflammation.

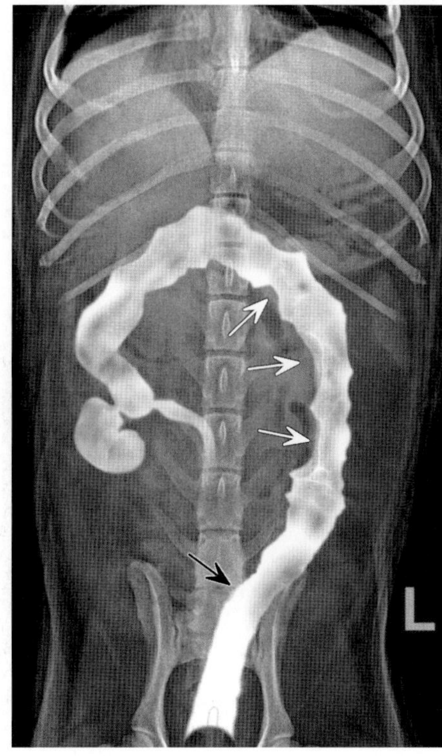

Figure 4.110 Severe colitis. VD view of a dog abdomen depicting a barium enema. Filling defects along the colon (white arrows) are due to granulomatous masses caused by chronic inflammation. The mucosal margin is less irregular in the distal colon (black arrow) where colitis is less severe.

A

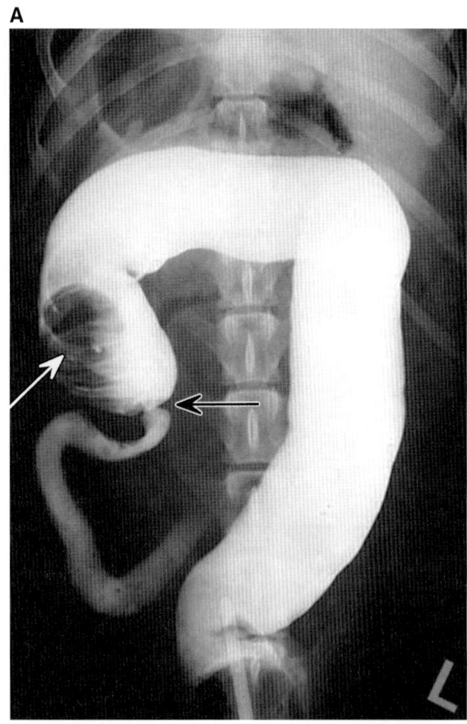

B

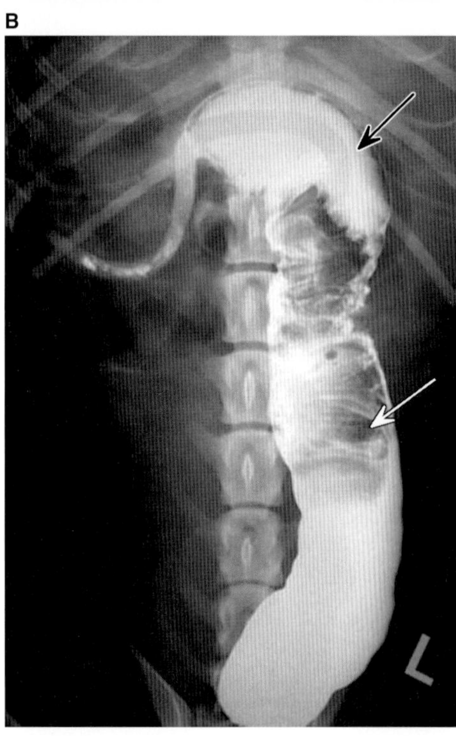

Figure 4.111 Cecal inversion. **A**. VD view of a dog abdomen depicting a colon that is moderately distended with barium. The cecum is absent from its normal location because it has prolapsed into the ascending colon, creating a filling defect (white arrow). The ileocolic junction is visible (black arrow). **B**. VD view of the same dog depicting a repeat barium enema made a few days later. Normal peristalsis pulls the cecum into the descending colon (white arrow) and the ileum follows (black arrow) resulting in an ileocolic intussusception.

A

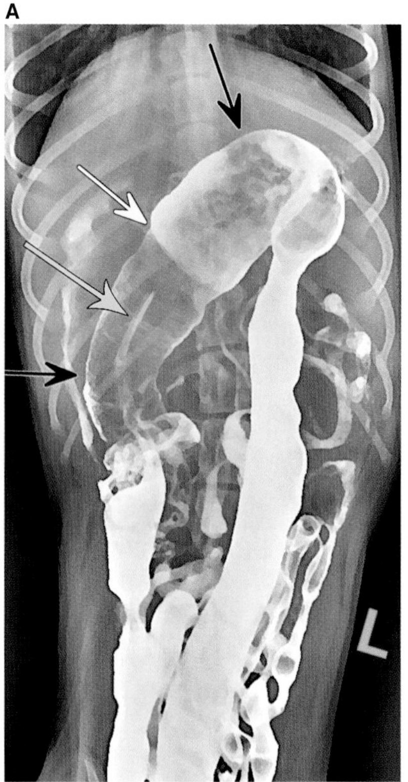

B

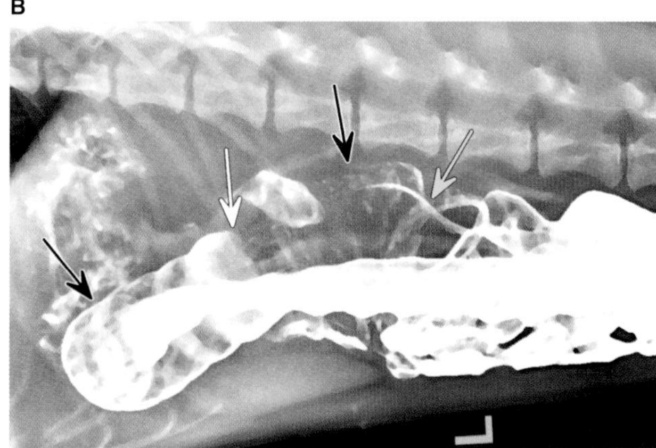

Figure 4.112 Ileocolic intussusception. VD view (**A**) and lateral view (**B**) of a dog abdomen depicting a barium enema with an upper GI study. The ascending and transverse colon are distended (black arrows). A thin line of barium is visible in the distended colon (yellow arrows), filling the narrow lumen of the intussusceptum. A curved barium:soft tissue interface marks the edge of the intussusception, sometimes called the "meniscus sign" (white arrow).

Urogenital tract

The urogenital tract includes the kidneys, ureters, urinary bladder, urethra, ovaries, uterus, vagina, prostate gland, and testicles. This text deals specifically with radiography, however, there are other imaging modalities which may yield additional diagnostic information about the urogenital tract (e.g., ultrasonography, computed tomography, endoscopy).

Kidneys and ureters

Normal radiographic anatomy

The kidneys and ureters are located ventral to the lumbar spine in the retroperitoneal space. The left kidney usually is caudal to the right, but both kidneys may be at same level and sometimes the right kidney is caudal to left. The ureters are not visible in radiographs due to their small size and similar opacity to the adjacent tissues.

Both kidneys should be similar in size, shape and opacity. Dog kidneys are oval or bean-shaped and cat kidneys tend to be more rounded. In dogs, the normal length of a kidney is about 2.5–3.5 times the length of the body of the L2 lumbar vertebra (Figure 4.113). The normal width of a canine kidney is about 2.0 times the length of L2. Cat kidneys measure about 2.0–3.0 times the length of L2 (Figure 4.114) and their normal width is about 3.0–3.5 cm. Feline kidneys tend to be smaller in neutered and older cats and larger and more rounded in intact cats.

Kidney size and shape are best assessed in a VD view, where there is no kidney overlap and both kidneys are equally magnified. In lateral views, the caudal pole of the right kidney commonly overlaps the cranial pole of the left kidney. Summation of the overlapped kidneys creates an area of greater opacity which may be mistaken for a mass. Sometimes the area of summation is mistaken for a small kidney. Kidney overlap tends to be less in a right lateral view than in a left lateral view.

The visibility of the kidneys depends on the amount of adjacent retroperitoneal fat and whether there is superimposition of the peritoneal viscera. Kidneys often are easier to see in cats and overweight dogs because there is more perirenal fat. Renal internal anatomy is not visible in survey radiographs (Figure 4.115).

Abnormal kidney position

In dogs, the right kidney is located at about the level of T13-L3. The left kidney is at about L1-5. In deep-chested dogs, the kidneys tend to be more cranial in position and may blend with the liver and spleen. In cats, the right kidney is at about L1-4 and the left kidney is at about L2-5. In overweight animals, the kidneys may be more ventral in position due to excess retroperitoneal fat. Cat kidneys tend to be more mobile than dog kidneys.

Non-visualization of a kidney may be because it is absent, obscured, or in an abnormal location. Absence of a kidney may be due to failure of the kidney to develop (renal aplasia or agenesis) or previous surgical removal (nephrectomy). In these cases, the remaining kidney usually is enlarged due to compensatory hypertrophy.

A

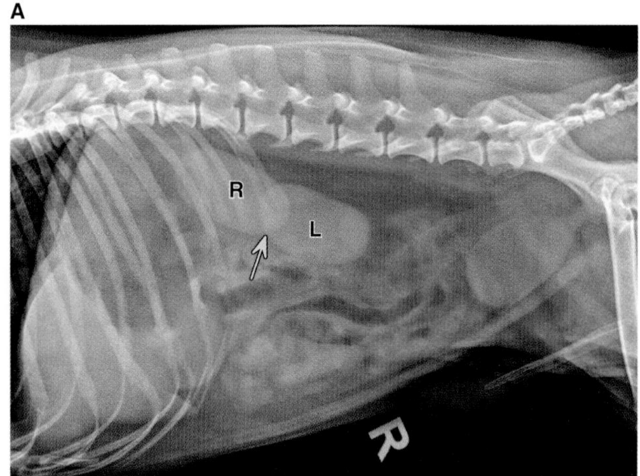

B

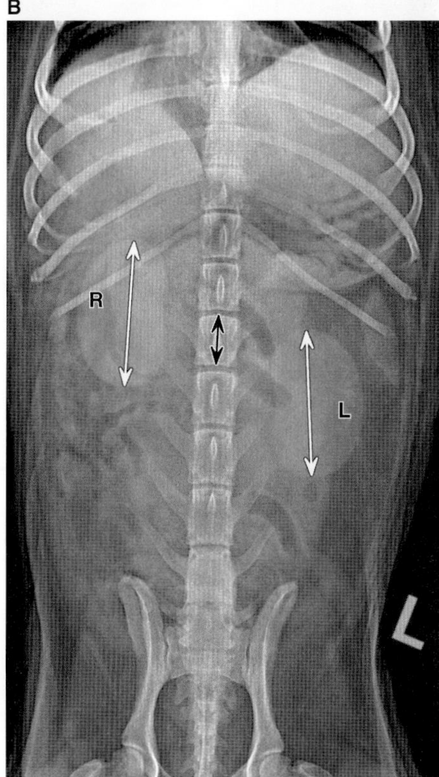

Figure 4.113 Normal canine kidneys. Lateral view (**A**) and VD view (**B**) of a dog abdomen depicting normal right (R) and left (L) kidneys. In the lateral view, the kidneys overlap to create an area of increased opacity (yellow arrow). In the VD view, the length of each kidney (white double-headed arrows) is compared to the length of the L2 lumbar vertebra (black double-headed arrow). Normal kidney size is 2.5–3.5 × L2.

A kidney may be obscured due to superimposition of adjacent structures (more common if the kidney is small) or lack of an opacity interface. The intestines frequently overlie the kidneys in a VD/DV view. When this is a problem, abdominal compression can be used to displace the bowel and better visualize a kidney (Figures 2.19 and 4.118). Rotation of the

A

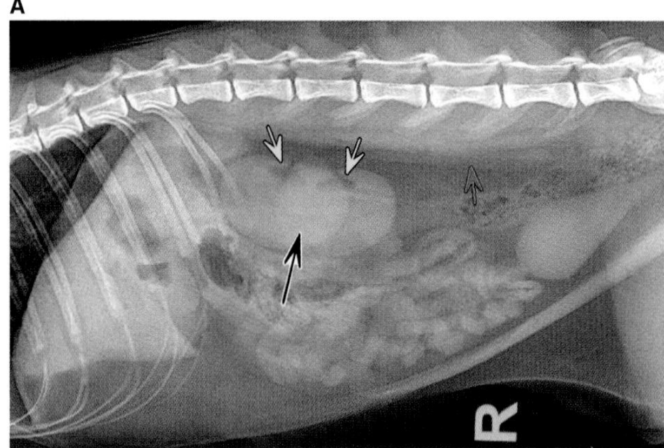

B

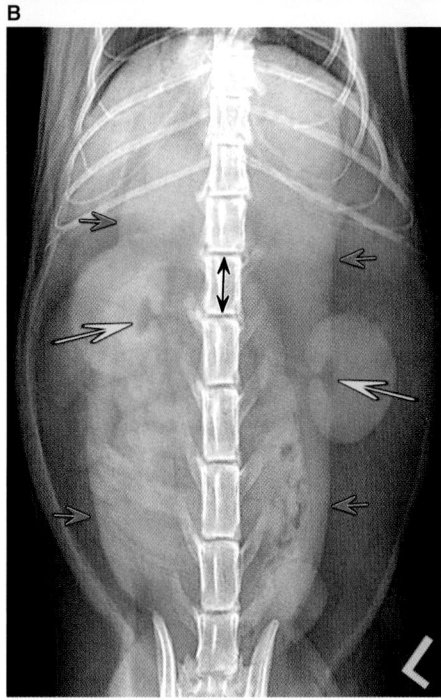

Figure 4.114 Normal feline kidneys. Lateral view (**A**) and VD view (**B**) of a cat abdomen depicting normal kidneys. In the lateral view, the caudal pole of the right kidney summates with the cranial pole of the left kidney to produce an area of increased opacity (black arrow). Fat in each renal pelvis (yellow arrows) is less opaque than the renal parenchyma. In the VD view, the length of each kidney is compared to the length of the L2 vertebral body (black double-headed arrow). Normal kidney size in cats is 2.0–3.0 × L2. The hypaxial muscles frequently are visible in abdominal radiographs of cats (red arrows).

patient during positioning for radiography can superimpose the spine or other body parts on a kidney. Visualization of renal margins relies on retroperitoneal fat for an opacity interface. Lack of fat or the presence of fluid in the retroperitoneal space may obscure one or both kidneys (e.g., emaciation, urine leakage, retroperitoneal inflammation, hemorrhage).

Renal ectopia is a rare congenital anomaly in which one or both kidneys develop in an abnormal location. An ectopic kidney may be normal in size, shape and function - or it may be small, rotated, or abnormal in shape. Ectopic kidneys frequently are located in the caudal abdomen, but they have been reported in the pelvic canal and in the thoracic cavity. To avoid mistaking an ectopic kidney for an intra-abdominal mass, be sure to systematically identify all of the organs in the abdominal cavity.

Displacement of a kidney may be due to a nearby mass effect, loss of abdominal integrity, or renal avulsion. As mentioned previously, a mass effect may result from organomegaly or an abnormal growth (e.g., tumor, abscess, cyst, others). Loss of abdominal integrity may be due to a diaphragmatic or body wall hernia or rupture. Avulsion of a kidney typically is the result of severe trauma and often is accompanied by retroperitoneal swelling.

Abnormal kidney size

One or both kidneys may be small or enlarged due to a congenital, physiologic, or pathologic condition. Note: abnormal kidney size may or may not correlate with abnormal renal function. In addition, normal kidney size does not rule out renal disease. Disorders such as renal inflammation, an early

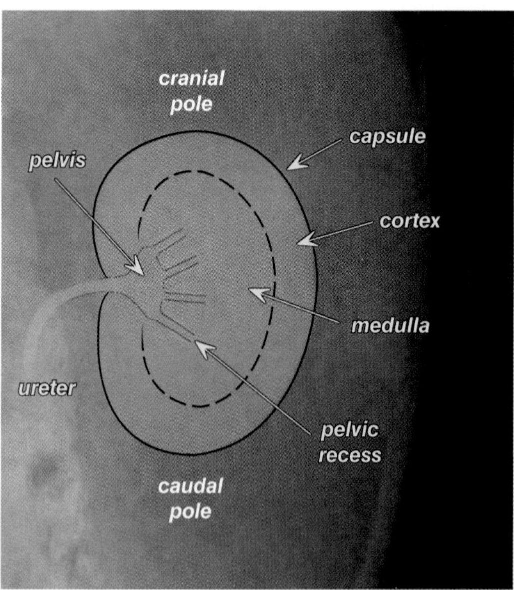

Figure 4.115 Normal renal anatomy. VD view of a cat abdomen illustrating the cross-sectional anatomy of a kidney. Urine is produced in the cortex and medulla. The urine flows into the pelvic recesses and pelvis, which are part of the renal collecting system. The renal capsule is a tough fibrous outer layer that surrounds the kidney. The capsule usually is covered with perirenal fat. The dashed line indicates the corticomedullary junction.

or partial kidney obstruction, and small renal masses may not initially alter the size or shape of the kidney. Patients with unilateral kidney disease may remain asymptomatic until disease becomes severe in the remaining kidney.

A **small kidney** is due to either *renal hypoplasia* or *renal fibrosis* (Figure 4.116). Again, renal size may or may not correlate with renal function. **Renal hypoplasia** is the abnormal development of a kidney that results in a small renal cortex. In survey radiographs, the margin of a hypoplastic kidney tends to be even and well-defined. In an excretory urogram, there typically is less renal parenchyma and a normal appearing renal collecting system. The collecting system may appear large due to the decreased corticomedullary ratio.

A

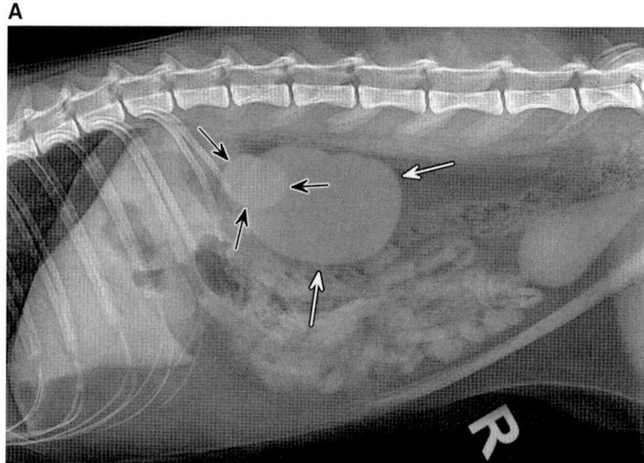

B

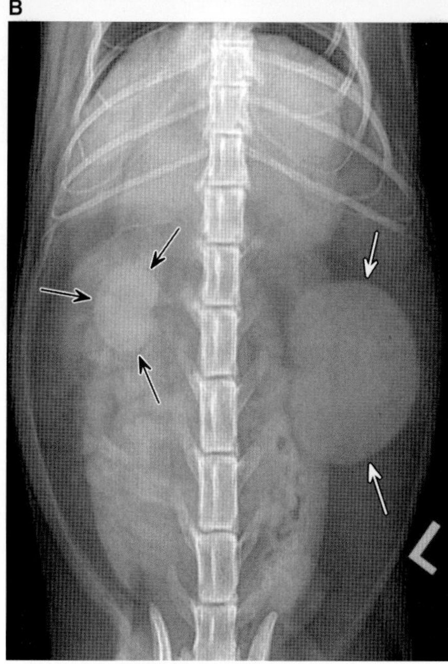

Figure 4.116 Small kidney. Lateral view (**A**) and VD view (**B**) of a cat abdomen depicting a small right kidney (black arrows). The left kidney is large (white arrows) due to compensatory hypertrophy.

Renal fibrosis usually is caused by chronic kidney inflammation. In survey radiographs, the margin of a fibrotic kidney often is irregular. In an excretory urogram, the nephrogram may appear inhomogeneous or patchy with a thin or uneven renal cortex. The cortex may be abnormal due to renal infarcts, which typically produce wedge-shaped filling defects. In the pyelogram, the renal pelvis may be dilated and irregular in shape with blunted pelvic recesses. Exudates in the renal collecting system can produce irregular filling defects.

Physiologic renomegaly occurs when one kidney hypertrophies to compensate the other kidney being other absent or non-functional. Bilateral renal hypertrophy may occur with a portosystemic vascular shunt because the kidneys will try to compensate for the diminished liver function. Hypertrophied kidneys often appear normal in shape and margination.

Pathologic renomegaly may be unilateral or bilateral (Figure 4.117). A kidney may enlarge due to widening of the renal parenchyma, dilation of the renal pelvis, or expansion of the renal capsule. Parenchymal widening most often is due to inflammation or infiltrative disease. One or more space-occupying lesions in a kidney(s) can lead to renomegaly and renal distortion (e.g., cysts, nodules, masses).

Dilation of the renal pelvis is *hydronephrosis*. Hydronephrosis most often is due to a urinary outflow obstruction, but the renal pelvis may dilate due to severe inflammation. Obstructions can be caused by congenital or acquired abnormalities. Congenital abnormalities include ectopic ureter and ureterocele. Acquired obstructions include calculi or other material in a ureter (see differential diagnoses).

Expansion of the renal capsule is caused by subcapsular accumulation of fluid. Fluid typically is either blood or a transudate, the latter occurs in a perirenal pseudocyst. Hemorrhage tends to be unilateral and may result from trauma or erosion of the renal cortex by a tumor or abscess. Pseudocysts often are bilateral.

Enlarged kidneys usually remain retroperitoneal, but they can sag ventrally and sometimes will overly the peritoneal space. The margin of a large kidney may be smooth or irregular, depending on the etiology (see differential diagnoses).

In cats, the kidneys tend to enlarge more in width than in length, resulting in a more rounded appearance than in dogs.

Abnormal kidney opacity

Kidneys normally are mostly soft tissue opacity. Fat sometimes is visible in the renal pelves, particularly in cats and overweight dogs (Figure 4.114). Gas, mineral, or metal opacity in a kidney is abnormal. Superimposition artifacts

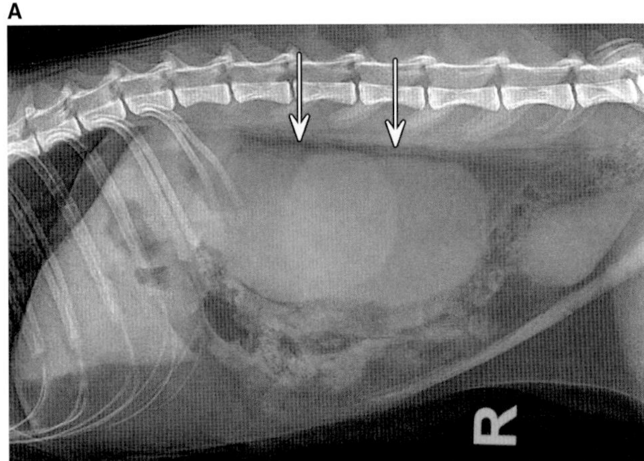

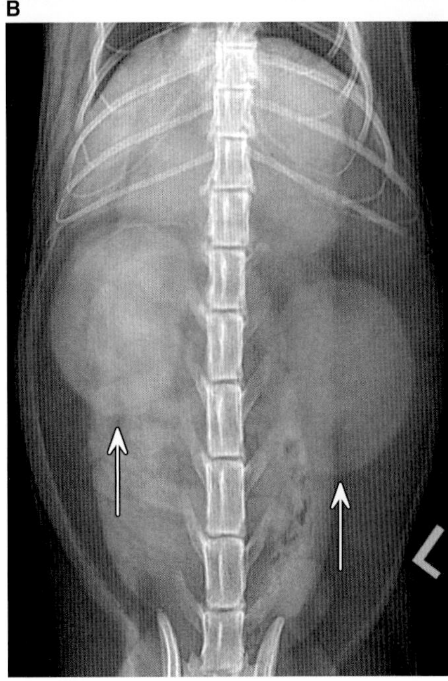

Figure 4.117 Bilateral renomegaly. Lateral view (**A**) and VD view (**B**) of a cat abdomen depicting enlargement of both kidneys (arrows). Renal margins are even and well-defined and the intestines are displaced ventrally. Possible etiologies include renal lymphoma, perirenal pseudocysts, bilateral hydronephrosis.

can mimic abnormal renal opacity (e.g., intestinal contents). Always confirm suspected lesions with orthogonal views or compression radiography.

Gas in one or both renal collecting systems most often is due to vesicoureteral reflux. Reflux of gas from the urinary bladder into the ureters, renal pelves, and pelvic recesses is common during pneumocystography (Figure 4.157). It can also occur in patients with emphysematous cystitis. Gas in the renal cortex may result from a penetrating wound or a gas-producing bacterial infection.

Mineral opacity in a kidney or ureter may represent urolithiasis or dystrophic mineralization (Figure 4.118). In a kidney, foci of mineralization in the renal pelvis are more likely to be calculi, whereas mineralization in the renal cortex is more likely to be dystrophic. Calculi are solid

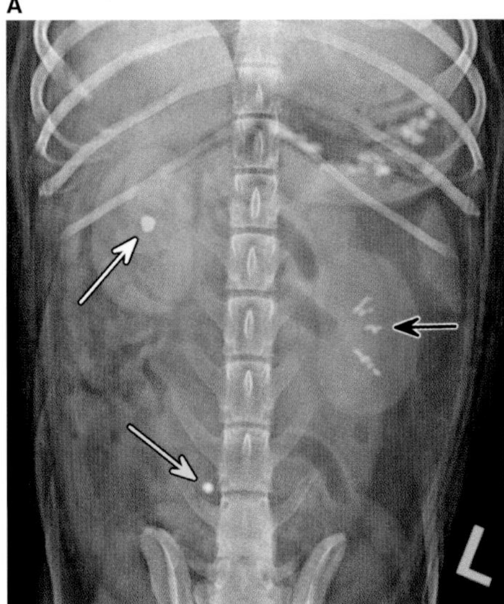

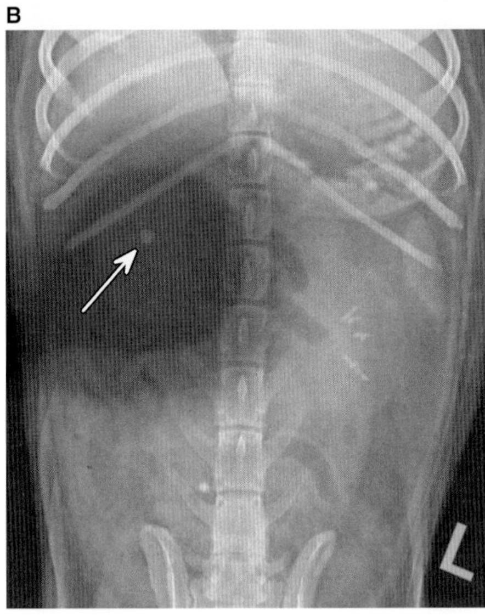

Figure 4.118 Renal mineralization. **A**. VD view of a dog abdomen depicting focal mineralization in the areas of the right kidney (white arrow), distal right ureter (yellow arrow), and left kidney (black arrow). The right cranial mineral opacity structure may be located in the kidney or in the overlying bowel. Notice there is mineral opacity material in the stomach, which means similar material may be present in the bowel. **B**. Follow-up VD view of the same dog made with abdominal compression. A wooden spoon is used to apply gentle pressure over the right kidney and displace the overlying bowel, revealing a renal calculus. Notice that the x-ray exposure was decreased to compensate for the reduced abdominal thickness.

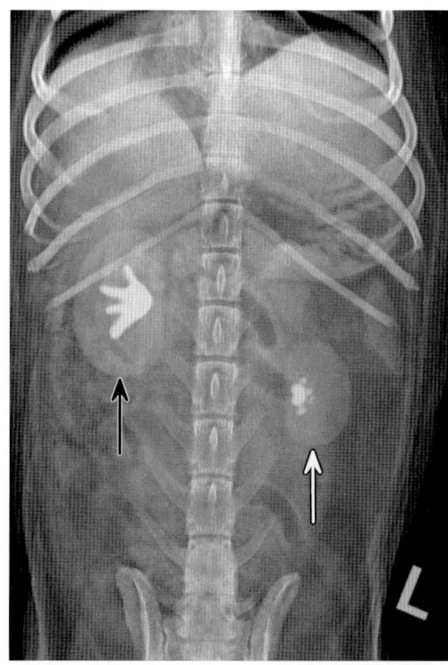

Figure 4.119 Renal calculi. VD view of a dog abdomen depicting a "staghorn calculus" in the right kidney (black arrow) and multiple mineral opacity calculi in the left renal pelvis (white arrow). The left kidney is small.

aggregations that can vary greatly in size, shape, number, and opacity. They can form anywhere in the renal collecting system of one or both kidneys. Larger calculi that conform to the shape of the collecting system are commonly called *staghorn calculi* (Figure 4.119). Renal calculi should be noted because they may eventually pass into a ureter or into the urinary bladder and cause obstruction or irritation.

Metal opacity in a kidney may be associated with a foreign object or contrast radiography. Most iodinated contrast agents are excreted via the kidneys, whether they are used to image the urinary tract or another body part. Similar to the vesicoureteral reflux of gas, positive contrast media can flow from the urinary bladder into the ureters and kidneys. Metallic foreign objects usually are readily identified in a radiograph, but confirming their location in a kidney requires orthogonal views.

Excretory urography

The procedure for excretory urography (EU), as well as its indications and contraindications, is described in the contrast radiography section of Chapter 2. An EU primarily is used to evaluate renal anatomy. It is not a very precise or reliable test of renal function. The degree and duration of urinary tract opacification depends on the dose of contrast medium, renal blood flow, and renal function. Patient hydration is important to maintain adequate renal perfusion. There are five phases to an EU. Each phase opacifies a different part of the urinary tract:

1. *Vascular phase*: renal vasculature is opacified.
2. *Nephrogram phase*: renal parenchyma is opacified.
3. *Pyelogram phase*: renal collecting system is opacified.
4. *Ureteral phase*: ureters are opacified.
5. *Bladder phase*: urinary bladder is opacified.

The **vascular phase** of an EU begins about 5 seconds after a rapid IV injection of a bolus of contrast medium as the arteries to each kidney are opacified (Figure 4.120). Sometimes two or more arteries may supply a kidney as a normal anatomic variation. During the vascular phase most of the contrast medium is in the blood vessels, which can lead to an overall increase in abdominal opacity. The aorta, renal artery and the arterial branches in each kidney tend to be particularly well-opacified.

The **nephrogram phase** of an EU begins about 10 seconds after injection, during which the renal parenchyma is opacified (Figure 4.121). The nephrogram persists for about 2 minutes and then gradually diminishes. Both kidneys should be similar in size, shape, and degree of opacification. Initially, the renal cortex is more opaque than the medulla because the contrast medium is filtered by the glomeruli

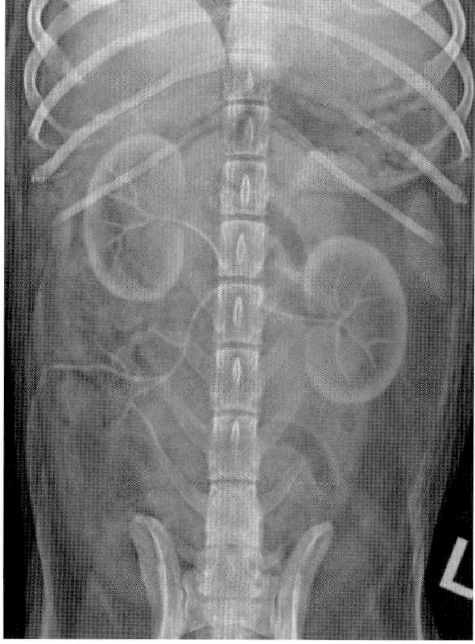

Figure 4.120 Vascular phase of EU. VD view of a dog abdomen depicting the appearance of the kidneys 5 seconds after rapid IV injection of contrast medium. The vascular supply to each kidney is visible and the renal cortices are beginning to opacity as the contrast agent is filtered from the blood.

A

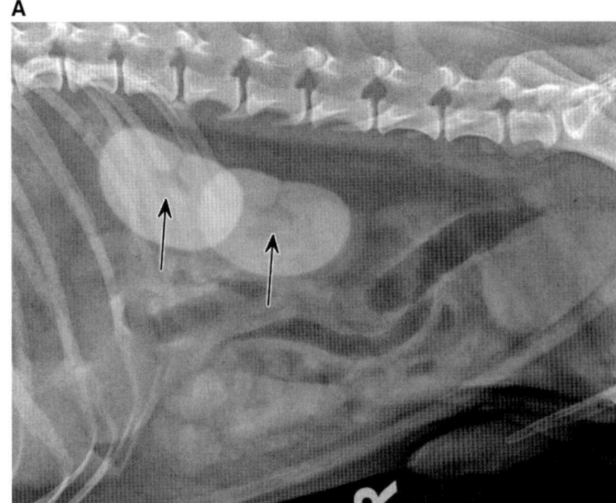

B

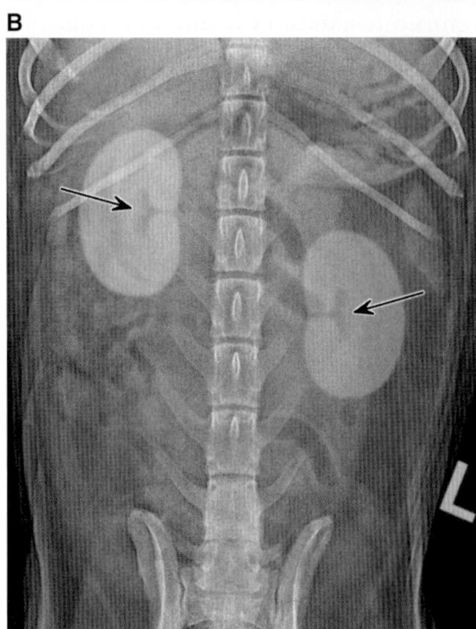

Figure 4.121 Nephrogram phase of EU. Lateral view (**A**) and VD view (**B**) of the same dog abdomen as in Figure 4.120, depicting the appearance of the kidneys 1 minute after IV injection of contrast medium. In each kidney, there is uniform opacification of the renal parenchyma. The renal pelves are less opaque (black arrows). Both kidneys are similar in size and shape with even, well-defined margins.

before entering the renal tubules. The parenchyma soon becomes more uniform in opacity and then slowly fades over time. Kidney function relies on glomerular filtration, working renal tubules, and a patent urine outflow.

Abnormal findings in a nephrogram include:

1. Only one kidney is opacified:
   a. Kidney is absent (e.g., aplasia, nephrectomy).
   b. Loss of blood supply to the kidney.
   c. Severe unilateral kidney disease.
2. Neither kidney is opacified:
   a. Insufficient dose of contrast medium.
   b. Poor renal blood flow and failure to deliver the contrast medium to the kidneys (e.g., heart failure).
   c. Severe bilateral kidney disease.
3. Faint nephrogram in one or both kidneys that fades without progressing to a pyelogram:
   a. Inadequate dose of contrast medium.
   b. Poor renal function.
4. Filling defects or heterogeneous opacification in one or both kidneys:
   a. Space-occupying renal lesions (e.g., tumors, cysts).
   b. Severe renal inflammation.
   c. Renal obstruction.
5. Only the peripheral rim of a kidney is opacified:
   a. Hydronephrosis; the renal collecting will be dilated in the pyelogram but may only be faintly opacified.
   b. Renal hypoplasia; the pyelogram usually is normal.
6. Nephrogram with a peripheral rim that is NOT opacified:
   a. Subcapsular accumulation of fluid (e.g., perirenal pseudocyst, hemorrhage).
7. Nephrogram that persists in serial radiographs and does not fade or that increases in opacity. The nephrogram does not progress to a pyelogram. There is no opacification of the renal pelves, ureters, or urinary bladder:
   a. Acute renal failure; patient requires immediate treatment, including fluid therapy.

The **pyelogram phase** begins about 1 minute after injection, during which the contrast medium fills the renal collecting system (Figure 4.122). The renal pelvis and pelvic recesses may remain opacified for several hours as the contrast medium is excreted by the kidneys. The normal renal pelvis occupies about one-third of the kidney. The pelvic recesses appear as thin, sharply-defined, parallel lines that radiate away from the pelvis and toward the renal cortex. Both of the renal collecting systems should be similar in size, shape, and opacity. The degree of opacification depends on the concentration of contrast medium in the urine and the volume of urine in the collecting system. The pyelogram normally is more opaque than the nephrogram because the kidneys resorb water and concentrate the contrast medium in the urine.

Abnormal findings in a pyelogram include:

1. Absence of pyelogram:
   a. Insufficient dose of contrast medium.
   b. Non-functional kidney(s).
2. Dilation of a renal collecting system (Figure 4.123):
   a. Recent fluid therapy or diuresis; mild dilation.
   b. Renal inflammation (e.g., pyelonephritis); mild dilation.

c. Abdominal compression was used to temporarily obstruct urinary outflow; mild dilation.
d. Ureteral obstruction (e.g., calculus, blood clot, tumor, ectopic ureter); mild to severe dilation.

3. Distortion or filling defects in renal collecting system:
   a. Debris or a mass in a pelvis or pelvic recess (e.g., tumor, calculus, polyp, blood clot).

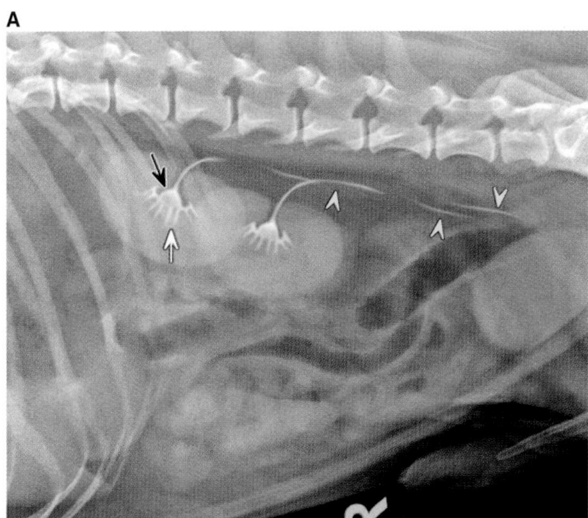

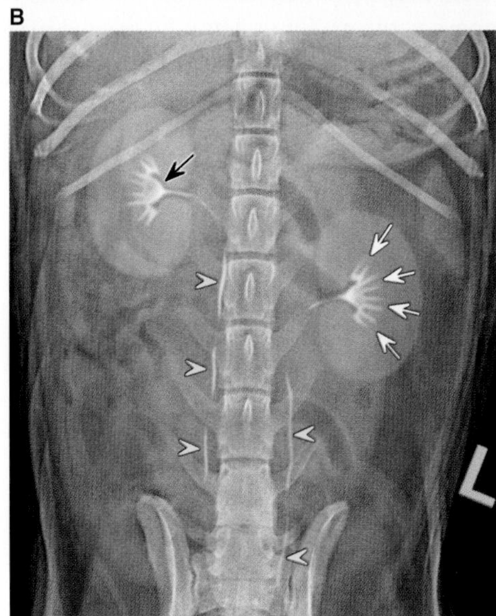

Figure 4.122 Pyelogram phase of EU. Lateral view (**A**) and VD view (**B**) of the same dog abdomen as in Figure 4.121, depicting the appearance of the urinary tract 5 minutes after IV injection of contrast medium. The nephrogram is fading and contrast medium fills each renal pelvis (black arrow) and the renal pelvic recesses (white arrows). The ureters are only partially opacified due to normal ureteral peristalsis (yellow arrowheads).

The **ureteral phase** of an EU begins with the pyelogram as urine and contrast medium flow into the ureters. There are normal peristaltic contractions in the ureters and quite often there is incomplete filling of the ureters. Ureteral contractions occur rapidly and frequently, so only small sections of a ureter are opacified at any one time. Temporary compression of the caudal abdomen will briefly block the flow of urine and increase ureteral filling, as described in the EU procedure in Chapter 2 and depicted in Figure 4.124. The normal ureters run caudally from each renal pelvis, through the retroperitoneal space, to the trigone of the urinary bladder. Near the trigone, each ureter curves cranially just before entering the bladder. An EU with a concurrent pneumocystogram enhances visualization of the vesicoureteral junction (Figure 4.125). This can be particularly useful when investigating ectopic ureters. Note: gas from a pneumocytogram can reflux into a ureter to produce bubble filling defects.

Abnormal findings in the ureters include:

1. Abnormal position of one or both ureters:
   a. Ectopic ureter.
   b. Traumatic avulsion.
   c. Displacement by an adjacent mass.
2. Dilation of a ureter:
   a. Distal obstruction (e.g., stricture, accidental ligation, external compression, tumor, polyp, lodged calculi, blood clot).
   b. Severe inflammation that leads to ureteral atony or ureteral ileus.
   c. Ureteral diverticulum; a focal dilation in a ureter; uncommon in dogs and cats.
   d. Ureteral rupture; dilatation of the affected ureter at the site of the rupture and proximally.
3. Lack of ureteral opacification:
   a. Insufficient dose of contrast medium.
   b. Proximal urinary outflow obstruction.
   c. Non-functional kidney.
   d. Ruptured ureter.
4. Filling defects in a ureter or irregular ureteral margins:
   a. Intraluminal mass (e.g., calculi, tumors, polyps, blood clots, gas bubble).
   b. Narrowing of the ureter (e.g., stricture, compression by adjacent mass).

The **bladder phase** of an EU is a positive contrast cystogram. Keep in mind that an excretory urography can be used to produce a cystogram when catheterization of the bladder is not possible.

Kidney inflammation

Signs of renal inflammation seldom are evident in survey radiographs (unless the inflammation is chronic and has

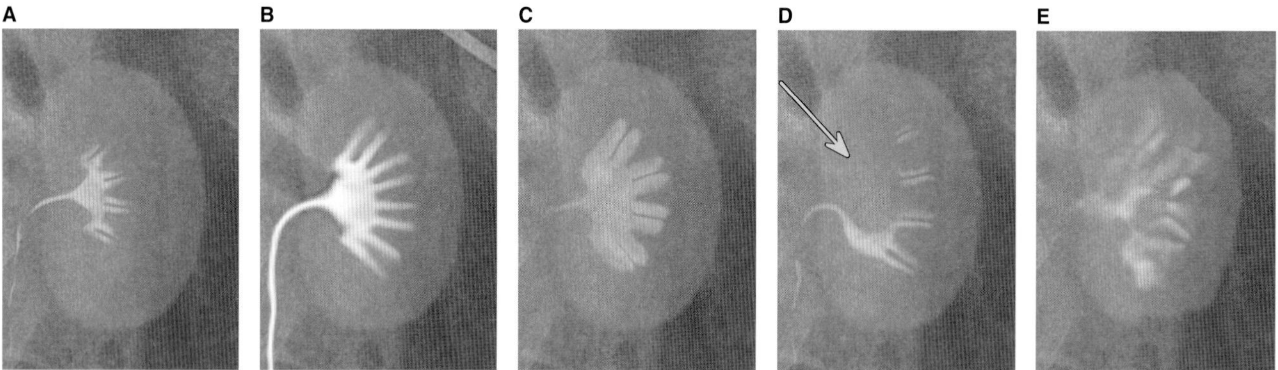

Figure 4.123 Pyelogram abnormalities. VD views of a dog abdomen with the left kidney isolated to depict various abnormalities in a pyelogram. **A**. Normal pyelogram for comparison. **B**. Mildly dilated renal collecting system; may be due to caudal abdominal compression, inflammation, or early obstruction. **C**. Dilated renal pelvis with wide, blunt pelvic recesses due to hydronephrosis. **D**. Large filling defect (arow) due to a mass in the renal parenchyma. **E**. Distorted renal collecting system with multiple filling defects due to infiltrative neoplasia.

progressed to renal fibrosis). Kidney inflammation most often is caused by an infection from the lower urinary tract. One or both kidneys may be involved. Other causes of nephritis include systemic infections, nephrolithiasis, and prolonged treatment with certain drugs (e.g., penicillin, cephalexin, aspirin, sulfa drugs).

The nephrogram phase of an EU often is normal in patients with renal inflammation. The pyelogram may reveal mild to moderate dilation of the renal collecting system (Figure 4.126), depending on the severity and duration of the inflammation. Inflammation in a ureter can lead to diminished peristalsis and varying degrees of ileus and ureteral dilation. Note: dilation of the renal collecting system or/and ureter can also be caused by recent fluid therapy or diuresis. Caudal abdominal compression is used to deliberately dilate the collecting system to enhance filling and opacification.

Kidney mass

Renal masses may be unilateral or bilateral, solitary or multiple. Kidneys with smaller or centrally located masses may appear normal in survey radiographs or only mildly enlarged.

Figure 4.124 Ureteral phase of EU. Lateral view of the same dog abdomen as in Figure 4.122, depicting the appearance of the renal collecting systems and ureters following the application and release of caudal abdominal compression. The renal pelves and pelvic recesses are mildly dilated and the ureters are visible in their entirety due to temporary blockage of urine flow. Both distal ureters are visible at the urinary bladder trigone (arrow). Notice that the ureters curve slightly cranially before entering the bladder.

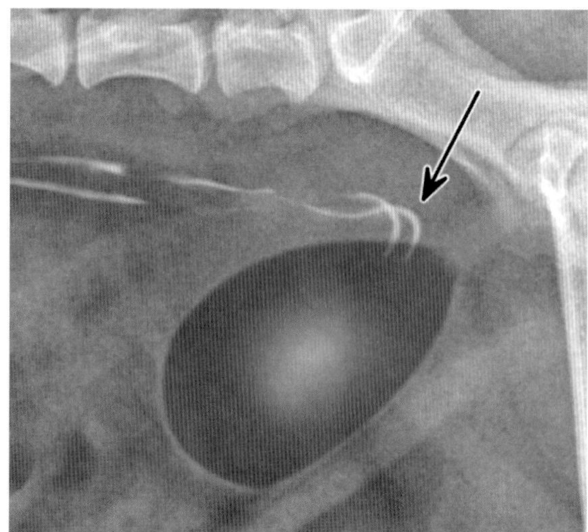

Figure 4.125 Vesicoureteral junction. Lateral view of a dog abdomen depicting a pneumocystogram combined with an EU. Performing both procedures concurrently can enhance visualization of the distal ureters as they enter the urinary bladder (arrow).

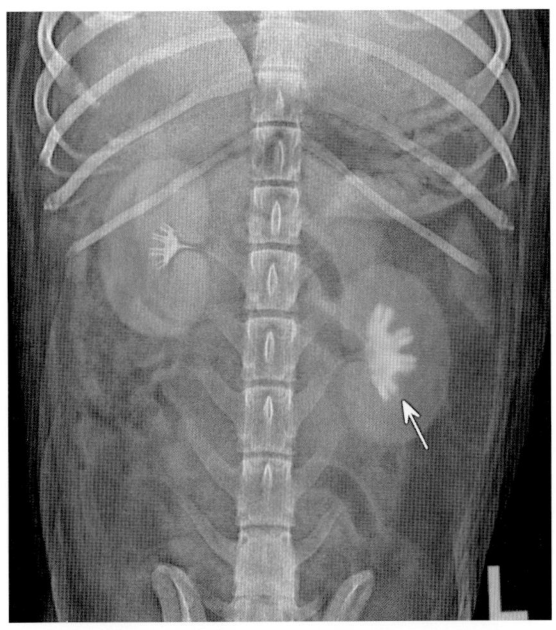

Figure 4.126 Left pyelonephritis. VD view of a dog abdomen depicting a pyelogram with a dilated left renal collecting system (arrow). The left renal pelvis is enlarged with less distinct edges and the pelvic recesses are widened and blunted. The right kidney is normal.

Larger masses and peripheral masses can both enlarge and distort the shape of a kidney (Figure 4.127). Types of renal masses include cysts, tumors, abscesses, hematomas, and others. However, the type of mass rarely can be determined from radiographs.

Cysts are fluid-filled cavities that usually develop in the parenchyma of a kidney. They may be congenital or acquired. Solitary and unilateral cysts often are asymptomatic and often inapparent in radiographs. They rarely communicate with the renal collecting system. Some cysts will enlarge over time and may eventually damage one or both kidneys.

Polycystic kidney disease (PKD) is a heritable disease in cats and dogs. It predominantly affects Persian and domestic long-haired cats and certain dog breeds (e.g., Cairn Terriers, Beagles, Bull Terriers). The cysts are present at birth and gradually enlarge over time. Animals with PKD may remain asymptomatic or the disease may progress to renal failure. When small, the cysts are difficult to detect with radiography. Larger cysts may be visible in a nephrogram as well-defined, rounded filling defects (Figure 4.128). More peripheral cysts can distort the border of a kidney. The pyelogram usually is normal, but large or numerous cysts can distort the renal collecting system.

Primary kidney tumors are uncommon in dogs and cats, but many are malignant. At the time of diagnosis, most renal tumors are large and distort the shape of the kidney. Long-standing tumors sometimes will mineralize. A nephrogram may reveal a round or irregular-shaped filling defect. Contrast medium sometimes will enter a tumor and persist after the rest of the nephrogram fades away. Large or multiple tumors can prevent a nephrogram and distort the pyelogram.

Perirenal pseudocyst

A perirenal pseudocyst is an abnormal accumulation of fluid around a kidney. The fluid may be either subcapsular or

A

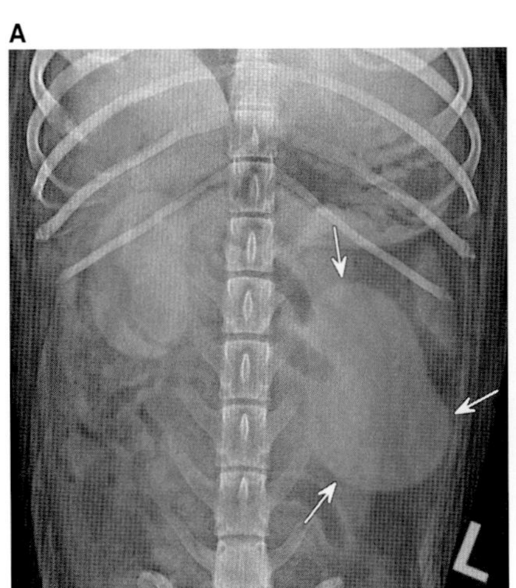

B

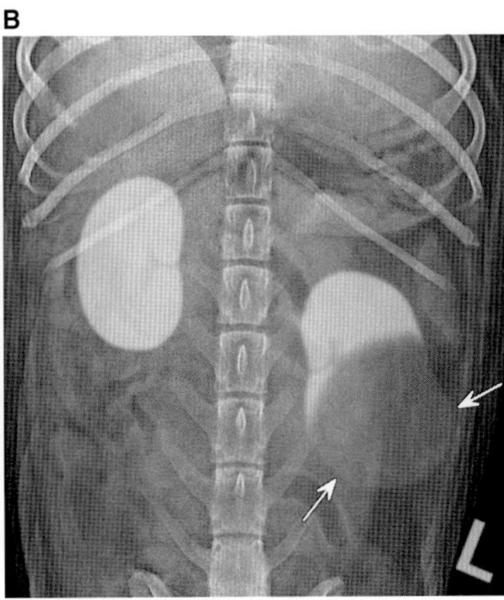

C

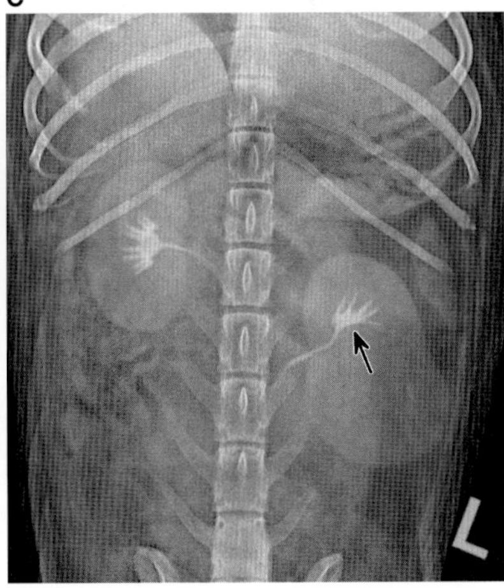

Figure 4.127 Renal mass. Three VD views of the same dog abdomen depicting an abnormal left kidney. **A**. Survey radiograph: the left kidney is enlarged and abnormal in shape (arrows). **B**. Nephrogram: there is a large filling defect in the caudal pole of the left kidney (arrows) caused by a mass. **C**. Pyelogram: the left renal collecting system is distorted (arrow) due to the mass in the caudal pole.

A

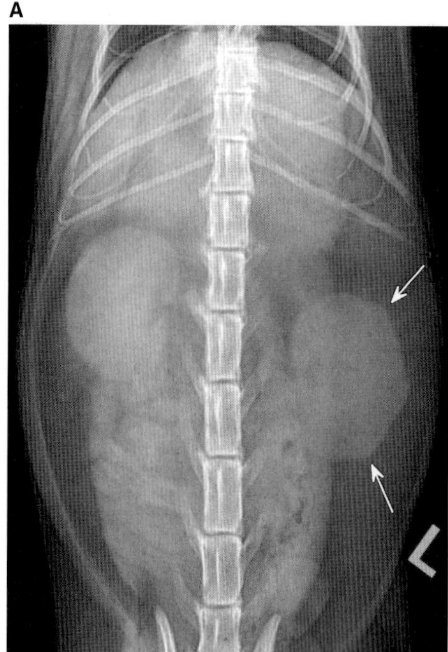

B

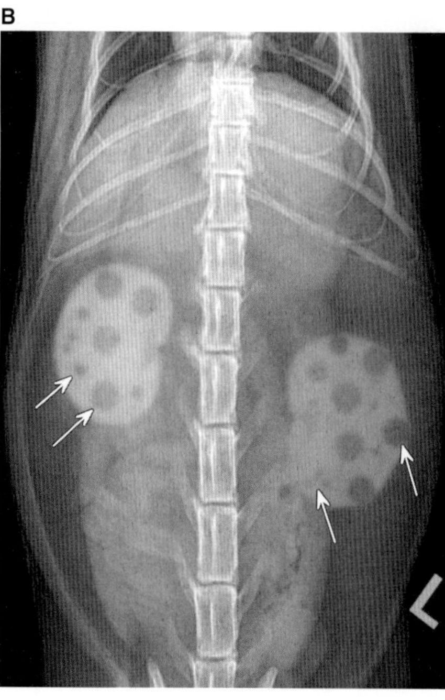

Figure 4.128 Polycystic Kidney Disease. Two VD views of the same cat abdomen. The survey radiograph (**A**) depicts bilateral renomegaly with several small bulges along the border of the left kidney (arrows). The nephrogram (**B**) depicts multiple, well-defined filling defects in the parenchyma of both kidneys (arrows). The round filling defects vary in size and may be caused by cysts or nodules.

extracapsular. In survey radiographs, the fluid and the kidney are the same opacity, so most perirenal pseudocysts are initially interpreted as renomegaly (Figure 4.129). Pseudocysts can become very large and may be unilateral or bilateral. They most often are reported in older cats. The margins of the pseudocyst generally are even and well-defined. The diagnosis usually is evident in an excretory urogram which reveals a kidney surrounded by non-opacified fluid. The nephrogram and pyelogram may be normal or pressure atrophy in a long-standing pseudocyst can lead to a small, irregular shaped kidney.

A

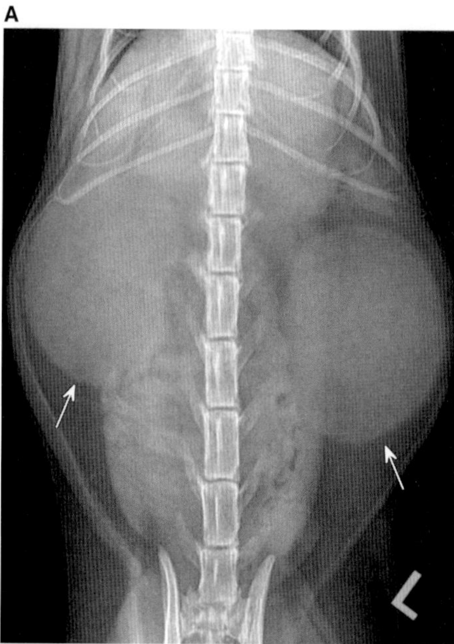

B

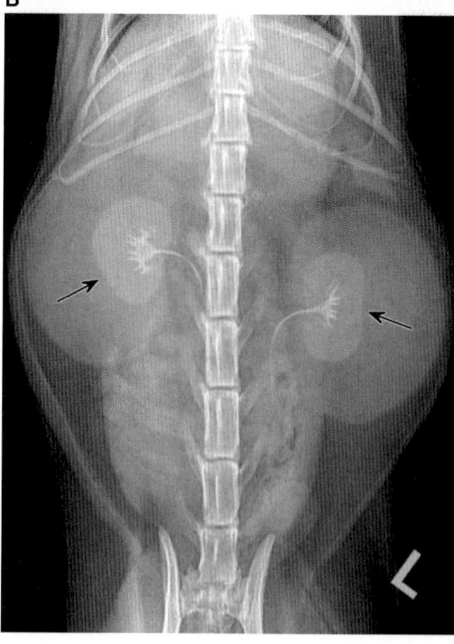

Figure 4.129 Perirenal pseudocysts. Two VD views of the same cat abdomen. The survey radiograph (**A**) depicts bilateral renomegaly (arrows). The excretory urogram (**B**) depicts opacification both kidneys (arrows). Each kidney is mildly irregular in shape and surrounded by non-opacified fluid.

Hydronephrosis

Dilation of the renal pelvis often leads to renomegaly, but it may or may not be evident in survey radiographs. It depends on the severity of the dilation, which is influenced by the degree and duration of the urinary outflow obstruction. An excretory urogram can help define the severity of the pelvic dilation and the site of the obstruction. The nephrogram frequently is normal during the early stages of hydronephrosis or with a mild, partial obstruction. If the obstruction persists or becomes more severe, the pelvis will continue to dilate and will gradually compress the renal parenchyma. Dilation widens the pelvic recesses and makes them appear blunted (Figure 4.130). In patients with severe hydronephrosis, the renal pelvis and pelvic recesses may be so distorted that they are unrecognizable. In cases of advanced hydronephrosis, only a thin rim of peripheral renal parenchyma may be opacified (Figure 4.131) or the kidney may not be opacified at all.

Ruptured kidney or ureter

Leakage of either urine or blood from a ruptured kidney (or urine from a ruptured ureter) leads to fluid accumulation in the retroperitoneal space. Fluid obscures retroperitoneal fat, making serosal margins less distinct and increasing retroperitoneal opacity. The affected kidney may appear irregular in shape or abnormal in position. Continued leakage of fluid enlarges the retroperitoneal space, which may displace the peritoneal structures ventrally (Figure 4.132). Peritoneal serosal margins remain distinct as long as the fluid is confined to the retroperitoneal space. Traumatic rupture of a kidney or ureter may be accompanied by concurrent bleeding in the peritoneal space and other signs of trauma (e.g., rib fractures, subcutaneous emphysema). Other causes of a ruptured kidney or ureter include chronic obstruction and erosion due to a calculus or tumor.

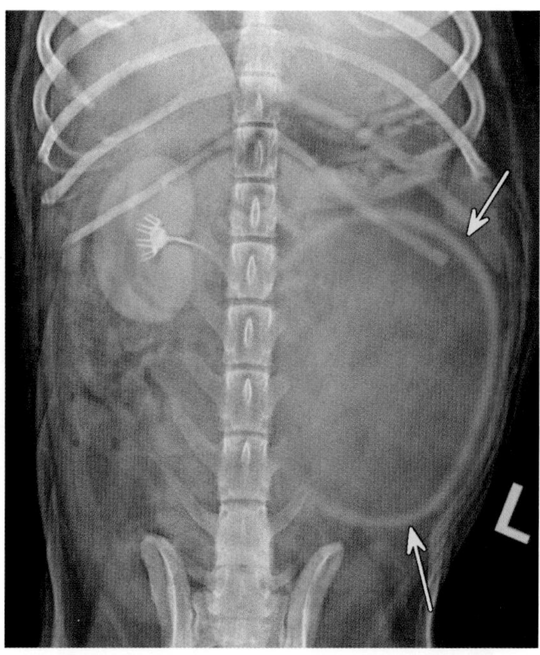

Figure 4.131 Severe hydronephrosis. VD view of a dog abdomen depicting the pyelogram phase of an excretory urogram. The left kidney is greatly enlarged with a thin rim of cortical opacification (arrows). The thin rim is the only remaining functional part of the kidney. Renal function is so severely diminished that there is no filling of the left renal collecting system. The right kidney is normal.

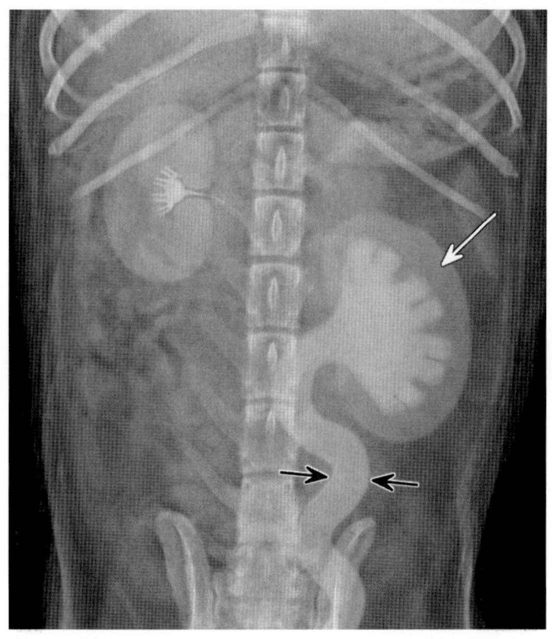

Figure 4.130 Hydronephrosis with hydroureter. VD view of a dog abdomen depicting the pyelogram phase of an excretory urogram. The left kidney is enlarged with a markedly distended renal pelvis and severely blunted pelvic recesses (white arrow). The left ureter is dilated and tortuous (black arrows). The right kidney is normal.

Excretory urography often is useful to evaluate a renal or ureteral rupture. The nephrogram of the affected kidney tends to be inhomogeneous due to parenchymal bleeding (Figure 4.133). If the renal artery is torn or obstructed, no nephrogram will be visible. The renal margin may be irregular or incomplete. The pyelogram may reveal a distorted renal pelvis due to a blood clot or an adjacent hematoma. The ureter sometimes is dilated due to abnormal peristalsis. If the renal pelvis is ruptured, contrast medium can enter and remain in the kidney parenchyma. Extravasation of contrast medium may be visible either under the renal capsule or flowing into the retroperitoneal space (Figure 4.134).

A

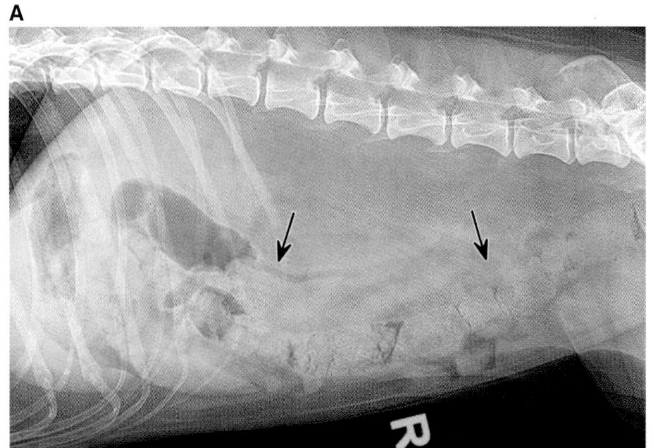

B

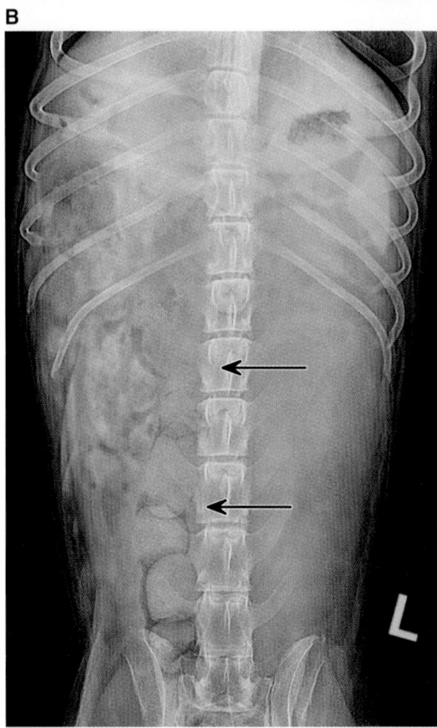

Figure 4.132 Retroperitoneal effusion. Lateral view (**A**) and VD view (**B**) of a dog abdomen depicting swelling of the retroperitoneal space. The peritoneal structures are displaced ventrally and to the right (arrows). Retroperitoneal serosal margins are indistinct; the margins of the kidneys and hypaxial muscles are not identified. Notice that the peritoneal serosal margins remain visible, indicating that the disease is confined to the retroperitoneal space. This patient's excretory urogram is depicted in Figure 4.133.

Ectopic ureter

Ectopic ureter is a congenital defect in which one or both ureters empties abnormally into the urethra or vagina. It is more common in dogs than in cats and more common in females than in males. An ectopic ureter may be *intramural* or *extramural*. Intramural is reported more often in dogs and occurs when the ureter enters the urinary bladder in the normal location but tunnels through the bladder wall to bypass the trigone. Extramural is more common in cats and occurs when the ureter completely bypasses the bladder to enter the urethra directly.

Survey radiographs often are unremarkable in patients with ectopic ureter. If both ureters are ectopic, the urinary bladder may be small due to disuse (i.e., *hypoplastic bladder*). The kidneys usually are normal in size. Small kidneys may result from chronic inflammation. Large kidneys can result from a distal ureteral obstruction and hydronephrosis.

A

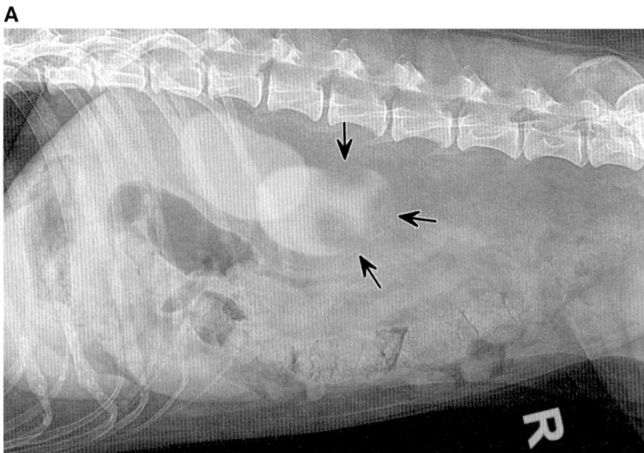

B

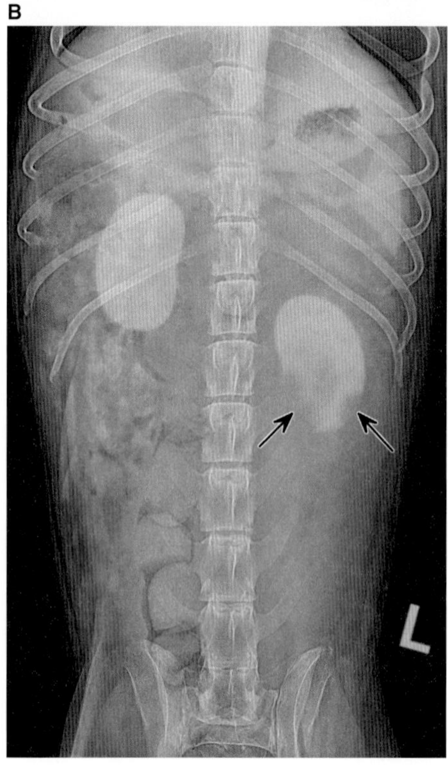

Figure 4.133 Retroperitoneal effusion. Lateral view (**A**) and VD view (**B**) of the same dog as in Figure 4.132 depicting a nephrogram with patchy filling defects in the left kidney (arrows). The filling defects are caused by parenchymal bleeding (see also Figure 4.134). The right kidney is normal.

During excretory urography, visualization of contrast medium in a structure other than the urinary bladder confirms the diagnosis of an ectopic ureter (Figure 4.135). Combining an EU with a pneumocystogram can enhance visualization of the vesicoureteral junction. Oblique views often are needed to further separate the ureters and to eliminate superimposition artifacts. Ureteral filling and opacification can be increased by temporarily compressing the caudal abdomen to restrict the flow of urine. Abdominal compression is not recommended with a pneumocystogram. In patients with ectopic ureter, contrast laden urine sometimes leaks onto the skin and hair coat, which can cover the area of interest with contrast medium, effectively ruining the radiographic study. This is especially problematic in females due to leakage from the vagina. Be ready for such an occurrence and take steps to prevent contamination of the field of view.

A

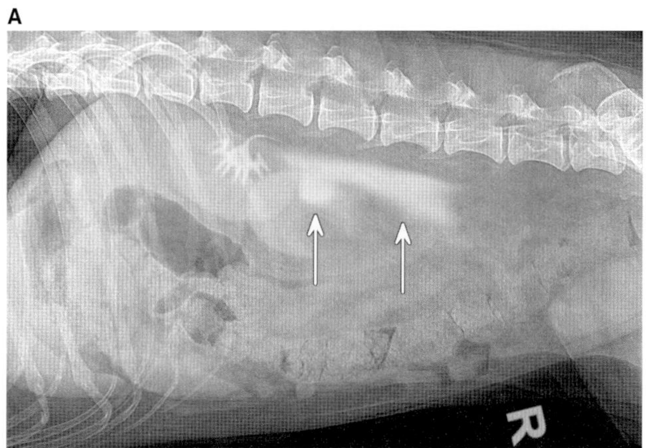

B

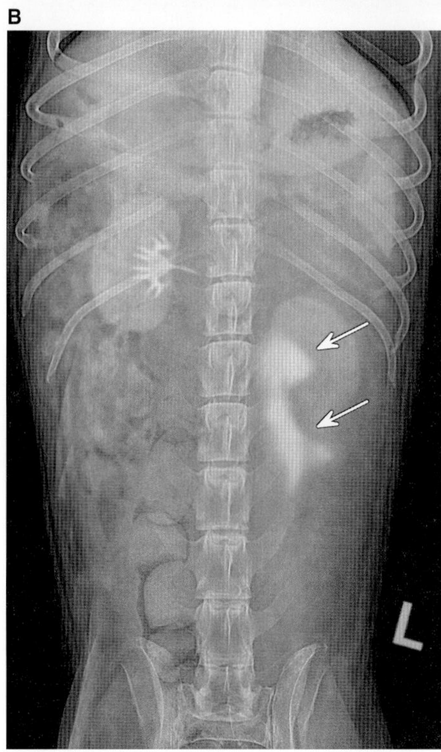

Figure 4.134 Retroperitoneal effusion. Lateral view (**A**) and VD view (**B**) of the same dog as in Figure 4.133 depicting a pyelogram. The left renal collecting system is indistinct and there is leakage of contrast medium into the retroperitoneal space (arrows). It is difficult to determine whether the leakage is from the kidney or the proximal ureter. The right kidney is again normal.

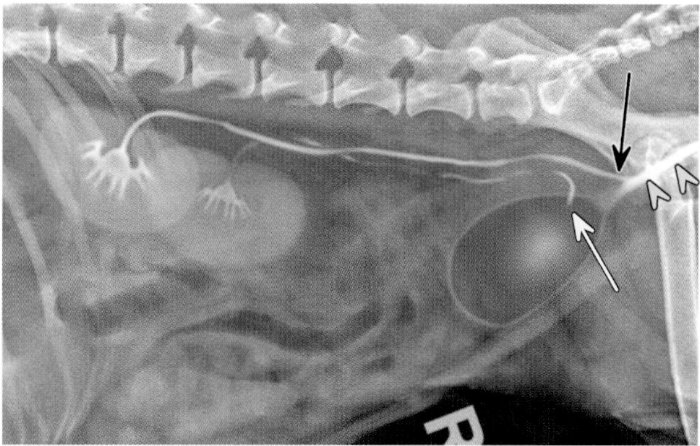

Figure 4.135 Ectopic ureter. Lateral view of a dog abdomen depicting a pyelogram with a pneumocystogram. The right ureter bypasses the urinary bladder to enter the urethra directly (black arrow). Contrast medium is visible in the urethra (yellow arrowheads) prior to any significant filling of the urinary bladder. The left ureter enters the bladder normally (white arrow). The right ureter is more completely opacified than the left and there is mild dilation of the right renal collecting system, possibly due to partial obstruction or inflammation.

An ectopic ureter may appear dilated (hydroureter) and more tortuous than normal due to inflammation and reduced peristalsis or due to a distal obstruction. Hydroureter may be accompanied by hydronephrosis or/and other ureteral abnormalities, such as a *ureterocele*.

A **ureterocele** is a congenital, cyst-like dilation in one or both distal ureters. Ureteroceles are uncommon in dogs and cats and may or may not block the flow of urine. They occur more often in females than in males. In an excretory urogram, the affected ureter terminates in a focal contrast-filled swelling (Figure 4.136). In a cystogram, a ureterocele produces a round, well-defined filling defect in the trigone region. When associated with an ectopic ureter, a ureterocele may be located in the urethra.

Urinary bladder

Normal radiographic anatomy

The urinary bladder generally is positioned between the pelvic inlet and the mid-abdomen (level of the umbilicus). Its size and shape can vary significantly depending on the volume of urine it contains. The serosal margin of the

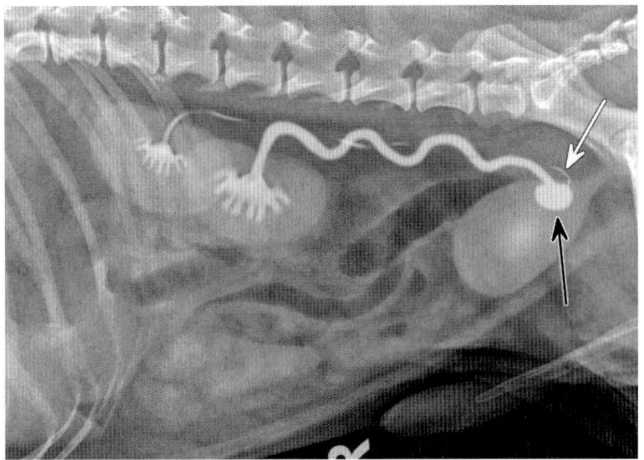

Figure 4.136 Ureterocele. Lateral view of a dog abdomen depicting a pyelogram. At the urinary bladder trigone, the left ureter terminates in a contrast-filled dilation (black arrow points to a ureterocele). The right ureter enters the bladder normally (white arrow). The ureterocele partially obstructs the flow of urine from the left kidney, leading to left hydroureter and hydronephrosis. The right ureter and renal collecting system are normal.

urinary bladder should be even and well-defined. Its mucosal margin is not visible in survey radiographs because urine and the mucosa are the same opacity. Bladder wall thickness, therefore, cannot be reliably assessed in survey radiographs.

For descriptive purposes, the urinary bladder is divided into three parts: *vertex*, *body*, and *neck*. The **vertex** is the cranial part, sometimes called the dome of the bladder. The **body** is the middle part of the bladder and the **neck** of the bladder joins the urethra. In dogs, the vesicourethral junction is typically located at the pelvic inlet. In cats, the junction may be several centimeters cranial to the pubis.

The **trigone** of the bladder is the area where the ureters enter. It is the triangular region along the caudal dorsal bladder that includes both the vesicoureteral junction and the vesicourethral junction (notice that the spelling is similar, but these are two different junctions).

In dogs, the urinary bladder is ovoid or teardrop-shaped with a tapered neck (Figure 4.137). The neck is about 1 to 2 cm in length. In cats, the bladder neck is relatively long (about 2 to 3 cm in length) which means the bladder tends to be more cranial in position than in dogs. The long neck of the feline bladder is sometimes called the pre-pelvic urethra.

Abnormal position of urinary bladder

Non-visualization of the urinary bladder is because it is either empty, ruptured, or displaced (see differential diagnoses). An **empty bladder** is small and may not be visible in survey radiographs because it obscured by overlying structures or because it is located within the pelvic canal. A "pelvic bladder" is sometimes seen in overweight dogs because the excess intra-abdominal fat can confine a small bladder to the pelvic canal. A "pelvic bladder" may also be due to a short urethra (Figure 4.139). A short urethra is a developmental abnormality that may or may not be clinically significant. It is reported more often in dogs than in cats and may predispose the patient to recurrent cystitis or incontinence.

A **ruptured bladder** sometimes is obscured in survey radiographs due to its small size or the loss of an opacity interface due to leakage of urine and blood. Urine leaking into the peritoneal cavity frequently leads to peritonitis and more widespread indistinct serosal margins. Avulsion of the bladder usually results in cranial displacement.

Displacement of the bladder most often is due to a nearby mass effect, either physiologic or pathologic. It may also result from a loss of abdominal integrity. A large colon,

A

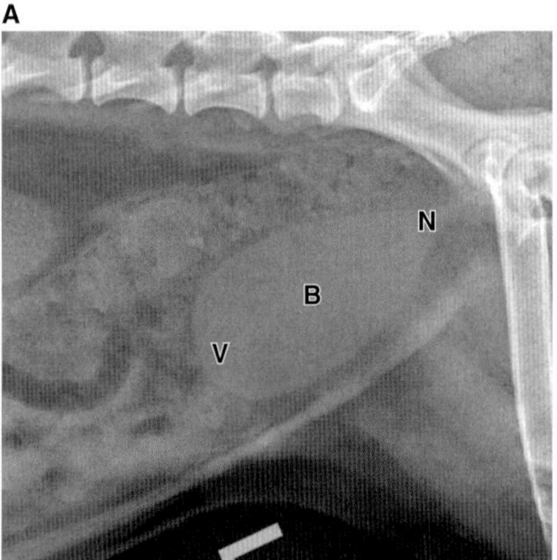

B

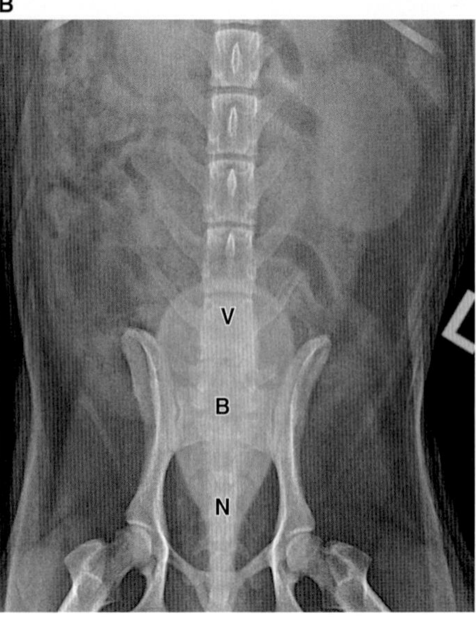

Figure 4.137 Normal canine urinary bladder. Lateral view (**A**) and VD view (**B**) of a dog abdomen depicting the urinary bladder and its three divisions: vertex (V), body (B), and neck (N).

A

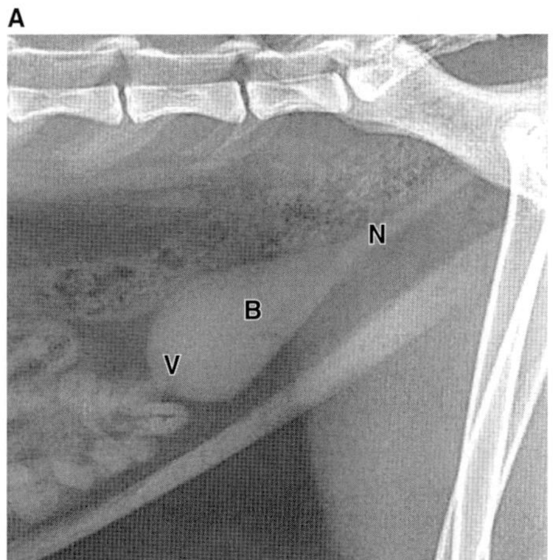

B

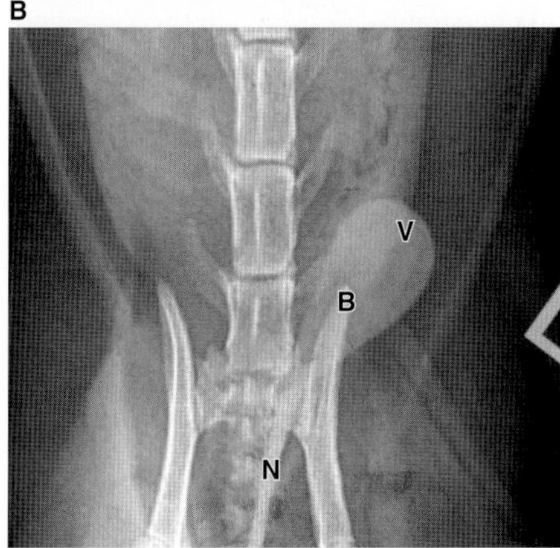

Figure 4.138 Normal feline urinary bladder. Lateral view (**A**) and VD view (**B**) of a cat abdomen depicting the urinary bladder and its three divisions: vertex (V), body (B), and neck (N).

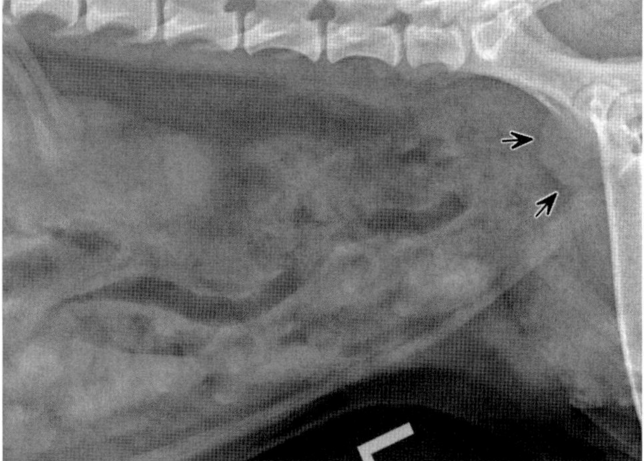

Figure 4.139 "Pelvic bladder". Lateral view of a dog abdomen depicting a urinary bladder that is located within the pelvic canal (arrows).

uterus, or prostate gland can easily displace the urinary bladder and may alter its shape. The bladder can become displaced through an abdominal or perineal hernia or due to a prolapse. Urinary **bladder prolapse** occurs when the bladder "flips over" and the vertex enters the pelvic canal. The bladder sometimes ends up in the perineal area, where it is unlikely to be identified in survey radiographs. Urinary bladder prolapse frequently leads to obstruction of the urethra and both ureters.

Abnormal size of urinary bladder

Evaluating the size of the urinary bladder tends to be a subjective assessment. A smaller than expected bladder may be due to recent voiding. A persistently small bladder may be due to an inability to expand, which can result from chronic inflammation and fibrosis of the bladder wall.

Even when full, a normal urinary bladder generally does not extend cranial to the level of the umbilicus. A larger than expected bladder may be due to a urinary outflow problem, neuromuscular disease, or voluntary retention (Figure 4.140).

Abnormal shape of urinary bladder

The shape of the urinary bladder is readily distorted by a mass or visceral crowding, especially when the bladder is not fully distended. The bladder wall may be indented by adjacent bowel (Figure 4.150). Abnormal bladder shape can also result from a lesion in the bladder wall or a very large mass in the bladder. Note: many bladder wall lesions are not evident in survey radiographs.

Abnormal opacity or content in the urinary bladder

Gas opacity and mineral opacity in the urinary bladder are abnormal and often visible in survey radiographs.

Gas in the urinary bladder may be iatrogenic or due to a gas-producing bacterial infection (*emphysematous cystitis*). Procedures such as cystocentesis and urethral catheterization allow air to enter the bladder lumen. Gas bubbles rise to the top of any urine in the bladder lumen and typically collect under its central curved "roof". Bubbles usually decrease in size and number in serial radiographs.

Emphysematous cystitis most often is associated with diabetes mellitus. It appears as multiple, coalescing gas bubbles that conform to the shape and location of the urinary bladder (Figure 4.141). Gas may be visible in the bladder wall, bladder lumen, or both. Gas can dissect through the bladder wall and into the adjacent tissues.

Mineralization in the urinary bladder may be dystrophic or it may be due to foreign material, but most often it represents calculi or sediment/debris in the bladder lumen. Dystrophic mineralization typically is associated with chronic

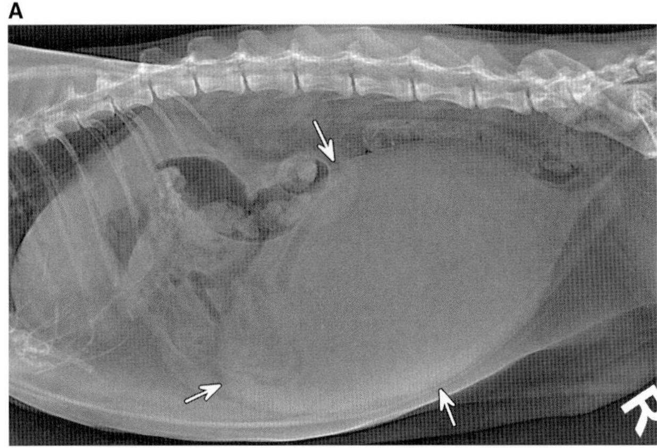

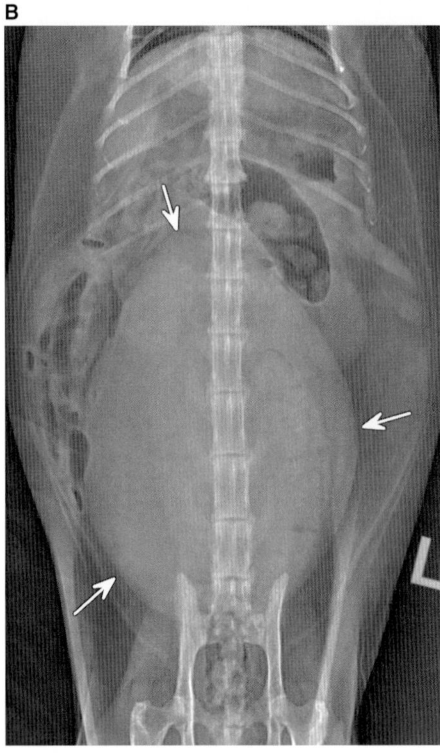

Figure 4.140 Large urinary bladder. Lateral view (**A**) and VD view (**B**) of a cat abdomen depicting a greatly distended urinary bladder (arrows). The intestines are displaced cranially, dorsally, and laterally by the large bladder. The cause is urethral obstruction.

inflammation or a long-standing blood clot or tumor. Foreign objects are uncommon in the urinary bladder (e.g., metal projectile, catheter fragment). Many foreign objects are freely moveable and change position in serial radiographs. Metal opacity objects in the bladder lumen can be concerning for heavy metal toxicosis.

A diffuse increase in bladder opacity may be due to contrast medium. Remember, the primary route of elimination for most iodinated contrast agents is via the urinary tract, regardless of the body part being imaged.

Cystic calculi, similar to renal calculi, can vary greatly in size, shape, number, and opacity (Figure 4.142). In general, the more calcium and phosphorous in a calculus, the greater its mineral opacity. However, the type or composition of urinary calculi cannot be reliably determined from radiographs. Calculi that contain little calcium or phosphorous may be soft tissue opacity, sometimes called "radiolucent." Soft tissue opacity calculi could be called "radiopaque" in a pneumocystogram.

Orthogonal views usually are needed to confirm cystic calculi. Superimposition of structures outside the urinary bladder, particularly intestinal contents, may be mistaken for bladder stones. When in doubt, empty the intestinal tract and repeat the radiographs or perform compression radiography or contrast radiography for clarification. Be sure to examine all radiographs for calculi in the kidneys, ureters or urethra (Figure 4.143).

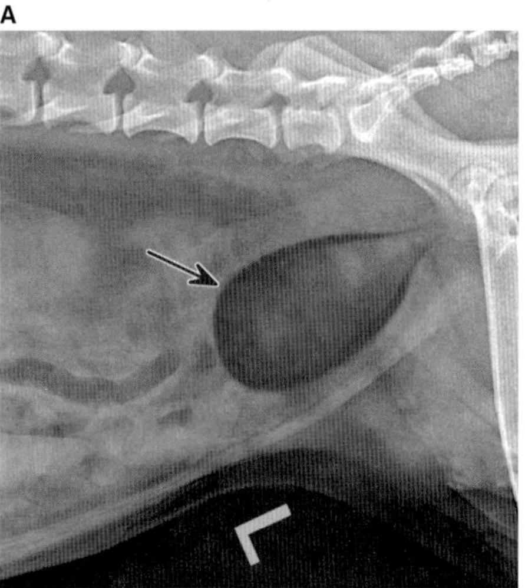

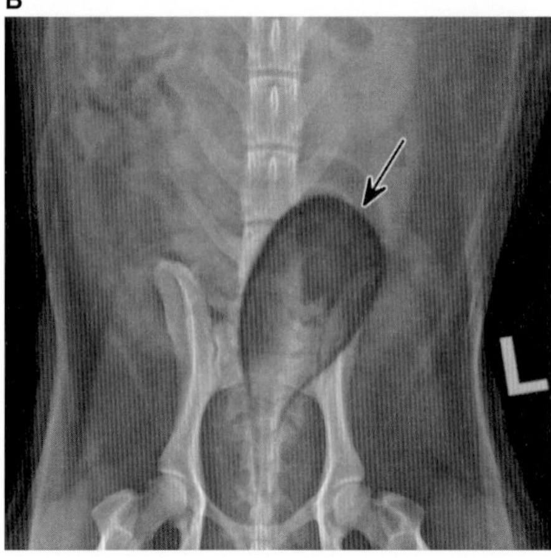

Figure 4.141 Emphysematous cystitis. Lateral view (**A**) and VD view (**B**) of a dog abdomen depicting a mottled pattern of gas bubbles in the wall and lumen of the urinary bladder (arrows).

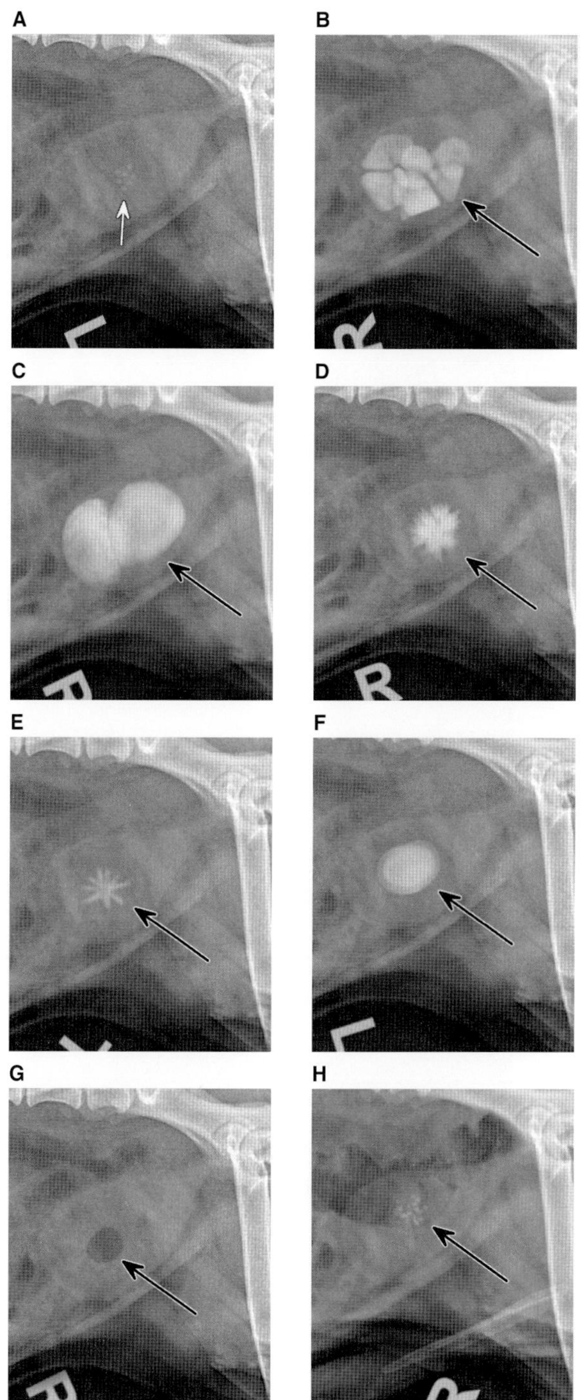

Figure 4.142 Cystic calculi. Lateral views of a dog abdomen depicting the radiographic appearance of various bladder stones (arrows). **A**. Tiny sand-like calculi. **B**. Multiple, smooth-bordered calculi. **C**. Two larger smooth bordered calculi. **D**. A stellate or star-shaped calculus. **E**. A spiculated calculus, similar to the stellate form. **F**. A layered calculus. **G**. A gas bubble which may be mistaken for a non-mineral opacity calculus. Note: most calculi are either soft tissue or mineral opacity. **H**. Superimposed intestinal content which may be mistaken for cystic calculi. Notice the similar content in the more proximal part of the descending colon. Abdominal compression could be used to displace the colon and better visualize the urinary bladder.

In lateral recumbency, most bladder stones fall to the dependent bladder wall and collect in the center of the bladder lumen. The larger mineral opacity calculi tend to be readily identified in radiographs, but cystography may be needed to detect the smaller and less opaque calculi. Tiny calculi may be more visible in a standing, horizontal beam lateral view because they tend to collect in the cranioventral curved part of the bladder and summation results in increased opacity.

When cystotomy is planned for the removal of bladder stones, it is important to make sure the calculi are present before surgery and that they are absent after surgery. Pre-operative radiographs are needed because bladder stones sometimes will dissappear prior to surgery, either because they passed during urination or because they dissolved. Post-operative radiographs are important because bladder stones sometimes are missed during surgery and because calculi can recur in a relatively short time after a cystotomy. Recurrance of bladder stones may be due to either migration of a calculus from the upper urinary tract or due to formation of a new calculus. With some clients it is essential to supply proof that all of the cystic calculi were removed.

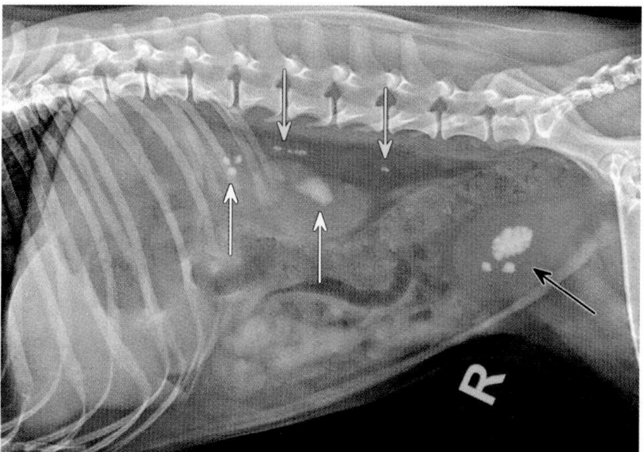

Figure 4.143 Urolithiasis. Lateral view of a dog abdomen depicting multiple mineral opacity calculi in the kidneys (white arrows), ureters (yellow arrows), and urinary bladder (black arrow).

Cystography

The procedure for cystography, as well as its indications and contraindications, is described in the contrast radiography section of Chapter 2. In a normal cystogram, the bladder lumen is homogeneous in opacity, the bladder wall is uniform in thickness, and the margin of the bladder mucosa is even (Figure 4.144).

The thickness of a normal bladder wall can vary considerably depending on the degree of bladder distention. The wall appears thicker with less bladder distention (which may be mistaken for a lesion) and thinner with greater distention (which can hide a lesion). In a moderately distended urinary bladder, the wall thickness is about 1 mm.

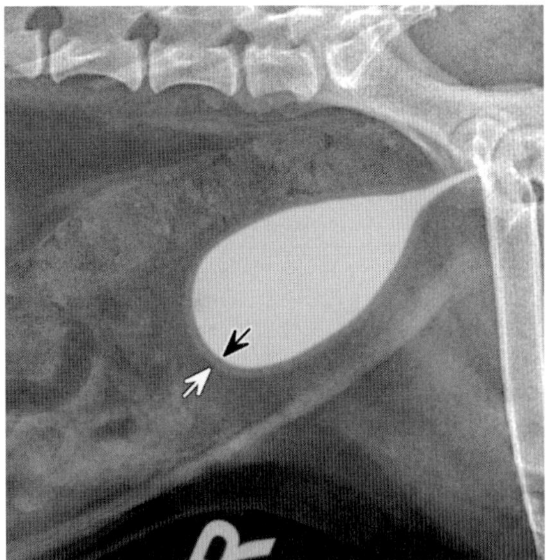

Figure 4.144 Normal cystogram. Lateral view of a dog abdomen depicting a positive contrast cystogram. Bladder wall thickness is measured from the mucosal margin (black arrow) to the serosal margin (white arrow) and normally is even and uniform.

Abnormal thickening of the bladder wall may be focal or diffuse. The most common causes are inflammation and neoplasia. The two are difficult to distinguish in radiographs. For the evaluation of bladder wall thickness, a positive contrast cystogram is preferred over a pneumocystogram because even a small volume of urine (or other fluid) in a gas-distended bladder can mimic a thickened bladder wall.

Radiographic signs of **cystitis** are non-specific. Characteristic findings in a cystogram include localized or diffuse thickening of the bladder wall, with or without an irregular mucosal margin (Figure 4.145). Thickening most often begins in the cranioventral part of the bladder. The thickened wall gradually thins further caudally to become more even and uniform. Subtle areas of thickening should be interpreted with caution because, as mentioned earlier, bladder wall thickness varies with the degree of bladder distention.

Chronic cystitis can lead to fibrosis of the bladder wall and loss of bladder distensibility. In these cases, the bladder often is persistently small and cystography must be performed with caution to avoid over-distending and rupturing the fibrotic bladder.

Filling defects in a cystogram can be caused by anything that prevents complete filling of the bladder lumen. In a positive contrast cystogram, a filling defect is an area of less opacity. In a pneumocystogram, a filling defect is an area of greater opacity. Causes of filling defects include gas bubbles, blood clots, calculi, masses, and polyps.

A

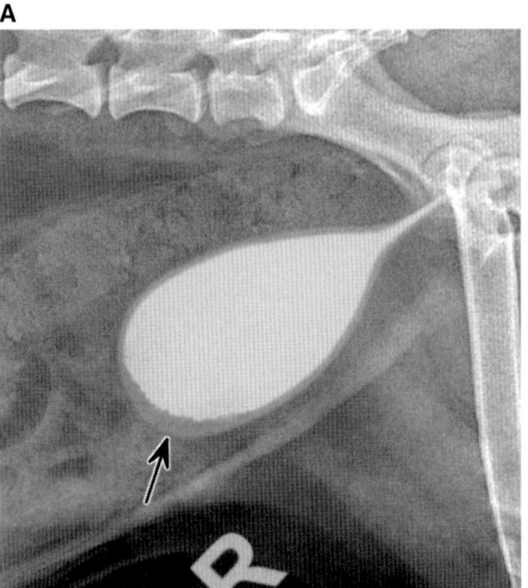

B

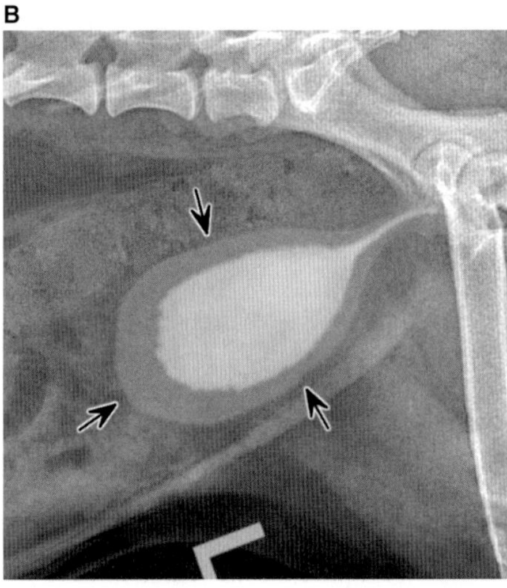

Figure 4.145 Cystitis. **A**. Lateral view of a dog abdomen depicting a positive contrast cystogram and thickening of the cranioventral bladder wall (arrow). The mucosal margin is slightly irregular. **B**. Lateral view cystogram of a different dog, depicting diffuse thickening of the bladder wall (arrows). The bladder mucosa is more irregular than in A. In both A and B, the bladder wall thickening is likely caused by inflammation, but neoplasia cannot be ruled out. In patients with chronic or recurrent cystitis the bladder wall can be many times normal thickness.

Gas bubbles in a positive contrast cystogram typically appear as round filling defects with distinct borders. Bubbles are freely moveable and tend to change position in serial radiographs. Gas may enter the bladder during catheterization or during infusion of contrast medium. To lessen the likelihood of introducing gas, the tip of the catheter should remain in the urethra rather than enter the bladder lumen. Gas bubbles float on top of any fluid in the bladder, typically moving to the periphery of the fluid. If the bladder is mostly fluid-filled, the bubbles will collect centrally, under the curved "roof" of the bladder (Figure 4.146). If the bladder is only partially filled with fluid, the bubbles likely will be at the edge of the fluid, similar to what happens with bubbles as you fill a glass with water. Numerous bubbles in the urinary bladder may produce a honeycomb pattern (Figure 4.147).

Blood clots generally produce filling defects that are irregular in shape with indistinct borders (Figure 4.149). Blood clots may be located anywhere in the bladder lumen, either attached to the bladder wall or freely movable in the lumen (some blood clots will float).

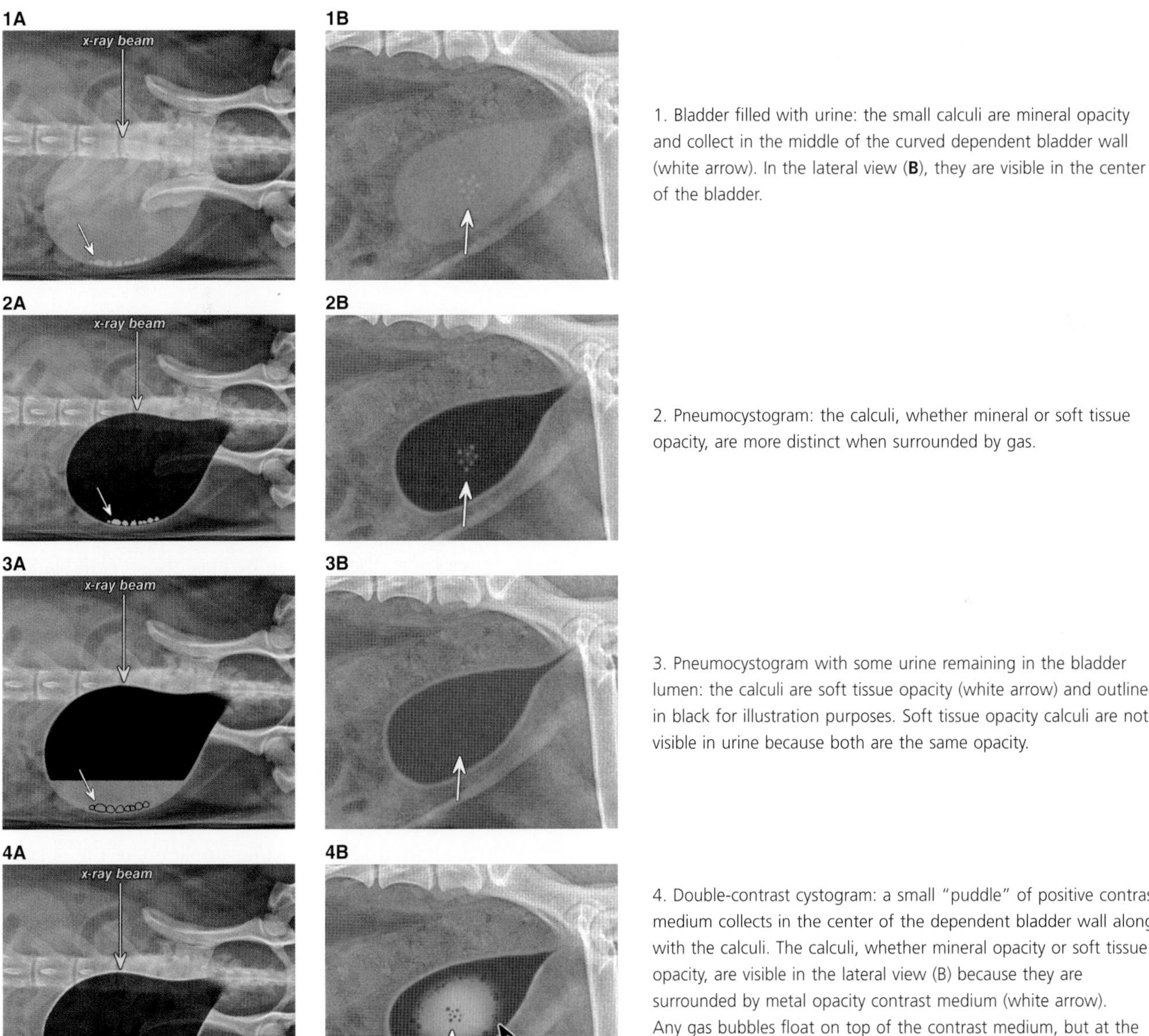

Figure 4.146 Cystic calculi and air bubbles. These images depict the distribution of calculi and gas in a urinary bladder that contains variable amounts of urine, gas, and contrast medium. Radiograph **A** in each example depicts a horizontal beam VD view of the abdomen made with the dog in right lateral recumbency. The direction of the x-ray beam is shown for the standard right lateral view of the same dog, which is depicted in radiograph **B**. Keep in mind that calculi are heavier than fluid and fall to the dependent part of the bladder. Gas bubbles float to the top of any fluid in the bladder lumen.

5A

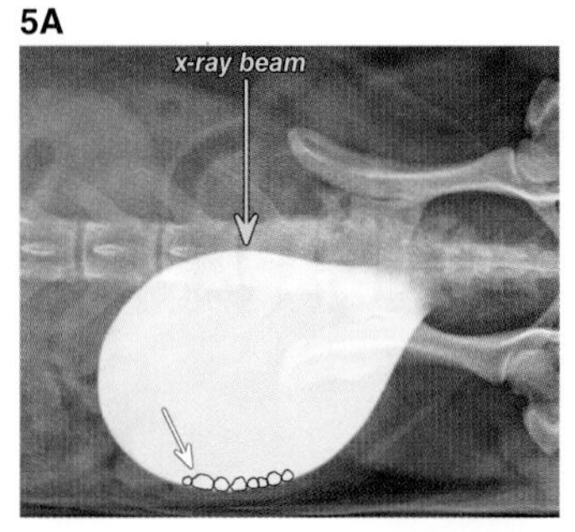

5B

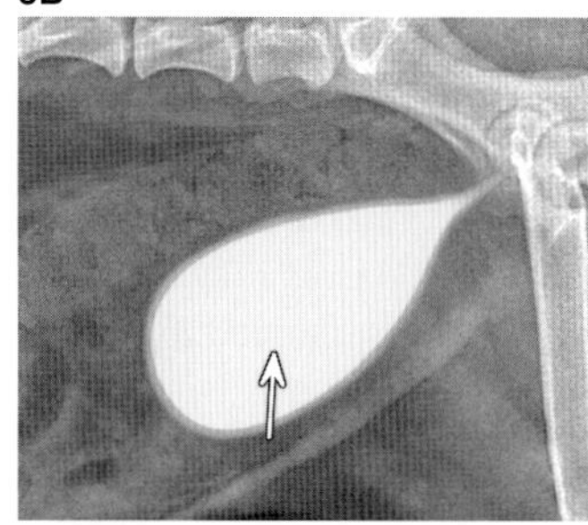

5. Positive contrast cystogram: small calculi are outlined in black (white arrow) because they are not visible in a bladder that is filled completely with positive contrast medium. Even mineral opacity calculi may be obscured by this degree of bladder opacification.

6A

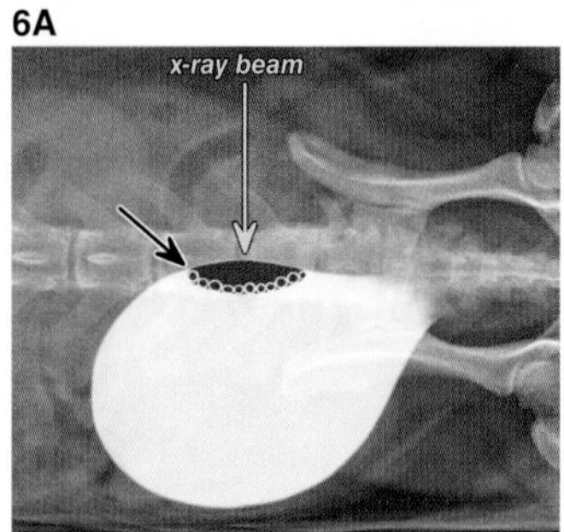

6B

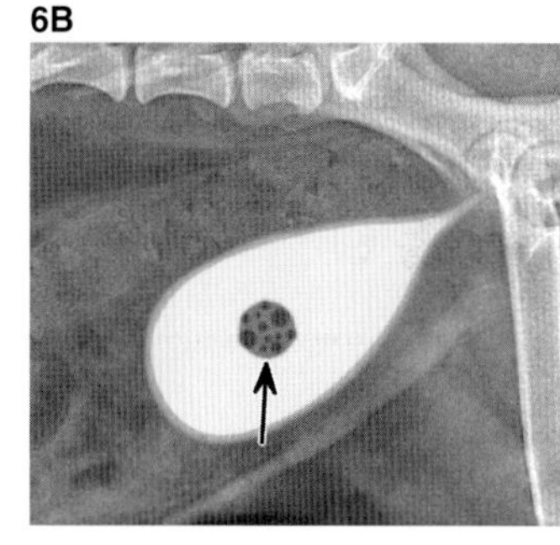

6. Positive contrast cystogram with gas bubbles: gas rises to the uppermost part of bladder and collects under the curved wall or "dome" of the bladder. In the lateral view, the bubbles are centrally located (black arrow) and may be mistaken for calculi.

Figure 4.146 (cont.) Cystic calculi and air bubbles. These images depict the distribution of calculi and gas in a urinary bladder that contains variable amounts of urine, gas, and contrast medium. Radiograph **A** in each example depicts a horizontal beam VD view of the abdomen made with the dog in right lateral recumbency. The direction of the x-ray beam is shown for the standard right lateral view of the same dog, which is depicted in radiograph **B**. Keep in mind that calculi are heavier than fluid and fall to the dependent part of the bladder. Gas bubbles float to the top of any fluid in the bladder lumen.

Cystic calculi that are not visible in survey radiographs may be detected with cystography. Most calculi are freely movable, but some will attach to the bladder wall. Filling defects caused by calculi can vary significantly in size, shape, and number. Filling defects may appear with smooth or irregular borders and sharp or indistinct margins. Mobile calculi move with gravity, often collecting in the center of the dependent, curved bladder wall (Figure 4.146). Bladder stones that are small or soft tissue opacity may not be visible in a positive contrast cystogram because the overall bladder opacity is too great, masking any opacity variation in that area (Figure 4.146). In these cases, the calculi often can be detected in a double contrast cystogram, because the bladder will be mostly gas-filled with only a thin pool of positive contrast medium around the calculi (Figures 4.146 and 4.148). The majority of bladder stones, even those that are mineral opacity, are less opaque than positive contrast media. Tiny calculi and soft tissue opacity calculi may also be missed in a pneumocystogram, because even a small volume of urine or other fluid adjacent to the calculi can eliminate the opacity interface. Here again, a double contrast cystogram may be the preferred study.

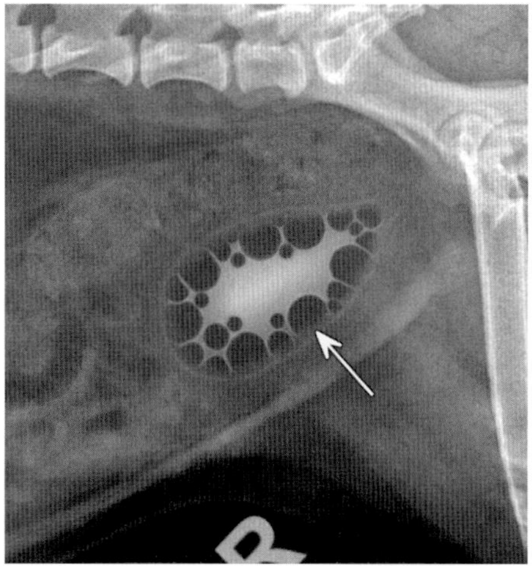

Figure 4.147 Gas bubbles in urinary bladder. Lateral view of a dog abdomen depicting a double contrast cystogram with multiple gas bubbles (arrow) due to iatrogenic introduction of air.

Masses in the urinary bladder usually produce filling defects that are fixed in position and accompanied by a thickened bladder wall. Examples of bladder masses include tumors, hematomas, and polyps. Many bladder masses are more visible when viewed in profile rather than *en face*.

Tumors most often arise in either the caudal or the cranial part of the urinary bladder (Figure 4.157). Most are malignant. Bladder tumors tend to be broad-based with irregular margins. The adjacent bladder wall usually is thickened. Caudal tumors can obstruct urine outflow, leading to abnormal bladder distention. Tumors in the trigone region can obstruct one or both ureters, leading to

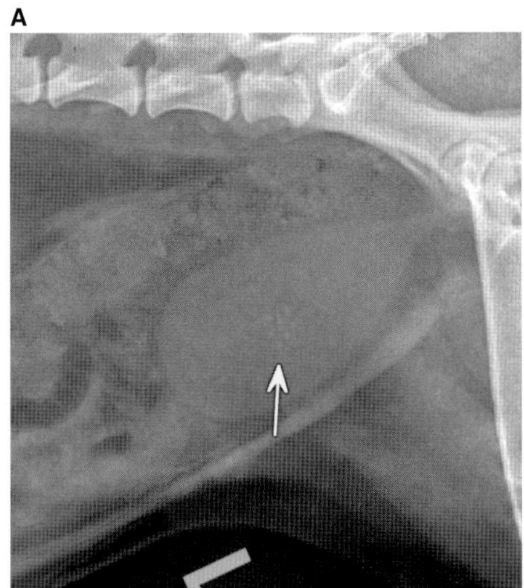

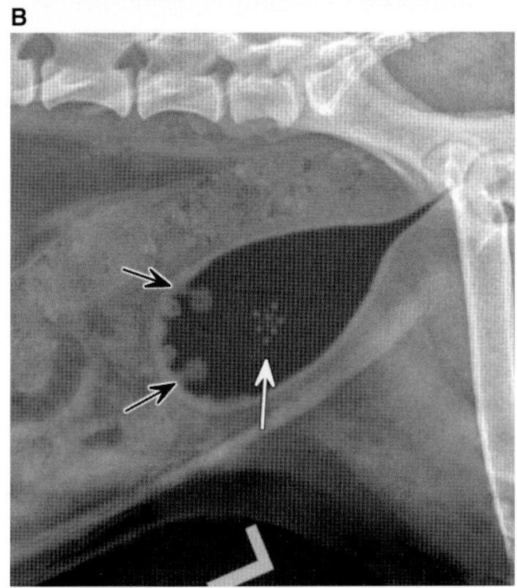

Figure 4.148 Pneumocystogram. **A**. Lateral view survey radiograph of a dog caudal abdomen depicting tiny, faint mineral opacity calculi in the urinary bladder (arrow). **B**. Pneumocystogram of the same dog enhances visualization of the calculi (white arrow) and reveals thickening and polypoid growths along the cranial bladder wall (black arrows).

hydronephrosis. Very large tumors can cause hypertrophic osteopathy. The most common urinary bladder tumor in dogs and cats is **transitional cell carcinoma**. This tumor frequently spreads to the sublumbar lymph nodes, the other urogenital structures, and to bones. Sublumbar lymphadenomegaly typically produces a retroperitoneal mass ventral to the L5–7 vertebrae. The sublumbar mass may be accompanied by a periosteal response along the ventrum of the lumbar vertebral bodies, sometimes extending to the pelvic bones.

Hematomas in the bladder wall usually produce smooth bordered filling defects that project into the lumen and taper at either end. A hematoma may be caused by trauma or it may be a complication of cystocentesis or catheterization. Hematomas can occur anywhere in the bladder wall.

Polyps appear as focal, pedunculated growths with smooth margins and thin attachments to the bladder mucosa (Figure 4.148). They typically measure about 1–3 mm in size. The adjacent bladder wall sometimes is thickened. Polyps may be solitary or multiple and can change in size and number in serial radiographs. They most often result from inflammation, but cannot be differentiated from neoplasia without histopathology.

Visceral crowding can distort the shape of the urinary bladder to produce a "pseudo-filling defect." For example, a partially filled bladder can be indented by the adjacent colon to produce a concave border with gradually sloping edges (Figure 4.150). This pseudo-filling defect may be eliminated by infusing additional contrast medium into the bladder lumen to more fully distend it.

Extravasation of contrast medium - contrast medium that projects beyond the lumen of the urinary bladder - may be due to a damaged bladder wall, a urachal abnormality, a fistula, or vesicoureteral reflux.

Damage to the bladder wall ranges from a mucosal injury to bladder rupture. Mucosal injuries may result from severe, chronic, or recurrent cystitis, neoplasia, or overdistention of the bladder. During cystography, high intraluminal pressure can push contrast medium through the damaged mucosa and into the subserosa (Figure 4.151). Contrast medium

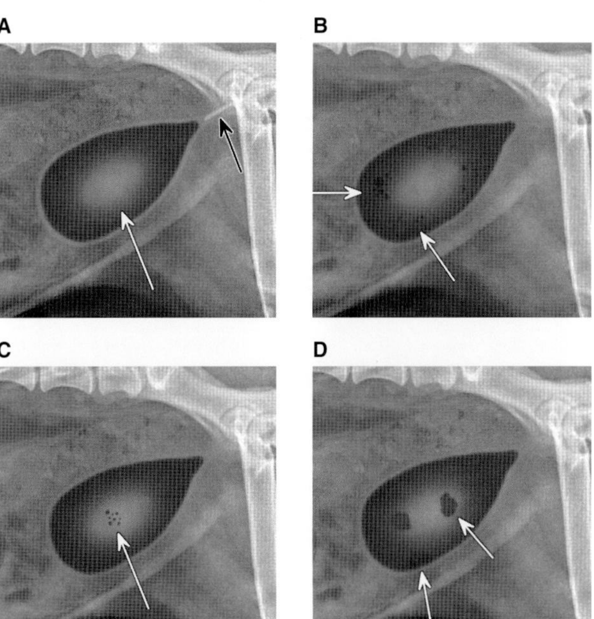

Figure 4.149 Double contrast cystography. Lateral views of a dog abdomen depicting various filling defects in double contrast cystograms. **A**. Normal study: the bladder is mostly gas-filled. There is a puddle of positive contrast medium in the center (white arrow). A catheter is visible in the urethra (black arrow). **B**. Gas bubbles are visible at the periphery of the contrast puddle (arrows). **C**. Tiny calculi can be seen the center of the contrast puddle (arrow). **D**. Blood clots are present in the contrast puddle and attached to the ventral bladder wall (arrows).

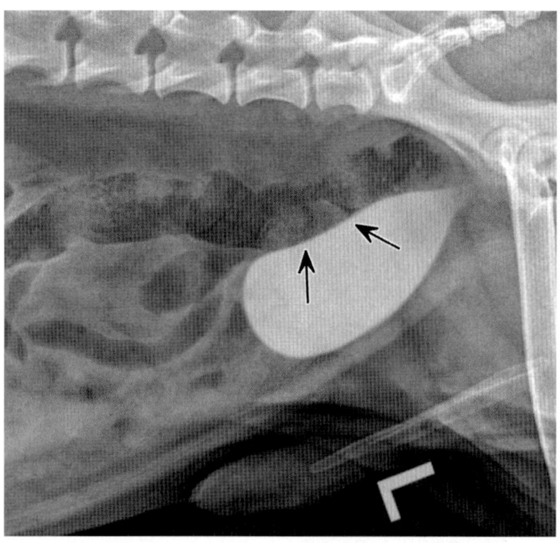

Figure 4.150 Pseudo-filling defect. Lateral view of dog abdomen depicting a positive contrast cystogram. The dorsal bladder wall is indented by the descending colon (arrows), which may be mistaken for thickening of the bladder wall.

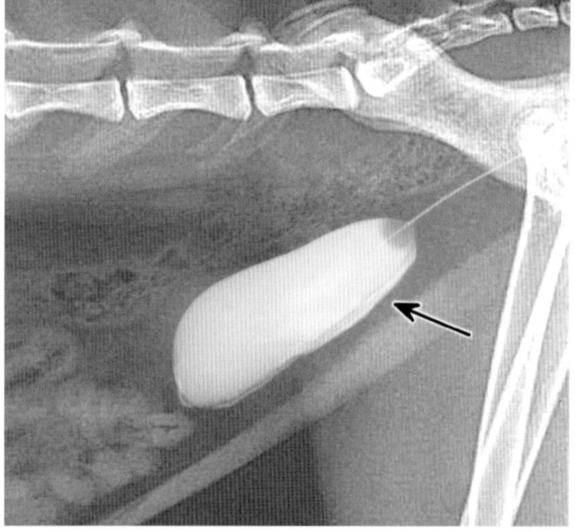

Figure 4.151 Subserosal leakage. Lateral view of a cat abdomen depicting a positive contrast cystogram with leakage into the bladder wall (arrow). Contrast medium is accumulating along the ventral subserosa due to a damaged mucosa.

may adhere to damaged mucosa, particularly if ulcers are present. Adherence of contrast medium usually is easiest to see in a double contrast cystogram. Ulcers in the bladder wall frequently are accompanied by blood clots in the lumen.

Rupture of the urinary bladder allows contrast medium to leak into the peritoneal space (Figure 4.152). A rupture may be caused by blunt force trauma, a penetrating wound, or a complication during cystocentesis or catheterization, particularly if the bladder is fully distended. Other causes of a rupture include chronic urinary outflow obstruction and erosion of the bladder wall due to neoplasia or severe inflammation.

When investigating a ruptured urinary bladder, positive contrast cystography is preferred over pneumocystography because small amounts of gas leaking into the peritoneal space are more difficult to detect or to differentiate from bowel gas. For cystography, if the contrast medium cannot be infused directly into the urinary bladder, as may be the case with an avulsed bladder, an excretory urogram can be performed to produce the cystogram.

A bladder with a small rupture (up to about 0.5 cm in size) may need to be moderately distended before contrast medium leaks out. Small leaks tend to dissipate quickly and are more likely to be detected when the cystogram is made during the infusion of the contrast agent. A bladder with a large rupture (2 cm or more in size) usually does not distend during infusion and the contrast medium flows directly into the peritoneal space. If too much contrast medium is infused before the radiograph is made, there may be confusion as to the origin of the leakage.

Urachal abnormalities result from failure of the urachus to close completely at birth. The urachus is the embryologic communication between the urinary bladder and the umbilicus. A *persistent urachal ligament* is a residual connection between the vertex of the bladder and the ventral body wall. The ligament may or may not be patent. Tension along this connection can distort the shape of the bladder and prevent complete filling and emptying. In radiographs, the

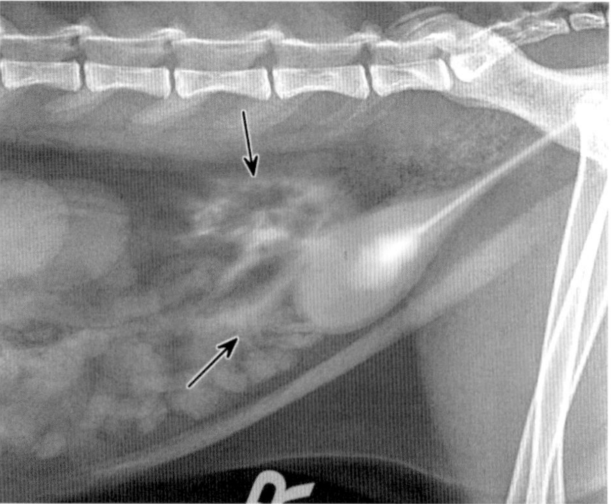

Figure 4.152 Ruptured urinary bladder. Lateral view of a cat abdomen depicting a positive contrast cystogram. The radiograph was made during active infusion of the contrast agent. Contrast medium is visible in the peritoneal space (arrows) as it leaks from a tear in the dorsal bladder wall.

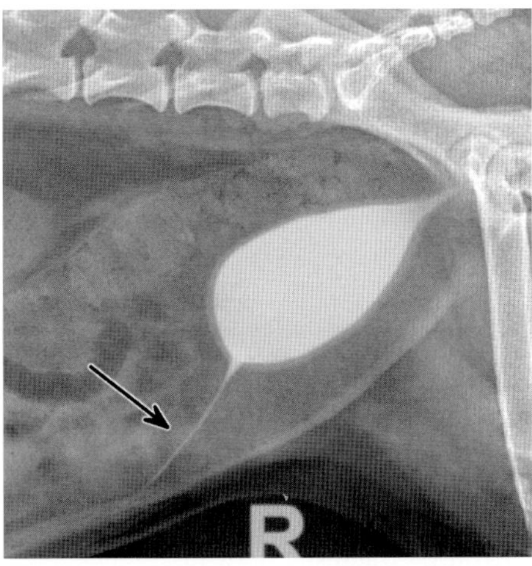

Figure 4.153 Persistent urachal ligament. Close-up lateral view of a dog abdomen depicting a positive contrast cystogram. Contrast medium fills most of a patent urachal remnant (black arrow) creating a thin opacified line that connects the bladder vertex to the ventral abdominal wall.

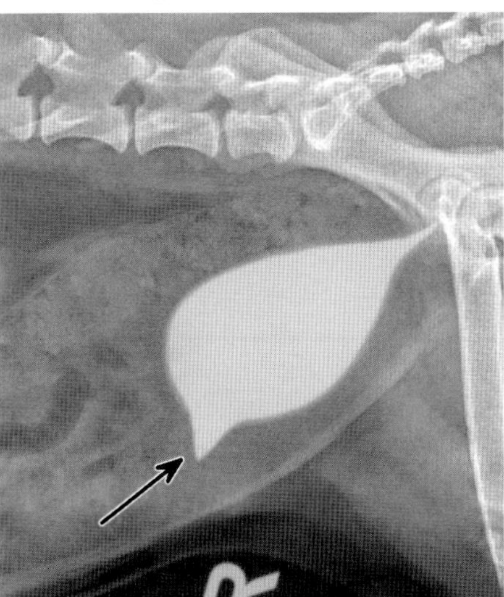

Figure 4.154 Urachal diverticulum. Close-up lateral view of a dog abdomen depicting a positive contrast cystogram. Contrast medium extends beyond the lumen of the urinary bladder (black arrow), filling an outpouch in the vertex that points toward the ventral body wall.

urinary bladder typically appears elongated with a pointed cranial end (Figure 4.153).

A *urachal diverticulum* is a partial remnant of the urachus. Urine may be retained in the diverticulum, leading to recurrent cystitis. In radiographs, it appears as a pointed projection that extends from the vertex of the bladder toward the umbilicus (Figure 4.154).

A *urachal cyst* is a fluid-filled cavity that forms in the remnants of the urachus. The cyst may or may not be patent with the bladder lumen or the ventral body wall. In radiographs, it appears as a persistent, stationary, soft tissue opacity "nodule" between the bladder and the umbilicus (Figure 4.155).

A urinary bladder **diverticulum** may also result from trauma or a developmental abnormality. The diverticulum is caused by protrusion of the bladder mucosa through a weak or torn muscle layer in the bladder wall (Figure 4.156).

As described earlier, **vesicoureteral reflux** during cystography can lead to contrast medium entering the ureters and renal collecting systems. Reflux can occur in a normal or diseased urinary bladder and can involve one or both ureters and kidneys (Figure 4.157).

A **fistula** is an abnormal communication between two or more separate structures. Fistulas involving the urinary tract

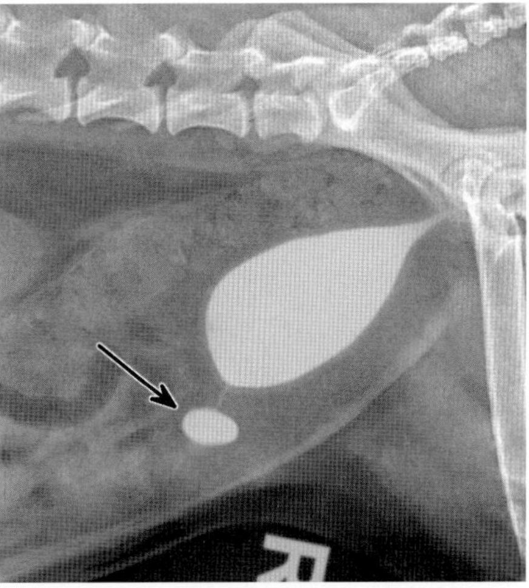

Figure 4.155 Urachal cyst. Close-up lateral view of a dog abdomen depicting a positive contrast cystogram. Contrast medium fills a dilated area in a urachal remnant (black arrow).

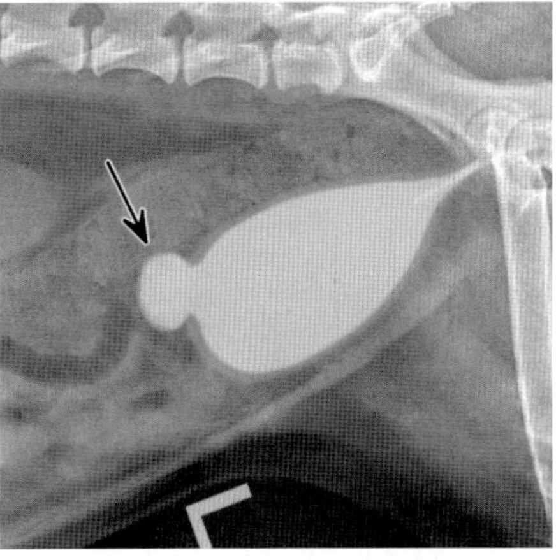

Figure 4.156 Diverticulum. Close-up lateral view of a dog abdomen depicting a positive contrast cystogram. Contrast medium extends beyond the bladder lumen (black arrow) to be contained in an outpouching along the cranial bladder wall. This diverticulum resulted from previous trauma.

A

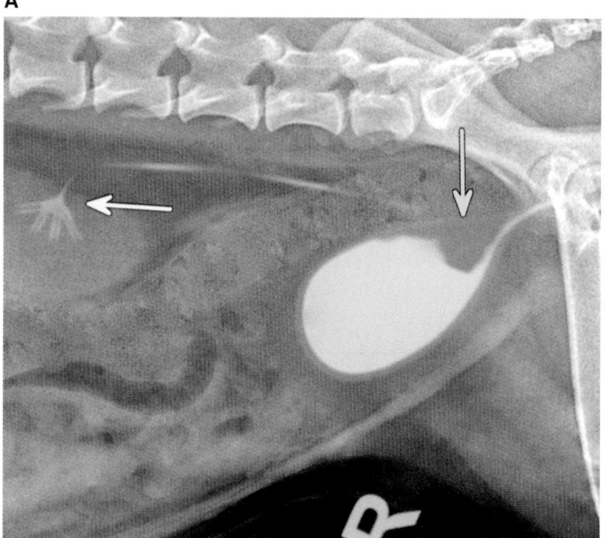

B

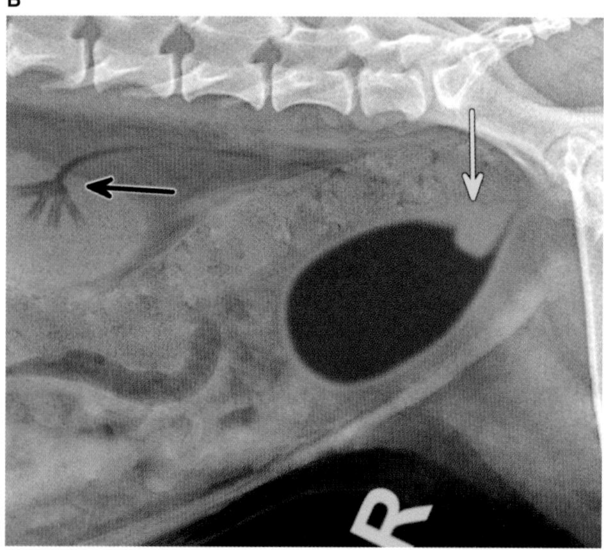

Figure 4.157 Urinary bladder tumor. **A**. Lateral view of a dog abdomen depicting a positive contrast cystogram with an irregular-shaped filling defect and a thickened bladder wall in the trigone region (yellow arrow). Vesicoureteral reflux results in contrast medium entering the ureter and renal collecting system (arrow). **B**. Lateral view of the same dog depicting a pneumocystogram. The same bladder lesion and similar vesicoureteral reflux are again present, but visible due to a gas opacity interface instead of a positive contrast interface.

are rare in dogs and cats, more often involving the urethra than the urinary bladder (Figure 4.168).

Urethra

Normal radiographic anatomy

The urethra runs caudally from the neck of the urinary bladder to the external urethral orifice. It is only a few centimeters long in cats and female dogs and longer in male dogs. The pre-pelvic part of the urethra is longer in cats than in dogs. Some authors consider the pre-pelvic urethra to be part of the bladder neck. The urethra is soft tissue opacity and visible in radiographs when surrounded by fat or filled with contrast medium.

The male urethra is divided into three parts: *prostatic, pelvic,* and *penile*. The prostatic urethra runs from the neck of the urinary bladder to the caudal edge of the prostate gland. It is the widest part of the urethra and completely encircled by the prostate gland. The pelvic urethra is located between the prostate gland and the ischial arch. The urethra is narrowest at the ischial arch. The penile urethra runs from the caudal edge of the pelvis to the tip of the penis. The *os penis* partially surrounds the distal urethra.

Abnormal appearance of the urethra

The position and size of the urethra rarely can be evaluated without urethrography. Urethral mineralization may be visible in survey radiographs (e.g., dystrophic mineralization, calculi). Dystrophic mineralization tends to appear thin and linear, whereas calculi usually are larger and more focal. Urethral mineralization may be obscured in radiographs by overlying skeletal structures. Rotating the patient and repositioning the pelvic limbs may eliminate some of these superimposition artifacts (Figure 4.158).

Urethrography

The procedure for urethrography, as well as its indications and contraindications, is described in the contrast radiography section of Chapter 2. When filled with contrast medium, the normal urethra appears as a continuous tubular structure with even, well-defined margins (Figures 4.159–4.162).

Filling defects in a urethrogram may appear as localized or diffuse narrowing of the urethral lumen or as a structure in the urethral lumen. Normal mucosal folds sometimes create linear or striated filling defects, depending on the degree of urethral distention. The urethral crest may produce a longitudinal filling defect in a mildly distended urethra (the urethral crest is a dorsal submucosal fold that runs longitudinally and contains muscular fibers).

Narrowing of the urethra may be transient due to normal peristalsis or a urethral spasm or it may be persistent due to pathology. Because a radiograph displays the appearance of the urethra only at the instant the image was made, serial radiographs sometimes are needed to confirm a lesion. Peristaltic contractions tend to be transient, evenly marginated, and variable in appearance between radiographs. They can be reduced or eliminated by sedating or anesthetizing the patient or by infusing lidocaine into the urethra prior to urethrography. Urethral spasms can persist longer than normal peristalsis. They occur more often at the ischial arch.

Pathologic narrowing of the urethra may be due to a stricture (Figure 4.163), thickening of the urethral wall, external compression, or material in the urethral lumen. Thickening of the urethral wall may be focal or diffuse, unilateral or circumferential, and most often is due to inflammation or infiltrative disease. The mucosal margin may be even or irregular, depending on the severity and duration of the disease (Figure 4.164). Material in the urethra may either narrow or widen the lumen.

A

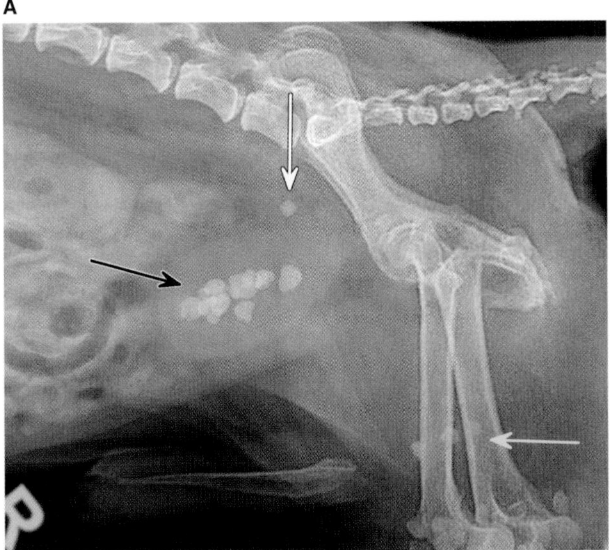

B

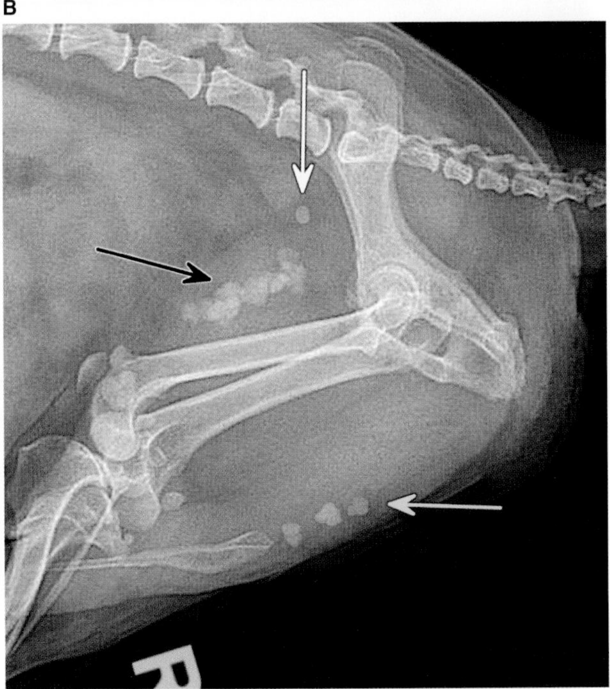

Figure 4.158 "Urethral view". **A**. Lateral view of a dog pelvis depicting mineral opacity calculi in the urinary bladder (black arrow) and distal ureter (white arrow). Calculi also are present in the penile urethra (yellow arrow), but they are partially hidden by the superimposed pelvic limbs. **B**. Flexed lateral view of the same dog eliminates superimposition of the pelvic limbs to better visualize the urethral calculi.

A

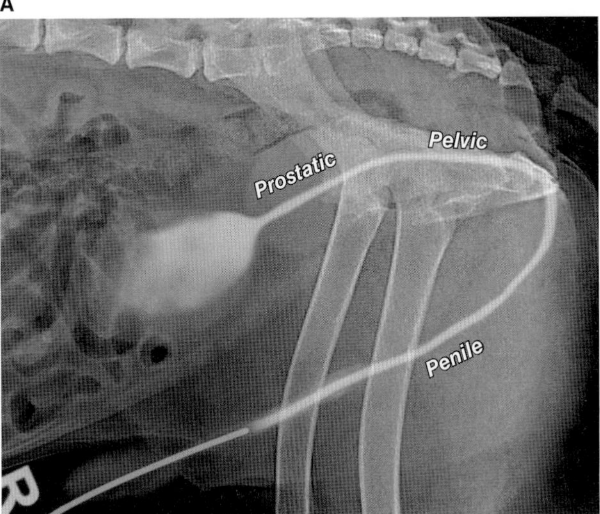

B

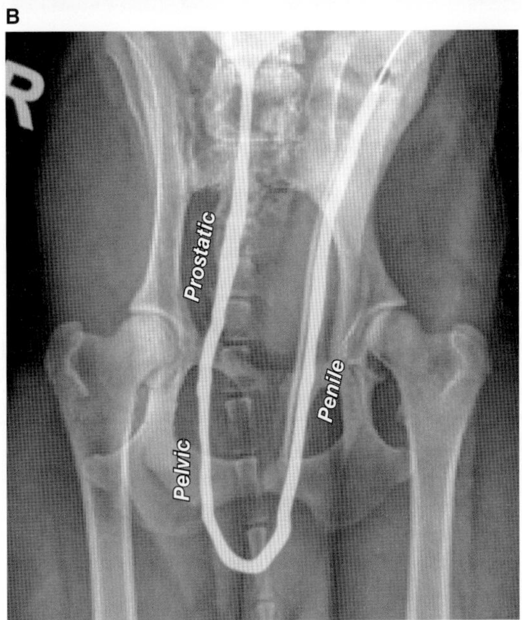

Figure 4.159 Normal urethra in a male dog. Lateral view (**A**) and VD oblique view (**B**) of a male dog depicting a normal retrograde positive contrast urethrogram. The radiographs were made during active infusion of the contrast medium to distend the urethra. The VD view is slightly obliqued to eliminate superimposition of the vertebrae.

Localized **urethral widening** is due to an intraluminal mass (e.g., calculus, blood clot, tumor, polyp). Diffuse widening (urethral dilation) is due to an outflow obstruction and increased intraluminal pressure. In male dogs, the normal prostatic urethra may be wider than other parts of the urethra.

Urethral calculi produce round or slightly irregular-shaped filling defects in a urethrogram, usually with well-defined margins. The urethral lumen may be narrowed or

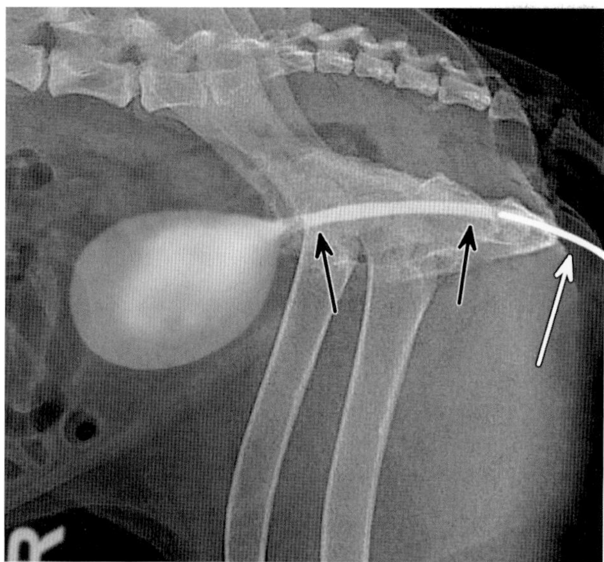

Figure 4.160 Normal urethra in a female dog. Lateral view of a female dog pelvis depicting a normal retrograde positive contrast urethrogram. The urethra is located entirely within the pelvic canal (black arrows). A catheter is visible in the caudal urethra (white arrow).

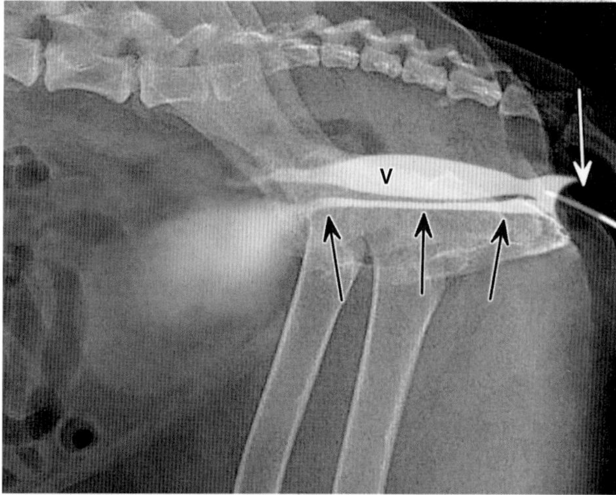

Figure 4.161 Vaginocystourethrogram. Lateral view of a female dog depicting retrograde infusion of positive contrast medium into the vagina (V). A balloon tip catheter is visible in the vestibule (white arrow). The radiograph was made near the end of infusion to visualize the urethra (black arrows) and contrast medium flowing into the urinary bladder.

widened at the calculus. Calculi tend to lodge more frequently in the os penis, at the ischial arch, and in the prostatic urethra. Soft tissue opacity calculi may only be visible in a urethrogram.

Blood clots tend to produce filling defects that are less distinct and more irregular in shape than those created by calculi. Blood clots may or may not be fixed in position and may focally widen or narrow the urethral lumen (Figure 4.165).

Gas bubbles in a urethrogram create distinct, round, or oval-shaped filling defects (Figure 4.166). They may be located anywhere in the urethra and readily change in size and position between radiographs. Gas bubbles conform to the size and shape of the urethral lumen and do not cause widening.

Urethral wall masses are fixed in position and project into the urethral lumen. The mucosal margin may be even or irregular and the adjacent urethral wall may or may not be thickened. **Polyps** tend to produce smooth-bordered filling defects without wall thickening, whereas **tumors** are more likely to create an irregular mucosal margin and a thickened urethral wall. Tumors generally narrow the urethral lumen initially, but with continued growth, they may

A

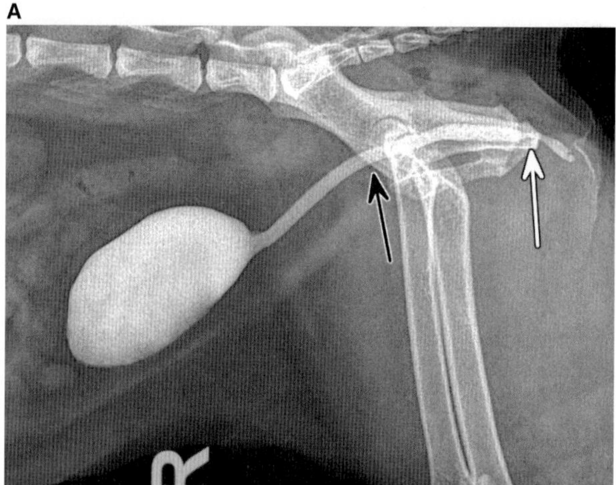

B

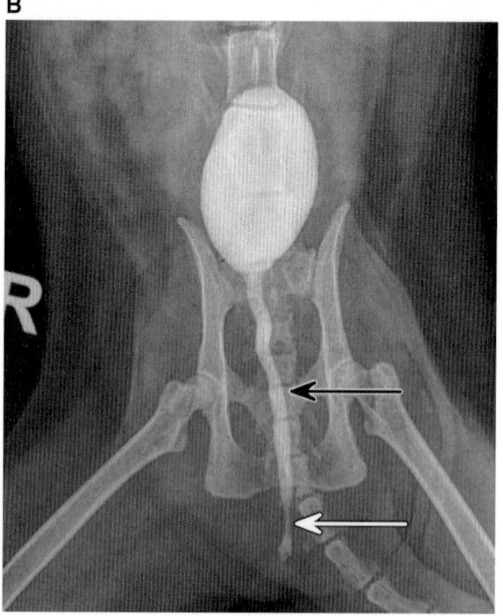

Figure 4.162 Normal urethra in a male cat. Lateral view (**A**) and VD view (**B**) of a male cat depicting a normal *voiding* or *antegrade* positive contrast urethrogram. The neck of the urinary bladder and the pre-pubic urethra (black arrow) are relatively long in cats. The penile urethra is slightly narrowed at the ischium (white arrow).

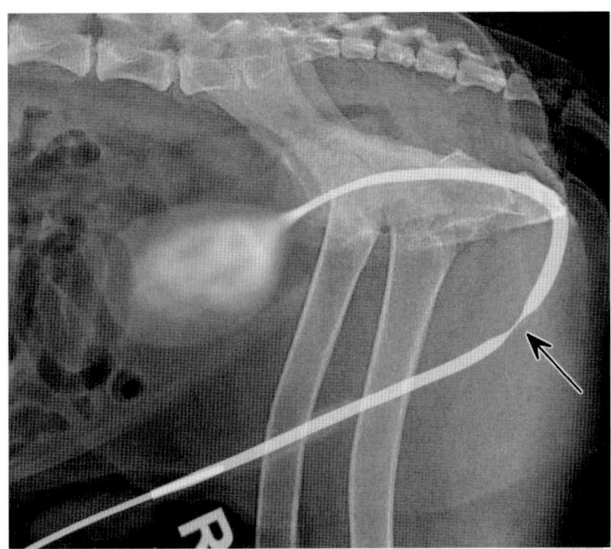

Figure 4.163 Urethral stricture. Lateral view of a male dog depicting a retrograde positive contrast urethrogram. Localized narrowing is visible in the penile urethra (arrow). Transient narrowing suggests a urethral spasm, whereas persistent narrowing is likely a stricture. Serial radiographs frequently are valuable to confirm pathology.

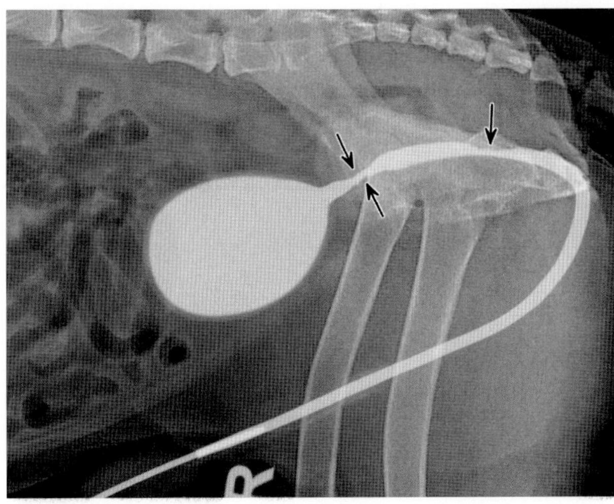

Figure 4.164 Urethral lesions. Lateral view of a male dog depicting a retrograde positive contrast urethrocystogram. Filling defects with irregular margins are visible in the prostatic and pelvic urethra (arrows). The urethral lumen is locally narrowed at the lesion sites. Possible etiologies include thickening of the bladder wall (e.g., neoplasia, chronic inflammation) and adhered blood clots.

cause widening and eventually lead to urethral obstruction. Long-standing or aggressive tumors can erode through the urethral wall, allowing contrast medium to leak into the adjacent tissues or into the tumor. Urethral tumors are rare in dogs and cats, most often reported in the distal urethra of females and in the prostatic urethra of males. Transitional cell carcinoma is the most common.

Compression of the urethra by an external mass produces an even, well-defined indentation that tapers at the edges. The urethra may also be displaced by the mass. Examples of periurethral masses include prostatomegaly, a displaced urinary bladder, and nearby tumors.

Contrast medium that extends beyond the limits of the urethral lumen may be due to urethral rupture, fistula formation, or reflux (see differential diagnoses).

Urethral rupture may result from trauma, pressure necrosis, or erosion. Traumatic ruptures may be due to blunt

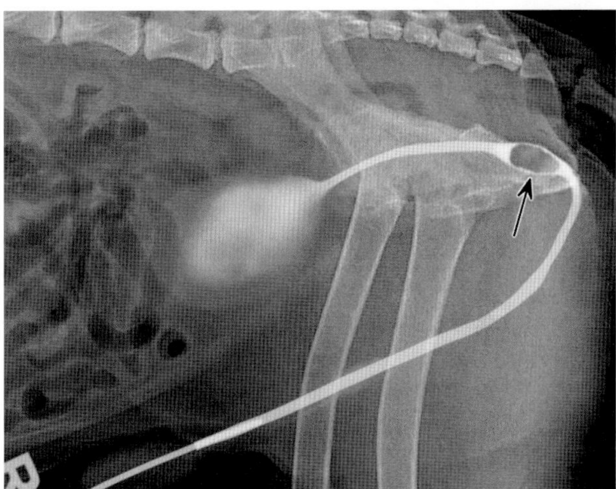

Figure 4.165 Urethral filling defect. Lateral view of a male dog depicting a retrograde positive contrast urethrogram. The filling defect in the pelvic urethra (arrow) is slightly irregular in margination and widens the urethral lumen. Possible etiologies include a blood clot, calculus, or mural mass such as a tumor.

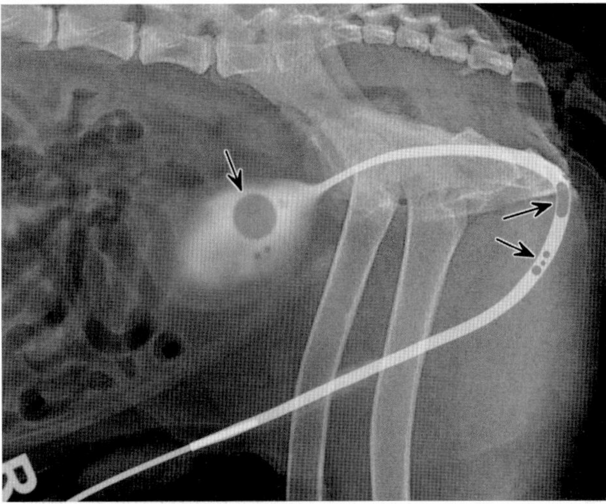

Figure 4.166 Gas bubbles in urethra. Lateral view of a male dog depicting a retrograde positive contrast urethrocystogram. Gas bubbles in the urethra and urinary bladder appear as well-defined, rounded filling defects in the penile urethra (arrows).

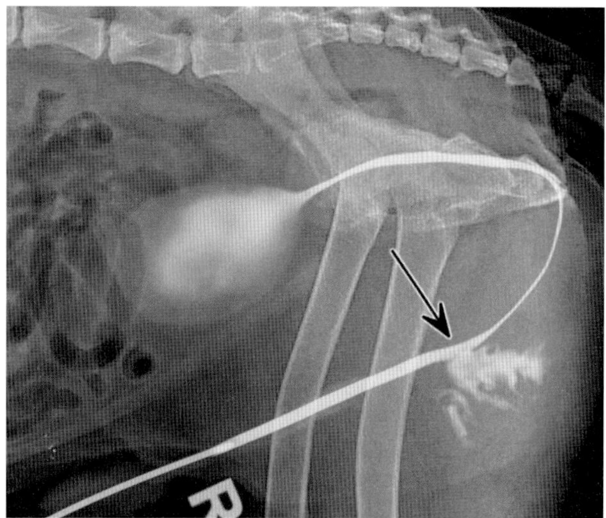

Figure 4.167 Urethral rupture. Lateral view of a dog abdomen depicting a retrograde positive contrast urethrogram. The radiograph was made during active infusion of the contrast agent to reveal leakage from the penile urethra (arrow).

force injuries or iatrogenic causes such as faulty catheterization. Pressure necrosis can result from a lodged calculus. Erosion of the urethra can be caused by neoplasia or severe inflammation. Urethral ruptures are easiest to identify in a urethrogram made during active infusion of the contrast medium. Note: high intraluminal pressure is more likely to cause contrast medium to leak into the adjacent tissues (Figure 4.167). Acute urethral ruptures typically present with soft tissue swelling and indistinct serosal margins at the leakage site. The urinary bladder often is normal size. Complete transection of the urethra typically results in cranial displacement of the bladder.

A **urethral fistula** is an abnormal communication between the urethra and either the rectum, vagina, uterus, or the external body wall. A fistula may be congenital due to a defect in the fetal cloaca or it may be acquired following a urethral rupture or urethral surgery. During urethrography, contrast medium flows simultaneously into the urethra and into the another body part (Figure 4.168). The fistula itself may be visible as a smooth-bordered projection, extending away from the urethra.

Reflux of contrast medium can occur in the prostate gland, an ectopic ureter, or in the adjacent vasculature (i.e., urethrocavernous reflux). Prostatic reflux is normal in dogs as long as the contrast medium remains in the prostatic ducts and does not enter the prostatic parenchyma. When opacified, the prostatic ducts appear as thin, well-defined, and linear structures (Figure 4.169). Contrast medium in the prostatic parenchyma is more diffuse and indistinct (Figure 4.170) and may occur with a prostatic tumor or abscess. However, not all prostatic lesions will communicate with the urethra and lack of prostatic opacification does not rule out severe prostatic disease.

Male genital system

Normal radiographic anatomy

Male genital structures often visible in survey radiographs include the prostate gland, penis, and testicles.

The **prostate gland** is an extra-peritoneal structure that is located just caudal to the urinary bladder. It is not visible in cats. In dogs, the prostate gland is a rounded, bilobed, soft tissue opacity structure with even margins. It is located

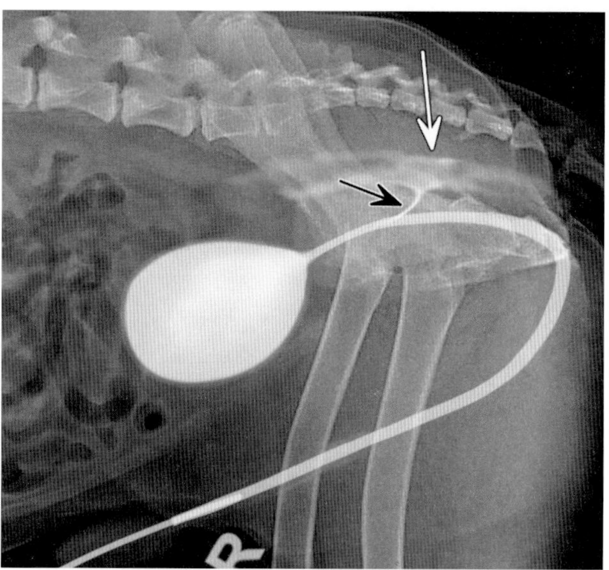

Figure 4.168 Urethrorectal fistula. Lateral view of a dog abdomen depicting a retrograde positive contrast urethrocystogram. Contrast medium extends beyond the urethral lumen through a thin communication (black arrow) into the rectum (white arrow).

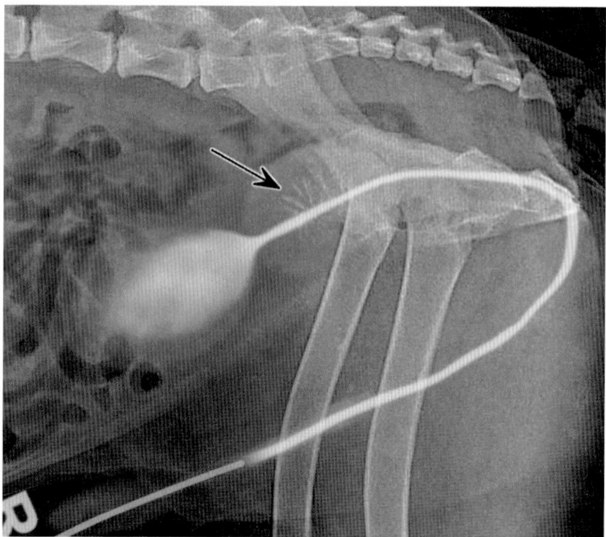

Figure 4.169 Prostatic reflux. Lateral view of a dog abdomen depicting a retrograde positive contrast urethrogram. Reflux of contrast medium into the prostatic ducts produces well-defined, linear opacification (arrow).

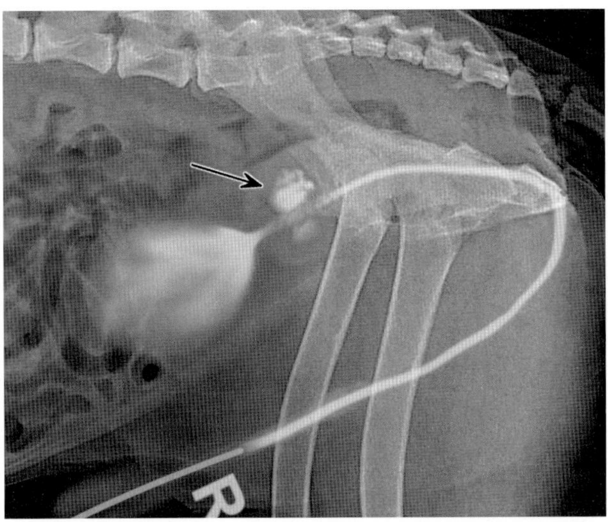

Figure 4.170 Leakage into prostatic parenchyma. Lateral view of a dog abdomen depicting a retrograde positive contrast urethrogram. Contrast medium entering the prostate gland is diffuse and ill-defined (arrow), suggestive of a prostatic tumor or abscess.

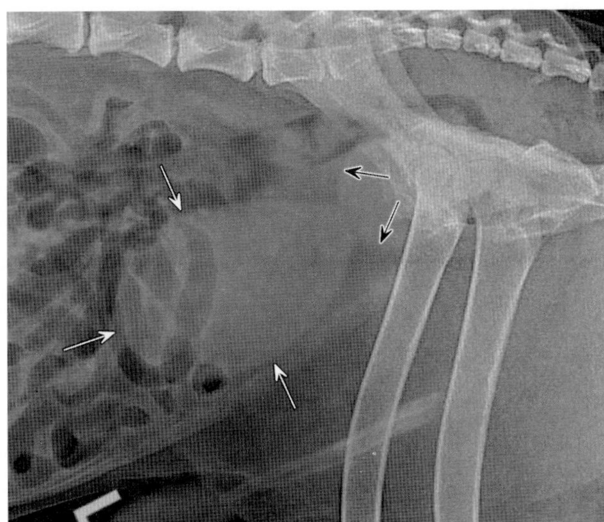

Figure 4.171 Normal prostate gland. Lateral view of a dog abdomen depicting the prostate gland and urinary bladder. The cranial border of the prostate gland projects from the pelvic inlet (black arrows) to blend with the neck of the urinary bladder. The borders of the bladder (white arrows) are partially obscured by overlying bowel.

mostly within the pelvic canal. In a lateral view, the cranial and ventral borders of the prostate gland often are visible as they protrude cranially from the pelvic inlet (Figure 4.171). The borders are visible because there is adjacent fat, including a triangular-shaped fat pad in the caudoventral abdomen (Figure 4.172). The dorsal border of the prostate gland often is effaced by the rectum and the caudal border usually is obscured by the overlying pelvis and hips. A full urinary bladder sometimes will pull the prostate gland further cranially and enhance its visualization. In a VD view, the prostate gland is located on midline and frequently it is hidden by the superimposed rectum, pelvis, and vertebrae. Its convex cranial border sometimes is identified just cranial to the pubis and its bilobed shape may be visible.

The **penis** of all dogs and some cats contains an *os penis*. The os penis is an extra-skeletal bone (a bone not attached to the skeleton). It sometimes develops from multiple secondary centers of ossification. Incomplete union of the ossification centers may be mistaken for a fracture in the os penis or a urethral calculus, especially at the proximal end.

The **canine os penis** is relatively large and usually visible in radiographs (Figure 4.173). In a VD/DV view, superimposition of the penis and prepuce can appear as a well-defined, fusiform structure which may be mistaken for an intra-abdominal mass. The margins of the prepuce, however, usually are more distinct than the intra-abdominal structures because it is outlined by air. In addition, the prepuce usually can be identified in the lateral view, at the same level as in the VD/DV view. The **feline os penis** is small and seldom identified in radiographs (Figure 4.174).

The **testicles** (or testes) develop within the abdominal cavity. They migrate to the scrotum during the first two to six months of age. Both testicles are located in the scrotum, ventral to the perineum, however, they seldom can be individually distinguished in radiographs (Figure 4.178).

Prostate gland abnormalities

Non-visualization of the canine prostate gland usually is because it is small. The prostate gland naturally is small in immature and neutered dogs.

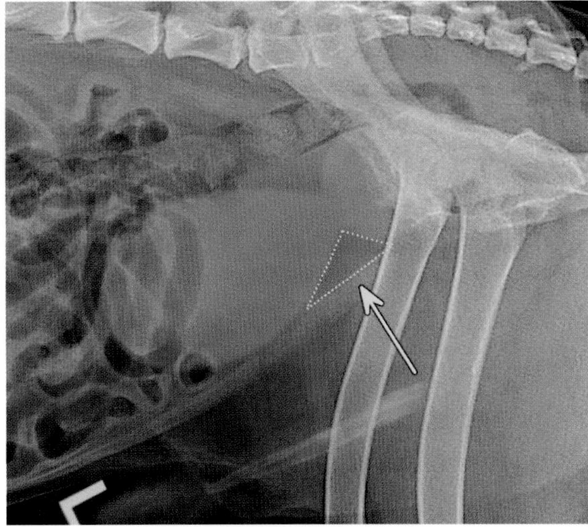

Figure 4.172 Normal prostate gland. Lateral view of the same dog as in Figure 4.171 depicting the triangular-shaped fat pad located between the urinary bladder and the prostate gland (arrow). Fat provides the opacity interface needed to visualize the serosal margin of the prostate gland.

A

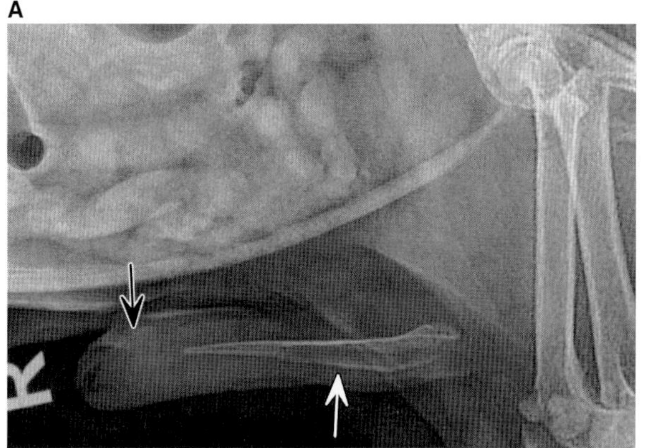

B

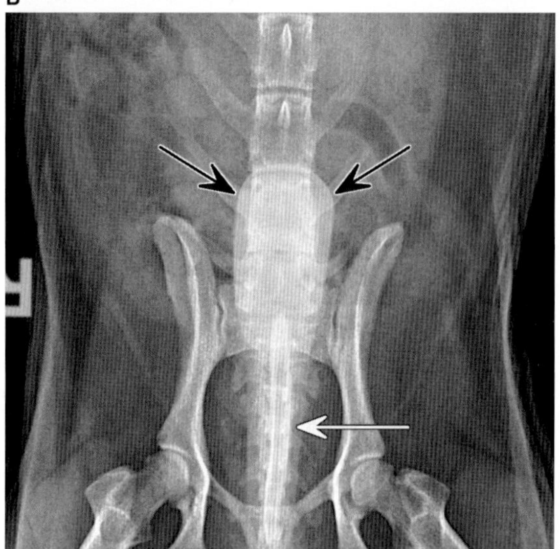

C

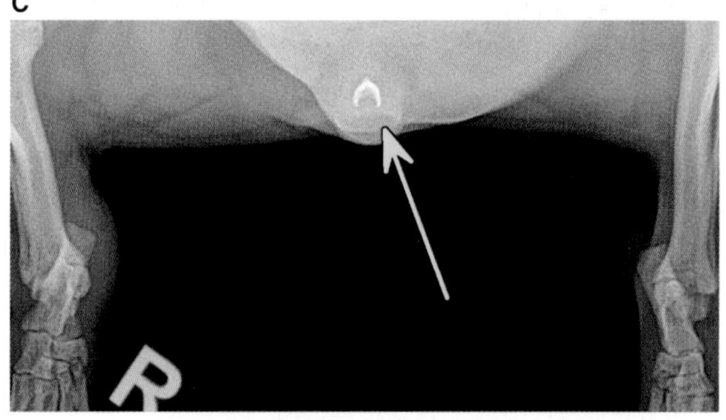

Figure 4.173 Dog os penis. Lateral view (**A**), VD view (**B**), and skyline view (**C**) of a dog penis. The os penis (white arrow) is easier to see in the lateral view. It often is obscured by superimposition of the vertebrae in the VD view. The prepuce (black arrows) in the VD view sometimes is mistaken for an abdominal mass. Notice, however, that the margin of the prepuce is surrounded by air and appears sharper than the margins of the intra-abdominal structures. In the skyline view, the os penis is viewed end on to reveal its arched shape (yellow arrow).

The **size of the prostate gland** is easiest to evaluate in a lateral view. The height of the prostate gland should not exceed about 70% of the height of the pelvic inlet (Figure 4.175). As the prostate gland enlarges, it typically protrudes further cranially and often displaces the urinary bladder and rectum (Figure 4.176). Displacement of the bladder usually is cranial, but it can be dorsal, ventral, or lateral depending on the degree of prostatomegaly and whether the enlargement is symmetrical or asymmetrical. Displacement of the rectum usually is dorsal and the rectum may be compressed. Compression and narrowing of the rectum can lead to constipation. Causes of prostatomegaly include hyperplasia, neoplasia, and inflammation (see differential diagnoses). Severe prostatomegaly (greater than 90% of pelvic inlet height) is suggestive of a prostatic mass (e.g., tumor, abscess, cyst).

Benign prostatic hyperplasia (BPH) is the most common cause of prostatomegaly in intact dogs. It is a progressive condition that is influenced by testosterone. BPH generally causes symmetrical prostatomegaly with even, well-defined margins. In some patients with BPH, cysts will form in the prostatic parenchyma (i.e., cystic hyperplasia). The cysts often are multiple and variable in size.

Prostatitis can cause variable degrees of prostatomegaly, often with a less distinct prostatic margin. Prostatic inflammation frequently is associated with BPH but may be caused by an infection. Prostate gland infections can progress to abscessation. Large abscesses can distort the shape of the prostate gland. Chronic or repeated episodes of prostatitis may lead to fibrosis and tissue contracture, which also can distort the shape of the prostate gland.

Prostatic neoplasia is uncommon in dogs and rare in cats. Tumors of the prostate gland occur more often in older, intact males, but can arise in castrated males. Slow-growing tumors tend to produce symmetrical prostatomegaly, whereas rapidly growing neoplasms are more likely to cause an asymmetric enlargement. Indistinct prostatic margins may be due to inflammation or extension of the tumor through the prostatic capsule. Prostate gland tumors often are malignant and can metastasize to the sublumbar lymph nodes, periprostatic tissues, and nearby skeletal structures

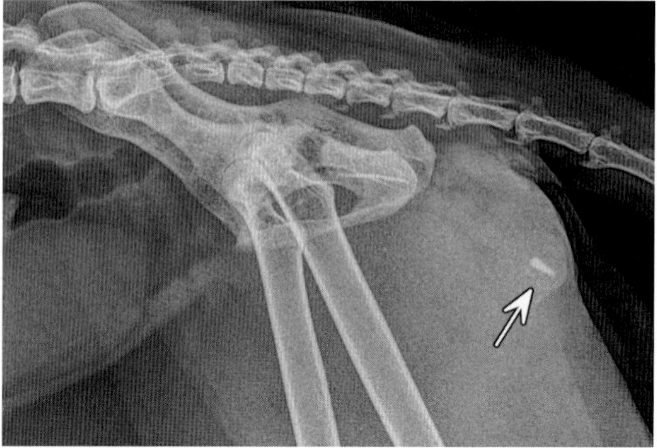

Figure 4.174 Cat os penis. Lateral view of a cat pelvis depicting the normal feline os penis (arrow).

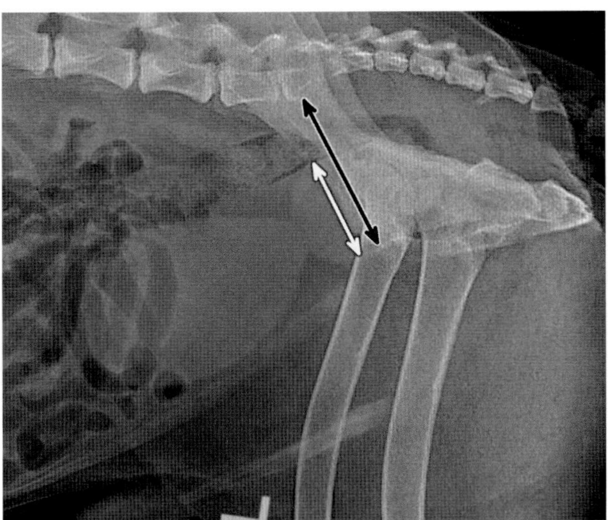

Figure 4.175 Normal prostate size. Lateral view of a male dog depicting the height of the prostate gland (white arrow) and the height of the pelvic inlet (black arrow). Pelvic inlet height is measured from the ventral edge of the sacrum to the tip of the pubis. A normal-size prostate gland generally does not exceed 70% of the height of the pelvic inlet.

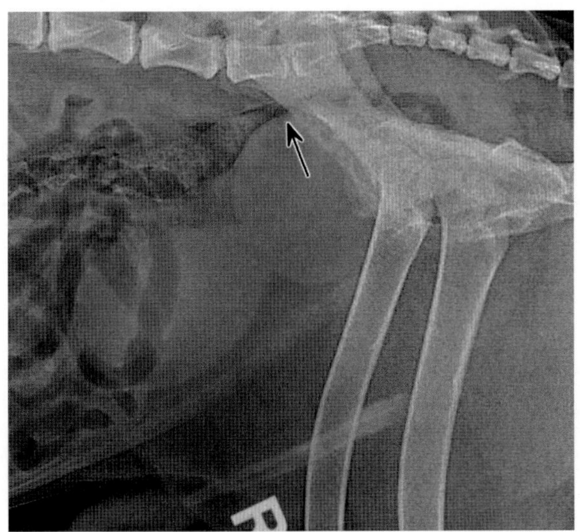

Figure 4.176 Prostatomegaly. Lateral view of a male dog depicting an enlarged prostate gland and narrowing of the rectum (arrow).

(Figure 4.25). Neoplasia is the most common cause of mineralization in the prostate gland.

Cysts can form within the prostate gland or next to it. Cysts that form next to the prostate gland are called (*paraprostatic* cysts). They develop from embryologic remnants that remain attached to the prostate gland. **Paraprostatic cysts** are uncommon, most often reported in older, intact dogs. They can vary greatly in size and may become quite large. Most paraprostatic cysts are sterile. If a cyst becomes infected, an abscess may form or the cyst may fill with blood to become a hemocyst. In radiographs, a paraprostatic cyst typically appears as a soft tissue opacity mass near the urinary bladder (Figure 4.177). The mass tends to be well-defined with an even border. It may be located caudal, dorsal, ventral, or lateral to the bladder. The prostate gland may or may not be enlarged. A large paraprostatic cyst may resemble the urinary bladder, a finding sometimes described as a "duplicate bladder." Some cysts blend with the prostate gland, effacing the borders of both the cyst and the prostate gland.

Mineral opacity in the prostate gland most often is due to neoplasia, but it can also result from chronic inflammation. The two cannot be reliably distinguished in radiographs. Both can produce solitary or multifocal areas of mineralization with distinct or indistinct margins (Figure 4.178). The prostate gland may or may not be enlarged. Mineralization due to neoplasia is reported more often in castrated males. Prostatic mineralization due to inflammation is more often reported in intact males. Long-standing prostatic or paraprostatic cysts sometimes develop a thin rim of peripheral mineralization along the edge of the cyst.

Prostatic calculi occasionally occur in the prostatic ducts, appearing as small, round, well-defined mineral opacity structures in the prostatic parenchyma.

Gas in the prostate gland may be caused by a gas-producing bacterial infection (Figure 4.179) or it may be iatrogenic, caused by reflux during pneumocystography.

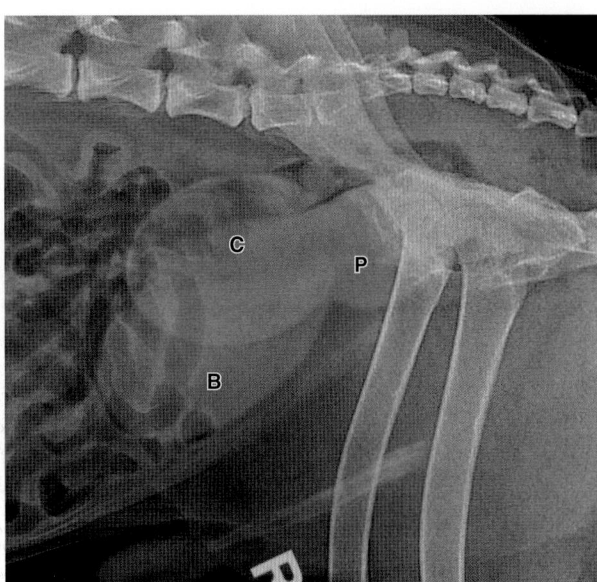

Figure 4.177 Paraprostatic cyst. Lateral view of a male dog depicting the typical appearance of a paraprostatic cyst (C). The cyst is located near the urinary bladder (B) and blends with the cranial border of the prostate gland (P). It is difficult to distinguish the bladder from the cyst without cystography or other diagnostics.

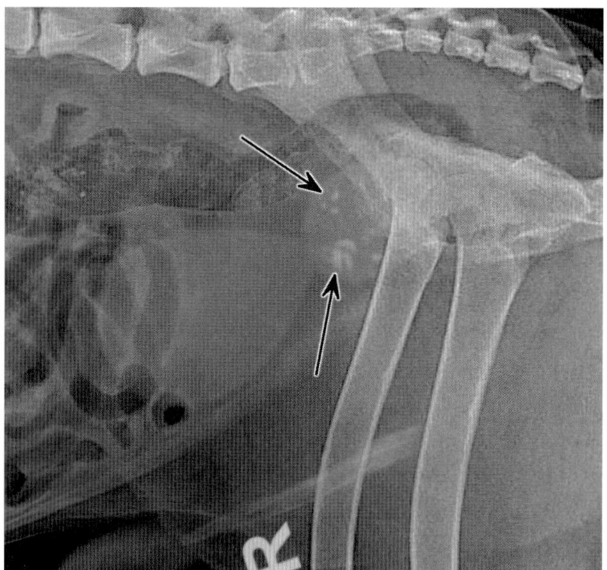

Figure 4.178 Prostate mineralization. Lateral view of a male dog depicting multifocal mineralization in the prostate gland (arrows). Possible etiologies include neoplasia and chronic inflammation.

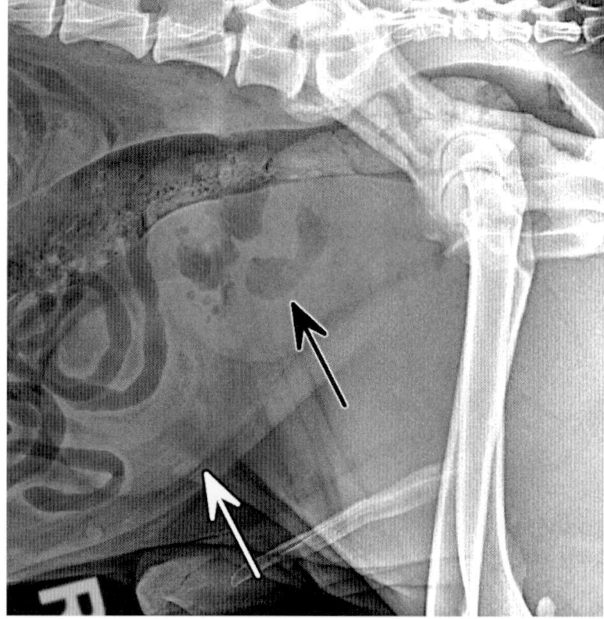

Figure 4.179 Prostatic abscess. Close-up lateral view of a dog abdomen depicting prostatomegaly with pockets of gas in the prostatic parenchyma (black arrow). The urinary bladder is displaced cranioventrally (white arrow). Possible etiologies include abscess or tumor in the prostate gland.

Testicle abnormalities

The testicles seldom can be adequately evaluated with radiographs. They appear as uniform soft tissue opacity structures, often without distinct borders (Figure 4.180). Enlargement of one or both testicles can produce a non-specific swelling in the scrotum. Scrotal swelling can also result from an inguinal or scrotal hernia or due to fluid in the scrotum (e.g., hydrocele). Testicular enlargement may be caused by inflammation, torsion, or neoplasia. Infection with *Brucella canis* sometimes is accompanied by vertebral osteomyelitis or discospondylitis.

Absence of the testes may be due to castration or failure of one or both testicles to descend, the latter is called *cryptorchidism*. A retained testicle may be located anywhere between the kidneys and the scrotum. Most often it is in the caudal abdominal cavity or in the inguinal canal. Undescended testicles often are small and soft tissue opacity. They seldom are identified in survey radiographs. Retained testicles that are larger than twice the diameter of the small intestine and those that are mineralized may be identified. Compression radiography can be useful to displace overlying bowel and improve visualization. Retained testicles, especially when enlarged, may move ventrally due to gravity.

Both the enlargement and the mineralization of retained testicles often is caused by neoplasia. Testicular torsion can also lead to enlargement due to venous congestion. The most common neoplasm in a retained testicle is a Sertoli cell tumor. Sertoli cell tumors that are functional can lead to hyperestrogenism, which can cause gynecomastia, atrophy of the other testicle, a pendulous prepuce, and alopecia. In the absence of a functional Sertoli cell tumor, most cryptorchid dogs have prostatomegaly.

Penile abnormalities

The dog penis usually is visible in a lateral view, but it often is obscured in the VD/DV view due to superimposition of the spine and pelvis. The cat penis seldom is identified in survey radiographs.

Pathology of the penis includes infection, neoplasia, and fractures, any of which can lead to osseous remodeling of the os penis. Acute pathology usually is accompanied by soft tissue swelling. Tumors that affect the penis may arise in the urethra, in the adjacent soft tissues, or rarely in the os penis.

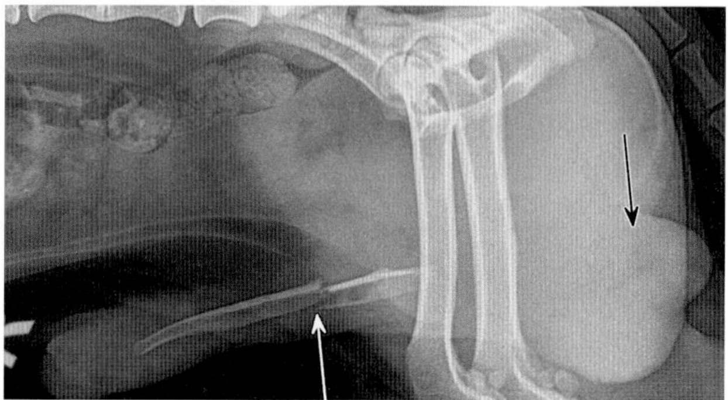

Figure 4.180 Os penis fracture. Close-up lateral view of a male dog depicting a mildly displaced fracture in the body of the os penis (white arrow). The scrotum and testicles are visible caudally (black arrow).

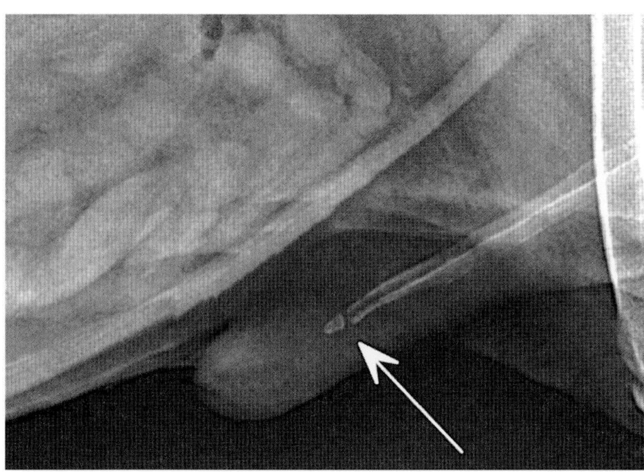

Figure 4.181 Os penis ossification center. Lateral view of a male dog depicting an united ossification center at the tip of the os penis (arrow). This normal anatomic variant may be mistaken for a fracture or urethral calculus.

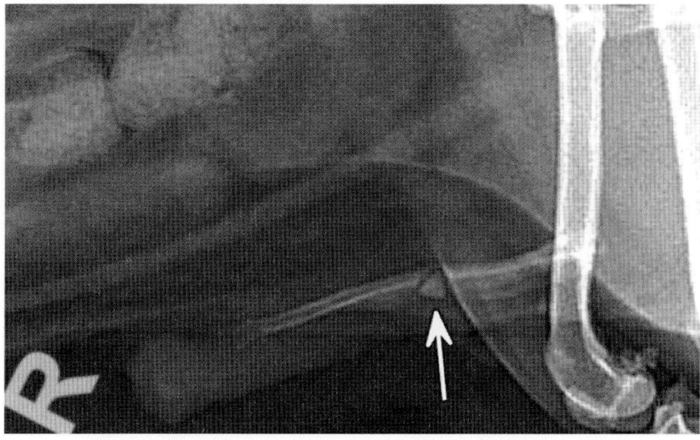

Figure 4.182 Urethral calculus in os penis. Lateral view of a male dog depicting a mineral opacity calculus lodged in the body of the os penis (arrow). Osteolysis surrounds the calculus due to pressure remodeling.

Fractures of the os penis most often are caused by trauma (Figure 4.180). The canine os penis frequently develops from separate centers of ossification, which sometimes fail to unite. As mentioned earlier, an united or accessory ossification center may be mistaken for a fracture or urethral calculus (Figure 4.181). Urethral calculi frequently lodge in or near the os penis (Figure 4.182).

Female genital system

Normal radiographic anatomy

The ovaries and uterus are located in the peritoneal space, not retroperitoneal. The **ovaries** are caudal and slightly ventral to each kidney. They normally are too small and similar in opacity to the adjacent structures to be distinguished in radiographs.

The **uterus** is a Y-shaped organ consisting of *right* and *left horns*, a *body*, and a *cervix*. The uterine horns each begin near an ovary and run caudally to where they unite as the uterine body near the pelvic inlet. The body of the uterus sometimes is visible in radiographs, particularly when surrounded by fat and without superimposition of the intestines. The uterine body can resemble an empty segment of small intestine, both in size and opacity, but it extends into the pelvic canal (Figure 4.183). The uterine body is located ventral to the descending colon and rectum and ends at the cervix. The cervix is located entirely within the pelvic canal and connects the uterus to the vagina.

Ovary abnormalities

The ovaries can become visible in radiographs when they are enlarged or mineralized. Unilateral or bilateral enlargement may be due to an ovarian cyst, an abscess, or a tumor. Most ovarian masses that are large enough to be seen are neoplastic. Ovarian tumors often are malignant and or may not secrete hormones.

Ovarian masses typically are located caudal to the ipsilateral kidney in the dorsal peritoneal space. Large ovarian masses can move with gravity to the ventral abdomen and may also pull the kidney slightly ventrally. Masses that remain stationary may displace the kidney cranially and laterally or invade the kidney. An excretory urogram sometimes is useful to distinguish an ovarian mass from a kidney and to investigate renal involvement. Concurrent uterine enlargement may be present due to estrus or pyometra.

Ovarian masses may mineralize, particularly teratomas. In spayed dogs and cats, incidental focal mineralization sometimes is seen in the area of the ovaries due to dystrophic mineralization in the remaining parts of the ovarian pedicles or in a suture granuloma.

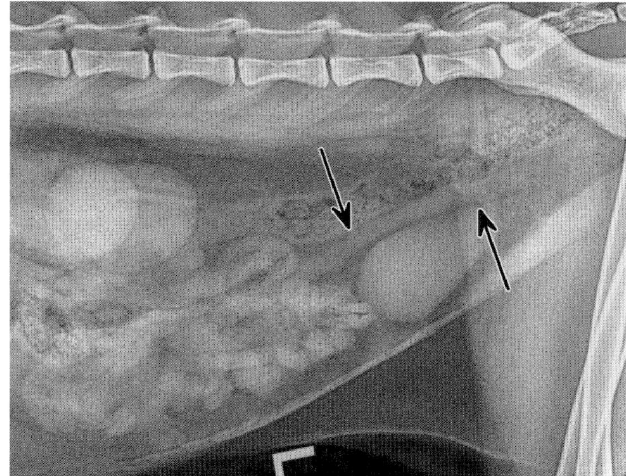

Figure 4.183 Normal uterus. Lateral view of a cat abdomen depicting a normal uterus, visible between the descending colon and urinary bladder (arrows).

Uterus abnormalities

The uterus is relatively fixed in position near the ovaries and at the pelvic inlet. The portion in between is movable and easily displaced. Abnormal position of the uterus may be due to a nearby mass effect or uterine prolapse through a hernia or ruptured body wall. A displaced uterus often is difficult to identify in radiographs unless it is enlarged or contains gas or mineral opacity.

Uterine enlargement seldom is evident in radiographs until it exceeds twice the size of the small intestine. Uterine width that is greater than twice the width of a segment of small bowel may be physiologic or pathologic, localized or generalized. Uterine enlargement due to pregnancy cannot be differentiate from enlargement due to disease until fetal ossification occurs. In general, a large uterus creates a mass effect in the caudal to mid-abdomen. If needed, compression radiography may improve visualization.

In a lateral view, enlargement of the uterine body (or the uterine stump in a spayed female) may displace the descending colon dorsally and the urinary bladder ventrally. Sometimes the bladder and the uterus are superimposed. A very large uterus can compress the urinary bladder and obstruct urine outflow.

Generalized uterine enlargement may be due to pregnancy, fluid in the uterus, or a thickened uterine wall. In radiographs, a dilated uterus appears as a convoluted, tubular, soft tissue opacity structure in the caudal ventral abdomen (Figure 4.184). In a VD view, the distended uterine horns may be lateral to the descending colon on the left and lateral to the small intestines on the right. The cranial part of a large uterine horn may be mistaken for a kidney.

Gas in the uterus (*physometra*) may result from a gas-producing bacterial infection or it may be iatrogenic following uterine catheterization or abdominocentesis. Gas-producing bacteria may be associated with fetal death (*fetal emphysema*), uterine torsion, or pyometra (Figures 4.188 and 4.189).

Mineralization in the uterus most often represents fetal ossification. Dystrophic mineralization may result from chronic inflammation, neoplasia, or a long-standing uterine mass or cyst.

Gravid uterus

The gestation period in dogs and cats is about 63 days (range: 57–72 days). Up to about 30 days of pregnancy, there generally is little radiographic evidence of uterine enlargement. Between 30 and 40 days, the uterus usually is wider than the small intestine and it may appear segmented with multiple mild dilations. After about 40 days, the uterus becomes more uniform in size with more even margins.

The **earliest radiographic signs** of fetal ossification may be visible at about 42–45 days. All fetuses should be similar in size and degree of development (Figures 4.185 and 4.186). The classic normal fetal position is a neutral, partially-flexed or C-shaped posture with the fetal mandible resting on the sternum and all limbs in flexion. This position may be considered a "comfortable" position, as opposed to an "uncomfortable" position, the latter raising concerns for the health of the fetus. Note: assessing fetal health often requires additional diagnostics or follow-up radiographs (see abnormal pregnancy in the next section).

When the purpose of radiography is to confirm pregnancy and to estimate litter size, it is recommended to make the **radiographs after 55 days gestation**. This is to minimize the harmful effects of radiation on the developing fetuses. The lateral view tends to be the most useful when counting the

A

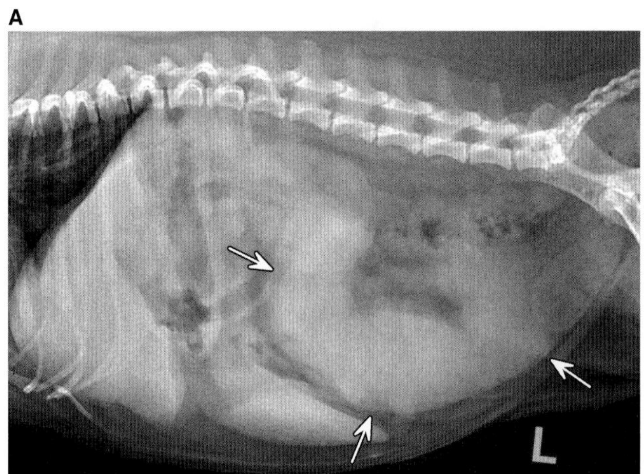

B

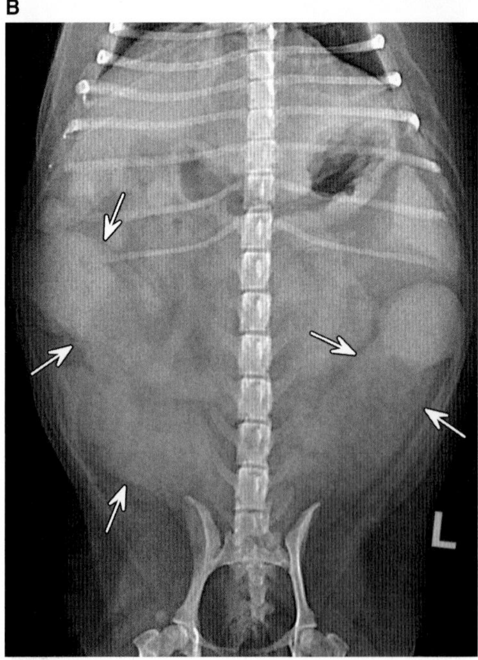

Figure 4.184 Large uterus. Lateral view (**A**) and VD view (**B**) of a dog abdomen depicting an enlarged uterus. The distended uterine body further separates the urinary bladder and descending colon. The two dilated and tortuous uterine horns are visible along the right and left lateral abdominal walls (arrows). Possible causes for the uterine enlargement include pregnancy, pyometra, mucometra, hydrometra, or neoplasia.

A

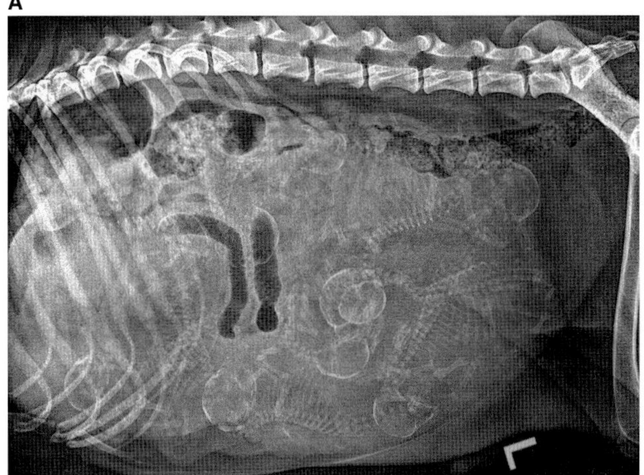

B

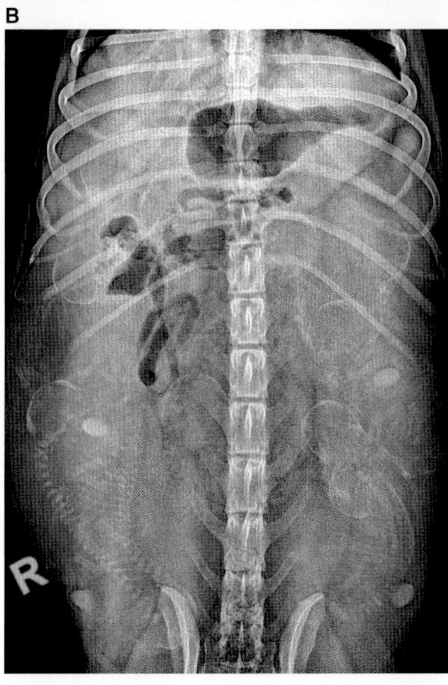

Figure 4.185 Canine pregnancy. Lateral view (**A**) and VD view (**B**) of a dog abdomen depicting multiple fetal skeletons, all similar in size and stage of development.

number of fetuses, however, orthogonal views frequently are needed when there is a large number of superimposed fetuses. To estimate fetal number, count the number of fetal skulls and the number of fetal spines; the two numbers should be equal. To avoid counting the same fetus more than once, mark each skull and spine on the film radiograph with a wax pen or use computer software to label each one in the digital images.

The **postpartum uterus** may remain large and radiographically visible for a week or more after delivery. It gradually involutes and becomes smaller over time, which can be monitored in serial radiographs if needed.

Radiographic findings can be useful to estimate the number of days to parturition (Figures 4.186 and 4.187). Different parts of the fetal skeleton ossify at different times during gestation. **Time to parturition** may be estimated by the initial appearance (onset of ossification) of the following fetal structures:

1. Skull, vertebrae: three to four weeks prior to parturition.
2. Humerus, femur: two to three weeks prior to parturition.
3. Radius, ulna, tibia: about two weeks prior to parturition.
4. Phalanges, tail: one to two weeks prior to parturition.
5. Teeth: less than one week to parturition.

Abnormal pregnancy

Radiographic signs of problems during pregnancy often are non-specific and must be interpreted in light of the patients clinical signs, results of physical examination, laboratory tests, and other diagnostic information. "Treat the patient, not the radiographs."

Dystocia is difficult birthing. It may result from maternal issues or fetal factors (see differential diagnoses). Radiographic signs that may indicate dystocia include no fetus near the pelvic canal in a patient that is near term (possible uterine inertia), a fetus that is in an abnormal presentation, and a larger than expected fetus.

Sometimes there is concern as to whether or not a large fetus will be able to pass through the pelvic canal. It is difficult to assess the width of the pelvic canal with radiographs because soft tissue structures in the canal are not distinguished. The pelvic canal may be narrower than the bones indicate. On the other hand, the pelvis relaxes physiologically during parturition to enlarge the canal. Radiographs are useful to determine whether the pelvic canal is abnormally narrowed due to fracture or malformation, otherwise physical examination and clinical signs tend to be more reliable.

Signs of **fetal death** are important radiographic findings. The earliest sign is a fetus in an "uncomfortable" position.

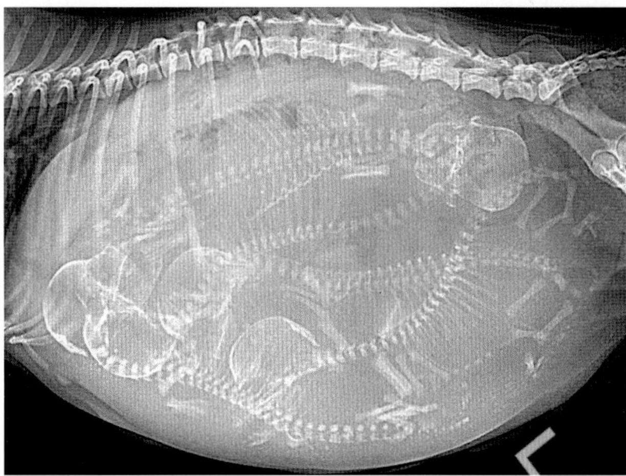

Figure 4.186 Canine term pregnancy. Lateral view of a pregnant dog abdomen depicting advanced fetal development.

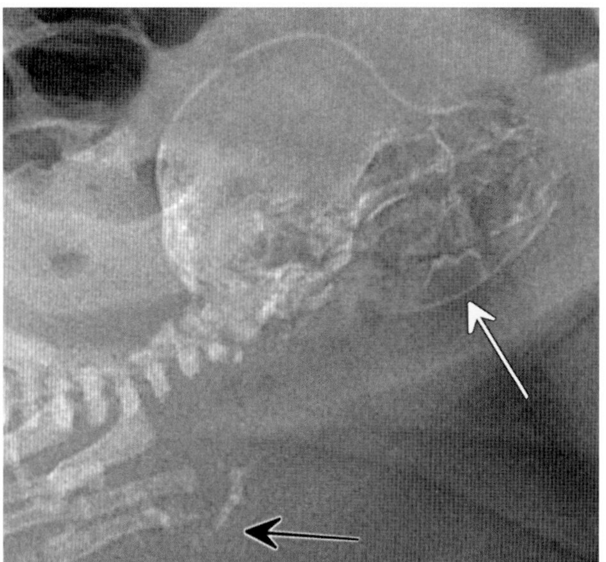

Figure 4.187 Canine term pregnancy. Lateral view of a term fetus depicting visualization of the teeth (white arrow) and digits (black arrow).

The body of the fetus may be straighter than expected (hyperextended) without the normal spinal curvature. The limbs may be extended rather than flexed. After fetal death, the bones of the skull may overlap, particularly the frontal and parietal bones, and the fetal skeleton may become less opaque due to osteolysis. Gas sometimes is seen in the fetus or uterus (Figure 4.188). Radiographic signs of fetal death typically require at least 24 hours to develop.

Fetal mummification appears as a small, abnormally shaped fetus with a severely contracted or "withered" skeleton. The uterus typically is small with little fluid surrounding the mummified fetus.

Ectopic pregnancy may be detected in radiographs if the pregnancy has progressed to fetal ossification. Typical findings include a tightly curled fetal skeleton that is separate from the uterus. An extrauterine fetus may be an asymptomatic finding. A skeleton in the GI tract of a patient that recently ingested a small animal (or fetus) may be mistaken for an ectopic fetus.

Vagina

Radiographic evaluation of the vagina usually requires vaginography (Figure 4.161), which is described in the contrast radiography section of Chapter 2. Filling defects in a vaginogram most often are caused by a mass (e.g., tumor, polyp) or vaginal prolapse. Large vaginal masses can displace the rectum dorsally and compress the urethra. A narrowed vagina may represent a developmental abnormality, such as vestibulovaginal stenosis, or a thickened vaginal wall due to edema or hyperplasia. Contrast medium outside the vagina can occur with ectopic ureters, rectovaginal fistulas, or traumatic damage to the vaginal wall.

Hermaphroditism

Hermaphroditism or *intersex* is a discrepancy between the external and internal genitalia. It can affect any breed of dog or cat. Hermaphroditism may be heritable; however, affected animals usually are infertile. **True** hermaphrodites

A

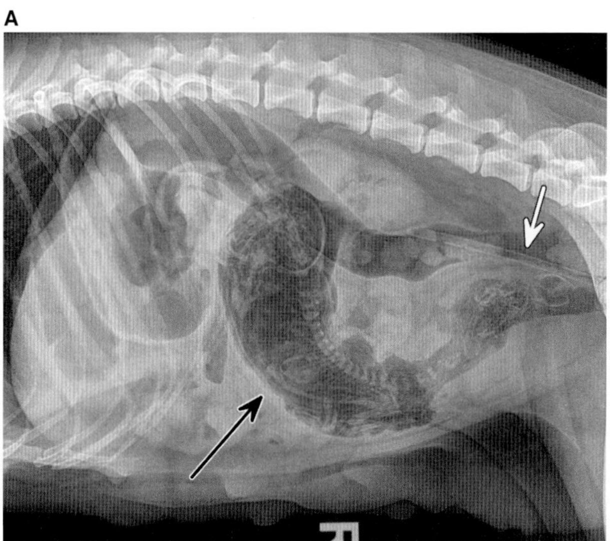

B

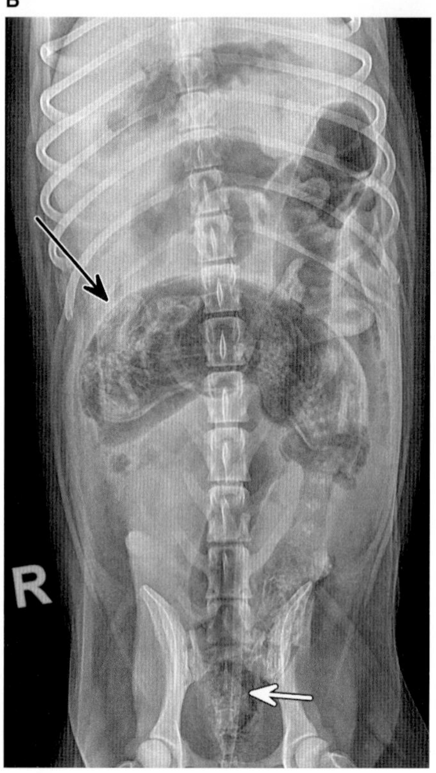

Figure 4.188 Fetal emphysema. Lateral view (**A**) and VD view (**B**) of a dog abdomen depicting gas in the uterus and gas in a contracted fetus (black arrow). Uterine gas extends to the pelvic canal. A pneumocolon was performed to identify the colon (white arrow).

A

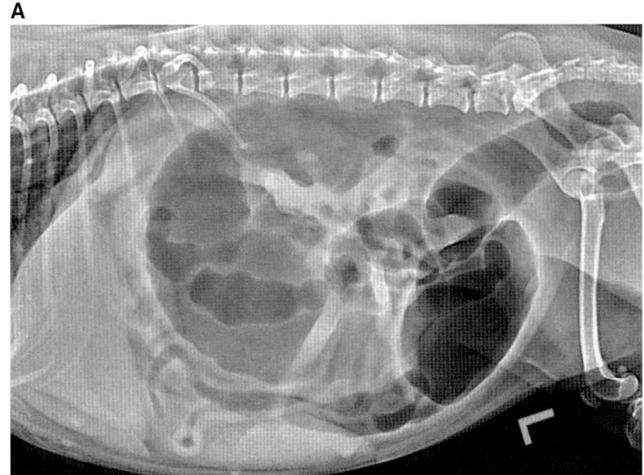

B

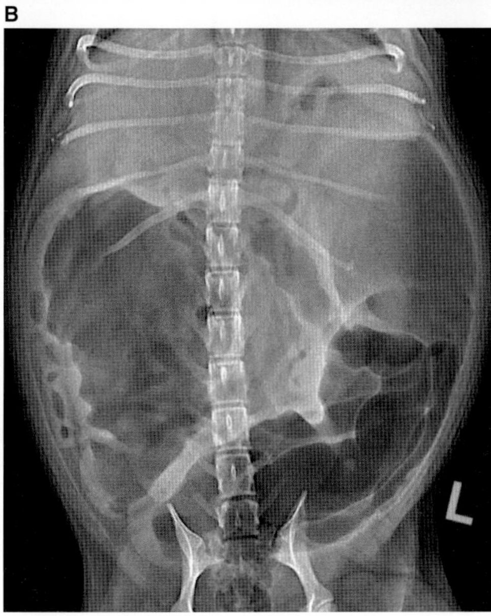

Figure 4.189 Emphysematous uterus. Lateral view (**A**) and VD view (**B**) of a dog abdomen depicting a large, gas-distended uterus.

have both ovarian and testicular tissues, either separate or merged together. **Pseudo**-hermaphrodites are either male or female, but with external genitalia that resemble the other gender.

Female pseudo-hermaphroditism is most common. The prostate gland may or may not be present and the os penis generally is small or absent. An os clitoris may be visible in radiographs. A uterus usually is present.

Male hermaphrodites can have a uterus masculinus. A **uterus masculinus** sometimes is large enough to be seen in survey radiographs. Enlargement may be due to cystic disease or infection. Compression radiography may aid visualization if needed. Rarely, a uterus masculinus will communicate with the urethra and fill with contrast medium during a retrograde urethrogram.

Adrenal glands

Normal radiographic anatomy

Each adrenal gland is situated just cranial, dorsal and medial to the corresponding kidney (*adrenal* means "near the kidney"). Both adrenal glands are retroperitoneal. They are not visible in radiographs unless enlarged or mineralized. The right adrenal gland is located near the caudal vena cava and the left adrenal gland is near the aorta.

Adrenal gland abnormalities

Small or absent adrenal glands are not diagnosed in radiographs; however, radiographic signs associated with low adrenal gland function may be present (see abnormal adrenal gland function later in this section). The most common radiographic finding with hypoadrenocorticism is hypovolemia, which may be evident as microcardia and small pulmonary vessels. Megaesophagus sometimes is present.

Adrenal gland enlargement may be due to hyperplasia or neoplasia. Hyperplasia usually is bilateral and results from a pituitary gland disorder. Neoplasia may be unilateral or bilateral. Whether due to hyperplasia or neoplasia, the enlarged adrenal gland(s) may become hyperfunctional, leading to an overproduction of cortisol, catecholamines, or sex hormones.

When large enough, adrenomegaly produces a mass effect near midline in the craniodorsal abdomen (Figure 4.190). A large adrenal gland can displace the corresponding kidney caudally and laterally. A large left adrenal gland may also displace the gastric fundus cranially and the transverse colon ventrally and caudally. Right adrenomegaly may also displace the duodenum laterally and ventrally. In general, the larger the adrenal gland, the more likely it is to be neoplastic. Adrenal tumors can grow quite large, even larger than a kidney, and may invade the nearby vessels (e.g., caudal vena cava, aorta, renal vasculature). Erosion through a blood vessel can lead to retroperitoneal hemorrhage, swelling, and loss of visualization of the retroperitoneal serosal margins.

Contrast radiography tends to be of limited value to evaluate the adrenal glands. During the vascular phase of an excretory urogram, the adrenal vasculature may be opacified and the outline of the adrenal glands may be visible. The nephrogram may reveal a deformed cranial pole caused by a large adrenal gland.

Mineralization in the adrenal glands may or may not be due to pathology. Orthogonal views are needed to confirm that the mineral opacity is actually associated with an adrenal gland and not due to a superimposition artifact (e.g., GI content, costochondral junction, other). In cats, adrenal gland mineralization is a frequent finding and generally considered to be incidental. It is seen more often in older animals and usually bilaterally. Mineralized adrenal glands in cats tend to be small and well-defined (Figure 4.191).

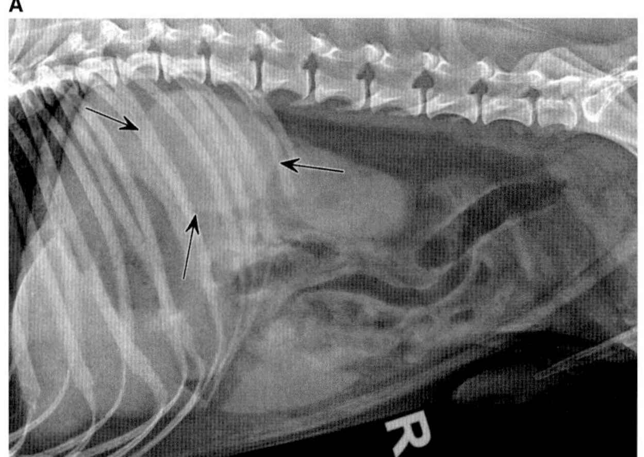

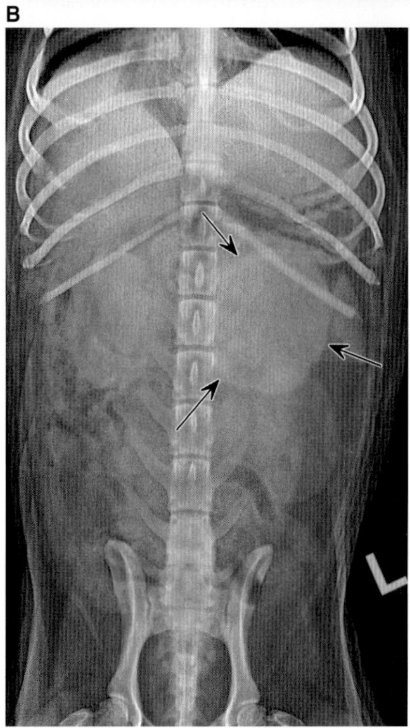

Figure 4.190 Adrenal gland tumor. Lateral view (**A**) and VD view (**B**) of a dog abdomen depicting a soft tissue opacity mass in the left craniodorsal aspect of the abdominal cavity (arrows). The left kidney is displaced caudally and the gastric fundus cranially. A mass in this area may be associated with the left adrenal gland, the spleen, the stomach, or the pancreas.

In dogs, adrenal gland mineralization is rare, usually unilateral, and most often associated with neoplasia. Mineralization tends to be patchy with indistinct margins (Figure 4.192). If the adrenal tumor is functional, other radiographic findings may be present, including hepatomegaly and a pendulous abdomen due to hyperadrenocorticism.

Abnormal adrenal gland function

Hyperadrenocorticism, the excess production of cortisol by the adrenal glands, is a common endocrine disease in dogs, but it is rare in cats. It most often is caused by a pituitary gland disorder that leads to bilateral adrenal gland hyperplasia. It can also result from a functional adrenal gland tumor.

Prolonged exposure to excess cortisol leads to hepatomegaly, weakened musculature, a pendulous abdomen, and clinical signs of polydipsia, polyuria, polyphagia, and others. Together these findings comprise **Cushing's syndrome**. Cushing's syndrome may also result from iatrogenic administration of corticosteroids.

Hypoadrenocorticism, the insufficient production of cortisol by the adrenal glands, is uncommon in dogs and rare in cats. It is caused by a loss of adrenal cortical tissue. Low cortisol leads to azotemia, electrolyte disturbances, generalized weakness, signs of GI disease, and bradycardia. Together these findings comprise **Addison's disease**.

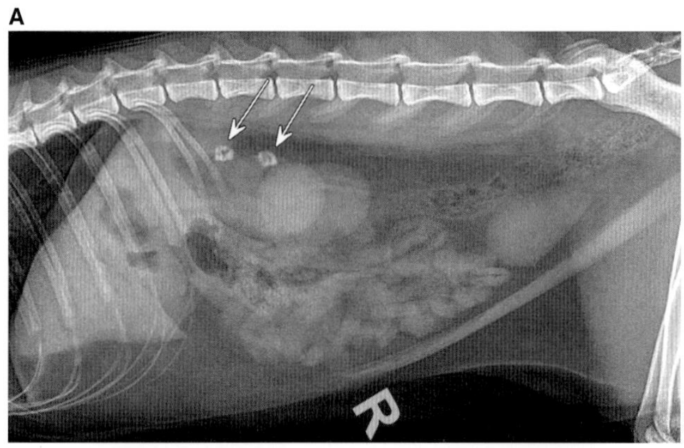

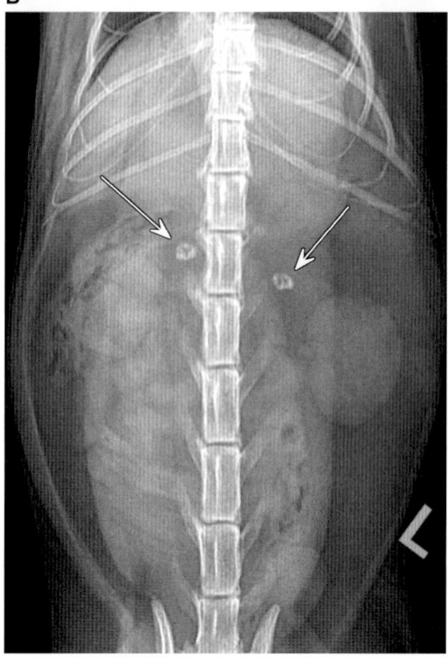

Figure 4.191 Adrenal gland mineralization. Lateral view (**A**) and VD view (**B**) of a cat abdomen depicting idiopathic adrenal gland mineralization just craniodorsal and medial to each kidney (arrows).

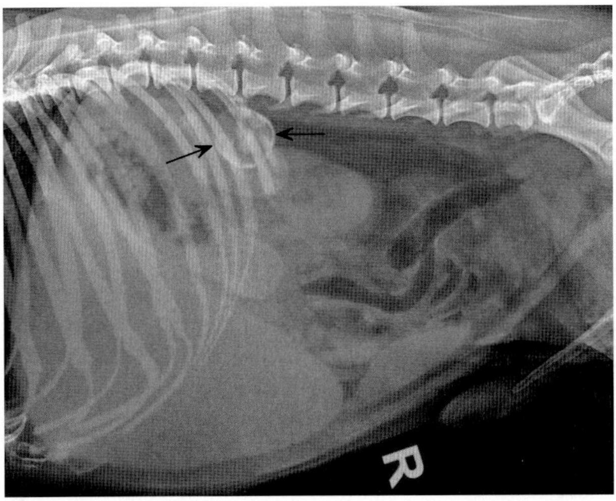

Figure 4.192 Adrenal gland mineralization. Lateral view of a dog abdomen depicting a mineralized mass in the area of the left adrenal gland (arrows). The liver is enlarged with rounded margins and the abdomen appears pendulous, consistent with a functional left adrenal tumor and hyperadrenocortism.

Radiographic signs of hyperadrenocorticism

1. Abdomen appears distended or pendulous, but peritoneal serosal margins are well-visualized without evidence of peritoneal effusion or inflammation.
2. Liver is enlarged with rounded margins.
3. Adrenal glands are not visible unless very large or mineralized.
4. Diffuse increase in lung opacity due to pulmonary fibrosis.
5. Cutaneous mineralization, especially along the dorsal thorax (*calcinosis cutis*).
6. Osteoporosis may be present in advanced cases.

Radiographic signs of hypoadrenocorticism

1. Hypovolemia is the most common finding: small cardiac silhouette, small pulmonary vessels, small aorta and caudal vena cava.
2. Megaesophagus sometimes is present.

Differential diagnoses for abdomen

All areas of each radiograph should be carefully examined in a systematic manner. Each anatomic structure must be scrutinized for abnormal position, size, shape, and opacity. Likely causes for radiographic abnormalities are listed below. Abnormalities caused by trauma frequently are accompanied by more signs of trauma such as soft tissue swelling, fractures, subcutaneous emphysema, free gas, or fluid in the abdominal cavity.

Types of masses or nodules

1. Tumor.
2. Abscess.
3. Granuloma.
4. Hematoma.
5. Seroma.
6. Cyst.
7. Lymphadenomegaly.
8. Nodular hyperplasia.
9. Organomegaly.

Abnormal position of a structure

(Structure is absent from its expected location.)

1. Developmental abnormality (e.g., ectopic location).
2. Mass effect causing displacement.
3. Loss of body wall integrity (e.g., hernia, rupture).
4. Volvulus or torsion (rotation on its axis).
5. Prior surgery.

Abnormal size of a structure

(Structure is smaller or larger than expected.)

1. Atrophy, hypoplasia.
2. Hypovolemia.
3. Fibrosis and contracture.
4. Hypertrophy, hyperplasia.
5. Inflammation, infection.
6. Neoplasia.
7. Obstruction.
8. Edema.

Abnormal shape of a structure

(May be associated with abnormal size.)

1. Trauma.
2. Necrosis, ulceration.
3. Loss of turgor (e.g., intestinal ileus).
4. Infiltrative disease (e.g., mass, cyst).
5. Fibrosis and contracture, infarct.
6. Prior surgery.

Abnormal number of a structure

1. Developmental abnormality (e.g., aplasia, duplication, supernumerary).
2. Prior trauma and loss of structure.
3. Prior surgery to remove or add structure (e.g., resection, transplant).

Abnormal opacity in a structure

1. Gas opacity (emphysema):
   a. Ruptured GI structure.
   b. Penetrating wound.

   c. Cavitary lesion.
   d. Migration of emphysema (e.g., tracheal rupture).
   e. Gas-producing bacterial infection.
   f. Iatrogenic (e.g., aspiration, recent surgery).
2. Fat opacity (e.g., obesity, lipoma).
3. Soft tissue opacity in a normally gas or fat opacity structure:
   a. Inflammation.
   b. Effusion or leakage of fluid (e.g., hemorrhage, ascites, urine)
   c. Mass.
   d. Foreign material.
4. Mineral opacity:
   a. Calculi.
   b. Foreign material.
   c. Dystrophic or metastatic mineralization.
   d. Neoplastic mineralization.
   e. Periosteal response.
5. Metal opacity:
   a. Foreign material.
   b. Contrast medium.
6. Loss of mineral opacity:
   a. Neoplasia.
   b. Infection.
   c. Nutritional disease.
   d. Metabolic disorder.
   e. Trauma with loss of tissue.
   f. Prior surgery.

Abnormal function of a structure

(Typically associated with GI or urogenital tract.)

1. Obstruction.
2. Inflammation, infection.
3. Trauma.
4. Neuromuscular disease.

Abdominal cavity

Abnormal size of the abdominal cavity

(May involve the peritoneal space, retroperitoneal space or both. When only one compartment is involved, the other is normal.)

Large or distended abdomen

1. Swelling in both, the peritoneal and retroperitoneal spaces:
   a. Excess fat (e.g., obesity); serosal margins remain distinct).
   b. Abnormal fluid (e.g., hemorrhage); serosal margins are indistinct.
2. Peritoneal swelling:
   a. Peritoneal effusion.
   b. Large mass.
   c. Organomegaly (e.g., liver, spleen).
   d. Dilated GI structure.
   e. Distended urinary bladder.
   f. Large uterus (e.g., pregnancy, pyometra).
3. Retroperitoneal swelling:
   a. Abnormal fluid; serosal margins are obscured:
      1) Urine leakage.
      2) Hemorrhage.
      3) Inflammation (e.g., migrating foreign object).
   b. Mass.
   c. Organomegaly (kidney, adrenal gland, lymph node).
4. Pendulous abdomen due to weak body wall muscles and ligaments (e.g., old age, hypercortisolism).

Small or contracted abdomen

1. Emaciation, cachexia. Both the peritoneal and retroperitoneal spaces are reduced in size. The ventral abdomen appears concave or "tucked-up."
2. Displaced viscera ("empty abdomen"):
   a. Hernia.
   b. Rupture of diaphragm or body wall.
3. Splinting of abdominal muscles (e.g., pain, patient struggling).
4. Severe dyspnea, inspiratory distress.
5. Concave deformity in body wall, either congenital or acquired (e.g., malformation, trauma, surgery).

Abnormal abdominal wall thickness or opacity

(Localized or diffuse thickening of the abdominal wall, with or without abnormal opacity.)

Thickened abdominal wall

1. Obesity; diffuse thickening due to subcutaneous fat.
2. Lipoma; localized fat opacity swelling.
3. Mass in body wall.
4. Hernia, ruptured body wall; intra-abdominal fat or organs displaced into subcutaneous tissues.
5. Iatrogenic (e.g., subcutaneous fluid therapy, injection site, recent surgery).
6. Fluid accumulation due to disease (e.g., edema, hemorrhage, cellulitis).
7. Surgical dehiscence.
8. Gynecomastia.

Mineral/metal opacity in abdominal wall

1. Calcinosis cutis; nodular or linear pattern of mineralization.
2. Hypercortisolism; mineral opacity in muscles.
3. Dystrophic mineralization (e.g., chronic inflammation, neoplasia).
4. Foreign material (e.g., projectile, microchip, sutures).
5. Superimposed dirt, debris, medication, contrast medium.

Gas opacity in abdominal wall

1. Penetrating wound (e.g., laceration, recent surgery).
2. Migration of pneumomediastinum.

3. Gas-producing bacterial infection.
4. Hernia containing a gas-filled GI structure(s).
5. Superimposition artifact (e.g., wet/dirty hair coat, topical medication or contrast agent, fascial plane).

Abnormal intra-abdominal opacity

(Diffuse or localized decrease or increase in peritoneal or/ and retroperitoneal opacity.)

Decreased intra-abdominal opacity

1. **Pneumoperitoneum**; free gas in peritoneal space:
   a. Post-operative gas; usually resorbed within a week, but can persist up to 4 weeks.
   b. Penetrating wound (e.g., gunshot, bite wound, laceration, recent surgery, abdominocentesis).
   c. Ruptured stomach or intestine:
      1) Ingested foreign material.
      2) Erosion of GI wall (e.g., tumor, ulcer).
      3) Necrosis of GI wall (e.g., chronic obstruction, torsion, thrombus).
      4) Surgical dehiscence.
   d. Gas-producing bacterial infection.
   e. Pneumoperitoneography.
2. **Pneumoretroperitoneum**:
   a. Extension of pneumomediastinum.
   b. Penetrating wound.
   c. Gas-producing bacterial infection.
3. **Pneumatosis**; gas in the wall or parenchyma of an organ:
   a. Pneumatosis coli; gas in the colon wall.
   b. Pneumatosis intestinalis; gas in the small bowel.
   c. Physometra; gas in the uterus (e.g., fetal death, gas-producing bacterial infection).
   d. Emphysematous cystitis (e.g., diabetes mellitus).
   e. Emphysematous cholecystitis.
   f. Cavitary abscess; in spleen, liver, mesentery.
4. Large volume of gas in the GI tract:
   a. Severe aerophagia.
   b. Intestinal ileus.
   c. Gastric dilation (e.g., GDV, gastric bloat).
   d. Negative contrast study.
5. Gas in urinary bladder:
   a. Recent catheterization or pneumocystogram.
   b. Emphysematous cystitis (diabetes mellitus, gas-producing bacterial infection).
   c. Pneumocystogram.
6. *Conditions that mimic decreased abdominal opacity*
   a. Overexposed radiograph.
   b. Superimposed subcutaneous emphysema.
   c. Large volume of gas in the GI tract (e.g., aerophagia, ileus).
   d. Obesity; excess fat in both the peritoneal and retroperitoneal spaces.
   e. Large lipoma; localized area of fat opacity, often producing a mass effect.
   f. "Empty abdomen"; displacement of abdominal contents due to hernia or ruptured body wall.

Diffuse increase in abdominal opacity

1. **Peritonitis**:
   a. Pancreatitis, pancreatic neoplasia.
   b. Penetrating wound.
   c. Infection; usually bacterial.
   d. Recent surgery.
   e. Ruptured hollow viscus; usually with concurrent pneumoperitoneum:
      1) Gall bladder rupture (bile peritonitis).
      2) GI rupture (e.g., ulceration, obstruction).
      3) Urinary bladder rupture.
2. Retroperitoneal inflammation:
   a. Penetrating wound.
   b. Migrating foreign object (e.g., grass awn).
   c. Extension from mediastinum or pelvic canal.
3. Steatitis in cats; serosal margins are obscured in areas of inflamed fat (e.g., falciform ligament, retroperitoneal space, inguinal region).
4. **Peritoneal effusion**; free fluid in the peritoneal space; type of fluid cannot be determined from radiographs. Abdomen may or may not be distended.
   a. Transudate:
      1) Hypoalbuminemia (renal or intestinal disease).
      2) Hepatic cirrhosis (portal hypertension).
      3) Portosystemic vascular shunt.
      4) Acute urine leakage (e.g., ruptured bladder).
      5) Tumor compressing venous return.
      6) Iatrogenic (e.g., peritoneal lavage, dialysis).
   b. Modified transudate:
      1) Right heart failure.
      2) Caudal vena cava obstruction (e.g., thrombosis).
      3) Pancreatitis; steatitis.
      4) Chronic active hepatitis.
      5) Torsion of an organ (e.g., spleen, liver).
      6) Peritoneal foreign material; walled-off abscess.
   c. Exudate:
      1) Hemorrhage (e.g., neoplastic erosion, trauma, coagulopathy).
      2) Ruptured spleen or liver (e.g., trauma, tumor, splenic torsion, severe inflammation).
      3) Bile leakage (e.g., trauma, tumor, obstruction, inflammation, ruptured mucocele, damage to duodenum).
      4) Chronic urine leakage (e.g., tumor, long term inflammation, obstruction).
      5) GI leakage (e.g., trauma, obstruction, severe inflammation, torsion/volvulus, tumor, foreign material, surgical complication).
      6) Feline infectious peritonitis (FIP).
      7) Neoplasia in peritoneal cavity.

d. Chylous effusion:
   1) Mesenteric disease (e.g., torsion, inflammation).
   2) Intestinal disease (e.g., lymphangiectasia).
   3) Lymphoma.
   4) Mass compressing the lymphatic vessels.

5. **Retroperitoneal effusion**:
   a. Urine leakage (e.g., ruptured kidney or ureter).
   b. Hemorrhage (e.g., trauma, tumor, coagulopathy).
6. Carcinomatosis; disseminated neoplasia.
7. *Conditions that mimic increased abdominal opacity*
   a. Underexposed radiograph.
   b. Low radiographic contrast:
      1) Scatter fog (e.g., thick abdomen, obesity).
   c. Weak opacity interface:
      1) Insufficient body fat (e.g., immature animal, emaciation, cachexia).
      2) Visceral crowding; summation of adjacent structures.
   d. Superimposed extra-abdominal structure (e.g., wet or dirty hair coat, blanket, positioning aid).

Mineral/metal opacity in the abdominal cavity

1. GI content (e.g., bones, foreign material).
2. Foreign material in abdominal cavity.
3. Iatrogenic (e.g., sutures, stent).
4. Contrast medium.
5. Dystrophic mineralization:
   a. Chronic or recurrent inflammation.
   b. Long standing mass.
   c. Biliary mineralization.
6. Metastatic mineralization (systemic disease):
   a. Hyperparathyroidism.
   b. Hypercortisolism.
   c. Uremia (e.g., gastric wall mineralization).
   d. Toxin (e.g., cholecalciferol).
   e. Hypervitaminosis D.
   f. Vascular mineralization; usually affects arteries (e.g., atherosclerosis, renal disease, thyroid disease).
7. Neoplastic mineralization (e.g., extra-skeletal osteosarcoma).
8. Benign osseous metaplasia; reported in liver, kidney, pancreas, mesentery.
9. Pregnancy (e.g., fetal ossification, ectopic fetus).
10. Nodular fat necrosis (Bate's body).
11. Calculi (e.g., uroliths, enteroliths, choleliths).
12. Adrenal gland mineralization:
    a. Cats: idiopathic aging change, incidental finding.
    b. Dogs: probable adrenal tumor.
13. *Conditions that mimic mineral/metal opacity in abdomen*
    a. Superimposition artifact:
       1) Prepuce, os penis (VD view).
       2) Wet/dirty hair coat; topical medication, spilled contrast agent.
       3) Mineralized skin lesion (e.g., calcinosis cutis, mammary tumor).
       4) Cutaneous/subcutaneous object (e.g., sutures, BB, pellet, shotgun pellets, microchip).
       5) Fabric between patient and image receptor (e.g., blanket).
       6) Monitoring equipment (e.g., ECG leads).
    b. End-on visualization of deep circumflex iliac artery (mimics a ureteral calculus).

Indistinct peritoneal serosal margins

(The edges of the soft tissue viscera appear hazy or they are not visible at all.)

1. Weak or absent opacity interface:
   a. Emaciation; insufficient body fat.
   b. Immature patient; lack of adult body fat.
   c. Peritonitis.
   d. Peritoneal effusion.
   e. Visceral crowding.
   f. Disseminated neoplasia (e.g., carcinomatosis).

Liver

Abnormal liver position

(Liver normally is located within the costal arch. The direction of displacement provides clues to etiology.)

Cranial displacement of liver

1. Deep-chested patient conformation.
2. Expiratory phase of respiration.
3. Diaphragmatic hernia or rupture.
4. Peritoneopericardial diaphragmatic hernia.
5. Large intra-abdominal mass (e.g., tumor, gastric distention, splenomegaly, advanced pregnancy).

Caudal displacement of liver

1. Wide or barrel-chested body conformation.
2. Inspiratory phase of respiration.
3. Pendulous abdomen due to weak or stretched ligaments (e.g., old age; hypercortisolism).
4. Hepatomegaly; liver margins are rounded.
5. Expanded thoracic cavity:
   a. Hyperinflated lungs.
   b. Severe pleural effusion or pneumothorax.
   c. Large intra-thoracic mass; severe cardiomegaly.

Dorsal displacement of liver

1. Excessive falciform fat; especially in obese cats.
2. Mass in falciform ligament or in ventral body wall.

Lateral or ventral displacement of liver

1. Loss of body wall integrity (e.g., hernia, rupture).

Abnormal liver size

- Small liver: occupies less than two intercostal spaces; liver does not extend to the costal arch; gastric pylorus is cranial to the fundus.
- Large liver: rounded margins; liver extends much caudal to the costal arch; stomach is displaced caudally and dorsally.
- Uneven liver size: liver mass; may distort shape of liver; uneven displacement of the stomach.

Small liver (microhepatia)

1. Hepatic cirrhosis:
   a. Infection (e.g., viral, leptospirosis).
   b. Toxins.
   c. Copper storage disease.
   d. Immune mediated.
   e. Idiopathic.
2. Portosystemic vascular shunt; kidneys may be large due to compensatory hypertrophy.
3. Hepatic fibrosis; reported in German Shepherd dogs.
4. Surgical removal of part of liver.

Conditions that mimic microhepatia

1. Cranial displacement of liver due to:
   a. Deep-chested body conformation.
   b. Expiratory phase of respiration.
   c. Diaphragmatic hernia or rupture.

Large liver (generalized hepatomegaly)

1. Endocrinopathy (e.g., hypercortisolism, diabetes mellitus, hypothyroidism).
2. Hepatic lipidosis; common in cats; also reported in young toy breed dogs (e.g., Chihuahua, Yorkshire Terrier); especially obese animals with sudden weight loss.
3. Neoplasia, primary or metastatic (e.g., lymphoma, hemangiosarcoma, carcinoma).
4. Right heart failure; venous congestion can cause concurrent splenomegaly and peritoneal effusion.
5. Caudal vena cava obstruction (*post caval syndrome, Budd-Chiari syndrome*):
   a. Thrombus.
   b. Diaphragmatic hernia.
   c. Large intra-thoracic mass.
6. Hepatitis (e.g., bacterial, mycotic, or viral infection); *Leptospirosis* carries zoonotic potential.
7. Nodular hyperplasia (e.g., chronic hepatitis).
8. Parasites; infection/migration can damage hepatobiliary system; parasites may be found in feces or blood:
   a. Liver flukes; reside in gall bladder and bile ducts leading to inflammation, fibrosis, and obstruction.
   b. Heartworm disease; right heart failure causes hepatic venous congestion.
   c. Intestinal parasites (e.g., *Toxocara*); migration through liver causes hepatitis, cholecystitis.
9. Malignant histiocytosis.
10. Amyloidosis.
11. Lymphocytic cholangitis (cats).

Localized hepatomegaly (liver mass)

1. Tumor, abscess, granuloma, hematoma.
2. Nodular hyperplasia.
3. Hepatic cysts; often benign and asymptomatic, but can become infected; may enlarge over time; large cysts can compress the biliary tree; cysts can rupture and hemorrhage:
   a. Biliary cyst; congenital dilation of bile duct.
   b. Biliary pseudocyst; caused by bile duct disease.
4. Biliary cystadenoma; a benign, usually solitary tumor that can become very large; more often reported in older cats.
5. Liver lobe torsion; uncommon cause of asymmetric liver enlargement; often accompanied by peritoneal effusion. Gas in the liver is due to necrosis and gas-producing bacterial infection.
6. Large gall bladder:
   a. Cholecystitis; bacterial infection secondary to intestinal reflux or hematogenous spread.
   b. Gall bladder outflow obstruction (e.g., tumor, cholelithiasis, chronic inflammation, pancreatic disease, duodenal disease).
7. Hepatic regeneration; asymmetric liver enlargement (e.g., following surgical removal of part of the liver).
8. Arteriovenous fistula; large tortuous vessels resulting in localized hepatomegaly.

Conditions that mimic general or local hepatomegaly

(Normal liver margins are sharp, not rounded.)

1. Immature animal; liver is relatively larger in juveniles than in adults.
2. Rotation of the patient during positioning for radiography; an oblique view of the liver can accentuate one side or make the liver edges appear rounded; the stomach may appear displaced.
3. Breed conformation: in wide-chested dogs, the stomach may be more caudal in position and the liver may extend caudal to the costal arch.
4. Summation of spleen with liver in lateral view; make the opposite lateral view to distinguish the two.
5. Obesity; a large, fat-laden falciform ligament may create a false impression of hepatomegaly, particularly in overweight cats.
6. Fluid-filled gastric pylorus in right lateral view may be mistaken for a liver mass; make a left lateral view to allow gas to enter the pylorus for identification (to add gas to

the stomach, allow the patient to drink a small amount of a carbonated beverage).
7. Expanded thoracic cavity; liver may extend caudal to the costal arch.
8. In cats, the right side of the liver normally appears larger than the left in a VD view.

Abnormal liver opacity

(Focal, multifocal or branching pattern of gas or mineral opacity in part or all of the liver. Gas or mineral may conform to shape and location of the gall bladder or/and bile ducts.)

Gas in liver

1. Emphysematous cholecystitis; usually associated with diabetes mellitus, but may be idiopathic.
2. Liver lobe torsion; abscess or tumor with a gas-producing bacterial infection.
3. Penetrating abdominal wound.
4. Recent abdominal surgery.
5. Reflux of gas from GI tract:
   a. Gastric dilation and volvulus.
   b. Gastric wall necrosis (e.g., GDV, gastric ulcer).
   c. Dysfunctional duodenal sphincter.
   d. Chronic bile duct obstruction.
6. Gas emboli.

Mineralization in liver

1. Cholelithiasis; gallstones may be asymptomatic.
2. Choledocoliths; calculi in common bile duct.
3. Bile duct mineralization; tree-like branching pattern; (e.g., chronic inflammation).
4. Dystrophic mineralization:
   a. Chronic cholangiohepatitis.
   b. Gall bladder wall (e.g., carcinoma, cystic mucinous hyperplasia).
   c. Long standing abscess, granuloma, hematoma.
   d. Parasitic cyst (e.g., echinococcus).
   e. Hepatic necrosis (e.g., liver lobe torsion).
5. Neoplasia (e.g., extra-skeletal osteosarcoma).
6. Idiopathic (age-related, older Yorkshire Terriers).
7. Recent contrast radiography procedure; iodinated media are partially excreted via the biliary system.

Conditions that mimic abnormal liver opacity

1. Superimposition artifact:
   a. Costal cartilage/costochondral junction.
   b. Debris or medication on skin or hair coat.
   c. Cutaneous mineralization (e.g., calcinosis cutis).
   d. Skin growth or nipple.
   e. Lung mineralization.
   f. Gastric content.
   g. Subcutaneous emphysema.
   h. Small pneumoperitoneum.

Spleen

Abnormal spleen position

(The spleen is not visualized in its expected location; especially the left craniodorsal abdomen.)

Non-visualization of spleen

1. Spleen is absent (e.g., prior splenectomy).
2. Spleen is small and obscured (see _small spleen_).
3. Lack of an opacity interface:
   a. Insufficient body fat (e.g., immature, emaciated).
   b. Peritoneal fluid (e.g., effusion, inflammation).
   c. Visceral crowding.
4. Poor radiographic technique (e.g., underexposure).
5. Spleen is displaced.

Cranial displacement of spleen

1. Deep-chested body conformation.
2. Microhepatia.
3. Caudal intra-abdominal mass.
4. Diaphragmatic hernia.

Caudal displacement of spleen

1. Hepatomegaly.
2. Distended stomach.

Lateral or ventral displacement of spleen

1. Gastric dilatation and volvulus.
2. Intra-abdominal mass.
3. Loss of body wall integrity (e.g., hernia, rupture).
4. Splenic torsion.

Abnormal spleen size

(Splenomegaly frequently is overdiagnosed; the key finding with an enlarged spleen is rounded margins.)

Small spleen

1. Hypovolemia.
2. Atrophy in aged animals.
3. Cats: normal spleen is proportionately smaller than in dogs.

Large spleen (generalized splenomegaly)

1. Breed variation; spleen is relatively large in certain dog breeds (e.g., German Shepherd, Greyhound, Scottish Terrier).
2. Pharmacologic response; certain drugs can cause smooth muscle relaxation and passive venous congestion in the spleen (common in dogs, but uncommon in cats):
   a. Phenothiazine sedation.
   b. Barbiturate anesthesia.
3. Physiologic response (e.g., patient stress).

4. Extra-medullary hematopoiesis in dogs (*splenic hyperplasia*):
   a. A response to red blood cell destruction (e.g., chronic anemia, hemolytic disorder, immune-mediated disease).
   b. A response to bone marrow insufficiency; spleen becomes responsible for red blood cell production (splenectomy in these cases can result in fatal anemia).
5. Right heart failure; venous congestion can lead to splenomegaly, hepatomegaly, peritoneal effusion.
6. **Splenic torsion** (reverse C-shaped spleen, ventrally and medially displaced, may be emphysematous); most often reported in large, deep-chested dogs:
   a. Associated with GDV.
   b. Idiopathic.
7. Inflammation/infection:
   a. Bacterial infection (e.g., septicemia, brucellosis, tuberculosis, ehrlichia, hemobartonella).
   b. Viral infection (e.g., FIP, canine hepatitis).
   c. Mycotic infection, granulomatous disease.
   d. Parasitic disease (e.g., toxoplasmosis, babesiosis, Leishmaniasis).
   e. Others (e.g., toxins, amyloidosis).
8. Portal hypertension (e.g., portal vein thrombus); leads to splenic venous congestion.
9. Hypereosinophilic syndrome; a rare blood disorder in cats.
10. Malignant histiocytosis; rare hereditary disease, most often reported in Bernese Mountain Dog.

Localized splenomegaly (splenic mass)

1. Nodular hyperplasia; may be asymptomatic in older dogs; uncommon in cats.
2. **Hematoma**; frequent finding in dogs:
   a. Trauma; look for other evidence of trauma.
   b. Idiopathic.
3. **Hemangiosarcoma**; most common splenic tumor; mostly large breed dogs (e.g., Great Dane, German Shepherd, Golden Retriever, Boxer); highly malignant tumor; readily metastasizes to liver, lung, and heart (latter can lead to pericardial effusion).
4. Lymphoma; may be accompanied by hepatomegaly and/or lymphadenomegaly.
5. Abscess; uncommon in dogs and rare in cats:
   a. Compromised splenic blood supply (e.g., splenic torsion, infarction); abscess may contain gas.

Conditions that mimic splenomegaly

(Normal spleen margins are sharp, not rounded.)

1. Visualization of a long portion of the spleen; tail of the spleen is further caudal than expected (may be near the urinary bladder).
2. Fluid-filled gastric pylorus in right lateral view may be mistaken for a splenic mass; make a left lateral view if needed for clarification.
3. Peritoneal mass (associated with pancreas, GI tract, mesentery).
4. Pedunculated hepatic mass that is caudal to the stomach.
5. Localized peritoneal inflammation or effusion.
6. Summation artifact (e.g., crowding of the small intestine); when in doubt, make both lateral views or use abdominal compression to displace the bowel.

Abnormal spleen shape

1. Splenic mass, solitary or multiple.
2. Nodular hyperplasia.
3. Extramedullary hematopoiesis.
4. Fibrosis with tissue contracture.
5. Diffuse neoplasia (e.g., lymphoma).
6. Trauma (recent or old).
7. Splenic torsion; spleen resembles a reverse C-shape.

Abnormal spleen opacity

1. Gas opacity in spleen:
   a. Gas-producing bacterial infection:
      1) Splenic torsion (most common).
      2) Long-standing splenic abscess.
   b. Gas emboli.
2. Mineral opacity in spleen:
   a. Chronic inflammation/infection.
   b. Long standing abscess, hematoma, tumor.
   c. Mycotic disease (e.g., histoplasmosis).
   d. Neoplasia (e.g., extra-skeletal osteosarcoma).

Conditions that mimic abnormal spleen opacity

1. Superimposition artifact:
   a. Debris or medication on skin or in hair coat.
   b. Cutaneous nodule.
   c. GI content.
   d. Subcutaneous emphysema.
   e. Small pneumoperitoneum.

Pancreas

Pancreatic disease

(Increased opacity and indistinct serosal margins in the area of the pancreas. A mass effect in this area can widen the gastroduodenal angle and displace the transverse colon caudally. A sentinel loop may be present in the duodenum or transverse colon.)

Pancreatitis (acute or chronic/recurrent)

1. Dietary indiscretion.
2. Obesity.

3. Certain drugs (e.g., aspirin, azathioprine, calcium).
4. Hypercortisolism.
5. Hyperlipidemia.
6. Recent surgery.
7. Trauma.
8. Anesthesia.
9. Parasites (e.g., liver flukes, toxoplasmosis).
10. Idiopathic.

Pancreatic mass

1. Neoplasia; pancreatic tumors often are primary; may be benign or malignant:
   a. Adenocarcinoma; can be aggressive and disseminate throughout the peritoneal space (i.e., *carcinomatosis*).
2. Abscess; may be a sequela to pancreatitis.
3. Pseudocyst; often a sequela to chronic pancreatitis.
4. Nodular hyperplasia.

Conditions that mimic pancreatic disease

1. Visceral crowding; in a VD/DV view, the right cranial abdominal quadrant often is more opaque and serosal margins are less distinct than in the left cranial quadrant.
2. Overstretching the patient during positioning for radiography can cause visceral crowding.
3. Intestinal obstruction (proximal bowel blockage).
4. Gastroenteritis or gastrointestinal mass.

Stomach

Abnormal stomach position

(Part or all of stomach is not visible in its expected location.)

Non-visualization of stomach

1. Empty stomach (e.g., anorexia, fasting, vomiting).
2. Loss of opacity interface:
   a. Insufficient body fat (e.g., immaturity, emaciation).
   b. Peritoneal fluid (e.g., inflammation, effusion).

Caudal displacement of stomach

1. Large liver (most common cause).
2. Expanded thorax with caudal displacement of diaphragm and liver:
   a. Severe pleural effusion.
   b. Severe pneumothorax.
   c. Hyperinflated lungs.
   d. Severe emphysema.

Cranial displacement of stomach

1. Small liver (e.g., hepatic cirrhosis, portosystemic vascular shunt).
2. Diaphragmatic hernia or rupture.
3. Gastroesophageal intussusception.
4. Deep-chested patient body conformation.
5. Mass effect (e.g., large transverse colon, late pregnancy, large intra-abdominal mass).

Lateral displacement of stomach

1. Splenomegaly, splenic mass.
2. Hepatomegaly, hepatic mass.
3. Pancreatic swelling or mass.
4. Gastric mass.
5. Loss of body wall integrity.

Abnormal size of stomach

(A larger than expected stomach often is a subjective assessment; serial radiographs can be useful to assess gastric emptying.)

Largely dilated stomach

1. Gluttony bloat; stomach is large with ingesta, but empties normally in serial radiographs.
2. Recent big drink of water; stomach is large with fluid opacity, but empties normally.
3. Severe aerophagia; stomach is large with gas, but empties normally in follow-up radiographs:
   a. Dyspnea.
   b. Patient is painful or struggling.
   c. Esophageal disease.
   d. Orogastric or endotracheal tube erroneously placed in esophagus.
4. Gastric outflow obstruction:
   a. Foreign material in stomach or proximal duodenum.
   b. Gastric dilatation and volvulus (GDV).
   c. Mass in stomach.
   d. Primary pyloric disease (e.g., spasm, hypertrophy, stenosis, fibrosis).
      1) Pyloric canal stenosis; congenital condition caused by smooth muscle hypertrophy (reported in Boston Terrier, Bulldog, Boxer and Siamese cats); clinical signs of vomiting begin shortly after weaning.

Abnormal stomach wall

(The gastric mucosal margin rarely is accurately identified without a gastrogram. Focal or diffuse thickening produces filling defects that repeat in serial radiographs; diseased stomach wall may appear "stiff"; mucosal margin may be irregular; rugal folds may be abnormal in width or number.)

Thin stomach wall

1. Gastric atrophy:
   a. Chronic or repeated episodes of gastritis.
   b. Idiopathic.

Gastric ulceration

1. Inflammation; acute or chronic gastritis.
2. Ingested irritant (e.g., rancid food, cleaning agent, petroleum product, foreign material).

3. Certain drugs (e.g., aspirin, corticosteroids, nonsteroidal anti-inflammatory drugs).
4. Eosinophilic gastritis (e.g., parasites, allergy).
5. Immune-mediated disease.
6. Chronic stress.
7. Systemic disease (e.g., renal failure, liver disease).
8. Infection (e.g., helicobacter).

Thickened stomach wall

1. Normal gastric peristalsis; transient wall thickening; seen more often when the stomach is empty.
2. Fluid accumulation in the stomach wall (e.g., edema, hemorrhage).
3. Hypertrophy/hyperplasia:
   a. Persistent vomiting.
   b. Severe or chronic inflammation/infection.
4. Granulomatous disease (e.g., mycotic infection).
5. Eosinophilic gastritis (allergic, parasitic, or immune-mediated disease).

Mass in stomach wall

1. Primary tumor:
   a. Adenocarcinoma: most common malignant tumor in dogs, frequently arising in the pylorus.
   b. Lymphoma: most common gastric tumor in cats; may produce local or diffuse thickening.
   c. Leiomyoma: benign tumor; tends to arise in the gastroesophageal area.
   d. Adenoma: benign gastric tumor.
2. Metastatic tumor (e.g., pancreatic carcinoma).
3. Polyp: a pedunculated nodule caused by chronic mucosal inflammation; rare in dogs and cats.
4. Abscess; infection, migrating foreign material.
5. Granuloma; mycotic infection (e.g., phycomycosis), parasites.
6. Cyst in stomach wall.

Abnormal stomach content or opacity

1. Mineral/metal opacity material in stomach lumen (certain metals in the stomach can lead to toxicosis):
   a. Ingested bones.
   b. Foreign material (e.g., needles, stones, fishhooks, dense rubber/plastic, some types of glass).
   c. Oral medications that contain bismuth or kaolin.
   d. Positive contrast medium; may persist in the gastric lumen if adhered to foreign material or to damaged mucosa or if re-ingested (coprophagia).
2. Mineralization in stomach wall:
   a. Chronic inflammation.
   b. Neoplasia.
   c. Chronic renal failure; thin, linear mineralization.
   d. Toxicity (e.g., cholecalciferol poisoning).
3. Gas in stomach wall:
   a. Gastric ulcer.
   b. Trauma to stomach wall:
      1) Mechanical irritation (ingested foreign material).
      2) Penetrating wound with perforation of the stomach.
      3) Blunt force to a distended stomach.
   c. Necrosis of the stomach wall:
      1) Altered blood flow to stomach (e.g., GDV, hypotension, shock, thromboembolism).
      2) Neoplasia (e.g., carcinoma, lymphoma, mast cell).
4. Soft tissue opacity in stomach lumen (may be recognized when surrounded by gas or due to a characteristic shape or pattern):
   a. Foreign material (e.g., fruit pits, many plastics, fabric/cloth, corn cob pieces).
   b. Trichobezoar.
   c. Mass.

Conditions that mimic abnormal gastric opacity or content

1. Normal fluid-filled pylorus in a right lateral view.
2. Superimposition artifact:
   a. Wet or dirty hair coat.
   b. Costochondral junction.
   c. Skin nodule/nipple.
   d. Hepatobiliary mineralization.
3. Food in stomach; in a gastrogram, ingesta creates filling defects that may be indistinguishable from abnormal content.
4. Gastric wall fat, particularly in overweight cats; submucosal fat may be mistaken for emphysematous gastritis.

Delayed gastric emptying

1. Insufficient volume of liquid in stomach lumen.
2. Certain drugs (e.g., anticholinergics, sedatives, atropine, narcotics, isoproterenol).
3. Patient disposition (e.g., stress, fear, pain, rage); allow the patient to rest for 15–30 minutes and repeat the radiographs.
4. Type of gastric content; solid/dry foods empty more slowly than liquids (solids in the stomach may require up to 12 hours to completely empty).
5. Type of contrast agent; the temperature, osmolarity, and consistency of the agent can affect the rate of gastric emptying.
6. Physical obstruction to gastric outflow (e.g., foreign material, mass, GDV).
7. Severe or chronic inflammation:
   a. Pancreatitis, peritonitis.
   b. Parvovirus, enterovirus, panleukopenia.
   c. Immune-mediated disease.
   d. Hypertrophic gastritis (small-breed dogs).
   e. Excessive gastrin secretion.
8. Recent stomach surgery (e.g., gastrotomy, gastropexy).
9. Ulceration in the gastric mucosa.
10. Granulomatous disease.
11. Systemic disease:

a. Uremia.
b. Hypothyroidism.
c. Hepatic encephalopathy).
d. Electrolyte disturbances (e.g., hypokalemia).

12. Nervous system dysfunction (e.g., dysautonomia, idiopathic gastric motility disorder).

Small intestine

Abnormal position of small intestine

(The small bowel is absent or displaced from its expected location or extends beyond the limits of the abdominal cavity.)

Non-visualization of small intestine

1. Underexposed radiographs.
2. Loss of opacity interface:
   a. Immature animal.
   b. Emaciation.
   c. Peritoneal effusion.
   d. Inflammation (e.g., peritonitis).
   e. Metastatic neoplasia (e.g., carcinomatosis).
3. Bowel is absent from the abdominal cavity:
   a. Hernia or rupture in diaphragm or body wall.
4. Short bowel syndrome:
   a. Congenital anomaly.
   b. Surgical removal.

Cranial displacement of small intestine

1. Deep-chested body conformation; bowel loops may be adjacent to the diaphragm.
2. Small liver.
3. Diaphragmatic hernia.
4. Peritoneopericardial hernia.
5. Caudal intra-abdominal mass effect:
   a. Mass (e.g., tumor, hematoma, lipoma).
   b. Large urinary bladder.
   c. Large uterus (e.g., pregnancy, pyometra).
   d. Large colon (e.g., constipation).

Caudal displacement of small intestine

1. Cranial intra-abdominal mass or organomegaly (e.g., large stomach, hepatomegaly, splenomegaly).
2. Empty urinary bladder and colon.
3. Inguinal hernia, perineal hernia.

Lateral displacement of small intestine (right or left)

1. Prolonged lateral recumbency, bowel is repositioned due to the effects of gravity.
2. Obesity; bowel usually is confined to the right ventral mid-abdomen.
3. Large colon (e.g., constipation, megacolon).
4. Intra-abdominal mass or organomegaly (e.g., kidney, spleen, liver, adrenal gland, ovary, others).
5. Loss of body wall integrity (e.g, hernia, rupture).
6. Medial displacement of descending duodenum can occur with a proximal small intestinal obstruction.

Ventral displacement of small intestine

1. Large colon, uterus, or kidney.
2. Retroperitoneal swelling (e.g., mass, fluid, fat).
3. Loss of ventral body wall integrity (e.g., umbilical hernia, surgical dehiscence).

Bunching of small intestine

1. Obesity: excessive intra-abdominal fat limits the available space for the small bowel; note: the intestines flow normally without tight turns.
2. Linear foreign material; bowel segments are plicated with sharp turns and crescent-shaped gas bubbles.
3. Adhesions between bowel segments (e.g., prior surgery, trauma, peritonitis).
4. Inflammation causing turgid bowel; increased bowel tonus, but no tight turns.

Abnormal enlargement of small intestine

(Abnormal bowel width may be due to dilation – obstructive or functional ileus – or due to thickening of the bowel wall. Accurate evaluation of bowel wall thickness usually requires contrast radiography.)

- One or more bowel segments is larger (wider) than twice the diameter (width) of the other bowel segments. Bowel width is measured from serosal margin to serosal margin.
- Bowel width is greater than twice the height of a lumbar vertebral body:
  - Dogs: bowel width exceeds 2 × L5.
  - Cats: bowel width exceeds 2 × L3 or L4.
- Cats: bowel width is greater than 12 mm.

Obstructive (mechanical) ileus

(Bowel segments proximal to the obstruction are dilated; distal segments may be normal size. Bowel segments may appear stacked or layered.)

1. Material or mass blocking the lumen:
   a. Foreign material.
   b. Constipation.
   c. Enterolith.
   d. Large parasite load.
   e. Linear foreign material.
   f. Tumor; may be benign or malignant; primary or metastatic; luminal, mural, or extraluminal:
      1) Adenocarcinoma (most common malignancy in dogs).
      2) Lymphoma (most common malignancy in cats).
   g. Abscess, granuloma, hematoma, polyp.

2. External mass compressing the bowel lumen.
3. Stricture.
4. Intussusception; more common in dogs than in cats (especially German Shepherd); usually young animals (less than 1 year old) but can occur at any age; previous history of GI disease is common; often a sequela to hypermotile intestines, which may be caused by:
   a. Parasites (e.g., hookworms, whipworms).
   b. Infection (e.g., bacterial, viral, protozoal).
   c. Foreign material (e.g., bones, plastic, rubber).
   d. Sudden dietary changes.
   e. Intestinal mass (e.g., tumor, polyp).
   f. Recent intestinal surgery.
   g. Idiopathic.
5. Hernia with trapped bowel.
6. Mesenteric volvulus; uncommon in dogs and cats; contributing factors may include:
   a. Tumor (e.g., ileocolic carcinoma).
   b. Gastric dilatation and volvulus (GDV).
   c. Inflammation (e.g., pancreatitis, enteritis, IBD).
   d. Obstruction (e.g., intussusception, foreign material).
   e. Blunt force abdominal trauma.
7. Intestinal torsion; rotation of a segment of small bowel along its longitudinal axis; a rare condition that leads to gas or fluid dilation in the affected segment.

Functional (paralytic) ileus

(Uniform dilation of bowel segments; often less severe distention than with obstructive ileus; no layering of bowel segments. Sentinel sign may be present.)

1. Severe inflammation.
2. Parasympatholytic drugs (e.g., atropine, narcotics).
3. Reflex ileus (associated with GDV).
4. Chronic obstructive ileus; long-term physical blockage leads to diminished peristalsis.
5. Bowel infarct (e.g., trauma, mesenteric thrombus); leads to ischemia and loss of blood supply to part or all of the intestine.
6. Recent surgery; physical handling of the bowel can lead to a temporary reduction in peristalsis.
7. Electrolyte imbalance (e.g., hypokalemia).
8. Neurologic disease (e.g., spinal cord trauma, dysautonomia).

Conditions that mimic dilated small bowel

1. Fluid in a bowel lumen that blends with the mucosal margins to mimic thickening of the bowel wall.
2. Colon mistaken for dilated small intestine; infuse a small volume of gas or positive contrast medium into the colon for identification. Conversely, a large amount of retained ingesta in the small bowel may be mistaken for feces in the colon.
3. Severe aerophagia, especially with patient anxiety or stress and during hot weather; large volume of gas in the small intestine, but the bowel is not abnormally distended; swallowed gas dissipates in follow-up radiographs.
4. Recent ingestion of large amount of food or water; make serial fasting radiographs to document passage of ingesta without obstruction.

Thickened bowel wall

1. Neoplasia.
2. Lymphangiectasia.
3. Enteritis:
   a. Bacterial infection (e.g., salmonella, *E. coli*, Rickettsia).
   b. Viral infection (e.g., parvovirus, rotavirus, coronavirus).
   c. Mycosis; endemic regions; may be accompanied by lymphadenopathy; disease usually is advanced at time of diagnosis (e.g., histoplasmosis, cryptococcus, pythiosis).
   d. Parasites (e.g., roundworms, hookworms).
   e. Protozoal infection (e.g., giardia).
   f. Dietary indiscretion (e.g., new type of food, foreign material).
   g. Overgrowth of intestinal bacteria.
   h. Hemorrhagic gastroenteritis: characterized by sudden onset of bloody diarrhea; more often in young, small-breed dogs.
   i. Infiltrative bowel disease (e.g., lymphoma).
   j. Genetics, breed predisposition (e.g., Basenji, German Shepherd, Shar-Pei, Siamese cat).
   k. Immune-mediated disease.
   l. Food allergy; may be accompanied by pruritis.
   m. Idiopathic; a common diagnosis in dogs and cats with chronic vomiting and diarrhea.

Abnormal transit through the small intestine

1. Rapid transit time (shorter time in small bowel):
   a. Inflammation (enteritis).
   b. Hypertonic contrast agent; ionic iodinated contrast media are irritating to the mucosa resulting in hyperperistalsis.
   c. Malabsorption syndrome; bowel lumen often is narrowed and peristalsis is diminished.
   d. Short bowel syndrome (e.g., prior surgical removal, congenital anomaly).
2. Delayed transit time (longer time in small bowel):
   a. Pharmacologic effect (e.g., atropine, sedatives, anesthetics, GI motility drugs).
   b. Ileus, functional or obstructive, partial or complete.
   c. Infiltrative or inflammatory bowel disease.
   d. Peritoneal inflammation (e.g., pancreatitis, peritonitis).

Abnormal opacity in small intestine

1. Mineral/metal opacity in small intestine:
   a. Ingested bones.
   b. Foreign material (e.g., stones, clay-based cat litter, gravel, wire, fishhook).
   c. Contrast medium.

   d. Medications containing bismuth, calcium, magnesium.
   e. Enterolith.
   f. Dystrophic mineralization:
      1) Renal disease; thin line of mineralization.
      2) Hypercalcemia.
      3) Toxins (e.g., cholecalciferol).
   g. <u>*Conditions that mimic bowel mineralization*</u>
      1) Superimposition artifact (artifact is often recognized in the orthogonal view):
         a) Colon contents (e.g., feces).
         b) Urolith (kidney, ureter, urinary bladder).
         c) Debris or medication on skin or hair coat.
         d) Cutaneous growth (e.g., mammary tumor, nipple).
2. Gas in small intestine:
   a. Aerophagia; usually abundant gas in stomach.
   b. Recent enema.
   c. Inflammation (e.g., enteritis, peritonitis).
   d. Partial obstruction.
   e. Debilitated, recumbent animal.
   f. Gas in bowel wall (*pneumatosis intestinalis*):
      1) Necrotizing enterocolitis.
      2) Volvulus and ischemic necrosis.
      3) Trauma (e.g., foreign object migration).
      4) Bacterial infection; more often in an immune-compromised animal.
      5) Repeated enemas.

Large intestine

Abnormal position of large intestine

(Colon is not visible in its expected location.)

<u>*Non-visualization of colon*</u>
1. Colon is empty; infuse a small volume of gas or positive contrast medium per rectum and repeat the radiograph to identify the colon.
2. Colon is obscured by overlying structures; repeat radiographs with abdominal compression or contrast medium in colon.

<u>*Ventral displacement of colon*</u>
1. Retroperitoneal swelling:
   a. Fat in an overweight patient.
   b. Fluid accumulation (e.g., blood, urine).
   c. Mass (e.g., tumor, lymphadenomegaly).
   d. Renomegaly.
   e. Lumbar spine pathology.
2. Normal redundant colon.

<u>*Dorsal displacement of colon*</u>
1. Large urinary bladder.
2. Splenomegaly.
3. Large uterus (e.g., pregnancy, pyometra, tumor).
4. Prostatomegaly.
5. Other large abdominal mass.

<u>*Lateral or medial displacement of colon*</u>
1. Normal redundant colon.
2. Obesity; fat restricts the position of the colon.
3. Large urinary bladder.
4. Organomegaly (e.g., spleen, kidney, adrenal gland, ovary, pancreas, uterine horn, prostate gland).
5. Mesenteric mass.
6. Congenital anomaly (rare); colon develops left of midline.

<u>*Caudal displacement of transverse colon*</u>
1. Large stomach (e.g., recent meal, gastric bloat).
2. Hepatomegaly.
3. Splenomegaly.
4. Left pancreatic mass.
5. Expanded thorax (e.g., pneumothorax, COPD).

<u>*Displacement of rectum*</u>
1. Mass in pelvic canal (e.g., urethra, prostate gland, vagina, lymph node).
2. Pelvic bone disease (e.g., tumor, infection, fracture).
3. Perineal hernia.
4. Prolapse of urinary bladder.

Abnormal size of large intestine

- Width of colon is greater than 3 times the width of the small intestine.
- Colon width is greater than 2 times the length of L7.

<u>*Narrowed colon*</u>

(Abnormal narrowing of the colon often requires a contrast study for verification. Pathologic narrowing persists in serial radiographs and usually is accompanied by constipation or obstipation.)

1. Normal peristalsis; transient narrowing.
2. Spasm; transient narrowing that persists longer than normal peristalsis; may be caused by mechanical irritation (e.g., enema, colonography).
3. Stricture (e.g., neoplasia, severe inflammation, scar tissue from previous trauma or surgery).
4. Compression by an extraluminal mass; colon often is displaced (e.g., sublumbar mass, large urinary bladder, large uterus).

<u>*Dilated (widened) colon*</u>
1. Large volume of feces:
   a. Type of diet, such as lots of bones.
   b. Lack of opportunity to defecate.
   c. Psychogenic factors resulting in refusal to defecate (e.g., pain, behavior, training, altered environment, inhibition of defecation reflex).

2. Acute **Megacolon**: transient functional dilation due to weak or absent peristalsis:
   a. Electrolyte imbalance (e.g., hypokalemia, hypercalcemia).
   b. Metabolic imbalance (e.g., hypothyroidism, hyperparathyroidism).
   c. Trauma.
   d. Toxins (e.g., lead poisoning, systemic infection).
   e. Pharmacologic effect (e.g., narcotics, diuretics, antihistamines, antacids, sedation, anesthesia).
3. Chronic **Megacolon**: permanent functional dilation due to weak or absent peristalsis:
   a. Neuropathic or myopathic disease.
      1) Spinal trauma.
      2) Sacrococcygeal agenesis in Manx cats.
      3) Spina bifida manifesta.
   b. Severe inflammation or infection.
   c. Hypertrophic megacolon: predisposed by lots of bones in diet and inactivity.
   d. Idiopathic:
      1) Cats: megacolon secondary to urethrostomy; can lead to perineal hernia.
4. Colon obstruction:
   a. Foreign material; either ingested or inserted.
   b. Narrowing of the pelvic canal; greater than 50% narrowing can lead to constipation/obstipation:
      1) Fracture, malunion fracture.
      2) Osseous neoplasia.
      3) Mass in pelvic canal.
   c. Compression of colon (e.g., prostatomegaly, sublumbar mass, large urinary bladder or uterus).
   d. Stricture (e.g., tumor, scar tissue).
   e. Perineal hernia; localized rectal distention that may be outlined caudally by crescentic gas shadow; usually with prostatomegaly.
   f. Rectovaginal fistula.
   g. Mass in colon or rectum.
   h. Abnormal developmental of anal membrane, rare (e.g., atresia ani, atresia coli, imperforate anus, rectal agenesis); the rectum terminates proximal to the anus. A fistula sometimes develops, allowing the patient to defecate through the vagina or urethra.
5. Colon torsion or volvulus (rare); colon rotates around its mesentery; usually large-breed dogs.

<u>Short colon</u>
1. Severe colitis.
2. Previous surgical resection.
3. Intussusception.
4. Developmental abnormality.

<u>Abnormal-shaped colon</u>
1. Redundant colon; a normal variation; there may be additional loops or bends in colon; the descending colon may appear kinked or tortuous.
2. Adhesions (e.g., chronic inflammation, trauma).
3. Infiltrative disease (e.g., neoplasia, immune-mediated).
4. Foreign material in the colon.
5. Mass in the colon.
6. Cecal inversion.

Abnormal content or opacity in large intestine
1. **Gas**, more than expected in the colon:
   a. Normal (e.g., recent defecation).
   b. Recent enema.
   c. Aerophagia.
   d. Rectal examination prior to radiography.
   e. Vigorous abdominal palpation.
   f. Inflammation/infection (e.g., parvovirus, whipworms).
   g. Obstructive or functional ileus.
   h. Intussusception or cecal inversion; may result from chronic inflammation (e.g., parasites, IBD) or a weak ligaments in ileocecocolic area.
   i. Colon volvulus or torsion.
   j. Gas in colon wall (*pneumatosis coli*); typically a linear or mottled pattern:
      1) Gas-producing bacterial infection.
      2) Ulcerative colitis.
      3) Ischemia (e.g., mesenteric thrombosis).
      4) Mucosal perforation caused by rectal exam, enema, endoscopy, foreign material, neoplasia.
2. **Soft tissue**, unusual shape or pattern of soft tissue in the colon:
   a. Ileocolic intussusception
   b. Tumor.
   c. Polyp.
   d. Foreign material.
   e. Cecal inversion.
3. **Mineral/metal**, unexpected opacity in the colon:
   a. Ingested bones.
   b. Foreign material.
   c. Dehydrated feces (e.g., obstipation).
   d. Contrast medium.
   e. Mineralization in colon wall (e.g., chronic inflammation, neoplasia, adherent feces).

<u>Conditions that mimic abnormal opacity in the colon</u>
1. Superimposition artifact:
   a. Small intestine content.
   b. Urinary bladder calculi or mineralized mass.
   c. Adjacent granuloma (e.g., uterine suture).
   d. Mineralized intra-abdominal cyst (e.g., nodular fat necrosis or "Bate's body").

Kidneys

Abnormal position of kidneys

- One or both kidneys is not seen in the expected location(s).
- Left kidney may be displaced by enlargement of the left adrenal gland, spleen, left limb of pancreas, descending colon.
- Right kidney may be displaced by enlargement of the adrenal gland, caudal vena cava, descending duodenum, right limb of pancreas, ascending colon.

Non-visualization of kidney

1. Underexposed radiograph.
2. Loss of opacity interface:
   a. Insufficient body fat (e.g., immature, emaciated).
   b. Adjacent fluid (e.g., inflammation, effusion).
3. Obscured by overlying structures:
   a. Small intestine; repeat the radiographs using abdominal compression to displace the bowel.
   b. Patient is rotated; repeat the radiograph, paying special attention to patient positioning.
4. Absence of a kidney:
   a. Renal aplasia; congenital failure of a kidney to develop; the associated ureter and ipsilateral reproductive tissues also may be absent; predisposed breeds include Beagle, Shetland Sheepdog, Doberman Pinscher.
   b. Surgical removal of a kidney.
5. Ectopic kidney; a developmental abnormality.

Cranial displacement of kidney

1. Expiratory radiograph; diaphragm and viscera may be further cranial than expected.
2. Normal anatomic variation; left kidney usually is caudal to the right, but sometimes it is at the same level or cranial to the right kidney.
3. Diaphragmatic hernia or rupture.
4. Microhepatia (e.g., hepatic cirrhosis, portal shunt).
5. Caudal retroperitoneal mass.

Caudal displacement of kidney

1. Inspiratory radiograph; diaphragm and viscera may be further caudal than expected.
2. Hepatomegaly, splenomegaly.
3. Large stomach.
4. Mass adjacent to kidney.
5. Loss of abdominal integrity (e.g., rupture, hernia).

Ventral displacement of kidney(s)

1. Excessive retroperitoneal fat (e.g., obesity, lipoma).
2. Large, displaced ovary pulling the kidney (e.g., ovarian tumor).
3. Retroperitoneal swelling (e.g., fluid, mass).

Abnormal size and shape of kidneys

- Kidney size (length) is compared to the length of the second lumbar vertebra in a VD view:
  - Dogs: normal range is 2.5–3.5 × L2.
  - Cats: normal range is 2.0–3.0 × L2.
- Kidneys sometimes appear relatively large in intact cats, especially older males.

Normal appearing kidneys with severe renal disease

1. Acute inflammation (e.g., nephritis, pyelonephritis).
2. Acute toxicity (e.g., ethylene glycol, gentamicin, cisplatin, snake venom).
3. Amyloidosis.
4. Early hydronephrosis.

Normal size kidneys with irregular renal margins

1. Peripheral cysts, nodules, or masses.
2. Renal infarcts.
3. Ruptured kidney (e.g., trauma, erosion).

Small kidneys

1. Renal hypoplasia.
2. Renal fibrosis.
3. Renal atrophy (reported in Samoyed).
4. Hydronephrosis (rare); a chronic partial urinary obstruction without renal backflow can lead to a small, irregular-shaped kidney.
5. Artifact: overlap of the kidneys in lateral view may be mistaken for a small kidney.

Unilateral renomegaly with smooth margin

1. Compensatory hypertrophy; the other kidney is non-functional and may be small or absent.
2. Acute inflammation (e.g., nephritis, pyelonephritis).
3. **Hydronephrosis**:
   a. Congenital obstruction:
      1) Ectopic ureter.
      2) Stenosis or atresia of lower urinary tract.
      3) Telangiectasia; aberrant blood vessels constricting urinary outflow.
      4) Ureterocele, a distal ureteral obstruction.
   b. Acquired obstruction:
      1) Urinary calculi.
      2) Tumor in bladder trigone or distal ureter.
      3) Retroperitoneal mass compressing a ureter.
      4) Chronic inflammation (e.g., pyelonephritis).
      5) Parasitic disease (*Dioctophyma renale*).
      6) Accidental ligation of a ureter.
      7) Adhesions from previous trauma or surgery.
      8) Radiation therapy.
4. Primary renal tumor:
   a. Adenocarcinoma (most common in dogs).
   b. Lymphoma (most common in cats, usually bilateral).

c. Squamous cell carcinoma, papillary carcinoma.
d. Nephroblastoma; young dogs, the affected kidney can become quite large.
e. Metastatic tumor in kidney (e.g., osteosarcoma, hemangiosarcoma, melanoma; mast cell tumor).
5. Large renal cyst, centrally located in a kidney.
6. Polycystic kidney disease with small or centrally located cysts.
7. Perirenal pseudocyst; more common in cats.
8. Perinephric abscess.
9. Subcapsular hematoma.

Unilateral renomegaly with irregular margin
1. Large peripheral renal mass.
2. Multiple smaller peripheral cysts or nodules in a kidney.

Bilateral renomegaly with smooth margins
1. Acute inflammation (e.g., nephritis, pyelonephritis).
2. Polycystic kidney disease with small or centrally located cysts.
3. Lymphoma; particularly in cats; usually bilateral and symmetrical renomegaly.
4. Feline infectious peritonitis (FIP).
5. Perirenal pseudocyst.
6. Amyloidosis.
7. Hydronephrosis; bilateral urinary outflow obstruction is less common than unilateral.
8. Parasite infection (*Dioctophyma renale*).
9. Portosystemic shunt; bilateral compensatory renomegaly in response to reduced liver function.
10. Caudal abdominal compression during excretory urography, temporary restriction to urine outflow.

Bilateral renomegaly with irregular margins
1. Lymphoma.
2. Feline infectious peritonitis (FIP).
3. Polycystic kidney disease with larger or more peripheral cysts.
4. Renal cystadenocarcinoma; heritable disease causing multiple tumors in both kidneys and cutaneous nodules on the head and legs (*dermatofibrosis*); reported in German Shepherds.

Abnormal number of kidneys
1. Absence of a kidney:
   a. Renal aplasia.
   b. Surgical removal.
   c. Renal ectopia.
2. Extra kidney; rare in dogs and cats:
   a. Congenital renal duplication.
   b. Renal transplant; in cats, the native kidney sometimes is not removed during the transplant.

Abnormal opacity in kidneys
1. Gas opacity in kidney:
   a. Gas-producing bacterial infection.
   b. Vesicoureteral reflux (e.g., emphysematous cystitis, pneumocystogram).
   c. Traumatic influx of air from an intra-abdominal or extra-abdominal source.
2. Mineral or metal opacity in kidneys:
   a. Calculi.
   b. Foreign material.
   c. Contrast medium.
   d. Metabolic disease (e.g., hypercalcemia, hyperparathyroidism, hypervitamin D).
   e. Chronic renal inflammation (e.g., glomerulonephritis).
   f. Nephrotoxic drugs (e.g., Gentamicin, Amphotericin B, Cisplatin).
   g. Toxin/poison (e.g., ethylene glycol, cholecalciferol).
   h. Long-standing renal mass or infarct.
   i. Telangiectasia.
   j. Vascular mineralization (usually older animals).
   k. Idiopathic.

Conditions that mimic abnormal renal opacity
1. Normal fat in renal pelvis mistaken for gas.
2. Summation of overlapping kidneys in a lateral view, may be mistaken for a renal mass.
3. Superimposition artifact (e.g., GI content, skin nodule, nipple, skin debris, medication on hair coat), artifacts often are identified with orthogonal views or using compression radiography.
4. Deep circumflex iliac artery mistaken for a ureteral calculus in a lateral view.

Urinary bladder

Abnormal position of urinary bladder
(Bladder is not seen in its expected location.)

Non-visualization of bladder
1. Underexposed radiograph.
2. Absence of opacity interface.
3. Empty bladder.
4. Short urethra syndrome or "pelvic bladder."
5. Obesity in dogs.
6. Bladder obscured by overlying structure (e.g., pelvic limb musculature, jejunum, colon).
7. Ruptured bladder.
8. Displaced urinary bladder:
   a. Inguinal hernia.
   b. Perineal hernia.

   c. Ruptured body wall.
   d. Prolapse of bladder.

Cranial displacement of urinary bladder
1. Obesity in cats.
2. Large colon or rectum (e.g., ileus, constipation).
3. Prostatomegaly.
4. Large uterus or uterine stump.
5. Pelvic/urethral mass.
6. Avulsion of bladder from urethra.
7. Caudal sublumbar mass.

Caudal displacement of urinary bladder
1. Obesity in dogs, bladder is confined to pelvic canal.
2. Empty bladder.
3. Short urethra syndrome or "pelvic bladder."
4. Hypoplastic bladder (e.g., bilateral ectopic ureters).
5. Perineal hernia; displacement may be intermittent.
6. Large mid-abdominal mass.

Ventral displacement of urinary bladder
1. Large colon (e.g., constipation, megacolon).
2. Large uterus (e.g., pregnant, pyometra).
3. Retroperitoneal swelling (e.g., mass, fluid).
4. Inguinal hernia.
5. Loss of ventral body wall integrity.
6. Persistent urachal ligament.

Dorsal displacement of urinary bladder
1. Caudoventral intra-abdominal mass.
2. Swelling along ventral body wall (e.g., edema, inflammation, tumor).

Conditions that mimic abnormal position of bladder
1. Paraprostatic cyst mistaken for urinary bladder.
2. Ectopic kidney mistaken for urinary bladder.
3. Other intra-abdominal mass mistaken for bladder; particularly if bladder is too small to be identified.

Abnormal size of urinary bladder

(Bladder is smaller or larger than expected.)

Small urinary bladder
1. Empty bladder, recent voiding of urine.
2. Cystitis; bladder tends to be small due to frequent voiding or non-distensible bladder wall.
   a. Bacterial infection.
   b. Chronic renal disease
   c. Trauma.
   d. Patient stress.
   e. Congenital abnormality (e.g., urachal remnant).
3. Ruptured bladder:
   a. Blunt force trauma, particularly when the bladder is full.
   b. Chronic urethral obstruction.
   c. Penetrating wound (e.g., gunshot, stabbing, bone fragments from a fractured pelvis).
   d. Erosive lesion (e.g., neoplasia, infection).
   e. Iatrogenic:
      1) Faulty catheterization.
      2) Overzealous abdominal palpation.
4. No urine production (e.g., renal failure, anuria).
5. Non-distensible bladder (e.g., severe chronic cystitis, bladder wall neoplasia).
6. Bladder hypoplasia (e.g., bilateral ectopic ureters).
7. Fistula (urethrorectal, urethrovaginal).

Large urinary bladder
1. Voluntary retention of urine (e.g., housebroken, anxious, stressed, nervous, painful urination).
2. Outflow obstruction (e.g., calculus, tumor, stricture).
3. Neurologic disease:
   a. Spina bifida.
   b. Damage to brain stem or spinal cord.
4. Loss of bladder tone due to overdistention.

Abnormal shape of urinary bladder

1. Bladder wall is indented by adjacent viscera or mass effect.
2. Tumor involving the bladder wall.
3. Urachal diverticulum.
4. Persistent urachal ligament.
5. Urachal cyst.
6. Chronic obstruction leading to loss of muscle tone and a flaccid bladder.
7. Rupture of bladder wall.
8. Diverticulum in bladder wall; traumatic diverticula and bladder wall contusions appear similar initially but contusions usually heal within 48 hours and the bladder then distends normally.
9. Adhesions pulling on bladder (e.g., prior surgery, previous trauma).
10. Spasm of bladder wall; typically caused by severe trauma, usually subsides within a few days.
11. Fistula; abnormal communication between bladder and another organ.
12. Structure adjacent to bladder, may mimic abnormal shape due to blending with the bladder margin (e.g., paraprostatic cyst).

Abnormal content or opacity in urinary bladder

1. Gas in urinary bladder:
   a. Iatrogenic; gas bubbles usually are located at the periphery of any fluid in the bladder lumen:
      1) Cystocentesis.
      2) Urethral catheterization.
      3) Pneumocystogram, double contrast cystogram.
   b. Emphysematous cystitis; often associated with diabetes mellitus.

2. Mineral or metal opacity in urinary bladder:
   a. Cystic calculi.
   b. Sludge; an amorphous crystalline debris.
   c. Dystrophic mineralization (e.g., chronic inflammation, neoplasia).
   d. Contrast medium.
   e. Foreign material:
      1) Metallic projectile.
      2) Catheter fragment.
3. Soft tissue opacity in urinary bladder:
   a. Calculi.
   b. Mass (e.g., tumor, hematoma, polyp, blood clot).

<u>Conditions that mimic abnormal bladder opacity</u>

1. Superimposition artifact:
   a. Intestinal content.
   b. Fascial plane, subcutaneous emphysema.
   c. Pneumoperitoneum.
   d. Cutaneous growth, nipple, prepuce.
   e. Suture granuloma from prior hysterectomy.
   f. Wet or dirty hair coat; medication on skin.

Thickened urinary bladder wall

(Cystography usually is needed to examine the bladder wall. Wall thickness in a moderately distended bladder seldom exceeds 2 mm.)

1. Chronic cystitis:
   a. Infection (e.g., *E. coli*, *Streptococcus*).
   b. Chronic renal disease.
   c. Patient stress.
2. Trauma; hemorrhage or edema in bladder wall.
3. Neoplasia.
4. Muscular hypertrophy secondary to chronic urinary outflow obstruction.
5. Ureterocele; may be in the bladder wall or lumen (*intravesicular* or *orthotopic* ureterocele) or in the bladder neck or urethra (*ectopic* ureterocele), latter is associated with an ectopic ureter.

<u>Conditions that mimic bladder wall thickening</u>

1. Inadequate distention of urinary bladder.
2. Blood clots adhered to bladder mucosa.

Extravasation of contrast agent during cystography

(Contrast medium extends beyond the bladder lumen.)

1. Ruptured bladder.
2. Damaged bladder mucosa; submucosal accumulation of contrast medium (e.g., trauma, iatrogenic).
3. Vesicoureteral reflux; contrast medium in ureter and renal collecting system.
4. Patent urachus.
5. Diverticulum (e.g., urachal, traumatic).
6. Fistula (rare); an abnormal communication between the urinary bladder and either the vagina, uterus, or rectum. Contrast medium appears simultaneously in the bladder and in the other organ.

Urethra

Abnormal size of urethra

(Urethrography reveals focal or diffuse narrowing or widening of the urethral lumen.)

<u>Narrowed urethra</u>

1. Normal peristalsis; transient narrowing.
2. Urethral spasm; transient, common in prostatic urethra; may be more frequent due to inflammation.
3. Thickened urethral wall:
   a. Inflammation, non-infectious; (e.g., trauma, tumor, calculi, faulty catheterization).
   b. Infection; often associated with disease in urinary bladder, prostate gland or vagina.
   c. Neoplasia (e.g., transitional cell carcinoma, transmissible venereal tumor); females more often are affected than males, usually mature animals.
   d. Granulomatous disease.
4. Intraluminal mass (localized narrowing):
   a. Calculus.
   b. Blood clot.
   c. Tumor.
   d. Polyp.
5. Stricture (e.g., chronic inflammation, neoplasia, trauma from calculi, surgery, catheterization).
6. External compression; periurethral mass effect:
   a. Prostatomegaly.
   b. Pelvic tumor.
   c. Lymphadenomegaly.

<u>Widened urethra</u>

1. Outflow obstruction (diffuse widening).
2. Intraluminal mass (localized widening):
   a. Calculus.
   b. Tumor.
3. Periurethral adhesions pulling on urethral wall.
4. Urethral diverticulum or fistula.
5. Iatrogenic (e.g., positive pressure during urethrography).
6. Pharmacologic effect (e.g., infused analgesic).

<u>Extravasation of urethral contrast medium</u>

1. Ruptured urethra:
   a. Trauma, faulty catheterization.
   b. Neoplastic erosion of urethral wall.
   c. Severe or chronic inflammation.

2. Prostatic reflux; normal if flow is into prostatic ducts, abnormal if into the prostatic parenchyma:
   a. Prostatic neoplasia.
   b. Prostatic abscess.
   c. Cystic hyperplasia.
3. Fistula; abnormal communication between urethra and rectum or vagina.
4. Ectopic ureter; reflux of contrast into ureter and sometimes into kidney.
5. Urethrocavernous reflux; contrast medium enters the adjacent vasculature or parenchyma of the penis.

Abnormal urethral opacity

1. Gas in urethra:
   a. Iatrogenic (e.g., catheterization).
   b. Trauma (e.g., penetrating wound).
   c. Gas-producing bacterial infection.
2. Mineralization in urethra:
   a. Calculi.
   b. Dystrophic mineralization (e.g., chronic inflammation, tissue necrosis).
   c. Neoplastic mineralization.
   d. Contrast medium in urethra (metal opacity).

Conditions that mimic abnormal urethral opacity

1. Os penis accessory ossification center; may be mistaken for a mineral opacity urethral calculus.
2. Vestigial os penis in hermaphrodite dogs.
3. Normal os penis in cats; typically a small and faintly mineralized structure.
4. Superimposition artifact (e.g., nodule, gas).

Prostate gland

Prostatomegaly

(Normal height of the prostate gland is about 70% of the height of the pelvic inlet in a lateral view.)

1. Benign prostatic hyperplasia (BPH); intact males.
2. Inflammation; infection (prostatitis).
3. Neoplasia:
   a. Adenocarcinoma (most common).
   b. Transitional cell carcinoma
   c. Leiomyosarcoma.
4. Androgen-producing testicular tumor.
5. Abscess.
6. Cyst in prostate gland.
7. Paraprostatic cyst.

Conditions that mimic prostatomegaly

1. Cranial displacement of normal prostate gland due to full urinary bladder or weakened ventral abdominal muscles (latter due to old age, hypercortisolism).
2. Superimposed pelvic limbs or colon.
3. Mass in pelvic canal or urethra.

Abnormal opacity in prostate gland

1. Gas in prostate gland:
   a. Iatrogenic introduction of gas (e.g., urinary catheterization, reflux during pneumocystogram).
   b. Gas-producing bacterial infection.
2. Mineralization in prostate gland:
   a. Neoplasia (most common).
   b. Chronic prostatitis.
   c. Cyst (prostatic or paraprostatic).
   d. Abscess.
   e. Prostatic calculi.

Conditions that mimic abnormal prostate opacity

1. Superimposition artifact: (e.g., subcutaneous emphysema, fascial plane).
2. Calculi in prostatic urethra.
3. Reflux of contrast medium into prostatic ducts during urethrography.
4. Superimposition artifact (e.g., wet or dirty hair coat, debris or medication on skin, cutaneous nodule).

Uterus

Non-visualization of the uterus

1. Normal, non-gravid uterus.
2. Peritoneal effusion.
3. Prolapse of uterus through a hernia or ruptured body wall.

Localized uterine enlargement

1. Early or asymmetric pregnancy.
2. Uterine mass.
3. Fluid trapped in one uterine horn (e.g., pyometra, mucometra, hydrometra, hematometra).
4. Torsion of a uterine horn.

Generalized uterine enlargement

1. Pregnancy; cannot be distinguished from disease in the uterus until fetal ossification.
2. Postpartum uterus; uterus can remain large and visible in radiographs for a week or more after delivery.
3. Pseudocyesis (false pregnancy).

4. Abnormal fluid in uterus:
   a. Pyometra; purulent fluid.
   b. Hydrometra; clear, aseptic fluid.
   c. Mucometra; aseptic mucoid fluid, often associated with cystic endometrial hyperplasia.
   d. Hematometra; aseptic bloody fluid.
5. Thickening of uterine wall (e.g., inflammation, endometrial hyperplasia).
6. Uterine torsion (rare); usually associated with pregnancy or pyometra.
7. Uterine adenomyosis; proliferation of uterine glands.
8. Obstructed uterus (e.g., hydrocolpos, congenital vaginal blockage, cystic uterine remnant).
9. Cystadenocarcinoma; uterine tumors in German shepherd dogs (i.e., multiple leiomyomas).

Conditions that mimic uterine enlargement

1. Small intestine ileus, bowel dilated with fluid.
2. Caudal intra-abdominal mass (e.g., tumor, abscess, granuloma, cyst) associated with spleen, intestine, mesentery, or lymph node.

Displacement of the uterus

(Uterus is readily displaced by an intra-abdominal mass effect. Note: the normal, non-gravid uterus seldom is identified in survey radiographs.)

1. Physiologic or pathologic enlargement of nearby viscera.
2. Prolapse through a hernia or ruptured abdominal wall.

Dystocia

1. Maternal issues that can cause dystocia:
   a. Uterine inertia; no uterine contractions or contractions stop before birthing is complete.
   b. Uterine displacement (e.g., hernia, uterine torsion).
   c. Narrow or obstructed birth canal (e.g., mass in canal, malunion pelvic fracture, juvenile pubic symphysodesis).
2. Fetal factors that can cause dystocia:
   a. Oversized fetus; common when there is only one or a few fetuses.
   b. Abnormal presentation of fetus to pelvic canal.
   c. Abnormal development of fetus.
   d. Death of fetus.

Abnormal opacity in uterus

1. Gas in uterus:
   a. Gas-producing bacterial infection:
      1) Fetal death
      2) Uterine torsion.
      3) Pyometra.
   b. Iatrogenic:
      1) Uterine catheterization.
      2) Abdominocentesis.
2. Mineral opacity in uterus:
   a. Fetal ossification.
   b. Chronic inflammation.
   c. Neoplasia.
   d. Long standing uterine mass or cyst.

Adrenal glands

Abnormal adrenal gland size

1. Adrenomegaly:
   a. Hyperplasia; due to pituitary gland disorder.
   b. Neoplasia; may be unilateral or bilateral:
      1) Adenocarcinoma; a primary adrenal tumor that can grow larger than a kidney; may or may not be functional.
      2) Pheochromocytoma; rare neuroendocrine tumor; more often reported in older animals; often functional (overproduction of catecholamines epinephrine and norepinephrine).
      3) Hemangiosarcoma in retroperitoneal space can secondarily invade adrenal glands.
      4) Spread of lymphoma.

Conditions that mimic adrenomegaly

1. A well-visualized proximal spleen may be mistaken for adrenomegaly, particularly in a lateral view.

Adrenal gland mineralization

1. Dogs: probable neoplasia; may be unilateral or bilateral; tumor may or may not be functional.
2. Cats: often idiopathic; usually bilateral; tends to be seen in older cats as an incidental finding.

5 Musculoskeleton

Radiography of the Dog and Cat: Guide to Making and Interpreting Radiographs, Second Edition. M.C. Muhlbauer and S.K. Kneller.

Companion website: www.wiley.com/go/muhlbauer/dog

Introduction to musculoskeletal radiography

Bone responds to diseases and injuries with either an increase in mineral or a decrease in mineral. Abnormal bone is either too light or too dark in radiographs. Different bone diseases often present with similar radiographic findings. In many cases, a definitive diagnosis is not possible from radiographs alone. Although you do not need patient history and results of laboratory testing to read the radiographs, this information often is useful to interpret your findings.

The musculoskeletal structures are evaluated for soft tissue abnormalities as well as abnormal position, size, shape, margination, and opacity of the bones. Knowledge of normal anatomy is essential. Comparison radiographs of the contralateral limb, or of a known normal limb, are helpful to differentiate normal variations from pathology. Also useful are reference materials such as radiology and anatomy textbooks, websites, and models, the latter including skeletons and bone specimens. At the end of this chapter is an appendix with lists of differential diagnoses for numerous radiographic findings. When describing bone lesions, it is important to note their distribution:

1. Monostotic (all in same bone).
2. Polyostotic (multiple bones affected).
3. Unilateral or bilateral.
4. Symmetrical or asymmetrical.
5. Epiphyseal, physeal, metaphyseal, diaphyseal.

Procedure for making musculoskeletal radiographs

1. Measure the thickest portion of the body part being imaged.
2. Center the x-ray beam on the bone or joint of interest.
3. Collimate the field-of-view as small as practical. When making radiographs of long bones, include the joints proximal and distal. Radiographs of joints should include the adjacent third of the long bones.
4. To maximize bone to soft tissue contrast, try to keep the kVp near 70.
5. The exposure technique used to image bones may need to be modified to evaluate soft tissues.

Standard views of musculoskeletal structures

1. A lateral view and the orthogonal craniocaudal (caudocranial) or dorsopalmar (dorsoplantar) view are standard for all orthopedic studies.
2. When making a lateral view, the limb of interest should be positioned closest to the image receptor to minimize distortion artifacts.
3. Isolate the limb of interest from other body parts to avoid superimposition artifacts.
4. Poor positioning can mimic or mask skeletal disease and is a common cause of misdiagnoses.

Supplemental views of musculoskeletal structures

1. Obliqued, flexed, extended, tangential, rotated, or skyline views can help visualize bony surfaces not well seen in standard views.
2. Comparison radiographs of the contralateral limb frequently aid in interpreting questionable findings.
3. Radiographs made with the patient fully weight bearing help to accurately assess joint space width.
4. Stress views are used to evaluate joint instability or subluxation when not evident in standard views. The radiograph is made while the bones proximal and distal to the joint are stabilized, and a force is applied against the joint (Figure 2.31).
5. Follow-up radiographs document the progression of disease, response to therapy and may reveal lesions not previously evident. Follow-up radiographs generally are made in 1–2 week intervals, sooner if clinically indicated.

Soft tissues

Soft tissue abnormalities frequently accompany and often precede active bone disease. Recognizing the presence or absence of soft tissue swelling is extremely useful when trying to decide whether the appearance of a bony structure represents a normal anatomic variation, an inactive lesion, or an active disease process. In some cases, the cause of pain or lameness is limited to the soft tissues, such as sprains (ligament injuries), strains (muscle injuries), bruises, inflammation, and others. Conditions that can mimic a soft tissue abnormality include bunching of the skin, superimposed skin folds, and dirt, debris, or fluid on the skin or in the hair coat.

Soft tissue swelling may be localized or diffuse. Localized swelling can be caused by a mass. Diffuse swelling often is caused by fluid (e.g., edema, hemorrhage, inflammation, others). Swelling may be identified by the displacement or effacement of the nearby fascial planes.

A **soft tissue mass** is a localized area of swelling with a defined margin. The margin may or may not be visible in radiographs, depending on the opacity interface with the adjacent tissues. A soft tissue mass in muscle or surrounded by fluid, for example, is not distinguished because the opacities are the same. A soft tissue mass must be large enough to distort the border of the muscle or displace a fascial plane to be identified. Types of soft tissue masses include tumor, hematoma, cyst, abscess, granuloma, and lymphadenomegaly, the latter occurring at a known location for a lymph node.

Lipomas are fat opacity masses, they often can be distinguished from soft tissue in survey radiographs (Figure 5.1). Many lipomas develop in fascial planes. Mixed opacity lipomas may result from fluid mixing with fat or due to a more aggressive type of lipoma such as dissecting lipoma or liposarcoma. The margins of liposarcomas tend to be indistinct.

An **arteriovenous fistula** is an abnormal communication between an artery and a vein, which can appear as a soft tissue opacity mass. They occur more often in a limb and may be accompanied by a periosteal response or pressure remodeling in the adjacent bone.

Lymphedema is an abnormal accumulation of lymphatic fluid in one or more limbs. Swelling typically is more severe in the distal part of the limb due to the effects of gravity. Unless the edema is due to trauma, the skeletal structures usually are normal.

A **loss or reduction of soft tissue** may be due atrophy or the physical absence of tissue. Atrophy generally results from disuse, which may be due to pain, immobilization, or paralysis. A physical deficit may be caused by severe trauma or surgical removal.

Gas in the soft tissues can result from a penetrating wound, migration of gas from a nearby damaged structure

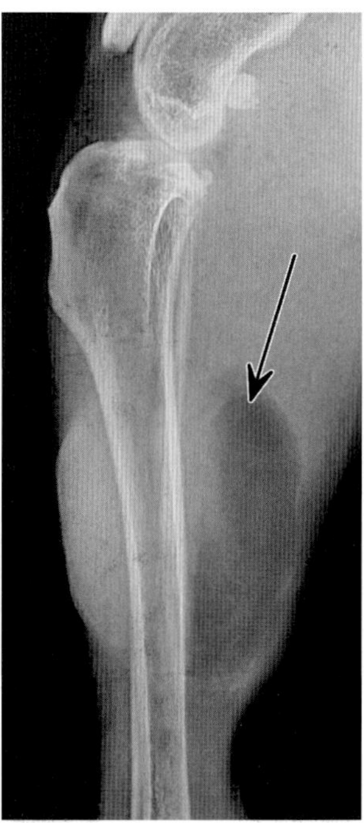

Figure 5.1 Lipoma. Lateral view of a dog crus depicting a fat opacity mass in the soft tissues caudal to the tibia (arrow).

(e.g., ruptured trachea), or a gas-producing bacterial infection. The gas may be localized or diffuse and usually produces a heterogeneous pattern due to multiple bubbles. Soft tissue emphysema can occur in the subcutaneous, intramuscular, or interfascial tissues. The volume of subcutaneous gas sometimes is quite large and widespread, displacing the skin away from the body and making the patient appear bloated. Conditions that may be mistaken for soft tissue emphysema include fat opacity in the soft tissues (e.g., fascial plane, lipoma) and superimposition of skin folds.

Mineralization in the soft tissues may be dystrophic, metastatic, neoplastic, or due to foreign material. There are several different mechanisms by which soft tissue structures can mineralize, but they are difficult to differentiate in radiographs. The location of the mineralization and results of laboratory testing sometimes provide clues to the etiology. Soft tissue mineralization ranges from disorganized to highly organized. Clinical signs usually are absent unless a secondary complication develops, such as interference with mobility, ulceration, or infection. **Dystrophic mineralization** occurs locally in damaged, degenerating, or dead tissue. Serum calcium and phosphorous usually are normal. **Metastatic mineralization** occurs in normal tissues away from the site of disease. It frequently is associated with abnormal serum calcium and phosphorous, but blood work sometimes is normal.

Calcinosis cutis is mineralization in the skin. It most often is associated with hypercortisolism, but it can result

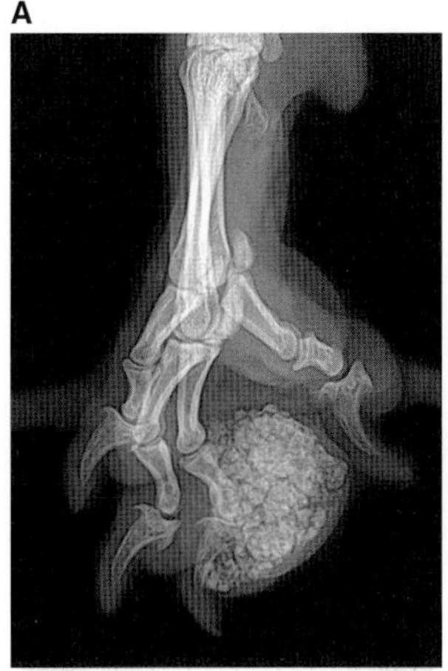

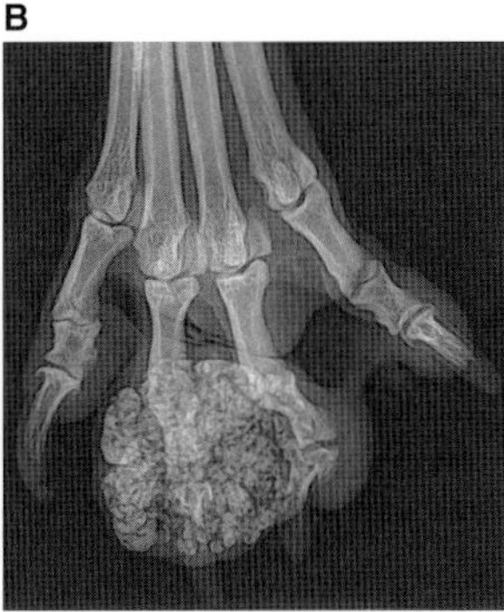

Figure 5.2 Calcinosis circumscripta. Lateral view (**A**) and dorsopalmar view (**B**) of a dog manus depicting a well-defined mass of heterogenous mineralization in the soft tissues near the third digit. Careful inspection reveals that the bones are not involved. The digits were gently separated using gauze tied around the toes.

from trauma, chronic inflammation, and others. In radiographs, calcinosis cutis typically appears as thin, linear mineralization near the skin surface. It may be focal or multifocal.

Calcinosis circumscripta is mineralization in the subcutaneous tissues. The etiology is unknown. It is uncommon in dogs and rare in cats, most often reported in young, large breed dogs. Calcinosis circumscripta tends to occur at bony prominences and under footpads. In radiographs, it appears as well-defined, rounded clusters of heterogeneous mineralization (Figures 5.2 and 5.3), sometimes called *tumoral calcinosis*. It often develops near a skeletal structure and may be mistaken for bone disease, but there is no periosteal response nor evidence of osteolysis.

Vascular mineralization occurs in the walls of blood vessels, usually arteries. In dogs, it most often is seen along the abdominal aorta and its major branches. In cats, particularly older animals, it more often occurs in the thoracic aorta. Vascular mineralization frequently is idiopathic, but it may be associated with a systemic or endocrine disease.

Mineral and metal opacity **foreign materials** usually are readily identified in radiographs, but they must be confirmed in orthogonal views to avoid misdiagnosing a superimposition artifact. Soft tissue opacity foreign materials seldom are distinguished unless adjacent to fat or gas (e.g., glass, wood, plastic, plant materials). A fistulogram may help locate a foreign object if a draining tract or site of entry is found.

Orthopedic anatomic considerations

Bone is approximately one-third organic material (*osteoid*) and two-thirds inorganic material (*mineral*). Osteoid is soft tissue opacity and not differentiated from the adjacent soft tissues. In most cases, only the mineral portion of bone is visible in radiographs.

The average number of bones in a dog is about 320 and the average number in a cat is about 240. A typical dog skeleton includes:

- 50 vertebrae
- 26 ribs
- 8 sternebrae
- 41 skull bones
- 9 hyoid bones
- 45 bones in each pectoral limb
- 48 bones in each pelvic limb
- 1 os penis in males (an extra-skeletal bone, not attached to the skeleton).

Types of bone

There are two general types of bone: cortical and cancellous. **Cortical bone** forms the outer layer or *cortex* of most bones, including all long bones. Cortical bone is also called *compact bone* and makes up about 80% of the total bone mass in the body. In radiographs, it is relatively uniform in appearance and homogeneous in opacity (Figure 5.4).

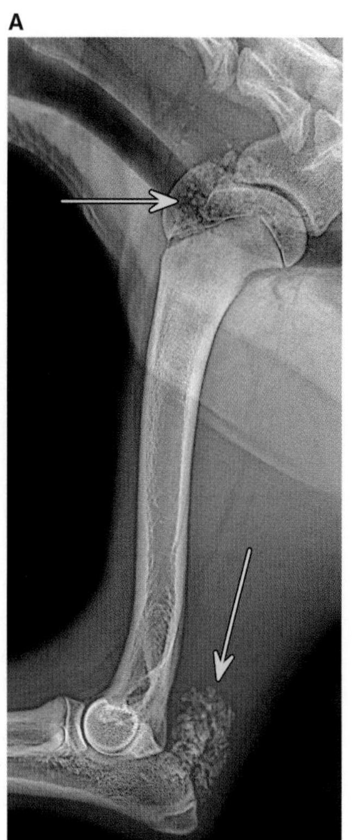

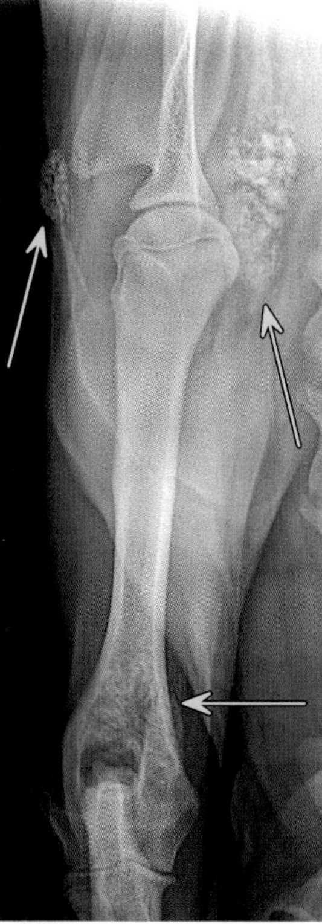

Figure 5.3 Calcinosis circumscripta. Lateral view (**A**) and caudocranial view (**B**) of a dog humerus depicting heterogenous mineralization in the soft tissues near the elbow and shoulder (arrows).

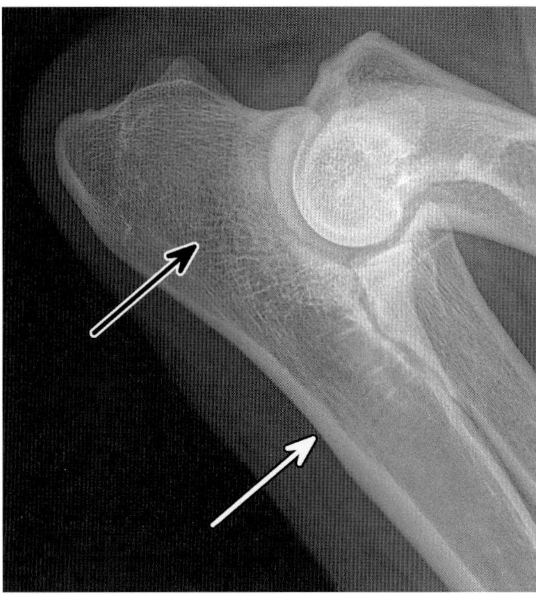

Figure 5.4 Cortical and cancellous bone. Lateral view of a dog elbow depicting the appearance of cancellous bone (black arrow) and cortical bone (white arrow).

Cancellous bone consists of a network of thin bony plates called *trabeculae* with many open spaces, or "pores", in between. Cancellous bone is also called *trabecular bone* and makes up about 20% of the skeletal mass. Because of the trabeculae, the surface area of cancellous bone is nearly 10 times that of cortical bone. Trabecular bone is found at the ends of long bones, in the vertebrae, and in flat bones. In radiographs, it is more porous and heterogeneous in opacity than cortical bone (Figure 5.4), sometimes described as sponge-like in appearance.

Shapes of bones

Bones commonly are classified as either long, short, flat, or irregular in shape. **Long bones** are longer than they are wide. They consist of a shaft and two ends. Long bones are found in the limbs (e.g., humerus, femur, radius, ulna, tibia) where they provide strength and mobility.

Short bones are as wide as they are long, sometimes described as *cuboidal*. They are found in the carpi and tarsi, where they provide stability and some movement.

Flat bones are relatively broad and flattened, as the name suggests. They are found in the head, ribs, and limb girdles (e.g., pelvis, scapula), where they provide protection for the internal structures.

Irregular bones are more complex in shape and do not fit into the other classifications. These include the vertebrae, many of the bones in the skull, and sesamoid bones.

Sesamoid bones are located in tendons where they help reduce strain near a freely moving joint. They are small and usually round or ovoid in shape. Some sesamoid bones are lined on one side with articular cartilage (e.g., patella, palmar sesamoids, plantar sesamoids).

Bone development

Most bones form via *endochondral ossification*, which means they develop in a cartilaginous frame. Some bones form via *intramembranous ossification*, which means they grow in connective tissue without an intervening cartilage model. Many of the bones in the skull form via intramembranous ossification.

During endochondral ossification, growing cartilage is systematically replaced by bone. The points in the cartilage frame where bone initially forms are called ossification centers.

Primary ossification centers develop in the shafts of long bones and in the bodies of short bones, irregular bones, and sesamoid bones. **Secondary ossification centers** develop at the ends of long bones and form bony prominences, which serve as attachment sites for ligaments, tendons, and other structures. There may be multiple secondary ossification centers in one bone. Secondary centers sometimes fail to fuse to the parent bone and instead develop into separate small, round or oval-shaped mineral opacity structures. These are called **accessory ossification centers** or *accessory ossicles*. The locations of many accessory ossicles are known (often they occur near a joint) and they are described and illustrated in this chapter. Knowledge of accessory ossification centers is important because they may be mistaken for pathology, such as avulsion fractures.

Long bones form in a cartilage frame. Longitudinal growth occurs at growth plates called **physes**, which are located near one or both ends of the bone. A physis appears in radiographs as soft tissue opacity band. The different parts of a long bone are named in relation to the physis (Figure 5.5).

The **diaphysis** is located "between the physes." It is the shaft of the long bone, the diaphysis appears in radiographs as homogenous cortical bone on either side of a less opaque medullary cavity. Although cortical bone completely encircles the medullary cavity, the bony cortex appears as two distinct divisions due to the summation of bone (Figure 5.6).

The **metaphysis** is located "next to the physis." It is the wider end of the shaft of a long bone and consists of mostly cancellous bone. Metaphysis also means "change next to the physis" because this is where the wider bone is actively remodeled to become the narrower shaft. This area of bone remodeling is called the **cut-back zone** and appears in radiographs as a part of the cortex with a less distinct margin. The cut-back zone sometimes is mistaken for pathology; however, there is no soft tissue swelling or pain with normal bone growth.

The **epiphysis** is located "upon the physis." It is the rounded end of a long bone that supports the articular cartilage. The epiphysis is mostly cancellous bone with a thin layer of dense subchondral bone. The subchondral bone appears in radiographs as a thin line of increased opacity at the articular border.

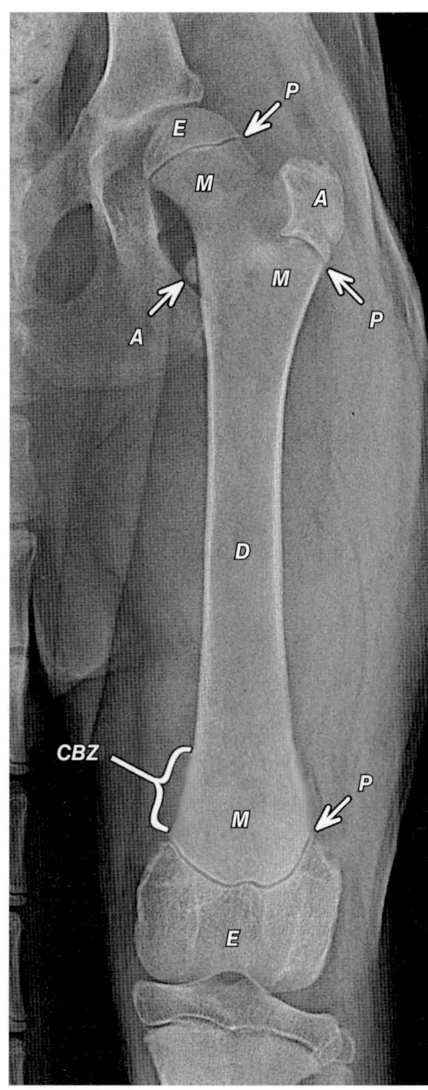

Figure 5.5 Parts of a long bone. Craniocaudal view of an immature dog femur depicting normal anatomy. P = physis, E = epiphysis, M = metaphysis, D = diaphysis, A = apophysis, CBZ = cut-back zone. Notice that the cortical margin is not as sharp in the cut-back zone.

An **apophysis** is a non-articular epiphysis. It forms a bony prominence that serves as an attachment site for a tendon, ligament, or joint capsule. Examples include the greater trochanter, greater tubercle, and tibial tuberosity. An apophysis sometimes is called a *traction epiphysis* because the structures that attach here exert a pulling force, whereas the structures at an epiphysis exert compressive forces due to weight bearing.

The parts of growing bones are not visible in radiographs until they ossify. Ossification centers become visible at predictable times in dogs and cats, and the secondary centers are expected to fuse with the parent bone within certain time intervals. These are listed in Table 5.1 and illustrated in Figures 5.7–5.13.

Bone growth ceases when cartilage growth stops. After the cartilage stops growing, the metaphyses and epiphyses gradually blend together and the physes become thinner and thinner until the physes "close." A "closed" physis appears in radiographs as a thin sclerotic line which is called a **physeal scar**. The physeal scar slowly fades as the animal matures and eventually disappears.

Nearly all bone surfaces are covered with a thin membrane called the **periosteum**. The articular surfaces and most of the sesamoid bones are not covered with periosteum. The periosteum consists of two layers, a tough fibrous outer layer and an inner layer that produces bone. The outer layer provides protection and connection, the latter because it blends continuously with tendons and ligaments at their attachment sites. The inner layer of the periosteum, called the *cambium layer*, is attached to the bone cortex by Sharpey's fibers. The periosteum contributes to the circumferential growth of long bones and aids in bone healing.

Bone response to disease or injury

Bone responds to disease with either an increase in mineral or a decrease in mineral, and often it is both. At least **30%–50%** of the mineral content must change before a bone lesion can be seen in a radiograph. This amount of change typically requires at least one to two weeks to occur.

A

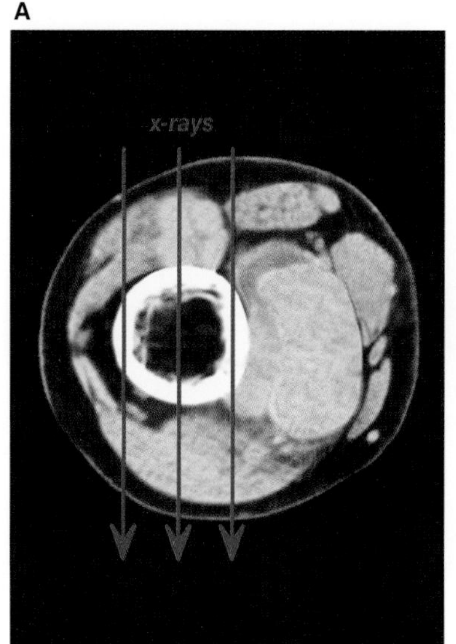

B

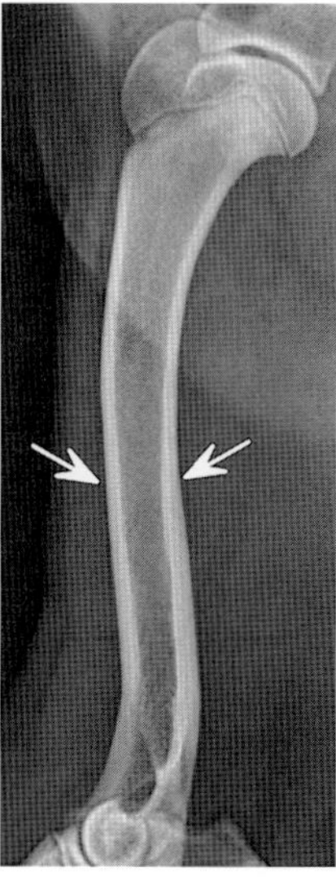

Figure 5.6 Long bone cortices. **A**. Cross-sectional CT image of a dog's long bone. Notice that the total thickness of bone through which the x-rays are passing (red arrows) is much less in the middle than on either side. The cortex is the same thickness all around the medullary cavity, but summation of bone will make parts of the cortex appear more opaque in a two-dimensional radiograph. **B**. Lateral view of a dog humerus depicting the more opaque cranial and caudal cortical bone (arrows).

Table 5.1 Epiphyses and apophyses: ages at appearance and fusion

Site	Appearance	Fusion (Dogs)	Fusion (Cats)
Scapula			
Supraglenoid tubercle	7–9 weeks	4–7 months	3–4 months
Humerus			
Greater tubercle	2–3 weeks	4 months (to humeral head)	
Proximal epiphysis (humeral head)	2 weeks	10–13 months	18–24 months
Distal epiphysis (humeral condyles)	(See condyles)	6–8 months (to diaphysis)	
Lateral condyle	2–3 weeks	6 weeks (to medial condyle)	3–4 months
Medial condyle	3–6 weeks	6 weeks (to lateral condyle)	3–4 months
Medial epicondyle	7–9 weeks	6 months (to medial condyle)	3–5 months
Radius			
Proximal epiphysis	3–5 weeks	5–11 months	6–7 months
Distal epiphysis	2–4 weeks	6–12 months	13–21 months
Ulna			
Olecranon (tuberosity of olecranon)	7–9 weeks	6–10 months	8–12 months
Anconeal process	12 weeks	4–5 months	
Distal epiphysis	7–8 weeks	7–12 months	13–24 months
Carpus			
Radial carpal bone	3–4 weeks		
Ulnar carpal bone	4–5 weeks		
Central carpal bone	4–5 weeks		
Intermediate carpal bone	2–4 weeks		
Accessory carpal bone (body)	2 weeks		3–5 months
Accessory carpal bone (epiphysis)	7 weeks	3–6 months	
First–fourth carpal bones	3–4 weeks		
Sesamoid bone	16 weeks		
Metacarpus/metatarsus			
Distal epiphysis (MC I)	5–7 weeks	6–7 months	
Distal epiphysis (MC II–V)	4–5 weeks	5–7 months	6–10 months
Phalanges			
Proximal epiphysis	6–8 weeks	4–6 months	
Dorsal sesamoids	4–5 months		4–5 months
Volar sesamoids	3–4 months		
Pelvis			
Ileum	Birth	4–6 months	
Ischium	Birth	4–6 months	
Acetabulum	7–11 weeks	4–6 months	

CHAPTER 5

Table 5.1 (Continued)

Site	Appearance	Fusion (Dogs)	Fusion (Cats)
Tuber ischii	3–5 months	8–10 months	
Symphysis pubis	5–12 months	60 months (5 years)	
Ischial arch	6 months	12 months	
Iliac crest	16 weeks	1–2 years (may remain open permanently)	
Femur			
Proximal epiphysis (femoral head)	2–4 weeks	8–12 months	7–10 months
Greater trochanter (major)	5–8 weeks	6–11 months	7–9 months
Lesser trochanter (minor)	5–10 weeks	8–13 months	8–10 months
Distal epiphysis	2–3 weeks	8–11 months (to diaphysis)	12–18 months
Medial and lateral condyles	2–3 weeks	3 months (medial to lateral condyle)	
Patella	7–9 weeks		
Tibia			
Lateral and medial condyles	2–3 weeks	6 weeks (medial to lateral condyle)	
Tibial tuberosity	7–9 weeks	6–8 months (to condyle)	12–18 months
		8–12 months (to diaphysis)	
Proximal epiphysis	3–8 weeks	8–12 months	12–18 months
Distal epiphysis	2–4 weeks	8–11 months (to diaphysis)	9–12 months
Medial malleolus	11–13 weeks	5 months	
Fibula			
Proximal epiphysis	7–10 weeks	8–12 months	13–17 months
Distal epiphysis	4–7 weeks	7–12 months	9–13 months
Tarsus			
Calcaneus	1 week		
Talus	1 week		
Intertarsal bones (central, I–IV)	3–4 weeks		
Tuber calcis (calcanean tuber)	6–8 weeks	3–8 months	7–12 months
Tarsal bones (central, I–IV)	2–4 weeks		
Sesamoids			
Patella	7–9 weeks		
Fabellae (stifle)	12 weeks		2–5 months
Popliteal (stifle)	12 weeks		4–5 months
Dorsal digits	20 weeks		
Plantar digits	8 weeks		
Phalanges			
Proximal epiphysis (II–V)		6–7 months	
Distal epiphysis			

A

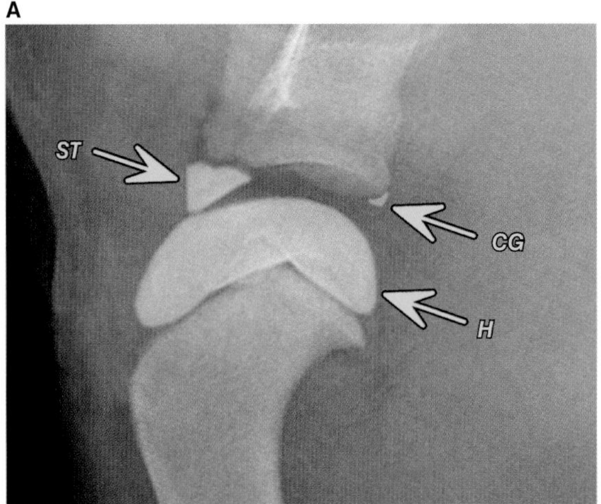

B

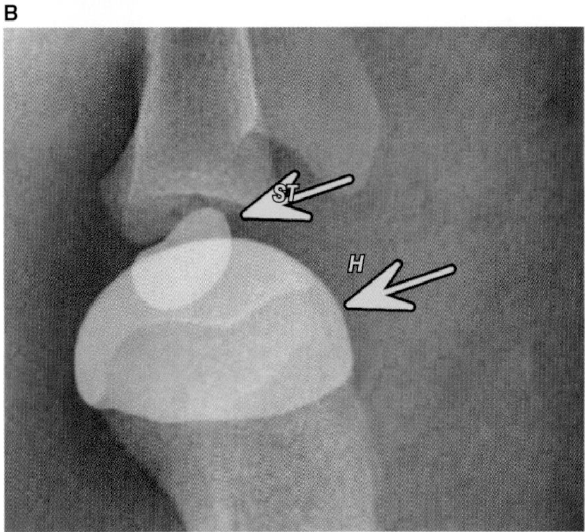

Figure 5.7 Normal shoulder epiphysis. Lateral view (**A**) and craniocaudal view (**B**) of an immature dog scapulohumeral joint depicting the humeral head (*H*), supraglenoid tubercle (*ST*), and caudal glenoid accessory ossification center (*CG*).

Bone production is a non-specific periosteal response to bone damage. The formation of new bone is an attempt to heal, not a "reaction" to any particular disease. Whenever the periosteum is separated from the cortex and maintains its blood supply, it will produce mineral to fill the space between the lifted periosteum and the cortex of the bone. Mineral is produced by the cambium layer and deposited along the fibrous and vascular tissues that remain connected to the cortex. The formation of new bone, therefore, is perpendicular to the periosteum. The further the periosteum is separated from the cortex, the larger and more irregular the new bone production because there is more space to fill. The stages of a periosteal response are illustrated in Table 5.2.

A

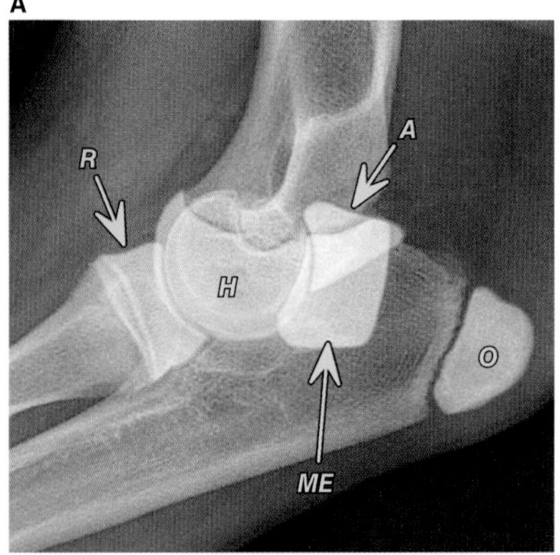

B

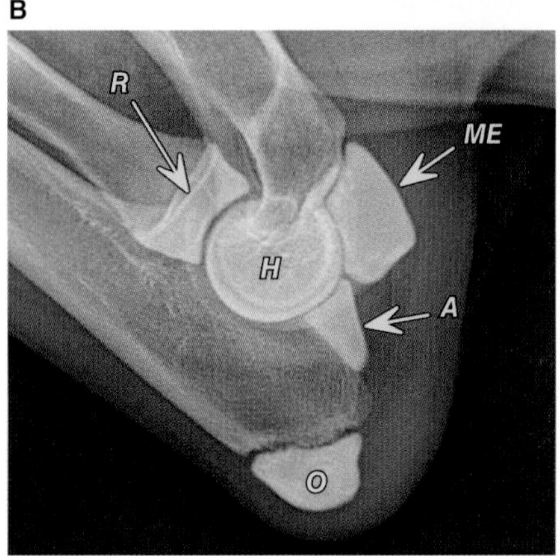

C

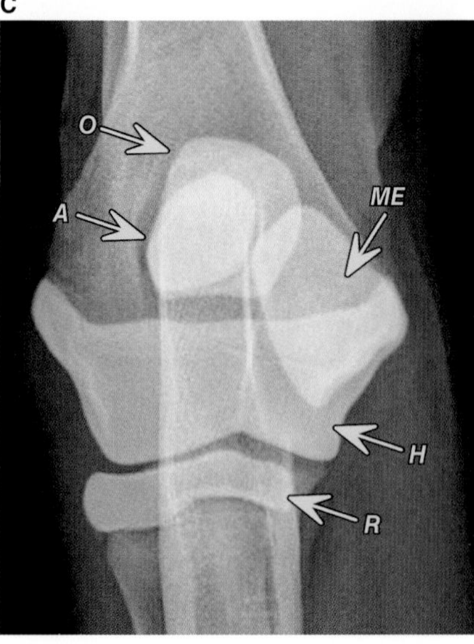

Figure 5.8 Normal elbow epiphyses. Lateral view (**A**), flexed lateral view (**B**), and craniocaudal view (**C**) of an immature dog elbow depicting the distal humeral condyle (*H*), medial epicondyle (*ME*), olecranon tuber (*O*), anconeal process (*A*), and radial head (*R*).

A

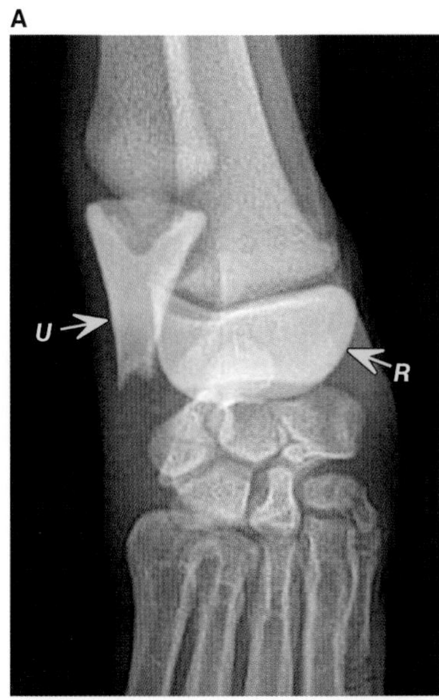

B

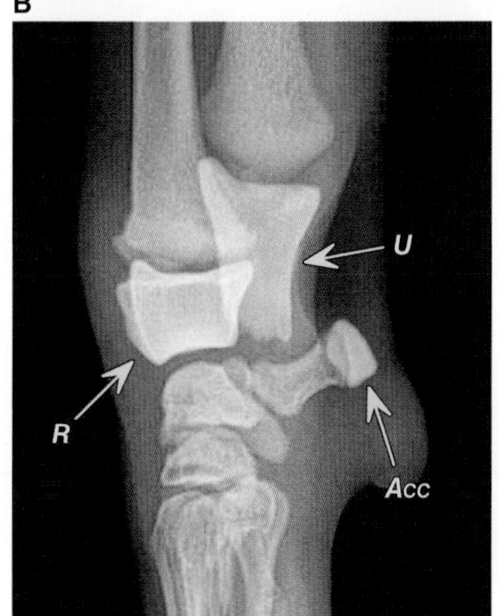

Figure 5.9 Normal carpal epiphyses. Lateral view (**A**) and dorsopalmar view (**B**) of an immature dog carpus depicting the distal radial epiphysis (*R*), distal ulnar epiphysis (*U*), and accessory carpal bone (*Acc*).

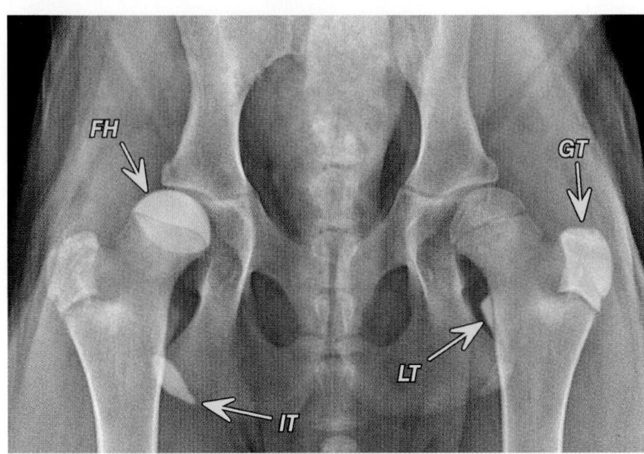

Figure 5.10 Normal pelvic epiphyses. VD view of an immature dog pelvis depicting the femoral head (*FH*), greater trochanter (*GT*), lesser trochanter (*LT*), and ischiatic tuberosity (*IT*).

A

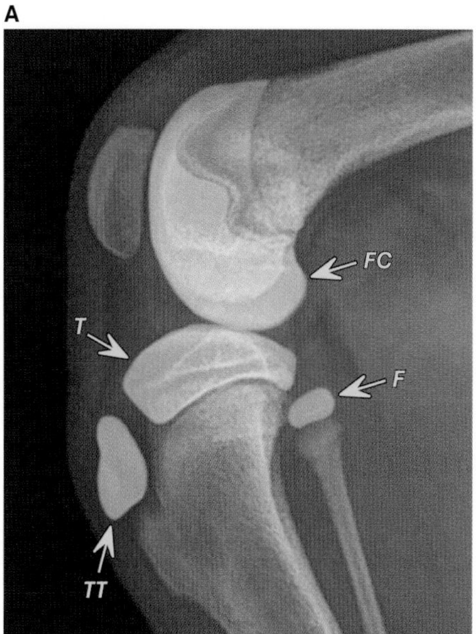

B

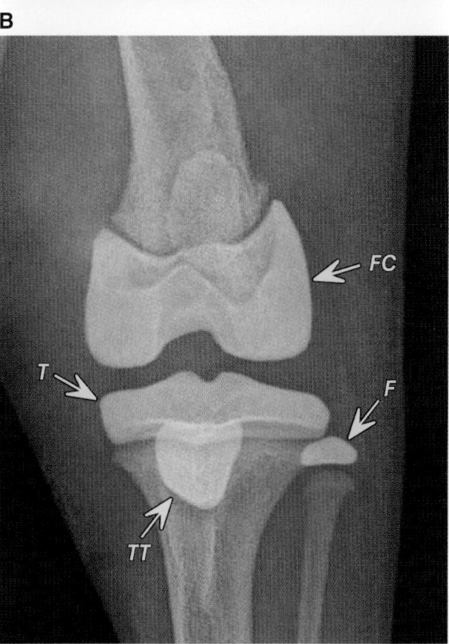

Figure 5.11 Normal stifle epiphyses. Lateral view (**A**) and Caudocranial view (**B**) of an immature dog stifle depicting the femoral condyle (*FC*), tibial plateau (*T*), tibial tuberosity (*TT*), and fibular head (*F*).

When you see a periosteal response, the first thing to determine is whether it is **active** or **inactive**. If it is active, you must deal with the bone disease now. If it is inactive, you can observe the lesion to see whether it remains inactive (i.e., a benign process). It is important to make sure an apparently benign lesion remains inactive before abandoning diagnostics or treatment. To determine whether new bone production is active or inactive, look at its margin. **The less distinct the margin, the more active the periosteal**

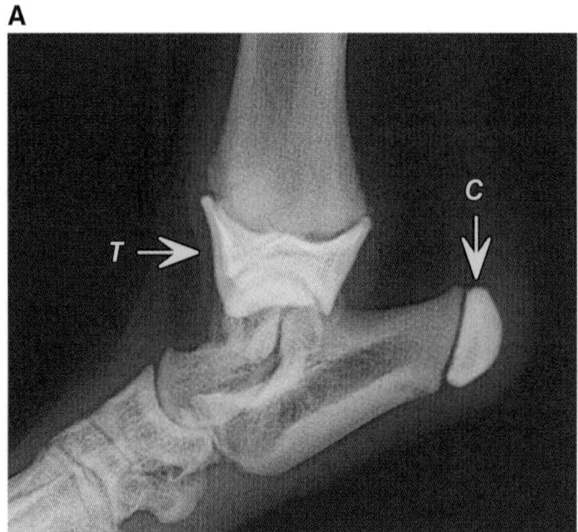

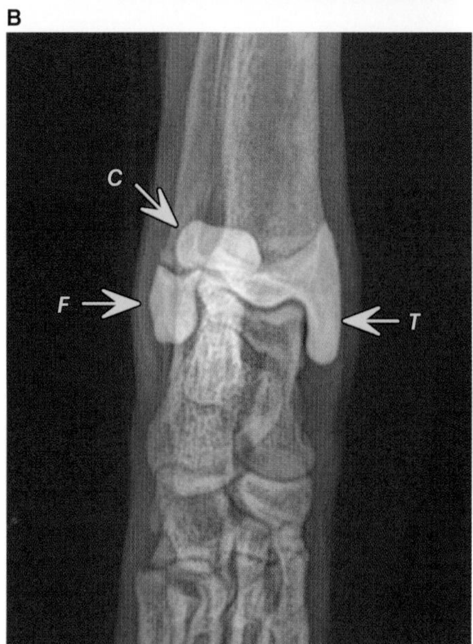

Figure 5.12 Normal tarsal epiphyses. Lateral view (**A**) and dorsoplantar view (**B**) of an immature dog tarsus depicting the distal fibular epiphysis (*F*, also called the lateral malleolus), the distal tibial epiphysis (*T*, also called the medial malleolus), and the calcaneal tuberosity (*C*, also called the tuber calcis).

response. The simplest way to evaluate a bony margin is to trace it with an imaginary pencil or stylus. If it is easy to draw a line along the edge of the new bone, it is well-defined and not very active. The more difficult it is to trace the margin, the more active the disease process.

Active disease processes continue to push the periosteum away from the cortex. The subperiosteal space may fill with blood, tumor cells, edema, or purulent material, any of which will prevent complete mineralization of the subperiosteal space. As long as the disease process is active, the edges of the new bone being produced will remain indistinct. A well-defined margin can only be established once the disease process has stopped and there is time for mineral deposits to fill the space. The better defined the margin, the less active the process.

It is essential to realize that **the definition or sharpness of the new bone margin has nothing to do with its size or shape**. New bone with an "irregular" border does not mean the margin is ill-defined, and new bone with a "smooth" border does not mean the margin is well-defined. Some periosteal responses are quite extensive, producing large amounts of new bone with irregular or uneven borders, but this does not tell us whether the disease is active or inactive. It may give us some idea about the severity of the bone damage, but we must evaluate the margin to determine whether further diagnostics or treatment are immediately needed.

The aggressiveness of a bone lesion is reflected by the degree of osteolysis. Osteolysis is the pathologic destruction of bone. The less distinct the margin around an area of osteolysis, the more aggressive the disease process. In addition to tracing the margin to determine its sharpness, look at the **zone of transition** between the abnormal bone and bone that appears normal. The longer and less defined the zone between abnormal and normal, the more aggressive the disease process.

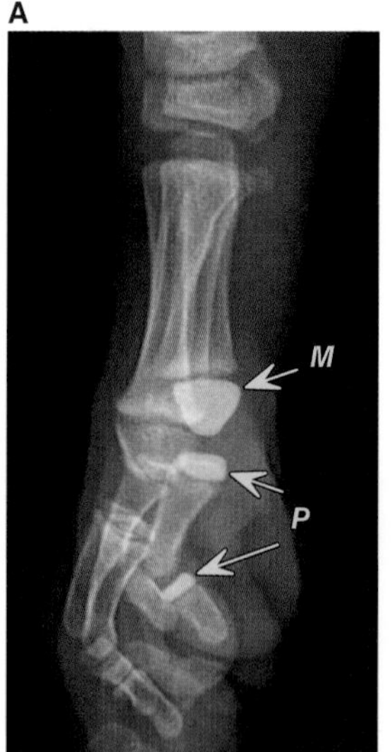

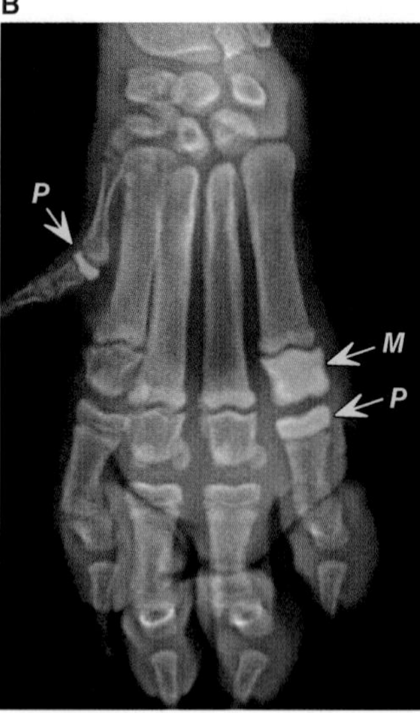

Figure 5.13 Normal digit epiphyses. Lateral view (**A**) of an immature dog pes and dorsopalmar view (**B**) of an immature dog manus. Depicted are the epiphyses in the metatarsal/metacarpal bones (*M*) and in the phalanges (*P*). Notice that there are only distal metacarpal and metatarsal epiphyses and only proximal phalangeal epiphyses. In the DP view, the first digit phalangeal epiphysis is labeled.

The aggressiveness of a bone lesion is also assessed by its **rate of change in serial radiographs**. The more rapid the change, the more aggressive the disease. Very aggressive bone diseases can produce visible osteolysis in 5–7 days. Bone production, however, usually takes at least 7 to 10 days to become visible in a radiograph, regardless of the cause of the periosteal response. Occasionally, periosteal new bone production is visible in less than 7 days in a young, rapidly growing animal. Note: a periosteal response does not tell us how aggressive the disease is, only how active.

The radiographic appearance of periosteal new bone also tells us something about its chronicity. New bone production initially is more opaque near the displaced periosteum because this is where it is being formed. As healing progresses and more mineral is deposited, the new bone increases in opacity and becomes more homogeneous. New bone gradually matures over the following weeks, becoming more organized and trabeculated. During the following months and years, normal stresses gradually remodel the bone until it eventually resembles the original size and shape. The change from unorganized mineral deposits to organized bone reveals the chronicity of the lesion. Knowing how long a lesion has been present is valuable for patient management and may provide clues to its etiology. With many bone diseases, it is a race between the pathologic process and the healing response. Serial radiographs help monitor the progression of disease and the patient's response to therapy.

Patterns of bone remodeling

Patterns of bone production and bone destruction have been used over the years in an attempt to narrow the list of differential diagnoses. Most patterns, however, are not diagnostic of any specific disease. Patterns sometimes are helpful to describe radiographic findings, and some of the classic patterns are discussed on the following pages. However, any aggressive disease process, regardless of etiology (e.g., malignant tumor, bacterial infection, severe trauma) can produce radiographic signs of aggressive bone disease. Likewise, any benign disease process, regardless of etiology (e.g., bone bruise, bone cyst, tumor) can produce radiographic signs of benign bone disease.

The value of radiography is to help determine the activity, aggressiveness, chronicity, and extent of bone disease. Bone lesions may be solitary or multifocal, monostotic or polyostotic, and may arise in the diaphyseal, metaphyseal, or epiphyseal region of a bone. It is important to remember that radiographs are snapshots in time. They depict the appearance of a lesion only at the moment the images were made. Serial radiographs often are needed to determine the true nature of a disease process. In addition, some diseases may be obscured by a pre-existing condition, such as degenerative joint disease masking a tumor.

Table 5.2 Stages of periosteal response

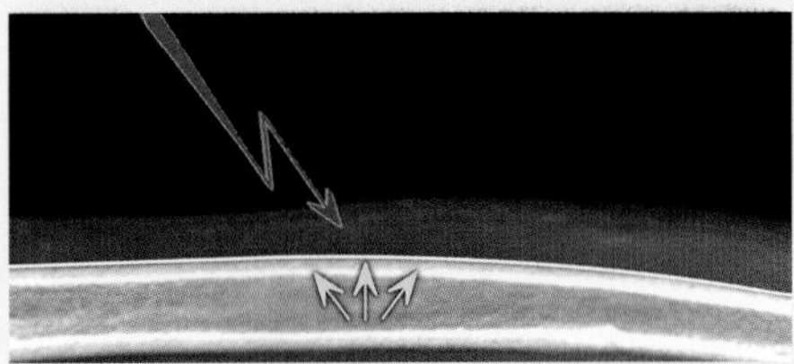

1. Bone disease results in separation of the periosteum from the cortex.

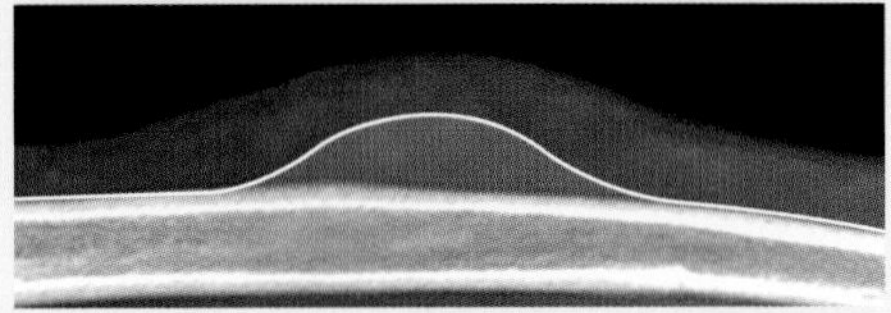

2. The periosteum is elevated due to subperiosteal accumulation of fluid or cells. Soft tissue swelling is present.

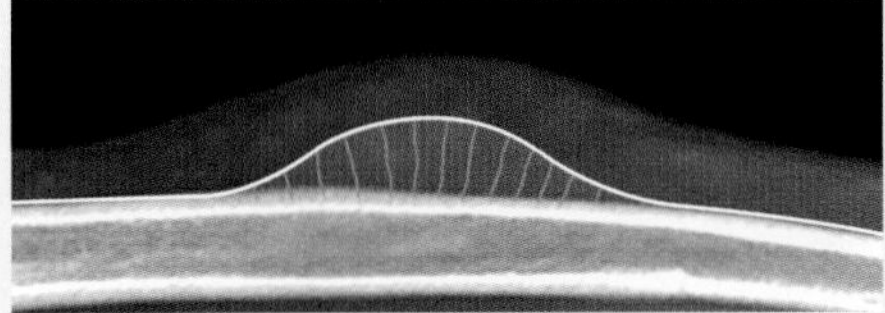

3. The elevated periosteum is connected to the underlying cortex by Sharpy's fibers and blood vessels, which extend perpendicular from the periosteum to the cortex.

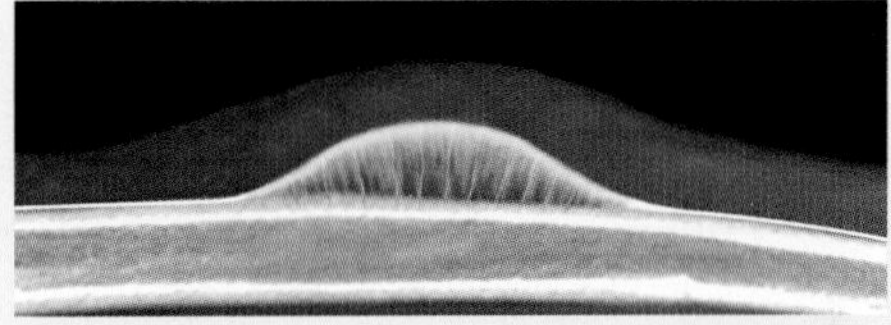

4. The cambium layer produces mineral to fill the subperiosteal space. The mineral is laid down along the perpendicular fibers and vessels from the periosteum to the cortex.

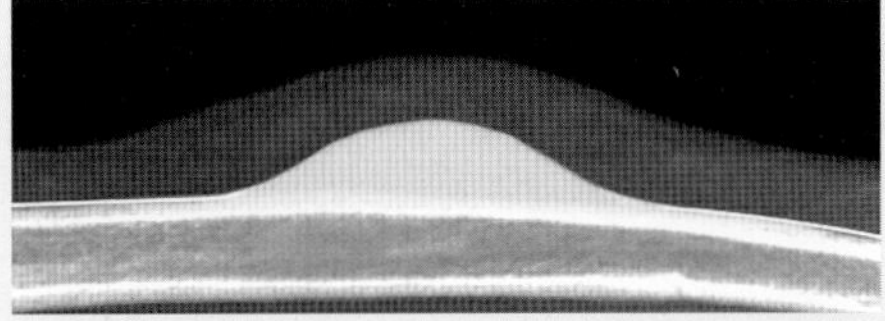

5. Mineral deposits continue until the subperiosteal space is completely filled.

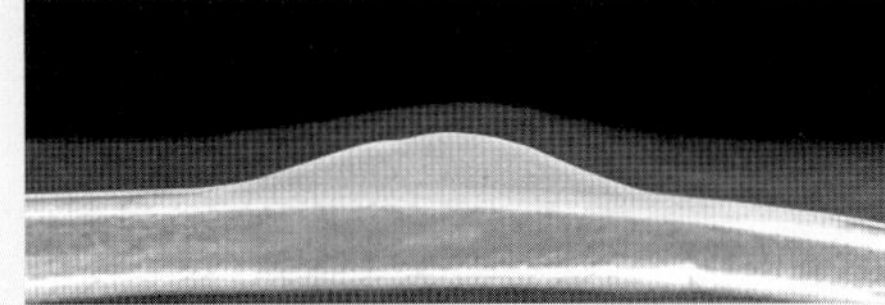

6. Mineral gradually matures into organized bone with a well-defined margin. Over time, normal stresses remodel the new bone until it gradually returns to original shape.

Patterns of periosteal response

Patterns of bone production tend to emphasize the shape of the new bone rather than its margination. Remember, the shape is not the same as the margination. In all of the patterns discussed below, the margins of the new bone may be well-defined or ill-defined, depending on how active the disease process was at the time of radiography. Note: it is the bony margin at the edge of the periosteal response, away from the underlying cortex, that must be evaluated to determine lesion activity. Lesion aggressiveness (i.e., osteolysis) is determined by evaluating the cortex and underlying bone.

Smooth bordered new bone production generally occurs when the periosteum was not separated very far from the cortex. This may occur with a slow-growing disease process or early in the course of a more aggressive disease. When the periosteum is only mildly elevated from the cortex, mineral can quickly fill the subperiosteal space to produce new bone with a smooth, even border. Again, the margin may be well-defined or ill-defined, depending on the activity of the disease process. **Uneven or irregular**-shaped new bone production occurs when at some point, the periosteum was separated a considerable distance from the cortex (Figure 5.14).

Multilayered new bone production occurs with diseases that grow intermittently, each time elevating the periosteum. New bone is produced in layers between growth episodes of the disease. The radiographic appearance has been described as *lamellar, laminated,* or *onion skin*. The shape of the new bone tends to be even and smooth-bordered (Figure 5.15). Again, the margin of the outer-most layer may be well-defined or ill-defined, depending on the current activity of the disease.

Brush border new bone production occurs when the periosteum is elevated along a broad expanse of cortex. Mineralization is perpendicular to the periosteum, creating an appearance which has been described as resembling the bristles of brush or "hairs-standing-on-end" (Figure 5.16). If the separation between the periosteum and the cortex is larger and more chronic, the new bone may be more organized and appear "columnar" or "palisading."

The **sunburst pattern** of new bone production occurs when the periosteum is separated from the cortex in all directions. This typically is caused by a rapidly growing lesion that originates at a single site. Periosteal mineral is produced perpendicular to the elevated and rounded periosteum and extends toward the cortex. The mineralization is not perpendicular to the cortex, rather it appears to radiate from the center of the lesion as numerous bony spicules that resemble a "sunburst" (Figure 5.17). A sunburst periosteal response most often is attributed to neoplasia, but it can occur with severe osteomyelitis or trauma.

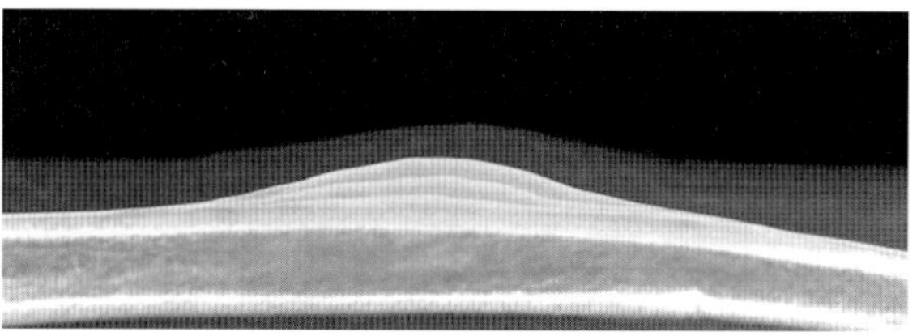

Figure 5.15 Lamellated periosteal response. Lateral view of a section of a long bone depicting layers of periosteal new bone production. The new bone is organized, indicating this is a chronic process. The outer margin is smooth and well-defined, indicating it is currently inactive.

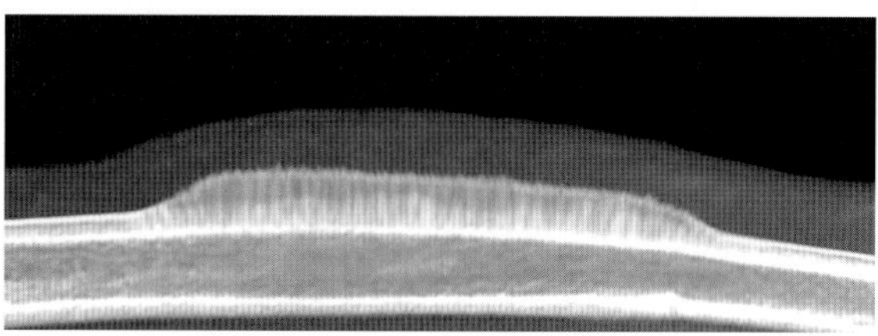

Figure 5.16 Brush border periosteal response. Lateral view of a section of a long bone depicting periosteal new bone that is perpendicular to the periosteum and cortex. The margin is indistinct indicating this is an active bone lesion.

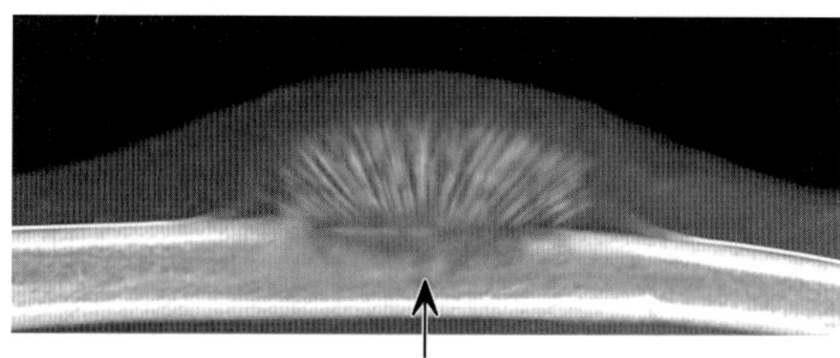

Figure 5.17 Sunburst periosteal response. Lateral view of a section of a long bone depicting spicules of mineralization appearing to radiate from a localized area in the diaphyseal region (arrow). The margins of the periosteal response are hazy and ill-defined and there is cortical destruction, indicating an active and aggressive bone lesion.

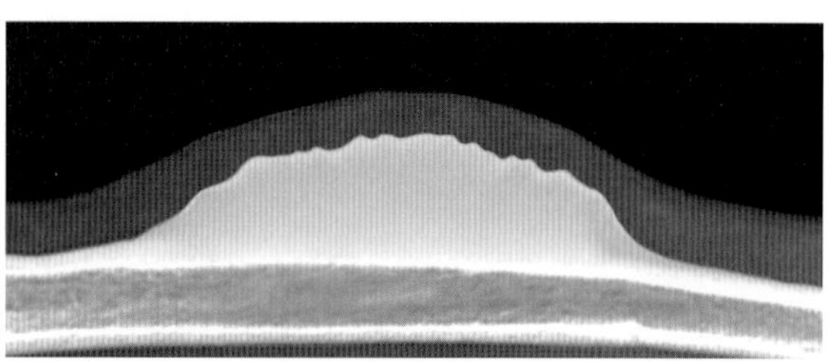

Figure 5.14 Irregular periosteal response. Lateral view of a section of a long bone depicting a large amount of homogeneous new bone production. The periosteum was separated a relatively long distance from the cortex. The new bone margin is irregular, but well-defined, indicating this is an inactive process.

Amorphous new bone production occurs with very rapidly growing disease processes that actually break through the periosteum. In these cases, the elevated periosteum is ruptured and discontinuous. Parts of the periosteum that retain a blood supply produce perpendicular mineralization which appears in radiographs as multiple mineral opacity foci without any form or organization (Figure 5.22). Amorphous new bone tends to develop further away from the cortex than most other periosteal responses. It most often is seen with aggressive tumors or severe trauma.

Codman's triangle is another finding that occurs with very rapidly growing disease processes and frequently is attributed to neoplasia. It is caused by continued growth of the disease that elevates the periosteum again, lifting the newly formed bone away from the cortex. Codman's triangle appears as a small, well-defined, wedge-shaped area of mineralization at the periphery of the lesion (Figure 5.18). The triangular-shaped mineralization may be separated from the cortex by soft tissue opacity material (e.g., fluid, cells) or the mineralization may extend to the cortex. Because the margin associated with Codman's triangle is well-defined, the disease process may be erroneously diagnosed as inactive. But the triangle occurs at the periphery of the actual lesion and does not represent the true character of the disease.

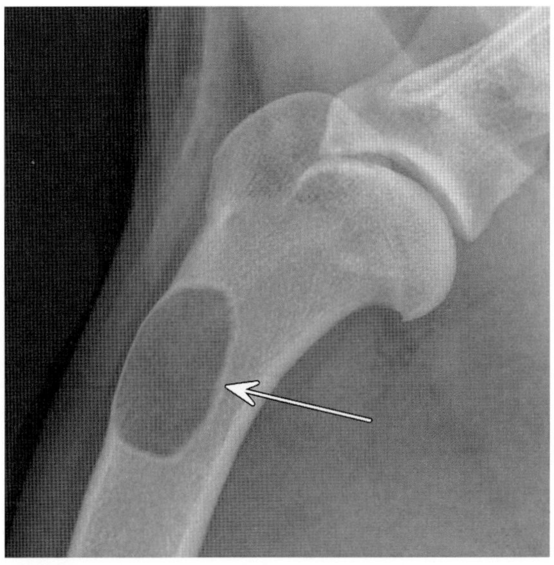

Figure 5.19 Geographic osteolysis. Lateral view of a dog shoulder depicting a large, solitary area of osteolysis in the proximal diaphyseal region of the humerus (arrow). The margins are well-defined with a short zone of transition between abnormal and normal bone. A thin rim of osteosclerosis surrounds the lesion. The adjacent cortex is thinned and expanded outward, but remains intact. There is no soft tissue swelling. This is a benign lesion, possibly a bone cyst.

Patterns of osteolysis

Patterns of bone destruction generally emphasize the sizes of the contiguous osteolytic lesions. However, it is the sharpness of the margins that is the key to determine aggressiveness. There are three classic patterns of osteolysis. From least aggressive to most aggressive, they are: *geographic, moth-eaten,* and *permeative*. In many bone lesions, there is more than one pattern present. The most aggressive pattern determines the true nature of the disease process.

A **geographic** pattern of osteolysis refers to a larger area of bone loss, over 10 mm in size (Figure 5.19). It often is caused by a benign condition but can result from aggressive disease. Benign is differentiated from aggressive by the sharpness of the margin and the zone of transition between abnormal and normal bone. A well-defined osteolytic margin suggests a slow-growing lesion (e.g., bone cyst, benign tumor, pressure remodeling). In these cases, the area of bone loss may be surrounded by osteosclerosis, indicating that the body actually is "reacting" to the disease. A slow-growing lesion may cause thinning or outward expansion of the adjacent cortex, but rarely will the cortex be disrupted. Geographic osteolysis with an ill-defined margin and a longer zone of transition generally results from the coalescence of moth-eaten and permeative osteolysis.

A **moth-eaten** pattern of osteolysis appears as multiple smaller areas of bone loss, each about 3–10 mm in size. The margins usually are indistinct with a longer zone of transition from abnormal bone to normal bone (Figure 5.20). A moth-eaten pattern tends to occur with more aggressive disease processes (e.g., neoplasia, osteomyelitis). The adjacent cortex may be thin and irregular in shape, sometimes with a disrupted border.

A **permeative** pattern of osteolysis appears as numerous, tiny areas of bone loss, 1–2 mm in size, with no clear distinction between normal and abnormal bone (Figure 5.21). These pinpoint lesions are caused by a very aggressive disease process (e.g., malignant neoplasia, severe osteomyelitis).

A

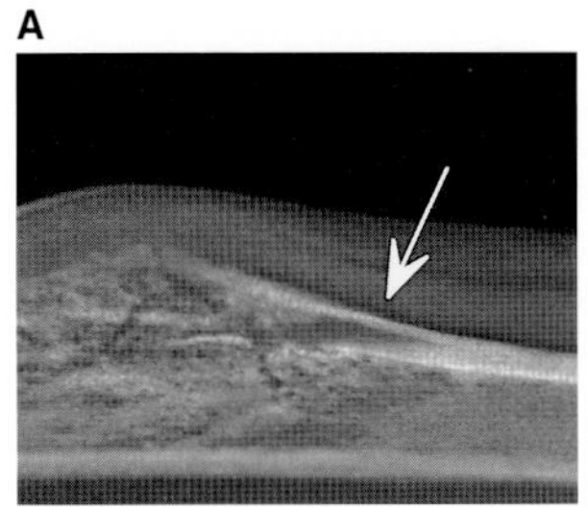

B

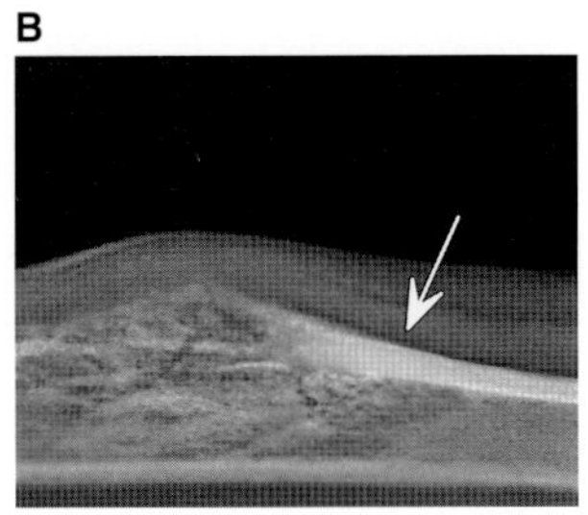

Figure 5.18 Codman's triangle. Lateral views of a section of a long bone depicting an aggressive lesion. Codman's triangle is visible at the periphery of the lesion (arrows) and may appear as elevated mineralization with soft tissue opacity underneath, as shown in **A**, or as mineralization that extends to the cortex, as shown in **B**.

They may be difficult to detect until a larger area of osteolysis has developed. The adjacent cortex often is thin and less distinct, or it may not be visible at all due to severe disruption by the disease.

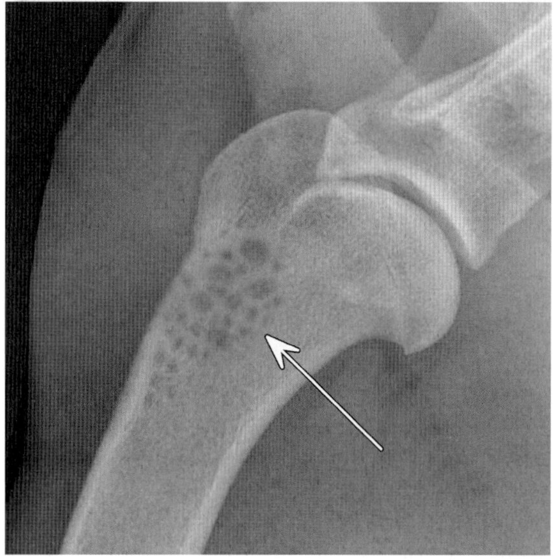

Figure 5.20 Moth-eaten osteolysis. Lateral view of a dog shoulder depicting multiple small areas of osteolysis in the metaphyseal region of the humerus (arrow). The margins are indistinct, and the adjacent cortex is thin and less opaque. There are soft tissues swelling. This is an aggressive lesion, possibly due to neoplasia or osteomyelitis.

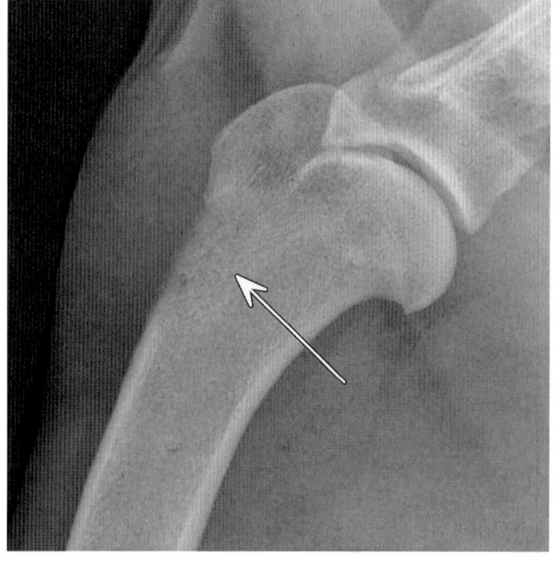

Figure 5.21 Permeative osteolysis. Lateral view of a dog shoulder depicting numerous, tiny foci of osteolysis in the proximal humerus (arrow). These foci are difficult to distinguish from normal bone until they coalesce to become larger osteolytic areas. The adjacent cortex is indistinct and diminished in opacity. The adjacent soft tissues are swollen. This is a very aggressive bone lesion due to malignant neoplasia or severe osteomyelitis.

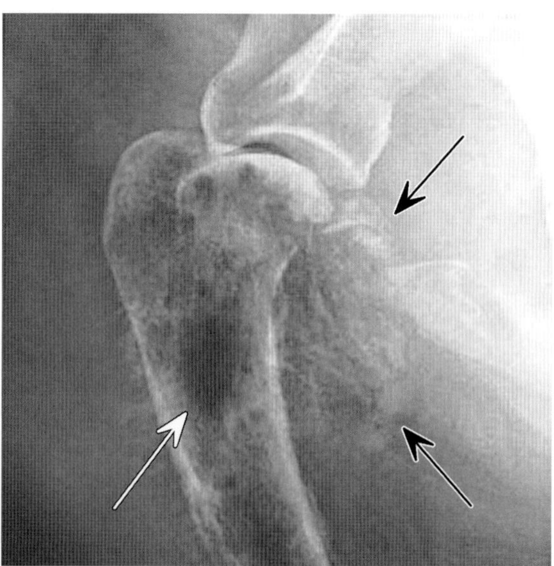

Figure 5.22 Mixed pattern of osteolysis and periosteal response. Lateral view of a dog shoulder depicting an active and aggressive bone disease in the humerus. Periosteal new bone production is amorphous and ill-defined (black arrows). There is a mixed pattern of osteolysis, including permeative, moth-eaten, and geographic areas of bone loss (white arrow) and extensive cortical destruction. This is a very aggressive disease process, most likely a malignant bone tumor or possibly severe osteomyelitis.

Mixed patterns of osteolysis are common, especially with aggressive diseases (Figure 5.22). In many cases, osteolysis is a continuum of patterns, with permeative progressing to moth-eaten and then to geographic bone loss. In the race between pathology and healing, one pattern may change to another as the disease process waxes and wanes over time. As long as the disease remains unchecked, bone destruction will continue, and margins will remain ill-defined with a longer zone of transition.

Bone production

The formation of new bone may be associated with growth, healing, or metabolic disease. In radiographs, new bone production appears as increased opacity. Bone growth and development have been discussed. Bone healing generally involves a periosteal response, which also has been discussed. It is worth mentioning that bone healing includes an **endosteal response**, which is similar to a periosteal response but occurs along the inner surface of the cortex. Endosteal bone production tends to be less evident in radiographs than periosteal bone production.

A frequently encountered type of bone production is an **exostosis**. An exostosis is any abnormal mineralized structure that extends outward from the surface of a bone. The term is not specific to any condition or disease; however, exostoses are important to recognize, and they must be differentiated from normal prominences. The most common exostoses are osteophytes and enthesophytes, which are discussed in greater detail with joint disease.

Osteosclerosis is new bone production within the bony matrix. It leads to thicker trabeculae and smaller spaces between them, both of which increase bone opacity (Figure 5.23). Osteosclerosis is caused by an increase in mineral deposit, a reduction in the resorption of mineral, or both. It may be a localized attempt to heal a lesion, as the body tries to wall-off or repair the damaged part of the bone, or it may be diffuse due to abnormal bone metabolism (i.e., osteopetrosis). In radiographs, localized osteosclerosis may appear as a rim of increased opacity adjacent to a bone lesion. It sometimes is seen in subchondral bone near a damaged joint. The presence of osteosclerosis can help differentiate osteomyelitis from osseous neoplasia because the body is much more likely to wall off an infectious agent than a tumor. Histopathology, however, usually is necessary for definitive diagnosis.

Osteopetrosis is a form of osteosclerosis that affects the entire skeleton. It results from decreased resorption of bone due to abnormal osteoclastic activity. In radiographs, the bones are relatively normal in length and profile but increased in opacity. The appearance has been described as "ivory," "marble," or "chalky" bones (Figure 5.24). The cortices are thickened and the medullary cavities are narrowed. The corticomedullary contrast is less distinct. In cancellous bone, the trabeculae become thickened and the spaces obscured by the increased mineral. Osteopetrosis is a rare congenital disease in dogs and cats. It results in brittle bones that lead to pathologic fractures and it causes anemia due to reduced bone marrow function.

Lead poisoning in young animals can produce thin, transverse lines of osteosclerosis in the metaphyseal regions of long bones. The lines form parallel to the physes and most often are seen in the distal radius and ulna. They also have been reported in the vertebrae. Chronic lead poisoning (*plumbism*) can lead to osteopenia.

Growth arrest lines are thin, transverse lines of osteosclerosis in the diaphyseal regions of long bones (Figure 5.25). They are caused by changes in the rate of growth in an immature bone, which may result from a systemic illness, dietary change, or other stressor. The lines are sharply-defined and seen most often in the femurs, usually bilaterally. There is no soft tissue swelling, periosteal response, or evidence of active bone remodeling. The importance of growth arrest lines is their potential to mimic pathology, such as a fracture, bone infarct, or panosteitis.

Bone infarcts appear in radiographs as distinct foci of osteosclerosis that are irregular in shape with well-defined margins (Figure 5.26). They most often are seen in the medullary region of a long bone, generally distal to the elbow or stifle. Bone infarcts usually are multiple and may be monostotic or polyostotic. They result from a localized loss of blood supply, typically caused by embolic disease (e.g., neoplasia, trauma, vasculitis, recent orthopedic surgery). Most infarcts are asymptomatic.

Bone loss

The loss of mineral from bone may be due to increased resorption, reduced deposition, or active bone destruction. Sometimes it is a combination of these. The term **osteopenia** means "too little bone" and is used to describe diminished

A

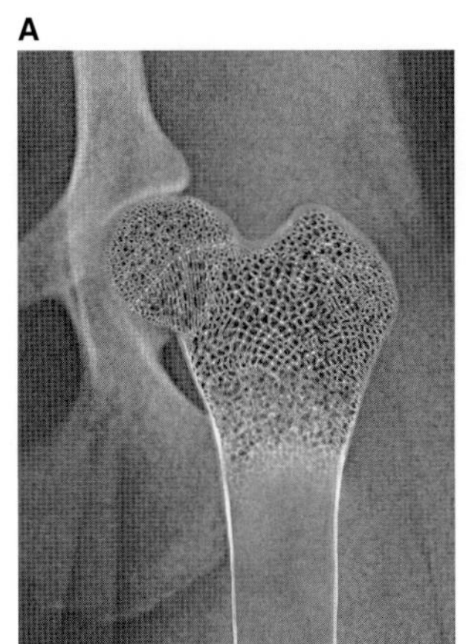

B

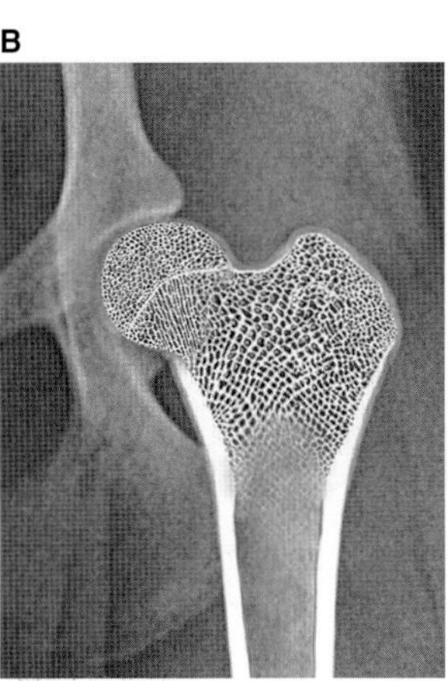

C

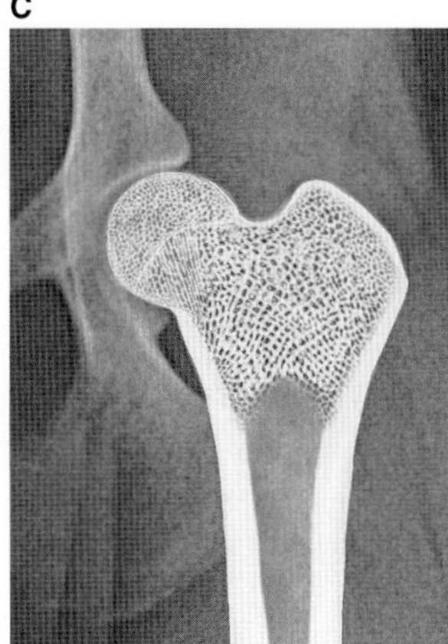

Figure 5.23 Osteoporosis and osteosclerosis. VD views of a dog proximal femur illustrating the appearance of (**A**) osteoporotic bone, (**B**) normal bone, and (**C**) osteosclerotic bone. Osteoporotic bone (**A**) is less opaque than normal with thin trabeculae, larger intertrabecular spaces, thin cortices, and less bone-to-soft tissue contrast. In osteosclerotic bone (**C**), the trabeculae are thicker, the intertrabecular spaces are smaller, the cortices are thickened, and the medullary cavity is smaller.

A

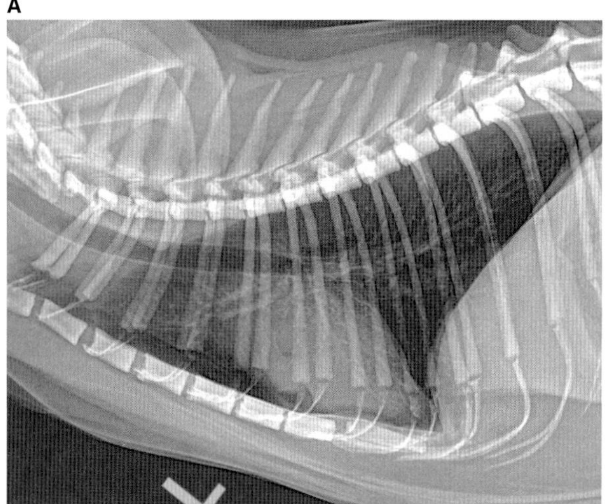

B

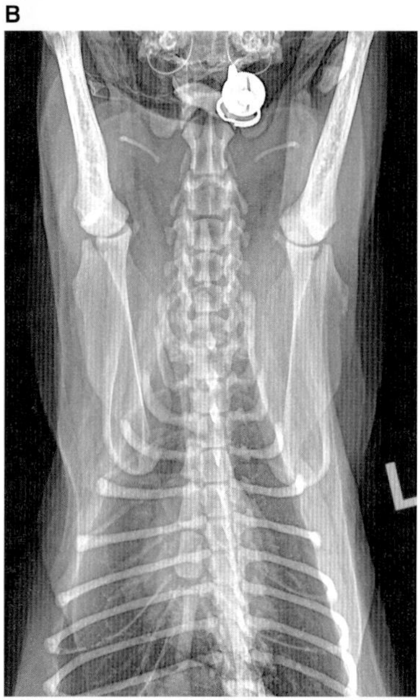

Figure 5.24 Osteopetrosis. Lateral view (**A**) and VD view (**B**) of a cat thorax depicting increased opacity and thickened cortices in the axial and appendicular skeleton (e.g., vertebrae, sternebrae, ribs, humeri).

bone opacity. Osteopenia may result from *osteolysis, osteoporosis,* or *osteomalacia.*

Osteolysis was discussed earlier as it pertains to the aggressiveness of bone lesions. Specifically, it is the pathologic destruction of bone that results in loss of both mineral and matrix. Causes of osteolysis include neoplasia, infection, and pressure necrosis.

Osteoporosis means "porous bone" and refers to the loss of bone mineral due to an imbalance between bone formation and bone resorption. Osteoporosis that affects the entire skeleton and is caused by a systemic disease, such as hyperparathyroidism. Osteoporosis in a single limb is caused by disuse (e.g., immobilization, pain, paralysis). Generalized osteoporosis tends to initially be more evident in the vertebrae, followed by the mandible and then the long bones. Osteoporosis in a single limb initially is more severe in the distal bones (e.g., distal epiphyses, cuboidal bones). Osteoporosis sometimes is called "bone atrophy" and leads

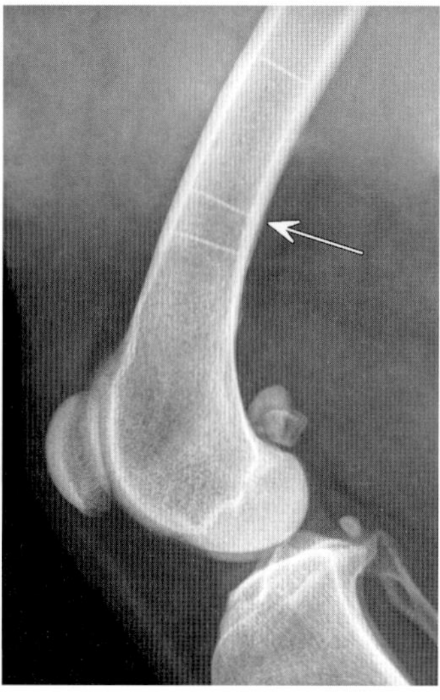

Figure 5.25 Growth arrest lines. Lateral view of a dog stifle depicting several thin, well-defined, transverse lines of osteosclerosis in the femur (arrow). Other names include *stress lines* and *growth retardation lines*.

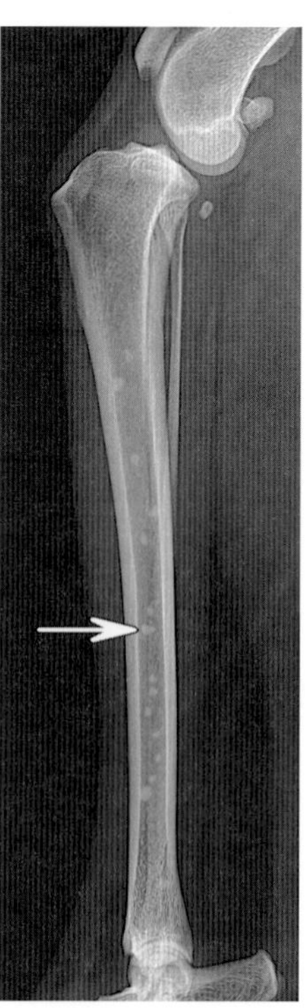

Figure 5.26 Bone infarcts. Lateral view of a dog crus depicting multiple, well-defined foci of mineral opacity in the medullary cavity of the tibia (arrow). The radiograph was made to evaluate a cranial cruciate ligament injury (note the cranial displacement of the tibia in relation to the distal femur) and the infarcts were an incidental finding.

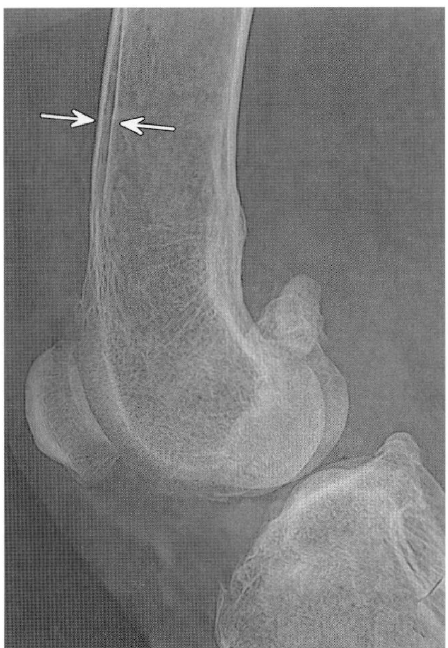

Figure 5.27 Osteopenic bones. Lateral view of a dog stifle depicting disuse osteoporosis. The bone opacity is diminished, the cortices are thin, there is less bone-to-soft tissue contrast, and there is a coarse trabecular pattern. A double cortical line is visible along the cranial border of the femur due to intracortical resorption of bone (arrows).

to thin, weak bones that are prone to pathologic fractures (Figure 5.23).

Osteomalacia means "soft bone" and refers to the loss of bone mineral due to faulty ossification. The most common cause is a dietary deficiency (e.g., Vitamin D, calcium, phosphorous). Osteomalacic bones are soft, but many affected dogs and cats do not exhibit orthopedic signs of disease. In immature animals, osteomalacia is called *rickets*.

Osteoporosis and osteomalacia rarely can be differentiated in radiographs. The term **osteopenia** applies to both. Osteopenic bones are less opaque and there is less contrast between bone and soft tissues (Figure 5.27). The cortices become thin and faint, sometimes developing a "double cortical line" due to intracortical resorption of bone. Cancellous bone becomes more porous in appearance due to the larger spaces and thinner trabeculae, commonly described as a "coarse trabecular pattern." Corticomedullary contrast is diminished.

Fractures

A fracture is a break or a discontinuity in a bone. It is caused by a physical force that exceeds the bone's structural capacity. Fractures are more likely in bone that has been weakened by disease. Soft tissue swelling usually accompanies a fracture, especially in the acute stages, which is helpful to distinguish pathology from normal anatomy or an imaging artifact. Knowledge of sesamoid bones, accessory ossification centers, nutrient foramina, growth plates, and the normal shapes of bones is essential to avoid a misdiagnosis. Nondisplaced fractures may not be evident in initial radiographs but may be detected in a follow-up study when a periosteal response develops or when the fracture line widens during healing or as a result of displacement. The radiographic description of a fracture should include the type of fracture, the parts of the bones involved, the degree of displacement and rotation, whether the fracture is articular, and an assessment of the adjacent soft tissues (Box 5.1).

Box 5.1 Radiographic description of a fracture

1. Type of fracture (e.g., incomplete or complete, simple or complex, closed or open).
2. Name and part of the bone involved (e.g., humeral condyle, femoral neck).
3. Direction and degree of bone fragment displacement (e.g., overriding, angled, mildly displaced). The position of the distal unfixed fragment is described in relation to the proximal fixed segment.
4. Direction of the fracture line:
   a. *Transverse* (90° to the long axis of the bone).
   b. *Short oblique* (45°–90° to the long axis of the bone).
   c. *Long oblique* (0°–45° to the long axis).
   d. *Spiral*: the fracture line wraps around the long axis of the bone; typically caused by a rotational force.
5. Whether or not the fracture is articular.
6. The appearance of the adjacent soft tissues (e.g., swelling, emphysema, tissue defects, presence of foreign material).
7. Radiographs of long bone fractures should include the joints proximal and distal to assess joint involvement and degree of fracture rotation.

Most fracture lines are less opaque than the adjacent bone. The fracture sometimes is more opaque than adjacent bone due to summation of overlying fracture fragments (e.g., compression fracture, folding fracture).

Incomplete fractures are those in which the cortex is broken on only one side and the bone is not in complete discontinuity. When the cortex is broken on the convex side, it is called a *greenstick* or *hairline fracture* (Figure 5.28). If the cortex is broken on the concave side, it is a *folding, torus*, or *buckling* fracture (Figure 5.29). An incomplete fracture in a fracture fragment is called a *fissure* fracture (Figure 5.31), which is important to identify because a fissure can become a complete fracture during reduction and repair. *Stress* or *fatigue* fractures are caused by repetitive cycling injuries that damage the bone at a rate faster than it can heal.

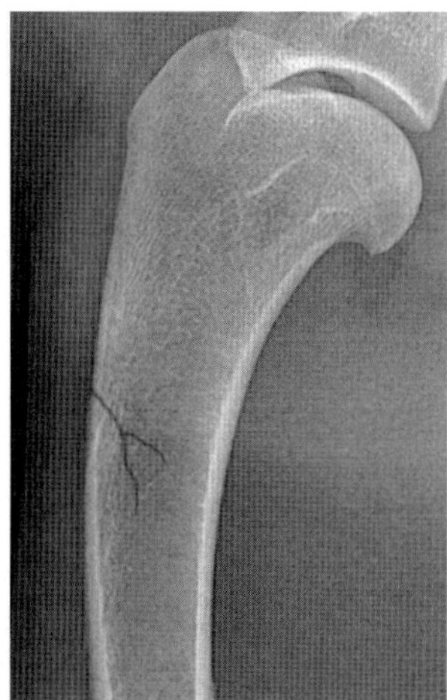

Figure 5.28 Greenstick fracture. Lateral view of a dog proximal humerus depicting an incomplete fracture on the convex side of the bone.

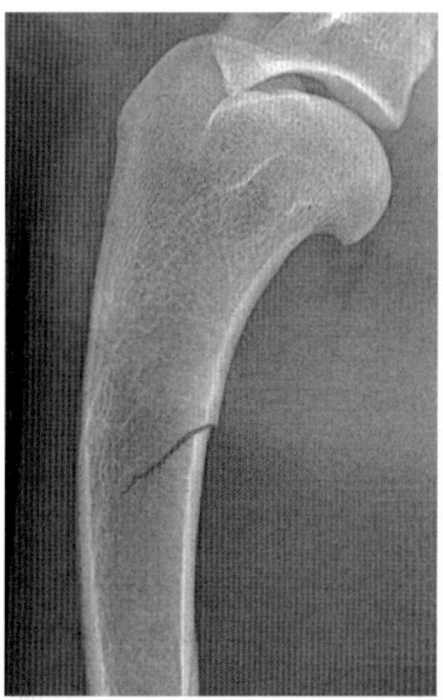

Figure 5.29 Torus fracture. Lateral view of a dog proximal humerus depicting an incomplete fracture on the concave side of the bone.

An incomplete fracture may not be visible in radiographs unless the x-ray beam is aligned with the fracture line.

Complete fractures are those in which the fracture line extends through the entire bone. A **simple** complete fracture consists of one fracture line and two fragments (Figure 5.30). In a **complex** complete fracture, there are multiple, non-continuous fracture lines and more than two fragments (Figure 5.31). The fracture is *comminuted* if all of the fracture lines communicate at a single point. Comminuted fractures consist of three or more fragments. More than five fragments is considered highly comminuted. Fragments that are wedge-shaped commonly are called "butterfly" fragments. In a *segmental* fracture, the fracture lines do not communicate and the result is one or more isolated segments of bone (Figure 5.32).

Fractures in paired long bones sometimes are accompanied by a luxation in the adjacent joint. A **Monteggia fracture**, for example, is a fracture in the proximal 1/3 of the ulna with a concurrent luxation of the radial head. It is important to identify the luxation prior to treating the fracture.

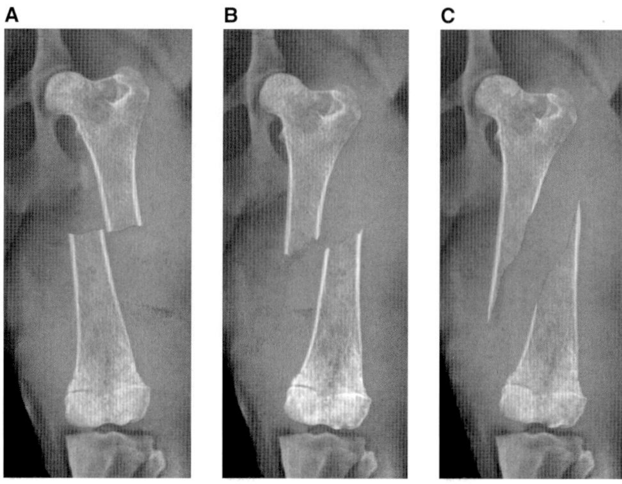

Figure 5.30 Simple complete fractures. Lateral views of a dog femur illustrating mid-diaphyseal fractures that are transverse (**A**), short oblique (**B**), and long oblique (**C**). The soft tissues are swollen.

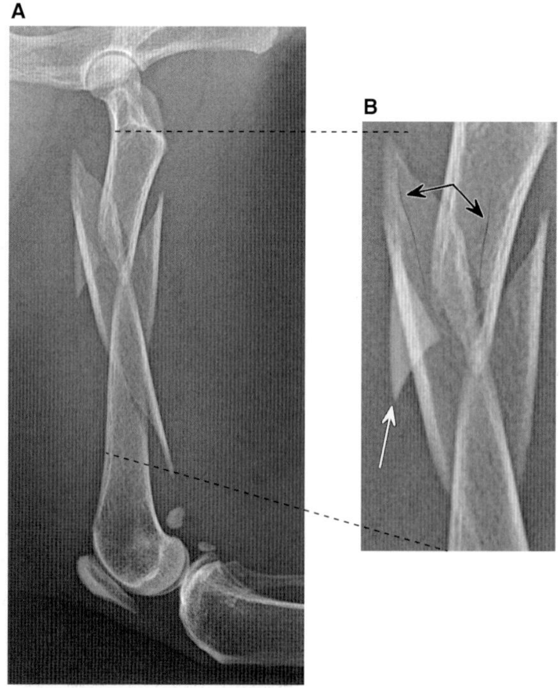

Figure 5.31 Comminuted fracture. **A**. Lateral view of a dog femur depicting a mid-diaphyseal fracture with multiple fragments. **B**. Enlarged image of the fracture in radiograph **A** highlighting a butterfly fragment (white arrow) and fissure fractures in the larger fragments (black arrows).

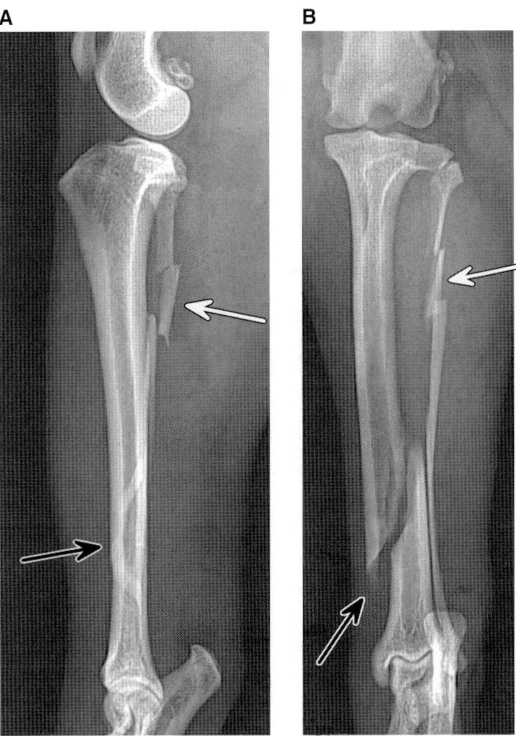

Figure 5.32 Spiral and segmental fractures. Lateral view (**A**) and craniocaudal view (**B**) of a dog crus depicting a spiral oblique fracture in the distal tibial diaphysis (black arrow) and a segmental fracture in the proximal fibular diaphysis (white arrow). In the lateral view, the tibial fracture line is more opaque than the adjacent bone due to summation of the ends of the fragments. Displacement of the fragments is not evident in the lateral view and the fracture may be missed without the orthogonal view.

Closed fractures are those in which the overlying skin and soft tissues are intact. **Open** fractures occur when the overlying tissues are perforated (also called *compound* fractures). Open fractures usually are accompanied by subcutaneous emphysema and are at increased risk for infection (Figure 5.33).

T or Y fractures describe fractures in which the bone splits both longitudinally and transversely (Figure 5.34).

Avulsion fractures occur at attachment sites for ligaments, tendons, or joint capsules. A piece of bone is pulled away from main bone (Figure 5.35). The origin or "bed" of an avulsed fragment may be visible as a similar-sized defect in the main bone.

Compression fractures are those in which the ends of the bone fragments are jammed into each other resulting in a shortened or collapsed bone. The fracture line may or may not be visible in radiographs. When visible, the line may be less opaque or more opaque than the adjacent bone. Compression or *impaction* fractures most often are seen in the vertebral bodies (Figure 5.210) and in the short bones in the carpus or tarsus.

Chip fracture is a descriptive term that means "knocking off a corner." A small fragment is displaced from the main bone. Chip fractures occur most often in a short bone in the carpus or tarsus. They usually are articular. The site of origin or bed for the fracture fragment may or may not be identified.

Slab fracture is a descriptive term that means "knocking off a chunk." As with chip fractures, they occur most often in a short bone in a tarsus or carpus. Slab fractures involve the articular surfaces on both ends of the bone. If the fracture involves only one articular surface, it is a chip fracture.

Shearing fractures are caused by severe friction or a glancing trauma, such as an animal being dragged on pavement. Also called *abrasion* fractures, these are open fractures due to loss of overlying soft tissue.

Pathologic fractures are caused by normal stresses on abnormal bone. They occur in bone that has been weakened by an underlying disease or a developmental defect. Disease may be systemic (e.g., osteoporosis) or localized (e.g., tumor, cyst). In radiographs, the bone opacity at or near the fracture site usually is diminished and a periosteal response may be present, earlier than expected for normal fracture healing (Figure 5.42). Pathologic fractures tend to occur at the periphery of the abnormal part of the bone.

Physeal fractures occur in immature bones. They are classified based on the degree of physeal, metaphyseal, and epiphyseal involvement using the popular method proposed by Salter and Harris (Table 5.3). The Salter–Harris classification ranks physeal fractures according to the increasing probability (from less likely to more likely) of a growth deformity during fracture healing.

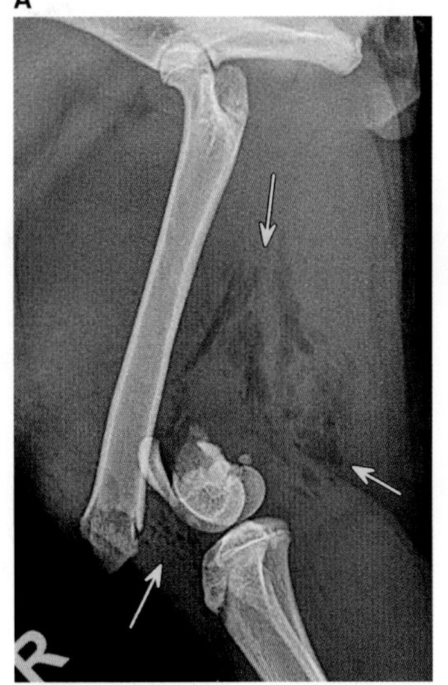

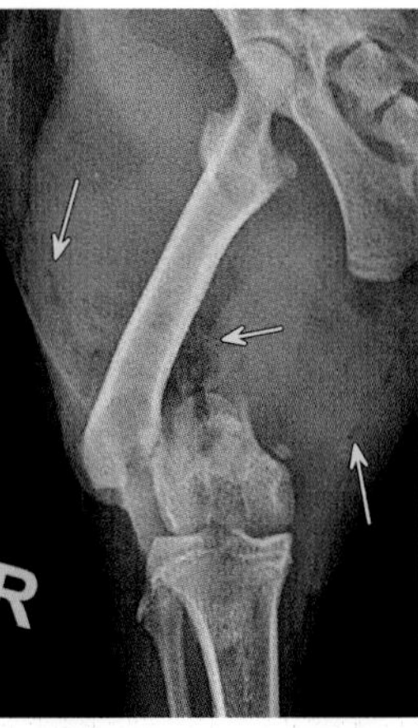

Figure 5.33 Open fracture. Lateral view (**A**) and craniocaudal view (**B**) of an immature cat pelvic limb depicting an open transverse fracture in the right femoral distal physis with caudal and medial displacement and override of the fracture fragments. There is moderate soft tissue swelling at the fracture site and gas in the soft tissues (arrows).

A 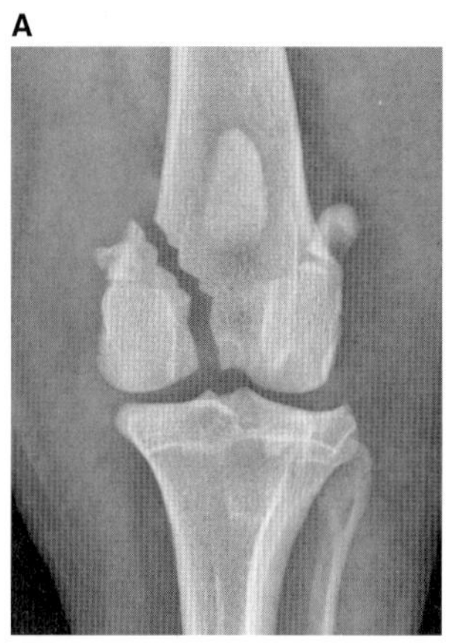

B 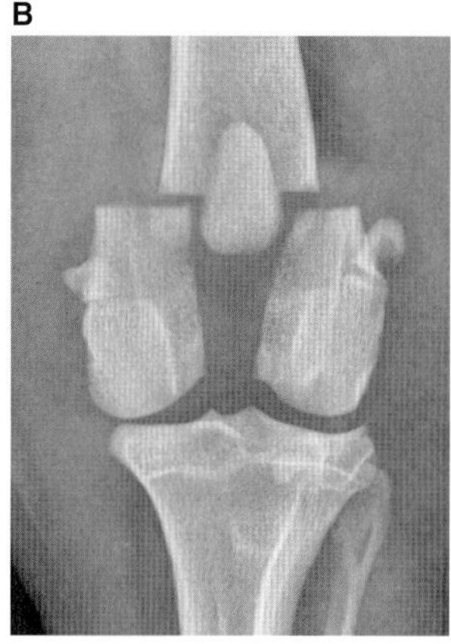

Figure 5.34 Condylar fractures. Craniocaudal views of dog stifles depicting a medial condylar fracture in the femur (**A**) and a "T" or "Y" fracture (**B**) that is both supracondylar and intercondylar.

Fracture healing

Fracture healing may be primary or secondary. **Primary** healing occurs when the fragments are in close apposition and the cortex is reestablished without the formation of a callus. This requires rigid stabilization and excellent anatomic alignment. **Secondary** fracture healing is more common and involves callus formation and subsequent remodeling (Table 5.4).

After a fracture occurs, bleeding from ruptured blood vessels results in a hematoma at the fracture site. The hematoma provides a temporary framework for subsequent healing. Within the framework, granulation tissue develops and a fibrocartilaginous callus forms, bridging the fracture fragments. This callus is soft tissue opacity and not visible in radiographs. It gradually becomes visible as mineral deposits are added from the periosteum and endosteum. The ends of the fracture fragments often become less distinct during early fracture healing due to active bone remodeling. The fracture line initially widens as bone is resorbed and then begins to narrow as bone is produced. As the fracture fills with mineral, it gradually disappears over the next 3–4 weeks. During this time, the callus continues to mineralize, increasing in opacity and making it better defined. Over the next few months, the new bone matures and develops trabeculation. The cortical margins become more distinct and the medullary cavity gradually is reestablished. The bone eventually resembles its normal appearance. Soft tissue swelling and emphysema that were present at the time of injury or introduced during open reduction and stabilization usually resolve during the first 5–10 days, unless there is an infection.

A fracture may be considered radiographically **healed** when the fracture line is no longer visible, the cortex is continuous and uninterrupted, and an ossified callus completely bridges the fracture fragments. Removal of fixation devices may be considered when there is radiographic evidence of a bridging bony callus.

Fracture complications

Multiple factors affect fracture healing, including the blood supply, the alignment and stability of the fracture fragments, and the overall health of the patient.

An adequate blood supply is important to callus formation and periosteal/endosteal bone production. A loss of blood supply may be due to severe tissue damage or removal of the hematoma. Intramedullary implants can disrupt endosteal blood supply and delay healing. Prolonged disuse of a fractured limb can lead to reduced blood flow and delayed healing.

A 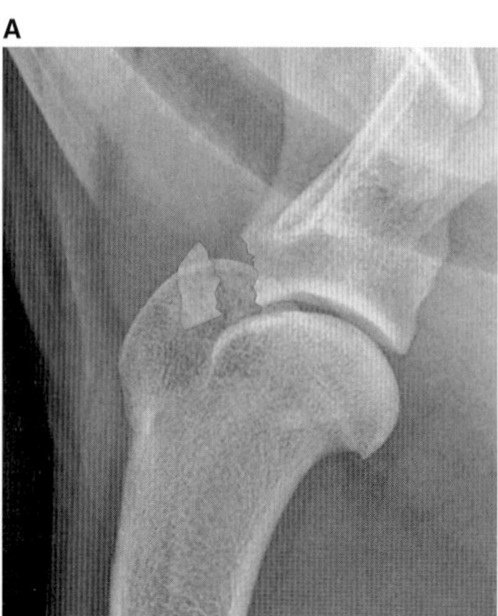

B 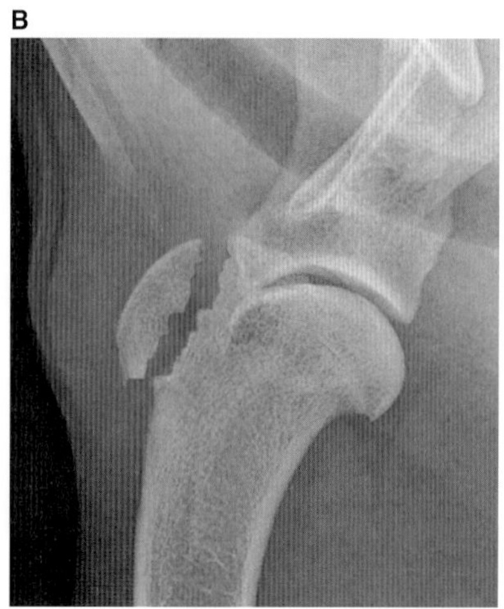

C 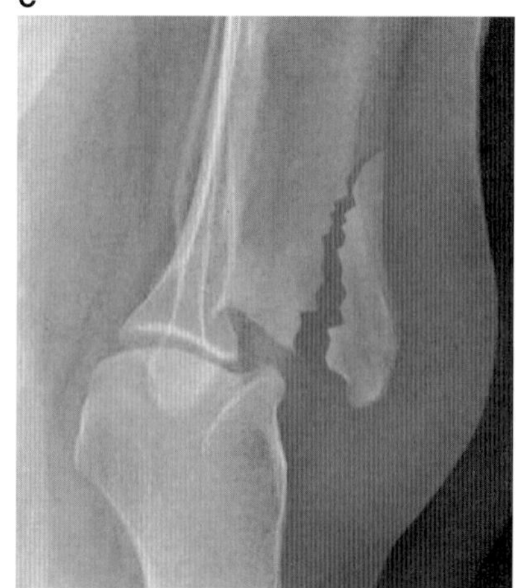

Figure 5.35 Avulsion fractures. **A**. Lateral view of a dog shoulder depicting an avulsion fracture in the scapular tuberosity. **B**. Lateral view of a dog shoulder depicting an avulsion fracture in the humeral greater tubercle with adjacent soft tissue swelling. **C**. Caudocranial view of a dog shoulder depicting an avulsion fracture in the spine of the scapula with adjacent soft tissue swelling.

Table 5.3 Salter–Harris classification of fractures

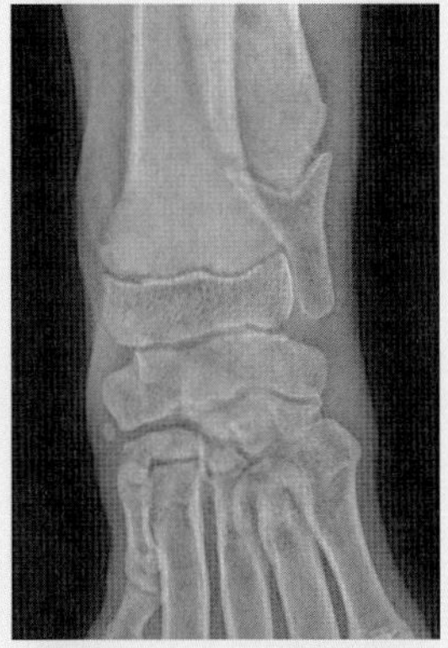 Dorsopalmar view of a normal immature dog carpus for comparison.	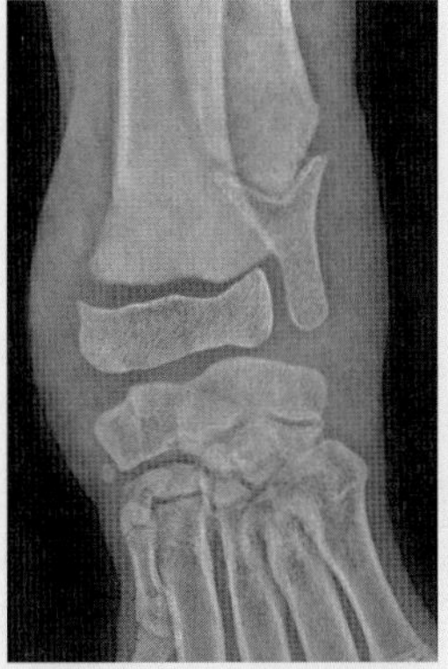 **Type I** physeal fracture involves only the physis; commonly called a "slipped physis."
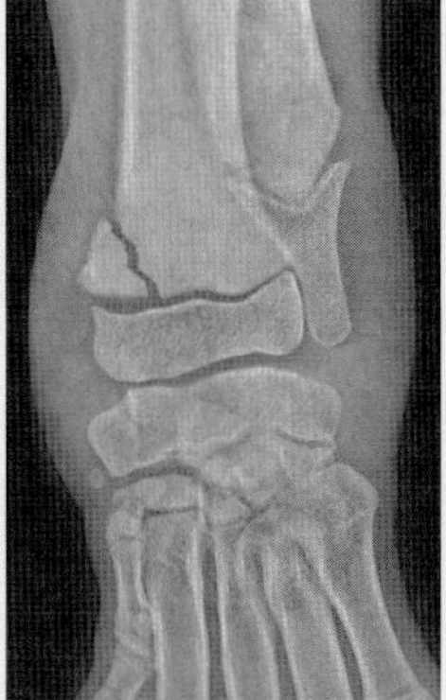 **Type II** physeal fracture involves the physis and the metaphysis.	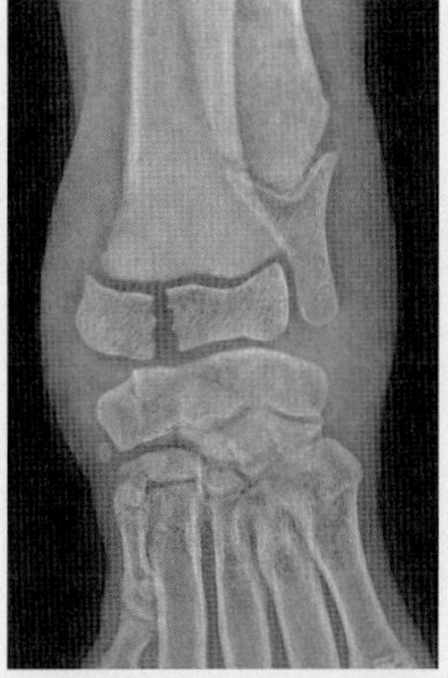 **Type III** physeal fracture involves the physis and the epiphysis; the fracture is articular.
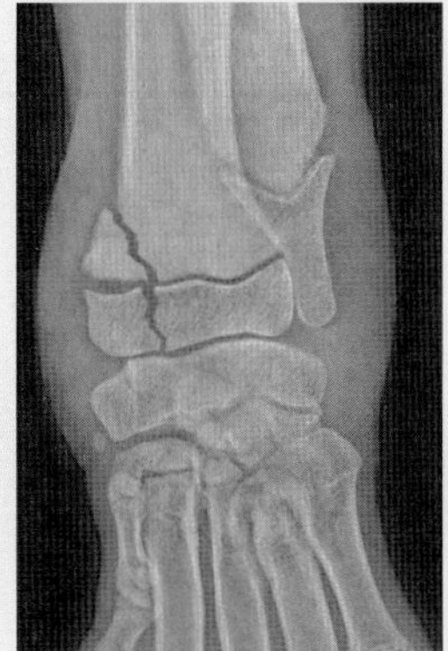 **Type IV** physeal fracture involves the physis, metaphysis, and epiphysis; the fracture is articular.	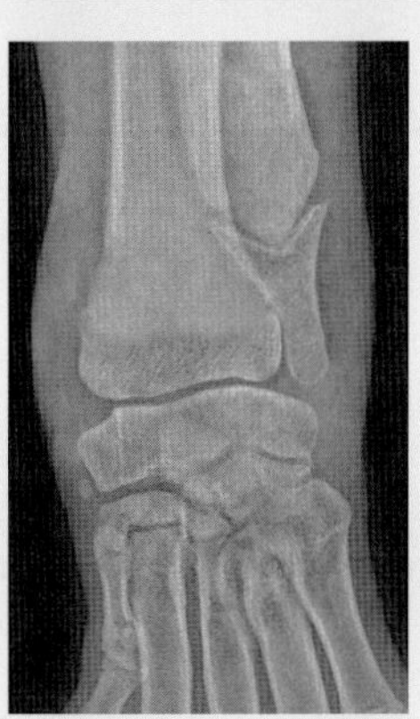 **Type V** physeal fracture is a compression fracture involving the entire physis.
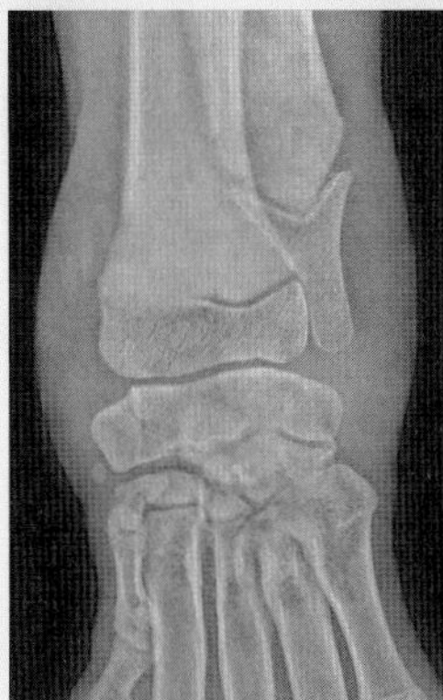 **Type VI** physeal fracture is a compression fracture involving only part of the physis; growth on the damaged side may slow or stop, while the other side grows normally.	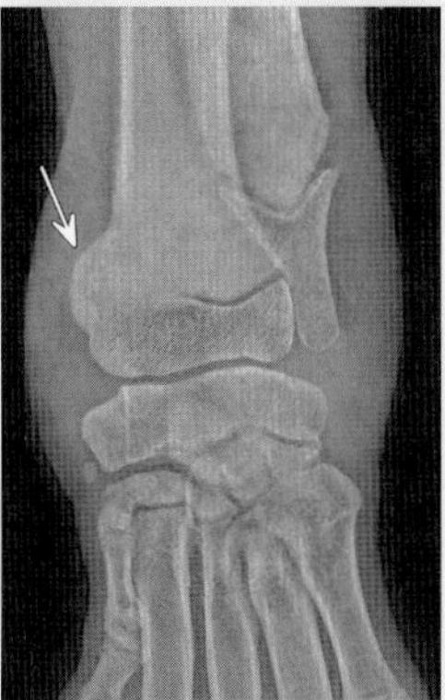 **Bony bridging** on one side of the physis (arrow) can restrict or stop growth on that side, similar to the Type VI physeal fracture described above.

Table 5.4 Stages of unncomplicated fracture healing

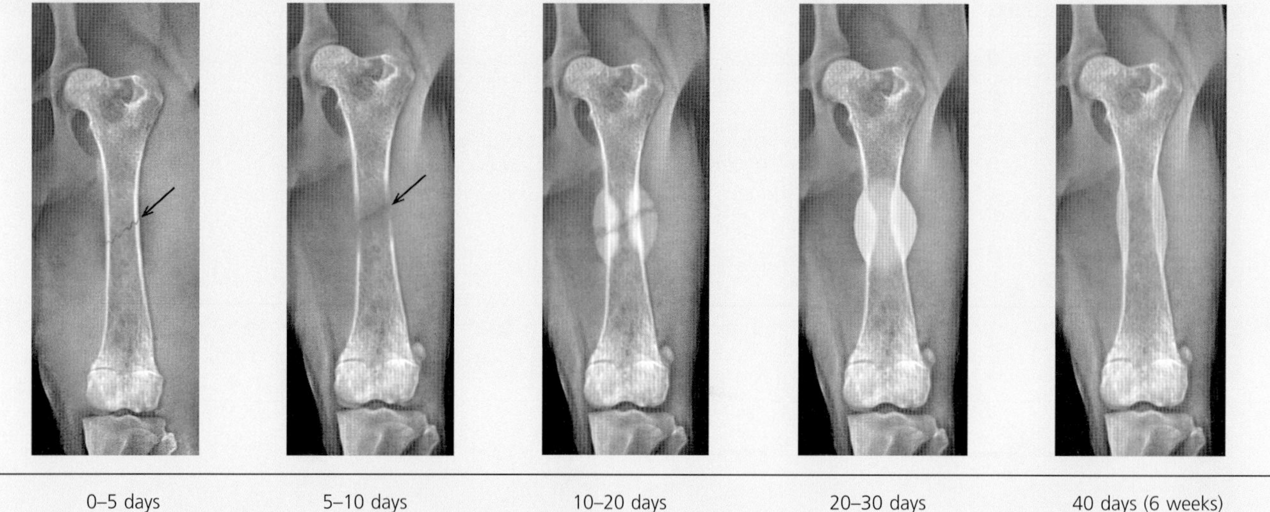

1. **0–5 days**: initial fracture with hemorrhage and soft tissue swelling; a hematoma forms.
2. **5–10 days**: the hematoma organizes into a soft tissue callus; the fracture line widens; the fracture ends are less distinct; soft tissue swelling diminishes.
3. **10–20 days**: mineral deposits from the periosteum and endosteum begin to mineralize the callus; the fracture line begins to narrow, but it is still visible; boney callus does not yet bridge the fracture fragments.
4. **20–30 days**: the fracture line is gradually disappearing; boney callus is more homogeneous and bridges the fracture site; the callus is becoming smoother with more defined margins.
5. **40 days (6 weeks)**: the fracture line is barely visible, if at all; the boney callus is smaller, better-defined, and nearly the opacity of the parent bone.
6. **90 days and more**: (no image) the boney callus matures and develops trabeculation; the medullary cavity is gradually reestablished; the cortical margins become more distinct. Over time, the bone continues to remodel and eventually resembles its original shape.

The apposition of the fracture fragments is important to healing. In general, at least 50% contact between bone fragments is needed for efficient healing. Spiral and oblique fractures tend to heal faster than transverse fractures due to the increased area of contact. The smaller the gap between fragments and the less movement at the fracture site, the quicker the bone will heal. Some bones naturally heal more slowly than others (e.g., distal radius, ulna, tibia).

Delayed union is fracture healing that takes longer than expected, but the bone eventually heals, both clinically and radiographically. Although no definite timetable exists, healing generally is considered delayed if bridging callus is not evident within 6–8 weeks (Figure 5.36).

Nonunion occurs when fracture healing stops before there is complete union. A fracture generally is considered a nonunion when there is no progression of callus formation after 6 months, and no further healing is expected unless intervention occurs. In radiographs, there is no evidence of active bone remodeling for several weeks; the fracture margins remain sharp and well-defined (Figure 5.37).

A **hypertrophic nonunion** results from chronic instability at the fracture site that prevents callus from bridging

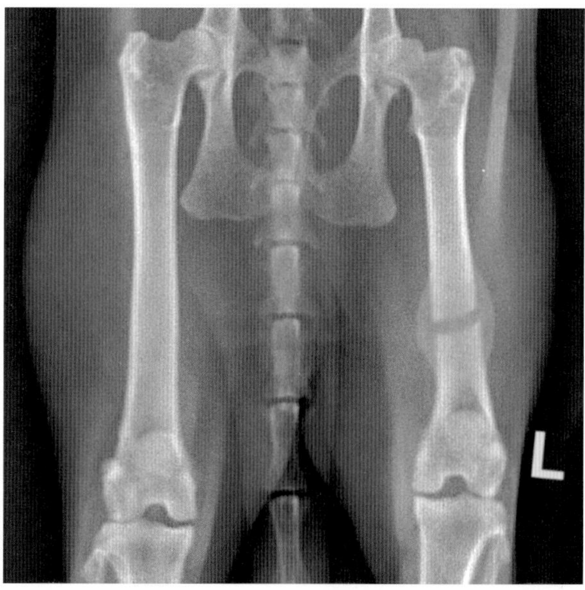

Figure 5.36 Delayed union fracture. VD view of a cat pelvis depicting a delayed union of a left femoral diaphyseal fracture. Callus is visible but less than expected. The fracture line remains distinct.

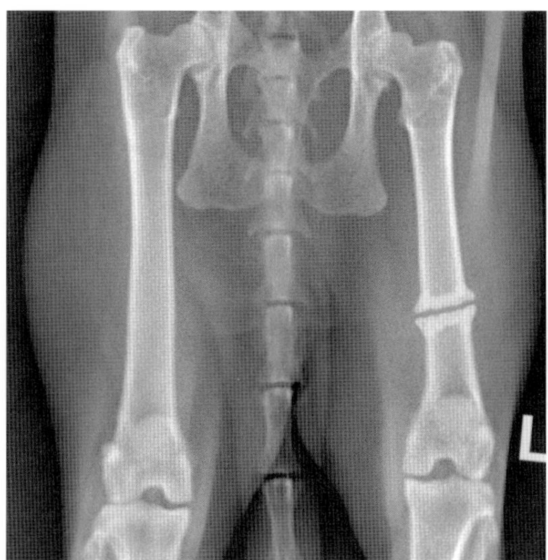

Figure 5.37 Nonunion fracture. VD view of a cat pelvis depicting a nonunion fracture in the left femoral diaphyseal region. A build-up of smooth, well-defined new bone is visible at each fragment end, but the new bone does not bridge the fracture gap. Fracture healing has ceased, bony margins are well-defined.

the fragments. Organized but inactive new bone builds up at the ends of the fracture fragments. The new bone tends to flair out from the cortical ends. In some cases, the ends of the fragments appear to "fit together" because of motion (e.g., one end becomes convex and the other concave) but there is a gap separating the fragments.

An **atrophic nonunion** occurs when the fracture fragments are chronically separated. There is no callus formation. The ends of the fragments appear thin and tapered due to bone resorption. Atrophic nonunions occur more often in small breed dogs and usually are accompanied by disuse osteopenia in the affected limb.

A **dystrophic nonunion** is caused by loss of blood supply to one or both fragments. The end of the affected fragment remains sharp, well-defined, and pointed due to a lack of bone remodeling. If the blood supply is only diminished and not completely lost, some remodeling may occur and the fracture ends may appear more rounded and sclerotic (called a *nonviable* nonunion). Complete loss of blood supply is called a *necrotic* nonunion.

Malunion fractures are those that are healed but with abnormal bone geometry (Figure 5.38). Abnormal geometry can lead to increased stress at the proximal or/and distal joint and may impair limb function. The healed bone fragments may be angled, rotated, shortened, or otherwise malaligned. Comparison radiographs of the contralateral limb may be useful to assess the degree of limb deformity.

A **sequestrum** is a fragment of bone that is no longer viable due to loss of its blood supply. It appears as a sharply-defined, sclerotic piece of bone that is not incorporated in the callus and exhibits little or no remodeling (Figure 5.39). A sequestrum may be located within its bone of origin or separate from it. Fragments that remain in the bone sometimes are located in a *lacuna*, which is a pocket of necrotic soft tissue. The lacuna often is surrounded by a rim of sclerotic bone called an **involucrum**. In some cases, a draining tract extends from the involucrum to the skin surface where it opens as a *cloaca*. The tract may be demonstrated in radiographs using fistulography (Figure 2.96). Sequestra are more likely to occur as a complication of osteomyelitis or in a necrotic nonunion, and rarely with neoplasia (i.e., osteosarcoma).

A **pseudoarthrosis** or "false joint" sometimes develops at a nonunion fracture site. It occurs when the fibrocartilage between the fracture fragments forms into a capsule that fills with serum. The pseudoarthrosis may allow the patient some use of the limb.

Occasionally a bone fragment will fuse to an adjacent bone. This is called a synostosis and can result in loss of movement.

Physeal injuries and limb deformities

Any physis in any bone can be injured and may lead to a growth deformity in the bone. The degree of the deformity depends on the age of the animal at the time of injury, which physis was affected, and the severity of the damage. Physeal injuries that lead to limb deformities may be unilateral or bilateral. Bilateral conditions may or may not be symmetrical.

Damage to a physis most often is due to trauma. The traumatic incident may or may not be known at the time of diagnosis. The younger the patient when the damage occurs, the greater the potential for limb deformity. In many cases, the

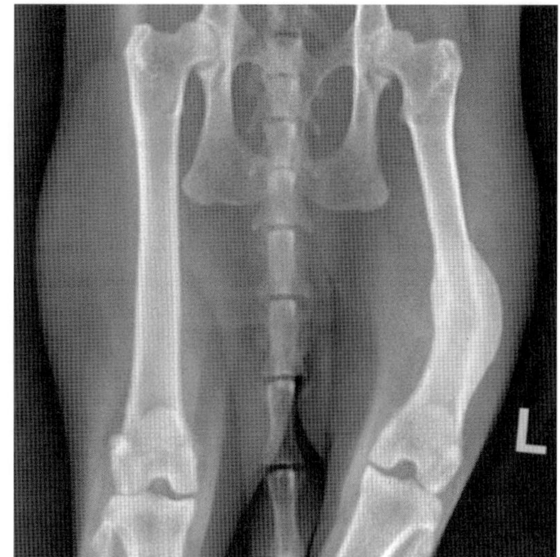

Figure 5.38 Malunion fracture. VD view of a cat pelvis depicting a malunion fracture in the left femoral diaphysis. The femur is healed, but it is abnormally angulated.

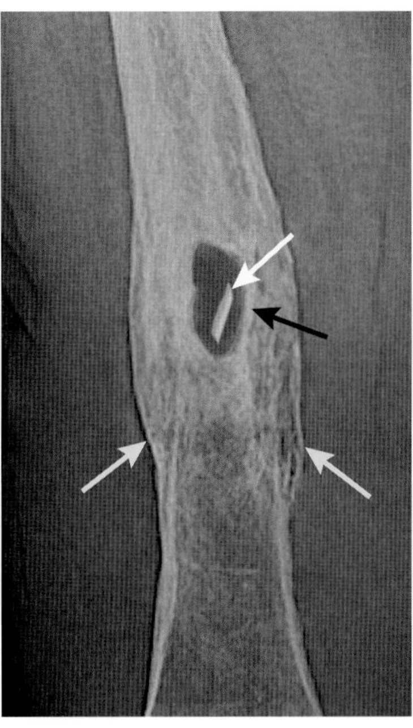

Figure 5.39 Bone sequestrum. Craniocaudal view of a long bone depicting a sharply marginated, sclerotic fragment of bone (white arrow) surrounded by sclerotic bone called an involucrum (black arrow). The sequestrum is surrounded by soft tissue opacity necrotic tissue. The periosteal new bone is well-defined (yellow arrows) consistent with a chronic and not very active lesion.

severity of physeal damage is not evident until bone growth stops (i.e., all the physes are closed). Therefore, the earlier a damaged physis is detected, the greater the possibility for successful treatment.

Physeal damage affects the **rate of bone growth**. If the entire physis is damaged, growth may either be delayed or stopped completely. If only part of a physis is damaged, that side may grow more slowly than the other. Abnormal rates of growth are most significant when paired bones are involved (i.e., radius and ulna, tibia and fibula). It is important to realize that complete cessation of long bone growth is not necessary to produce a limb deformity, merely a differential in the rate of growth between the two bones. **Asynchronous growth** can lead to abnormal shortening, bowing, and angulation of one or both bones. Limb deformities can lead to abnormal joint stresses, subluxation, and degenerative joint disease. Clinical signs tend to be more significant in young, large, and giant breed dogs due to their greater and faster bone growth. Certain dog breeds are deliberately bred to exhibit asynchronous growth as a desired trait (e.g., Bassett Hound, Dachshund).

In radiographs, the damaged part of a physis may or may not be visible. When visible, the damaged physis typically appears thinner and more opaque than the other physes, a finding commonly referred to as "premature closure" of the physis. Note: be cautious when interpreting subtle signs of a thinner, more opaque than expected physis because the normal physes can vary in appearance, even when comparing contralateral limbs. Experience is needed to recognize normal physeal variations and avoid overdiagnosis. Serial radiographs sometimes are needed. The important point is to carefully inspect the physes in a deformed limb to determine whether physeal damage and asynchronous growth might be the cause of the deformity. Asynchronous growth is discussed in greater detail in this chapter with Congenital and Developmental Abnormalities. If a physis is not visible at all, it likely is "closed," and no further growth should be expected from that site.

Osteomyelitis

Inflammation of bone tissue is called osteitis. If inflammation includes the medullary cavity, it is called osteomyelitis. Inflammation sometimes starts in the medullary cavity, especially if the cause is hematogenous in origin. If due to a penetrating wound, inflammation can start anywhere from the skin to the medullary cavity.

Osteomyelitis most often is caused by an **infection**, either bacterial, mycotic, or protozoal. Infection may be monostotic (all lesions in one bone), regional (all lesions in one limb), or polyostotic (lesions in multiple bones and multiple limbs).

The earliest radiographic sign of osteomyelitis is soft tissue swelling. Bone lesions may become visible after about 1–2 weeks, sometimes sooner in very young animals. Bone lesions caused by active inflammation typically appear as an ill-defined periosteal response. Osteolysis may develop if inflammation remains active and unchecked by either body defenses or appropriate therapy. Bone weakened by osteolysis is susceptible to pathologic fracture. In chronic cases, osteosclerosis surrounds the lytic areas as the body attempts to wall-off the infection. Osteomyelitis, whether due to a bacterial or mycotic infection, rarely extends into the joints.

Bacterial osteomyelitis tends to stimulate a greater periosteal response than a mycotic infection or a tumor.

Elevation of the periosteum is caused by subperiosteal accumulation of fluid (e.g., purulent, hemorrhagic, serous). In radiographs, the subperiosteal fluid may separate the periosteal new bone from the underlying cortex. Bacterial infections tend to result in a more rapid accumulation of subperiosteal fluid which can spread proximally and distally along the diaphyses of the long bones (Figure 5.40). In some cases, the entire diaphysis will be involved.

Bacterial osteomyelitis typically affects a single limb, but multiple bones in that limb may be involved (Figure 5.41). Bacterial infection can result from a penetrating wound, extension of an infection in the adjacent tissues, or hematogenous spread. Polyostotic bacterial infections are less common, typically resulting from a systemic infection.

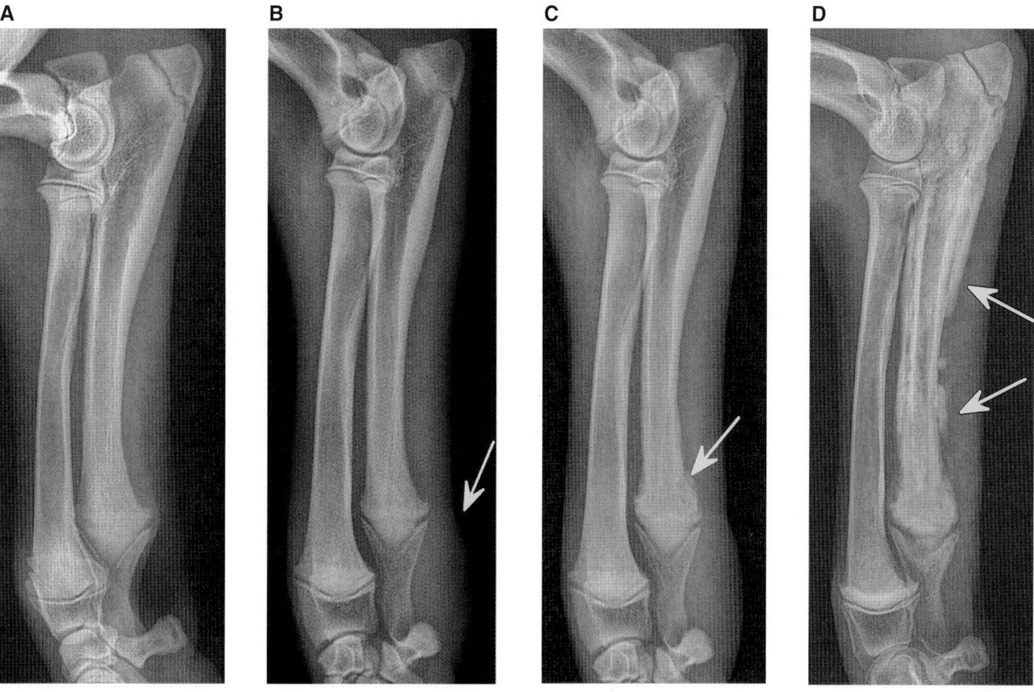

Figure 5.40 Bacterial osteomyelitis. Lateral views of the same dog antebrachium depicting progression of osteomyelitis. **A**. Normal radius and ulna. **B**. Soft tissue swelling is visible at the distal ulna (arrow). **C**. A periosteal response has developed at the distal ulnar metaphysis (arrow). **D**. The periosteal new bone has extended along the ulnar diaphysis (arrows).

Lesions can occur in any part of any bone, but they are more likely in areas with a rich blood flow, such as the metaphyses in immature animals and the vertebrae and ribs in older animals. Occasionally a bone abscess develops, appearing as a focal, sharply marginated area of decreased opacity. Chronic infections can lead to development of a fistulous tract.

Mycotic osteomyelitis usually is hematogenous in origin and polyostotic in distribution. Mycosis in a single bone is uncommon, but when it occurs the ends of the bone (metaphyseal or epiphyseal region) are more likely to be affected. Mycotic infection at the end of a bone often is indistinguishable from a bone tumor, although mycoses tend to more osteoproductive and neoplasms more osteolytic. Mycotic osteomyelitis tends to produce a smaller and better defined periosteal response that bacterial infections and rarely involves the entire diaphysis, as often is seen with bacterial infections. Fungal infections typically grow more slowly and periosteal elevation is more gradual.

Mycotic osteomyelitis is more common in endemic regions. It is reported more often in dogs than in cats, particularly in young adult, large-breed dogs used for hunting. Animals that are immunocompromised are at increased risk.

Protozoal osteomyelitis is uncommon in dogs and cats. Parasites that may infect bone include *hepatozoonosis*, *leishmaniasis*, and *neosporosis*. Protozoa may enter bone via hematogenous spread or from the adjacent soft tissues. Lesions usually are polyostotic and aggressive. Any bone may be affected, but the long bones most often are involved. Periosteal new bone may be ill-defined (active process) or well-defined (inactive disease) and varies in appearance from smooth and laminar to very irregular and proliferative.

A B

Figure 5.41 Osteomyelitis. Dorsoplantar views of a dog's right and left tarsus. There is soft tissue swelling in the right tarsus and a periosteal response along the lateral margins of the right distal calcaneus, the fourth tarsal, and the proximal fifth metatarsal bones (arrows). The left tarsus is normal (the left tarsal radiograph is oriented to match the right for ease of comparison).

Table 5.5 General considerations comparing neoplasia and osteomyelitis*

Characteristic	Neoplasia	Bacterial Osteomyelitis	Mycotic Osteomyelitis
Signalment	Older, larger animals	Younger animals	Younger animals
Location	Usually metaphyseal	Often diaphyseal	Metaphyseal or epiphyseal
Distribution	Usually monostotic	Often polyostotic	Polyostotic or monostotic
Lesion size	More focal	More diffuse	More focal
Lytic or productive	Mostly osteolytic	Mostly osteoproductive	Mostly osteoproductive
Periosteal response	More irregular and less distinct	Larger, better defined	Chronic, more organized, sharper margins
Cortical destruction	May be severe	Less common	Uncommon
Codman's triangle	More likely	Less likely	Unlikely
Rate of change in serial radiographs	More rapid change (days)	Less change (weeks)	Little change (weeks to months)
Sequestrum	Unlikely	More likely	Unlikely
Body defense	No defense	Strong defense	Variable defense

*A primary difference between a bone tumor and a bone infection is that the body does not react to a tumor, it only responds to the elevation of the periosteum and the destructive forces of the tumor. The body does, however, react to infection by mounting a defense against the etiologic agent. It is sometimes difficult for the body to curtail bacterial infections and they can spread up and down the diaphysis of the bone(s). Mycotic infections are slower growing, giving the body more time to limit their spread and confine them to a more focal area of bone. Tumors also are focal, but tumors tend to be more osteolytic than mycoses; mycoses tend to be more osteoproductive.

Osseous neoplasia

Neoplasia can involve any part of any bone. Most bone tumors are both osteolytic and osteoproductive, but they tend to be more lytic and less productive than bone infections. Unlike with an infection, the body does not react to a neoplasm (Table 5.5). No defense is mounted against a bone tumor. The body only responds to the separation of the periosteum, which is caused by the tumor physically elevating it. That said, differentiating osseous neoplasia from osteomyelitis often is difficult using radiographs alone. It has been taught traditionally that bone tumors do not cross a joint and infections can cross a joint. This may be true much of the time, but not always. In radiographs of any particular patient, you cannot be sure whether the lesion you are seeing is a tumor that did cross the joint or an infection that did not. Histopathology usually is needed for definitive diagnosis. Serial radiographs are useful to assess the rate of disease progression, especially when the initial findings are equivocal.

Primary bone tumors originate in bone. They rarely extend directly into an adjacent bone. Larger, advanced tumors can irritate a nearby bone and cause a periosteal response, but the response is much less severe than at the primary site and there is no cortical destruction. Primary tumors in the axial skeleton may be purely osteolytic, purely osteoproductive, or a combination of both. They most often are reported in the skull, followed by the ribs, pelvis, and then the vertebrae.

Osteosarcoma is the most common malignant bone tumor in dogs and cats. Most osteosarcomas arise as a solitary lesion, typically in the metaphyseal region of a long bone; rarely are they diaphyseal or epiphyseal. Most osteosarcomas present with an aggressive pattern of osteolysis, an irregular and ill-defined periosteal response, and variable degrees of soft tissue swelling (Figure 5.22). In some cases, osteolysis is the only radiographic finding; the periosteal response may be amorphous or not evident in the images. The aggressive nature of osteosarcoma leads to a wide and indistinct zone of transition between abnormal and normal bone. Cortical destruction is a frequent finding and Codman's triangle often is present. Osteosarcoma may be associated with bone infarcts. A classic "sunburst" pattern occurs in approximately one-third of osteosarcomas. Osteosarcoma most often is reported in older, large, and giant breed dogs. Common site predilections are "away from the elbow" and "toward the knee," which includes the proximal humerus, the distal radius and ulna, the distal femur, and the proximal tibia. Clinical signs of pain and lameness may be acute or their onset may be gradual and progressive. Pathologic fractures are common (Figure 5.42).

Parosteal osteosarcomas arise from the surface of cortical bone as opposed to most osteosarcomas which arise in

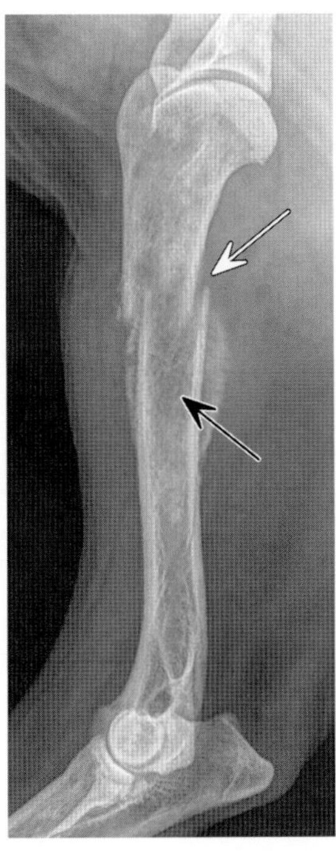

Figure 5.42 Pathologic fracture. Lateral view of a dog humerus depicting a diaphyseal fracture (white arrow) at the proximal aspect of an area of geographic osteolysis (black arrow). A periosteal response is present, sooner than expected for fracture repair, indicating that a disease process was present before the fracture.

cancellous bone. They typically appear as a smooth-bordered, lobulated, mineral opacity mass extending outward from the border of a long bone. The bony mass usually is sclerotic with a well-defined margin. There often is little or no osteolysis. Over time, the mass may eventually invade the cortex and extend into the medullary cavity. Parosteal osteosarcomas, or *juxtacortical osteosarcomas*, are uncommon in dogs and cats. They tend to be slower growing and carry a better prognosis than typical osteosarcomas, but they can metastasize. In cats, parosteal osteosarcomas tend to arise in the humerus or femur, whereas in dogs, they are more likely to occur near the stifle. Although more common in long bones, they have been reported in a frontal bone and a mandibular ramus.

Giant cell tumors are rare in dogs and cats. They most often are reported in the metaphyseal or epiphyseal region of a long bone, particularly the distal ulna. They are slow growing and usually benign. In radiographs, giant cell tumors typically produce an expansile area of geographic osteolysis with a septated or multiloculated center and a well-defined margin. In most cases, there is no visible periosteal response. If a response is present, rule out osteosarcoma. A giant cell tumor may resemble a bone cyst, but the tumor tends to grow, which often is evident in serial radiographs.

Secondary bone tumors originate elsewhere in the body and spread to bone. They are uncommon in dogs and cats. However, any malignant tumor can involve bone by direct extension or metastasis. Examples of soft tissue tumors that can invade bone include a squamous cell carcinoma that invades the mandible or the digits and a synovial cell sarcoma that invades the adjacent bones. Soft tissue tumors also can cause pressure remodeling or a periosteal response in an adjacent bone without directly invading it.

Malignant tumors that arise in bone, lung, prostate gland, and mammary glands tend to metastasize to bone more often than those arising in other tissues. Metastasis usually is polyostotic and often involves the diaphyseal and metaphyseal regions of long bones. Lesions typically are aggressive with some degree of cortical destruction. The initial periosteal response often is small, smooth bordered, and well-defined, particularly in the ribs, but can become much more active.

Multiple myeloma and **lymphoma** tend to produce multiple osteolytic foci with little or no periosteal response (Figure 5.43). These often occur at sites not typical for primary neoplasia. Lymphoma may produce medullary osteosclerosis.

Digital tumors may originate in bone or in the adjacent soft tissue. The typical radiographic findings are osteolysis in the affected digit, adjacent soft tissue swelling, and little to no visible periosteal response (Figure 5.121). Most digital tumors are subungual and confined to the third phalanx. They rarely cross the joint, but they can. Infection in a digit that leads to osteomyelitis is more likely to cross a joint, but not always. Again, histopathology usually is needed for diagnosis.

Subungual tumors are reported most often in older, large-breed dogs, particularly those with black hair coats. They are

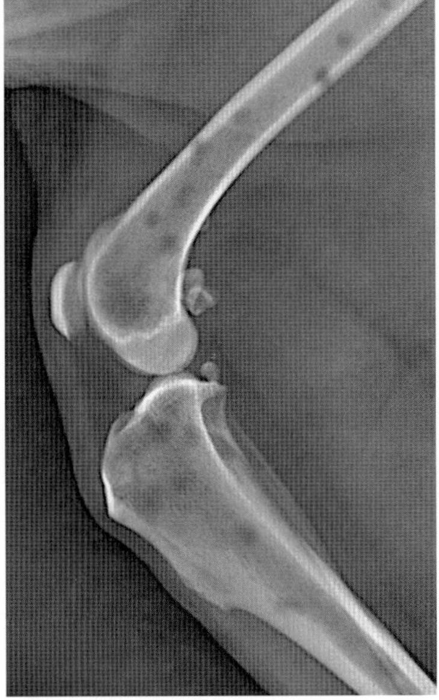

Figure 5.43 Metastatic osseous neoplasia. Lateral view of a dog stifle depicting multiple focal areas of osteolysis in the femur and tibia due to multiple myeloma.

uncommon in cats. Usually, only a single digit is involved, but tumors can arise in multiple digits and in multiple limbs.

Benign conditions of bone

Benign bone diseases change slowly over time and rarely involve other tissues. They are uncommon in dogs and cats, more often reported in young, large breed dogs. Any suspected benign lesion must be proven to be benign with serial radiographs. A malignant bone tumor is much more likely that a bone cyst or a benign tumor. Most benign bone diseases are difficult to differentiate with radiographs. Some will grow and may eventually interfere with limb or joint function, but most remain asymptomatic. Larger lesions can impinge on an adjacent structure or weaken the bone and predispose it to a pathologic fracture. Occasionally a skeletal deformity is present at the site of a benign lesion.

A **bone cyst** is a cavity within a bone. The cavity often is filled with fluid. In radiographs, a bone cyst appears as an area of geographic osteolysis with a well-defined margin (Figure 5.44). The center often is septated. The adjacent cortex may be thinned or displaced, but it remains intact. If the cortex becomes too thin, however, a pathologic fracture may occur. A periosteal response is rare and soft tissue swelling often is minimal or absent. Most bone cysts are monostotic and develop in the diaphyseal or metaphyseal region of a long bone. They more often are reported in the distal radius or ulna, but can affect any bone. In the spine, bone cysts are more likely to be located in a dorsal spinous process than in a vertebral body. The etiology of most bone cysts is unknown. A simple or solitary bone cyst (*unicameral* cyst) sometimes develops from a hematoma that formed following a traumatic event. An aneurysmal bone cyst may result from the arteriovenous shunting of blood that causes expansile remodeling in the bone. An odontogenic bone cyst is associated with teeth that are devitalized, malformed, impacted, or unerupted.

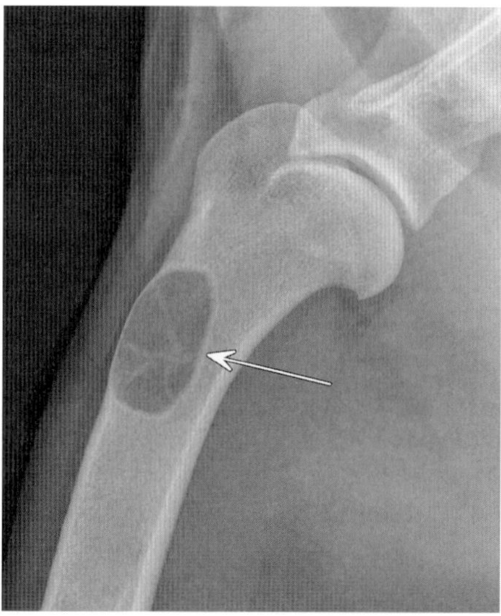

Figure 5.44 Bone cyst. Lateral view of a dog shoulder depicting a well-defined area of geographic osteolysis with a septated center in the proximal humerus (arrow). The adjacent cortex is thin and slightly expanded outward.

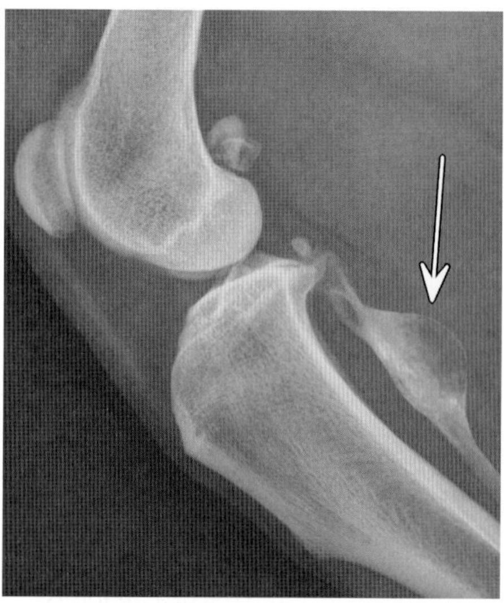

Figure 5.45 Enchondroma. Lateral view of a dog stifle depicting a well-defined, expansile area of soft tissue opacity in the proximal fibula (arrow). No periosteal response nor soft tissue swelling is evident.

Enchondromas and **osteochondromas** are benign cartilaginous tumors that develop from displaced growth cartilage. The cartilage continues to grow in the abnormal location and functions similar to a physis. These tumors are typically soft tissue opacity due to their cartilage content. Some may contain mineralized tissue, often in the form of a thin rim of bone. Differentiating enchondroma from osteochondroma using radiographs often is difficult and may be clinically unimportant.

An **enchondroma** is derived from the actively proliferating cartilaginous tissue of the physis. Its typical location is the endosteal surface of the bone where it causes an expansile lesion that thins the adjacent cortex (Figure 5.45). Usually, there is no periosteal response or significant soft tissue swelling. The center of the lesion may contain bony trabeculae. Enchondromas typically form in the metaphyseal or diaphyseal region of one or more long bones, most often in a distal limb. Multiple sites of enchondroma is called *enchondromatosis*.

An **osteochondroma** is derived from aberrant physeal cartilage that separates from the edge of a normal growth plate. As the patient grows, the separated piece of cartilage also grows, but in an abnormal location. Osteochondromas can arise in any bone that develops from cartilage. They appear as well-defined expansile lesions without evidence of osteolysis, soft tissue swelling, or an active periosteal response. In the early stages, an osteochondroma may appear separate from the underlying cortex, sometimes resembling calcinosis circumscripta. Osteochondromas may be solitary or multiple, monostotic or polyostotic. The presence of multiple osteochondromas is called *osteochondromatosis* or *multiple cartilaginous exostosis*.

In dogs and cats, osteochondromas may be found anywhere but most often in two specific locations: the distal radius and the femoral shaft. In the distal radius, they typically appear as a broad-based growth, sometimes interfering with the ulna to cause pain and lameness. In the femur, they typically appear as a spur-shaped growth extending from the caudal border of the midshaft (Figure 5.46). Osteochondromas usually stop growing at skeletal maturity. Rarely, a symmetrical or annular osteochondroma at the physis will lead to limb shortening or deformity. Although uncommon, osteochondromas can develop in the trachea, in joints, and sometimes in flat or irregular bones. They have been reported in the pelvis, spine, and skull, particularly in cats, but tend to be less organized in these areas than in long bones. Spinal osteochondromas more often occur in the cervical or thoracic spine, usually near a spinous process.

Osteomas are benign, slow-growing tumors that arise from the surface of a bone. They may be difficult to differentiate from parosteal osteosarcomas. The typical appearance of an osteoma is a very opaque bony mass extending away from the cortex. The margins of the mass tend to be smooth and well-defined without evidence of osteolysis and with little to no soft tissue swelling. Osteomas more often involve

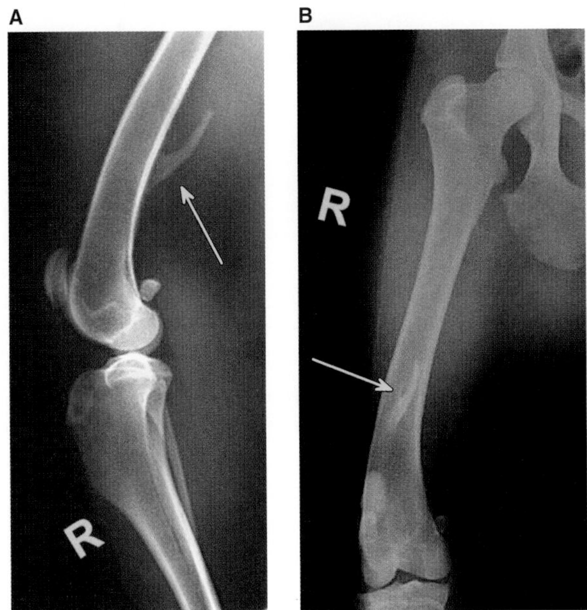

Figure 5.46 Osteochondroma. Lateral view (**A**) and caudocranial view (**B**) of a dog femur depicting a spur-shaped growth on the caudal border of the right femur (arrow).

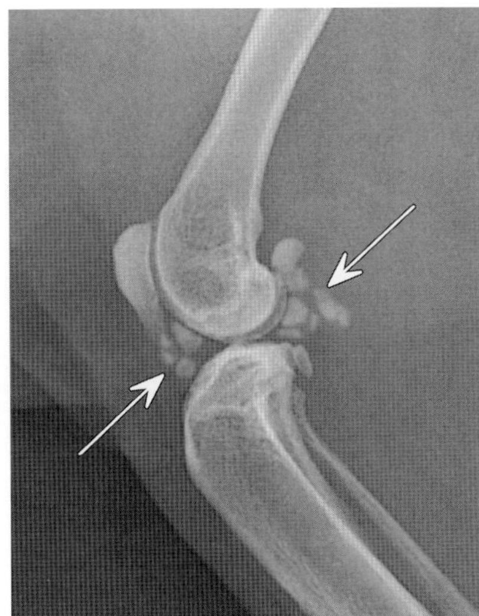

Figure 5.47 Synovial osteochondromatosis. Lateral view of a cat stifle depicting mineral opacity structures in the femorotibial joint (arrows).

the cranial vault, a mandible, or a sinus. Other than a firm swelling, most affected animals are asymptomatic.

Chondromas are benign, slow-growing tumors of cartilage. They arise in flat bones, such as the ribs, more often than long bones. In radiographs, a chondroma appears as a well-defined, expansile, soft tissue opacity mass in the bone. Any periosteal response usually is minimal with smooth, well-defined margins and little soft tissue swelling. Chondromas typically are less mineralized than osteochondromas.

Synovial osteochondromas appear as one or more well-defined, mineral opacity structures in a joint (Figure 5.47). They may be round or irregular in shape and often occur bilaterally (radiographs of the contralateral joint are recommended). The etiology of synovial osteochondromas often is unknown. They are seen more often in cats than in dogs, particularly in mature animals. Osteochondromas nourished by synovial fluid can continue to grow. In cats, the joints most often involved are the stifles, elbows, shoulders, and digits. In dogs, it is the hips, stifles, and elbows. In dogs, synovial osteochondromas are more common in larger breeds and with chronic osteochondritis dissecans. When multiple joints are affected, the condition is called *synovial chondromatosis*.

Congenital and developmental abnormalities

Abnormal number of bones

Congenital absence of bones is uncommon in dogs and cats. Supernumerary bones are more common, particularly in the digits. Some conditions may be heritable.

Ectrodactyly is the abnormal development of bones in a limb. It most often occurs in the metatarsus or metacarpus

A

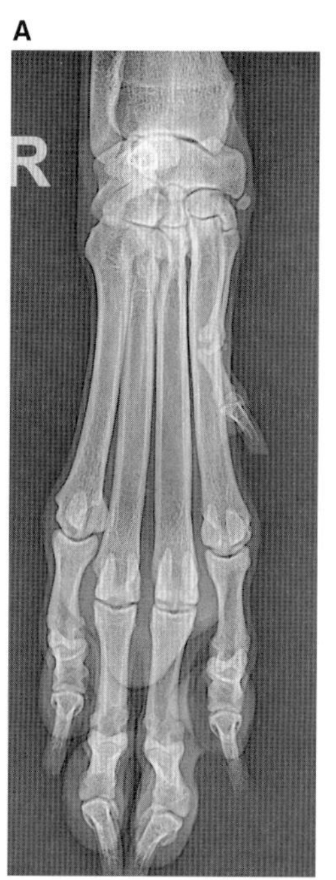

B

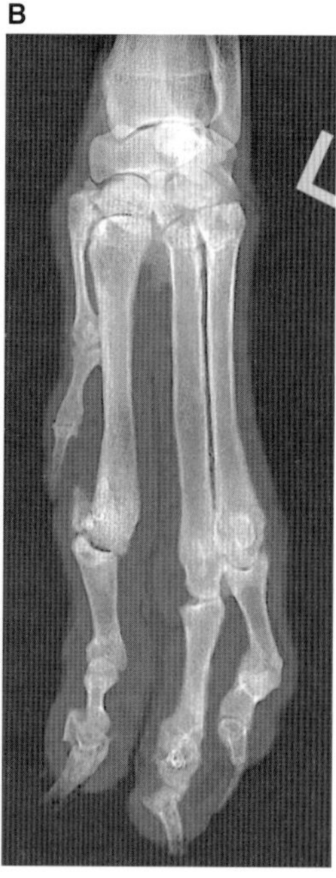

Figure 5.48 Ectrodactyly. DP views of a dog right manus (**A**) and left manus (**B**) depicting absence of the left third metacarpal bone and its associated phalanges.

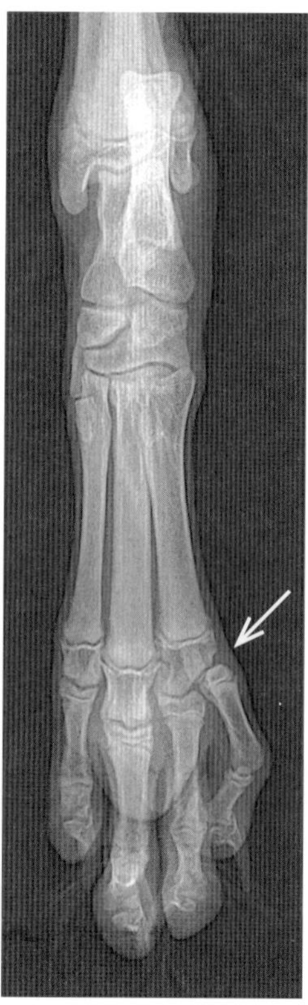

Figure 5.49 Ectrodactyly. Dorsoplantar view of a dog pes depicting absence of a metatarsal bone. The extra digit at the fifth metatarsal bone makes the ectrodactyly less evident at first glance.

where one or more of the central digits is absent or reduced in size (Figures 5.48 and 5.49). The remaining digits may be further separated than normal or fused together, commonly called *split hand deformity* or *lobster-claw syndrome*. The condition usually is unilateral. The ipsilateral elbow may be subluxated or luxated.

Hemimelia is the partial or complete absence of a normally paired bone (i.e., radius/ulna or tibia/fibula). Most often, it is the radius or tibia that is affected. The existing paired bone tends to be larger in diameter with thicker cortices than normal due to stress remodeling (Figure 5.50). The joints proximal and distal may be subluxated or luxated.

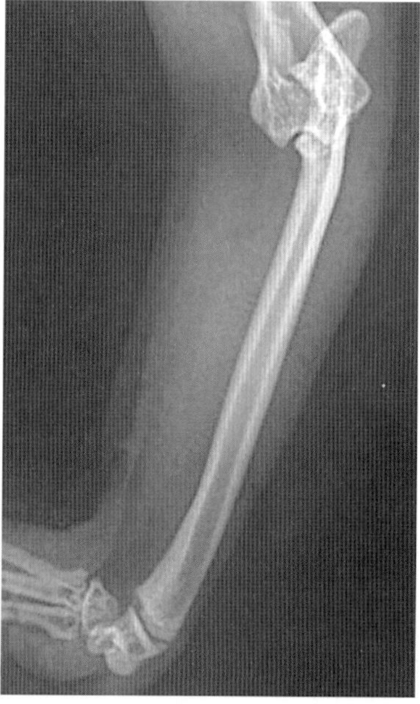

Figure 5.50 Hemimelia. Craniocaudal oblique view of a dog antebrachium depicting absence of the radius. The ulna is larger than normal and the carpus is luxated.

Polydactyly is an increase in the number of digits on one or more limbs. It is a common inherited trait in cats and certain dog breeds (e.g., Great Pyrenees). More than one extra digits may be present (Figure 5.51). The development of the extra digit(s) may be partial or complete and may also include extra metacarpal or metatarsal bones or just extra phalanges.

Syndactyly is the bony or soft tissue fusion of two or more adjacent digits. The bones may either blend together as a bony union or they may remain separate but in close apposition with one another due to a fibrous union.

Chondrodysplasia

Commonly called *dwarfism*, chondrodysplasia is a skeletal deformity caused by abnormal endochondral ossification.

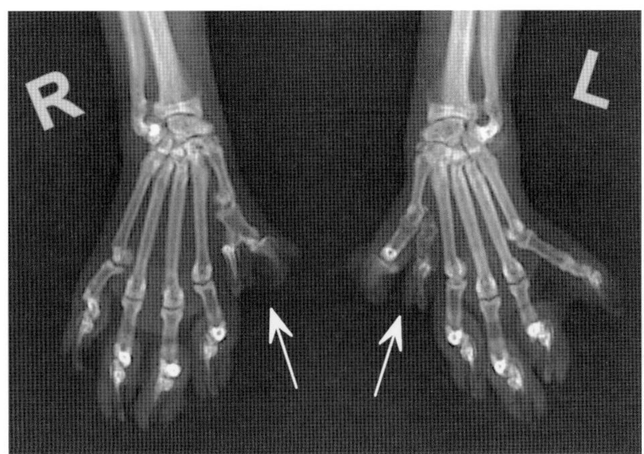

Figure 5.51 Polydactyly. Dorsopalmar view of a cat right and left manus depicting partial development of extra digits in the medial aspect of each foot (arrows).

It may be *proportionate*, affecting all bones in the skeleton equally, or it may be *disproportionate*, leading to abnormalities in some bones but not in others. Chondrodysplasia is deliberately bred into certain breeds of dogs and cats (e.g., Dachshund, Basset Hound, Bulldog, Pug, Pekinese, Lhasa Apso, Welsh Corgi, Munchkin cats).

Proportionate dwarfism is usually caused by inadequate growth hormone, which often is a pituitary problem. Affected animals are diminutive in stature and slow to grow. They tend to retain their juvenile hair coats, though symmetrical alopecia and hyperpigmentation often develop later in life. In radiographs, all bones are smaller than normal but proportionate in size. Formation of ossification centers and physeal closure times tend to be similar or slightly delayed compared to non-chondrodystrophic animals.

Disproportionate dwarfism can result in numerous skeletal abnormalities, including stunted bone growth, asynchronous growth of paired bones, varus or valgus limb deformities, hemivertebrae, joint subluxations, and others. Many affected animals also suffer stenotic nares and elongated soft palates. In radiographs of immature animals, the epiphyses may appear mottled due to delayed ossification, a condition called **epiphyseal dysplasia** (Figure 5.52). Epiphyseal dysplasia may be visible up to about 4 months of age, after which ossification usually has progressed to the point that the mottling is no longer evident. Mottling tends to be more evident in the humeral condyles, carpi, and tarsi, but the femurs, metacarpi/metatarsi, and vertebrae usually are also involved. Closure of the physes frequently is delayed leading to wider and more irregular growth plates. The metaphyses may be widened or "flared" and increased in opacity.

In the appendicular skeleton, disproportionate dwarfism causes abnormal shortening of the bones in the extremities. The thoracic limbs tend to be more severely affected than the pelvic limbs. Asynchronous growth of the radius and ulna is common, leading to radius curvus and pes valgus deformities. Endochondral cartilage sometimes is retained, most often in the distal ulnar metaphysis. Development of the coronoid process, medial humeral condyle, and anconeal process may be delayed or incomplete due to chondrodysplasia. The carpal and tarsal bones may be misshapen. With maturity, the epiphyseal, physeal and metaphyseal abnormalities often regress; however, the long bone deformities are permanent. Secondary degenerative joint disease is common in affected animals, as is hip dysplasia.

In the axial skeleton, abnormalities due to chondrodysplasia are less common. The vertebrae may be shortened, which affects body length, and fusion of the vertebral endplates to the vertebral bodies may be delayed. The ventral vertebral margins may appear irregular, sometimes described as "lipping" or "pleating." The ends of the ribs may be flared and concave or "cupped" at the costochondral junctions.

Congenital hypothyroidism or *cretinsim* can result in disproportionate dwarfism. Low levels of thyroid hormone during growth may be due to hypoplasia or aplasia of the

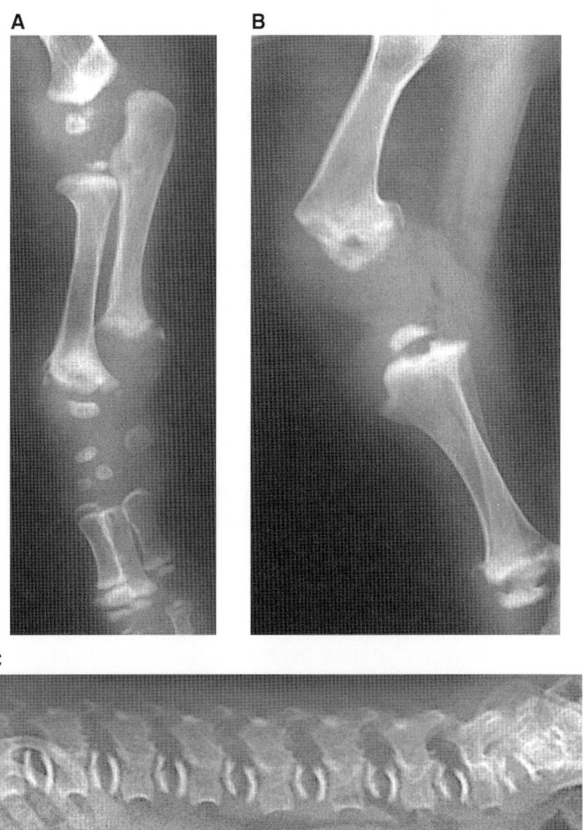

Figure 5.52 Epiphyseal dysplasia. Lateral views of a puppy thoracic limb (**A**), pelvic limb (**B**), and lumbar spine (**C**) depicting delayed epiphyseal ossification. The visible epiphyses appear mottled and irregular. The distal ulnar and femoral epiphyses should be visible, but are not.

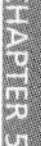

thyroid gland, defective thyroid hormone synthesis, or an iodine deficiency. If hypothyroidism occurs after cessation of bone growth, no dwarfism or skeletal changes develop. Congenital hypothyroidism most often is reported in Boxers and sometimes in other breeds. Affected dogs present with short, bowed limbs and long bodies. Radiographic findings include epiphyseal dysplasia, delayed physeal closures, and delayed ossification. Many of the long bones are short and bowed with thick cortices, particularly the proximal tibia, distal femur, and distal humerus. The medullary canals may be increased in opacity. Secondary degenerative joint disease is common. The vertebrae frequently are abnormal in shape and shortened due to endplate dysplasia, often leading to spinal kyphosis. The skull usually is shorter and broader than normal due to delayed closure of the fontanelles and shortened facial bones. Dental eruption usually is delayed. Concurrent hydrocephalus may be present.

Hyperparathyroidism

The abnormal, excessive production of parathyroid hormone leads to loss of calcium from the skeleton and generalized osteoporosis. In radiographs, bone is less opaque, there is less bone-to-soft tissue contrast, bone cortices become thin, and there is a coarse trabecular pattern. Osteoporosis commonly leads to pathologic fractures. Long bones may be deformed and in various stages of fracture healing. Malunion fractures frequently are present.

One of the earliest radiographic signs of hyperparathyroidism often is loss of the dental lamina dura. In advanced cases of osteoporosis, fibrous osteodystrophy develops and the teeth may appear to "float" in soft tissue due to the severe loss of bone opacity. There are three types of hyperparathyroidism: *primary*, *secondary*, and *pseudo-hyperparathyroidism*.

Primary hyperparathyroidism is caused by disease in one or more of the parathyroid glands, often a tumor. **Secondary hyperparathyroidism** is caused by an imbalance in the body's calcium to phosphorous ratio; usually due to either excess dietary phosphorous or abnormal retention of phosphorous due to chronic renal disease. Both of these conditions can result in the overproduction of parathormone. **Pseudo-hyperparathyroidism** is associated with a malignant tumor that causes hypercalcemia as part of a *paraneoplastic syndrome*. It has been reported with lymphoma, multiple myeloma, and others. The parathyroid glands are normal but overactive.

Osteogenesis imperfecta

Osteogenesis imperfecta presents as generalized osteoporosis due to a rare defect in collagen production. It may be confused with hyperparathyroidism. Growth deformities can occur in young animals, and pathologic fractures are common. Affected animals may exhibit some degree of dwarfism. The rib cage typically is small and may compress the intrathoracic viscera.

Rickets

Rickets is a disease of growing bones caused by a dietary deficiency, usually a lack of vitamin D. It is rare in dogs and cats. Rickets, sometimes called *juvenile osteomalacia*, results in abnormal ossification that leads to softening and weakening of the bones. In radiographs, the physes appear wider and more irregular than normal (Figure 5.53). The metaphyses often are widened or flared and concave or "cupped" with more pointed edges. The epiphyses, however, are normal, which helps differentiate rickets from other causes of skeletal dysplasia. There is little or no soft tissue swelling. Rickets affects all bones, but abnormalities tend to be more severe in the distal radius, ulna, and tibia. Untreated cases can progress to long bone deformities.

Mucopolysaccharidosis

This is a group of heritable diseases characterized by a buildup of mucopolysaccharides (MPS), also called *glycosaminoglycans*. MPS are long-chain sugar molecules that must be degraded by lysosomal enzymes for normal growth to occur. If the enzymes are abnormal, MPS can accumulate in the body and damage the musculoskeletal, circulatory, and neurologic systems. The type of damage varies with the type of enzyme deficiency but usually progresses as the animal ages.

Mucopolysaccharidosis can cause disproportionate dwarfism, which usually is evident by 8 weeks of age. Skeletal abnormalities include epiphyseal dysplasia, flared metaphyses, and short, deformed limbs. The diaphysis often are enlarged. Fascial dysmorphism is common with a large skull,

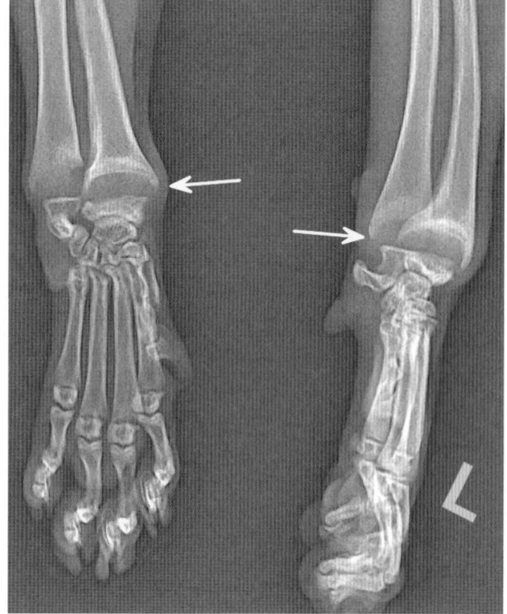

Figure 5.53 Rickets. Dorsopalmar oblique view of an immature cat thoracic limbs depicting widened physes with flared, concave metaphyses (arrows).

short maxillary, incisive, and mandibular bones, small or absent frontal sinuses, and abnormal teeth. The vertebrae may be fused, shortened, and/or misshapen, sometimes cuboid in appearance, especially along the cervical and lumbar spine. The odontoid process (dens) may be hypoplastic or fragmented. The vertebral body endplates frequently are sclerotic. Degenerative changes may be present along the dorsal vertebral articulations. The clavicles and distal ends of the ribs may be widened. Pectus excavatum often is present. Many affected animals have hip dysplasia and other appendicular joints may be deformed. Degenerative joint disease is common. Generalized osteoporosis usually is present, varying from mild to severe.

Mucopolysaccharidosis is uncommon in dogs and cats, most often reported in Siamese cats. In addition to skeletal deformities, the disease may lead to cardiac anomalies, hydrocephalus, paresis or paraplegia, and ocular abnormalities.

Canine leukocyte adhesion disorder (CLAD)

CLAD is rare inherited condition that impairs the function of granulocytes. Affected animals exhibit stunted growth and often suffer recurrent bacterial infections. Bony abnormalities include a moderate to severe periosteal response along the mandible (may resemble craniomandibular osteopathy), increased opacity in the frontal sinuses, and widening or flaring of the metaphyses. Metaphyseal bone may appear heterogenous, sometimes described as stippled. Osteomyelitis often is present.

CLAD has been reported in several dog breeds, including Irish Setter, Irish Red and White Setter, Doberman Pinscher, and Weimaraner. The disease is invariably fatal, with most animals dying at a few months of age.

Asynchronous growth and limb deformity

As mentioned earlier, the physes are susceptible to injury and the distal ulnar physis in dogs is particularly vulnerable due to its unique conical shape. Damage to a physis can lead to abnormal bone growth and a limb deformity, especially when it results in disproportionate or asynchronous growth between paired bones (e.g., radius and ulna, tibia and fibula). The greater the damage and the younger the animal, the more severe the limb deformity. Early diagnosis is crucial to successful treatment, which can minimize future problems with the leg. Serial and comparison radiographs often are useful for diagnosis. When investigating a thoracic limb deformity, make the following evaluations:

1. Measure and compare the lengths of the right and left radius and the right and left ulna.
2. Compare the widths of the joint spaces at both ends of the antebrachium.
3. Determine the direction of any diaphyseal bowing or curvature.
4. Note any angulation at the carpus.
5. Examine the relationship between the ulnar medial coronoid process and the articular margin of the radial head in the lateral view.
6. Look for degenerative joint disease in the elbow and carpus.

Damage to the **distal ulnar physis** that results in asynchronous growth with the radius leads to radius curvus, elbow subluxation, and carpal valgus. The abnormally shortened ulna causes the radial diaphysis to curve cranially and medially. The abnormal curvature is called "bowing" due to the "bowstring" effect of the ulna, which is fixed at the carpus and humerus. The radial cortex thickens along the concave side due to stress remodeling. Shortening of the ulna also can lead to widening of the humeroulnar joint space, making the space more wedge-shaped (Figures 5.54 and 5.55). The ulnar medial coronoid process moves distal to the radial head, creating a "stair step" along the radioulnar articular border (Figure 5.56). The normal radioulnar border is smooth. Greater than 2 mm displacement is significant. At the carpus, the shortened ulna causes the manus to deviate laterally because the ulnar styloid process is further proximal than normal. Severe disproportionate growth may lead to a very short ulna and luxation of the humeroradial joint with lateral displacement of the radial head (Figure 5.57). Abnormal stress on the anconeal process may prevent fusion or deform or fracture the process. A very short ulna also can lead to luxation of the radiocarpal joint.

Damage to the **distal radial physis** that results in asynchronous growth often leads to elbow subluxation and carpal varus. The abnormally shortened radius can cause widening of the humeroradial and radiocarpal joint spaces (Figure 5.58). The manus may deviate laterally because the ulnar styloid process is further distal than normal. Damage that affects only part of the distal radial physis can result in one side of the physis growing slower than the other side (Figure 5.59). In this situation, the manus deviates toward the damaged side and the radial diaphysis may curve or bow toward the normal side (concave side of diaphysis toward the damaged side of the physis). The humeroradial joint space may be widened.

Damage to **both** the distal radial and distal ulnar physes that results in abnormal growth can lead to shortening of both the radius and ulna. The elbow or carpus may be subluxated depending on the degree of damage to each physis. Damage to the proximal radial physis that results in abnormal growth leads to shortening of the radius and findings similar to those seen with damage to the distal radial physis, but usually not as severe. Similar to physeal damage, fusion of the radius and ulna in an immature animal can result in asynchronous growth (Figure 5.60).

Hypertrophic osteodystrophy (HOD)

Hypertrophic osteodystrophy is a systemic disease that affects the metaphyses of immature long bones (HOD

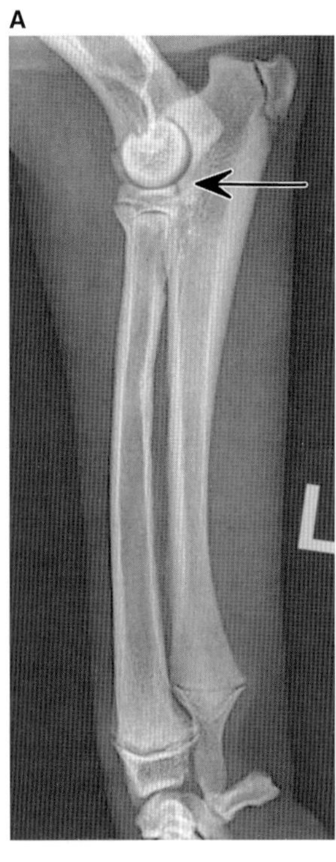

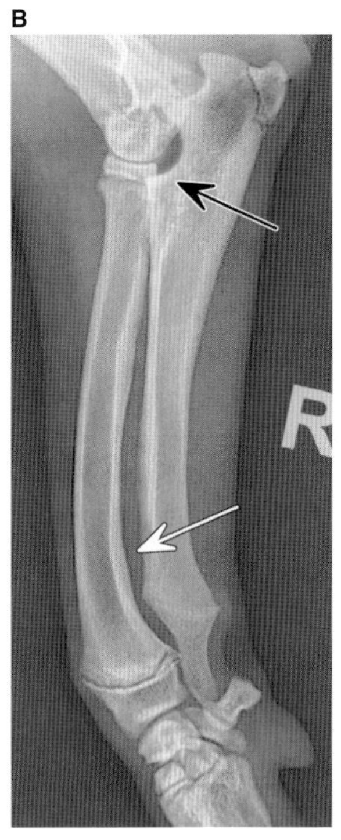

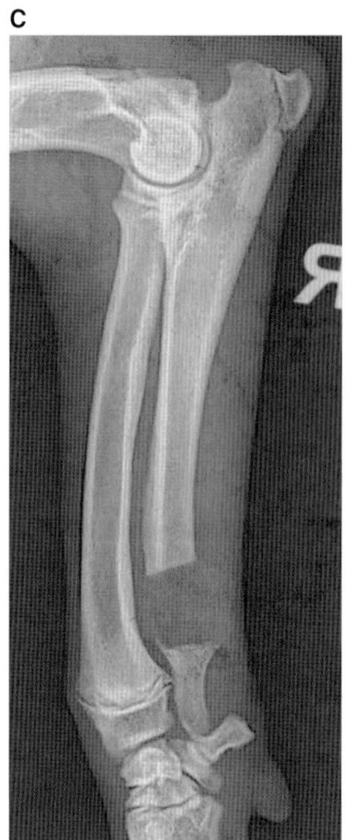

Figure 5.54 Asynchronous growth. **A**. Lateral view of an immature dog's left antebrachium. The limb is normal. The articular margin of the ulnar trochlear notch is continuous with the radial head, forming a smooth articulation with the humeral head (black arrow). **B**. Lateral view of the same dog's right antebrachium. There is a disproportionate rate of growth between the radius and the ulna. The distal ulnar physis is closed, which stops further growth. The radial physis is still open and the radius continues to lengthen. The abnormally shortened ulna leads to cranial bowing of the radius (white arrow) and humeroulnar subluxation (black arrow). Notice the "stair step" between the proximal radius and ulna compared to the same area in the normal left limb. **C**. Postoperative radiograph made following a distal ulnar ostectomy. The humeroulnar luxation is reduced.

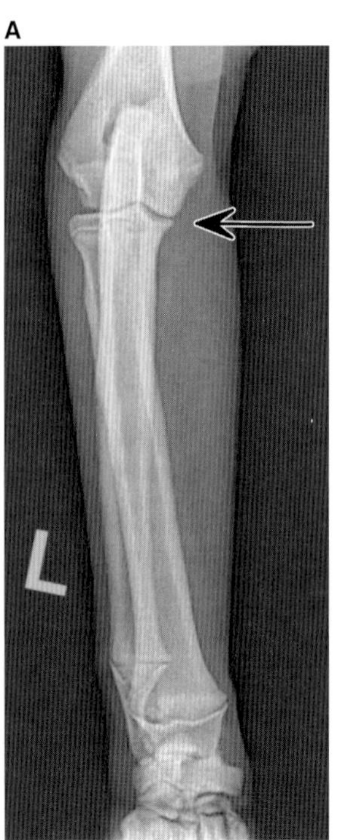

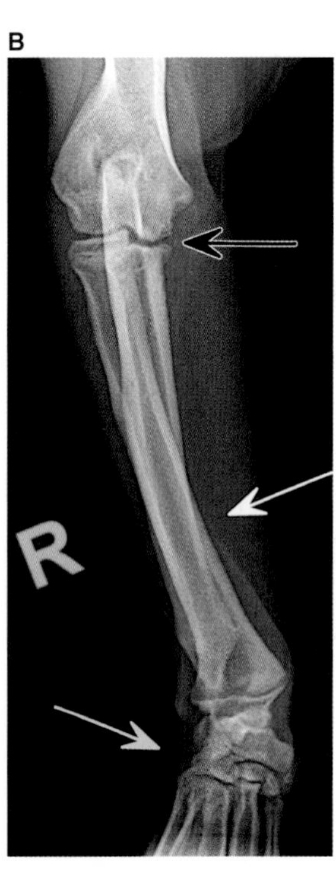

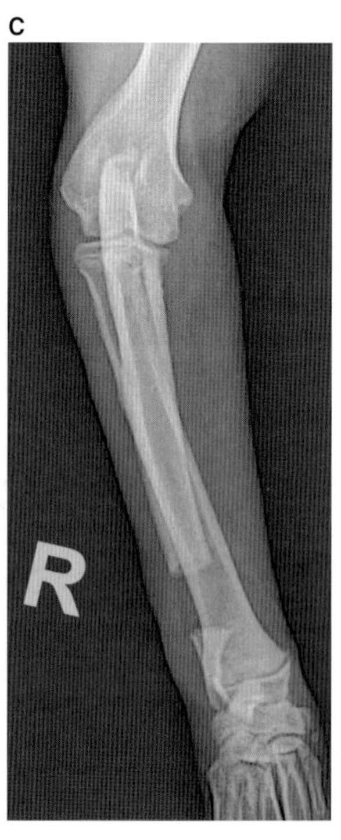

Figure 5.55 Asynchronous growth. **A**. Craniocaudal view of the left antebrachium of the same dog as in Figure 5.54. The limb is normal. The ulnar medial coronoid process is even with the radial head, forming a continuous articulation with the humeral condyle (black arrow). **B**. Craniocaudal view of the same dog right antebrachium. Premature closure of the distal ulnar physis results in an abnormally shortened ulna. Continued growth at the radial physis leads to lateral bowing of the radius (white arrow), lateral deviation of the carpus (yellow arrow), and humeroulnar subluxation (black arrow). Again, notice the "stair step" between the proximal radius and ulna compared to the same area in the normal left limb. **C**. Postoperative view made after a distal ulnar ostectomy. The humeroulnar luxation is reduced and the carpus is less deviated.

sometimes is called *metaphyseal osteopathy*). Any metaphysis in any long bone can be affected, but lesions tend to be most severe in the distal radius and ulna. Lesions usually are bilateral and relatively symmetrical. The long bones distal to the carpus and tarsus often are spared. Rarely, HOD can affect the mandible, cranium, or ribs.

The etiology of HOD is unknown. The initial radiographic sign of HOD is a thin line of soft tissue opacity near the physis (Figure 5.61), sometimes called a "double physis" sign. The line is caused by bleeding in the metaphyseal zone of provisional calcification that prevents mineralization in a thin band of trabecular bone. Bleeding also extends under

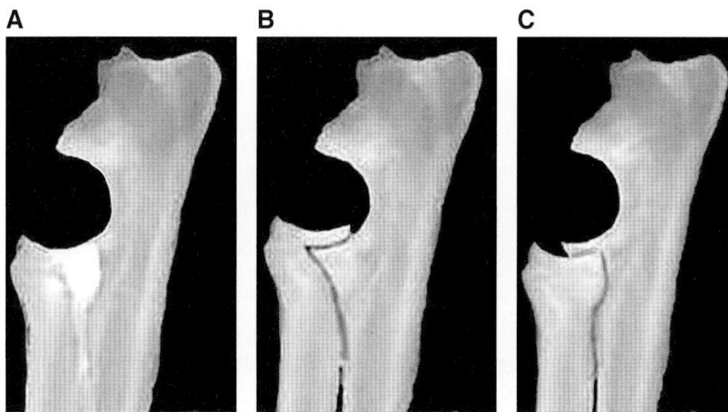

Figure 5.56 Elbow subluxation. **A**. Illustration showing the normal alignment along the radioulnar articular border. **B**. Subluxation caused by asynchronous growth with an abnormally shortened ulna. There is a misalignment or "stair-step" along the radioulnar border with the ulnar medial coronoid process distal to the radial head. **C**. Subluxation caused by asynchronous growth with an abnormally shortened radius There is a "stair-step" because the medial coronoid is proximal to the radial head.

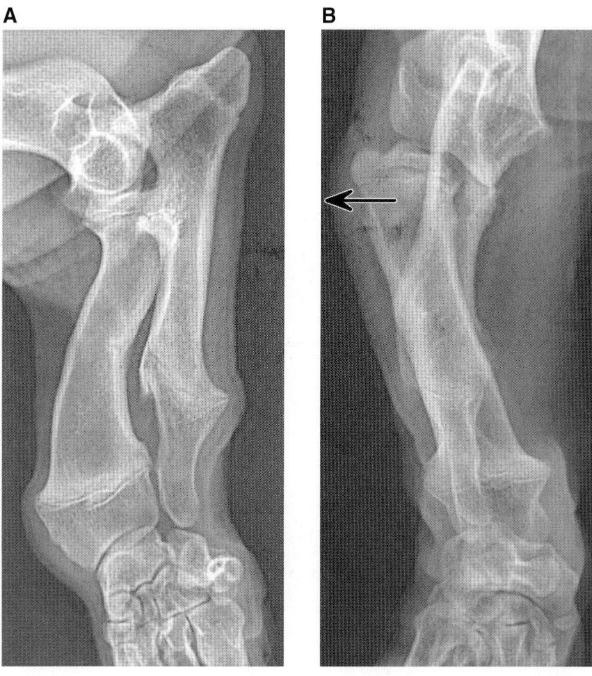

Figure 5.57 Asynchronous growth. Lateral view (**A**) and craniocaudal view (**B**) of a dog antebrachium with severe disproportionate growth of the radius and ulna. Depicted in these radiographs is an abnormally shortened ulna that lead to radius curvus, carpal valgus, lateral luxation of the radial head (arrow indicates direction of displacement), and humeroulnar subluxation.

the periosteum, separating it from the cortex. Typically, swelling develops in the adjacent soft tissues. A periosteal response produces mineral in the subperiosteal space, appearing in radiographs as a "cuff" or "sleeve" of new bone around the metaphysis. The subperiosteal space continues to fill with mineral over the next week or two, enlarging the "cuff" and making it more homogeneous. The metaphysis may appear more opaque due to summation of periosteal new bone (Figure 5.62). In chronic cases, the periosteal cuffing can extend to the physis and may bridge the physis to restrict bone growth and possibly lead to a limb deformity.

HOD most often is reported in young, rapidly growing, large, and giant breed dogs. It often begins around 4 months of age. Affected animals typically present with swollen, painful metaphyses, which may be mistaken for joint swelling. Factors that may contribute to the development of HOD include vitamin C deficiency (HOD sometimes is called *skeletal scurvy*) and infection with canine distemper virus.

HOD usually is a self-limiting disease. Most cases resolve completely after a few weeks. Pain management sometimes is difficult. During resolution, the soft tissue swelling subsides and the metaphyseal "cuffs" gradually remodel and become smaller. Very severe cases of HOD occasionally are accompanied by septicemia and pneumonia, which rarely can be fatal.

As we've discussed, HOD lesions occur in the area of the metaphyseal cutback zone. The normally irregular and indistinct margins in this area may be mistaken for pathology. Note: there is no soft tissue swelling or pain with normal growth.

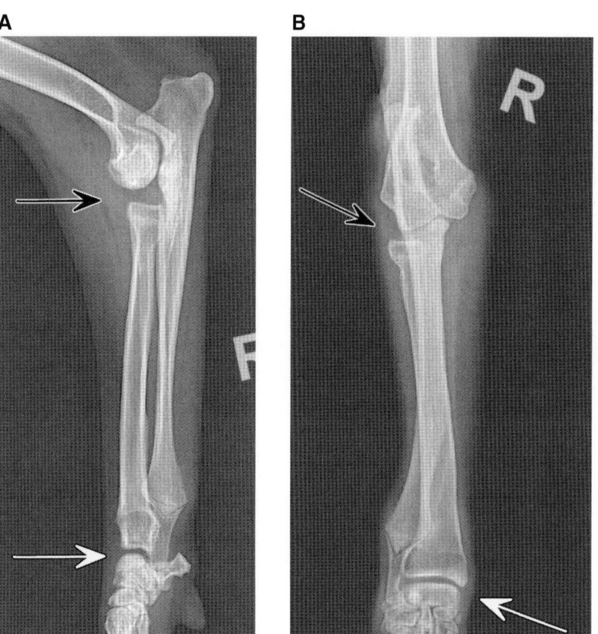

Figure 5.58 Asynchronous growth. Lateral view (**A**) and craniocaudal view (**B**) of a dog antebrachium depicting an abnormally shortened radius that resulted in widening of the humeroradial and radiocarpal joint spaces. The distal radial physis is closed; no further growth will occur here. The ulnar physis is still open so the ulna continues to lengthen normally, leading to the humeroradial and radiocarpal subluxations.

A B

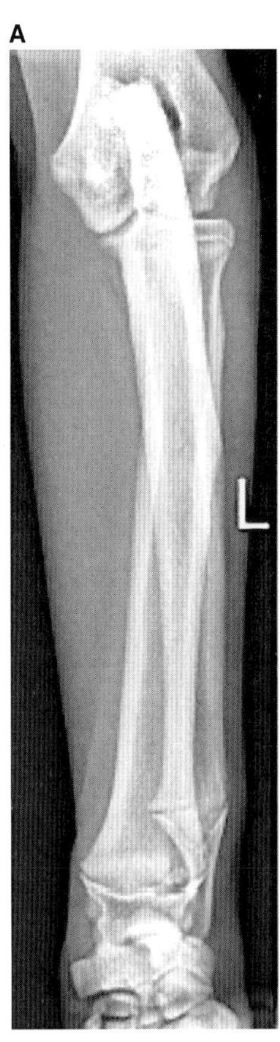

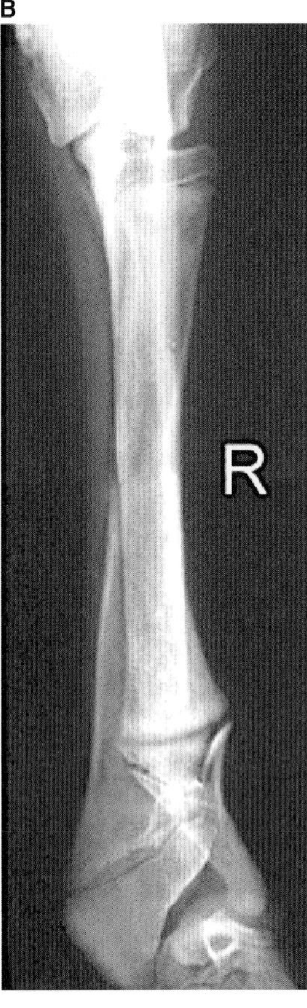

Figure 5.59 Asynchronous growth. Craniocaudal views of an immature dog right antebrachium (**A**) and left antebrachium (**B**) depicting abnormal growth in the right distal radius due to partial damage of the physis. There is less or slower growth at the lateral aspect of the damaged physis than at the medial aspect. Continued growth at the medial aspect leads to carpal valgus and humeroradial subluxation. The left limb is normal.

Hypertrophic osteopathy (HO)

Hypertrophic osteopathy is a periosteal response that occurs secondary to a mass-effect in the thoracic or abdominal cavity. The most common cause of HO is intra-thoracic disease, particularly large lung tumors. HO has also been seen with infection in the thoracic or abdominal cavity, severe cardiomegaly, and secondary to certain tumors and large masses in the abdomen.

The mechanism of HO is unknown, but periosteal new bone forms along the diaphyses of multiple long bones. Usually, all four limbs are involved. HO typically begins in the digits and progresses proximally. New bone formation tends to be bilateral, symmetrical, and progressive, typically with a palisading appearance (Figure 5.63). The margins of the new bone generally are ill-defined during active production and become better defined over time. Margins usually are well-defined in chronic cases (Figure 5.64). Soft tissue swelling is present in most cases, more severe during active bone production. The long bone cortices remain intact without evidence of osteolysis. If disease is unchecked, all long bones in all legs eventually will be affected. Rarely, other bones are involved (e.g., carpi, tarsi, vertebrae, pelvis).

HO most often is reported in middle-aged to older dogs but can occur in any age, breed, or gender. If the primary lesion is removed or otherwise resolved, the bone lesions gradually regress.

Retained cartilage core (distal ulna)

Endochondral cartilage sometimes is retained in the metaphysis of a long bone due to failure of ossification. This occurs most often in the distal ulna, but it has been reported in the distal radius and in the lateral femoral condyle. In radiographs, the retained cartilage appears as a triangular or cone-shaped area of soft tissue opacity in the metaphysis (Figure 5.65). The triangle or cone is widest at the physis and tapers toward the diaphysis. The cartilagenous core may be surrounded by a rim of osteosclerosis. Retention of cartilage sometimes is bilateral and radiographs of the contralateral limb are recommended.

Retained cartilage cores most often are reported in young, rapidly growing, large and giant breed dogs (e.g., Great Dane, Saint Bernard, Setters). The retained cores in many

A B

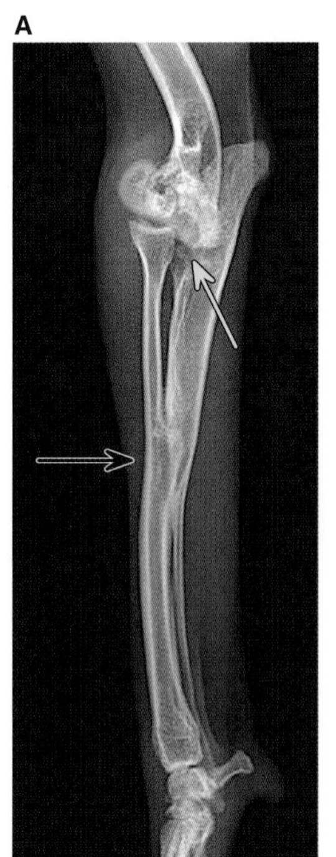

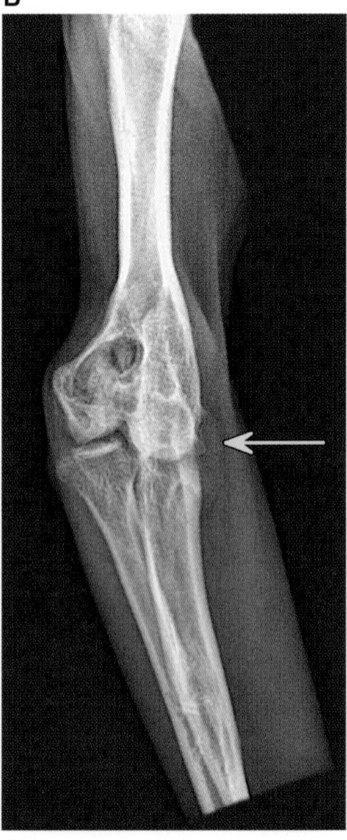

Figure 5.60 Asynchronous growth due to synostosis. **A**. Lateral view of a dog antebrachium depicting a diaphyseal fusion between the radius and ulna (black arrow). The fusion restricted lengthening of the ulna and resulted in elbow subluxation (yellow arrow). **B**. Craniocaudal view of the same dog elbow depicting the elbow subluxation (arrow).

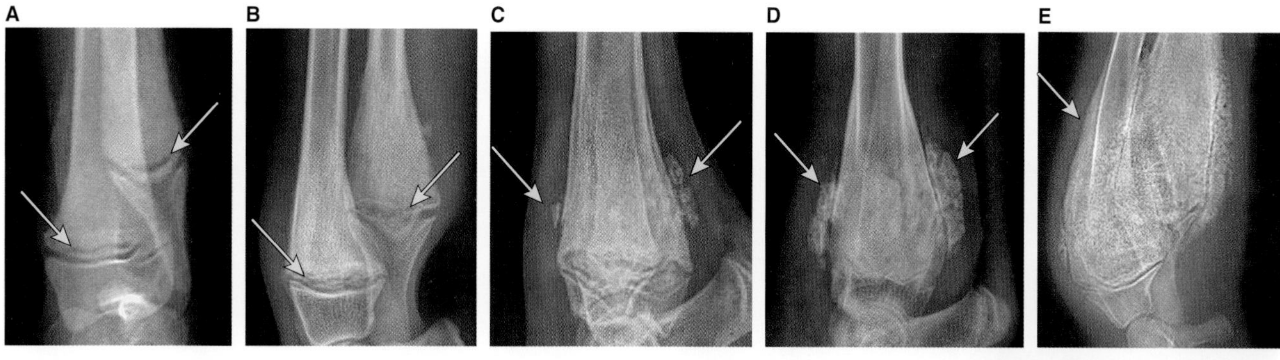

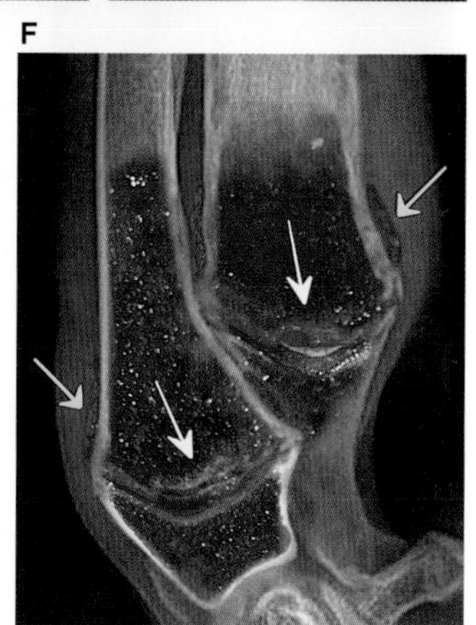

Figure 5.61 Hypertrophic osteodystrophy. **A**. Craniocaudal view of a dog distal antebrachium depicting lines of decreased opacity in the metaphysis, parallel to the physes (arrows). This is sometimes called a "double physis" sign. **B**. Lateral view of the same dog 2 days later with wider soft tissue opacity lines (arrows), more soft tissue swelling, and a minimal amount of mineralized subperiosteal hemorrhage. **C**. Lateral view of the distal crus (same dog a few days later) depicting mineralization of subperiosteal hemorrhage (arrows) and soft tissue swelling. The "double physis" sign is less distinct, but still present. **D**. Lateral view of the same dog later in the disease depicting larger cuffs of new bone around the metaphysis (arrows). The "double physis" sign is no longer evident (typically it only lasts a couple of weeks). **E**. Lateral view of a dog distal antebrachium depicting periosteal new bone filling the space between the elevated periosteum and the cortex (arrow). The new bone is smooth, well-defined, and beginning to organize and blend with the mineralized subperiosteal hemorrhage. **F**. This image depicts superimposition of a pathology specimen on a radiograph of the distal antebrachium to illustrate the appearance of hemorrhage near the physis (white arrows) and under the periosteum (yellow arrows).

cases are temporary, but some are permanent. Retained cartilage sometimes is seen in long bones that are slow growing and may or may not be the cause of the abnormal growth rate. Most retained cartilages are asymptomatic and may even be a variation of normal.

Panosteitis

Panosteitis is a painful bone disease of unknown etiology. Lesions due to panosteitis appear in radiographs as patchy areas of increased medullary opacity in one or more long bones (Figure 5.66). Lesions may resolve in one bone and manifest in another, appearing to "move" from bone to bone. More than one lesion may be present in a bone. Panosteitis usually is bilateral but not symmetrical. It tends to predominantly affect the larger long bones (e.g., humerus, femur, radius, ulna, tibia), but sometimes will involve the metacarpal and metatarsal bones. The areas of increased medullary opacity generally are irregular in shape with ill-defined margins. They usually begin near a nutrient foramen. At the lesion sites, the bony trabeculae often appear hazy and sclerotic, and there is less corticomedullary contrast. In severe cases, lesions may occupy the majority of the diaphyseal region. A thin, smooth-bordered periosteal response sometimes is present, typically with an ill-defined margin during the active stages of panosteitis and a well-defined margin

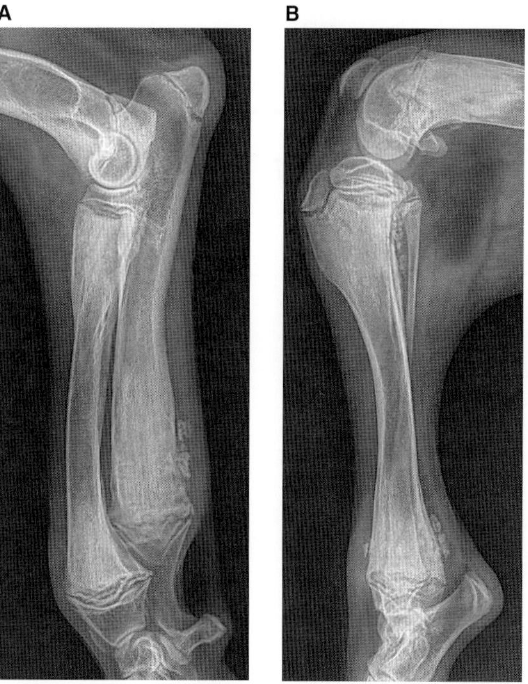

Figure 5.62 Hypertrophic osteodystrophy. Lateral views of a dog forelimb (**A**) and hindlimb (**B**) depicting the distibution of HOD lesions at the ends of the long bones. Notice the increased opacity in the metaphyseal regions due to summation of periosteal new bone.

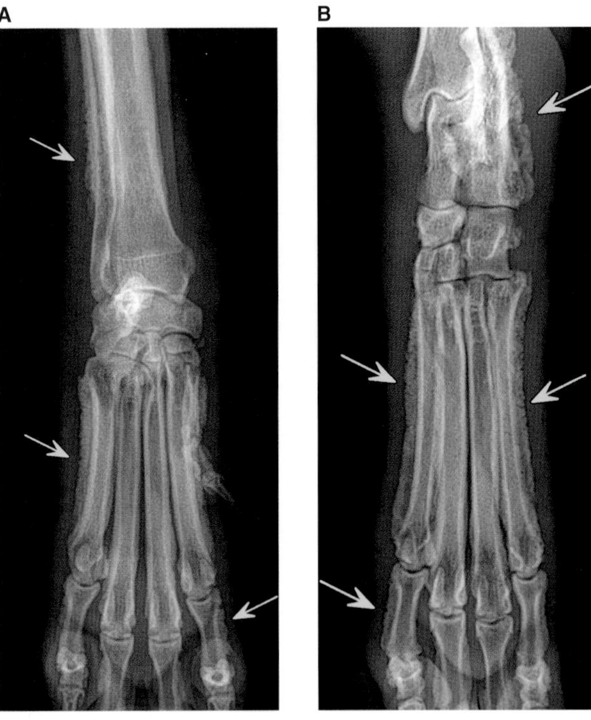

Figure 5.63 Hypertrophic osteopathy. Dorsopalmar view of a dog carpus (**A**) and dorsoplantar view of the same dog tarsus (**B**) depicting an irregular, well-defined, periosteal response along the distal ulna, the metacarpal and metatarsal bones, and the phalanges (arrows). There is diffuse, mild soft tissue swelling. Notice the medullary regions of the long bone diaphyses appear increased in opacity due to summation of periosteal new bone (may be mistaken for panosteitis).

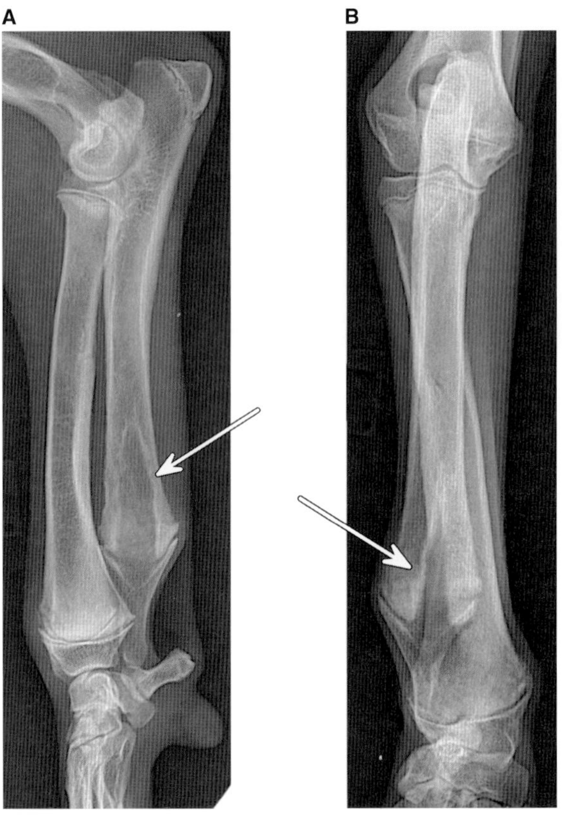

Figure 5.65 Retained cartilage core. Lateral view (**A**) and craniocaudal view (**B**) of an immature dog antebrachium depicting a cone-shaped soft tissue opacity area in the distal ulnar metaphysis, extending into the diaphysis (arrows). The physes and epiphyses are normal.

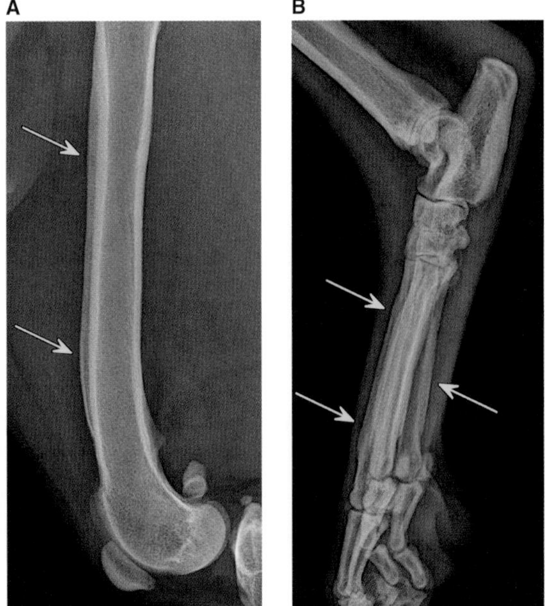

Figure 5.64 Chronic hypertrophic osteopathy. Lateral view of a dog femur (**A**) and tarsus (**B**) depicting a smooth-bordered, well-defined, periosteal response along the cranial border of the femur and the dorsal and plantar borders of the metatarsal bones (arrows).

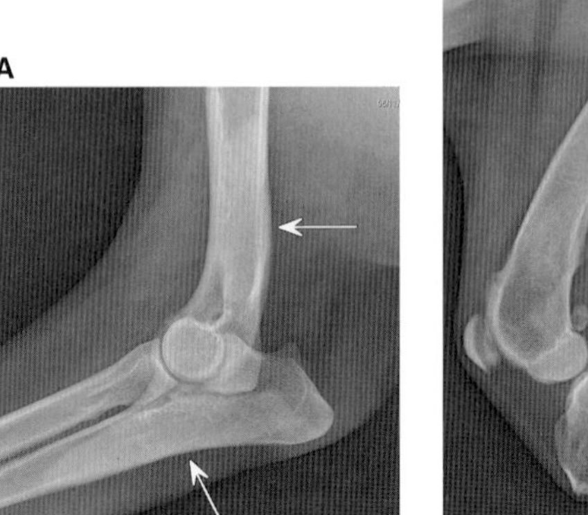

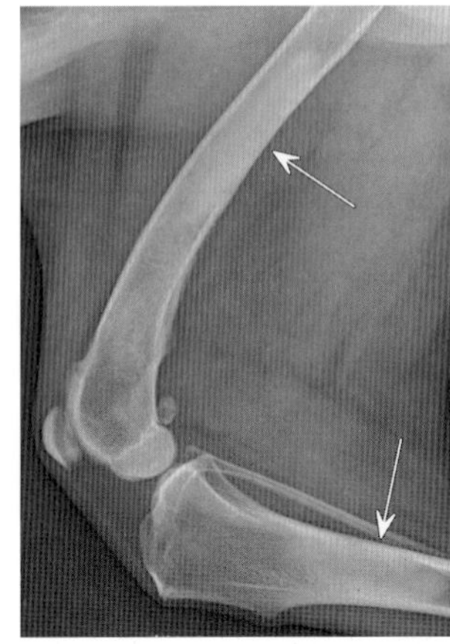

Figure 5.66 Panosteitis. Lateral views of a dog elbow (**A**) and stifle (**B**) depicting increased medullary opacity in the distal humerus, proximal ulna, femur, and proximal tibia (arrows).

when disease is inactive. Soft tissue swelling usually is minimal or absent.

Panosteitis most often is reported in young, large and giant breed dogs (German Shepherds and Bassett Hounds are overrepresented). It occasionally is seen in older animals. Males more often are affected than females. Panosteitis is a self-limiting disease characterized by a sudden onset of shifting leg lameness. Lameness may be protracted over several months and may involve a single limb or multiple limbs, either simultaneously or sequentially. The severity of the radiographic findings may not correlate with the severity of the clinical signs.

During recovery from panosteitis, lesions regress and the bones eventually resume a normal appearance. In some cases, sclerotic lines may persist in the diaphyses. These narrow, transverse lines may resemble growth arrest lines. Another cause of medullary osteosclerosis that may mimic panosteitis is a bone infarct. Bone infarcts, however, are more focal and the margins tend to be sharper (Figure 5.26). Summation of periosteal new bone may be mistaken for increased medullary opacity, particularly in patients with HO or HOD. Determining the distribution of the lesions is helpful to differentiate panosteitis from HO and HOD (Box 5.2).

Box 5.2 Panosteitis vs HO and HOD

- HO and HOD are nearly always bilateral and symmetrical.
- Panosteitis often is bilateral and not symmetrical.
- HO is diaphyseal.
- HOD is metaphyseal.
- Panosteitis is medullary.

Joints

Normal radiographic anatomy

A joint consists of two or more bones united by soft tissue structures. There are three main types of joints, categorized by the type of soft tissue that connects the bones: *synovial*, *fibrous*, and *cartilaginous*. Some joints are combinations of these. For example, the sacroiliac and tibiofibular joints comprise both synovial and fibrous types of joints.

Synovial joints, or *diarthrodial joints*, provide the greatest range of movement. They allow flexion, extension, adduction, abduction, circumduction, and rotation. Synovial joint configurations may be ball-and-socket, hinged, condylar, or pivotal. All synovial joints include a capsule that encloses a cavity that contains synovial fluid and articular cartilage. A meniscus and ligaments may also be present. The joint capsule is composed of an outer fibrous layer and an inner synovial membrane. The synovial membrane produces synovial fluid which nourishes and lubricates the joint. Examples of synovial joints include:

1. Extremity joints (e.g., shoulder, stifle, elbow, tarsus).
2. Facet joints between vertebrae.
3. Atlantoaxial joint.
4. Costovertebral joints: unite the ribs with the thoracic vertebrae.
5. Sternocostal: unite the costal cartilages with the sternebrae.
6. Temporomandibular joints.

Fibrous joints, or *synarthrodial joints*, are the least movable joints. They lack a joint cavity and seldom are visible in radiographs. Sometimes, when the x-ray beam is perpendicular to the joint, a fibrous joint is seen as a thin, soft tissue opacity space between bones. Examples of fibrous joints include:

1. Sutures that unite the flat bones of the skull.
2. Syndesmoses: interosseous ligaments that unite the hyoid bones; unite the tibia with the fibula; and unite the radius with the ulna.
3. Gomphoses: periodontal ligaments that unite the teeth with the underlying alveolar bone.

Cartilage joints unite two or more bones with either hyaline cartilage (*synchondroses*) or fibrocartilage (*amphiarthroses*). Fibrocartilage joints contain an intervening plate of cartilage, which may or may not ossify over time. Examples of cartilage joints include:

1. Parts of the fetal skeleton.
2. Physes: unite the epiphyses with the metaphyses.
3. Costochondral junctions in immature animals.
4. Symphyses in the mandible and pelvis.
5. Intervertebral and intersternebral discs.

Abnormal joint apposition

Abnormal alignment or separation of joined bones may be either a partial or a complete dislocation. A partial dislocation – or subluxation – describes the partial loss of contact between the articular surfaces. A complete dislocation – or luxation – describes the total loss of contact between articular surfaces. Subluxation and luxation can occur with any joint.

The width of a synovial joint space, as seen in most radiographs, primarily represents the thickness of the articular cartilage, as opposed to the volume of fluid in the joint. Both cartilage and synovial fluid are soft tissue opacity. To accurately assess joint space width, weight-bearing radiographs are needed with the x-ray beam directed perpendicular to the joint. A widened synovial joint space in a non-weight-bearing image usually is due to increased joint fluid, but may be caused by an intra-articular mass or loss of subchondral bone. A narrowed synovial joint space most often is due to loss of articular cartilage.

Joint swelling

Soft tissue swelling associated with a synovial joint may be intra-capsular or extra-capsular, focal or diffuse. **Intra-capsular swelling** most often is caused by joint effusion. The type of fluid cannot be determined from radiographs. Swelling due to effusion is restricted by the joint capsule. The edges of the expanded capsule may be visible when outlined by fat in nearby fascial planes. Displacement of the fascial planes is an important sign of joint swelling. The joint space may or may not be visibly widened. Causes of excess fluid in a synovial joint include inflammation, infection, and hemorrhage (see differential diagnoses).

Blood in a joint (*hemarthrosis*) may result from trauma or coagulopathy. Chronic or repeated episodes of hemarthrosis can lead to villonodular synovitis and may erode the articular cartilage. Loss of articular cartilage often leads to a narrowed joint space with irregular and sclerotic subchondral bone.

Villonodular synovitis is abnormal hyperplasia of the synovial tissues, most often caused by repeated episodes of trauma or hemarthrosis. It is uncommon in dogs and cats. The thickened synovium can cause pressure remodeling and osteolysis in the adjacent bone. In radiographs, the osteolytic lesion typically is smooth-bordered and well-defined, sometimes resembling a bone cyst (Figure 5.67). Villonodular synovitis has been reported in the stifle, coxofemoral joint, and carpus of dogs.

Extra-capsular joint swelling tends to be more diffuse than joint effusion and may efface the fascial planes. It typically results from injury to the supporting structures of the joint (e.g., muscles, ligaments, tendons, joint capsule). Types of injuries range from overstretching to complete tearing.

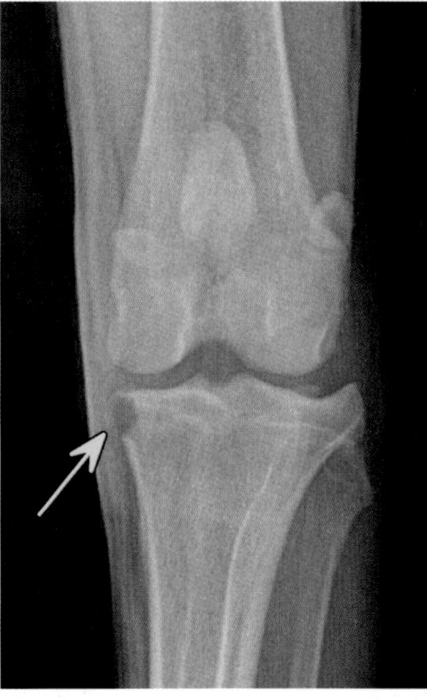

Figure 5.67 Villonodular synovitis. Caudocranial view of a dog stifle depicting a focal area of decreased opacity at the edge of the proximal tibia (arrow) caused by pressure remodeling due to synovial thickening.

Radiographic findings include soft tissue swelling and varying degrees of abnormal joint alignment. Placing the joint in flexion, extension, or stressing the joint during radiography often is helpful to identify laxity and instability. Patients with chronic soft tissue injuries may present with disuse osteoporosis, muscle atrophy, and secondary degenerative joint disease.

Joint swelling due to neoplasia or infection may be intra-capsular, extra-capsular or both. Serial radiographs often are helpful to monitor the progression of disease. Radiographic signs of osteolysis sometimes develop quickly in patients with joint tumors (e.g., synovial cell sarcoma).

Joint mineralization

Mineralization sometimes is seen in arthritic joints. Intra-articular mineral opacity structures often represent fragments of articular cartilage that subsequently mineralized. If such fragments appear to be separate from other mineralized structures, they commonly are called "joint mice." The problem is that without sequential radiographs that prove a fragment is mobile, a free mineral opacity structure cannot be differentiated from an attached mineral opacity structure or mineralization in a meniscus or in the joint capsule.

Gas in joints

Causes of intra-articular gas include a gas-producing bacterial infection, recent arthrocentesis and arthrography. Occasionally, intra-articular gas results from the **vacuum phenomenon**. The vacuum phenomenon occurs when negative pressure is created in a joint, allowing nitrogen gas to emerge from the joint fluid. Negative pressure sometimes is created by pulling on a limb during positioning for radiography. It has been reported in shoulder joints, hip joints, between vertebrae, and between sternebrae. Intra-articular gas due to the vacuum phenomenon is not directly indicative of joint disease, but it happens more often in abnormal joints. Of interest, the vacuum phenomenon has been used as a "contrast procedure" to visualize the articular cartilage in human hip joints.

Joint diseases

There are numerous causes of joint disease, including congenital and developmental abnormalities, metabolic diseases, trauma, inflammation, neoplasia, and others (see differential diagnoses). Radiographic findings often are nonspecific and they can vary considerably, depending on the severity and duration of the underlying disorder (Boxes 5.3 and 5.4). A definitive diagnosis may not be possible from radiographs alone.

Congenital and developmental malformations

Joint deformities that occur at birth or during growth often are permanent. A deformity may be genetic or it may result

Box 5.3 Radiographic description of joint disease

Distribution of lesions:

1. Monoarticular = 1 joint.
2. Oligoarticular = 2–5 joints
3. Polyarticular = 6 or more joints
4. Unilateral or bilateral.
5. Symmetrical or asymmetrical.
6. Confined to specific limbs or parts of limbs:
   a. Thoracic limbs or pelvic limbs only.
   b. Tarsi and/or carpi only.

Soft tissues:

1. Swelling, intracapsular or extracapsular
2. Atrophy
3. Mineralization, intra-articular or extra-articular.
4. Emphysema.

Bone:

1. Osteolytic, osteoproductive, or both.
2. Subchondral bone, sclerotic, lytic, cystic.

Box 5.4 Radiographic signs of joint disease

1. Malalignment of bones (may be mimicked by poor positioning)
2. Joint capsule distension (e.g., joint effusion, synovial thickening)
3. Altered width of joint space (widened or narrowed)
4. Osteophytes (form at edges of articular margins)
5. Enthesophytes (form at attachment sites)
6. Subchondral osteosclerosis or osteolysis
7. Soft tissue mineralization (periarticular or intra-articular)
8. Intra-articular gas (vacuum phenomenon)

from trauma, a nutritional deficiency, or a metabolic disorder. The articulating bones sometimes are abnormal in shape, alignment, or number. Bone malformations can cause abnormal joint stresses, which often lead to pain, an abnormal gait, and an earlier onset of degenerative joint disease. However, some affected animals remain asymptomatic.

Valgus limb deformities are those in which the distal portion of the limb turns outward and the toes point laterally.

Varus deformities are those in which the distal limb turns inward and the toes point medially.

Genu varum is "knock-kneed"; the stifles angle inward, toward each other, and the tarsi become further separated when the stifles are moved together.

Genu valgum is "bow-legged"; the stifles bend outward, away from each other, and the stifles do not touch when the tarsi are moved together.

Genu recurvatum describes a hyperextended stifle; the stifle "bends backward" due to abnormal muscle contracture.

Degenerative joint disease (DJD)

Degenerative joint disease is the most common arthropathy in dogs and cats. It is the end result of all unchecked joint diseases. DJD is often called *arthritis, osteoarthritis,* and *osteoarthrosis*. The development of DJD begins with inflammation (Table 5.6). Inflammation leads to joint effusion which widens the joint space and diminishes the lubricating properties of synovial fluid. Swelling and pain make the joint stiff and decrease its range of motion. Over time, the reduced range of motion leads to greater pressure in the weight-bearing areas of articular cartilage and less pressure at the peripheral, non-weight-bearing areas. In addition, less joint movement reduces the pumping action of joint fluid and decreases nutrition to the articular cartilage. All of this leads to cartilage degeneration. The weight-bearing cartilage becomes thinner due to fibrillation, resulting in a narrower joint space and subjecting the underlying bone to greater stress. Loss of the protective cartilage leads to microfractures in the subchondral bone and osteosclerosis. In severe cases the microfractures can progress to osteolysis, erosive lesions and tiny cyst-like areas. Continued loss of cartilage can result in bone-touching-bone. The cartilage in the non-weight-bearing areas proliferates and becomes thicker. Blood vessels soon extend into this hypertrophied cartilage, leading to mineralization and osteophyte formation. The osseous changes associated with DJD are permanent and irreversible. Progression of DJD sometimes can be slowed with appropriate therapy.

Osteophytes are the most common and specific radiographic sign of DJD. They sometimes appear within a few weeks of joint damage. Osteophytes appear as well-defined, bony projections at the periphery of articular cartilage (Figures 5.68 and 5.69). Similar in appearance to osteophytes are enthesophytes.

Enthesophytes are well-defined exostoses that occur at the attachment sites of tendons, ligaments, and joint capsules. They result from chronic stress or trauma at the attachment and form in the direction of the pull or tension. Enthesophytes frequently develop at arthritic joints, but they are not specific for DJD. An enthesophyte may develop following any episode of abnormal stress or trauma to an attachment.

Both osteophytes and enthesophytes commonly are called "bone spurs," but they must be differentiated from each other and from normal anatomy. It is important to know where cartilage ends and where structures attach, even when not visible in radiographs. For example, some of the bony prominences seen in normal chondrodystrophic patients differ from what might be expected and may be mistaken for bone spurs.

Arthritis

The most common type of "arthritis" in dogs and cats is actually degenerative joint disease. This differs from the "arthritis"

Table 5.6 Stages of degenerative joint disease

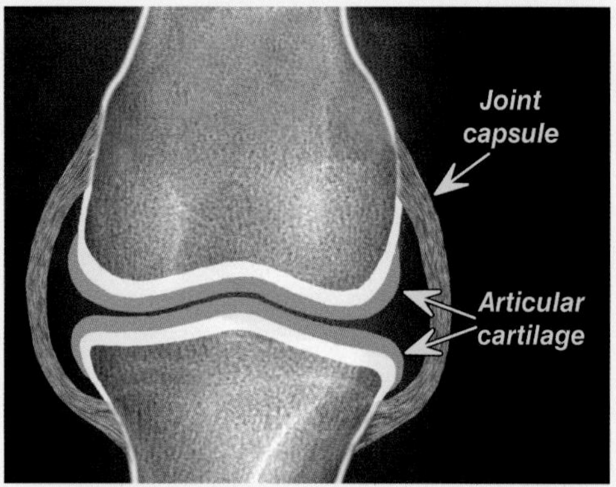

Illustration of a synovial joint. The joint capsule, synovial fluid, and articular cartilage are all soft tissue opacity and would not be distinguished in an actual radiograph. They are displayed here in different shades of gray for illustration purposes. Notice that the space separating the bones is mostly articular cartilage. The lighter shaded area adjacent to the articular cartilage is cortical bone, also called subchondral bone.

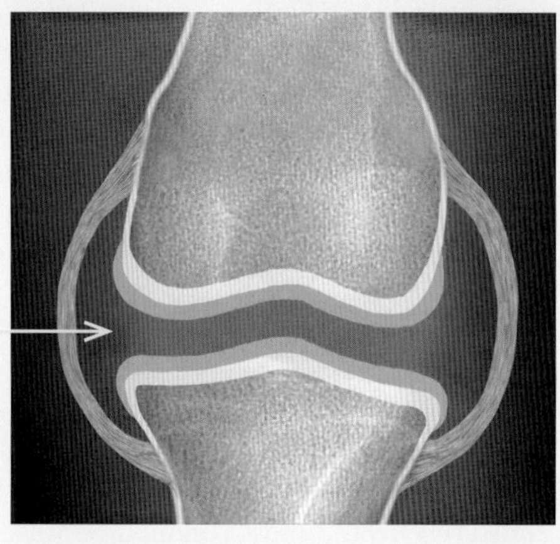

1. Injury to the joint leads to inflammation and joint effusion. Effusion widens the joint space (arrow) and makes the synovial fluid less lubricating. Swelling and pain diminish joint motion which alters weight distribution and reduces nutrition to articular cartilage.

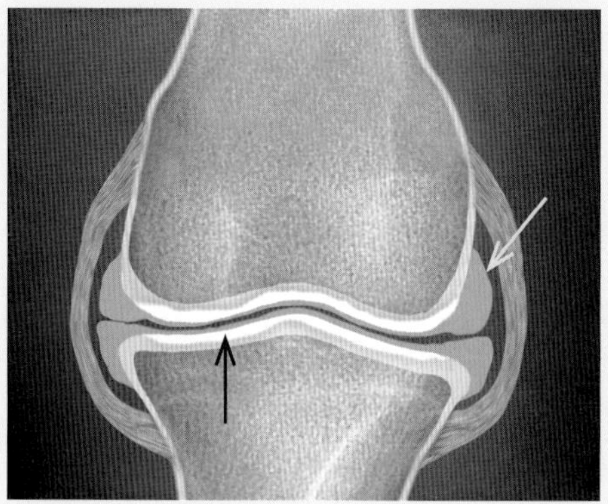

2. The weight-bearing cartilage becomes thinner due to fibrillation, which leads to a narrow joint space and subchondral osteosclerosis (black arrow). The peripheral, non-weight-bearing cartilage hypertrophies (yellow arrow).

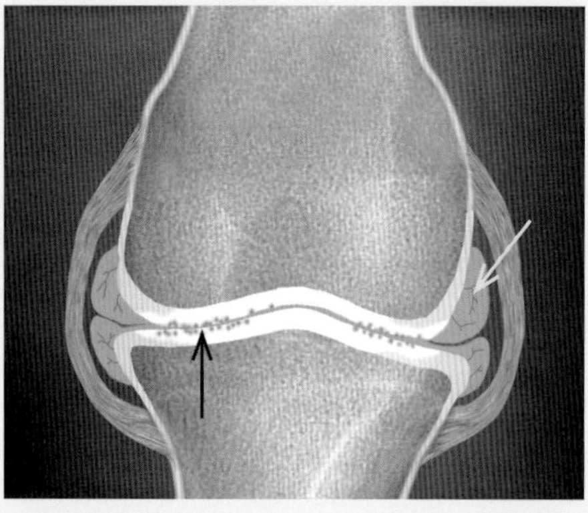

3. Microfractures in the subchondral bone lead to foci of osteolysis (black arrow). Blood vessels enter the hypertrophied peripheral cartilage (yellow arrow), leading to mineralization and osteophyte formation.

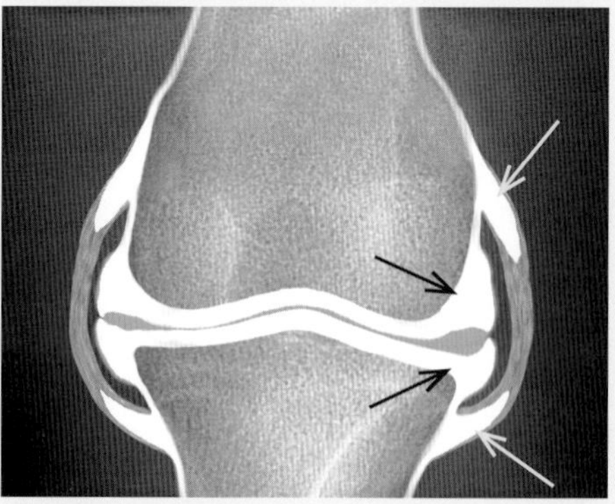

4. Osteophytes develop at the edges of the articular cartilage (black arrows) in non-weight-bearing areas. Enthesophytes form at the attachment sites of the joint capsule (yellow arrows).

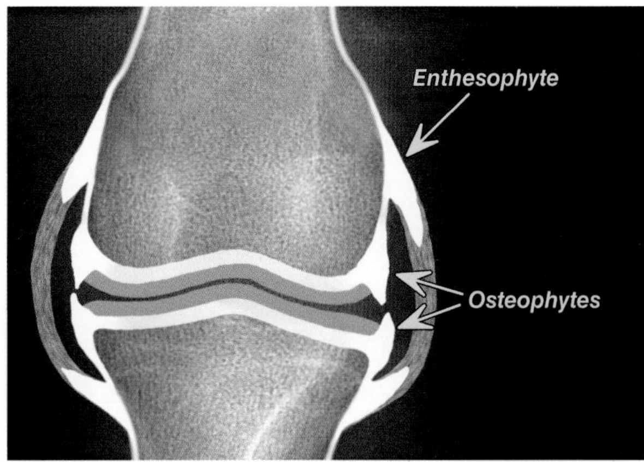

Figure 5.68 Osteophytes and enthesophytes. Illustration of a synovial joint with DJD. Osteophytes form at the periphery of the articular cartilage, in the non-weight-bearing areas. Enthesophytes form at attachment sites (in this case, at the joint capsule attachments). Compare this illustration with the normal synovial joint in Table 5.6.

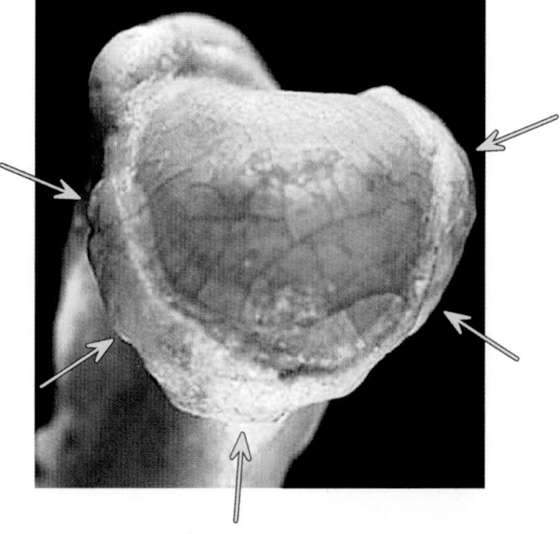

Figure 5.69 Osteophytes. Photograph of a dog humeral head specimen depicting periarticular osteophytes (arrows).

generally described in people, which often is immune-mediated. True arthritis in dogs and cats (not DJD) may be broadly classified as either erosive or non-erosive and either infectious or non-infectious. A third category is immune-mediated. Radiographs frequently are normal during the initial stages of arthritis. Joint effusion and/or periarticular soft tissue swelling are the earliest radiographic findings and may be the only findings, unless the arthritis becomes erosive or progresses to DJD.

Erosive arthritis is characterized by damage to the articular cartilage, to the subchondral bone, and to the supportive structures around the joint. Radiographic signs, however, seldom are evident until the later stages of disease (Figure 5.70). Destruction of the articular cartilage leads to a narrowed joint space and lesions in the subchondral bone. Subchondral osteolysis appears as small "punched out" defects along the articular border. Most erosive arthritides are progressive. In severe or chronic cases there may be marked osteolysis in the long bone epiphyseal regions and

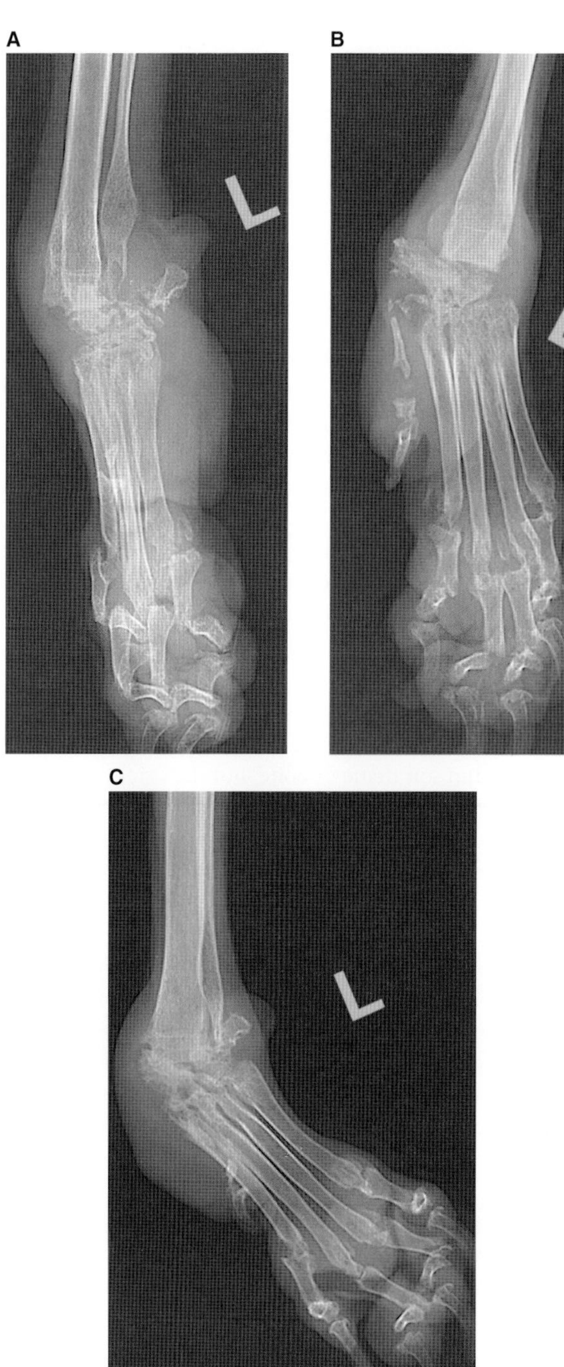

Figure 5.70 Erosive arthritis. Lateral view (**A**), dorsopalmar views (**B** and **C**) of a cat manus depicting extensive subchondral osteolysis in the metacarpophalangeal and interphalangeal joints with joint swelling, collapse of the joint spaces, and weakening of the supportive ligaments.

along the articular borders of the small bones. Osteolytic lesions also may develop at the attachment sites of tendons, ligaments, and joint capsule. Degradation of the joint capsule and supporting ligaments results in joint laxity, subluxation, and luxation. Mineralization sometimes is seen in the supporting structures. Disuse muscle atrophy and osteopenia are common in affected limbs.

Infectious arthritis may be bacterial, mycotic, viral, or parasitic. The causative agent may enter the joint via hematogenous spread, direct extension from an adjacent infection, or a penetrating wound. Blood-borne agents tend to affect multiple joints (polyarticular). Unchecked infections can extend into the subchondral bone causing osteomyelitis. Chronic infection leads to secondary degenerative joint disease. Viral arthritis often is associated with a systemic infection and tends to be polyarticular. Swelling at the joints may be the only radiographic finding. Most viral arthritides resolve within about a week after the systemic disease ends, without any residual joint disease.

Immune-mediated arthritis usually is polyarticular. The etiology often is unknown and a number of complexes or syndromes have been described. Some syndromes are specific to certain breeds of dogs or cats and may be complicated by inflammation in other parts of the body (e.g., myositis, meningitis). Immune-mediated arthritis tends to be more severe in the smaller joints of the distal extremities.

Neoplasia of joints

Tumors are uncommon in the joints of dogs and cats. They may arise from soft tissue or bone, but the origin and type of tumor rarely can be determined from radiographs. Joint swelling is common, usually with an extracapsular component. The joint space may be widened and mineralization may be present in the joint, the latter appearing as either an amorphous, multifocal, or linear pattern. Most tumors that involve a joint are malignant, including **synovial cell sarcomas**, which arise from the synovium in either the joint, bursa, or tendon sheath. Synovial cell sarcomas tend to be aggressive, producing osteolysis in bones on both sides of the joint (Figure 5.71). Usually, there is little to no periosteal response. Synovial sarcomas are uncommon in dogs and rare in cats. They can affect any joint but most often are reported in the stifle or elbow. Tumors in the stifle may displace the patella cranially.

Bone tumors, both primary and metastatic, rarely involve joints. That said, there are reports of osteosarcoma extending into a joint and feline lymphosarcoma involving joints.

Osteochondrosis

Osteochondrosis is a disorder of growing bones in which subchondral bone fails to ossify normally. Abnormal ossification can lead to thickened areas of cartilage that are relatively weak. Normal stresses or minor trauma can soften, collapse, or create fissures in the cartilage. The lesions typically appear in radiographs as flattened or concave defects along the articular margin of the affected bone (Figure 5.72). The bone adjacent to the lesion may appear lytic, sclerotic, or both, depending on the duration and severity of the lesion. Varying degrees of joint effusion usually are present. Sometimes a flap of cartilage becomes separated from the underlying bone, in which case the condition is called **osteochondritis dissecans** or **OCD**. The flap is not visible in radiographs unless it is mineralized. Cartilage flaps may remain attached,

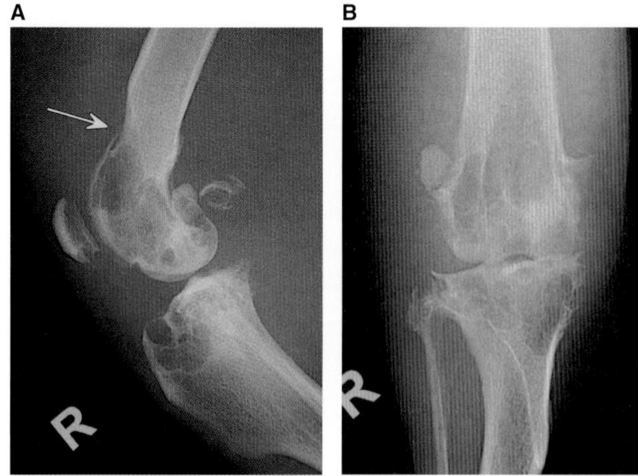

Figure 5.71 Synovial cell sarcoma. Lateral view (**A**) and caudocranial view (**B**) of a dog stifle depicting geographic and permeative osteolysis in the distal femur and proximal tibia. There is a concave defect along the cranial cortex of the distal femur due to pressure remodeling caused by the tumor (arrow).

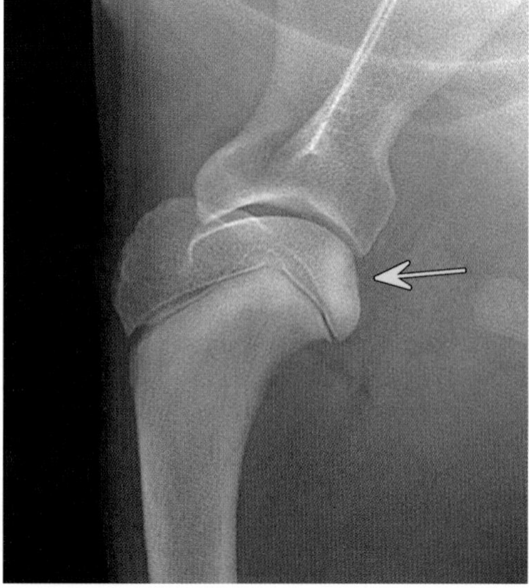

Figure 5.72 Osteochondrosis. Lateral view of a dog shoulder depicting a flattened, osteosclerotic area in the caudal aspect of the humeral head (arrow).

dissolve, or become a free fragment in the joint. A mineralized free fragment commonly is called a "joint mouse." Intra-articular pieces of cartilage, nourished by synovial fluid, may grow and form synovial osteochondromas, which are discussed later in this chapter.

Osteochondrosis lesions can occur in any synovial joint. They are most common in the shoulder, elbow, stifle, and tarsus at the sites described below:

1. Shoulder: caudal aspect of the humeral head.
2. Elbow: humeral condyle, anconeal process, coronoid process.
3. Tarsus: trochlea of the talus.
4. Stifle: femoral condyles.

Osteochondrosis lesions often are bilateral, but clinical signs may only be apparent in one leg. Radiographs of both limbs are recommended. Osteochondrosis is suspected to contribute to other developmental abnormalities of the skeleton, including:

1. Ununited anconeal process in the elbow.
2. Fragmented medial coronoid process in the elbow.
3. Traction apophysitis of the tibial tuberosity.

Osteochondrosis most often is reported in rapidly growing, large, and giant breed dogs. Males more often are affected than females (2 : 1). Multiple factors may contribute to the development of osteochondrosis, including genetics, blood supply to developing bones, and nutrition.

Appendicular skeleton

The positioning guide in Chapter 2 of this book illustrates many of the radiographic views used to image musculoskeletal structures. Radiographs of long bones should include the proximal and distal joints. Radiographs of joints should include the adjacent one-third of each of the articulating bones. Standard orthogonal views of an extremity include lateral and craniocaudal/caudocranial or dorsopalmar/dorsoplantar views. Supplemental views may be needed to further evaluate a structure or to confirm a lesion. Supplemental views are described with each body part in this chapter. Comparison radiographs of the contralateral limb frequently are helpful. Arthrography may be useful to delineate an articular margin or to reveal defects not evident in survey radiographs. The procedure for arthrography, as well as its indications and contraindications, are discussed in Chapter 2, Contrast Radiography. However, the increased availability of arthroscopy, CT, and MRI has largely replaced the need for arthrography.

Shoulder

Normal radiographic anatomy

The scapulohumeral joint is a ball and socket type of synovial joint, able to move in virtually any direction. The primary motions in dogs and cats are flexion and extension. The anatomy of the shoulder is illustrated in Figures 5.73–5.78.

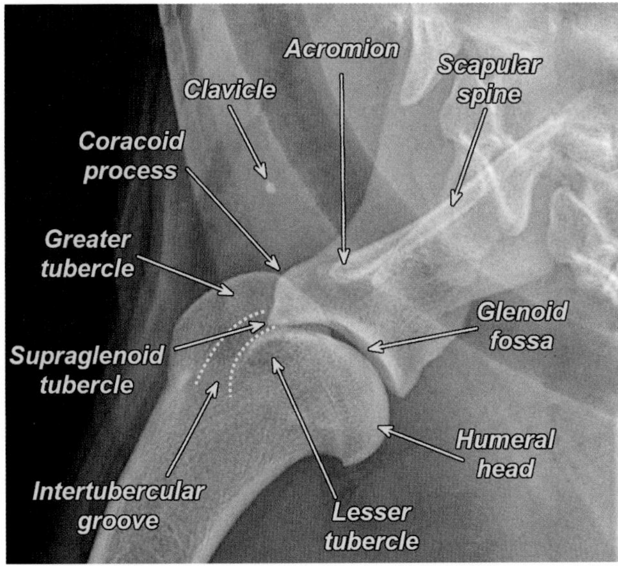

Figure 5.73 Normal shoulder. Lateral view of a dog scapulohumeral joint depicting normal anatomy.

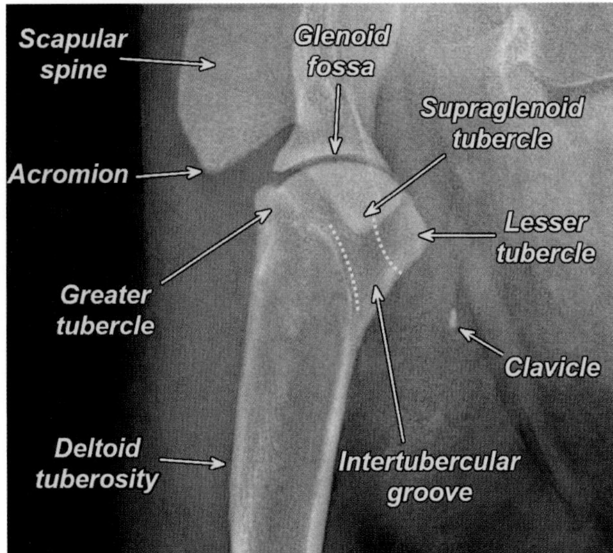

Figure 5.74 Normal shoulder. Craniocaudal view of a dog scapulohumeral joint depicting normal anatomy.

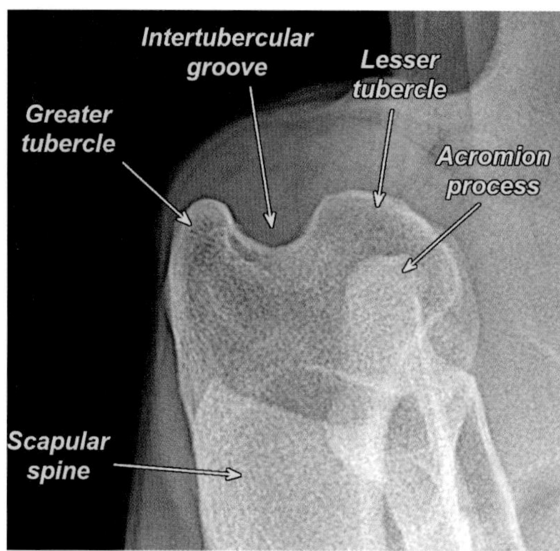

Figure 5.75 Normal shoulder. Skyline view of a dog humerus depicting normal anatomy.

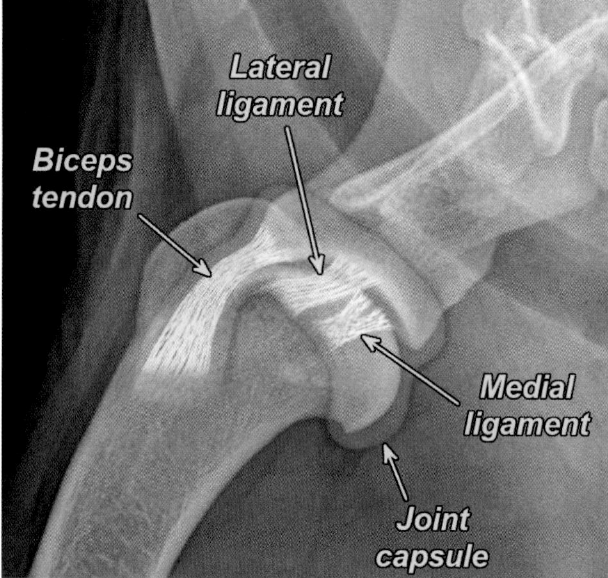

Figure 5.76 Normal shoulder. Lateral view of a dog scapulohumeral joint depicting the attachment sites for the joint capsule and the intra-articular ligaments, the latter including the biceps tendon and the medial and lateral glenohumeral ligaments.

The **clavicles** are located just cranial and medial to each proximal humerus, near the greater tubercles. They are well visualized in cats, but small and only partially mineralized or non-mineralized in dogs (Figure 5.79).

An **accessory ossification center** sometimes is present on the distal scapula, at the caudal aspect of the glenoid (Figure 5.80). It more often is seen in medium to large breed dogs. In many dogs this is an asymptomatic finding, but in some cases it may contribute to shoulder pain and lameness.

The **caudal circumflex humeral artery** frequently is seen end-on in a lateral view (Figure 5.83). It is located near the caudal part of the scapulohumeral joint and when surrounded by fat may be mistaken for a mineral opacity structure in the joint.

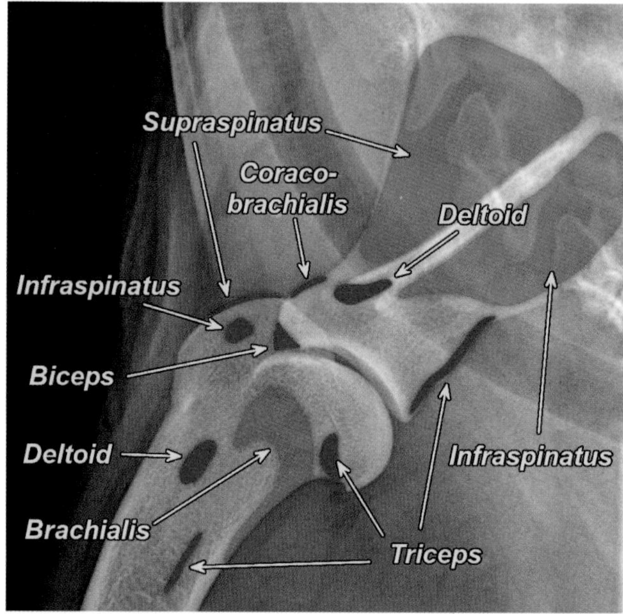

Figure 5.77 Normal shoulder. Lateral view of a dog scapulohumeral joint depicting the attachment sites for muscles and their tendons.

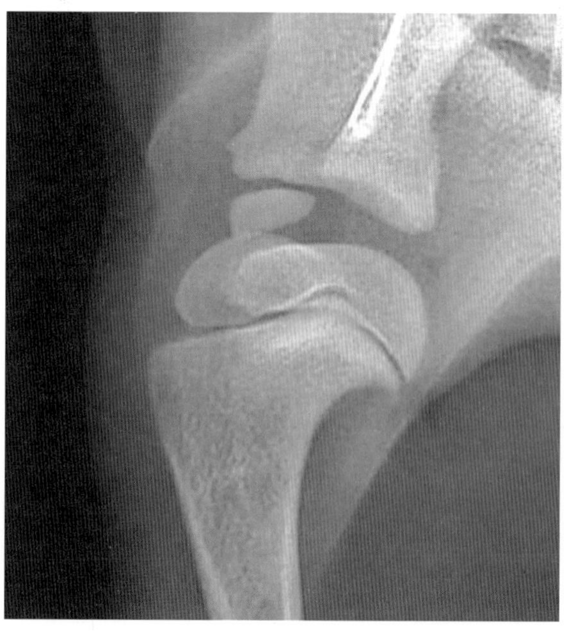

Figure 5.78 Normal immature canine shoulder. Lateral view depicting a puppy scapulohumeral joint.

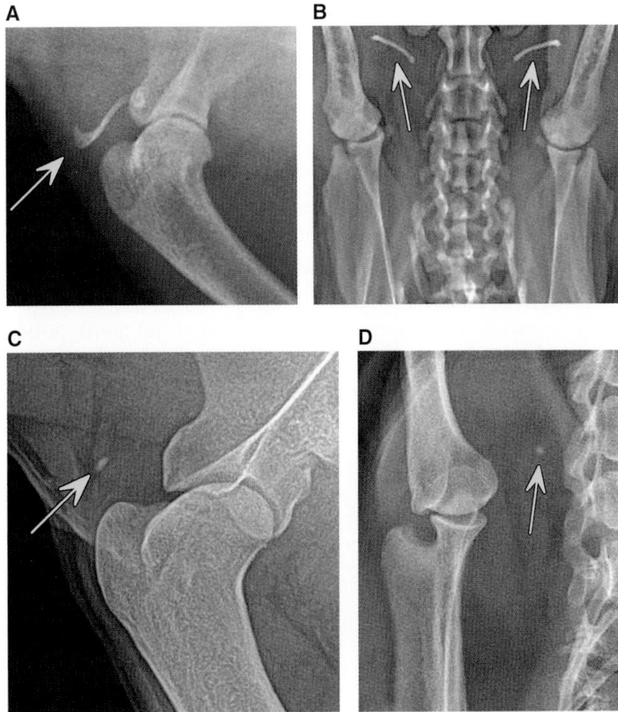

Figure 5.79 Normal clavicle. Cat: lateral view (**A**) and caudocranial view (**B**) of a cat shoulder depicting the relatively large and curvilinear feline clavicles (arrows). Dog: lateral view (**C**) and caudocranial view (**D**) of a dog shoulder depicting the relatively small and incompletely mineralized canine clavicle (arrows).

Radiographic views of the shoulder

1. **Lateral** view (Figure 2.21).
2. **Caudocranial** view (Figure 2.23).
3. **Pronation/supination**: a lateral view made with the limb slightly supinated or pronated to visualize more of the caudal articular margin of the humeral head; often valuable to detect osteochondrosis lesions.
4. **Skyline** view: a cranioproximal–craniodistal flexed view used to better visualize the bicipital or intertubercular groove (Figure 2.24).
5. **Traction** view: a lateral view made while pulling the limb away from the body to evaluate joint laxity. A significant change in the width of the scapulohumeral joint space between no-traction and traction suggests joint laxity which may be due to medial shoulder joint instability. Bear in mind, however, that the shoulder is a relatively loose joint and widening of the joint space can be misinterpreted. Experience and comparison radiographs of the opposite limb help avoid misdiagnosis.

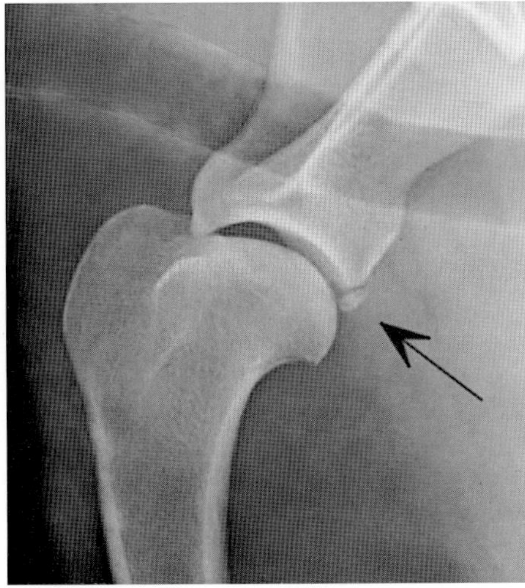

Figure 5.80 Accessory caudal glenoid ossification center. Lateral view of a dog shoulder depicting a focal mineral opacity at the caudal margin of scapular glenoid (arrow).

Shoulder degenerative joint disease

Radiographic signs of DJD in the scapulohumeral joint often are easiest to see in the lateral view. Osteophytes develop at the edges of the articular cartilage, including the bicipital groove (Figure 5.81). Osteophytes in the bicipital groove typically appear as linear mineralization superimposed on the greater tubercle in a lateral view (Figure 5.85). Conditions that may be mistaken for osteophytes include an accessory caudal glenoid ossification center, the normal scapular glenoid in chondrodystrophic dogs, and tendon mineralization.

Shoulder fractures

Soft tissue swelling is common at the fracture site, both intra-capsular and extra-capsular. Avulsion fractures may occur at the scapular tuberosity, the greater tubercle of the humerus, or at the acromion (Figure 5.33). Scapular fractures in the blade or spine of the scapula often are difficult to recognize due to summation of adjacent structures. These fractures sometimes are more evident in a caudocranial radiograph that is centered on the scapula (Figure 2.24), made with the limb extended and the sternum slightly rotated toward the opposite limb.

Shoulder luxation

Luxation of the scapulohumeral joint may be due to trauma or a developmental abnormality. Traumatic luxations generally are unilateral, whereas developmental malformations tend to be bilateral. The proximal humerus may be displaced medially or laterally in relation to the distal scapula. Medial displacement is more likely in small-breed dogs and lateral displacement is more common in large-breeds. Cranial displacement occasionally is seen and caudal luxations are rare. In a lateral view, a luxated shoulder may appear as a narrowed scapulohumeral joint space or the joint space may not be visible due to overlap of the scapula and humerus. Soft tissue swelling is common with traumatic luxations. Swelling sometimes is difficult to see due to superimposition of adjacent structures. Some luxations will spontaneously reduce while the patient is being positioned for radiography.

A

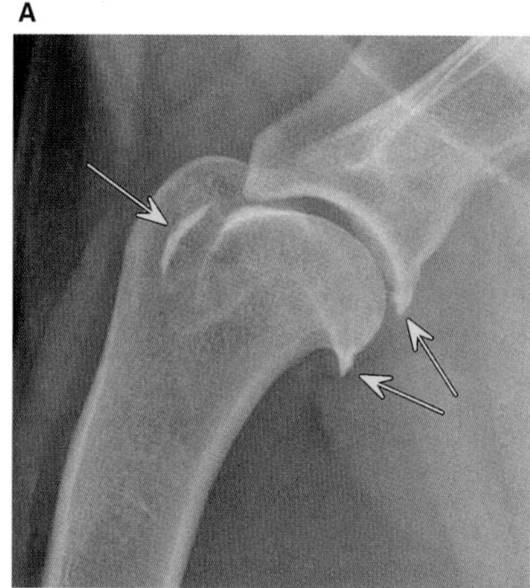

B

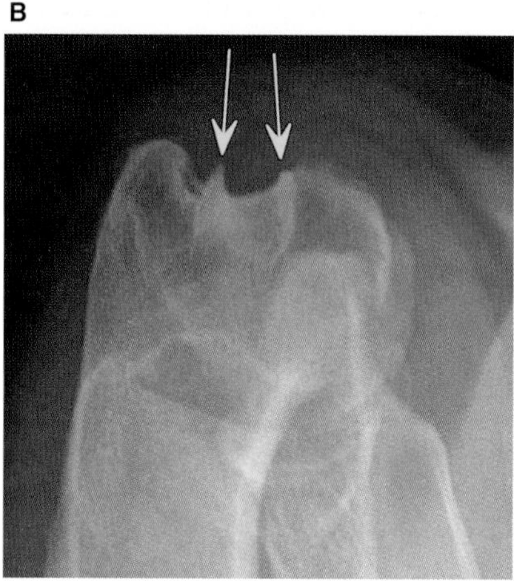

Figure 5.81 Shoulder DJD. Lateral view (**A**) and skyline view (**B**) of a dog shoulder depicting osteophytes on the caudal articular margins of the humeral head and scapular glenoid and along the bicipital groove (arrows).

With chronic shoulder luxations, the bones tend to progressively remodel due to abnormal stresses and may be misshapen (Figure 5.82). Degenerative joint disease is a common sequela. Misshapen bones also occur with developmental abnormalities, particularly in small-breed dogs (e.g., Yorkshire Terrier, Miniature Poodle, Miniature Schnauzer, Japanese Spitz, Pomeranian). Underdevelopment of the glenoid leads to a flattened glenoid fossa. Malformation also is reported in chondrodystrophic breeds (e.g., Dachshund, Bassett Hound), typically appearing as a small, flattened humeral head with an abnormal slope and a shallow glenoid fossa. Misshapen bones generally prevent a successful reduction of the luxation.

Shoulder osteochondrosis

The classic radiographic finding of scapulohumeral osteochondrosis is a flattened or concave defect along the caudal articular margin of the humeral head (Figure 5.83). The lesion often is easiest to see in a lateral view. Sometimes the affected limb needs to be rotated to visualize more of the humeral head to see the lesion. This is accomplished by making lateral views of the shoulder with the limb in supination and then in pronation. Osteochondrosis often is bilateral and radiographs of both shoulders are recommended.

As mentioned earlier, osteosclerosis may surround the defect and sometimes a flap of mineralized cartilage is seen at the lesion site. When present, intra-capsular mineralized fragments typically localize in the caudal joint compartment (Figure 5.84) or sometimes in the bicipital tendon sheath. End-on visualization of the caudal circumflex humeral artery may be mistaken for a mineralized fragment in the caudodistal joint pouch (Figure 5.83). Intra-articular gas occasionally is seen in the scapulohumeral joint due to the vacuum phenomenon.

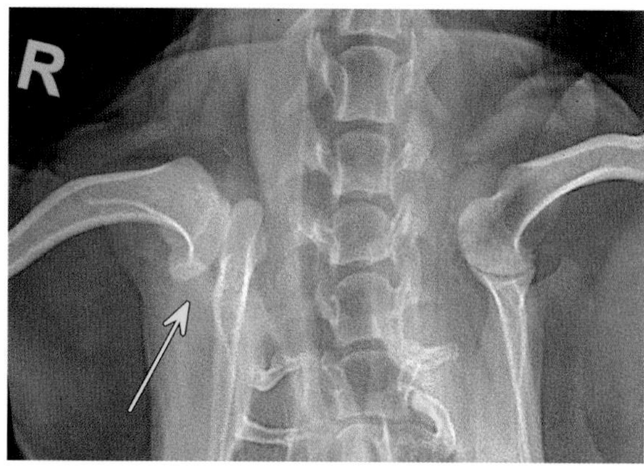

Figure 5.82 Scapulohumeral luxation. Caudocranial view of the shoulders of a dog depicting chronic luxation of the left scapulohumeral joint with remodeling of the humeral head and distal scapula (arrow). The left scapulohumeral joint is normal.

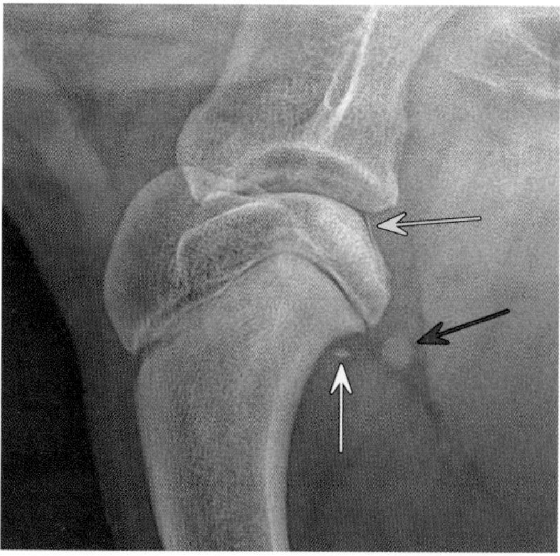

Figure 5.83 Osteochondrosis. Lateral view of an immature dog shoulder depicting flattening of the caudal humeral head with subchondral osteosclerosis and a thin flap of mineralized cartilage (yellow arrow). A mineralized fragment is visible in the caudal joint pouch (white arrow). The deep circumflex humeral artery is seen end-on (red arrow), visible because it is surrounded by fat.

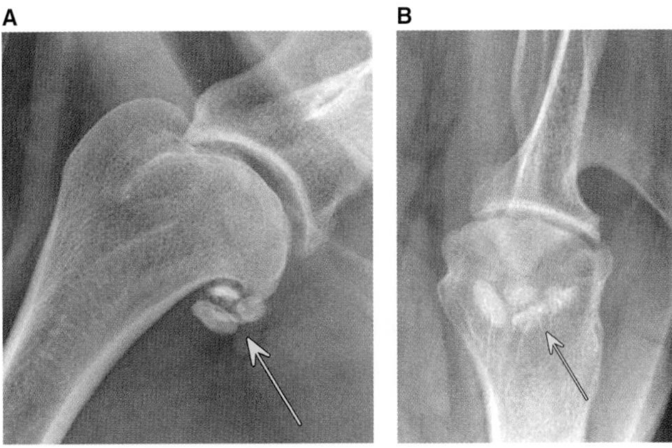

Figure 5.84 Mineralized intra-articular structures. Lateral view (**A**) and caudocranial view (**B**) of a dog shoulder depicting well-defined, mineralized fragments in the caudal joint pouch (arrows).

Shoulder tendinopathy

Tendon pathology may result from acute trauma or chronic inflammation. Acute trauma may result in a partial or complete tear or an avulsion fracture. Shoulder tendon injuries most often are reported in middle-aged, large breed dogs (e.g., Labrador Retriever, Rottweiler). Chronic inflammation often is caused by repetitive, low-grade trauma. Tendon damage may lead to mineralization, which usually is easiest to see in a lateral view (Figure 5.85). Of course, the craniocaudal view should be included for complete evaluation and to help rule out other diseases. Adding a skyline view aids in localizing mineralization relative to the bicipital (intertubercular) groove. Keep in mind that the bicipital groove is lined with articular cartilage and that the bicipital tendon sheath communicates with the scapulohumeral joint. Mineralization in the bicipital groove may be associated with the biceps tendon, its tendon sheath or it may represent osteophytosis.

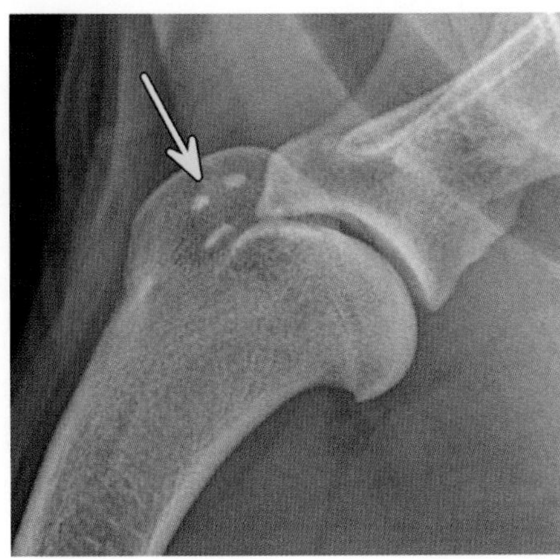

Figure 5.85 Shoulder mineralization. Lateral view of a dog scapulohumeral joint depicting foci of mineralization in the area of the greater tubercle (arrow). Mineralization in this area may represent osteophytes along the bicipital groove or it may be associated with the supraspinatus, infraspinatus, or biceps muscle tendon or joint capsule. Occasionally, sesamoid bones are present in this area. Note: mineralization occurs over time and may or may not be associated with current lameness.

The **biceps tendon** originates on the supraglenoid tubercle. Chronic inflammation can lead to an irregular and indistinct bony margin or enthesopathy at the tubercle. In an arthrogram (Figure 2.95), the margin of a chronically inflammed biceps tendon may be irregular. Filling defects may be seen in the tendon sheath or joint due to free fragments or iatrogenic introduction of gas bubbles. Fibrosis or synovial hyperplasia may limit filling of the bursa.

The **supraspinatus** and **infraspinatus tendons** are very short. Radiographic evidence of tendinopathy most often is seen at their insertions. The supraspinatus inserts on the medial aspect of the greater tubercle and the infraspinatus inserts on the lateral aspect. Injuries to these tendons may appear as focal, rounded areas of decreased opacity in the greater tubercle. Tendon mineralization may be visible near the proximal aspect of the greater tubercle (Figure 5.86).

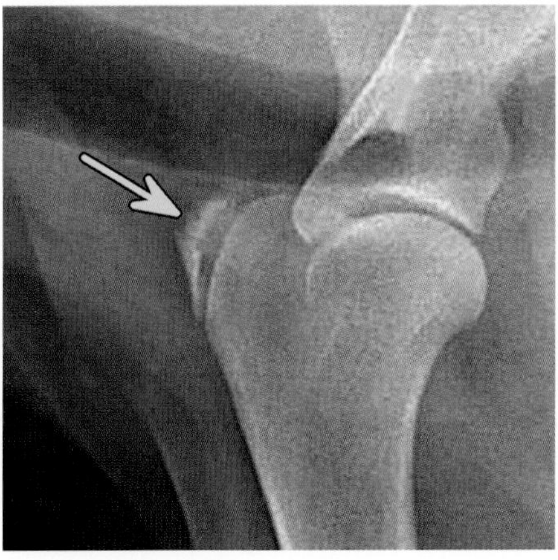

Figure 5.86 Supraspinatus tendinopathy. Lateral view of a dog shoulder depicting mineralization along the cranial border of the greater tubercle (arrow), in the area of insertion of the supraspinatus muscle tendon.

Elbow

Normal radiographic anatomy

The elbow is a hinged synovial joint that is a composite of two articulations: the *humeroradial* joint and the *humeroulnar* joint. The **humeroradial** joint is formed by the humeral condyle and the radial head. It transmits most of the weight supported by the limb and allows rotation of the antebrachium. The **humeroulnar** joint is formed by the humeral condyle and the trochlear notch of the ulna. It stabilizes the elbow, restricting movement to the sagittal plane. Both joints share a common joint capsule. Elbow anatomy is illustrated in Figures 5.87–5.95. In cats there is a supracondylar foramen on the lateral aspect of the distal humerus (Figure 5.90), located proximal to the humeral condyle. The brachial artery and median nerve pass through this opening.

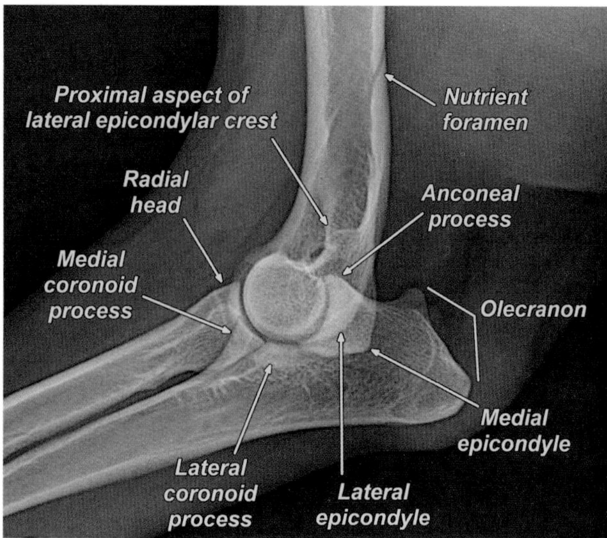

Figure 5.87 Normal elbow. Lateral view of a dog elbow depicting normal anatomy.

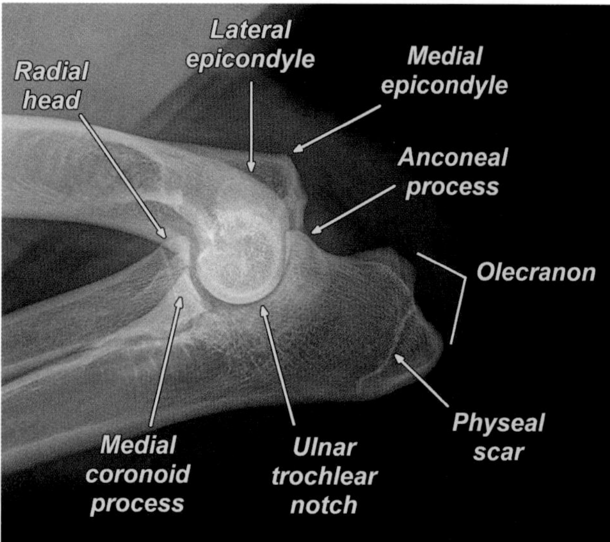

Figure 5.88 Normal elbow. Flexed lateral view of a dog elbow depicting normal anatomy. The trochlear notch of the ulna is also called the **semilunar notch**.

At the proximal end of the ulna there are three important prominences: the oleranon, the anconeal process, and the coronoid process.

The **olecranon** is the "head of the ulna."

The **anconeal process** is the part of the ulna that fits in the olecranon fossa of the humerus. It develops from a secondary ossification center that becomes visible in radiographs at about 11 weeks of age. The anconeal process normally fuses with the olecranon by about 20 weeks of age.

The **coronoid process** serves to increase the articular surface area of the elbow. It is divided into a prominent medial extension that articulates with the radius and a smaller lateral extension that articulates with the distal humerus.

A **sesamoid bone** frequently is present lateral to the elbow, especially in cats and larger dogs. It usually is bilateral, located near the head of the radius in the tendon of the supinator muscle or sometimes in the annular ligament (Figure 5.89).

Radiographic views of the elbow

1. **Lateral** view (Figure 2.25).
2. **Craniocaudal** view (Figure 2.27).
3. **Flexed lateral** view: lateral view made with the elbow in extreme flexion to better visualize the anconeal process by eliminating superimposition of the humeral medial epicondyle (Figure 2.26)
4. **Craniolateral-caudomedial oblique** view: a craniocaudal view made with the limb in a neutral, slightly inwardly rotated position instead of fully extended to better visualize the medial coronoid process (Figure 2.28).
5. **Craniodistal-caudoproximal** view: a craniocaudal view made with the x-ray beam angled 20° to enhance visualization of the elbow joint space (Figure 2.27).
6. **Stress view**: a craniocaudal view made with the distal humerus and proximal antebrachium stabilized while a medial-to-lateral or lateral-to-medial force is applied to the elbow to assess joint laxity and integrity (Figure 2.31).

Elbow degenerative joint disease

DJD in the elbow most often is a sequela to a congenital elbow condition, many of which are discussed below. It may

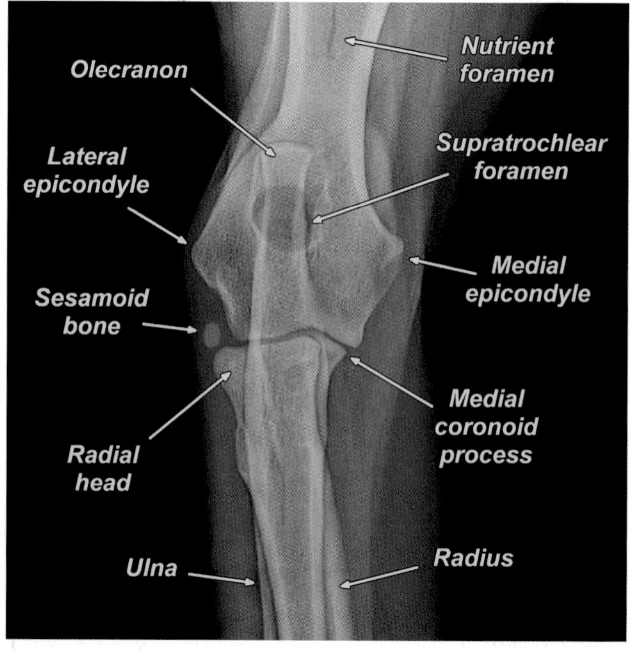

Figure 5.89 Normal elbow. Craniocaudal view of a dog elbow depicting normal anatomy.

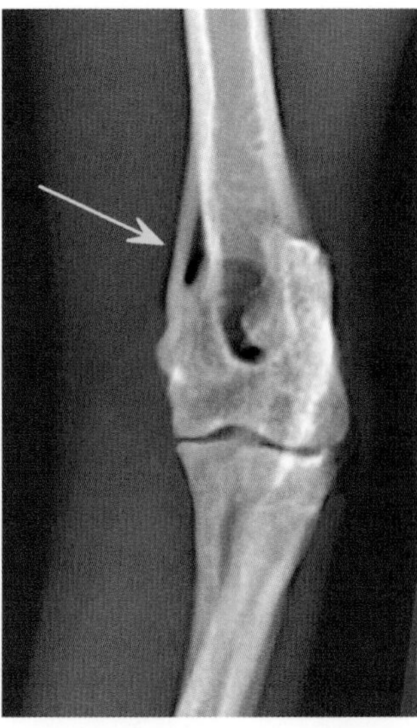

Figure 5.90 Supracondylar foramen. Craniocaudal oblique view of a cat elbow depicting the normal foramen on the lateral aspect of the distal humerus (arrow).

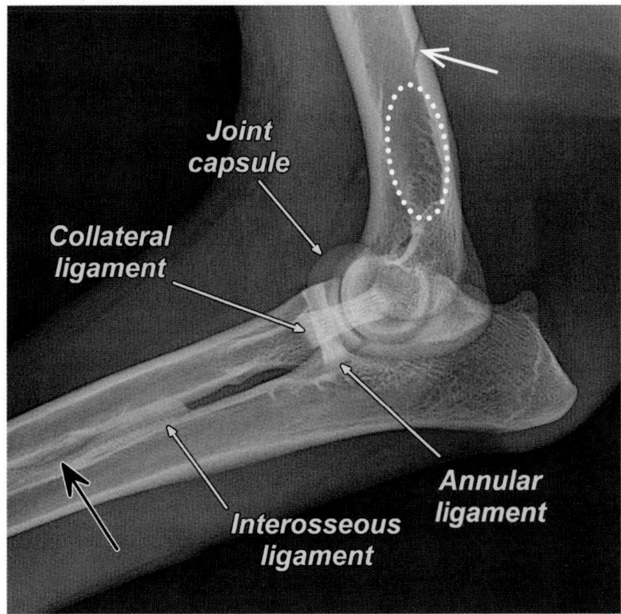

Figure 5.91 Normal elbow. Lateral view of a dog elbow depicting the attachment sites for ligaments and the joint capsule. The black arrow points to enthesopathy at the attachment of the interosseous ligament. This is a common and usually asymptomatic finding. There is no osteolysis and the amount of interosseous mineralization can vary considerably between individuals. The white dotted oval indicates the normally less opaque part of the humeral medullary cavity, located distal to the nutrient foramen (white arrow). This part of the distal humerus is a common area for panosteitis lesions. If this area is not relatively less opaque, consider panosteitis as the cause.

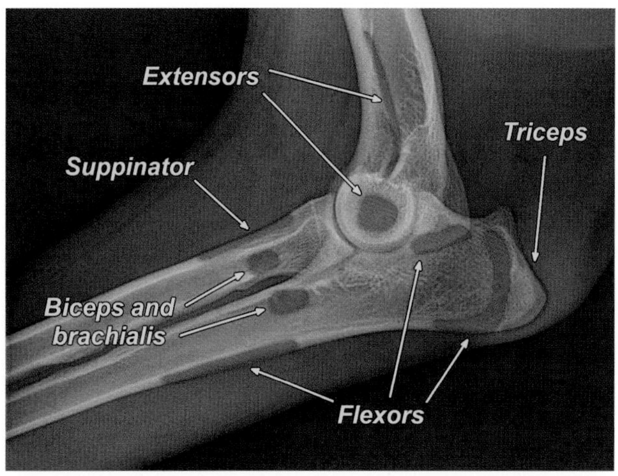

Figure 5.92 Normal elbow. Lateral view of a dog elbow depicting the attachment sites for muscles and their tendons.

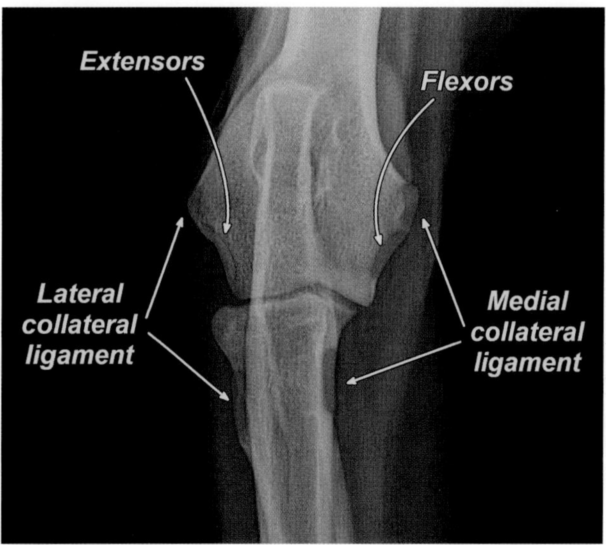

Figure 5.93 Normal elbow. Craniocaudal view of a dog elbow depicting attachment sites for the collateral ligaments and the origins of the flexor and extensor muscle tendons.

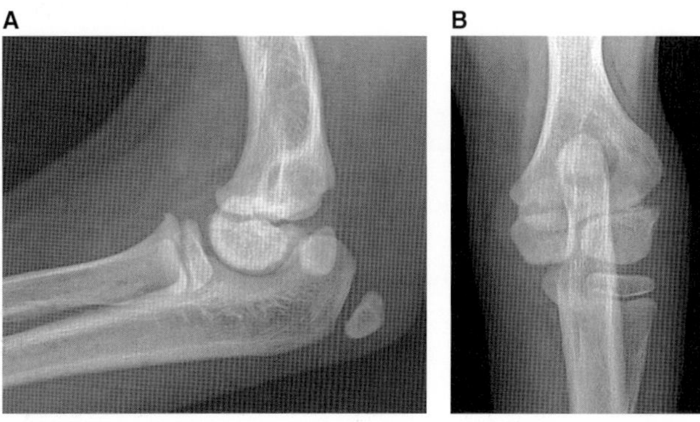

Figure 5.94 Normal immature canine elbow. Lateral view (**A**) and craniocaudal view (**B**) depicting a puppy elbow.

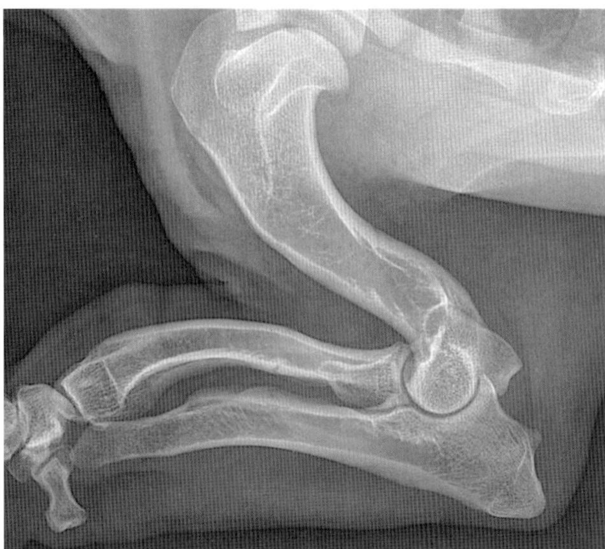

Figure 5.95 Chondrodystrophic forelimb. Lateral view of the thoracic limb of an adult Corgi with no evidence of lameness.

also follow elbow trauma or chronic inflammation. DJD usually is bilateral but not necessarily symmetrical (Figure 5.96).

An **enthesophyte** in the flexor tendon is sometimes seen extending distally from the caudal border of the medial epicondyle (Figure 5.97). It commonly is called *flexor enthesopathy* or a *medial epicondylar spur*. The enthesophyte often is an asymptomatic finding, but occasionally it is associated with mild lameness. It may be accompanied by additional mineralization in the flexor tendon, located further distal and more medial to the epicondyle. Flexor enthesopathy is seen more often in large-breed dogs and may be unilateral or bilateral.

Elbow dysplasia

The term "elbow dysplasia" was introduced several years ago to help understand a group of elbow abnormalities that are now recognized as the following six conditions:

1. Asynchronous growth of the radius and ulna (discussed earlier with congenital and developmental abnormalities).
2. Fragmented medial coronoid process.
3. Ununited anconeal process.
4. Elbow incongruity.
5. Osteochondrosis.
6. Ununited medial humeral epicondyle.

Each of these disorders is discussed in more detail below. They can occur independently or in conjunction with one another. Elbow dysplasia most often is reported in young, medium to large breed dogs. Males more often are affected than females. Clinical signs of pain and lameness typically develop between 4 and 18 months of age, but some dogs remain asymptomatic for years. Lameness tends to be worse after exercise. In severe cases, the thoracic limbs may rotate inward and the elbows rotate outward (relative to their normal orientation). Elbow dysplasia often is bilateral, but clinical signs may be unilateral. Radiographs of both elbows are recommended. Degenerative joint disease is a common sequela to elbow dysplasia, and it is progressive. Signs of DJD may be evident as early as 7 months of age.

A

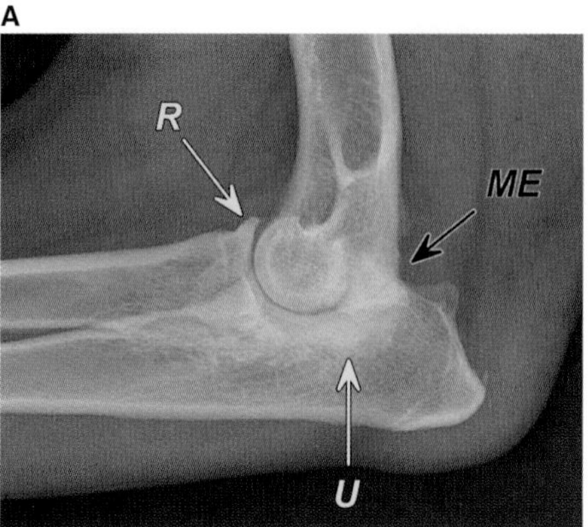

B

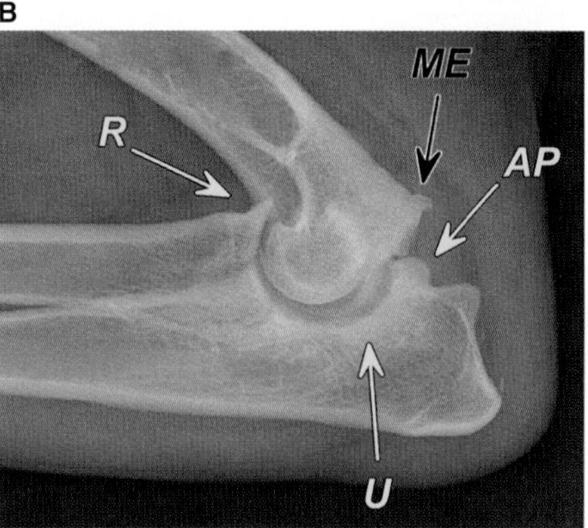

C

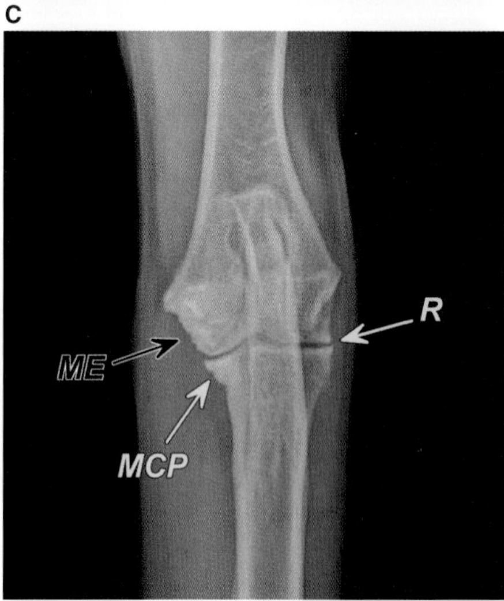

Figure 5.96 Elbow DJD. Lateral view (**A**), flexed lateral view (**B**), and craniocaudal view (**C**) of a dog elbow depicting osteophytes on the radial head (R), medial coronoid process (MCP), along the ulnar trochlear notch (U), and at the anconeal process (AP) as indicated by the yellow arrows. The black arrows point to enthesophytes on the medial epicondyle (ME). The bone spurs on the medial epicondyle and anconeal process are not well visualized in the lateral view (**A**) due to summation. The lesions are readily identified in the flexed lateral view (**B**).

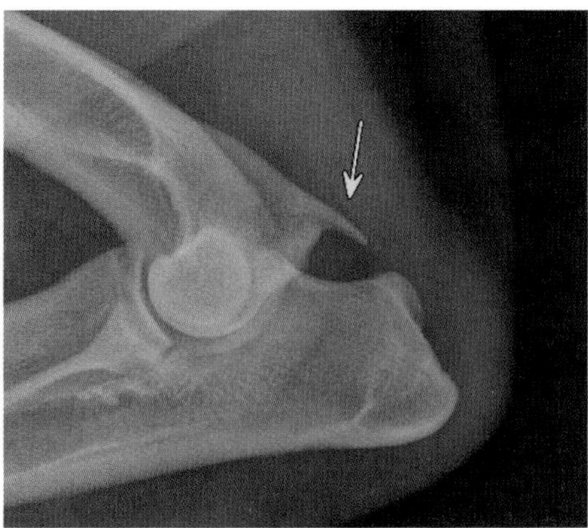

Figure 5.97 Elbow enthesophyte. Lateral view of a dog elbow depicting a bone spur on the medial epicondyle (arrow).

Fragmented ulnar medial coronoid process

The medial coronoid process is easiest to see in a craniolateral-caudomedial oblique view. A normal process is sharply marginated and triangular in shape. A fragmented process typically appears less distinct than the adjacent bone with a blunted, rounded, or irregular shape (Figure 5.98).

Fragmented medial coronoid process is the most common elbow disorder in dogs. It occurs in many breeds, most often reported in Bernese Mountain Dog, Labrador Retriever, Golden Retriever, Rottweiler, Newfoundland, and German Shepherd. Although it is most common, a fragmented medial coronoid process is difficult to diagnose with certainty from radiographs because an actual fragment seldom is seen. The fragment may not be completely separated from the ulna or it may fail to mineralize and remain soft tissue opacity cartilage. Essentially, if there is osteophyte or enthesophyte formation or indistinct bony margins on the medial aspect of the elbow joint with no other abnormalities, the radiographic findings are most likely due to fragmented medial coronoid process.

Sometimes a small, concave defect (a focal area of osteolysis) is seen immediately opposite the medial coronoid process, on the medial articular margin of the humeral condyle (Figure 5.98). This defect commonly is called a "kissing lesion". It may be difficult to distinguish from an osteochondrosis defect (Figure 5.107).

In some patients with fragmented medial coronoid process, osteophytes develop on the proximal margin of the anconeal process (Figure 5.96). The new bone is easiest to see in an extreme flexed lateral view. It is important to note that in some dogs the edge of the ulnar trochlear notch is visible dorsal to the border of the anconeal process and may be mistaken for pathology (Figures 5.99–5.103).

Ununited anconeal process

An anconeal process is considered ununited if it fails to fuse with the ulna by 20 weeks of age. In German Shepherds, it should fuse by 22 weeks of age. Failure to fuse leads to elbow instability and progressive DJD.

In radiographs of an united anconeal process, a line of soft tissue opacity usually is visible between the process and the olecranon (Figure 5.104). The line represents the physis and it may be partial or complete. Note: if any part of the physis remains open after about 5 months of age it is abnormal. If the patient is near 5 months old, repeat the radiographs in 1 or 2 weeks to be sure the anconeal process is abnormal. An united anconeal process may or may not be visibly displaced. It often is best evaluated in an extreme flexed lateral view, which eliminates superimposition of the medial epicondyle. This is particularly important in immature dogs where the

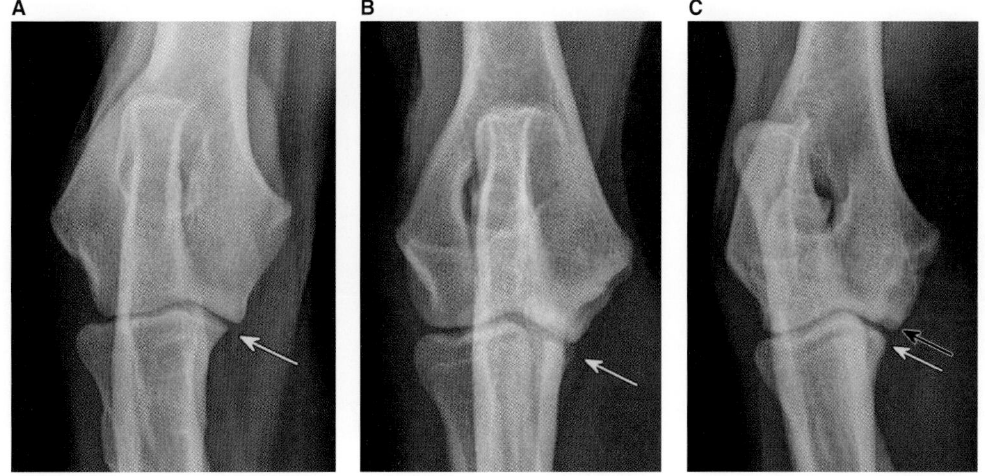

Figure 5.98 Fragmented medial coronoid process. **A**. Craniocaudal view of a dog elbow depicting the normal appearance of the medial coronoid process (arrow). **B**. Craniocaudal view of a different dog elbow depicting a blunted, rounded medial coronoid process (arrow). The process is not well visualized due to superimposition of the ulna. **C**. Craniocaudal oblique view of the same dog as in (**B**). Rotation of the elbow eliminates superimposition of the ulna to improve visualization of the blunted medial coronoid process (yellow arrow) and reveals a focal area of osteolysis in the distal humerus (a "kissing lesion", black arrow).

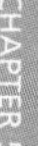

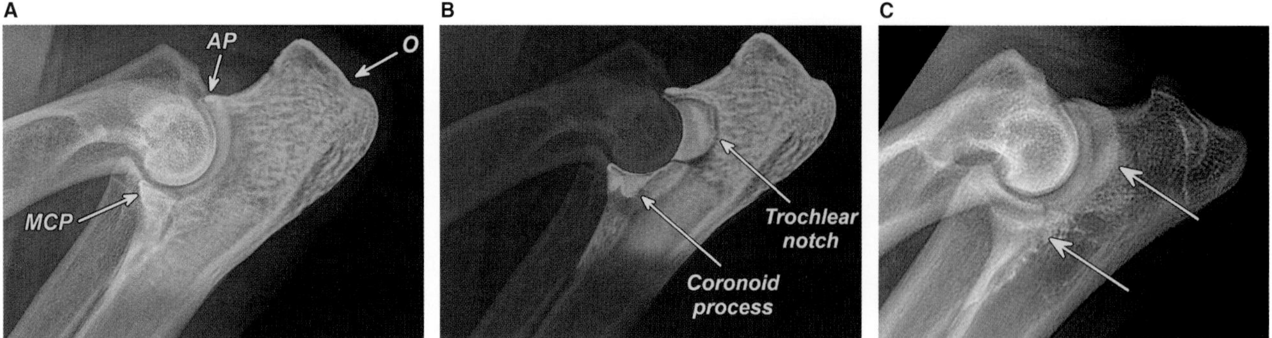

Figure 5.99 Ulnar articular surfaces. **A**. Flexed lateral view of a dog elbow illustrating the medial coronoid process (MCP), anconeal process (AP), and olecranon (O). **B**. Same specimen as **A**, but the ulna is highlighted and the other bones faded to show the articular surfaces of the ulnar coronoid process (medial and lateral projections) and trochlear notch. **C**. An actual radiograph with the same ulnar articular surfaces highlighted (arrows).

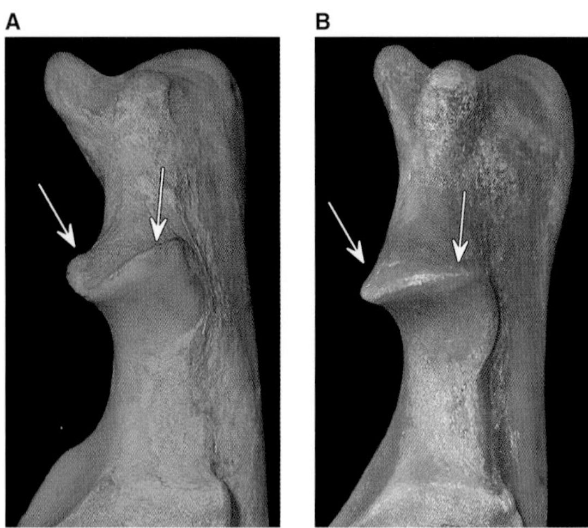

Figure 5.100 Ulnar trochlear notch. Photographs of two different canine bone specimens that demonstrate a normal variation in the appearance of the ulnar trochlear notch (arrows). The articular edges in **A** extend further proximally than in **B**.

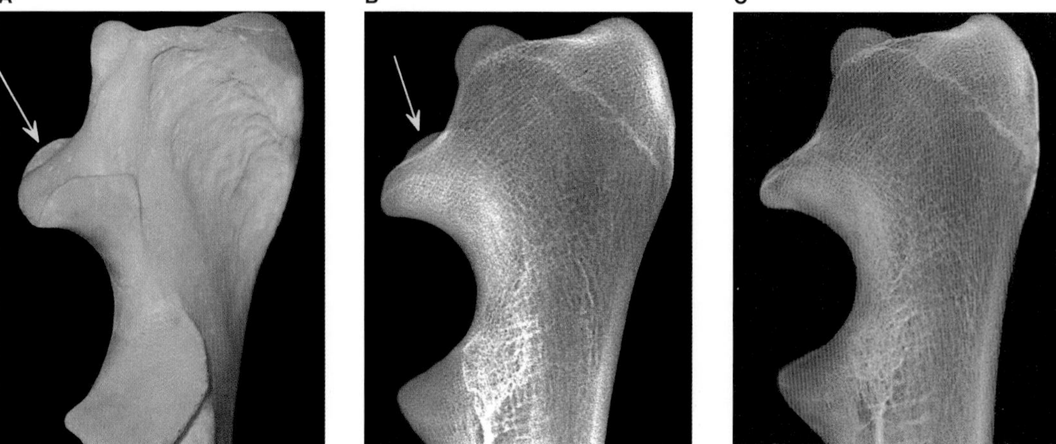

Figure 5.101 Ulnar trochlear notch. **A**. Photograph of the same ulna as in Figure 5.100A, but from a different angle. The articular border of the trochlear notch is visible above (proximal to) the anconeal process (arrow). **B**. Lateral radiograph of an ulna in which the articular border of the trochlear notch projects proximal to the anconeal process (arrow). **C**. Lateral radiograph of a different ulna in which the articular border of the trochlea is not visible proximal to the anconeal process.

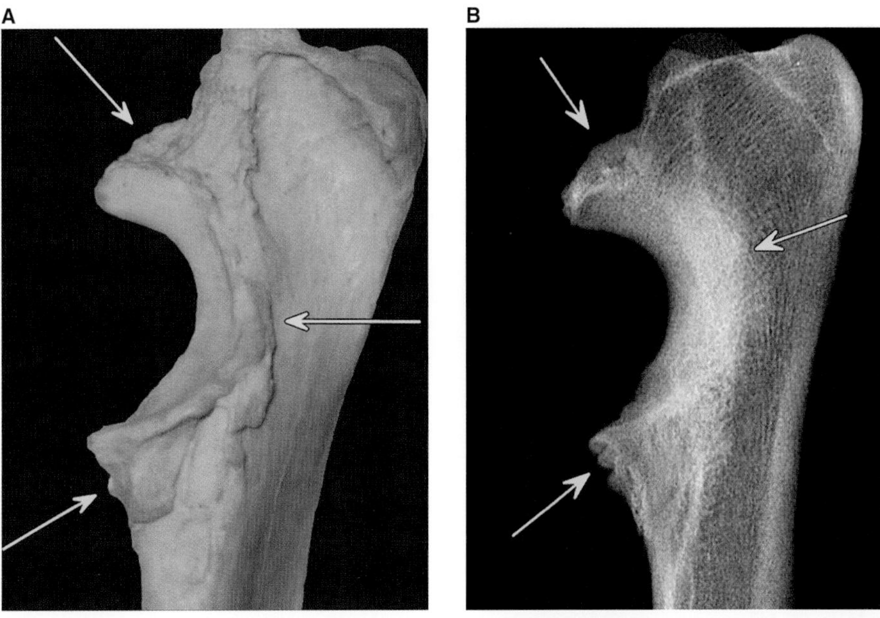

Figure 5.102 Ulnar degenerative changes. **A**. Photograph of an ulna bone specimen with osteophytes along the trochlear notch and anconeal process (arrows). **B**. Lateral radiograph of the ulna bone specimen (arrows point to osteophytes). Compare with the normal ulna bone specimen and radiographs in Figure 5.100.

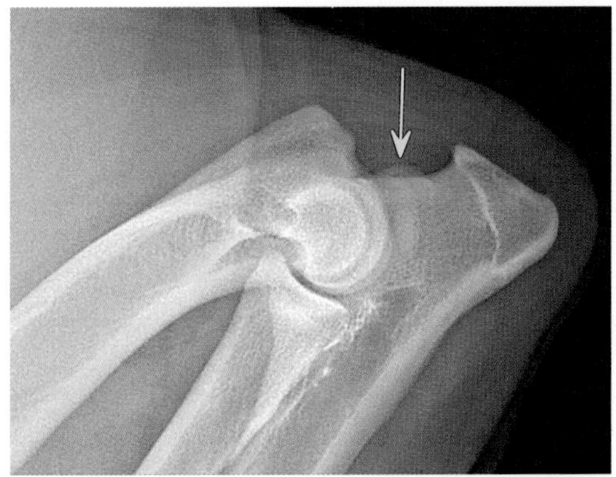

Figure 5.103 Elbow "bump". Flexed lateral view of a dog elbow depicting a smooth, well-defined bony margin extending proximal to the anconeal process (arrow). The dog is asymptomatic and there are no other signs of degenerative joint disease, no soft tissue swelling, or other signs of an elbow abnormality in this radiograph. The elbow, including the medial coronoid process, was normal in the orthogonal view, suggesting that this elbow "bump" likely is a normal anatomic variation caused by the articular border of the ulnar trochlear notch.

physis of the humeral medial epicondyle often is superimposed on the anconeal process in a lateral view (Figure 5.105).

Ununited anconeal process occurs in many dog breeds, but German Shepherds are overrepresented. It is bilateral in about a third of affected dogs. Factors that contribute to an ununited anconeal process include abnormal bone development (e.g., genetics, nutrition), asynchronous growth of the radius and ulna, and trauma.

Elbow incongruity

The term "incongruity" can be confusing. Some use it to describe any bad alignment between the bones in a joint. In the elbow, however, incongruity is an actual disorder. Elbow incongruity is a developmental abnormality in which the humeral condyle and the ulnar trochlear notch do not fit together properly (Figure 5.106). Usually, the trochlear notch is too small.

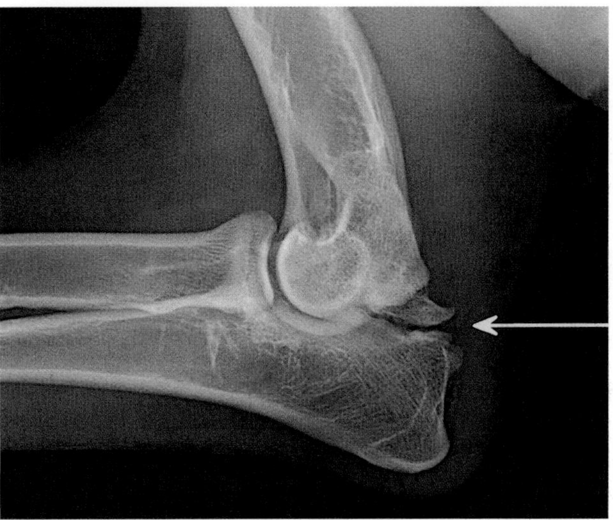

Figure 5.104 Ununited anconeal process. Lateral view of a dog elbow depicting a line of soft tissue opacity at the base of the anconeal process (arrow).

A

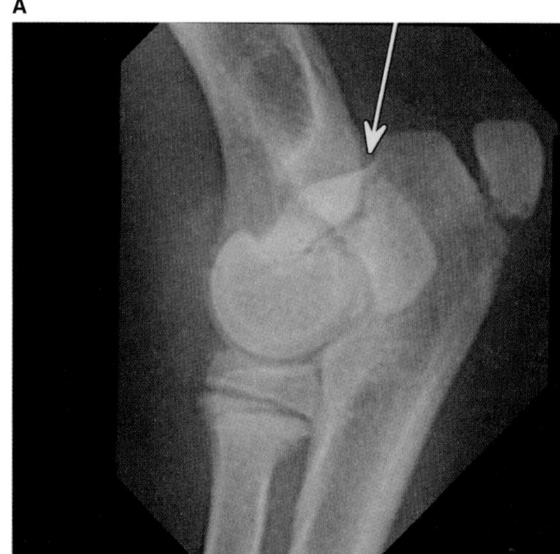

B

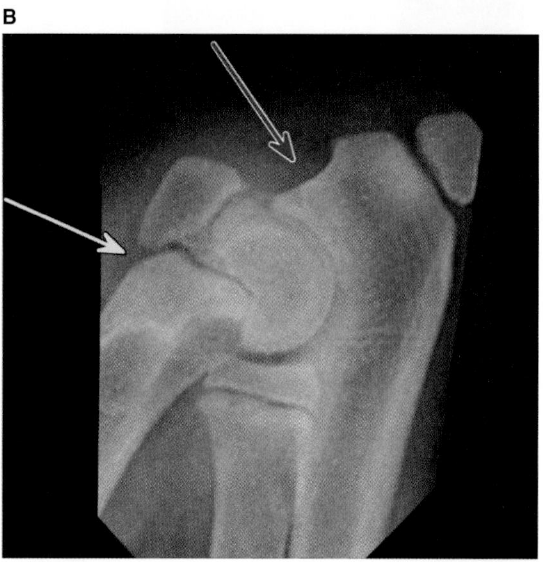

Figure 5.105 Normal elbow. **A**. Lateral view of an immature dog elbow depicting superimposition of the physis of the medial humeral epicondyle (arrow) on the anconeal process. Superimposition of the physis may be mistaken for an ununited anconeal process. **B**. Flexed lateral view of the same dog, eliminating superimposition of the physis (yellow arrow) and revealing a normal anconeal process (black arrow). The physis of the medial epicondyle generally remains visible until about 6 months of age.

Asynchronous growth of the radius and ulna frequently is confused with elbow incongruity. Both of these disorders create abnormal stresses in the elbow, which may lead to an ununited anconeal process or a fragmented medial coronoid process. With asynchronous growth, however, humeroulnar subluxation results from an abnormally shortened ulna, which sometimes is amenable to surgical treatment. This is not the case with elbow incongruity; no satisfactory treatment has been developed for true elbow incongruity. It is important to differentiate these two conditions.

Radiographic signs of elbow incongruity include an abnormally shaped ulnar trochlear notch; usually more elliptical than the normal semicircular appearance. The humeroulnar joint space often is uneven and may appear wedge-shaped, both proximally and distally. Subchondral osteosclerosis sometimes is present.

Poor patient positioning can easily mimic elbow incongruity. If you are unsure of your radiographic findings,

A

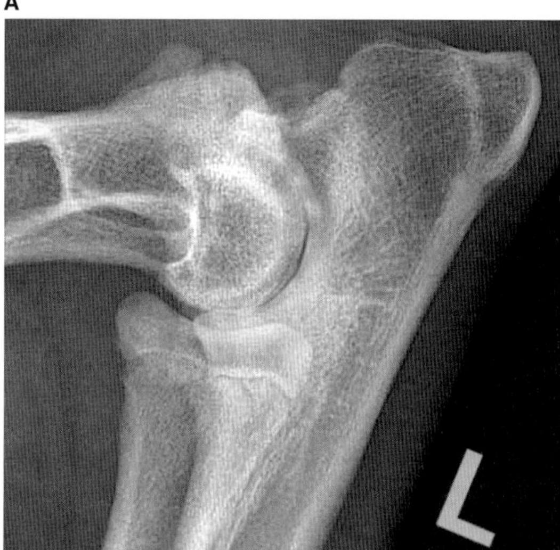

B

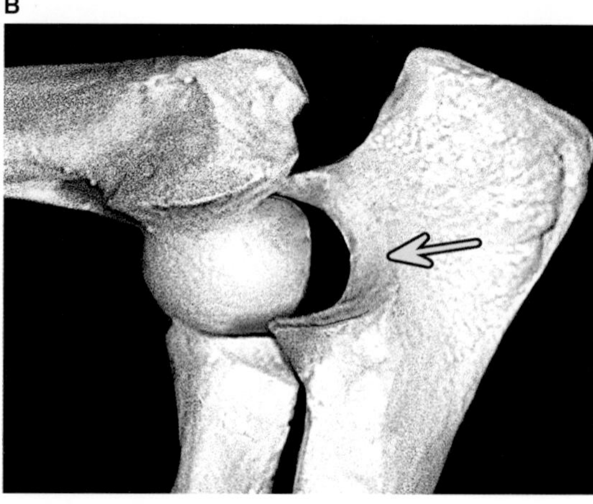

Figure 5.106 Elbow incongruity. Lateral view of a dog elbow (**A**) and an illustration of a dog elbow (**B**), both depicting abnormal fit between the humeral condyle and the ulnar trochlear notch. The trochlear notch is too small (arrow).

repeat the radiograph paying particular attention to positioning of the elbow.

Elbow osteochondrosis

In the elbow, the most common site for an osteochondrosis lesion is on the medial aspect of the humeral condyle. Occasionally a lesion is seen on the lateral aspect of the condyle. The lesion usually is easiest to see in a craniocaudal view, appearing as a focal, concave defect along the articular margin of the condyle (Figure 5.107). Rarely, a mineralized flap or mineralized fragment is visible in the joint.

Ununited medial humeral epicondyle

The distal humerus develops from three ossification centers. The centers normally fuse by 6 months of age. Failure of the medial epicondylar ossification center to unite humeral condylar ossification centers can result in a discrete mineral opacity structure located in the soft tissues medial and caudal to the elbow joint (Figure 5.108). The structure tends to be easiest to see in a craniocaudal view. Sometimes more than one mineralized structure is present.

Ununited medial epicondyle may be unilateral or bilateral. It is uncommon in dogs, most often reported in Labrador Retrievers, German Shepherds, and English Setters. Other possible causes for a mineralized structure caudomedial to the elbow include flexor tendinopathy and traumatic avulsion. With an united medial humeral epicondyle, soft tissue swelling is absent and the medial border of the humeral condyle is well defined. The condyle may be irregular, but there is no evidence of active bone disease. Unless there is swelling or an active periosteal response, a separate mineral opacity structure in this area is likely an inactive or chronic, incidental finding.

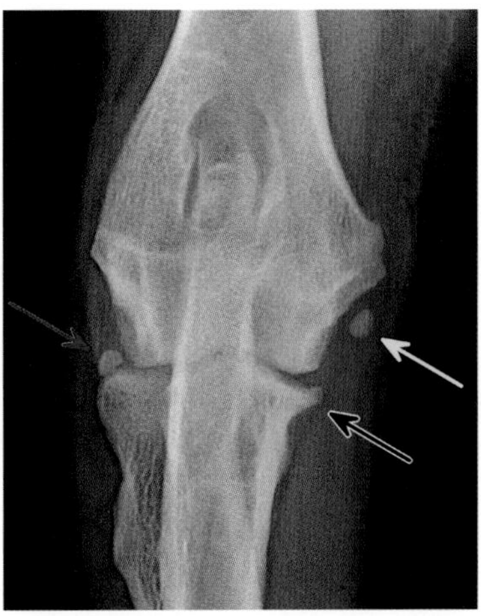

Figure 5.108 Ununited medial humeral epicondyle. Craniocaudal view of a dog elbow depicting a mineral opacity structure in the soft tissues medial to the humeral medial epicondyle (yellow arrow). There is no soft tissue swelling or evidence of active bone remodeling. The margin of the medial epicondyle is slightly irregular, but well defined. An osteophyte is visible on the medial coronoid process (black arrow). A normal sesamoid bone is present near the radial head (red arrow).

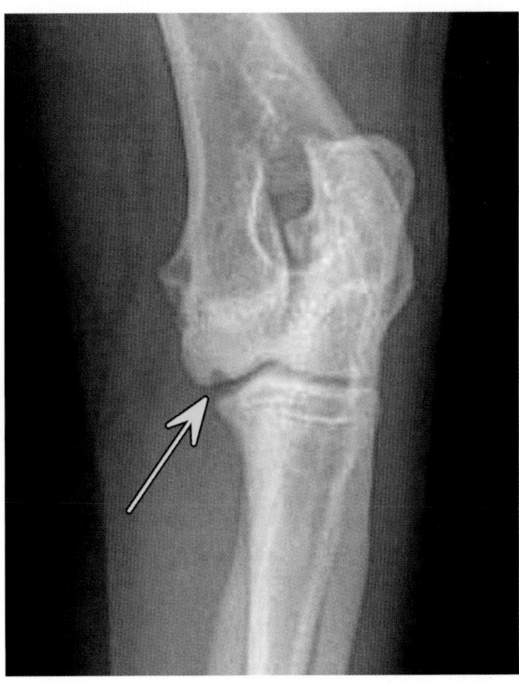

Figure 5.107 Osteochondrosis. Craniocaudal oblique view of a dog elbow depicting a focal area of decreased opacity on the medial articular margin of the humeral condyle (arrow). This subchondral defect is consistent with an OCD lesion, however, a similar finding may be seen due to focal osteolysis adjacent to a fragmented medial coronoid process (i.e., "kissing lesion").

Elbow Fractures

Most elbow fractures are caused by trauma (e.g., blunt force injury, animal suspended by its limb). Sometimes a fracture is predisposed by a developmental abnormality, such as incomplete ossification of the humeral condyle, or disease in the elbow that leads to a pathological fracture.

Distal humeral fractures tend to occur more often in the lateral part of the condyle than in the medial part. The fracture may be T or Y-shaped. A fracture in the proximal ulna sometimes is accompanied by a cranial luxation of the radial head, which is called a *Monteggia* fracture. Olecranon fractures may or may not be articular.

Incomplete ossification of humeral condyle

The humeral condyle is formed by lateral and medial centers of ossification that normally fuse by 3 months of age. Failure of the centers to completely unite results in a weak area that is predisposed to fracture. In a craniocaudal view, incomplete ossification of the humeral condyle typically appears as a vertical line of soft tissue opacity near the middle of the condyle (Figure 5.109). The line may be very small and difficult to see. Sometimes the elbow needs to be slightly rotated so the x-ray beam is aligned with the non-mineralized cartilagenous line and to eliminate superimposition of the olecranon. Note: summation of the ulna may be mistaken for a line of incomplete ossification.

Incomplete ossification of the humeral condyle most often is reported in Spaniels (may be hereditary) and small, chondrodystrophic dog breeds. It usually is bilateral, but lameness may be unilateral (make radiographs of both limbs). In some affected dogs, the humeral supratrochlear foramen is absent due to abnormal development.

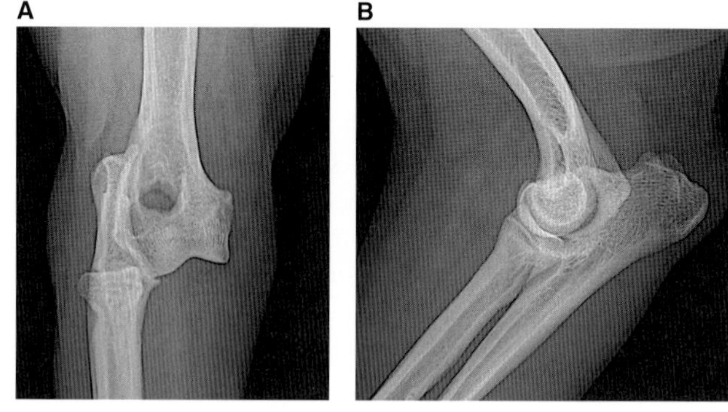

Figure 5.110 Elbow luxation. Craniocaudal view (**A**) and lateral view (**B**) of a dog elbow depicting a lateral luxation of the humeroantebrachial joint. The luxation could easily be missed in the lateral view alone.

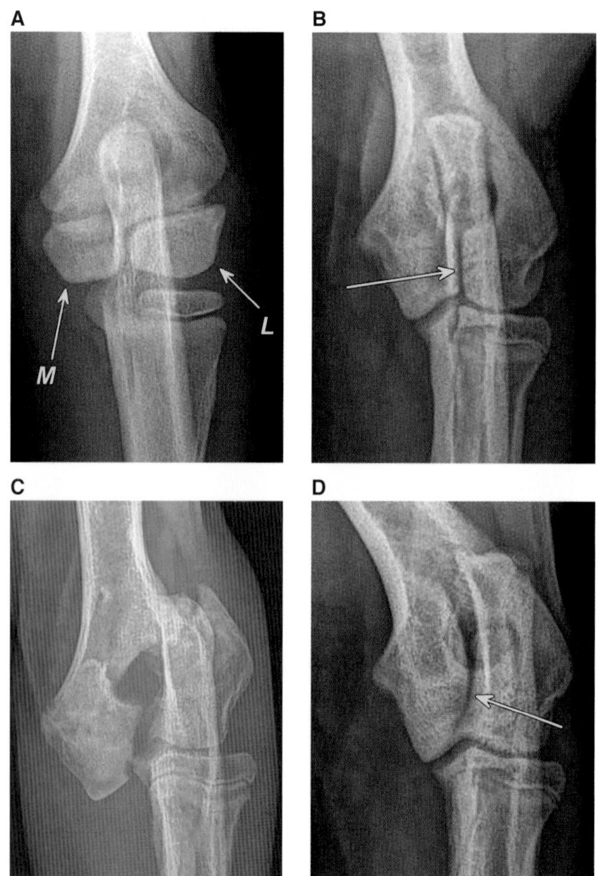

Figure 5.109 Incomplete ossification of humeral condyle. **A**. Craniocaudal (CrCa) view of an immature dog depicting the normal medial and lateral ossification centers (M and L) that fuse to form the humeral condyle. **B**. CrCa view of a different immature dog depicting a soft tissue opacity line in the humeral condyle (arrow) due to incomplete mineralization of the cartilage between the ossification centers. **C**. CrCa view of a dog elbow depicting a laterally displaced lateral humeral condylar fracture. **D**. CrCa view of a normal dog elbow depicting an artifact in the humeral condyle caused by summation of the ulna (arrow). This artifact may be mistaken for incomplete ossification of the humeral condyle.

Elbow luxation and subluxation

Dislocation of the elbow may be congenital or acquired. Congenital luxations tend to be bilateral and without any history of trauma. Acquired luxations usually are unilateral and most often caused by trauma (Figure 5.110). Traumatic luxations usually are accompanied by soft tissue swelling and often by fractures. Small avulsion or chip fractures may result from a ligamentous pull or because the elbow bones fit together in such an intricate manner. Always look for chip fractures in a luxated elbow as these can complicate subsequent treatment.

Congenital elbow luxations may involve either the humeroradial or humeroulnar joint, and sometimes both. Soft tissue swelling may or may not be present. A chronically luxated radial head often appears rounded due to lack of normal joint forces. Congenital elbow luxation most often is reported in small dogs (e.g., Pug, Dachshunds, Miniature Poodle, Pekingese). Secondary degenerative joint disease is common.

Subluxation of the elbow often is associated with asynchronous growth of the radius and ulna or elbow incongruity. It may be unilateral or bilateral. If bilateral, subluxation may or may not be symmetrical. Damage to the elbow supporting structures can lead to elbow instability and subluxation. Stress view radiographs sometimes are needed to demonstrate laxity and subluxation (Figure 5.111).

Patella cubiti

Patella cubiti is a rare congenital condition in which the proximal ulnar epiphysis and metaphysis, which would normally form the olecranon, are separated from the ulnar diaphysis and pulled proximally by the triceps muscle. The result is a misshapen proximal ulna and a mineral opacity structure located caudal to the distal humerus. The mineralized structure represents the separated part of the olecranon and often is shaped like a patella, thus the name of the condition. Patella cubiti may be unilateral or bilateral and most often is reported in Doberman Pinschers. It may be difficult to distinguish from a chronic, ununited fracture without patient history. The term *patella cubiti* sometimes is used to describe ectopic sesamoid bones near the elbow.

Radioulnar ischemic necrosis (RUIN)

RUIN is a rare condition in dogs characterized by osteolysis and new bone production along the interosseous ligament of the radius and ulna. The etiology is unknown, but the ischemia may be associated with damage to the interosseous ligament or neoplasia. Lesions typically begin in the proximal third of the radius and ulna, near the nutrient foramina. They typically appear as concave foci of osteolysis with a localized periosteal response along the opposing borders of one or both bones (Figure 5.112). Because the normal appearance of the interosseous area is so variable, serial radiographs often are helpful. Active lesions produce increased osteolysis over a 2–3 week interval, whereas healing lesions typically develop better-defined margins associated with the new bone production. RUIN is difficult to differentiate from neoplasia and mycosis in radiographs. Histopathology and culture usually are needed to confirm the diagnosis. Although some patients recover with rest, surgical intervention often is recommended.

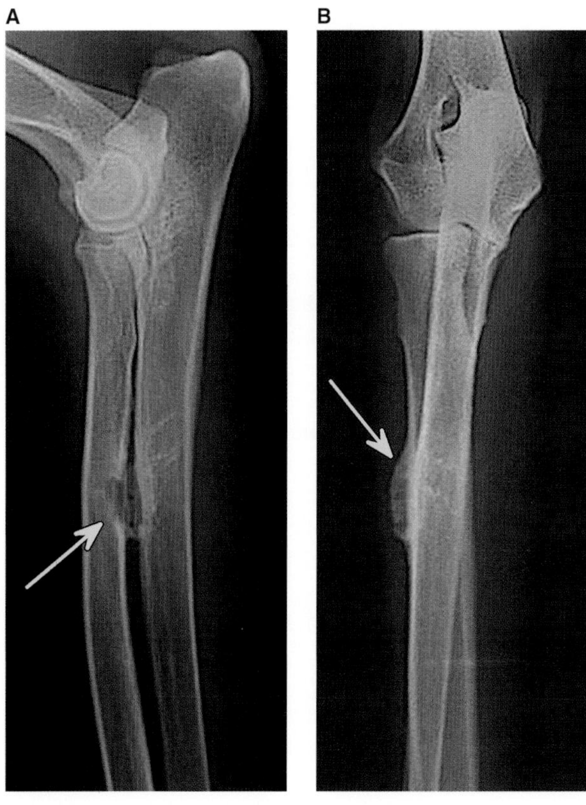

Figure 5.112 RUIN. Lateral view (**A**) and craniocaudal view (**B**) of a dog antebrachium depicting focal osteolysis and a periosteal response in the interosseous space between the radius and ulna (arrows).

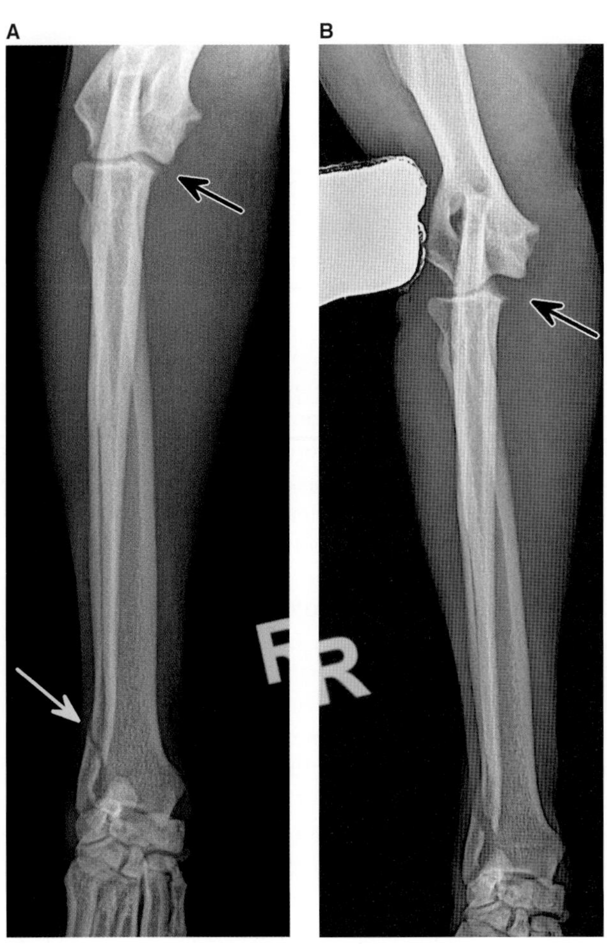

Figure 5.111 Elbow subluxation. **A**. Craniocaudal view of a dog antebrachium depicting very subtle, slight widening of the humeroulnar joint space (black arrow) and a minimally displaced oblique fracture in the distal ulna (yellow arrow). **B**. Stress view crca view of the same dog depicting more severe widening of the joint (black arrow) due to application of a lateral-to-medial force at the elbow, documenting abnormal elbow joint laxity. Notice that the distal ulnar fracture is also widened in this view.

Carpus

Normal radiographic anatomy

The carpus is a composite synovial joint consisting of three major articulations: *antebrachiocarpal, middle carpal,* and *carpometacarpal*. The middle carpal joint comprises the two rows of carpal bones. The *intercarpal* joints are between the individual carpal bones, which are called *short* or *cuboidal* bones. The carpal bones are supported by a flexor retinaculum and palmar fibrocartilage. No collateral ligaments span all three major carpal joints. Carpal flexion and extension primarily occur at the antebrachiocarpal and middle carpal joints. Little movement occurs at the carpometacarpal joint. The term **Manus** refers to the distal part of a thoracic limb and includes the carpus and the digits. Carpal anatomy is illustrated in Figures 5.113 and 5.114. An immature canine carpus is depicted in Figure 5.119 and an immature feline limb in Figure 5.120.

A sesamoid bone frequently is present medial to the carpometacarpal joint. Another sesamoid bone sometimes is seen medial to the distal radius, located in the radiocarpal ligament. Sesamoid bones are visible when mineralized and they usually are bilateral, but not always.

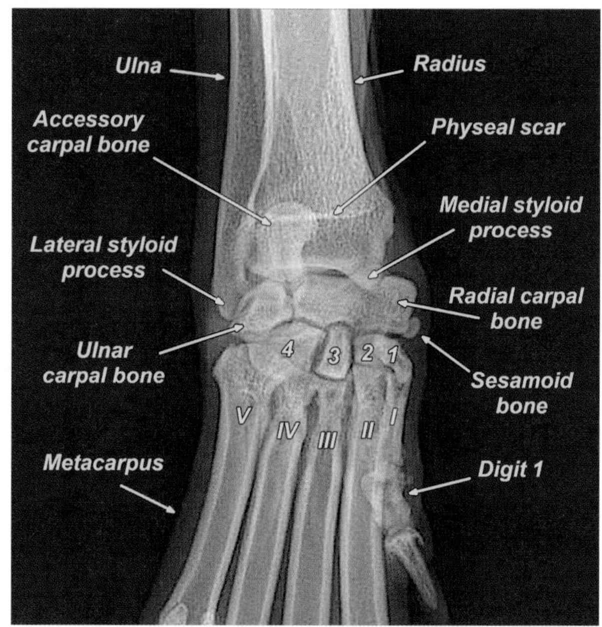

Figure 5.114 Normal carpus. Dorsopalmar view of a dog carpus depicting normal anatomy. The accessory carpal bone is superimposed on the distal radius The distal row of carpal bones are numbered 1–4 and the metacarpal bones are numbered I–V. A fifth carpal bone may be present in some dogs.

Radiographic views of the carpus

When making carpal radiographs, most patients are less likely to resist positioning when the limb is pushed forward at the elbow rather than pulled by the foot. The radiographer also is safer using this method, both from radiation and from an aggressive patient.

Radiographic views of the carpus include:

1. **Lateral** view (Figure 2.29).
2. **Dorsopalmar** view (Figure 2.30).
3. **Supplemental** lateral and DP views made with the carpus in pronation, supination, flexion, or extension to see more of the osseous borders of the multiple carpal bones.
4. **Skyline** view: a flexed proximodorsal-distodorsal view of the carpus to evaluate the dorsal margins of the carpal bones (Figure 2.30).
5. **Standing** views: standard views made with the patient weight-bearing on the limb to more accurately evaluate the width of the joint space.
6. **Stress** views: stabilize the distal antebrachium and the proximal metacarpus and apply a force to the carpus to assess joint integrity (force can be medial-to-lateral, lateral-to-medial, or rotational) (Figure 2.31).

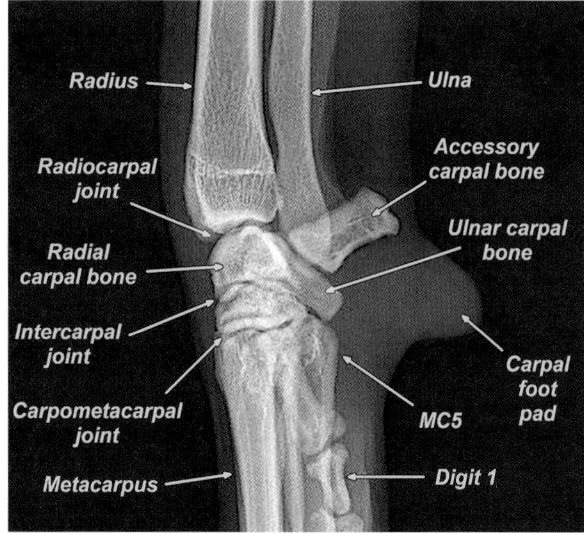

Figure 5.113 Normal carpus. Lateral view of a dog carpus depicting normal anatomy. The fifth metacarpal bone (MC5) is identified because it is positioned immediately distal to the ulnar carpal bone. The other metacarpal bones, as well as the distal row of carpal bones, are summated in this view and not individually recognized.

Carpal luxation and subluxation

Subluxation typically results from carpal laxity and instability which may be caused by repetitive low-grade trauma, an angular limb deformity, or chronic inflammation that weakens the supporting ligaments. Aged, overweight, large-breed dogs are predisposed. Damage to collateral ligaments can lead to medial or lateral instability, whereas palmar instability typically is caused by hyperextension of the carpus that tears the palmar and accessory carpal ligaments (i.e., jumping from a height). Joint swelling usually is present with acute injuries and may be intracapsular, extracapsular, or both. In radiographs of a subluxated or luxated carpus, the articulating bones are malaligned and the joint spaces may be widened (Figure 5.115). Articular or periarticular fractures may be present (e.g., avulsion, compression, chip). Stress views sometimes are needed to diagnose joint instability and to demonstrate the severity of the luxation. Comparison radiographs of the contralateral limb may be useful to avoid over or under diagnosis. Sometimes, however, subluxations are bilateral. Note: poor positioning of the carpus can mimic a subluxation.

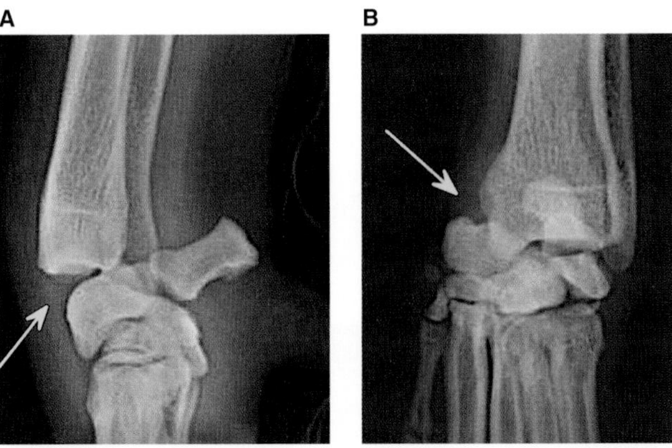

Figure 5.115 Carpal luxation. Lateral view (**A**) and dorsopalmar view (**B**) of a dog carpus depicting a medial luxation of the antebrachiocarpal joint (arrows). Bandaging material is visible peripheral to the skin in the lateral view.

Carpal fractures

Most fractures of carpal bones are chip, slab, or avulsion types. Carpal fractures may also involve the distal radial or ulnar styloid process or the proximal metacarpus. The supporting structures may be damaged as well, including ligaments, joint capsule, and others.

Developmental abnormalities and disease in the carpus can predispose to fractures. The radial carpal bone, for example, develops from three ossification centers and incomplete fusion can lead to weak areas in the bone. Incomplete fusion has been reported in Boxers and may be bilateral. Accessory carpal bone fractures most often occur in very active or athletic dogs (e.g., racing Greyhounds). Identification of carpal fractures may require oblique and skyline views. Stress views with the carpus in flexion, extension, or rotated may aid in diagnosis and assessment of joint laxity.

Carpal stenosing tenosynovitis

Chronic inflammation in the tendon of the abductor pollicis longus muscle can lead to localized fibrosis and restriction of tendon movement. Radiographic findings include soft tissue swelling at the medial aspect of the carpus and a well-defined enthesophyte on the dorsomedial aspect of distal radius (Figure 5.116). The enthesophyte develops at the site of origin of the abductor pollicis longus.

Stenosing tenosynovitis most often is reported in large breed dogs. It typically results from overuse and repetitive low-grade injuries. Clinical signs include variable lameness and a firm swelling at the medial aspect of the carpus. Lameness tends to be more severe after rest and following strenuous exercise. Flexion of the carpus may cause pain and demonstrate restricted mobility.

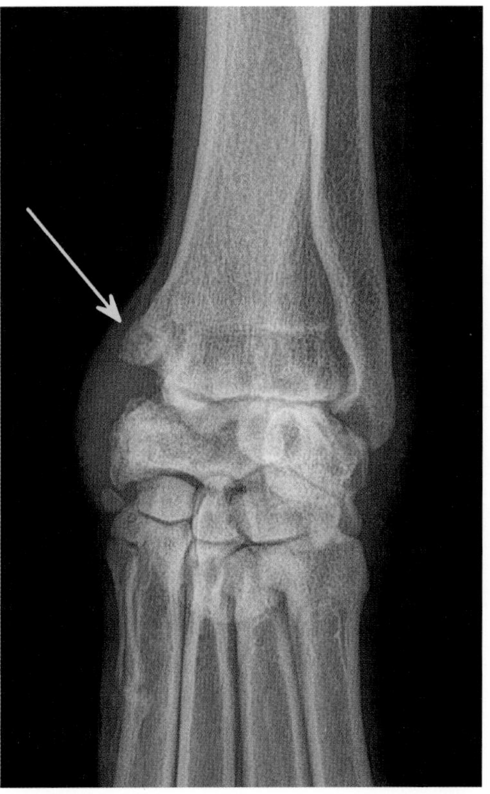

Figure 5.116 Stenosing tenosynovitis. Dorsopalmar view of a dog carpus depicting localized soft tissue swelling along the medial carpus and an enthesophyte on the medial aspect of the distal radius (arrow).

Digits

Normal radiographic anatomy

The digits include the metacarpal or metatarsal bones and the phalanges. The feet of most dogs and cats contain five digits, numbered 1 through 5 from medial to lateral. The first digit is non-weight-bearing and commonly called the **dewclaw**. It includes a metacarpus and only 2 phalanges. In digits 2 through 5 there are three phalanges. Digital anatomy is illustrated in Figures 5.117–5.120.

Each metacarpal/metatarsal bone develops from only two ossification centers: one in the diaphysis and the other in the distal epiphysis. The proximal and middle phalanges also develop from two ossification centers: one in the diaphysis and one in the proximal epiphysis. The distal phalanx develops from a single ossification center.

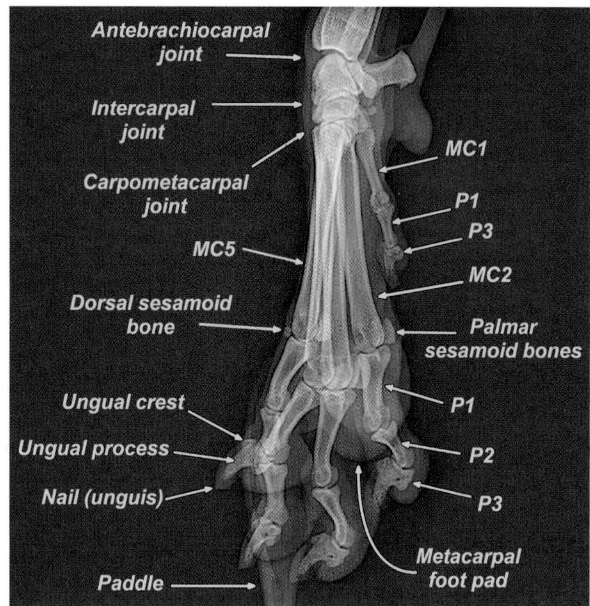

Figure 5.117 Normal foot. Lateral view of a dog manus depicting normal anatomy. The digits are separated by using gentle compression applied with a plastic paddle. The first digit or "dewclaw" is shorter than the others and includes the first metacarpal bone (MC1), a proximal phalanx (P1), and a distal phalanx (P3). The second digit is identified because it is adjacent to the first and includes MC2, a proximal phalanx (P1), a middle phalanx (P2), and a distal phalanx (P3). The dorsal border of the fifth metacarpal bone (MC5) is identified because digit 5 is shorter than digits 3 and 4 (digit 2 also is shorter than digits 3 and 4).

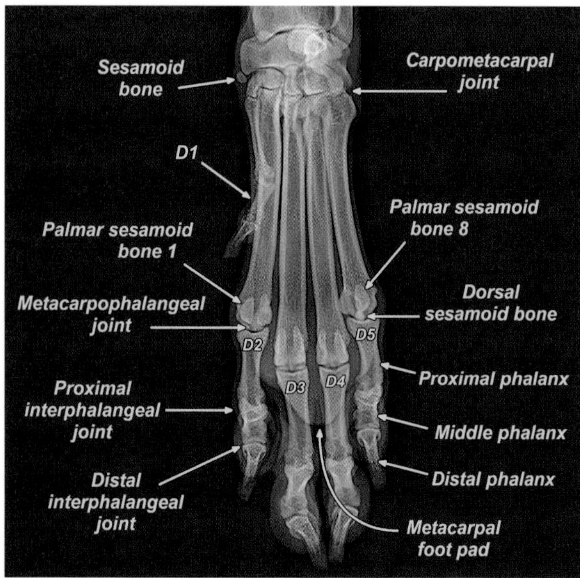

Figure 5.118 Normal foot. Dorsopalmar view of a dog manus depicting normal anatomy. The medial carpal sesamoid bone is located in the tendon of the abductor pollicis longus muscle. Digits 1 through 5 are labeled D1-D5. The palmar sesamoid bones are numbered from medial to lateral 1-8. The metacarpal foot pad is superimposed on the digits.

In digits 2–5 there are three **sesamoid** bones at each metacarpophalangeal and metatarsophalangeal joint: a single dorsal sesamoid and paired palmar/plantar sesamoids. The palmar/plantar sesamoids are numbered 1 through 8 from medial to lateral. **Bipartite** and **multipartite** sesamoids are common in dogs and usually incidental findings. Digits 5 and 2 most often are affected. Multipartite sesamoid bones appear as two or more variably sized, well-defined, mineral opacity structures in the area of a sesamoid bone. They may be differentiated from fractures by a lack of soft

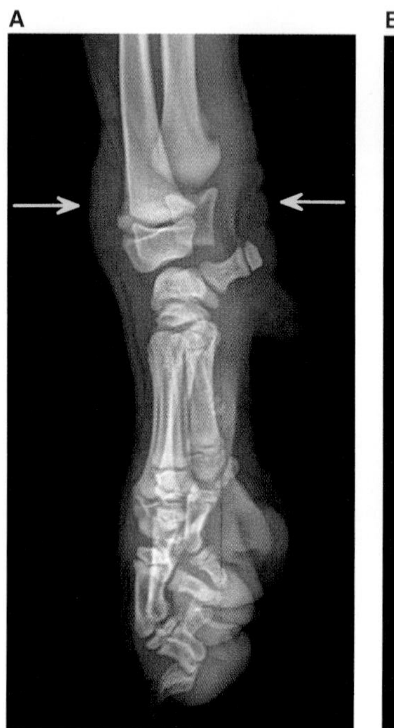

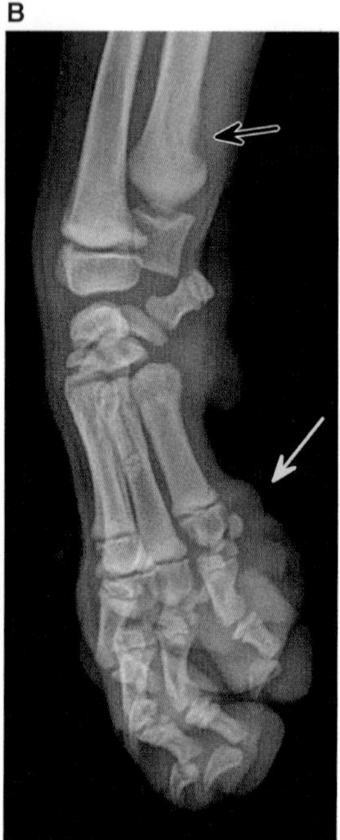

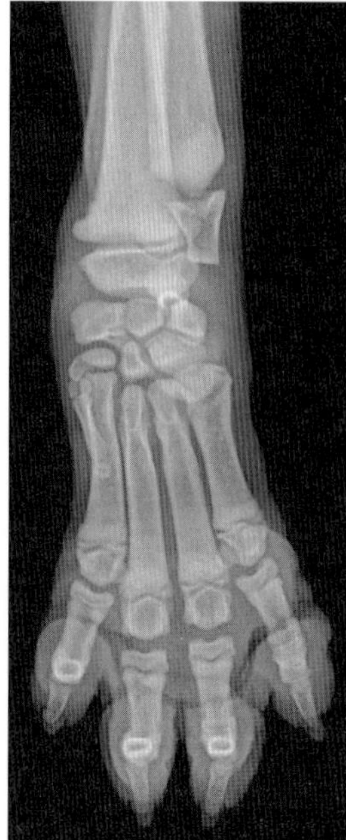

Figure 5.119 Normal immature canine manus. Lateral view (**A**), lateral oblique view (**B**), and dorsopalmar view (**C**) of a puppy carpus and digits. The yellow arrows point to bunching of the skin caused by wrapping a tie around the limb to aid in positioning. The black arrow points to the cut back zone in the radial metaphysis.

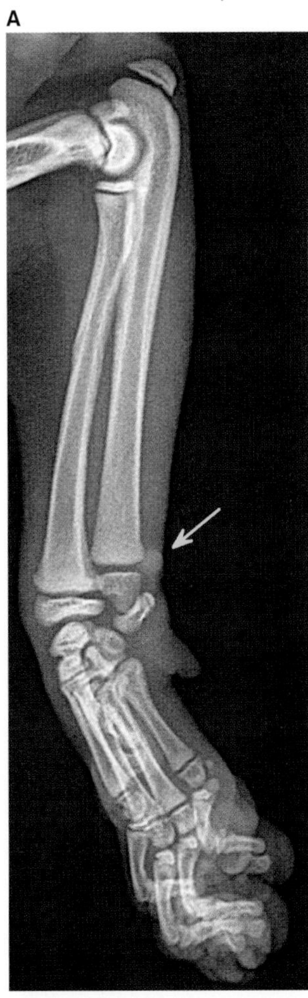

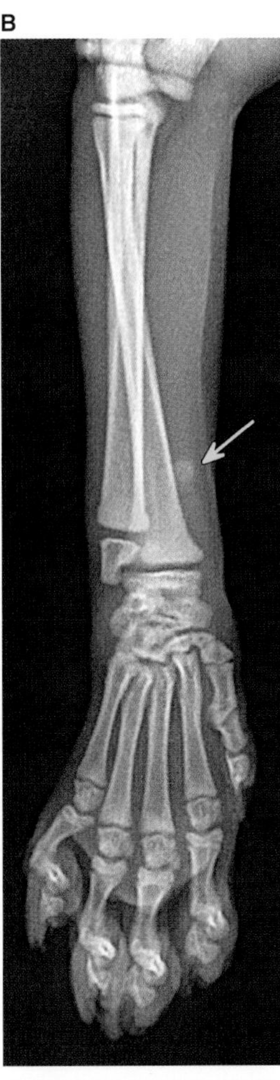

Figure 5.120 Normal immature feline forelimb. Lateral view (**A**) and craniocaudal view (**B**) depicting a kitten thoracic limb. The arrow points to the supracarpal foot pad which appears as a soft tissue opacity nodule in the caudomedial aspect of the distal antebrachium. It sometimes is mistaken for a lesion. Notice that in cats, the distal ulna is relatively larger than in dogs and the distal ulnar physis is transverse as opposed to conical in shape.

tissue swelling, no active bone remodeling, and they do not change in appearance in serial radiographs.

The metacarpophalangeal, metatarsophalangeal, and interphalangeal articulations are examples of "saddle-type" synovial joints. The dorsal interphalangeal joint capsules are thick and unite with the extensor tendons.

Digit radiographs

As described with the carpus, positioning the foot often is easier when pushing the elbow (or tarsus) rather than pulling the foot. Radiographs of a manus or pes include:

1. **Lateral** view (Figures 2.29).
2. **Dorsopalmar/dorsoplantar** view (Figure 2.33).
3. **Oblique** views: lateral and DP views with the limb slightly rotated in whichever direction is needed to better visualize the bony margin of interest.
4. **Compression** or **traction** views: lateral and DP views are made while gently compressing the digits with a plastic or wooden paddle to separate them (Figure 2.32). Digits also may be separated using gauze, tape, or string.

Digit fracture or luxation

Fractures, luxations, and subluxations in digits most often are caused by trauma. Soft tissue swelling usually is present. Open fractures and penetrating wounds may be accompanied by subcutaneous emphysema. Some fractures are articular. Sesamoid bone fractures typically result from hyperextension injuries, particularly in large dogs, with palmar sesamoids 2 and 7 most often affected.

A digital subluxation may spontaneously reduce during positioning for radiography, but soft tissue swelling usually remains to indicate an abnormality. Positioning artifacts can mimic subluxation. Superimposition artifacts can mimic fractures (e.g., footpad, wet or dirty hair). Most superimposition artifacts are identified with orthogonal views or close inspection that reveals the artifact line extending beyond the limits of the bone.

Digit neoplasia

Tumors in digits may originate in bone or soft tissue. Usually only one digit is involved, but sometimes multiple digits on one or more feet are affected. Most digital tumors are subungual (under the nail) and confined to the distal phalanx. Lesions tend to be primarily osteolytic with minimal or no periosteal response. Localized soft tissue swelling or a mass often is visible adjacent to the lytic bone, except where limited by the nail (Figure 5.121). Bone tumors rarely cross the joint, but they can.

Digit tumors are reported more often in dogs than in cats, particularly older large-breed dogs with black hair coats (e.g., Labrador Retriever, Standard Poodle). In dogs, squamous cell carcinoma is most common and melanoma is second. In cats, fibrosarcoma is most common. Bronchial adenocarcinoma in cats can metastasize to the digits. Osteosarcoma can involve a digit (Figure 5.122).

Digital osteomyelitis

Osteomyelitis may involve one or more digits. Typical radiographic findings include soft tissue swelling and an active periosteal response. Osteomyelitis often produces a more severe periosteal response than neoplasia and may involve the adjacent joint(s). Erosive arthritis sometimes is present, particularly in the distal interphalangeal joint. Digit osteomyelitis may result from a penetrating wound, migrating foreign material, or systemic infection. Mineral or metal opacity foreign materials usually are readily identified.

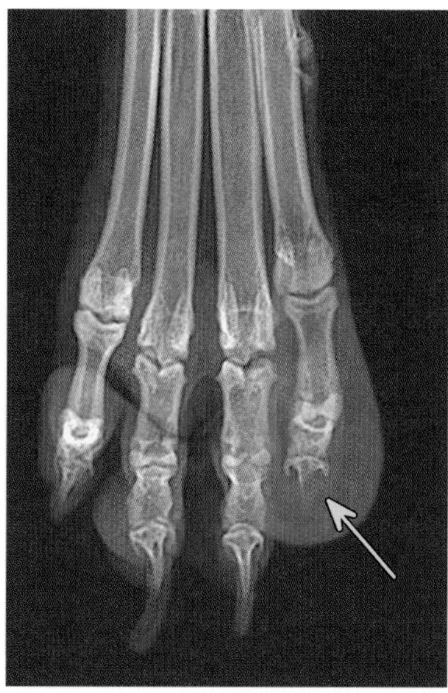

Figure 5.121 Digital neoplasia. Dorsopalmar view of a dog foot depicting soft tissue swelling and osteolysis associated with the distal phalanx in the second digit (arrow). There is no visible periosteal response and no evidence that the lesion involves the joint or any other bone.

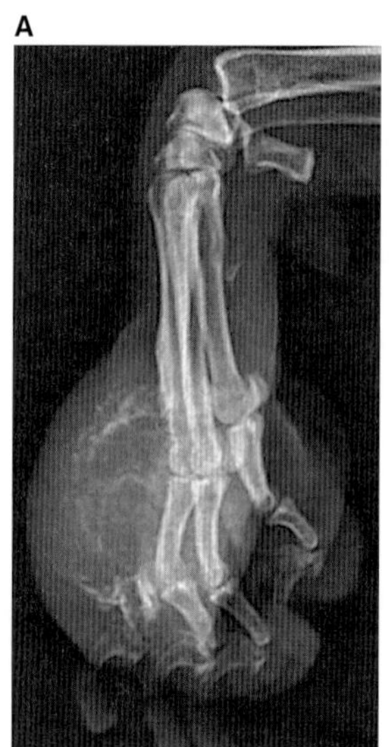

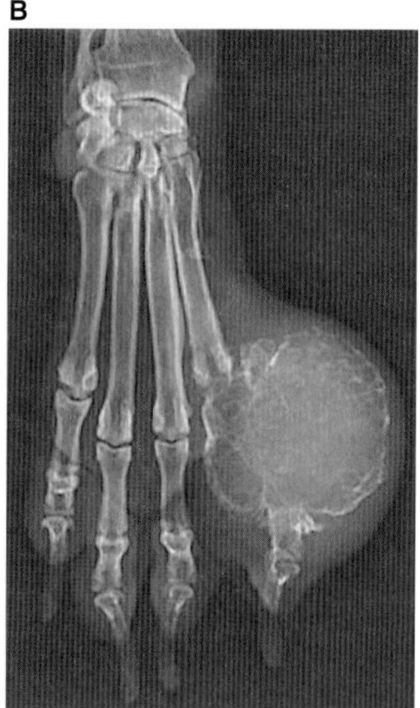

Figure 5.122 Digital lesion. Lateral view (**A**) and dorsopalmar view (**B**) of a dog manus depicting an aggressive, expansile, osteolytic lytic lesion in the proximal phalanx of the second digit. The final diagnosis was osteosarcoma.

A draining tract may be present, in which case fistulography may yield additional diagnostic information.

Digit intraosseous epidermoid cyst

Sometimes called a "pseudotumor," an intraosseous cyst appears as a well-defined, focal area of osteolysis in the ungual process of a third phalanx. The cyst may be surrounded by a rim of osteosclerosis. Soft tissue swelling may be present, but a periosteal response is absent unless the cyst becomes infected or fractured. The origin of an intraosseous cyst may be congenital or acquired secondary to trauma. Usually only one digit is involved. Affected animals may experience pain. Similar cysts have been reported in the skull and vertebrae.

Pelvis

Normal radiographic anatomy

The pelvis is formed by the union of two halves or *hemipelves*, linked together by a cartilaginous joint called the pubic symphysis. Each hemipelvis is composed of ilial, ischial, acetabular, and pubic bones, all of which normally fuse by 6 months of age. The acetabulum is formed at the junction of these four bones. Each ilium is attached to the sacrum by a sacroiliac joint, which is a combination synovial and cartilaginous joint. At each sacroiliac joint the ilium and sacrum are lined with articular cartilage and united by a thin joint capsule. Pelvic anatomy is illustrated in Figures 5.123–5.128.

The pelvic bones develop from multiple ossification centers. **Accessory centers** are common and must be recognized to avoid misdiagnosing an avulsion fracture. Described below are the more frequently seen pelvic secondary and accessory centers:

1. Ischiatic tuberosities: small, rounded, mineral opacity structures that can remain separate from the ischium until about 10 months of age (Figure 5.128, lateral view).
2. Caudal aspect of the pubic symphysis: a triangle-shaped bone structure that may be visible in the ischial arch up to about a year of age (Figure 5.124).
3. Ileal wings: a crescent-shaped ossification center along the craniodorsal border which may not fuse to the ilium for many years or it may never fuse.
4. Lateral aspect of the cranial acetabulum rim: a tiny triangle of bone that may be seen at the junction of the cranial and dorsal acetabular rims in a VD view (Figure 5.129).
5. Iliopubic eminence: an ossification center that occasionally develops in the tendon of the psoas minor muscle, just cranial to the eminence (Figure 5.129).
6. Femoral lesser trochanter: a rounded mineral opacity structure sometimes is present in the tendon of the iliopsoas muscle, medial to the lesser trochanter (Figure 5.129).
7. Femoral greater trochanter: one or more rounded, mineral opacity structures may be visible in the gluteal muscle tendon, located just proximal to the trochanter in a VD view; most often seen in large dogs (Figure 5.129).

The **coxofemoral joint** or **hip joint** is a ball-and-socket synovial joint that is highly mobile. Flexion and extension of

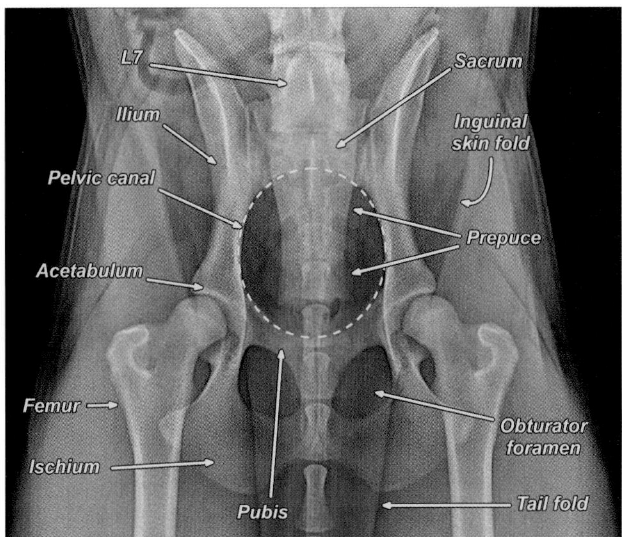

Figure 5.123 Normal pelvis. VD view of a dog pelvis depicting normal anatomy and superimposition artifacts; the latter includes the prepuce, tail folds, and inguinal skin folds.

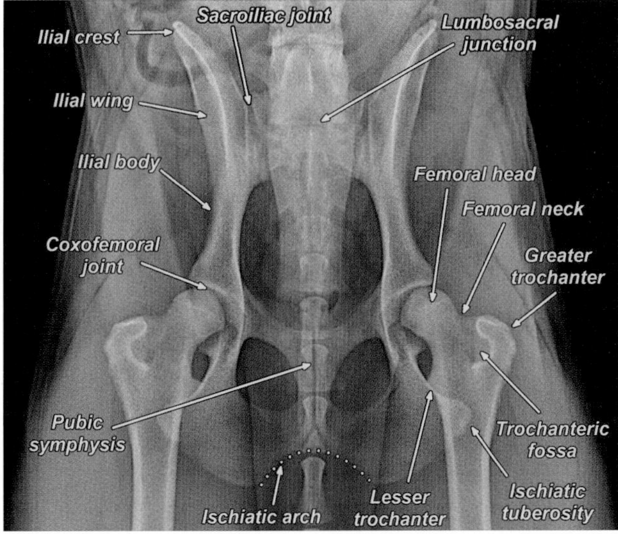

Figure 5.124 Normal pelvis. VD view of a dog pelvis depicting normal anatomy (same radiograph as Figure 5.123, but additional structures are labeled). Notice the triangle shaped bone structure at the caudal aspect of the pubic symphysis (it should not be mistaken for a fracture).

the limb are the primary motions. There is an intra-capsular ligament between the head of the femur and the acetabular fossa called the *round ligament,* sometimes referred to as the *teres ligament* or *ligament of femoral head*. The ligament originates from a flattened area on the femoral head called the *fovea capitus*. The normal flattened fovea capitus sometimes is mistaken for pathology.

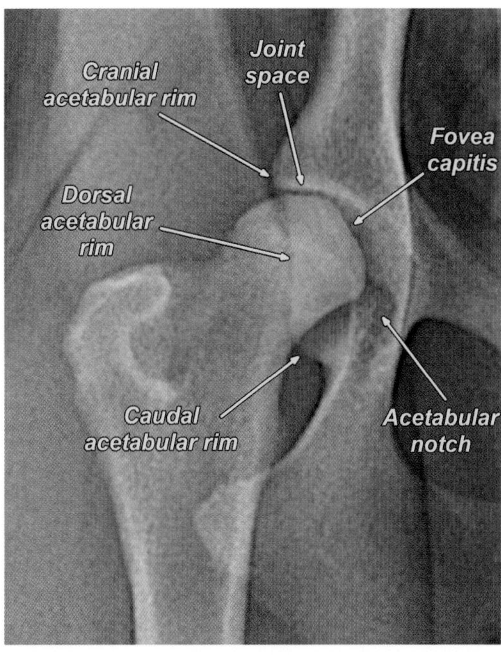

Figure 5.125 Normal coxofemoral joint. Close-up VD view of a dog pelvis depicting normal anatomy. The "joint space" arrow points to the cranial third of the acetabulum, which is the part of the joint space that should be evaluated for evidence of subluxation. Don't evaluate the middle third because of the fovea capitis and don't evaluate the caudal third because of the acetabular notch. Note: the acetabular notch is a non-weight bearing part of the coxofemoral joint and therefore a common site of osteophyte formation in cases of DJD.

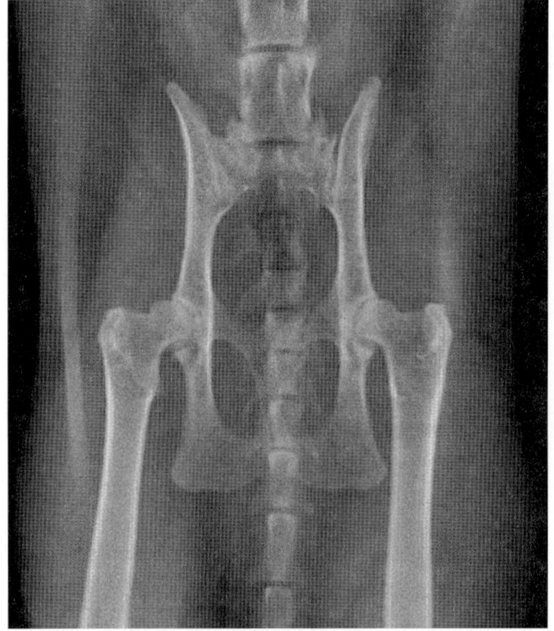

Figure 5.126 Normal feline pelvis. VD view of a cat pelvis. Compared to dogs, the feline pelvis is more rectangular in shape with relatively longer ischii.

Radiographic views of the pelvis

1. **Lateral** view (Figure 2.34).
2. **Extended ventrodorsal** view (Figure 2.35).
3. **Frog-leg view**: a flexed ventrodorsal view to assess acetabular depth, evaluate coxofemoral fit, and detect minimally displaced fractures in the femoral head and neck (Figure 2.36).
4. **Half-axial** view: an extended VD view made with the limbs half extended instead of fully extended (thus the name "half" axial) and a fulcrum placed between the thighs (above the stifles) to distract the hips and investigate coxofemoral joint laxity (Figure 2.37).
5. **Dorsal acetabular rim** view: a DV view with the hips flexed to assess acetabular depth and hip joint laxity (Figure 2.38).
6. **PennHIP** views: extended, compressed, and distracted VD views to investigate coxofemoral joint laxity. A PennHIP custom-designed distraction device is required. Veterinarians who want to use this method must be specially trained and certified by PennHIP and must submit all radiographs to PennHIP for analysis.

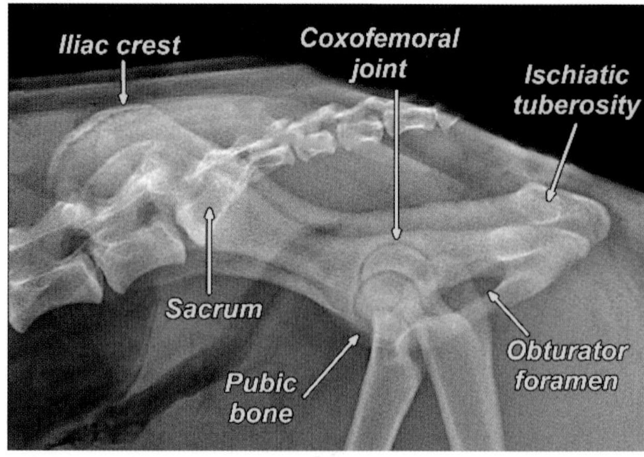

Figure 5.127 Normal pelvis. Lateral view of a dog pelvis depicting normal anatomy. The radiograph is slightly obliqued to eliminate superimposition of the hemipelves and coxofemoral joints. The iliac crests may never completely fuse to the ilial wings.

A

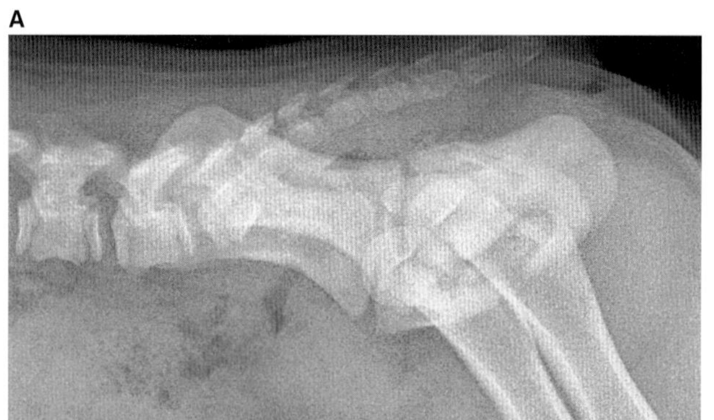

B

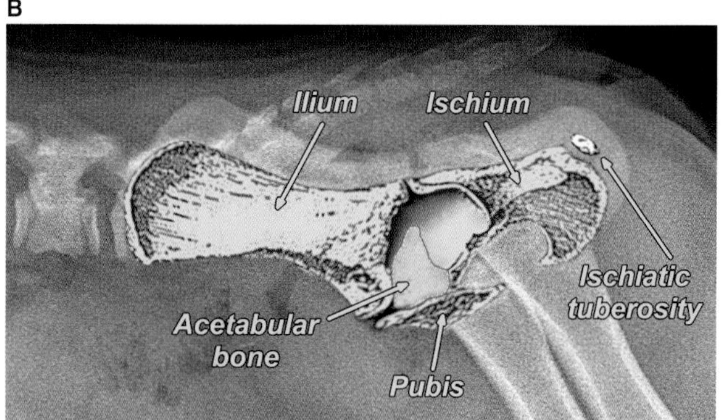

C

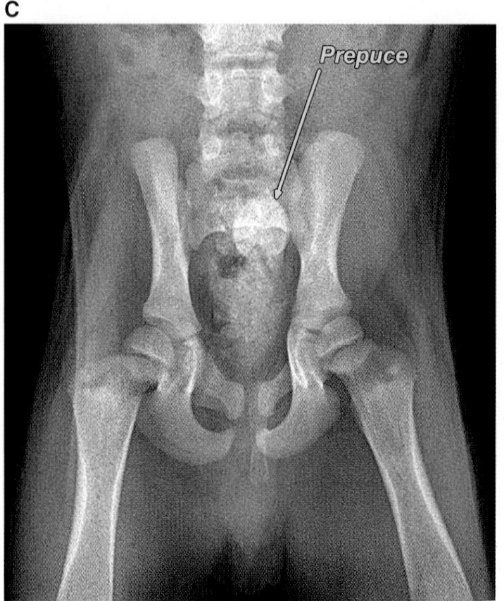

Figure 5.128 Normal immature canine pelvis. Lateral view (**A**), illustrated lateral view (**B**) and VD view (**C**) depicting a normal puppy pelvis. The triangular-shaped acetabular bone normally fuses with the ilium and ischium by about 8 weeks of age. In male dogs, the prepuce frequently is seen superimposed over the caudal abdomen in a VD/DV view and may be mistaken for a lesion.

Avascular necrosis of the femoral head

Loss of blood supply to the developing femoral head results in necrosis and collapse of the bone. The cause may involve trauma or genetics, but many cases are idiopathic. The initial radiographic finding is increased opacity in the femoral head, but this seldom is seen because radiographs rarely are made during the early stages. Progression of disease leads to bone resorption and a mottled decrease in opacity in the epiphyseal and metaphyseal regions of the proximal femur. An adjacent area of osteosclerosis may be present in the metaphysis. Both extended and flexed VD views of the pelvis may be needed to see the lesion. Collapse of the bone results in an irregular-shaped femoral head (Figure 5.130) and widening of the coxofemoral joint space. The acetabulum may be shallow or flattened due to abnormal joint stresses. Chronic disease frequently leads to disuse atrophy in the limb. Secondary degenerative joint disease is common.

Avascular necrosis is also called *ischemic necrosis of the femoral head* and *Legg–Calves Perthes disease*. It most often is reported in immature toy and small-breed dogs (e.g., Yorkshire Terrier, Toy Poodle, West Highland White Terrier, others) and may be heritable in some breeds. The lesions usually are unilateral. Although clinical signs may abate, the femoral head remains misshapen.

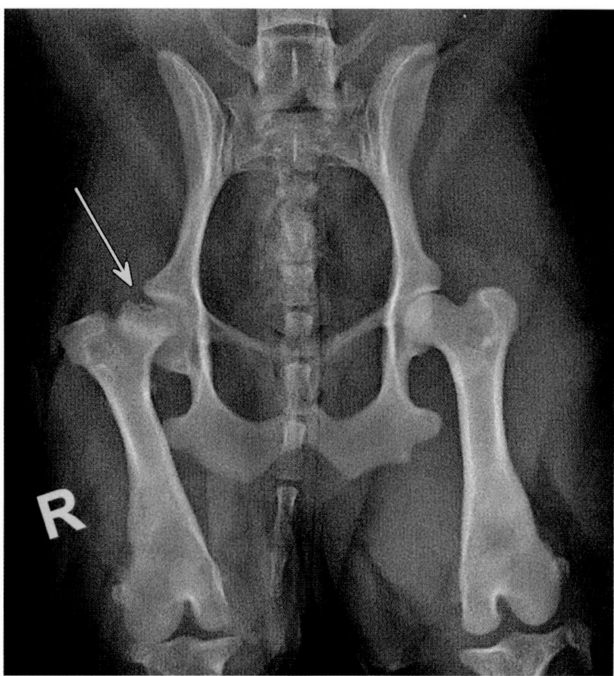

Figure 5.130 Avascular necrosis of femoral head. VD view of a dog pelvis depicting a misshapen right femoral head (arrow). The femoral head is diminished in opacity and there is adjacent osteosclerosis in the femoral neck.

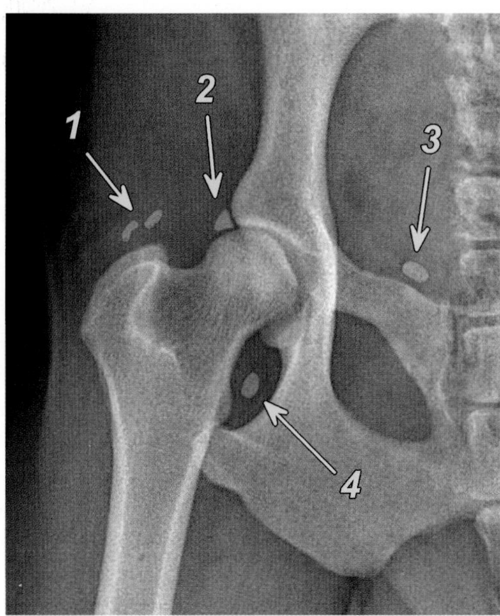

Figure 5.129 Pelvic accessory ossification centers. VD view of a dog pelvis depicting (**1**) mineralization in the gluteal muscle tendon; (**2**) an ossicle on the cranial acetabular rim; (**3**) sesamoid bone in the psoas minor muscle tendon, located near the iliopectineal eminence; (**4**) sesamoid bone in the iliopsoas muscle tendon.

Coxofemoral degenerative joint disease

The most common cause of coxofemoral DJD is hip dysplasia, and it usually is bilateral. Osteophytes tend to be most visible along the femoral neck and dorsal acetabular rim, but they also form in the acetabular notch (Figure 5.131). In mild or early cases, osteophytes on the femoral neck typically appear as a thin, mineral opacity line parallel with the physeal scar (Figure 5.132). Enthesophytes frequently form at the insertion of the joint capsule on the femoral neck, creating another thin line of mineral opacity just distal to the osteophyte line (the enthesophyte line is sometimes called "Morgan's line"). Remodeling of the femoral heads and necks may occur in advanced cases of DJD, but the apparent so-called "flattening" of the femoral head usually is due to a build-up of bone on the femoral neck rather than actual flattening of the head (Figure 5.139). Pelvic limb muscles may be atrophied and bones may be osteopenic due to disuse. Coxofemoral joint subluxation is not part of DJD, but frequently is present due to hip dysplasia.

Normal mineral opacity lines on the femoral neck that may be mistaken for osteophytes or enthesophytes include the physeal scar and a positive Mach band. A Mach band is an optical illusion created by x-rays passing through curved structures (Figures 5.133 and A38, the latter in the Artifacts

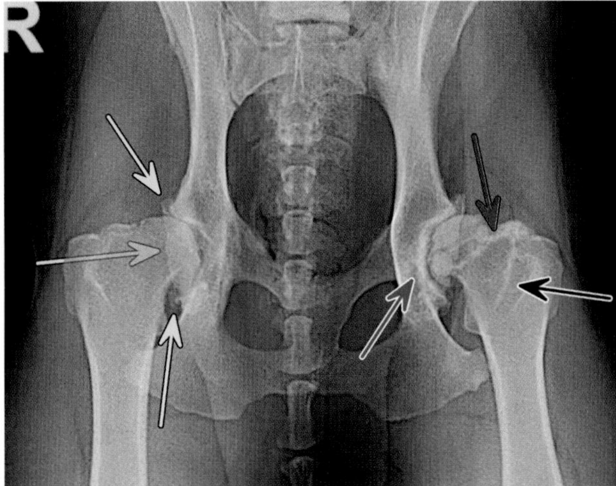

Figure 5.131 Hip DJD. VD view of a dog pelvis depicting bilateral osteophyte formation on the acetabular rims (yellow arrows point to osteophytes on the cranial, dorsal, and caudal aspects of the right acetabular rim), along the femoral necks (red arrow), and at the acetabular notch (blue arrow). Enthesophytes are present at the attachment sites of the joint capsule (black arrow).

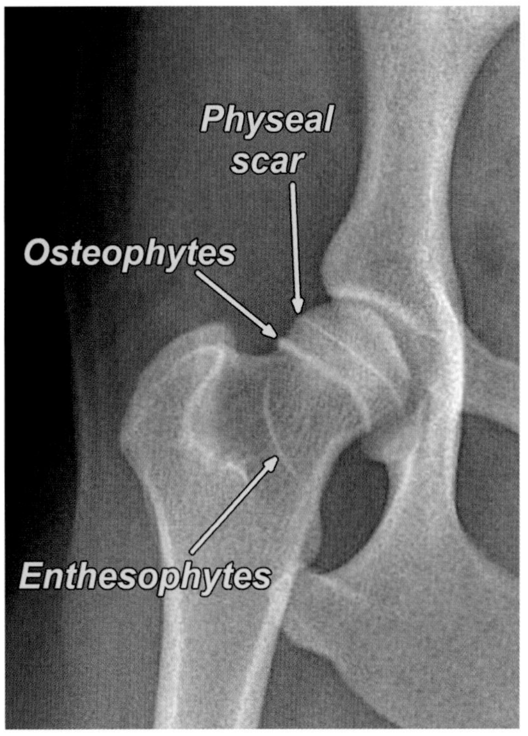

Figure 5.132 Femoral head and neck "lines". VD view of a dog pelvis depicting mineral opacity lines that often are seen on the proximal femur. The physeal scar is intra-articular. Osteophytes form at the edges of the articular cartilage. Enthesophytes form at the attachment of the joint capsule.

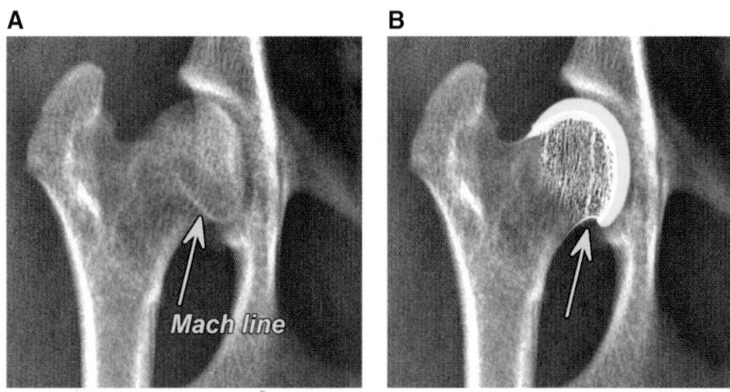

Figure 5.133 Mach line. **A**. VD view of a dog pelvis depicting a line of increased opacity along the femoral neck (arrow). This line is an artifact caused by the Mach phenomenon (Figure A38 in Chapter 2, Artifacts). **B**. In this image, a pathology specimen is superimposed on the radiograph to illustrate the tight "undercut" curve at the junction of the femoral head and neck (arrow). This curve is responsible for the positive Mach line. Notice that the Mach line does not extend outside or beyond the femoral neck, whereas osteophytes often do. Sometimes making additional views with the limbs in slightly different positions helps make the distinction.

section of Chapter 2). Positive Mach bands tend to be particularly prevalent in radiographs of chondrodystrophic dogs and Boxers.

Hip dysplasia

Hip dysplasia results from abnormal development of the coxofemoral joints. As mentioned earlier, it is the most common cause of DJD in the hips of dogs and cats. The key radiographic finding of hip dysplasia is joint laxity, which is recognized as subluxation of the coxofemoral joint(s). Other radiographic findings are secondary to hip subluxation and include a shallow acetabulum and DJD. Well-positioned radiographs are essential for accurate early diagnosis. Poor patient positioning can mask or mimic hip dysplasia.

Evidence of hip laxity and subluxation most often are obtained from an extended VD view of the pelvis (Figure 5.134). In a normal hip, the width of the joint space is even. The margins of the femoral head and acetabular rim are equally spaced from each other. Hip laxity allows the femoral head to move laterally, which produces a wedge-shaped joint space (Figures 5.135 and 5.136). The width of the joint space is evaluated in the cranial third of the joint (Figure 5.125). The middle third normally is uneven because it includes the acetabular notch and fovea capitus. In the caudal third, the ventral acetabulum is a continuation of the acetabular notch and the acetabular rim is more difficult to identify. Again, good patient positioning is essential because any hip joint that is "loose" can be radiographed in a normal or abnormal position. A distraction view often is helpful when findings are equivocal (Figures 2.37, 5.136, and 5.137).

When assessing the severity of hip dysplasia, the shape of the acetabulum must be considered. In an extended VD view

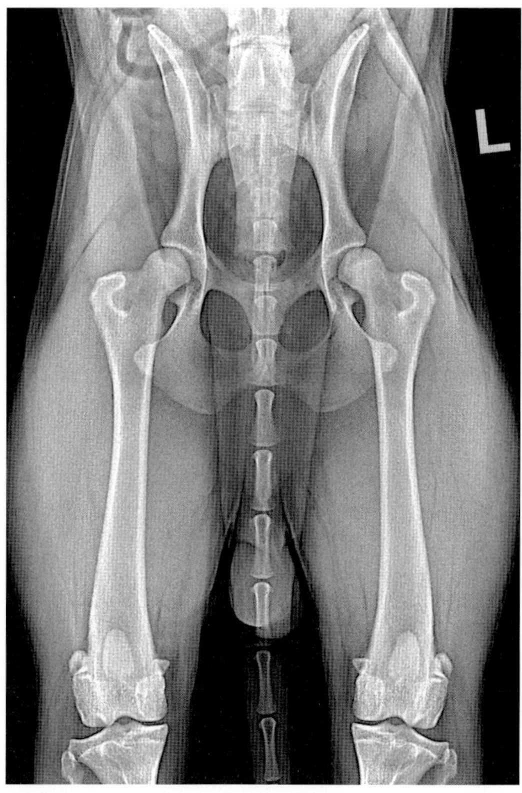

Figure 5.134 Extended VD view of the pelvis. VD view of a dog pelvis depicting the proper patient positioning for evaluation of hip dysplasia.

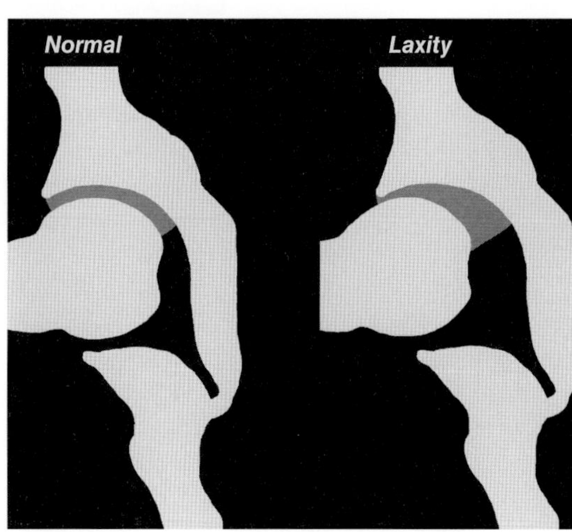

Figure 5.135 Coxofemoral joint "fit". This illustration depicts a normal coxofemoral joint on the left and a "loose" joint on the right. On the left, the cranial joint space is even (shaded area). On the right, the cranial joint space is wedged because the femoral head is subluxated (the head has moved away from the acetabular fossa). The concave area on the femoral head represents the normal fovea capitus.

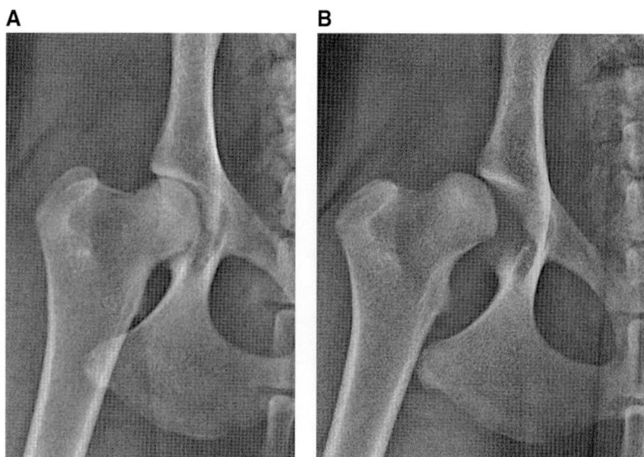

Figure 5.136 Distraction. A. VD view of a dog pelvis depicting a normal appearing coxofemoral joint. B. VD view of the same dog pelvis with distraction. The femoral head is displaced laterally (subluxated) indicating joint laxity.

of a normal hip, the acetabular fossa is C-shaped and the dorsal acetabular rim covers more than half of the femoral head. A shallow or "flared" acetabulum is a common finding in patients with hip dysplasia, often resulting in less than 50% coverage of the femoral head. Note: errors in patient positioning can mimic a shallow acetabular fossa (Figure 5.138). Rotation of the patient may make one acetabular fossa appear more shallow than actual and the other appear deeper than actual.

A truly abnormally shaped femoral head sometimes is seen in patients with severe hip dysplasia, but most apparently misshapen femoral heads appear that way due to osteophytosis. Large osteophytes on the femoral neck can give the false impression of a "flattened" femoral head. The buildup of bone on the neck may be mistaken for remodeling of the femoral head (Figure 5.139).

Coxa valga or coxa vera can occur with hip dysplasia, but these conditions frequently are overdiagnosed. Rotation of the femur readily mimics an abnormal femoral neck angle (Figure 5.140).

Hip dysplasia can occur in any breed of dog or cat. In many affected animals the hips will appear normal at birth and develop signs of dysplasia over time. The etiology of hip dysplasia is multifactorial. Both environmental and genetic factors play important roles.

In cats, the most common signs of hip dysplasia are subluxation and osteophytes on the dorsal acetabular rim. Osteophytes on the femoral neck are less common in cats than in dogs.

Coxofemoral joint laxity is considered to be the earliest clinical and radiographic sign of hip dysplasia. In many dogs, the hips are more lax during estrus and pregnancy. In these situations, consider postponing the investigation of hip dysplasia until at least 1 month after estrus or weaning

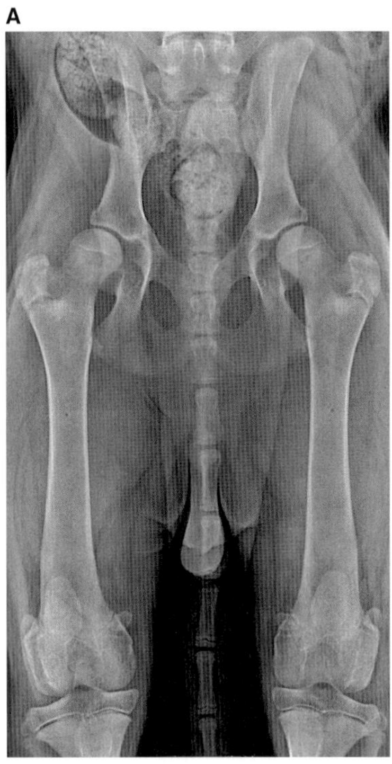

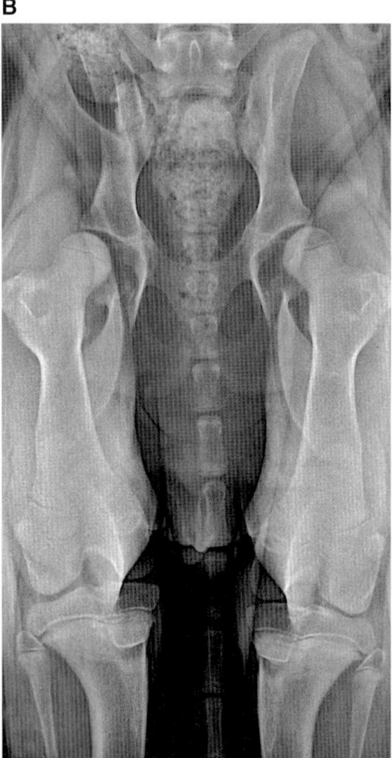

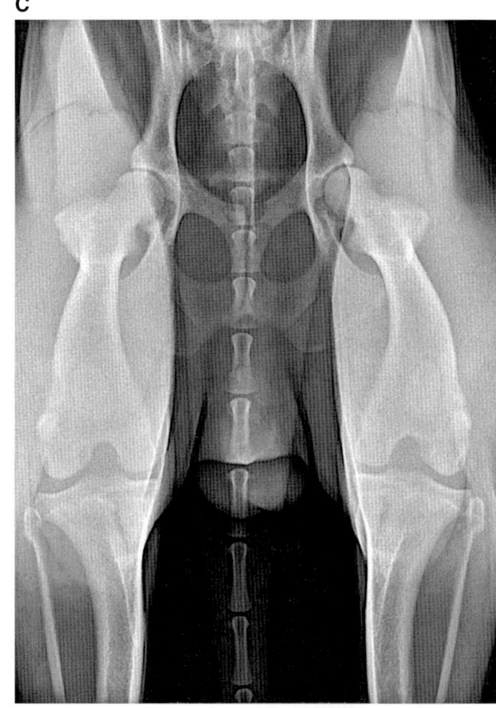

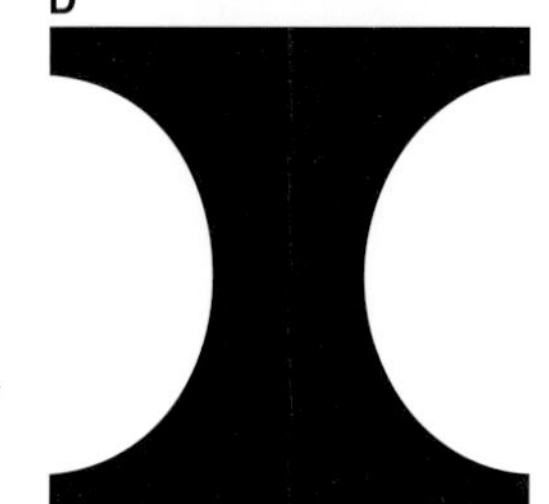

Figure 5.137 Half axial views. **A**. VD extended view of a dog pelvis with normal appearing coxofemoral joints. **B**. VD half-axial view of the same dog, but both hips are now subluxated, as indicated by the cranial wedging of the coxofemoral joints. Lateral distraction of the femurs reveals th hip laxity in this dog. **C**. VD half-axial view of a different dog pelvis for comparison. This dog has no evidence of hip laxity; the femoral heads remain well-seated in the acetabular fossae during distraction. **D**. An illustration of the distraction device that was placed between the patient's thighs to make the half-axial views. This device acts as a fulcrum to distract the hips when the tarsi are moved together (see also Figure 2.37).

a litter. Prolonged periods of physical inactivity also can lead to greater hip laxity (e.g., illness, confinement, weather conditions).

Hip dysplasia usually is bilateral, but occasionally it is unilateral. Distraction views and/or clinical hip palpation should be employed before accepting a diagnosis of unilateral hip dysplasia. Unilateral hip dysplasia appears to occur more often in certain genetic lines and seems to repeatedly involve the same side hip in that line. The incidence of unilateral disease, however, is independent of the overall rate of hip dysplasia in that breed.

Radiographic findings may not correlate with clinical signs. Some animals with obvious radiographic signs of hip dysplasia remain asymptomatic for years. However, animals with hip dysplasia should not be used for breeding.

Registry groups-hip dysplasia certification

Several groups exist worldwide to collect data about the prevalence of hip dysplasia and to certify dogs and cats. Radiographs are submitted and graded to assess coxofemoral joint conformation and the presence or likelihood of developing or transmitting hip dysplasia (Table 5.7). Some of these groups include the *Orthopedic Foundation for Animals* (**OFA**), the *Pennsylvania Hip Improvement Program* (**PennHIP**), the *Federation Cynologique Internationale* (**FCI**), and the *British Veterinary Association/Kennel Club* (**BVA/KC**).

The extended VD view of the pelvis was adopted by the American Veterinary Medical Association (AVMA) in 1961 for the detection of hip dysplasia. This view is used in many countries throughout the world for grading hips. A properly positioned VD view includes the following:

1. The entire pelvis, the two most caudal lumbar vertebrae, the femurs, and the stifles are all visible.
2. The pelvis and femurs are symmetrical.
3. Both ilial wings are equal in width.
4. The obturator foramina are equal size.
5. Both femurs are extended, parallel with each other, and parallel with the ilia.
6. Each patella is superimposed in the middle of the femur.

A

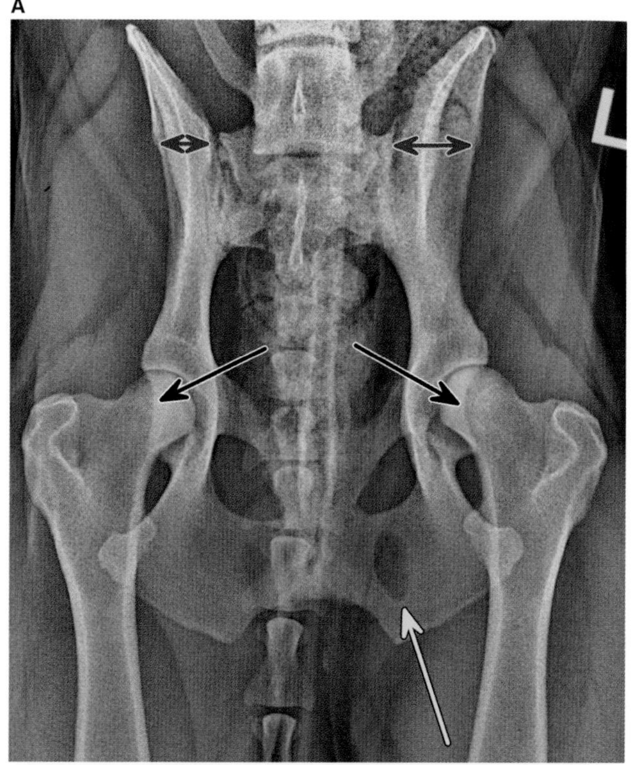

B

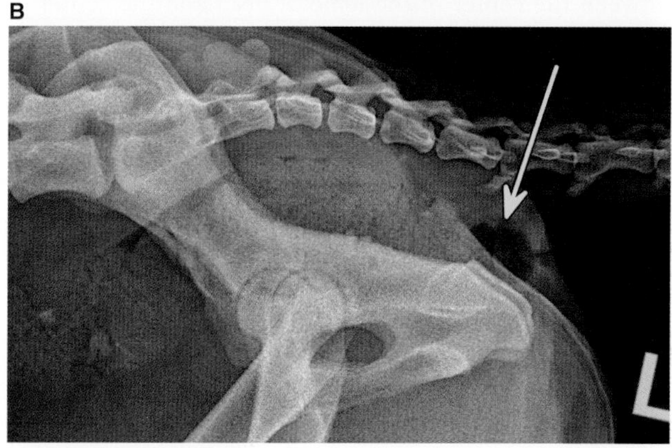

Figure 5.138 Rotated pelvis. VD view (**A**) and lateral view (**B**) of a dog pelvis. In the VD view, the left ilial wing appears wider than the right ilial wing (red double-headed arrows). Also in the VD view, the left obturator foramen appears smaller than the right obturator foramen. These findings indicate that the pelvis is slightly rotated. Pelvic rotation alters the apparent coverage of the femoral heads by the dorsal acetabular rims (black arrows). Notice that there appears to be less coverage of the left femoral head than the right. This is a positioning artifact that may be mistaken for a shallow left acetabular fossa. The acetabulum on the side with the wider ilial wing may appear abnormally shallow (memory tip: "wider = worse") and the acetabulum on the side with the bigger obturator foramen may appear deeper than actual size (memory tip: "bigger = better"). Notice in the VD view that there is a well-defined area of less opacity in the left ischium (yellow arrow). This is an artifact caused by superimposition of anal gland gas, as can be seen in the lateral view (arrow).

The **OFA** was established in 1966 as a hip registry for dogs. Cats are now also included. Each radiograph submitted to the OFA is independently reviewed by three board-certified veterinary radiologists. A consensus opinion is provided to both the owner and the referring veterinarian. Dogs that are at least 2 years of age receive one of seven grades, based on the radiographic appearance of the hips

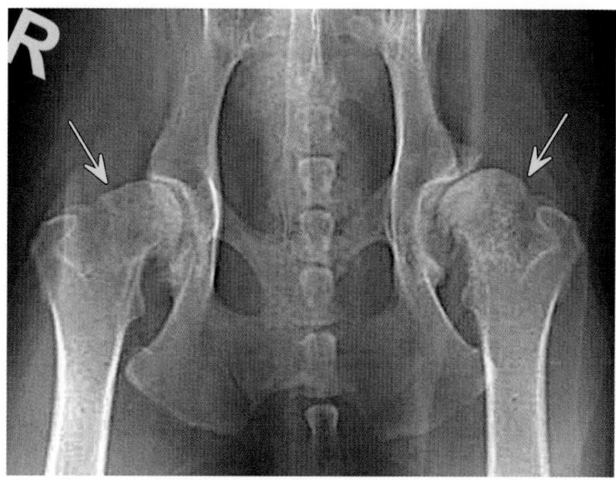

Figure 5.139 "Flattening" of the femoral heads. VD view of a dog pelvis depicting bilateral hip dysplasia with coxofemoral joint subluxation and advanced degenerative joint disease. The apparent "flattening" of the femoral heads, particularly in the left hip, is due to the extensive buildup of new bone on the femoral necks (arrows).

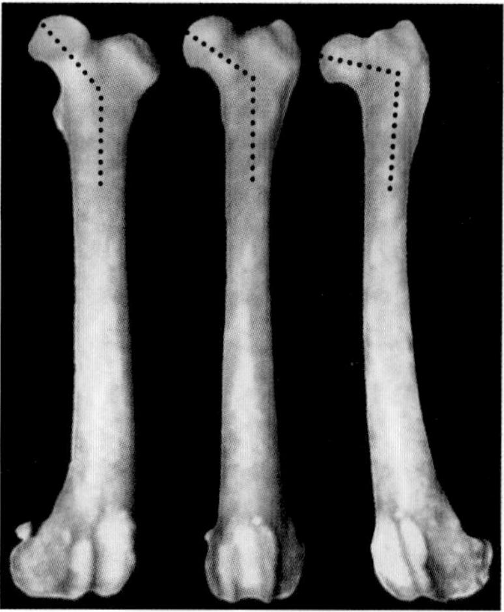

Figure 5.140 Angle of femoral neck. These photographs of the same bone specimen illustrate the different appearances of the femur depending on the point of view. Notice that the angle between the femoral neck and the femoral shaft (dotted lines) appears to vary as the femur is rotated. On the left, the angle appears increased (coxa valga); in the middle the angle is normal (the femur is viewed en face); and on the right, the angle appears decreased (coxa vara).

Table 5.7 Hip dysplasia registry grading scales (approximate)

	OFA	FCI (European)	BVA (UK/Australia)	SV (Germany)	PennHIP DI	Norberg Angle
Normal	Excellent	A-1	0–4	Normal	<0.3	≥105°
	Good	A-2	5–10	Normal		
Transitional	Fair	B-1	11–18	Normal		100°–105°
	Borderline	B-2	19–25	Fast Normal		
Dysplastic	Mild	C-1	26–30	Noch Zugelassen	>0.3	100°
		C-2	31–35			
	Moderate	D-1	36–45	Mittlere		90°–100°
		D-2	46–50			
	Severe	E-1	51–70	Schwere		≤90°
		E-2	71–106			

compared to normal dogs with similar signalment (Figure 5.141). The seven grades are:

1. **Excellent:** superior hip conformation characterized by a well-formed, C-shaped acetabulum, a deeply seated femoral head with greater than 75% coverage by the dorsal acetabular rim, and a uniform, thin, and even joint space.
2. **Good:** characterized by a well-formed, C-shaped acetabulum, 60%–75% coverage of the femoral head by the dorsal acetabular rim, and a well-seated, even joint.
3. **Fair:** minor irregularities and a slightly uneven joint space; the bones may not be ideally aligned, but they are not subluxated; the dorsal acetabular rim may be slightly concave; there is at least 50% coverage of the femoral head by the dorsal acetabular rim.
4. **Borderline:** no clear consensus for a grade due to either (1) nonspecific or questionable findings, (2) poor positioning, or (3) technique artifacts. Radiographs usually are repeated within 6–8 months.
5. **Mild** hip dysplasia: slight joint wedging and partial subluxation, a shallow and slightly flared acetabulum (less C-shaped); only 40%–50% coverage of the femoral head by the acetabular rim; the joint space is widened; early or mild degenerative joint disease is present.
6. **Moderate** hip dysplasia: significant joint wedging and subluxation; the acetabular fossae are shallow with only 25%–40% coverage of the femoral head; there is moderate degenerative joint disease.
7. **Severe** hip dysplasia: severe subluxation or the hips are completely luxated; the acetabular fossae are very shallow with less than 25% coverage of the femoral head; there is a large amount of degenerative joint disease.

PennHIP was established in the 1980s and requires two VD views of the pelvis for evaluation: one with the hips compressed and another with the hips distracted. The radiographs are objectively evaluated to provide a quantitative measurement of hip laxity which is called a distraction index (DI). The DI is calculated by measuring the distance between the center of the femoral head and the center of the acetabulum and dividing that number by the radius of the femoral head (Figure 5.142). The DI compares the degree of laxity in each hip during compression and distraction. Veterinarians who want to use this technique must be specially trained and certified by PennHIP. Any radiographs made must be submitted to the PennHIP Analysis Center for evaluation. Puppies as young as 16 weeks can be evaluated. DI ranges between 0.0 and 1.0. The lower the number the tighter the hip. A DI of 0.3 or less is considered normal. DI greater than 0.4 suggests a higher probability of developing secondary DJD.

The **FCI** is a group of more than 80 national kennel authorities in Europe, Russia, South America, and Asia that provide evaluations of hip conformation in dogs. Each extended VD radiograph is evaluated by one "scorer." No special certification is required to be a scorer. Dogs must be at least 1 year of age. The criteria used to score each hip include:

1. Norberg angle (illustrated in Figure 5.143).
2. Degree of subluxation.
3. Shape and depth of the acetabulum.
4. Signs of degenerative joint disease.

Each hip receives one of five possible grades:

A. **Normal**.
B. **Near normal**: the hip is congruent with a Norberg angle less than 105° or it is slightly incongruent with a Norberg angle of 105°.

C. Mild hip dysplasia: the hip is incongruent with a Norberg angle near 100°; the craniolateral acetabular rim is flattened (shallow); there is mild DJD.
D. Moderate hip dysplasia: the hip is obviously incongruent and subluxated; the Norberg angle is 90°–100°; the acetabular fossa is flattened (shallow); DJD is present.
E. Severe hip dysplasia: the hip is distinctly subluxated or luxated, the Norberg angle is less than 90°, the femoral head is deformed (flattened or mushroom-shaped); there is advanced DJD.

The **BVA/KC** is the hip grading method used in Britain, Ireland, Australia, and New Zealand. Hip scores are based on nine criteria; five of which deal with acetabular shape and depth, two with hip laxity and subluxation, and two with DJD. Each criterion is graded between 0 (ideal) and 6 (worst). The final score ranges from 0 to 53 for each hip or 0 to 106 for both hips. Scoring is done by three panelists from a group of radiologists or surgeons.

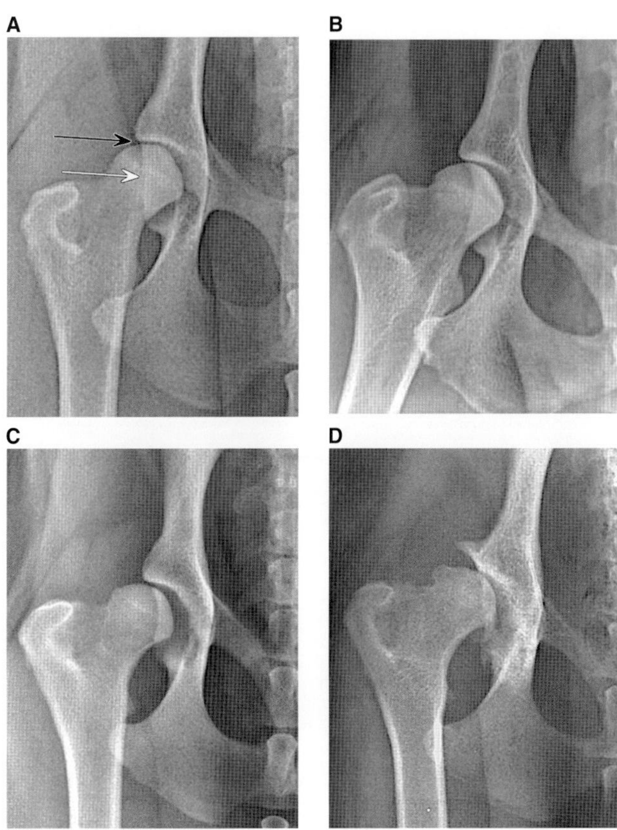

Figure 5.141 Grades of hip dysplasia. **A**. VD view of a dog pelvis depicting normal hip joint conformation. Notice the amount of coverage of the femoral head by the dorsal acetabular rim (white arrow) and the uniformly even coxofemoral joint space (black arrow). Remember to evaluate the cranial part of the joint space. **B**. VD view depicting mild hip dysplasia with slight cranial wedging of the coxofemoral joint space and less than 50% coverage of the femoral head by the dorsal acetabular rim. **C**. VD view depicting moderate hip dysplasia with more severe subluxation, less coverage of the femoral head, and osteophytes on the femoral neck. **D**. VD view depicting severe hip dysplasia with subluxation, a flattened acetabular fossa, and a large amount of osteophytosis.

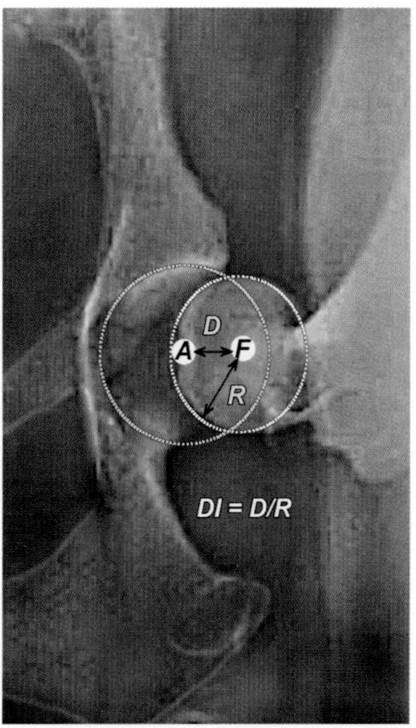

Figure 5.142 PennHIP. VD view of a dog made during distraction and illustrating the measurements used to calculate the Distraction Index (DI). DI is the distance (D) between the femoral head center (F) and the acetabular center (A) divided by the radius of the femoral head (R).

Pelvic fractures and luxations

Most pelvic fractures result from blunt force trauma and involve more than one pelvic bone. If only one bone appears to be fractured, look for a concurrent sacroiliac luxation. Supplemental views may be needed to identify all fractures in a damaged pelvis. Fracture lines associated with non-displaced or overlapping fractures may be more opaque than the adjacent bone due to summation of the ends of the fragments. Be sure to look for damage in other structures such as the urethra, urinary bladder, rectum, sciatic nerve, vertebrae, and retroperitoneal space.

Femoral head and neck fractures sometimes are only minimally displaced and difficult to recognize in an extended VD view. These fractures often become apparent in a flexed VD or "frog-leg" view because the bones are viewed from a different perspective and the adjacent tissues may become more relaxed, allowing the fragments to separate.

Many femoral neck fractures are intra-capsular. They may be unilateral or bilateral. Chronic or incomplete fractures sometimes present with an "apple core" appearance due to

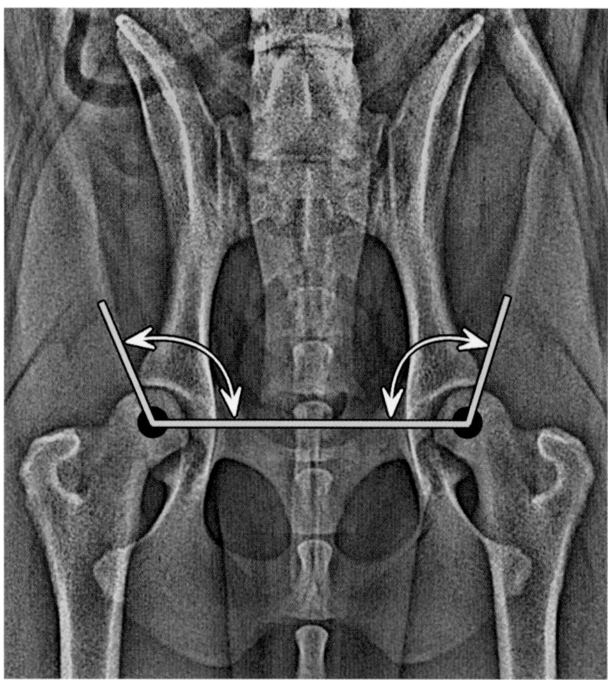

Figure 5.143 Norberg angle. VD view of a dog pelvis illustrating the Norberg measurement technique. The Norberg angle is a numerical assessment of hip joint laxity. To make the measurement, you first locate the center of each femoral head (black dots). Second, draw a line between the centers (yellow line). Third, draw a line from each center to the cranial acetabular rim (white lines). The intersection of a white line with the yellow line determines the Norberg angle for that hip. An angle greater than 105° is considered normal, an angle between 90° and 105° is borderline abnormal, and an angle less than 90° is abnormal.

bone resorption (Figure 5.144). At one time, an "apple core" femoral neck was thought to be a permanent lesion that was expected to lead to a complete fracture, however, many cases can resolve with proper care.

Capital physis fractures occur in immature animals and involve the proximal femoral physis and sometimes the femoral neck (Salter–Harris type I or II). In cats, capital physis fractures may result from a syndrome called **feline capital physeal dysplasia**. The etiology of this syndrome is unknown, but trauma rarely is reported. Osteonecrosis of the femoral neck leads to a pathologic fracture at the capital physis (Figure 5.145). The syndrome is also called *proximal femoral metaphyseal osteopathy*. It most often is reported in young male cats, less than 2 years old, especially overweight animals. Fractures can occur in any breed, but Siamese are overrepresented. Fractures may be unilateral or bilateral. If unilateral, the contralateral limb often is affected within 6–12 months.

An **avulsion fracture** sometimes is seen at the insertion of the gluteal tendon on the greater trochanter. A fracture here must be differentiated from the more frequently seen incidental tendon mineralization (Figure 5.129). With a fracture, there usually is soft tissue swelling and a site of origin for the fracture fragment. A fracture fragment also tends to be more irregular in shape than incidental mineralization.

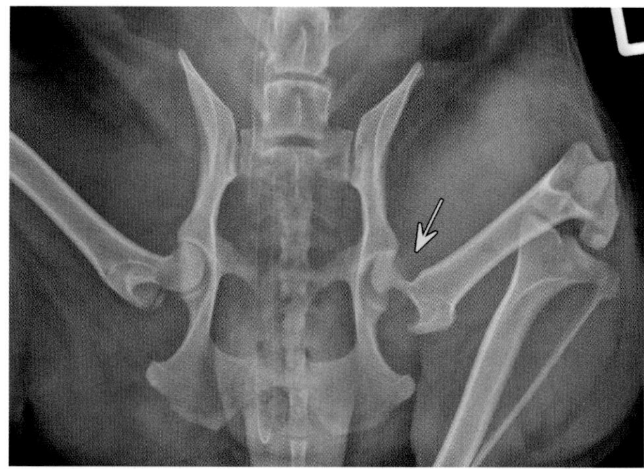

Figure 5.144 *Apple-core* lesion. Flexed VD view of a dog pelvis depicting a narrowed left femoral neck with an irregular, indistinct margin (arrow).

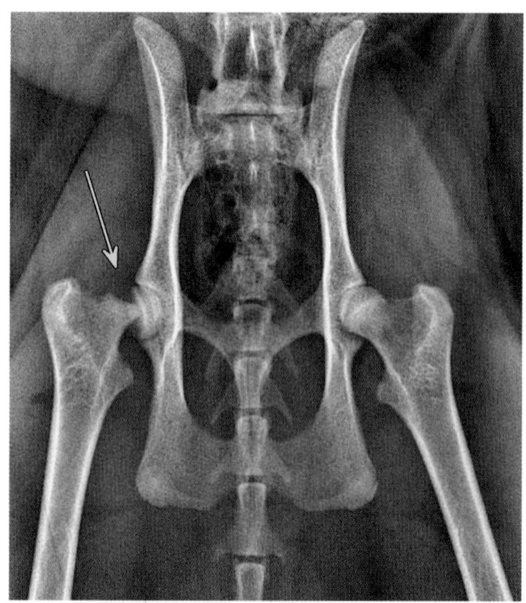

Figure 5.145 Feline capital physeal dysplasia syndrome. VD view of a cat pelvis depicting a displaced fracture in the right femoral proximal physis (arrow).

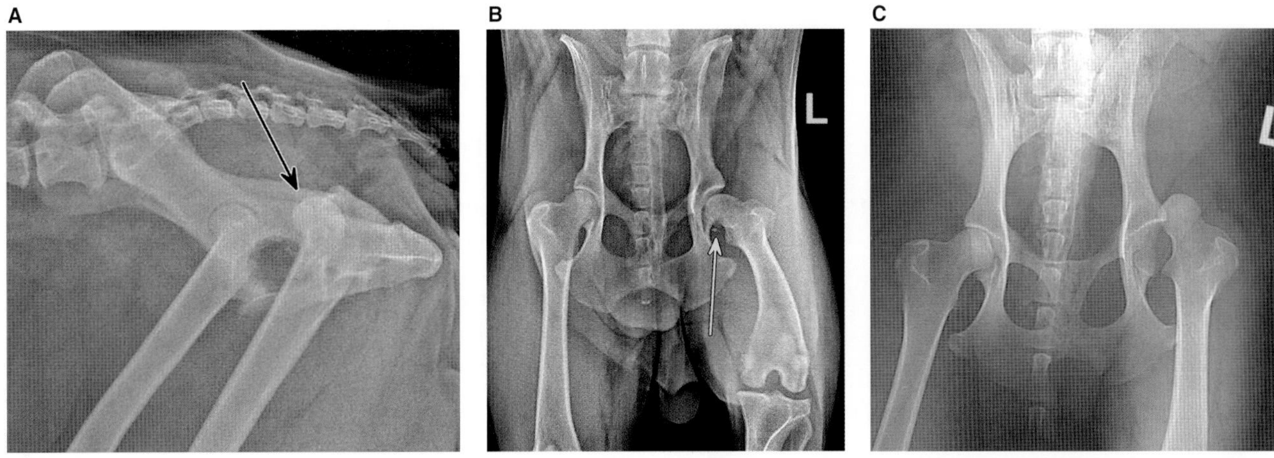

Figure 5.146 Coxofemoral luxation. **A**. Lateral view of a dog pelvis depicting dorsal displacement of the left femur (arrow). **B**. VD view of the same dog; the coxofemoral luxation is not as evident because the femoral head is superimposed on the acetabular fossa. The arrow points to a small chip fracture just caudal to the left femoral head. **C**. VD view of a different dog pelvis depicting cranial luxation of the left hip.

Coxofemoral luxation

Common causes of a dislocated hip include hip dysplasia and blunt force trauma. Most hip luxations are cranial and dorsal (Figure 5.146). Caudoventral luxations are less common, but they do occur. Medial luxation requires a concurrent acetabular fracture. A hip luxation may include a fracture, either in the femoral head, femoral neck, or acetabulum. Lateral oblique and flexed VD views frequently are useful to detect fracture fragments that are not apparent in standard views. An avulsion fracture at the insertion of the round ligament typically produces a small mineral opacity structure in the acetabular fossa. A fracture fragment in the acetabulum must be ruled out before attempting closed reduction of a luxated hip. A closed reduction also may fail if there is damage to the supporting structures or formation of a hematoma in the joint.

Sacroiliac luxation

In a VD view, the sacroiliac arch is formed by the medial borders of the ilia and the caudal border of the sacrum. The margin normally is continuous and smooth. A sacroiliac (SI) luxation interrupts the arch, creating a "stair-step" due to displacement of the ilium (Figure 5.147). SI luxations may be unilateral or bilateral. Unilateral luxations often are accompanied by one or more pelvic fractures. A common misdiagnosis of SI luxation occurs when the x-ray beam is aligned with a normal sacroiliac joint, making the normal separation between the ilium and sacrum appear wider or more "open" than in the other joint. This can be seen in Figure 5.147 where the normal pelvis is slightly rotated to make the right sacroiliac joint more visible than the left. The key to accurate diagnosis of SI luxation is to identify a stair-step in the sacroiliac arch.

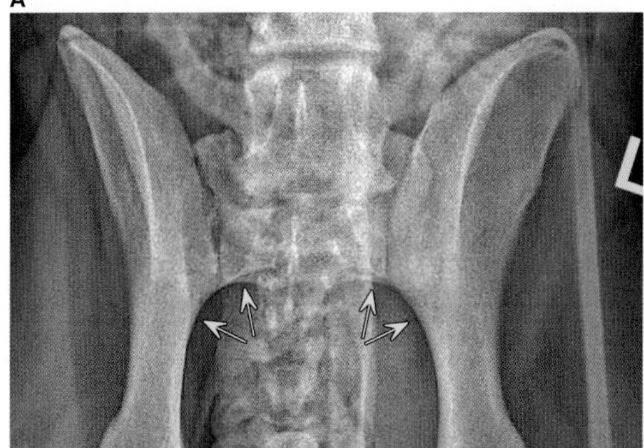

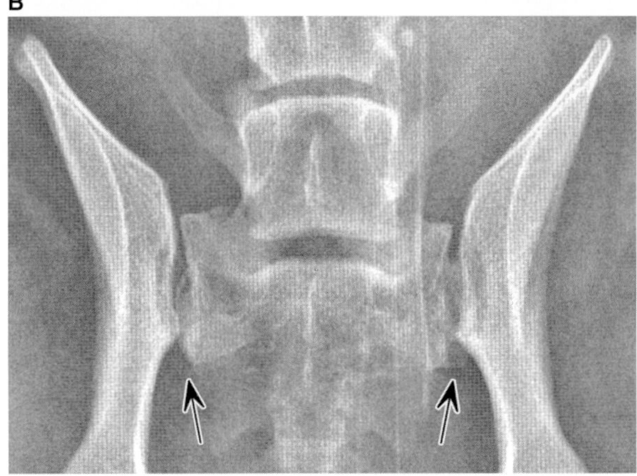

Figure 5.147 Sacroiliac luxation. **A**. VD view of a normal dog pelvis. The arch formed by the inner borders of each ilium and the sacrum is continuous and even (arrows). **B**. VD view of a sacroiliac luxation. There is a discontinuity or "stair-steps" in the arch (arrows) due to cranial displacement of the ilia.

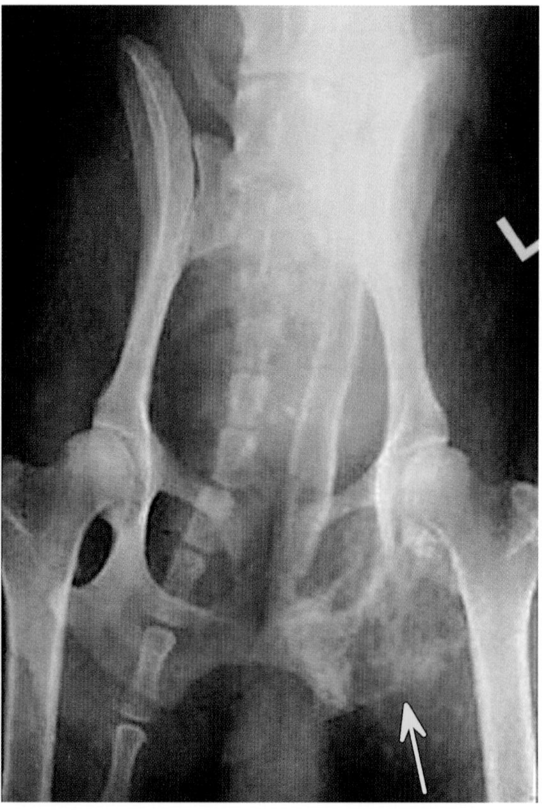

Figure 5.148 Pelvic neoplasia. VD view of a dog pelvis depicting aggressive osteolysis with an amorphous periosteal response in the left ischium (arrow).

Pelvic neoplasia

Pelvic tumors are uncommon in dogs and cats. Osteolysis tends to predominate, accompanied by variable degrees of periosteal new bone production and soft tissue swelling (Figure 5.148).

Stifle

Normal radiographic anatomy

There are two joints in the stifle: *femorotibial* and *femoropatellar*. The femorotibial is a condylar synovial joint and the femoropatellar is a gliding synovial joint. The anatomy of the stifle is illustrated in Figures 5.149–5.154.

In the cranial part of the femorotibial joint, there is a triangular-shaped body of fat called the *infrapatellar fat pad*. The fat pad is located between the patellar ligament, the distal femur, and the proximal tibia. Caudal to the femorotibial joint, a fat opacity fascial plane usually is visible near the gastrocnemius muscle belly. This plane is a valuable landmark to assess joint swelling.

Four sesamoid bones are present in the stifle: *patella, lateral fabella, medial fabella,* and *popliteal*. Knowledge of their normal locations avoids mistaking them for avulsion fractures and aids in diagnosing various soft tissue abnormalities. The **patella** or "kneecap" is the largest sesamoid. It is located in the tendon of the quadriceps muscle, cranial to the distal femur. The part of the quadriceps tendon between the patella and its insertion on the tibia is called the *patellar ligament*. In dogs, the patella is ovoid in shape. In cats, it is more tapered distally, sometimes described as shaped like a "teardrop" or "baseball cap." The caudal surface of the patella is lined with articular cartilage. The **fabellae** are sesamoid bones in the lateral and medial tendons of the gastrocnemius muscle. They are located caudal to the femoral condyles. The medial fabella tends to be smaller than the lateral fabella and may not ossify in some animals. It sometimes is seen more distal than the lateral fabella, in which case it may be mistaken for a tendon avulsion. One or both fabellae may develop from multiple ossification centers resulting in bipartite or multipartite sesamoid bones. These usually are asymptomatic and may be differentiated from fractures by the lack of soft tissue swelling and no active bone remodeling. Multipartite fabella are rounded with smooth and well-defined borders and do not change in appearance in serial radiographs (Figure 5.169). The **popliteal** sesamoid is located in the tendon of the popliteal muscle, caudal to the lateral part of the proximal tibia. It sometimes fails to ossify.

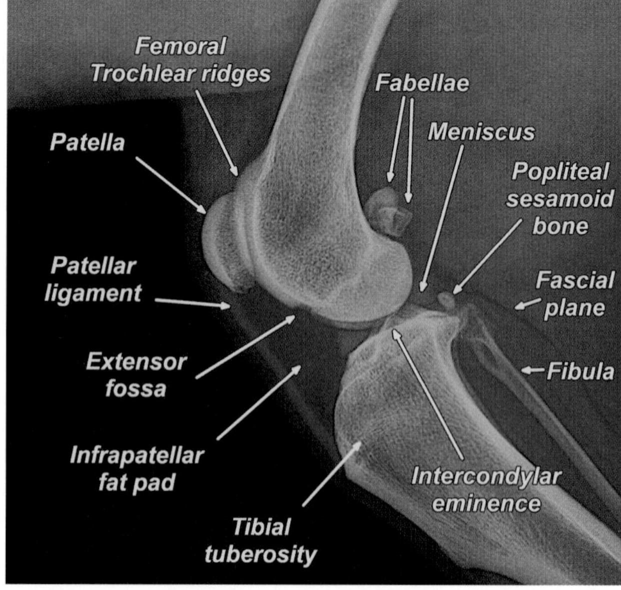

Figure 5.149 Normal stifle. Lateral view of a dog stifle depicting normal anatomy. Notice that the cranial portion of the meniscus is visible as the soft tissue opacity triangle caudal to the infrapatellar fat pad.

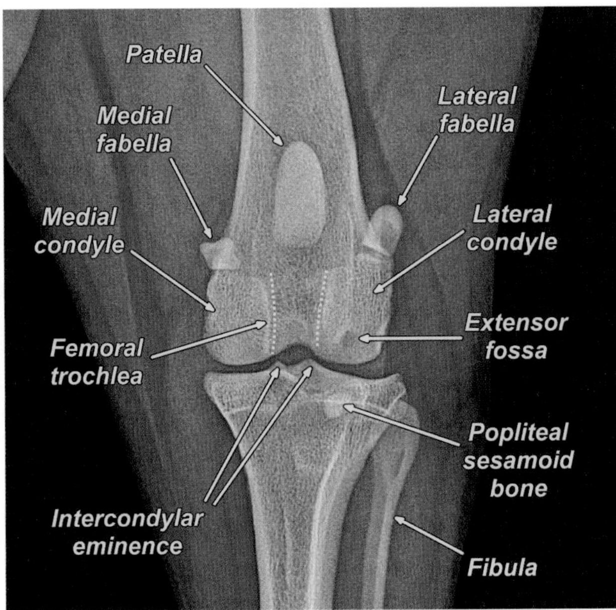

Figure 5.150 Normal stifle. Caudocranial view of a dog stifle depicting normal anatomy. The intercondylar eminence consists of lateral and medial tubercles that project into the intercondylar fossa of the femur. The femoral trochlea is also called the patellar groove. Notice that the lateral portion of the meniscus is visible as a soft tissue opacity triangle at the lateral aspect of the femorotibial joint space. The medial portion is thin and seldom visible.

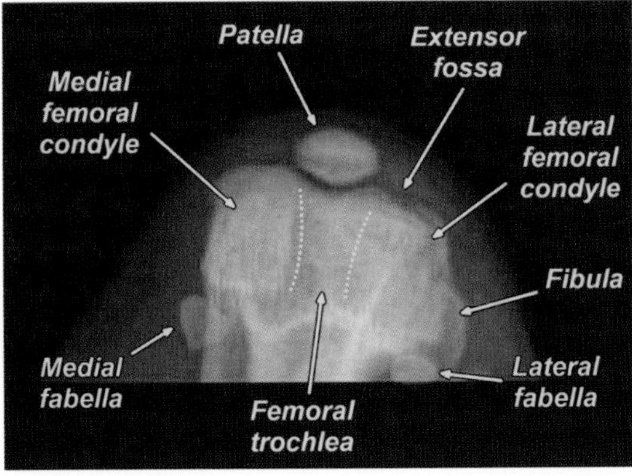

Figure 5.151 Normal stifle. Skyline view of a cat stifle depicting normal anatomy.

Radiographic views of the stifle

1. **Lateral** view (Figure 2.39).
2. **Caudocranial** view (Figure 2.40). In properly positioned lateral and caudocranial views, the intercondylar eminence of the tibia is centered with the femoral condyles.
3. **Tibial compression** view: a lateral view made with both the stifle and the tarsus flexed to assess stifle joint laxity caused by cranial cruciate ligament injury. The sensitivity and specificity of this view is reported to be superior to physically performing a cranial drawer test (Figure 2.41).
4. **Skyline** view: a flexed cranioproximal-craniodistal view to further evaluate the patella and patellar groove (Figure 2.42).
5. **Craniocaudal** view: less desirable than a caudocranial view due to greater magnification distortion of the stifle; however, extending the stifle while the patient is in dorsal recumbency may be preferred to doing so in ventral recumbency.

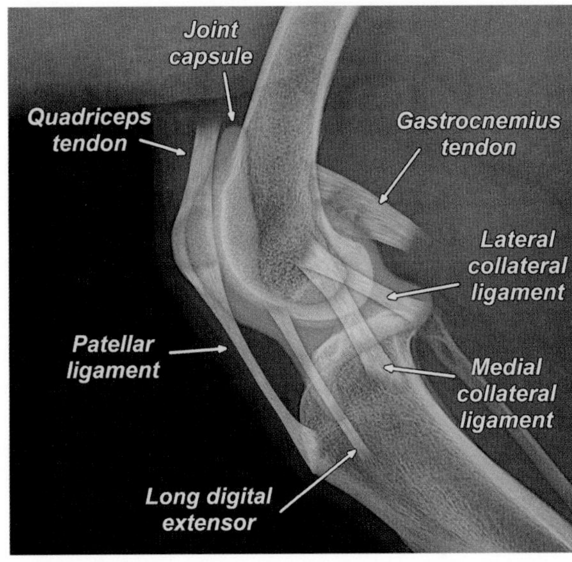

Figure 5.152 Normal stifle. Lateral view of a dog stifle illustrating the attachment sites of the joint capsule, ligaments, and tendons at the stifle.

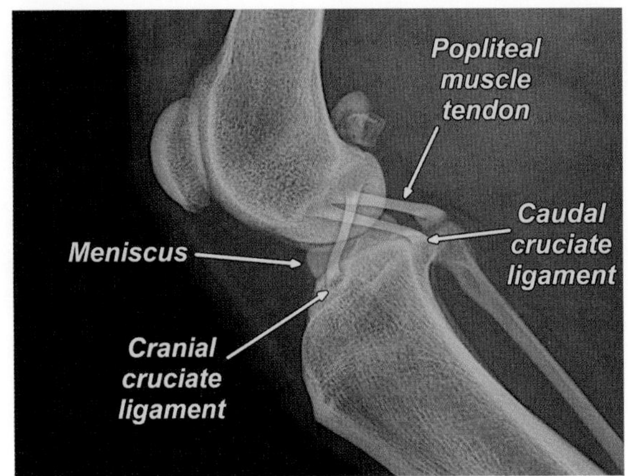

Figure 5.153 Normal stifle. Lateral view of a dog stifle illustrating the attachment sites of the cruciate ligaments.

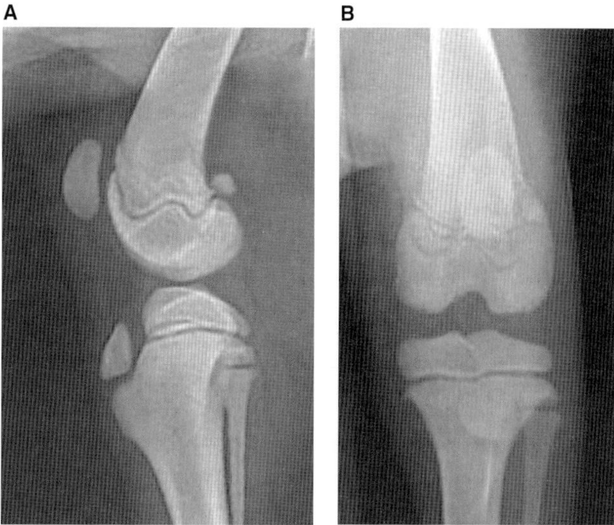

Figure 5.154 Normal immature canine stifle. Lateral view (**A**) and caudocranial view (**B**) depicting a puppy stifle.

Stifle degenerative joint disease

Stifle DJD often is a sequela to cranial cruciate ligament damage, particularly in larger dogs. It usually is bilateral. Other causes of stifle DJD include osteochondrosis, chronic patellar luxation, and previous trauma. Osteophytes typically appear first along the trochlear ridge, the patella, and at the extensor fossa (Figures 5.155 and 5.156). They later develop on the condyles, fabellae, popliteal sesamoid bone, and proximal tibia. Joint swelling is common due to joint effusion, synovial thickening, or swelling in the periarticular tissues. Focal, rounded areas of osteolysis may be seen in the intercondylar fossa of the femur in a caudocranial view. These subchondral bone cysts are a frequent finding with chronic DJD.

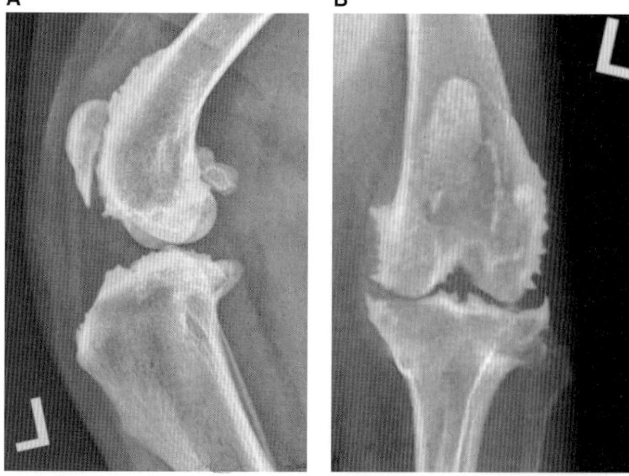

Figure 5.155 Stifle DJD. Lateral view (**A**) and caudocranial view (**B**) of a dog stifle illustrating the sites where osteophytes may form. Look for osteophytes in the peripheral areas of non-weight bearing articular cartilage, including the femoral trochlear ridges (patellar groove) and the tibial intercondylar eminence.

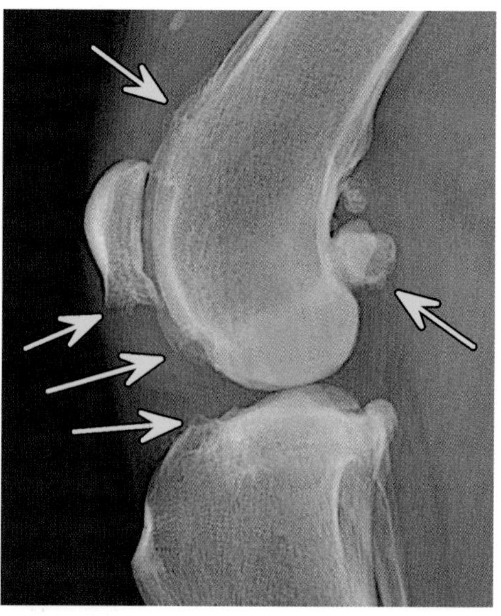

Figure 5.156 Stifle DJD. Lateral view of a dog stifle depicting osteophytes on the trochlear ridge of the femur, distal patella, extensor fossa, tibial plateau, and fabellae (arrows).

Stifle cruciate ligament injuries

Partial or complete tearing of a cruciate ligament usually leads to femorotibial joint instability, joint effusion, and eventually to DJD. Damage to the cranial cruciate ligament is much more common than damage to the caudal cruciate ligament.

Cranial cruciate ligament injury

A torn cranial cruciate ligament (CCL) allows the proximal tibia to move cranial in relation to the distal femur. This movement may be palpable as the *cranial drawer sign*. Lack of a cranial drawer sign, however, does not rule out a cranial cruciate ligament injury.

In radiographs, cranial displacement of the tibia is identified when the intercondylar eminence of the tibia is positioned cranial to the center of the femoral condyles (Figure 5.157). This finding may or may not be evident in a standard lateral view. When findings are equivocal, a tibial compression view may demonstrate the displacement (Figure 2.56). Whether making a standard view or a compression view, the stifle must be in a true lateral position to accurately assess femorotibial alignment. Rotation of the stifle can mimic or mask abnormalities. With many patients, the patella needs to be slightly rotated toward the image receptor to make a true lateral view. Another finding frequently associated with cranial displacement of the proximal tibia is distal displacement of the popliteal sesamoid bone.

Stifle joint effusion is common with cruciate ligament injuries. It appears as increased opacity in the femorotibial joint (Figure 5.158). Joint effusion distends the joint

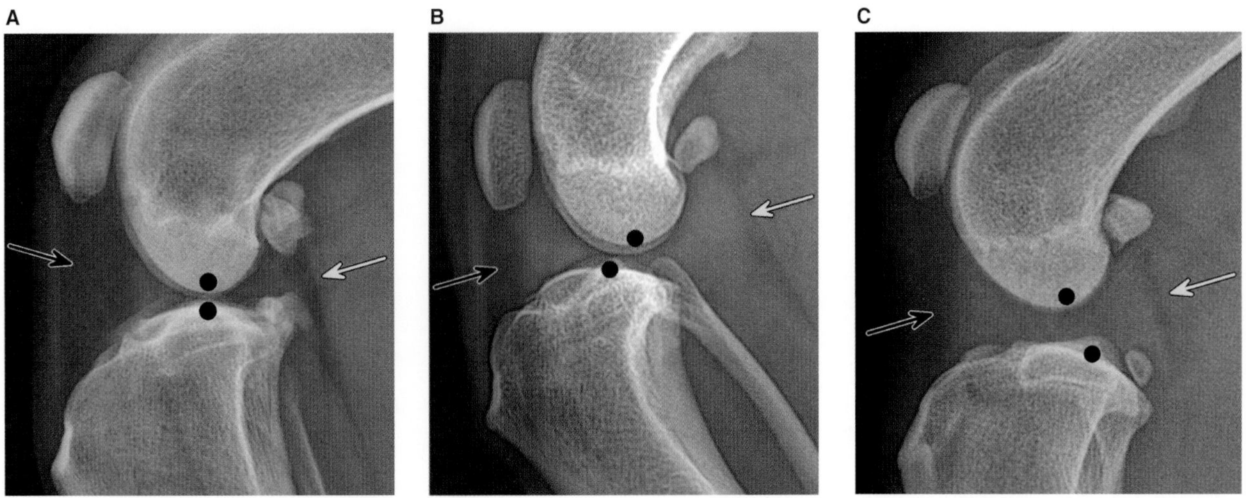

Figure 5.157 Cruciate ligament injuries. Lateral views of dog stifles. The black dots in each radiograph designate the center of the femoral condyles and the center of each tibial intercondylar eminence. The black arrows point to the infrapatellar fat pads. The yellow arrows point to a fat opacity fascial plane. **A**. Normal stifle with good alignment between the proximal tibia and the distal femur, a normal fat pad, and a normal fascial plane. **B**. The proximal tibia is cranially displaced in relation to the distal femur due to a rupture of the cranial cruciate ligament. Joint effusion distends the femorotibial joint capsule, partially effacing the fat pad and pushing the fascial plane caudally. **C**. The proximal tibia is caudally displaced in relation to the distal femur due to a caudal cruciate ligament rupture. Joint effusion again effaces the fad pad, reducing its apparent size, and pushes the fascial plane caudally.

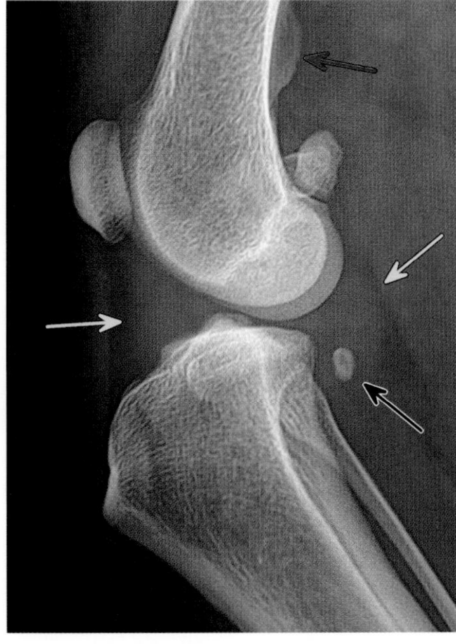

Figure 5.158 Cranial cruciate ligament rupture. Lateral view of a dog stifle depicting cranial displacement of the proximal tibia in relation to the distal femur. Joint effusion causes the joint capsule to distend, partially effacing the infrapatellar fat pad and pushing the caudal fascial plane further caudally (yellow arrows). The popliteal sesamoid bone is displaced caudally and distally (black arrow). The well-defined, smooth bordered bone along the caudal border of the distal femur is a normal attachment site for the origin of the gastrocnemius muscle tendons (red arrow). The size and appearance of this attachment site is variable between animals.

capsule, pushing the caudal fascial plane further caudally and reducing the apparent size of the infrapatellar fat pad. The fat pad appears smaller due to partial effacement and some degree of cranial displacement. Other causes of stifle joint effusion must be differentiated from a cranial cruciate ligament injury (e.g., infection, osteochondrosis, torn meniscus, tumor).

Rarely, an injury to the cranial cruciate ligament is accompanied by an avulsion fracture at an insertion of the ligament. It is more likely in younger animals. The avulsed fragment typically is seen in the intercondylar region of the distal femur. It may be difficult to differentiate from other mineralized intra-articular structures.

Factors that can contribute to cranial cruciate ligament injuries include hip dysplasia, old age, obesity, and patellar luxation. Cruciate ligament injuries may be unilateral or bilateral. Bilateral injuries may clinically mimic disease in the hips or spine.

Stifle fractures and luxations

Stifle trauma usually is accompanied by soft tissue swelling. Swelling may be due to joint effusion or thickening of the soft tissues near the trauma site, or both. The presence or absence of soft tissue swelling often helps differentiate pathology from normal anatomic variation or an imaging artifact. Comparison radiographs of the contralateral limb or a known normal limb also can aid with interpretation of radiographic findings.

Stifle avulsion fractures

An avulsion fracture generally presents as a separate mineral opacity structure located near the attachment site of a ligament or tendon. A bed for the fracture fragment sometimes is identified. Avulsion fractures usually are unilateral, but sometimes they are bilateral. They are more likely to occur in larger, immature dogs.

The **gastrocnemius** muscle tendons originate on the caudal aspects of the lateral and medial femoral condyles. A tendon avulsion typically results in caudal and distal displacement of the affected fabella (Figure 5.159). Displacement sometimes is more evident in radiographs made with the tarsus flexed. An avulsed bone fragment from the femur may also be present, typically located proximal to the displaced fabella. During healing the affected fabella may thicken and become irregular in shape. An enthesophyte may develop on the caudal femoral condyle at the site of injury. Dystrophic mineralization can occur in the adjacent soft tissues. Remember that the fabellae normally vary in position and to correlate radiographic findings with clinical signs (e.g., pain, swelling) to confirm an avulsion.

The origin of the **long digital extensor** tendon is the extensor fossa of the lateral femoral condyle. A tendon avulsion may displace a bone fragment from the femur to the cranial compartment of the femorotibial joint (Figure 5.160). When this happens, the extensor fossa typically is visibly enlarged due to loss of the bone fragment. Comparison radiographs of the contralateral limb may be useful for diagnosis. The long digital extensor tendon is closely associated with the femorotibial joint capsule and joint effusion may be present.

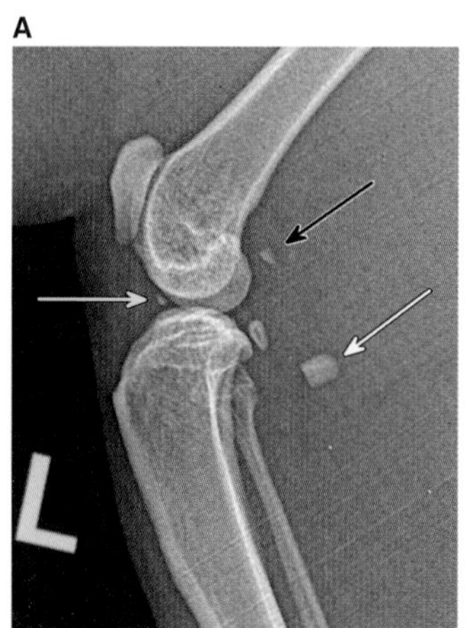

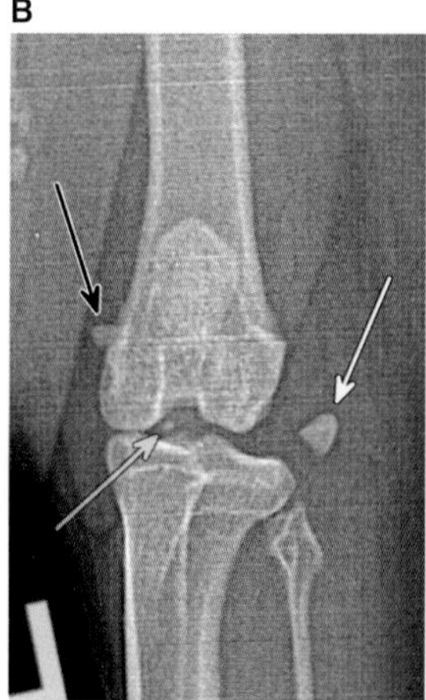

Figure 5.159 Gastrocnemius tendon avulsion. Lateral view (**A**) and caudocranial view (**B**) of a cat stifle depicting caudal and distal displacement of the lateral fabella (white arrow) due to tearing at the origin of the lateral branch of the gastrocnemius muscle tendon. The smaller medial fabella is normal in position (black arrow). The focal mineral opacity structure in the femoropatellar joint is likely associated with the meniscus (yellow arrow). These "meniscal ossicles" are a frequent, asymptomatic finding in cats. The mottled background pattern in these radiographs is caused by the canvas stretcher on which the cat was lying during radiography.

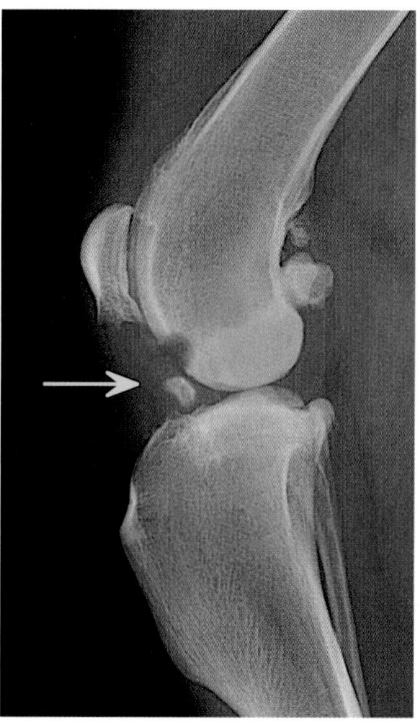

Figure 5.160 Avulsion of long digital extensor tendon. Lateral view of a dog stifle depicting an avulsed bone fragment that is displaced distally from the extensor fossa (arrow). There is joint effusion. Osteophytes and enthesophytes are visible, particularly on the patella and patellar groove.

The **popliteal** muscle originates on the caudal aspect of the lateral femoral condyle. A popliteal tendon avulsion sometimes is associated with damage to the cranial cruciate ligament. Avulsion of the tendon often leads to distal displacement of the popliteal sesamoid bone.

Avulsion of the tibial tuberosity

Tibial tuberosity avulsions occur in immature dogs and cats, prior to fusion of the tuberosity to the tibia. These usually are Salter–Harris type I fractures and they most often are caused by hyperflexion of the stifle. The fractured tuberosity is displaced proximally and may be rotated clockwise in relation to the proximal tibia (Figure 5.161). The severity of displacement and the degree of rotation depends on the amount of pull from the quadriceps tendon and whether the proximal tibial physis is also fractured. A fracture in the proximal tibial physis typically is identified by the caudal displacement of the proximal tibial epiphysis relative to the tibial shaft. The width of the fractured physis usually is uneven, wider on one side and narrower on the other. If the tuberosity is avulsed and the proximal tibial physis is not fractured, the space between the two may be wedge-shaped. In some cases, the fracture in the proximal tibial physis involves the metaphysis or/and epiphysis (Salter–Harris type II, III, or IV).

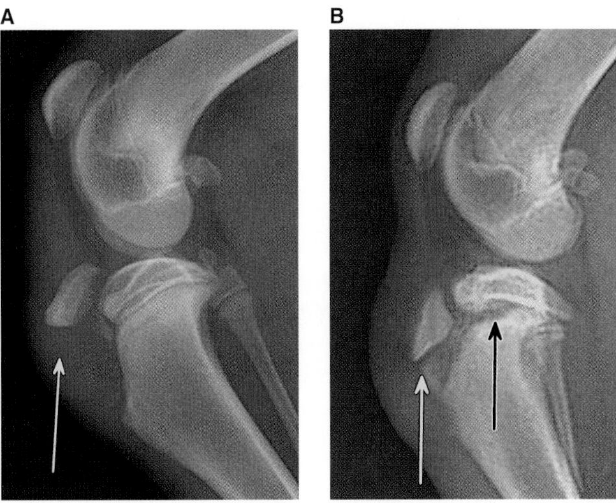

Figure 5.161 Avulsion fracture of tibial tuberosity. **A**. Lateral view of an immature dog stifle depicting proximal displacement and clockwise rotation of the tibial tuberosity fragment (yellow arrow) and moderate soft tissue swelling. **B**. Lateral view of a different immature dog stifle depicting less severe avulsion of the tibial tuberosity (yellow arrow) and a fracture in the proximal tibial physis, the latter resulting in caudal displacement of the proximal epiphysis (black arrow).

Another radiographic signs of tibial tuberosity avulsion is a patella that is positioned further proximally than expected. The patellar ligament frequently is thickened and may be less distinct.

In immature animals, there usually is a considerable amount of soft tissue opacity cartilage distal to the bone opacity tuberosity. This apparent "space" distal to the tuberosity may be mistakenly thought to be due to tuberosity avulsion. Soft tissue swelling helps differentiate an avulsion fracture from the normal appearance of an incompletely ossified tibial tuberosity. Avulsions usually are unilateral and comparison radiographs of the contralateral limb often are helpful. Follow-up radiographs generally reveal osseous remodeling if a lesion was present and not evident in the initial images. Tibial tuberosity avulsions may be idiopathic or they may be a form of osteochondrosis in certain dog breeds (e.g., Greyhound, English Bull Terrier, Staffordshire Terrier).

An incomplete avulsion of the tibial tuberosity may result from repetitive low-grade trauma or overuse. These injuries can lead to a condition called *traction apophysitis* or, as it is called in humans, *Osgood–Schlatter disease*. In these cases there is no displaced fragment, only soft tissue swelling. The margin of the tibial tuberosity may more irregular and less defined, and the pattern of ossification may be more heterogenous, but these tend to be subtle findings.

Patellar ligament rupture

Rupture of the patellar ligament typically causes two types of soft tissue swelling: thickening of the ligament and swelling in the adjacent tissues (Figure 5.162). The two often blend together and may not be separable in radiographs. The infrapatellar fat pad may be caudally displaced. The patella is positioned further proximally than normal, especially when the stifle is flexed. Rupture may be caused by blunt trauma or hyper-contraction of the quadriceps muscles. A patellar fracture sometimes is present. During healing, an enthesophyte may develop on the proximal tibial tuberosity.

Unrelated to a patellar ligament injury, an enthesophyte sometimes is seen on the distal tibial tuberosity in the area of attachment of the cranial tibial muscle tendon (Figure 5.170). Usually, there is no soft tissue swelling and it is an incidental finding.

Asynchronous growth of the tibia and fibula

Damage to the proximal tibial physis can lead to premature closure and a disproportionate rate of growth between the tibia and the fibula. In most cases, the tibial plateau develops abnormally (a condition called *tibial plateau deformans*). The most common type of damage is a Salter-Harris type V or VI fracture. The typical radiographic finding is a tibial plateau that slopes caudally and distally, often accompanied by bowing of the fibula (Figure 5.163). Tibial plateau deformans may resemble a chondrodystrophic tibia. Femorotibial joint effusion may be present. Abnormal growth of the tibia may lead to genu varum ("bow-legged") and a predisposition to cranial cruciate ligament injury. Secondary degenerative

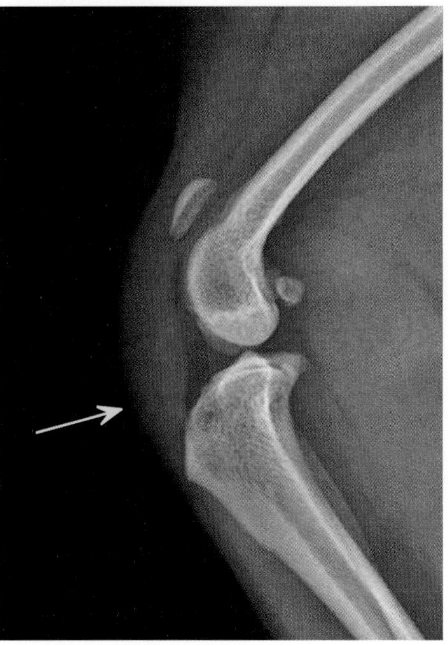

Figure 5.162 Ruptured patellar ligament. Lateral view of a cat stifle depicting soft tissue swelling associated with the patellar ligament (arrow) and proximal displacement of the patella. Soft tissue swelling blends with the patellar ligament because they are the same opacity with no different opacity between them.

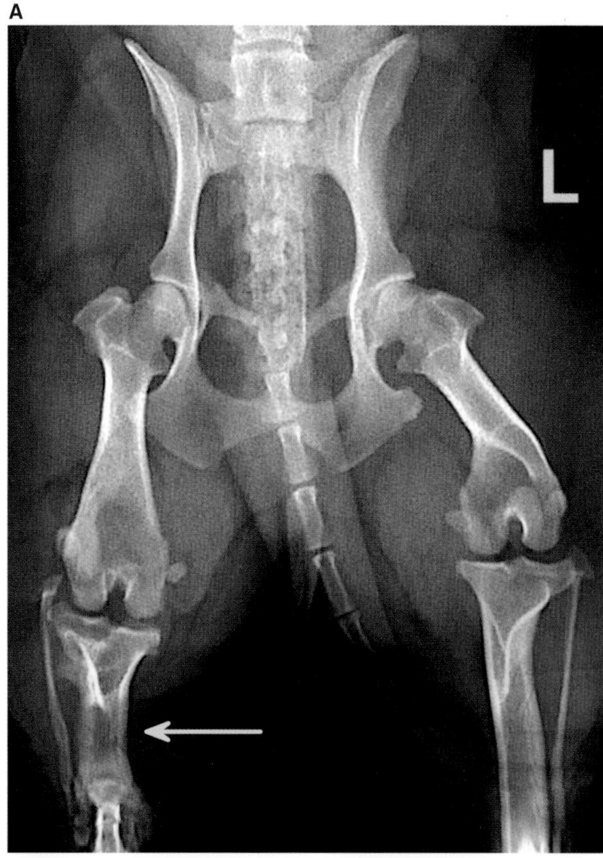

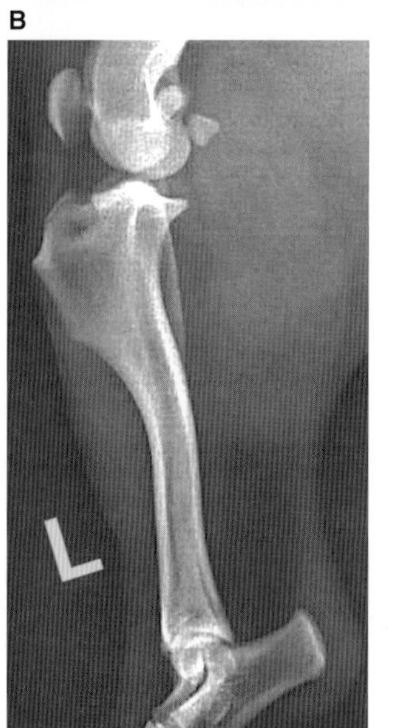

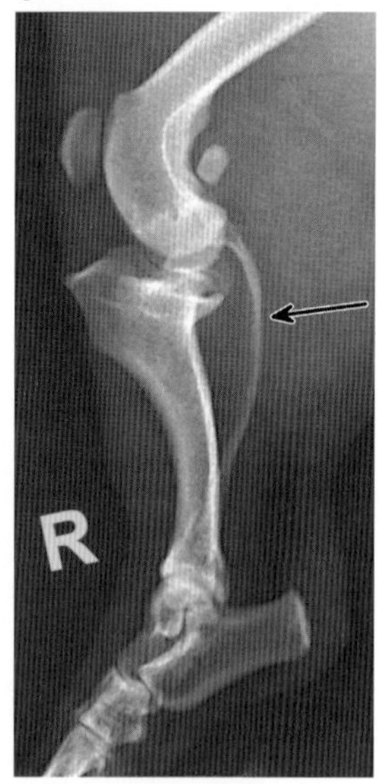

Figure 5.163 Damaged proximal tibial physis. VD view of the pelvis (**A**), lateral view of the left pelvic limb (**B**), and lateral view of the right pelvic limb (**C**) of the same dog depicting an abnormally shortened right tibia (yellow arrow) with a bowed right fibula (black arrow). The right tibial plateau slopes caudodistally and the right fibular head is luxated. The left leg is normal.

joint disease is common. Damage to the proximal tibial physis most often is reported in West Highland White Terriers and Rough Coated Collies. In severe cases, the patient may be unable to extend the stifle and may exhibit a crouching rear leg stance.

Stifle luxation

Dislocation of the stifle is reported more often in cats than in dogs. It typically is caused by traumatic ruptures of the collateral and cruciate ligaments. Malalignment of the bones may only be visible in one view, making orthogonal radiographs essential. Stress views sometimes are needed to determine the full extent of the damage and the degree of joint laxity. Injury severe enough to luxate the stifle frequently damages the menisci, joint capsule, nerves, and blood supply. Damage to vessels or nerves may limit successful treatment.

Patellar luxation

Patellar luxation usually is a clinical diagnosis. Radiographs often are useful to document secondary changes and to determine whether other disorders are present. In many cases, patellar luxation is intermittent and the position of the patella may or may not be abnormal at the time of radiography. In a caudocranial view, a displaced patella may be located medial or lateral to the femoral trochlea (Figure 5.164). In a lateral view, a luxated patella often is superimposed on the distal femur. Medial patellar luxation is much more common than lateral luxation. Medial luxations are most often reported in small dogs, particularly toy and miniature breeds. Lateral luxations more often are seen in large breed dogs. Both medial and lateral luxations usually are bilateral.

Factors that contribute to patellar luxation, and can be assessed with radiographs, include a shallow femoral trochlea (patellar groove), hip disease (e.g., dysplasia, aseptic necrosis), limb deformities (e.g., genu varum, genu valgum, pes varum, pes valgum), and trauma. A skyline view radiograph is useful to assess the depth of the femoral trochlea (Figure 5.164). Note: oblique positioning of the stifle can mimic a limb deformity (Figure 5.165).

Tibial cartilage rest

In the immature tibia, the proximal epiphysis is contiguous with the tibial tuberosity apophysis. Both the epiphysis and the apophysis are cartilagenous structures that normally ossify as the animal matures. In some dogs, part of the cartilage does not completely ossify, leaving a soft tissue opacity spot between the tibial plateau and the tibial tuberosity (Figure 5.166). This is an asymptomatic variation called a "cartilage rest", but it may be mistaken for a lytic lesion. Cartilage rests usually are bilateral. Radiographs of the opposite stifle may be helpful for diagnosis, but the two tibias may not be identical in appearance.

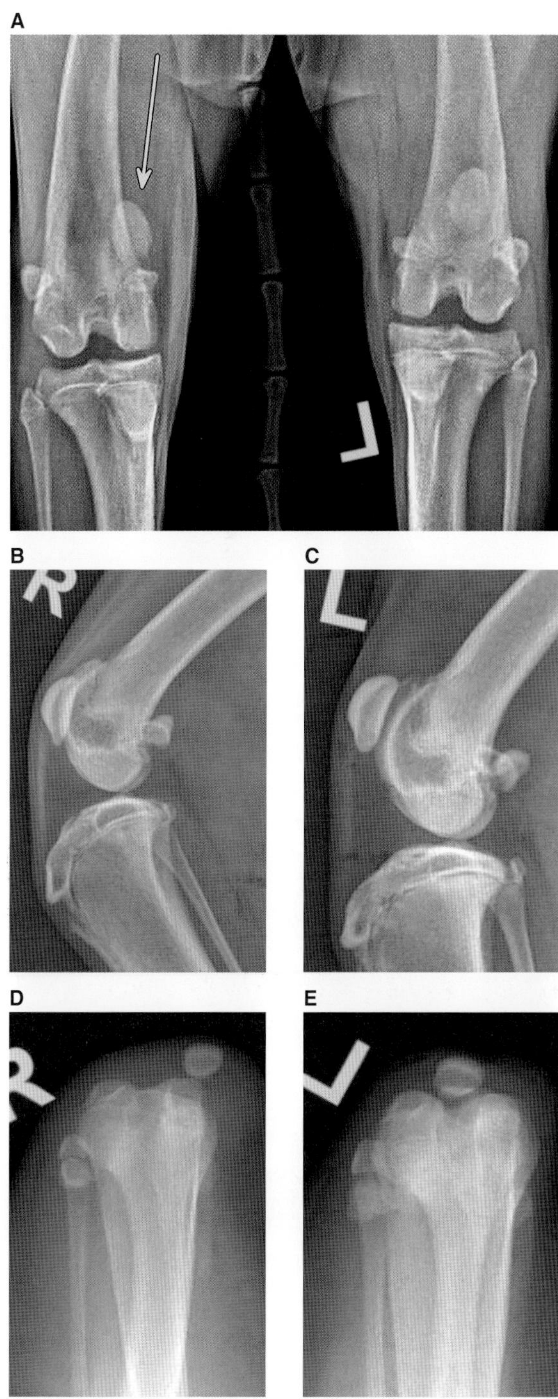

Figure 5.164 Medial patellar luxation. Craniocaudal view (A), lateral views (B and C), and skyline views (D and E) of an immature dog's right and left stifles depicting medial luxation of the right patella (arrow in A). The right patella partially overlies the femur in the lateral view (C). The left stifle is normal.

Stifle neoplasia

Many of the tumors that involve the stifle are primarily osteolytic with a variable periosteal response (Figure 5.71). Joint effusion is common and a soft tissue mass sometimes can be identified, often with lobulated margins. Stifle tumors usually are aggressive and most often reported in older, medium to large breed dogs (e.g., Rottweiler, Golden Retriever). Tumors that have been reported in the stifle include osteosarcoma, synovial cell sarcoma, fibrosarcoma, and chondrosarcoma.

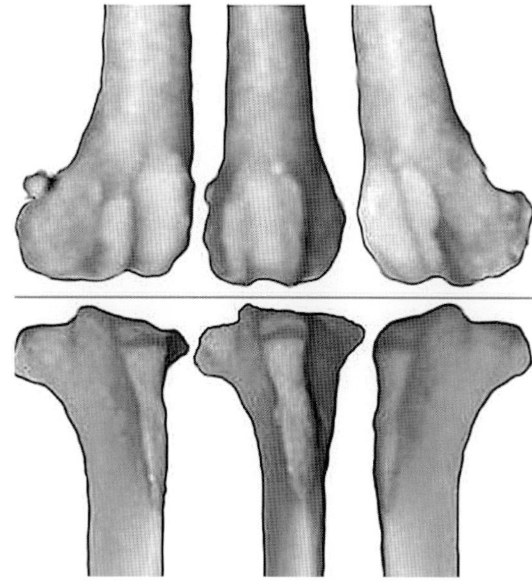

Figure 5.165 Effects of stifle positioning. These photographs of the same bone model illustrate the appearance of the distal femur and proximal tibia due to stifle rotation and different points of view.

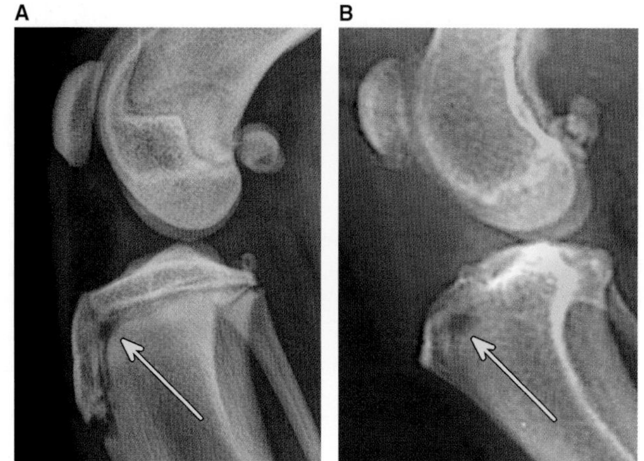

Figure 5.166 Tibial cartilage rest. A. Lateral view of a normal immature dog stifle depicting the cartilage junction between the physes in the proximal tibia and the tibial tuberosity (arrow). B. Lateral view of a normal adult dog stifle depicting a cartilage rest (arrow); a focal area of soft tissue opacity between the tibial plateau and the tibial tuberosity.

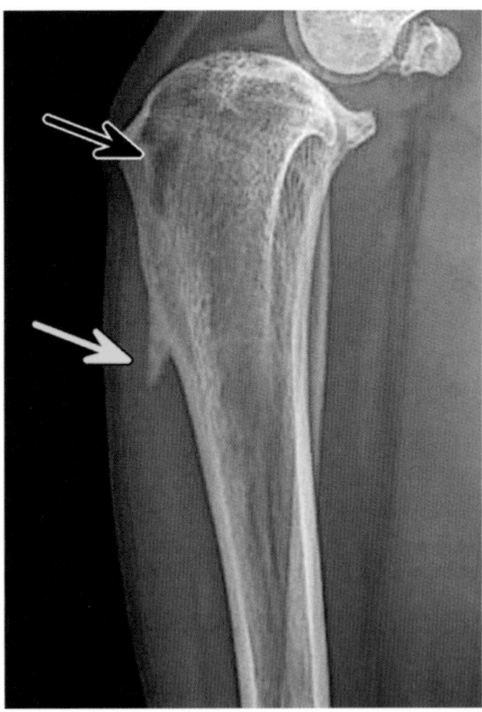

Figure 5.167 Incidental findings. Lateral view of a dog tibia depicting an enthesophyte in the cranial tibial muscle tendon, extending distally from the tibial tuberosity (yellow arrow). There is no soft tissue swelling or active bone remodeling. The black arrow points to decreased opacity in the proximal tibia due to cartilage rests (cartilage that did not completely ossify during bone development).

Stifle osteochondrosis

In the stifle, osteochondrosis lesions occur most often in the distal femur. Common sites include the medial aspect of the lateral femoral condyle, the medial femoral condyle, and the lateral trochlear ridge. Lesions typically appear as circular defects or flattened areas along the articular border (Figure 5.168). They may be surrounded by osteosclerosis. Joint effusion is common. Osteochondrosis is less common in the pelvic limbs than in the thoracic limbs. Mineralized fragments sometimes are present in the femorotibial joint. Mineralized flaps rarely are seen in the stifle. Secondary degenerative joint disease is a frequent finding. Osteochondrosis usually is bilateral, but lameness may be unilateral.

The normal extensor fossa on the cranial border of the lateral femoral condyle may be mistaken for an osteochondrosis lesion. The fossa, however, is located proximal to the articular margin.

Multipartite sesamoid bones

The patella and the fabellae develop from two or more ossification centers. Failure of the centers to unite results in a bipartite or multipartite sesamoid bone. In radiographs, this appears as two or more rounded, smooth-bordered, well-defined mineral opacity structures in the area of the patella or a fabella (Figures 5.169 and 5.170). Multipartite sesamoid

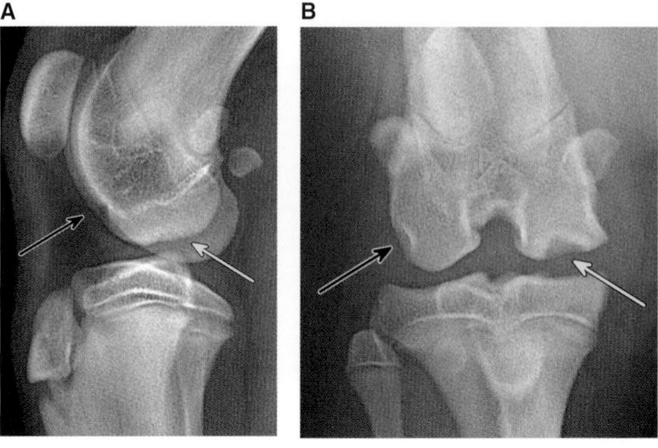

Figure 5.168 Stifle osteochondrosis. Lateral view (**A**) and caudocranial view (**B**) of an immature dog stifle depicting a flattened area on the articular border of the medial femoral condyle (yellow arrows). The rounded defect in the condyle is surrounded by osteosclerosis. The black arrows point to the normal extensor fossa which may be mistaken for a lesion.

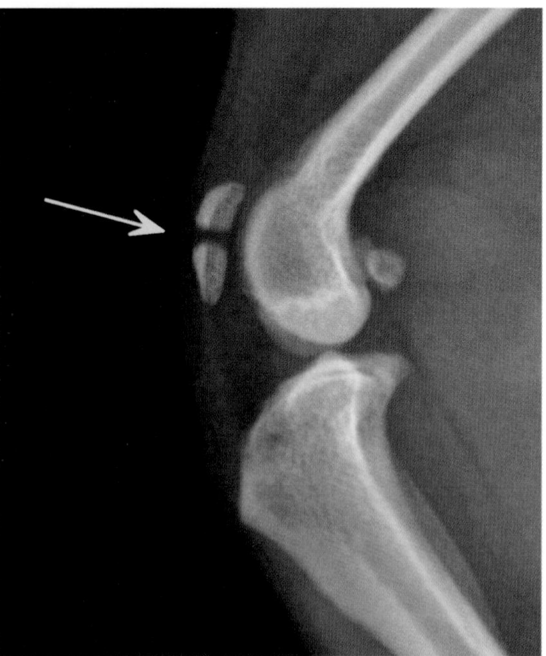

Figure 5.169 Bipartite patella. Lateral view of a cat stifle depicting two well-defined mineral opacity structures in the area of the patella (arrow). There is no soft tissue swelling. This finding is consistent with a bipartite patella; however, a chronic, non-union fracture of the patella may be similar in appearance.

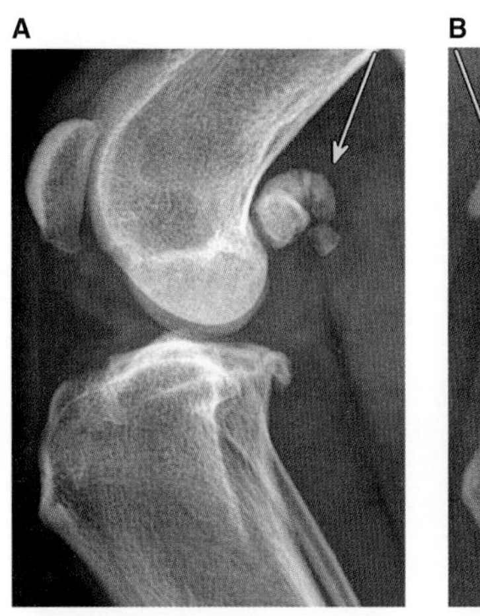

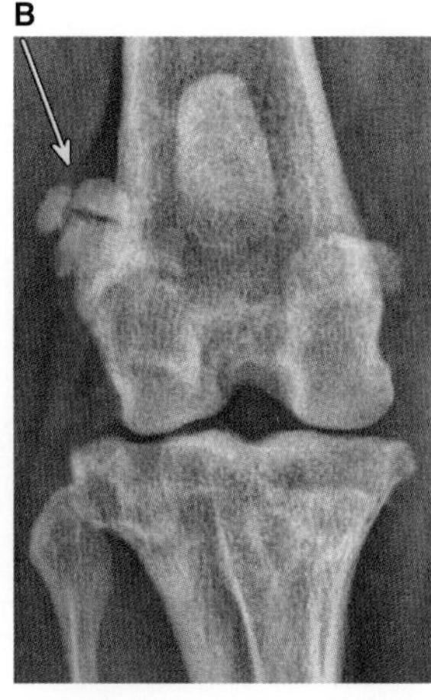

Figure 5.170 Multipartite fabella. Lateral view (**A**) and caudocranial view (**B**) of a dog stifle depicting multiple mineral opacity structures in the area of the lateral fabella (arrows). This is an incidental finding. There is, however, cranial displacement of the proximal tibia relative to the distal femur and moderate joint effusion indicating cranial cruciate ligament damage.

bones may be unilateral or bilateral and do not change in appearance in serial radiographs. Multipartite patella is reported more often in cats than in dogs. It is an uncommon condition that usually can be differentiated from a patellar fracture by the absence of soft tissue swelling and no active bone remodeling.

Tarsus

Normal radiographic anatomy

The tarsus is a composite synovial joint composed of four major articulations: tibiotarsal, proximal intertarsal, distal intertarsal, and tarsometatarsal. Other names for the tibiotarsal joint include: the tarsocrural joint, the talocrural joint, and the ankle. Most of the movement in the tarsus occurs at the tibiotarsal joint.

Crus refers to the lower part of the pelvic limb, between the stifle and the tarsus. Some frequently seen artifacts in this area are depicted in Figure 5.171. **Pes** refers to the distal part of the pelvic limb, which includes the tarsus and the digits. In most dogs and cats, there are four digits in each pes. The first digit usually is absent. Normal tarsal anatomy is illustrated in Figures 5.172–5.174.

There are multiple short or cuboidal bones in the tarsus. The most medial bone is the **talus** or tibiotarsal bone, which articulates with the tibia via two large trochlear ridges. The talus also articulates with both the lateral malleolus of the fibula and the medial malleolus of the tibia. The most lateral tarsal bone is the **calcaneus** or fibulotarsal bone, which is the largest and longest tarsal bone. A large process called the *tuber calcis* or *calcanean tuber* extends proximally from the calcaneus. The *common calcanean tendon* (Achilles tendon) attaches to the tuber calcis. The **central** tarsal bone is located distal to the talus and articulates with all of the other tarsal bones. The **fourth** tarsal bone is located distal to the calcaneus and spans both the proximal and distal intertarsal joints. One or two sesamoid bones may be visible plantar to the distal tarsus in the lateral and medial parts of the tarsometatarsal fibrocartilage. The lateral sesamoid bone tends to ossify more often than the medial sesamoid.

The medial collateral ligament of the tarsus runs from the medial malleolus to the first tarsal and metatarsal bones. The lateral collateral ligament runs from the lateral malleolus to the fifth metatarsal bone. Plantar ligaments extend from the calcaneus to the proximal metatarsus.

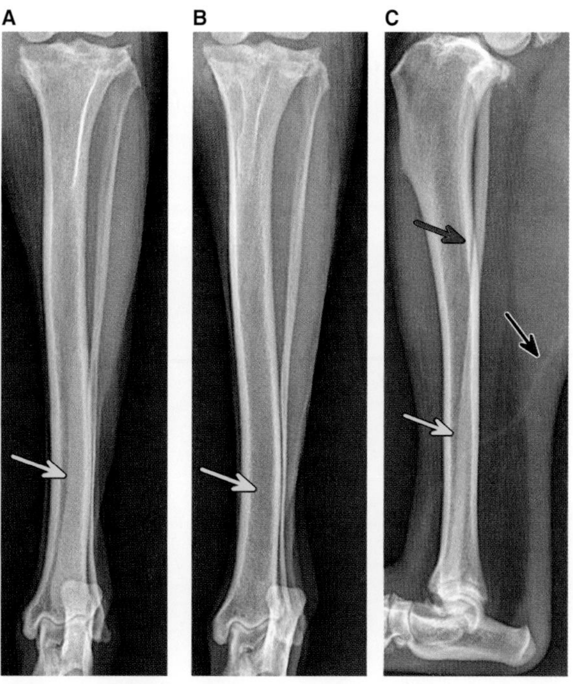

Figure 5.171 Summation artifacts. **A**. Craniocaudal view of a dog tibia depicting superimposition of the Achilles tendon on the medullary region of the distal tibia (arrow). The artifact may be mistaken for a fracture line. **B**. Craniocaudal view of the same tibia, but slightly obliqued to eliminate superimposition of the Achilles tendon. **C**. Lateral view of the same tibia depicting superimposition of the fibula, which also may be mistaken for a fracture line (yellow arrow). In addition, there appears to be a line of decreased opacity where the fibula crosses the caudal cortex of the tibia (red arrow). This is an optical illusion called a negative Mach line, another artifact which may be mistaken for a fracture or a nutrient foramen. The black arrow points to the saphenous vein.

Radiographic views of the tarsus

As mentioned earlier with the carpus and digits, the tarsus may be more easily positioned by pushing the stifle rather than pulling the foot.

1. **Lateral** view (Figure 2.43)
2. **Dorsoplantar** (DP) view (Figure 2.44).
3. **Oblique** views: lateral and DP views made with the limb slightly rotated to reduce superimposition of tarsal bones.
4. **Flexed DP** view: flexing the tarsus eliminates superimposition of the tuber calcis to enhance visualization of the tibiotarsal joint space (Figure 2.45).
5. **Standing** views: lateral and DP views made during full weight-bearing to more accurately evaluate joint space width.
6. **Stress** views (Figure 2.47): DP view made to assess joint integrity. The distal tibia and the proximal metatarsus are stabilized and a force is applied; the force may be medial-to-lateral, lateral-to-medial, or rotational, depending on the purpose of the study.

Tarsal common calcanean tendon injury

Damage to the Achilles tendon most often occurs near its attachment on the tuber calcis (Figure 5.175). Typical

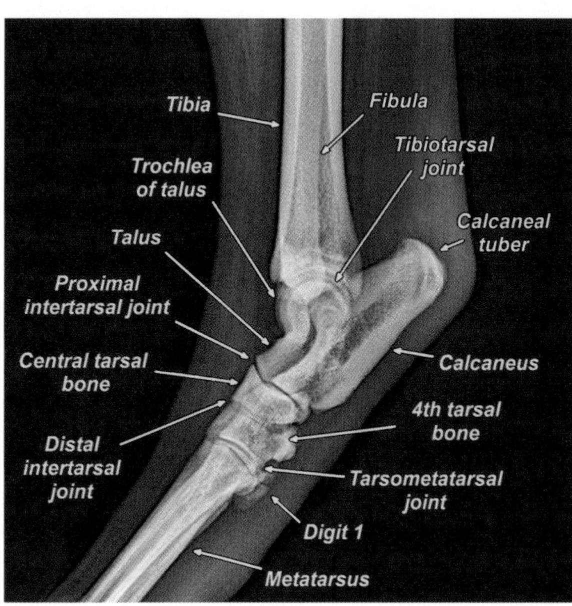

Figure 5.172 Normal tarsus. Lateral view of a dog tarsus depicting normal anatomy. The fibula is superimposed on the tibia (arrow points to the caudal edge of the fibula). The appearance of the first digit is quite variable. The central tarsal bone is identified because it is located immediately distal to the talus (arrow points to the dorsal border of the central tarsal bone).

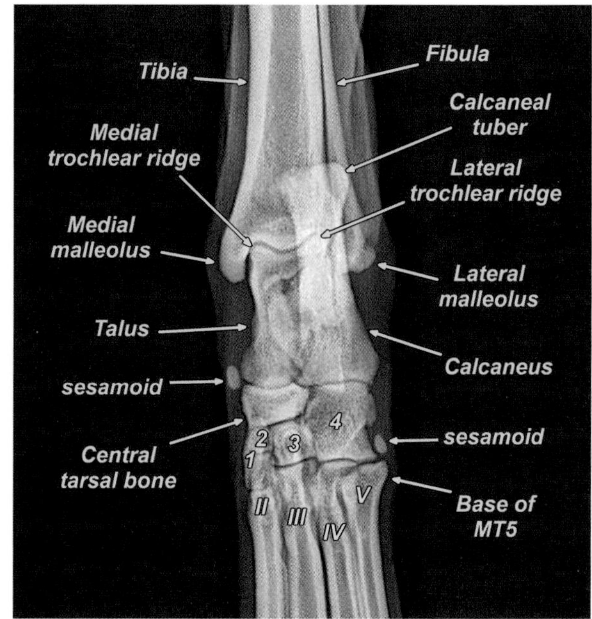

Figure 5.173 Normal tarsus. Dorsoplantar view of a dog tarsus depicting normal anatomy. The base of the fifth metatarsal bone (MT5 or V) is larger laterally, which is a useful landmark to determine the lateral side of the foot. The fourth tarsal bone spans the distal intertarsal joint space. The first tarsal and metatarsal bones are quite variable in appearance and are not present in all dogs. Sesamoid bones may be present on the medial and lateral aspects of the tarsus as shown. What we are calling a lateral sesamoid bone may in some dogs be a fifth tarsal bone. In cats, both the base of MT5 and the lateral malleolus tend to be relatively larger than in dogs.

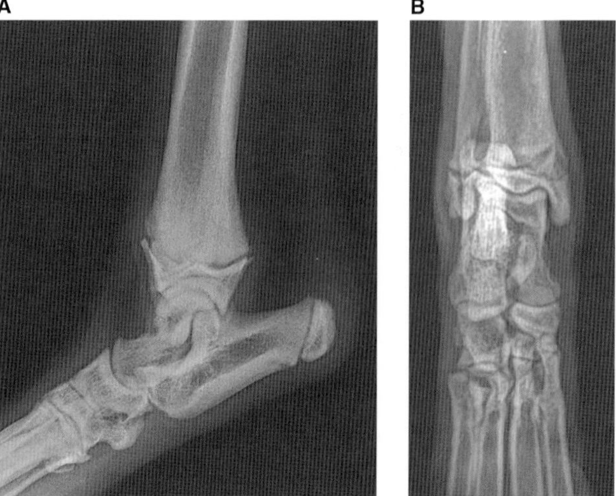

Figure 5.174 Normal immature canine tarsus. Lateral view (**A**) and dorsoplantar view (**B**) depicting a puppy tarsus.

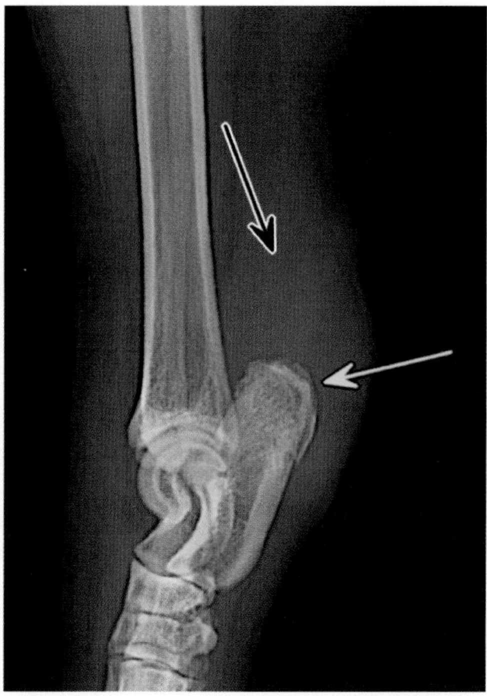

Figure 5.175 Common calcanean tendon injury. Lateral view of a dog tarsus depicting soft tissue swelling in the distal Achilles tendon (black arrow) and an irregular, but well-defined margin on the calcanean tuber (yellow arrow), the latter suggestive of a chronic condition.

radiographic findings include soft tissue swelling and less distinct margins along the injured part of the tendon. Avulsed bone fragments sometimes are present proximal to the tuber calcis (Figure 5.176). In chronic cases, mineralization may occur in the tendon and an enthesophyte may form on the tuber calcis. The margins of the tuber may be irregular and ill-defined during active disease and better defined as healing progresses. Acute injuries may be caused by a sudden impact, hyperflexion of the tarsus, or a laceration. Most are unilateral. Chronic injuries typically result from tendon degeneration due to overuse or overweight and often are bilateral.

Tarsus degenerative joint disease

Tarsal osteophytes and enthesophytes tend to be easiest to see on the dorsal aspects of the central and third tarsal bones (Figure 5.177). They also form on the plantar aspects of the talus and distal tibia, but can be difficult to identify due to superimposition of adjacent bones. Tarsal DJD often is accompanied by soft tissue swelling, either intra-capsular, extra-capsular, or both. DJD may be a sequela to trauma, osteochondrosis, or immune-mediated arthritis.

Tarsal fractures and luxations

Fractures involving the lateral or medial malleolus often are accompanied by subluxation or luxation of the tibiotarsal joint (Figure 5.178). Fractures in the central tarsal bone and calcaneus may result from extreme activity (e.g., racing Greyhounds). Central tarsal bone fractures typically are slab or sagittal types and may or may not be displaced.

Calcanean fractures may be simple or comminuted. The fragments usually are proximally displaced due to traction from the Achilles' tendon (Figure 5.176). Calcanean fractures may be articular and sometimes are accompanied by fractures in other tarsal bones.

Intertarsal and tarsometatarsal dislocations can result from acute trauma or degeneration of the plantar ligaments (Figure 5.179). Degeneration typically is caused by chronic low-grade trauma or immune-mediated arthritis. Degeneration is reported more often in obese, middle-aged dogs (particularly Collie breeds and Shetland Sheepdogs) and usually is bilateral. Stress view radiographs of both tarsi often are useful to evaluate joint laxity and subluxation.

Tarsal trauma in immature animals may damage the distal tibial physis, which can lead to abnormal growth. The lateral

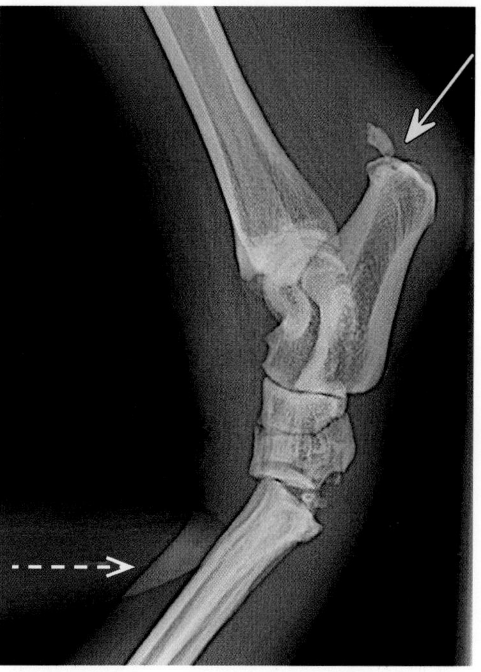

Figure 5.176 Tarsal trauma. Lateral view of a dog tarsus made while applying a dorsal-to-plantar stress at the proximal metatarsus (white dashed arrow). The radiograph depicts tarsometatarsal laxity and subluxation and tiny chip fractures at the joint. An avulsion fracture fragment is visible at the tuber calcis (yellow arrow).

part of the physis often is more severely affected and may result in a tarsal valgus limb deformity in which the toes point laterally and the distal tibias are close together ("cow-hocked" conformation). Certain dog breeds may be predisposed to this injury (e.g., Rough Collie).

Tarsal osteochondrosis

Osteochondrosis in the tarsus may be unilateral or bilateral. Lesions typically occur on the trochlear ridge of the talus, usually on the medial ridge, but occasionally on the lateral ridge. In radiographs, the affected ridge generally appears

A

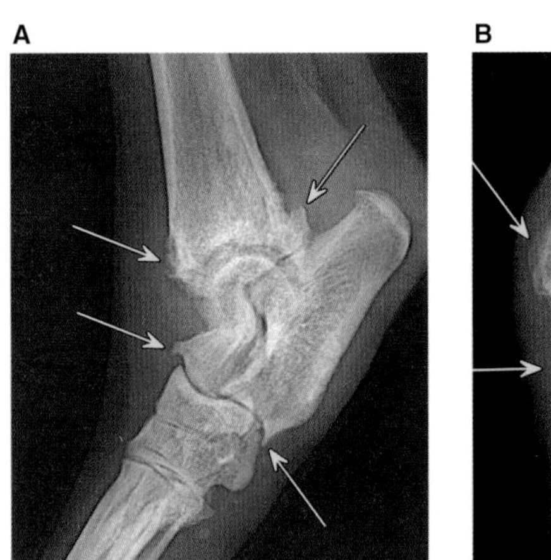

B

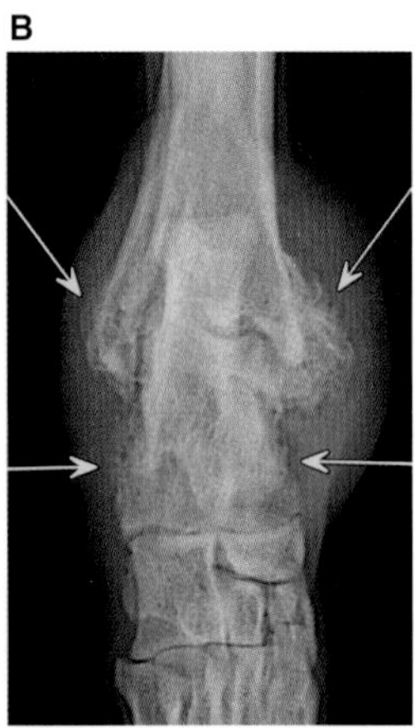

Figure 5.177 Degenerative joint disease in the tarsus. Lateral view (**A**) and DP view (**B**) of a dog tarsus depicting osteophytes on the distal tibia, fibula, talus, and calcaneus (arrows). There is moderate joint effusion.

A

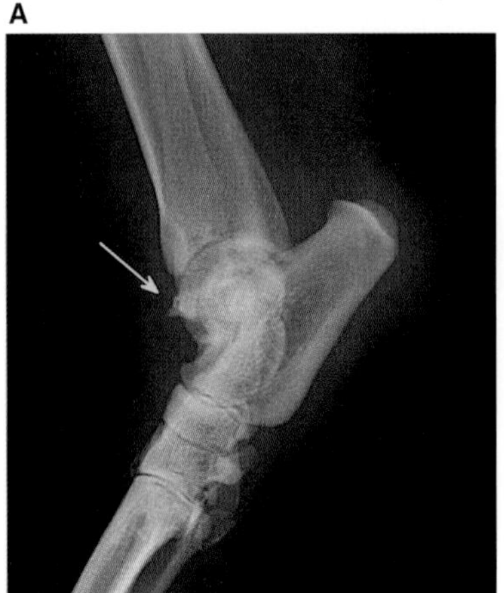

B

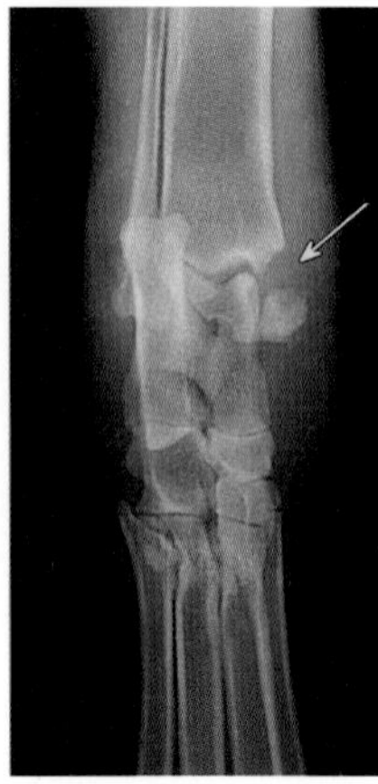

Figure 5.178 Fractured medial malleolus. Lateral view (**A**) and dorsoplantar view (**B**) of a dog tarsus depicting a distally displaced, short oblique fracture in the tibial medial malleolus (yellow arrow). In the DP view, the tibiotarsal joint space is widened medially due to ligamentous damage and subluxation.

A

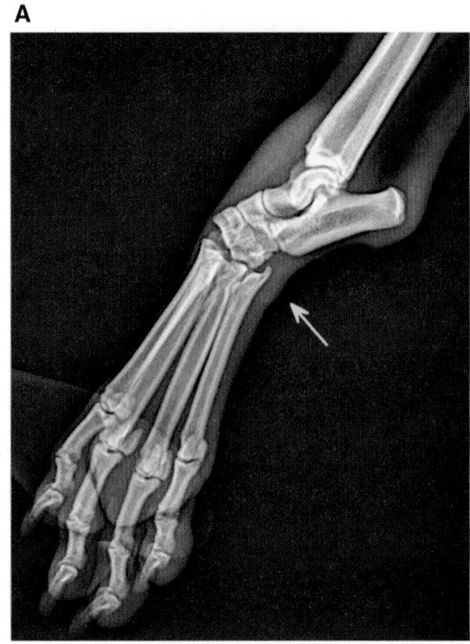

B

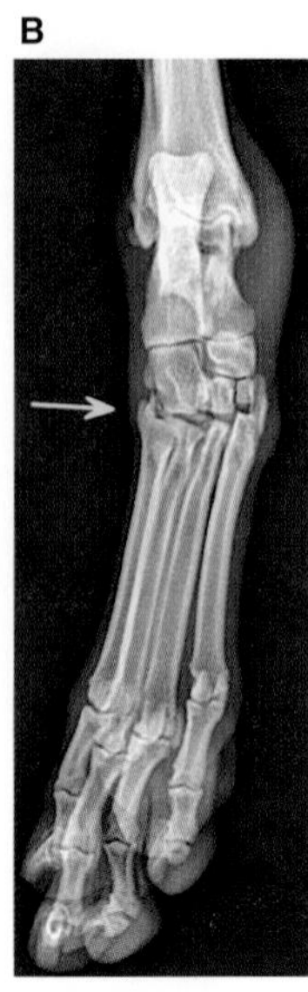

Figure 5.179 Tarsometatarsal luxation. Lateral oblique view (**A**) and dorsoplantar view (**B**) of a dog tarsus depiciting widening and malalignment at the tarsometatarsal joint, which is made evident by the application of a stress during radiography (arrows). The radiograph was made to investigate the proximal soft tissue swelling.

irregular with a flattened or concave articular border (Figure 5.180). The tibiotarsal joint space may be widened at the lesion site. Secondary DJD is common and frequently present at the time of radiography. Mineralized free fragments may be present in the tibiotarsal joint.

Osteochondrosis lesions on the talus may be difficult to identify due to superimposition of adjacent bones. Joint effusion usually is present and often is the most evident radiographic sign. **Tibiotarsal joint effusion** usually is easier to identify in a lateral view. In a normal tarsus, there is a less opaque area in the soft tissue between the distal tibia and the calcaneus because this area is quite thin, often composed of only 2 layers of skin (Figure 5.180). Joint effusion creates a soft tissue opacity bulge that is convex caudally and cranially, displacing periarticular fat away from the joint.

Supplemental views of the tarsus often are helpful to evaluate the trochlear ridge of the talus. DP oblique views made with the tarsus rotated to the right and then to the left and a flexed dorsoplantar view (skyline view, Figure 2.45) can be used to reduce superimposition artifacts.

Tarsal osteochondrosis is seen more often in young large-breed dogs. It is reportedly the most common cause of pain and swelling in the tarsus of young Rottweilers and Labrador Retrievers. Osteochondrosis should be a primary rule out in these patients. An uncommon condition reported in Rottweilers that may be related to osteochondrosis is fragmentation of the medial malleolus.

A

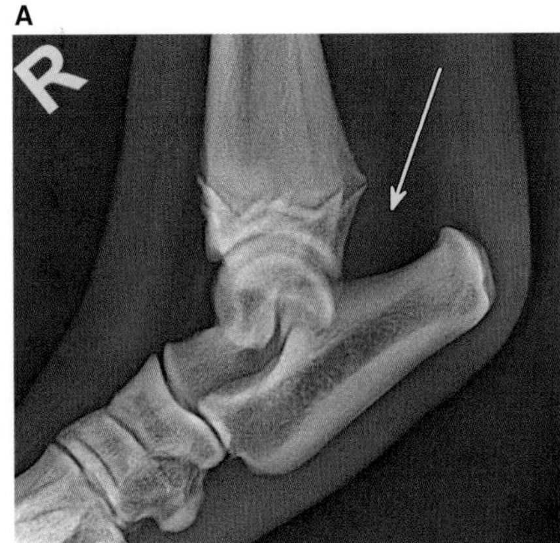

B

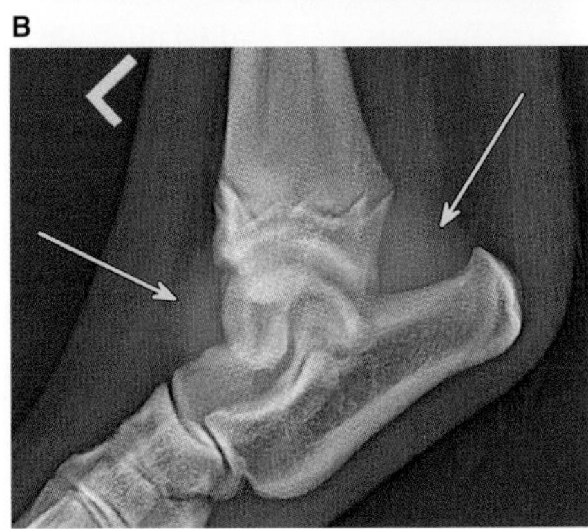

C D

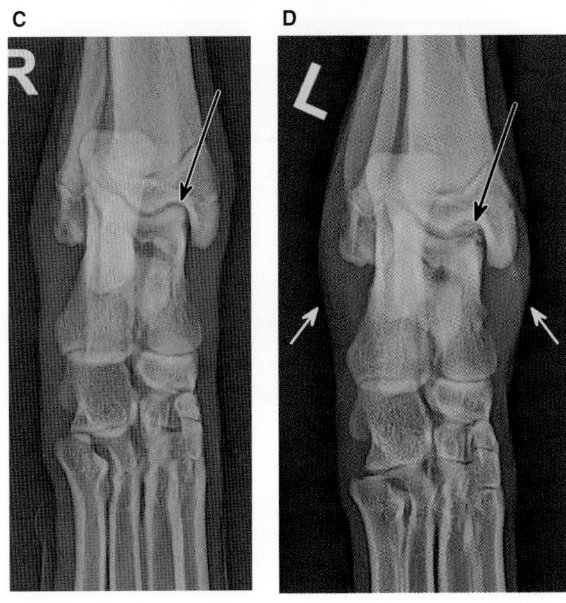

Figure 5.180 Tarsal osteochondrosis. **A**. Lateral view of a dog's right tarsus depicting the normal area of less opacity between the distal tibia and the calcaneus (arrow). **B**. Lateral view of the same dog's left tarsus depicting tibiotarsal joint effusion (arrows). **C**. Dorsoplantar (DP) view of the dog's right tarsus depicting the normal medial trochlear ridge of the talus (arrow). **D**. DP view of the dog's left tarsus depicting an osteochondrosis lesion on the talus (black arrow) and soft tissue swelling due to joint effusion (yellow arrows). The articular border of the medial trochlear ridge of the talus is flattened and the joint space widened. Note: radiographs C and D are oriented the same way for ease of comparison.

Axial skeleton

Although advanced imaging modalities such as computed tomography (CT) and magnetic resonance imaging (MRI) are used extensively to image the spine and skull, radiography is still useful. The axial skeleton consists of many complex and irregular shaped bones, requiring high-quality radiographs and careful evaluation. Proper patient positioning is essential and often requires sedation or anesthesia.

Vertebral column

Normal radiographic anatomy

Normal canine and feline vertebral anatomy is illustrated in Figures 5.181–5.190. Each vertebra develops from primary and secondary ossification centers. Primary centers form the vertebral bodies and the vertebral arches, which shape the spinal canal. Secondary centers form the vertebral endplates and the spinous processes (dorsal, transverse, and articular processes). All ossification centers normally fuse during the first year of life. The vertebral column is divided into five regions:

1. Cervical, consisting of 7 vertebrae (C1–7).
2. Thoracic, consisting of 13 vertebrae (T1–13)
3. Lumbar, consisting of 7 vertebrae (L1–7).
4. Sacral, consisting of 3 fused vertebrae (S1–3).
5. Caudal, consisting of 6–20 vertebrae (Cd1–20).

Cervical vertebrae

The cervical vertebrae are some of the most irregular-shaped bones in the body (Figures 5.181 and 5.182). **C1** is called the **atlas** because it "holds up the head." It is characterized by large lateral or transverse spinous processes (commonly called "wings" of C1) and no dorsal spinous process.

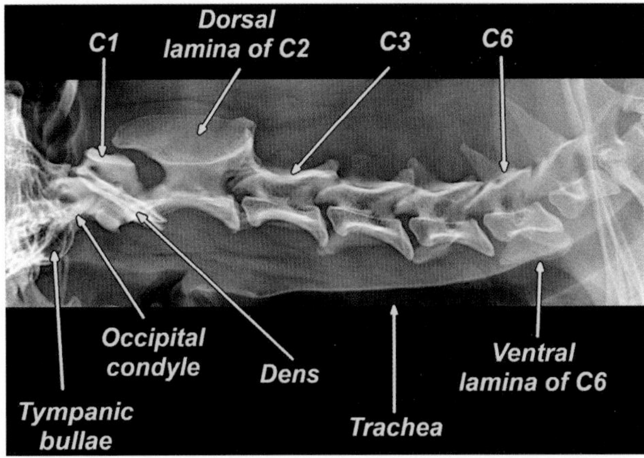

Figure 5.181 Normal cervical vertebrae. Lateral view of a dog cervical spine depicting normal anatomy.

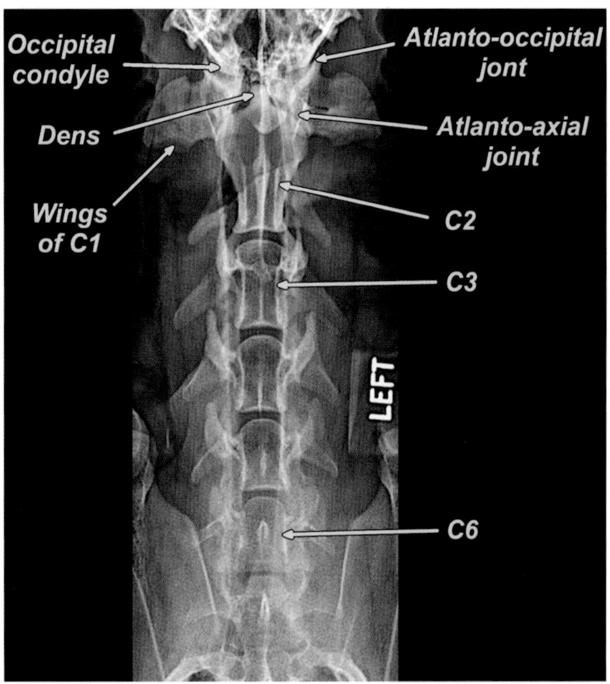

Figure 5.182 Normal cervical vertebrae. VD view of a dog cervical spine depicting normal anatomy.

The articulation between C1 and the skull is called the *atlanto-occipital joint*. This joint is commonly called the "yes" joint because it enables the up and down movements of the head.

C2 is called the **axis** because it allows the head to rotate. It is characterized by a large dorsal spinous process that partially overlaps C1. The C1–C2 articulation is called the *atlantoaxial joint*. The *odontoid process* or *dens* is a unique feature of C2 that allows side-to-side movements of the head (the atlantoaxial joint is commonly called the "no" joint). The dens projects into the spinal canal of C1 and is anchored to the body of C1 by the transverse ligament. There is no intervertebral disc at C1–2.

Other notable features in the cervical spine include: the body of **C3** is relatively shorter than the bodies of the more caudal cervical vertebrae. The transverse processes of **C6** are relatively large and project further ventrally than other transverse processes (sometimes called the *ventral lamina* of C6). They may be mistaken for an abnormality, such as an esophageal foreign object. The intervertebral disc spaces at **C2–3** and **C7–T1** often are narrower than the adjacent spaces.

Thoracic vertebrae

The thoracic vertebrae are characterized by large dorsal spinous processes (Figures 5.183 and 5.187). **T11** is called the **anticlinal** vertebra because it marks a transition in the thoracolumbar spine: the dorsal spinous processes cranial to T11 slope caudally (slant backward) and those caudal to T11 slope cranially (slant forward). The dorsal spinous process at T11 is nearly perpendicular to the vertebral body. Because of this transition, the **T10–11** intervertebral disc space normally is narrower than the adjacent spaces. Rarely, the anticlinal vertebra is located at T12 and the T11–12 intervertebral disc space is narrowed.

Lumbar vertebrae

The lumbar vertebrae are characterized by short dorsal spinous processes and large transverse processes (Figures 5.184–5.186). In cats, the lumbar vertebrae are relatively longer than in dogs and the lumbar spine tends to curve slightly ventrally compared to dogs (Figure 5.188). In dogs, the lumbar spine tends to be straighter or it curves slightly dorsally. The ventral margins of **L3** and **L4** often are less distinct than the adjacent vertebrae due to normal anatomic variations and the attachments of the diaphragmatic crura. The indistinct ventral borders may be mistaken for a periosteal response. The body of **L7** often is shorter than the bodies of the other lumbar vertebrae, but L7 can vary significantly in length.

Sacral vertebrae

The sacrum is composed of three vertebrae that are fused together without any intervertebral disc spaces. As a normal

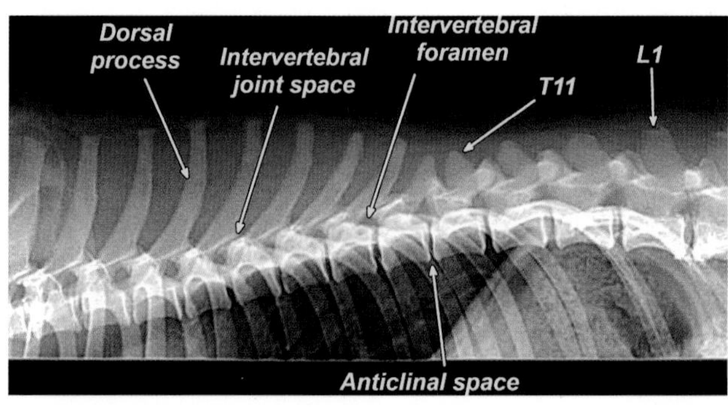

Figure 5.183 Normal thoracic vertebrae. Lateral view of a dog thoracic spine depicting normal anatomy.

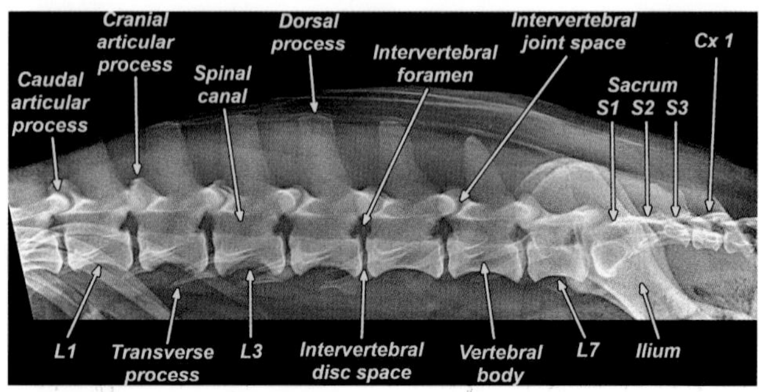

Figure 5.184 Normal lumbar vertebrae. Lateral view of a dog lumbar spine depicting normal anatomy.

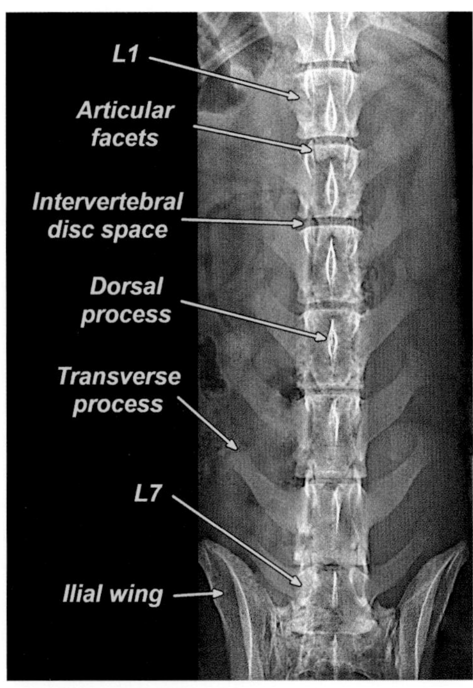

Figure 5.185 Normal lumbar vertebrae. VD view of a dog lumbar spine depicting normal anatomy.

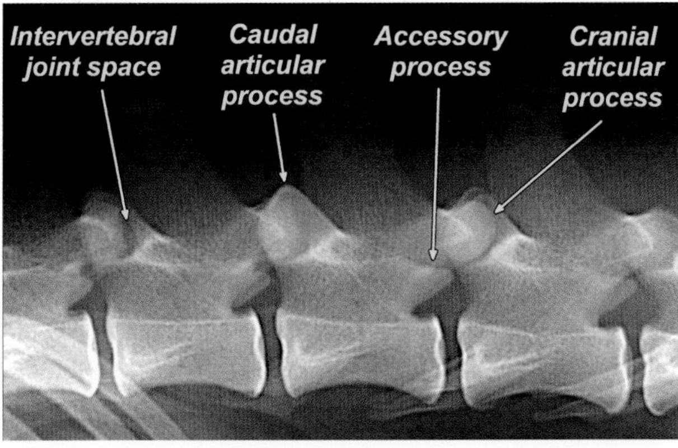

Figure 5.186 Normal lumbar vertebrae. Lateral view of a dog lumbar spine depicting normal anatomy. The spinous processes are highlighted for illustration purposes. Accessory processes begin at about T11 and get progressively larger caudal to L6. Because they overlie the intervertebral foramen, they may be mistaken for herniated disc material.

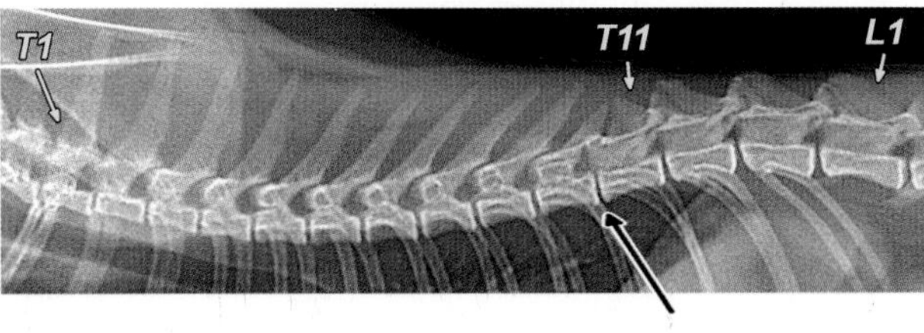

Figure 5.187 Normal thoracic vertebrae. Lateral view of a cat thoracic spine depicting normal anatomy. The black arrow points to the relatively narrower intervertebral disc space at the anticlinal junction.

anatomic variation, one or more of the sacral vertebrae may not completely fuse with the others.

Caudal vertebrae

Formerly called *coccygeal* vertebrae, the number of caudal vertebrae is quite variable due to breed characteristics. The number may be decreased due to tail amputation, which frequently is performed for cosmetic reasons. Ventral to the first few caudal vertebrae in many dogs and cats are small V-shaped or Y-shaped bony structures called *hemal arches* or *chevron bodies* (Figure 5.189). These structures sometimes are too small to be seen in radiographs or they may be incompletely mineralized. When visible, they may be mistaken for fracture fragments.

Cervicothoracolumbar spine

Between each pair of adjacent vertebrae is an **intervertebral foramen**. The foramina are actually the spaces between the adjacent vertebrae (Figures 5.183 and 5.184).

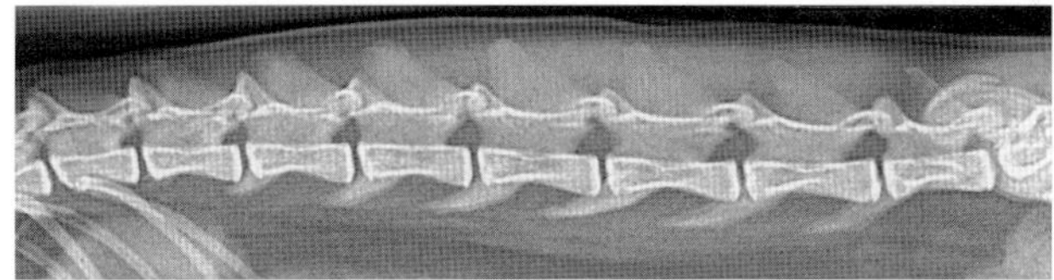

Figure 5.188 Normal lumbar vertebrae. Lateral view of a cat lumbar spine depicting normal anatomy (compare with Figure 5.184). The lumbar vertebrae in cats are relatively longer than in dogs.

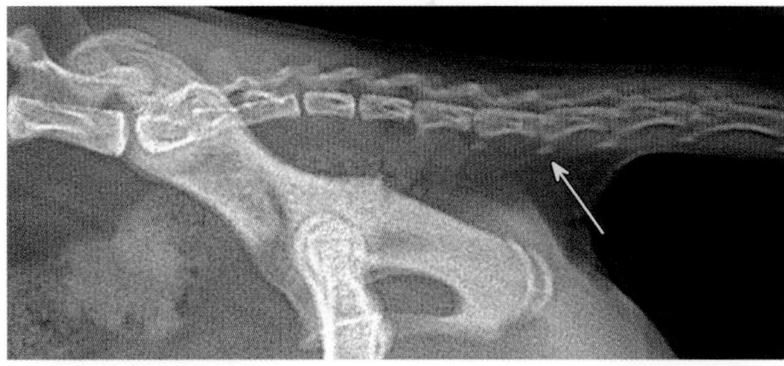

Figure 5.189 Normal caudal vertebrae. Lateral view of a cat pelvis and cranial tail depicting normal anatomy. The arrow points to a hemal arch.

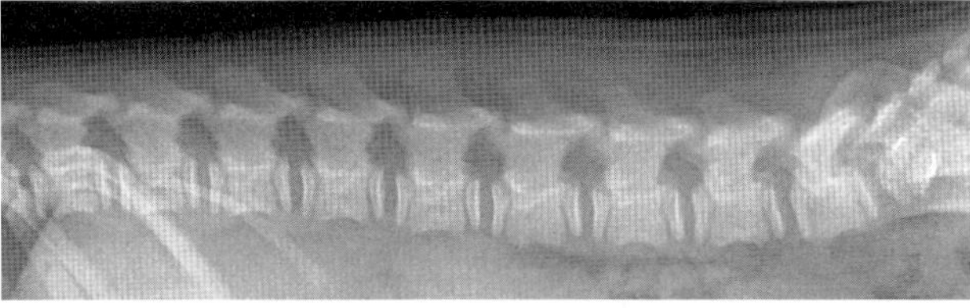

Figure 5.190 Normal immature dog spine. Lateral view of a 3-month-old puppy lumbar spine depicting the normal appearance of the vertebrae. The vertebral endplates have not yet fused with the vertebral bodies; the physes are still open.

In radiographs, the intervertebral foramina are visible ventral to the articular processes and dorsal to the intervertebral disc spaces. Each foramen serves as an exit point for spinal nerves. In the lumbar spine, the shapes of the foramina resemble "horse heads" or "Scotty dog heads" (the imaginary noses point cranially). The size and opacity of the adjacent foramina should be similar. The thoracic intervertebral foramina often are obscured by superimposed ribs.

Adjacent vertebrae articulate dorsally with each other via cranial and caudal articular processes (Figure 5.186). These articulations are synovial joints and are subject to degenerative joint disease. Articular processes normally are smooth-bordered with well-defined margins. The articular facet is the articulating surface of each process. The joint spaces should be similar in width between adjacent joints.

Intervertebral discs are located between all adjacent vertebral bodies except C1–2 and in the sacrum. The intervertebral discs act as shock absorbers and form cartilagenous joints that help hold the vertebral column together and allow slight movement between vertebrae. Each intervertebral disc space should be similar in width to the adjacent spaces. An intervertebral disc is composed of an *annulus fibrosus* and *nucleus pulposus* (Figure 5.191). The annulus is a tough outer layer of fibrocartilage that attaches the disc to the vertebral body endplates. The annulus is thinner dorsally, which is why intervertebral disc herniation is more likely to occur dorsally than in other directions. The nucleus pulposus is the gelatinous material located inside each disc.

The vertebral column is supported by dorsal and ventral **longitudinal ligaments**. The dorsal ligament runs along the floor of the spinal canal from the dens of C2 to the caudal vertebrae. It is thicker in the cervical region and thinner in the thoracolumbar area. The ventral ligament runs along the ventral borders of the vertebral bodies with attachments to each vertebra from C2 to S1. The ventral ligament is thinner in the cervical region and thicker in the caudal thoracic and lumbar regions.

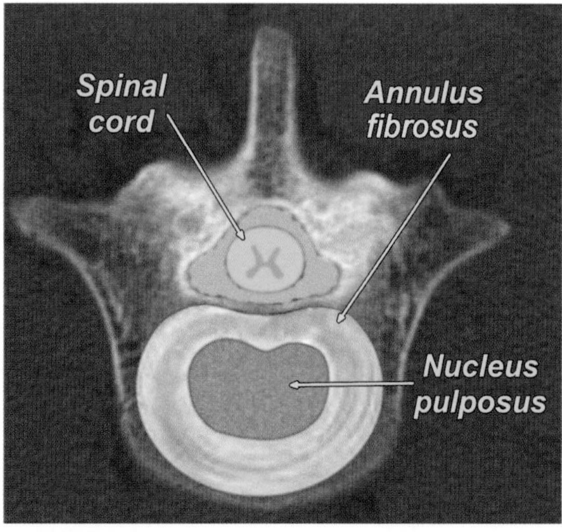

Figure 5.191 Normal vertebra. Cross-sectional CT image of a vertebra illustrating the spinal cord surrounded by fat, the nucleus pulposus, and the annulus fibrosis.

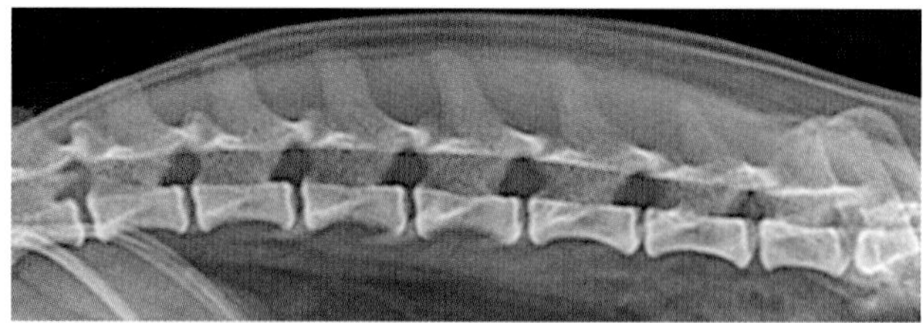

Figure 5.192 Lumbar intumescence. Lateral view of a dog lumbar spine illustrating the normal widening of the spinal canal between L3 and L5 (highlighted in red).

Intercapital ligaments pass between paired right and left rib heads. They are located dorsal to each intervertebral disc and provide an additional layer to resist dorsal intervertebral disc herniation from T2 to about T10.

Spinal cord

The spinal cord begins at the foramen magnum and ends at about L6. In large dogs, the spinal cord may end further proximally, sometimes at L4. In cats and small breed dogs, the spinal cord may extend to S1. The size of the spinal cord relative to the size of the spinal canal is larger in cats and small dogs than in medium and large dogs. This is one reason why intervertebral disc protrusions tend to produce more severe clinical signs in small dogs.

Spinal intumescences are parts of the spinal cord that are wider than other parts. These are areas where the peripheral nerves originate and the spinal canal widens to accommodate the larger diameter of the spinal cord (Figure 5.192). There are two intumescences, cervical and lumbar. The spinal cord is largest at the cervical intumescence, about C5–C7, due to the brachial plexus. The lumbar intumescence is at about L3–L5. The cervical spinal canal is wider from about C4–T1 and the lumbar canal it is wider from about L2–L6.

The spinal cord is surrounded by membranes, fluid, and fat (Figure 5.193). The **central canal** is a narrow space filled with cerebrospinal fluid that extends the length of the spinal cord. It communicates with the ventricular system of the brain.

Radiographic views of the spine

All parts of the spine that may be a location for the cause of the patient's clinical signs should be examined. Multiple radiographs often are needed, each centered on an area of interest and tightly collimated to include only 2–3 vertebrae cranial and caudal to the area of interest. Using a larger field-of-view results in significant distortion of the peripheral vertebrae and intervertebral disc spaces due to divergence of the x-ray beam.

Measure the thickest part of each spinal region and make the spine parallel with the image receptor. It is important to straighten any parts of the spine that curve or sag by placing foam wedges or towels under the patient to support and straighten the spine (Figures 5.194 and 5.215). Align the sternum and vertebral column in the same anatomical plane to eliminate rotation (Figure 5.195).

1. **Lateral** view: the right and left vertebral transverse processes should be aligned (superimposed). The same is true for the intervertebral foramina, the rib heads, and the ilial wings (Figures 2.59, 2.61, 2.63).
2. **VD** view: spine and sternum are superimposed, dorsal spinous processes are centered on the vertebral bodies, ilial wings are symmetrical (Figures 2.60, 2.62, 2.64).
3. **Oblique** views: lateral or VD view with the patient slightly rotated to the right or to the left. These views are used to visualize boney margins not well seen on standard views or to eliminate superimposition of adjacent structures.
4. **Flexion and extension** views: lateral views made with the spine flexed or extended to assess spinal stability and to diagnose compression of the spinal cord. These views are made cautiously because they can cause a more serious injury.

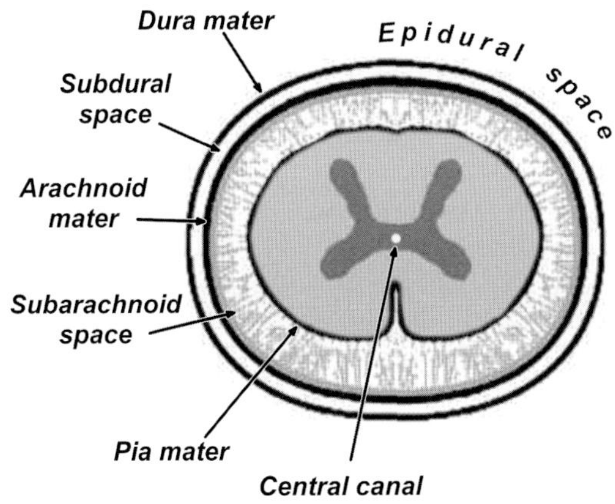

Figure 5.193 Cross-section of the spinal cord. The anatomy of the spinal cord meninges is illustrated. The *pia mater* covers the spinal cord; it is thin and delicate but impermeable to fluids. The *arachnoid mater*, named for its spiderweb like appearance, surrounds the pia mater and spinal cord, forming a loose sac. The *subarachnoid space* contains the cerebrospinal fluid. The *dura mater* is a tough outer layer. The *subdural space* is a potential space located between the dura and arachnoid. It can enlarge with fluid following trauma. The *epidural space* surrounds the dura mater and spinal nerve roots. Lymphatics, blood vessels, and fatty tissue are located in the epidural space.

A

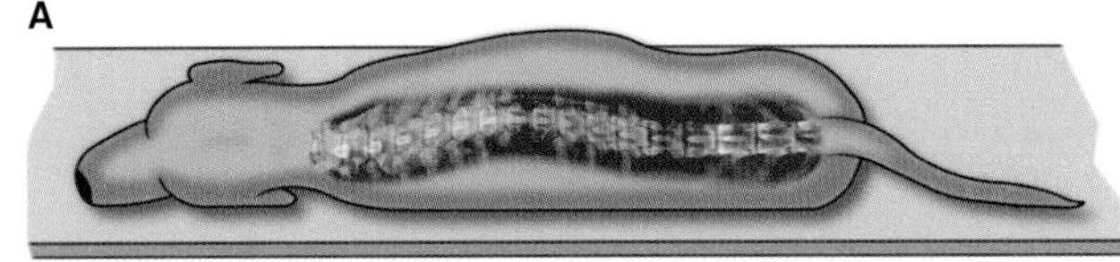

B

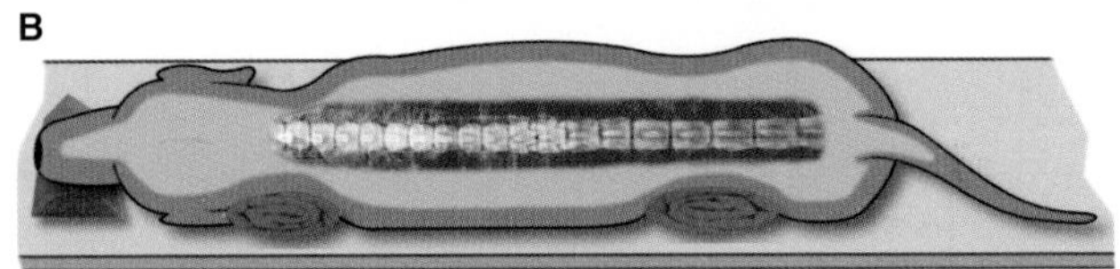

Figure 5.194 Positioning for lateral view of the spine. **A**. With the patient in lateral recumbency, the cervical and lumbar spinal regions normally sag, which can cause distortion and superimposition artifacts in the radiograph. **B**. Placing a foam wedge under the patients nose and small towels under the cervical and lumbar regions helps support the spine to better align the vertebrae.

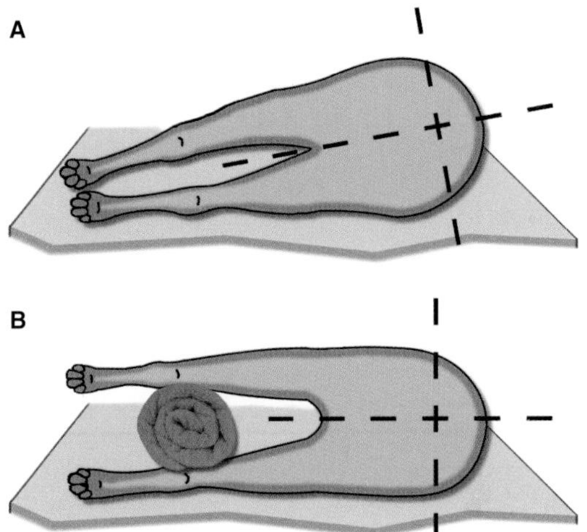

Figure 5.195 Rotation of the spine in a lateral view. These illustrations depict a patient in right lateral recumbency. The viewpoint is from the caudal aspect of the patient. The dotted lines represent the horizontal and vertical planes of the lumbar vertebrae. **A**. Without supporting the pelvic limbs, the lumbar planes naturally rotate as shown. **B**. Adding support, such as a rolled towel, between the pelvic limbs helps correct the rotation.

Spinal abnormalities

Radiographs of the spine should be carefully examined for abnormalities in the shape and alignment of the vertebrae, the number of vertebrae, the size and opacity of the spinal canal, and any swelling or abnormal opacity in the adjacent soft tissues. Evaluate the intervertebral disc spaces and dorsal articulations for abnormal width, margination, and opacity. During your evaluation, keep in mind that positioning artifacts can mimic or mask lesions. Always take positioning into account when interpreting radiographic findings.

Abnormal alignment of the spine

Lateral curvature of the spine is called *scoliosis*, ventral curvature is *lordosis*, and dorsal curvature is *kyphosis*. Causes of abnormal alignment include congenital malformation of the vertebrae, vertebral fractures, and vertebral subluxations or luxations. Again, poor positioning may be mistaken for an abnormal spinal curvature.

Abnormal number of vertebrae

An increase or decrease in the number of vertebrae may represent an actual change or an apparent change. An example of an actual change would be a patient with 6 or 8 lumbar vertebrae instead of 7 (which is not unusual in cats, Dachshunds, and other animals). Apparent changes in the number of vertebrae most often are due to transitional vertebrae and abnormal rib development. For example, the absence of ribs on T13 may be interpreted as twelve thoracic vertebrae and eight lumbar vertebrae. Similarly, extra ribs on L1 may be construed as 14 thoracic and 6 lumbar vertebrae. Whether actual or apparent, an altered number of vertebrae often is without clinical significance. It is, however, important to recognize the variation because the vertebrae commonly are used as anatomic landmarks in surgical and advanced imaging procedures.

Abnormal spinal canal

The normal spinal canal is relatively uniform in width with slight widening at the cervical and lumbar intumescences as described. Abnormal widening of the canal may result from pressure remodeling due to a mass (e.g., spinal cord tumor). Abnormal narrowing may represent a congenital or acquired stenosis, luxation, or fracture. Mineral opacity in the spinal canal usually is due to herniated intervertebral disc material or dural ossification. Summation of adjacent new bone production may be mistaken for mineral opacity in the canal (e.g., spondylosis, DJD).

Dural ossification is the formation of bony plaques in the dura mater. It appears as one or more thin, mineral opacity lines in the spinal canal (Figure 5.196). In a lateral view, the lines may be visible in the ventral or dorsal part of the spinal canal or both. They usually are easier to see at an intervertebral foramen where there is less summation of bone. The etiology of dural ossification is unknown. It is reported more often in the cervical and lumbar regions of older, large breed dogs and generally is considered to be an incidental finding. Extensive dural ossification can outline the spinal cord, mimicking a partial myelogram.

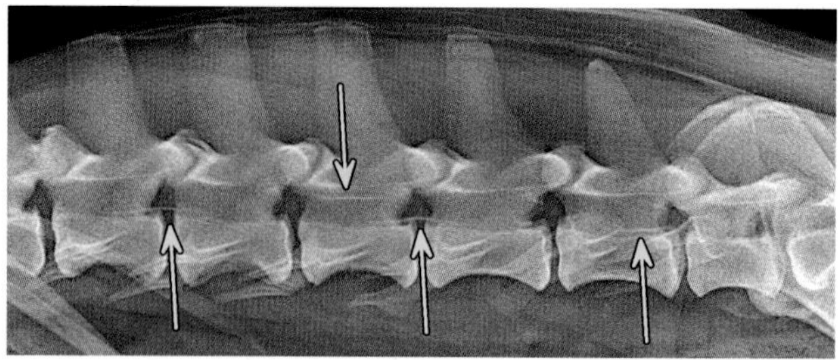

Figure 5.196 Dural ossification. Lateral view of a dog lumbar spine depicting thin mineral opacity lines along the ventral and dorsal spinal canal (arrows).

Abnormal vertebral opacity

Increased or decreased vertebral opacity may be generalized (e.g., osteoporosis, osteopetrosis) or localized (e.g., tumor, infection). Increased opacity is due to increased mineral, which may result from the following conditions, each of which is discussed further on the following pages:

1. Calcinosis circumscripta
2. Osteochondroma
3. Spinal DJD
4. Dural ossification
5. Hypervitaminosis A
6. Spondylosis deformans
7. DISH
8. Spondylitis

Calcinosis circumscripta

Calcinosis circumscripta appears as well-circumscribed areas of heterogeneous mineralization in the soft tissues adjacent to one or more vertebrae. It typically occurs near a dorsal or transverse spinous process. Again, the mineralization is in the soft tissues not in the vertebrae. There is no osteolysis or periosteal response (see Figures 5.2 and 5.3). Calcinosis circumscripta often is an asymptomatic finding.

Osteochondroma

Osteochondroma lesions in the spine appear as spherical, smooth-bordered, mineralized masses with well-defined, sometimes sclerotic margins. They tend to develop near a vertebral spinous process, most often in the cervical or thoracic spine. Masses may be solitary or multiple, monostotic or polyostotic, and may initially appear separate from the underlying bone (may resemble calcinosis circumscripta).

Spinal degenerative joint disease

Spinal DJD is characterized by osteophytes and subchondral osteosclerosis at the intervertebral articulations (Figure 5.197). It is seen more often in the cervical and lumbar regions of older animals. Many affected animals are asymptomatic; however, performance animals may exhibit a decrease in their ability to function as desired. Spondylosis deformans is often seen concurrently with spinal DJD (Figure 5.198).

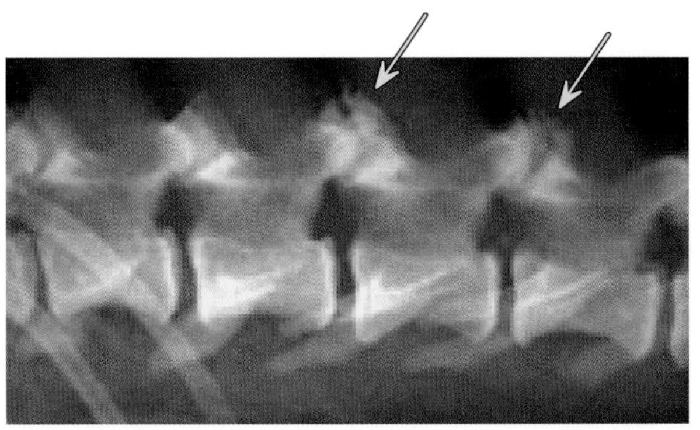

Figure 5.197 Spinal DJD. Lateral view of a dog lumbar spine depicting osteophytosis at the intervertebral joints (arrows).

Hypervitaminosis A

Excessive intake of vitamin A can lead to prolific new bone production along the spine, the long bones, and at the joints. Vitamin A toxicosis (also called *nutritional osteodystrophy*) most often is reported in cats fed a diet that consists primarily of liver. Affected cats also may suffer nutritional secondary hyperparathyroidism and generalized osteoporosis.

New bone production along the spine primarily involves the cervical and cranial thoracic regions. Vertebral lesions may resemble severe ventral and lateral spondylosis deformans with prolific new bone production at the dorsal vertebral articulations. On the long bones, new bone typically appears layered or laminar with smooth, well-defined margins. Bone production can bridge the limb joints to cause ankylosis at the hips, shoulders, elbows, and stifles.

Spondylosis deformans

Spondylosis deformans is a degenerative change characterized by new bone formation along the ventral and lateral aspects of one or more vertebral bodies. Bone initially forms at the edges of the vertebral body endplates and at the attachment sites of the ventral longitudinal ligament (Figure 5.198). It varies in appearance from small, curved, "beak-like" exostoses (enthesophytes) to large, solid, bony proliferations. The margins of the new bone are smooth and well-defined. Interdigitation of adjacent exostoses often form bony bridges between vertebrae.

Spondylosis is common in older dogs and cats, but it can begin as early as 2 years of age. The exostoses usually increase in number, size, and extent as the animal ages. Spondylosis tends to more severe along the midthoracic, lumbar, and lumbosacral spine. The vertebral body endplates are not involved, which helps differentiate spondylosis from other vertebral abnormalities. Spondylosis is non-inflammatory; there is no osteolysis, no active bone remodeling, and no soft tissue swelling. Superimposition of spondylosis may be mistaken for narrowing of an intervertebral disc space or mineralization in a disc space or in the spinal canal.

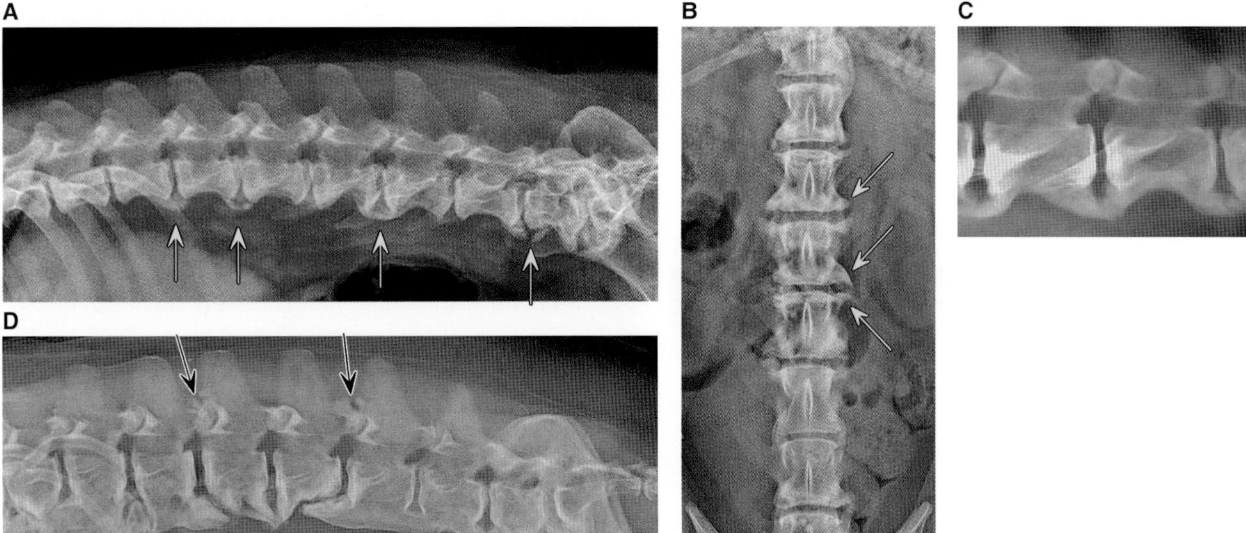

Figure 5.198 Spondylosis deformans. **A**. Lateral view of a dog lumbar spine depicting well-defined, smooth-bordered new bone production along the ventral aspects of multiple vertebral bodies (arrows). **B**. VD view of the same dog depicting well-defined exostoses along the lateral aspects of the lumbar vertebral bodies (arrows). **C**. Lateral view of a dog lumbar vertebrae depicting interdigitation of the exostoses along the ventral vertebral bodies, bridging the intervertebral disc spaces. Spondylosis does not involve the vertebral body endplates. However, it does begin very near the endplates at the attachments of the ventral longitudinal ligament. **D**. Lateral view of a dog lumbar spine depicting severe spondylosis with DJD (arrows point to osteophytes at the vertebral articulations).

In most animals, spondylosis deformans is an asymptomatic finding. In some cases, large amounts of bone production may limit the flexibility of the spine and in rare cases it may impinge on an emerging spinal nerve root. Spondylosis tends to be more severe in animals with congenital vertebral abnormalities, healing spinal fractures or luxations, and in patients with chronic conditions such as intervertebral disc disease, discospondylitis, and others.

Disseminated idiopathic skeletal hyperostosis (DISH)

DISH is characterized by extensive new bone production that bridges multiple vertebral bodies (Figure 5.199). It resembles severe spondylosis deformans. Radiographic findings include:

1. Continuous new bone production along the ventral and lateral aspects of three or more contiguous vertebrae.
2. Normal intervertebral disc spaces.
3. Osteophytes at the dorsal vertebral articulations.
4. Pseudoarthroses between the dorsal spinous processes.
5. Sclerosis and ankylosis at the sacroiliac joints and pubis.
6. Enthesophytes on the long bone tuberosities and trochanters.

The etiology of DISH is unknown. It usually is progressive and most often reported in young, large and giant breed dogs, particularly Boxers, Great Danes, and Bulldogs. There are a couple of other spinal conditions which may represent forms of DISH. These include *syndesmitis ossificans*, which is an extensive ossification of the ventral longitudinal ligament, and *Baastrup's disease*, with is a bony proliferation that is limited to the dorsal spinous processes. Both of these conditions have been reported in Boxers.

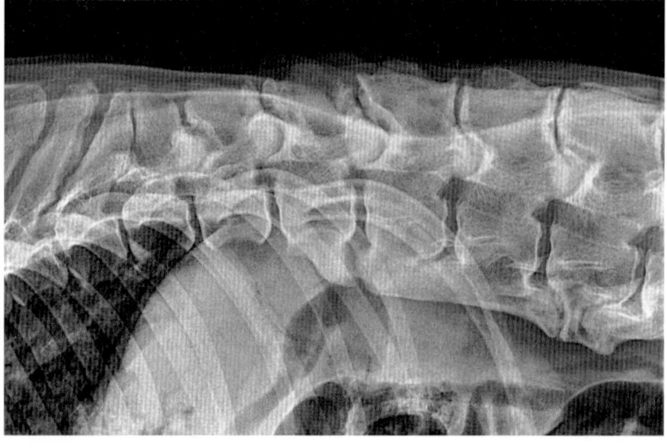

Figure 5.199 DISH. Lateral view of a dog thoracolumbar spine depicting extensive new bone production along the ventral and dorsal aspects of multiple vertebrae with pseudoarthrosis along the dorsal spinous processes.

Spondylitis

Vertebral inflammation generally is caused by an infection. Bacterial infection is most common. Other causative agents include mycotic and parasitic organisms. Radiographic findings typically include an active, proliferative, and ill-defined periosteal response involving one or more vertebral bodies. Lesions tend to be most evident along the ventral margins. Soft tissue swelling usually is present. Lumbar spondylitis may be accompanied by retroperitoneal swelling. Severe or chronic infections can progress to osteomyelitis or discospondylitis. Spondylitis generally results from extension of an adjacent soft tissue infection. Frequent causes of infection near the spine include a penetrating wound, a surgical complication, or a migrating foreign object. Foreign objects such as plant awns that either are inhaled, penetrate the skin, or are ingested can migrate along paths of least resistance to reach the paraspinal tissues.

Spinal neoplasia

Spinal tumors can arise in bone or soft tissue. Tumors in the spinal cord, spinal nerves, and meninges rarely are identified in survey radiographs unless there is secondary bone remodeling. The spinal canal may be widened due to expansile pressure remodeling or erosion of a lamina or pedicle. Nerve root tumors may enlarge an intervertebral foramen. Making both right and left lateral oblique views sometimes is useful to compare the sizes of the right and left intervertebral foramina.

Benign vertebral bone tumors rarely produce an active periosteal response. An osteoma typically appears as a well-circumscribed bony mass. Osteochondromas tend to be expansile and smoothly marginated with a well-defined sclerotic border.

Primary **malignant** bone tumors frequently involve only one vertebra. They usually are aggressive and both osteolytic and osteoblastic (Figures 5.200 and 5.201). Soft tissue swelling is variable. Pathologic fractures can occur, resulting in collapse and shortening of the vertebral body. Primary vertebral tumors rarely involve an intervertebral disc space.

Metastatic vertebral tumors usually involve more than one vertebra plus other parts of the skeleton (Figure 5.202). They may be osteolytic, osteoproductive, or both. Carcinomas originating from structures in the pelvic canal (e.g., prostate gland, urinary bladder, urethra, rectum) can spread via lymphatics to the sublumbar lymph nodes. They frequently cause a periosteal response along the ventral borders of the lumbar vertebral bodies. Periosteal new bone forms in the middle of the bodies as opposed to spondylosis deformans which forms toward the ends of the vertebral bodies. These tumors also may cause a periosteal response on the sacrum, pelvis, and femurs.

If surgery is planned, a myelogram may provide valuable information regarding the type and degree of spinal cord compression. Intramedullary compression may be caused by a spinal cord tumor. Intradural and extramedullary

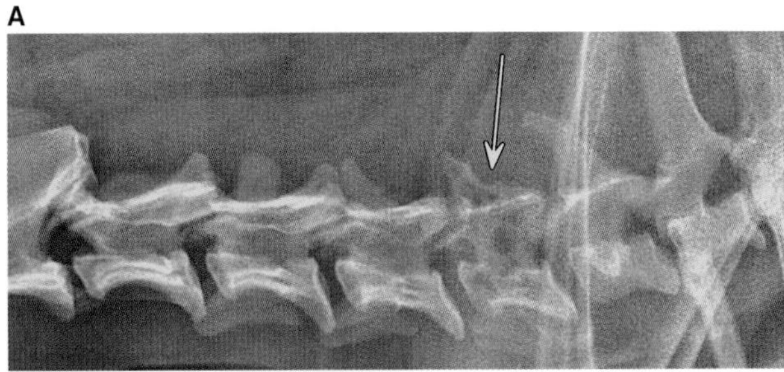

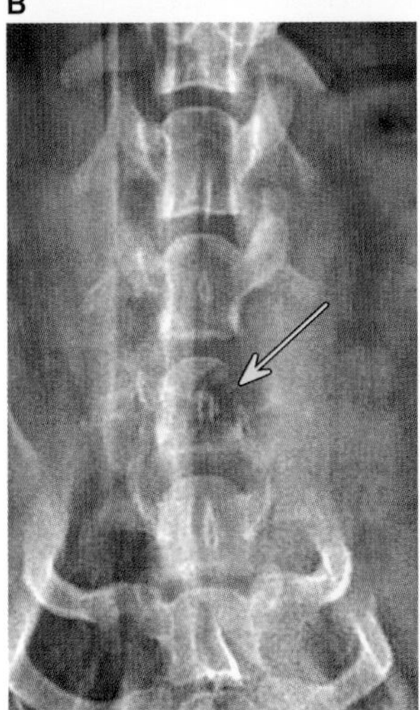

Figure 5.200 Vertebral neoplasia. Lateral view (**A**) and VD view (**B**) of a dog cervical spine depicting a moth-eaten pattern of osteolysis in the sixth cervical vertebra (arrow).

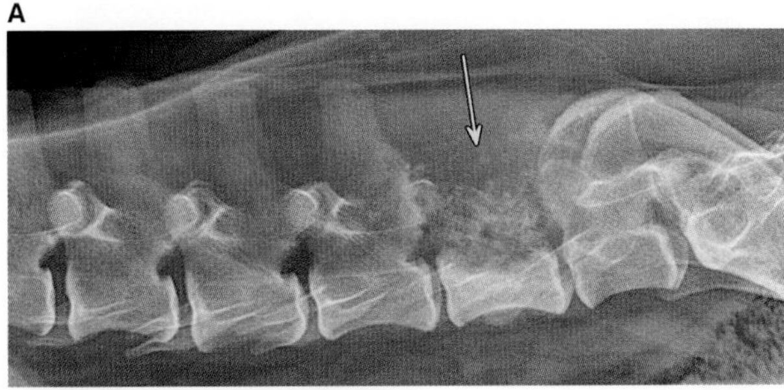

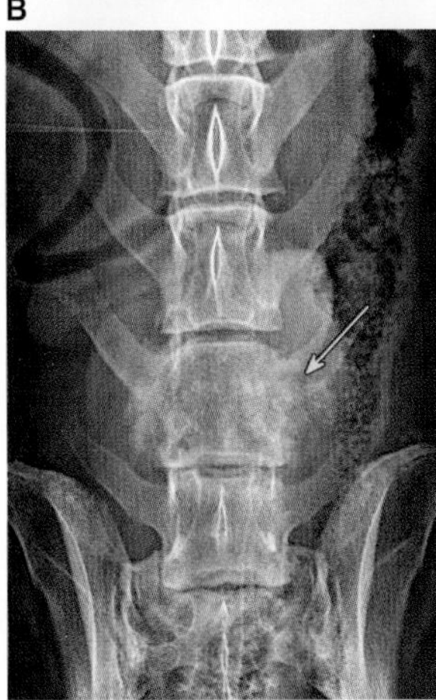

Figure 5.201 Vertebral tumor. Lateral view (**A**) and VD view (**B**) of a dog lumbar spine depicting marked osteolysis in the dorsal part of the sixth lumbar vertebra with an amorphous periosteal response (arrow). The vertebral body is increased in opacity, which sometimes is an early but non-specific radiographic finding with vertebral neoplasia.

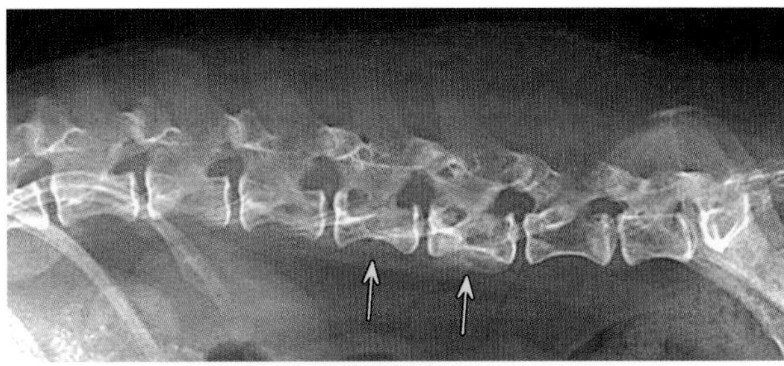

Figure 5.202 Multiple myeloma. Lateral view of a dog spine depicting multiple foci of osteolysis in multiple vertebrae, most severe in L4 and L5 (arrows).

compression may be caused by a nerve root tumor. Extradural compression may be due to a vertebral tumor, meningioma, or metastatic tumors.

Abnormal vertebral shape

One or more abnormally shaped vertebrae may be due to abnormal development or an acquired condition such as a fracture or tumor. Many developmental abnormalities are asymptomatic, but it is important to identify them because they may be the cause of abnormal spinal curvature or vertebral malalignment. Abnormal spinal curvature can make it difficult to properly position a patient for radiography. Vertebral malalignment may also create abnormal stresses in the adjacent vertebrae, predisposing the patient to intervertebral disc disease and degenerative joint disease.

Developmental vertebral abnormalities

All or part of a vertebra may be abnormally formed or it may be fused to another part of the skeleton. Rib abnormalities frequently are concurrent with vertebral abnormalities.

Hemivertebrae are partially formed vertebrae, often wedge-shaped in radiographs. They are seen most often in the thoracic region and caudally in the tail. The vertebral body end-plates tend to be normal in thickness and margination. The presence of hemivertebrae can lead to abnormal angulation of the spine, ranging from minimal to severe (Figure 5.203). The intervertebral disc spaces adjacent to a hemivertebra generally are normal in width but conform to the abnormal shape or angulation of the vertebra. Hemivertebrae rarely are symptomatic. They most often are reported in "screw-tail" breeds (e.g., English Bulldog, French Bulldog, Pug, Boston Terrier) and may be inherited in certain breeds (e.g., German Short-haired Pointer, Yorkshire Terrier, Manx cat). "Dorsal" hemivertebrae develop with a narrowed ventral portion which can lead to spinal kyphosis. "Ventral" hemivertebrae develop with a narrowed dorsal portion and can cause spinal lordosis. "Lateral" hemivertebrae develop with a narrowed right or left side which can lead to spinal scoliosis. "Butterfly" hemivertebrae develop without a central portion, resulting in a cleft through the vertebral

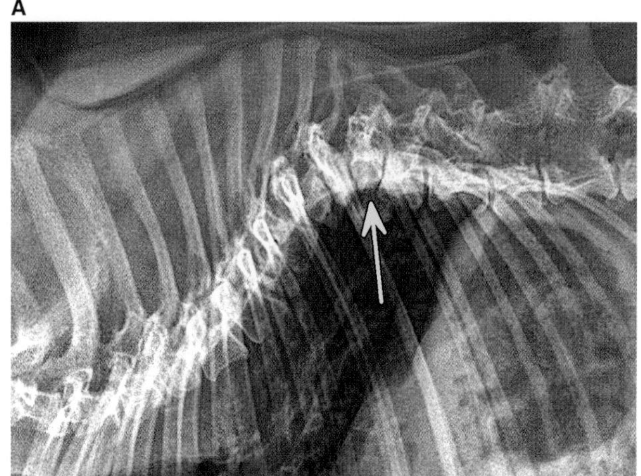

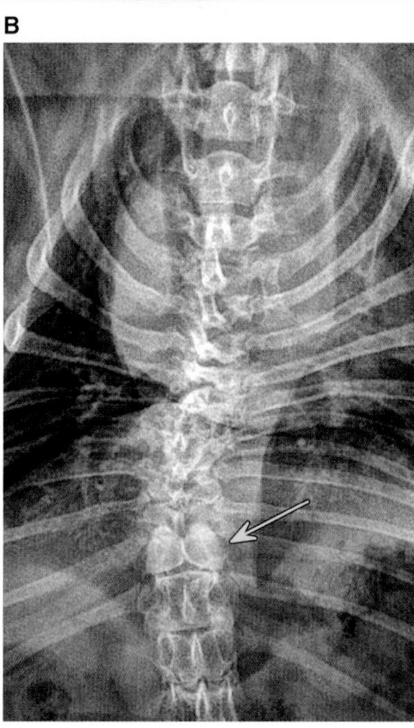

Figure 5.203 Hemivertebrae. Lateral view (**A**) and VD view (**B**) of a dog thoracic spine depicting scoliosis due to multiple hemivertebrae. Arrows point to a ventrally wedged vertebra in the lateral view and a "butterfly-shaped" vertebra in the VD view.

body and triangular-shaped ends that appear "butterfly-shaped" in a VD view (Figure 5.203).

Transitional vertebrae exhibit characteristics of two adjacent spinal regions (Figures 5.204 and 5.205). They typically occur at a spinal junction, either cervicothoracic, thoracolumbar, or lumbosacral. Transitional vertebrae are common in dogs and cats and rarely cause clinical signs. That said, a transitional vertebra at the lumbosacral junction can lead to abnormal stresses on the skeleton, which may predispose to degenerative disc disease, cauda equina syndrome, or to early DJD in the ipsilateral hip. Various types of transitional vertebrae are described below:

"Occipitalization" of C1 occurs when the atlas partially or completely fuses with the skull.

"Cervicalization" of T1 occurs when the first thoracic vertebra lacks one or both ribs, creating the appearance of 8 cervical vertebrae.

"Thoracization" of C7 occurs when ribs develop on the last cervical vertebra, either unilaterally or bilaterally.

"Thoracization" of L1 occurs when ribs develop at the first lumbar vertebra, either unilaterally or bilaterally, creating the appearance of 6 lumbar vertebrae.

"Lumbarization" of S1 occurs when the first sacral vertebra fails to fuse with the other sacral vertebrae, creating the appearance of 8 lumbar vertebrae. A unilateral or bilateral transverse process may develop on S1, and may or may not fuse with the ilium, either partially or completely.

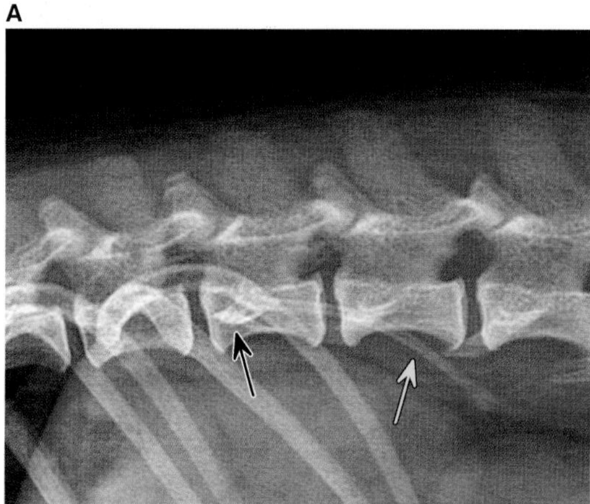

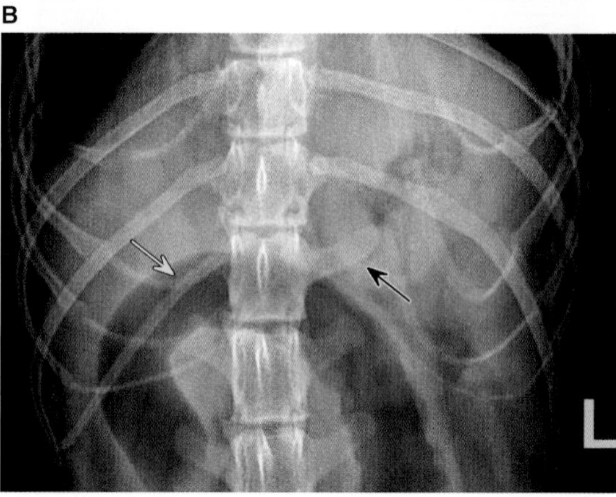

Figure 5.204 Transitional vertebra. Lateral view (**A**) and VD view (**B**) of a dog thoracolumbar spine depicting "lumbarization" of T13. There is a partially formed rib on the right side (yellow arrow) and a transverse spinous process on the left (black arrow).

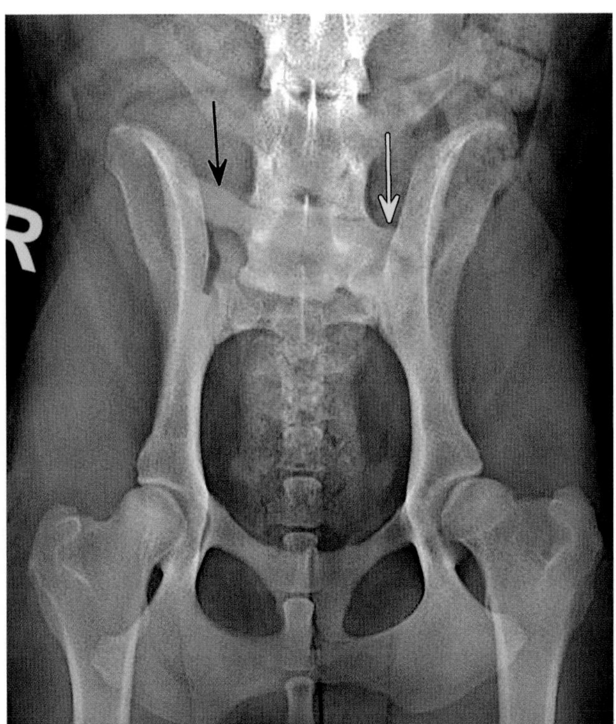

Figure 5.205 Transitional vertebra. VD view of a dog pelvis depicting "sacralization" of the seventh lumbar vertebra. The left side of L7 is partially fused with the left ilium to form part of a sacroiliac joint (yellow arrow). On the right side of L7 is a transverse process (black arrow).

"Lumbarization" of T13 occurs when the last thoracic vertebra lacks one or both ribs, either due to agenesis or hypogenesis (Figure 4.177), creating the appearance of 12 thoracic vertebrae and 8 lumbar vertebrae. Rib hypogenesis typically appears as a thin, linear, mineral opacity structure in the soft tissues, nearly parallel with the caudal ribs.

"Sacralization" of the first caudal vertebra (Cd1) occurs when Cd1 partially or completely fuses with the last sacral vertebra.

"Sacralization" of L7 occurs when the last lumbar vertebra fuses with the first sacral vertebra. Complete fusion creates the appearance of 6 lumbar vertebrae. Partial fusion occurs when a transverse process of L7 unites with the sacrum, sometimes articulating with the ilium. Partial fusion may be unilateral or bilateral.

Block vertebrae result from the congenital fusion of two or more adjacent vertebral bodies (*congenital synostosis*). Each fused vertebrae may be normal in length. The intervertebral disc spaces usually are absent or only partially developed (Figure 5.206). Block vertebrae rarely result in clinical signs. They occur more often in the cervical and lumbar regions. Note: the sacrum is a normal block vertebra. Block vertebrae occassionally will alter the curvature of the spine which can predispose the adjacent spine to intervertebral disc disease due to abnormal stresses. The spinal canal sometimes is narrowed at a block vertebra.

Abnormal development of the dens or its transverse ligament can lead to instability between the first and second cervical vertebrae. The dens or *odontoid process*, forms from a separate ossification center and normally fuses with C2 by 9 months of age. Abnormal development may present as a separate bony structure (failure of the dens to fuse), a small dens (hypoplasia), or no dens (aplasia). Instability between C1 and C2 may lead to atlantoaxial subluxation. **Atlantoaxial subluxation** can compress the spinal cord and lead to severe neurological problems or death. In addition to a developmental abnormality, trauma can cause AA subluxation due to fracture of the dens or rupture of the transverse ligament. C1–2 subluxation is identified in a lateral view as widening of the space between the dorsal border of C1 and the dorsal spinous process of C2 (Figure 5.207). Abnormal widening tends to be a subjective assessment based on experience. Widening may not be evident without some degree of cervical flexion, however, you must use extreme caution when manipulating the patient's head and neck in suspected cases to avoid exacerbating the clinical signs. An abnormal dens is an important radiographic finding; it may be absent, small, or fractured. An intact dens suggests the transverse ligament may be damaged or absent. The dens may be adequately visualized in a VD or lateral oblique view, but some studies require an open mouth rostro-caudal view with the x-ray beam centered on C1–2 (Figure 2.55).

Atlantoaxial subluxation most often is reported in young, miniature and toy breed dogs (e.g., Yorkshire Terrier, Chihuahua, Toy Poodle, others). Congenital abnormalities involving the dens have been reported in some large-breed dogs (e.g., Rottweiler, Doberman Pinscher). The atlantooccipital joint may be malformed in some patients. Congenital abnormalities usually lead to clinical signs of pain and neurologic disease at less than 1 year of age. Signs may be acute, chronic, or episodic, depending on the degree of subluxation.

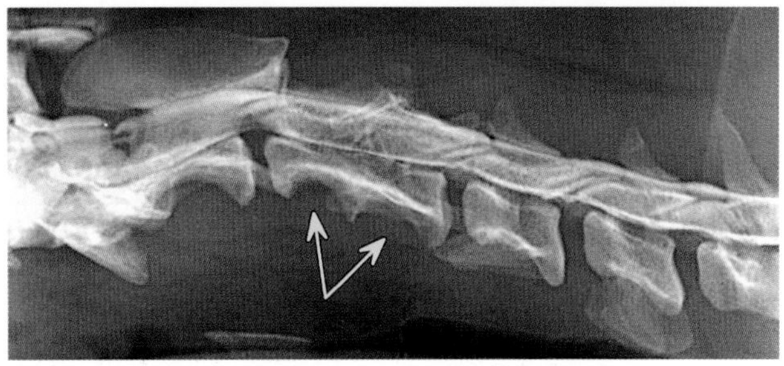

Figure 5.206 Block vertebra. Lateral view of a dog cervical spine depicting congenital fusion of the third and fourth cervical vertebrae (arrows). There is no intervertebral disc space between them. A myelogram had been performed on this dog and is normal.

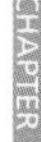

A

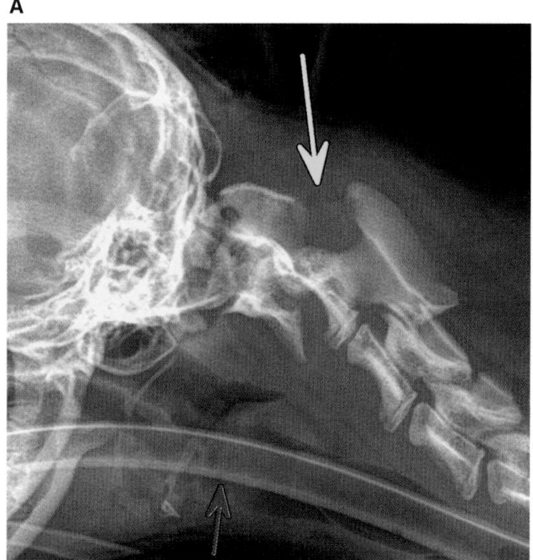

B

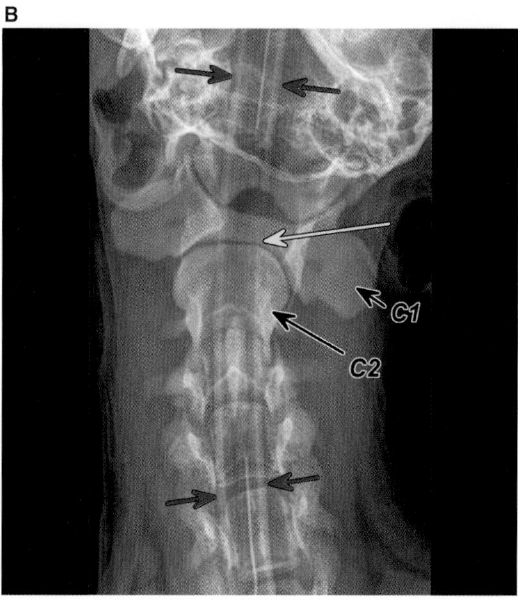

Figure 5.207 Atlantoaxial subluxation. Lateral view (**A**) and VD view (**B**) of a dog cervical region depicting dorsal displacement of C2 in relation to C1. There is widening of the space between C1 and C2 (yellow arrow in **A**). The dens is absent (yellow arrow in **B**). The red arrows point to the endotracheal tube.

Mucopolysaccharidosis is an inherited disease that can cause a variety of skeletal abnormalities (particularly in Siamese cats). Spinal abnormalities include short and misshapen vertebrae, primarily in the cervical and lumbar regions, and fusion of vertebrae (Figure 4.111). Degenerative changes often are present, including DJD and spondylosis deformans. The dens may be hypoplastic or fragmented.

Sacrocaudal dysgenesis is the absence of one or more of the caudal and sacral vertebrae. The result is a short or absent tail. Sacrocaudal dysgenesis may be accompanied by other vertebral and spinal cord abnormalities including hemivertebrae, block vertebrae, meningocele, syringomyelia, and shortening of the spinal cord. It is an inherited trait in Manx cats. Clinical signs of neurologic and urinary dysfunction may be present.

Spina bifida is a developmental abnormality in which the lateral vertebral arches fail to fuse dorsally. The result is an absent or split dorsal spinous process, sometimes called a *cleft spinous process* (Figure 5.208). In severe cases, the vertebral body or the entire vertebra is incompletely fused and may appear partially separated. The spinal canal frequently is widened at the affected vertebra. Spina bifida can occur anywhere along the spine but most often in the lumbar, sacral, and caudal regions. It is more common in "screw-tail" dog breeds (e.g., Bulldogs, Pug, Boston Terrier) and in Manx cats. Other spinal abnormalities may also be present (e.g., hemivertebrae, sacrocaudal dysgenesis, malformed spinal cord).

Spinal fractures and luxations

When severe spinal trauma is suspected, minimal movement of the patient is recommended. Horizontal beam radiography may be useful to make an orthogonal view with less risk to the patient (Figures 2.29 and 2.30). Most spinal fractures and luxations caused by trauma occur at the junctions of relatively mobile and less mobile parts of the spine (e.g., atlantooccipital, atlantoaxial, cervicothoracic,

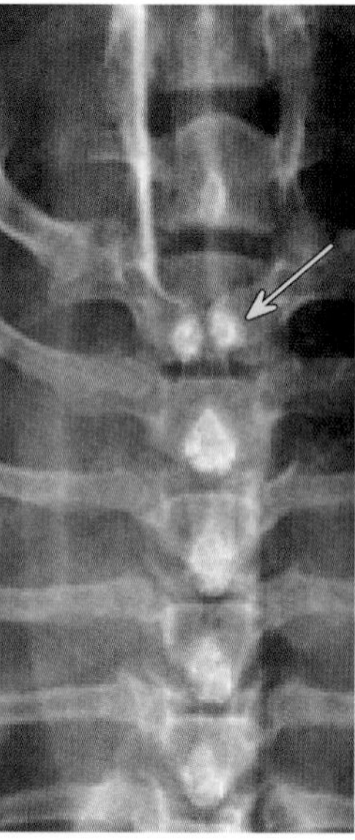

Figure 5.208 Spina bifida. Close-up VD view of a dog cervicothoracic spine depicting an incompletely fused dorsal spinous process on T1 (arrow).

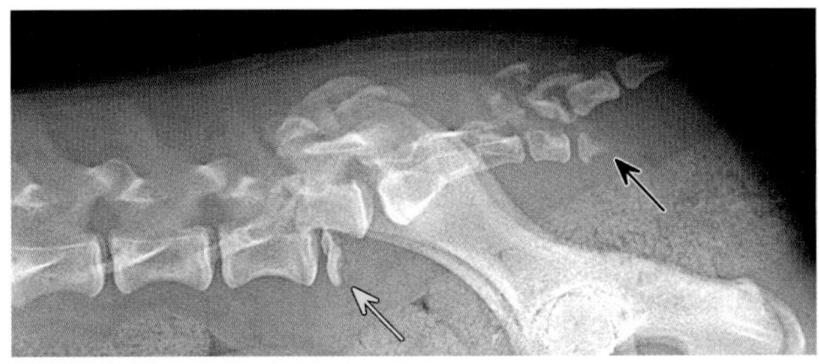

Figure 5.209 Overriding fractures. Lateral view of an immature dog lumbosacral spine depicting a fracture through the physis of the cranial endplate of L7 (yellow arrow) and through the second caudal vertebra (black arrow). The fractures are dorsally and cranially displaced and overriding.

thoracolumbar, lumbosacral). Fractures may be multiple and overriding (Figure 5.209). Pathologic fractures may result from neoplasia, nutritional deficiency, or severe infection.

Vertebral body fractures typically appear as an abrupt abnormal angulation in the spine. Compression fractures can result in abnormal vertebral length or shape (Figure 5.210). The lateral, ventral, and/or dorsal border of the fractured vertebra may be discontinuous. The articular facets may be separated from the vertebra. The adjacent intervertebral disc spaces may be widened or narrowed. Chip fractures sometimes are present at the ventral or dorsal margins of the fractured vertebral body. Swelling is common in the adjacent soft tissues or/and in the retroperitoneal space.

Fractures of the **spinous processes** more often are seen along the thoracic and lumbar vertebrae. Fractures often are multiple and sequential. Fracture lines in the dorsal spinous processes tend to be horizontal. Transverse process fractures often are unilateral and longitudinal. Concurrent signs of trauma in the thoracic or abdominal cavity are common.

Epiphyseal fractures occur in immature animals and may be complete or partial. The damaged physis may be wider and more irregular than the physes in the adjacent vertebrae. Displacement of an epiphyseal fragment may be dorsal or ventral depending on whether the injury was caused by hyperflexion or overextension.

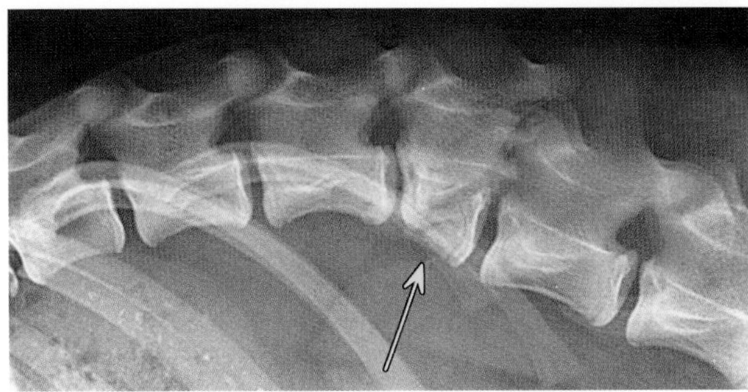

Figure 5.210 Compression fracture. Lateral view of a dog thoracolumbar spine depicting a compression fracture in the second lumbar vertebra (arrow).

Spinal osteochondrosis

Osteochondrosis lesions are uncommon in the spine. The typical radiographic appearance is an irregularly shaped osseous defect in a vertebral body endplate. The defect often is surrounded by osteosclerosis. A small fragment of bone may be present near the defect. The affected vertebra may be shortened. Lesions have been reported at the lumbosacral junction, typically involving the craniodorsal aspect of the body of S1 (Figure 5.211). Vertebral osteochondrosis most often is reported in large-breed dogs, particularly young German Shepherds. Clinical signs may be similar to cauda equina syndrome.

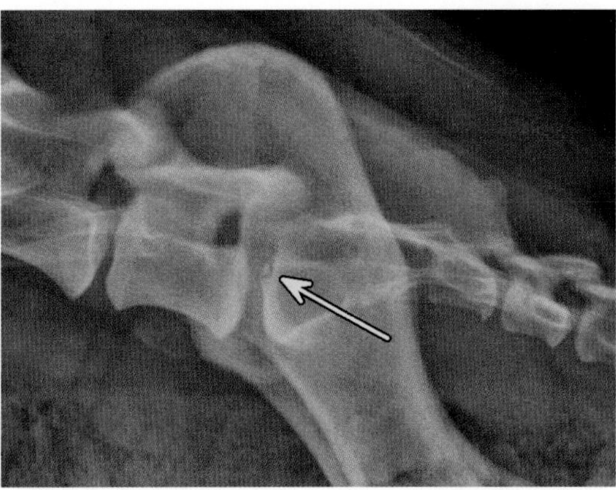

Figure 5.211 Osteochondrosis. Lateral view of a dog lumbosacral junction depicting a focal defect and a small mineralized fragment at the craniodorsal aspect of the first sacral vertebra (arrow).

Abnormal intervertebral disc spaces

Recall that the normal intervertebral disc spaces at the periphery of a radiograph naturally appear more narrow than those in the center due to divergence of the x-ray beam. Also, the disc spaces at C2–3, C7–T1, and T10–11 normally are more narrow than the adjacent spaces.

Increased opacity in an intervertebral disc space most often is caused by a mineralized disc. Decreased opacity may represent gas, which sometimes is caused by the vacuum phenomenon.

Intervertebral disc disease

Intervertebral disc disease (IVDD) refers to the protrusion or extrusion of disc material into the spinal canal that results in irritation or compression of the spinal cord or nerve roots and leads to neurological symptoms. The most common causes of IVDD are degenerative disc disease and trauma. IVDD can occur in any disc, but it most often is seen at C2–4 and T12–L7. It is less likely to occur at T2–12 because the

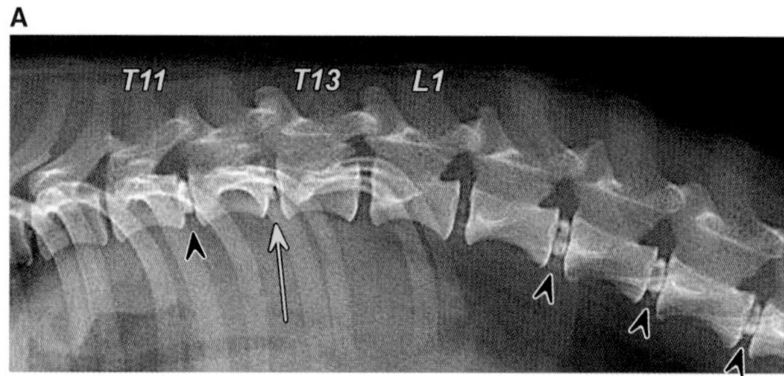

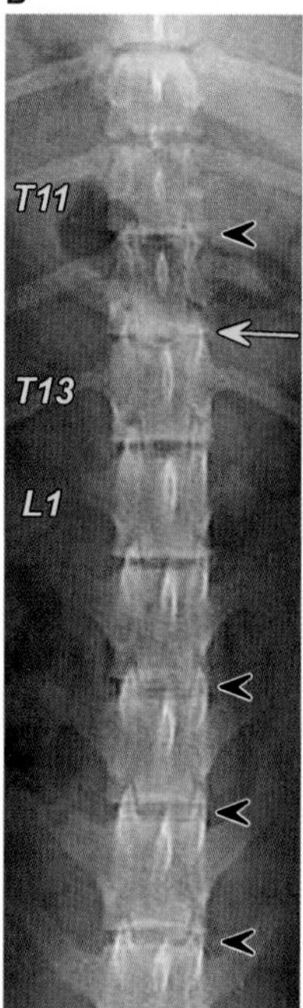

Figure 5.212 Intervertebral disk herniation. Lateral view (**A**) and VD view (**B**) of a dog thoracolumbar spine depicting a narrowed intervertebral disc space at T12-13 (yellow arrow). There is increased opacity in the intervertebral foramen at this site. Multiple in situ mineralized intervertebral discs are visible (black arrowheads). A myelogram was performed on this dog and is shown in Figure 5.213).

intercapital and conjugal ligaments along the ventral spinal canal provide an additional barrier to dorsal disc protrusion. The characteristic radiographic findings of IVDD are listed below and depicted in Figures 5.212 and 5.214. Keep in mind that normal-appearing radiographs do not rule out IVDD and poor positioning can mimic or mask IVDD (Figure 5.215).

1. Persistent narrowing of an intervertebral disc space as seen in multiple radiographs. Narrowing may or may not be uniform. Narrowing sometimes is more severe dorsally because the thicker ventral annulus remains intact.
2. Abnormal size, shape, or opacity of the intervertebral foramen compared to the adjacent foramina.
3. Narrowed space between articular facets (intervertebral joint space) compared with the adjacent joint spaces.
4. Focal soft tissue or mineral opacity material in the spinal canal. The margins of acutely extruded disc material tend to be indistinct initially, but often become better defined over time.

Mineralized intervertebral discs is a common finding in dogs and cats. Mineralization in an intervertebral disc space does not mean there is disc herniation. The most common cause is age-related disc degeneration. Mineralized in situ discs are seen frequently in radiographs of asymptomatic animals. What may be significant is the absence of in situ mineralization along a series of mineralized discs, because the absence may be the result of disc herniation. Heterogeneous mineralization may be caused by a disc breaking apart. Occasionally mineralization appears shell-like because the inner portion of the disc is absent.

Disc herniations have been classified as Hansen type I or type II (Figure 5.216). Type I is an acute or semi-acute rupture of the nucleus, while type II is a more chronic rupture that may progress over an extended period of time. Type I most often is reported in middle-aged chondrodystrophic dogs. In these breeds, disc degeneration can begin as early as 2 months of age and may be complete by 1 year of age. Type II disc herniations tend to occur in non-chondrodystrophic animals and instead of the nucleus herniating acutely and putting sudden

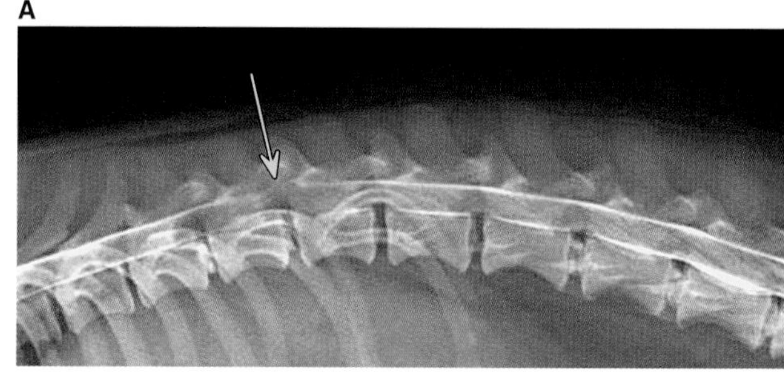

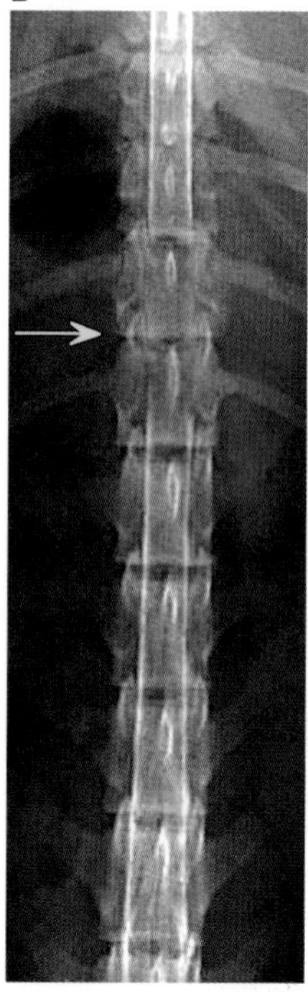

Figure 5.213 Intervertebral disk herniation. Lateral view (**A**) and VD view (**B**) of the same dog as in Figure 5.212. Contrast medium outlines the spinal cord except at T12–13, where there is little to no filling of the subarachnoid space (arrow). In this area, the spinal cord is swollen and/or compressed by herniated intervertebral disc material.

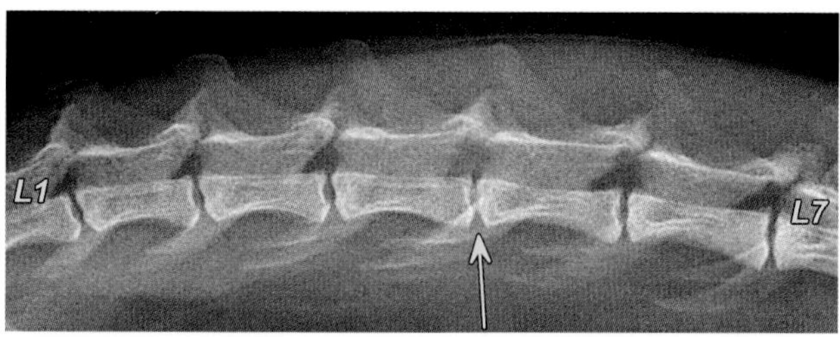

Figure 5.214 Intervertebral disc herniation. Lateral view of a cat lumbar spine depicting a narrowed intervertebral disc space at L4–5 (arrow). Notice the increased opacity in the intervertebral foramen at this site.

A

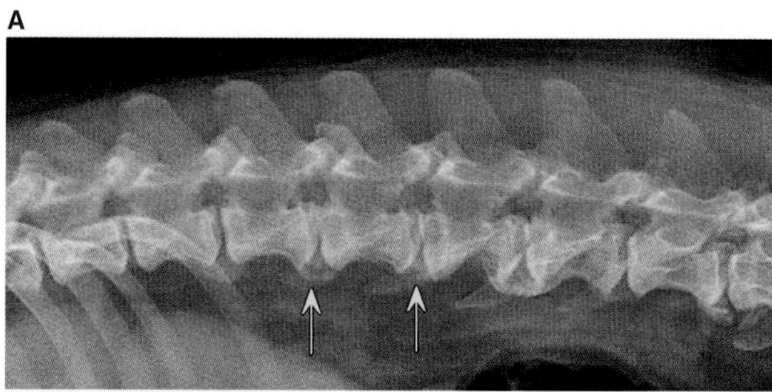

B

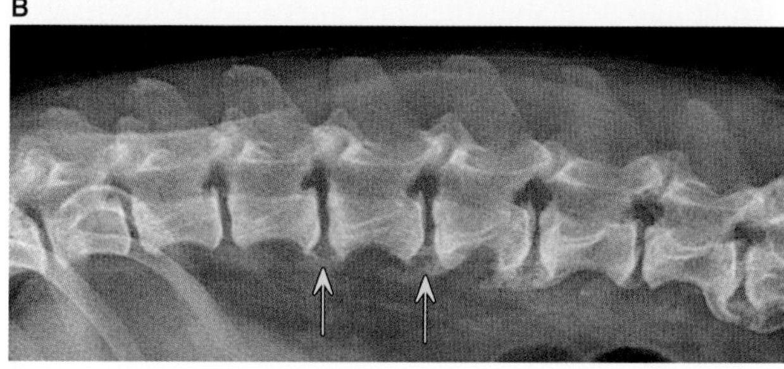

Figure 5.215 Spine positioning. Two lateral views of the same dog lumbar spine depicting the appearance of the vertebrae when the spinal column sags (**A**) and when it is supported (**B**). Compare the appearances of the L2–4 intervertebral disc spaces and foramina (arrows) in **A** and **B**.

pressure on the spinal cord, the annulus gradually degenerates causing progressive compression or irritation to the spinal cord and/or nerve roots. Spondylosis deformans is a frequent finding in patients with IVDD.

Myelography to evaluate IVDD should be performed only if surgery is planned (if a surgical lesion is found). In a myelogram, a protruding intervertebral disc or extruded material creates a filling defect due to an extradural lesion that displaces the spinal cord away from the lesion (Figure 5.213). The spinal cord may be swollen due to edema or hemorrhage, creating an intramedullary lesion that extends either cranially, caudally, or both from the lesion site. Cord swelling may be present with or without a visible extradural lesion.

Lumbosacral disease

Various disorders at the lumbosacral junction can lead to compression of the caudal spinal nerve roots and neurological symptoms. Congenital malformations, vertebral instability, and degenerative changes all can injure the cauda equina. Characteristic radiographic findings include:

1. Narrowing or dorsal wedging of the lumbosacral intervertebral disc space (Figure 5.217).
2. Narrowing of the spinal canal at the lumbosacral junction; the dorsoventral dimension may be decreased either due to congenital malformation or new bone formation at the vertebral facets.
3. Ventral displacement of the sacrum in relation to the last lumbar vertebra; sacral subluxation typically creates a "stair-step" at the dorsal aspect of the lumbosacral vertebral bodies as well as ventral displacement of the dorsal margin of the sacrum, which results in narrowing of the effective spinal canal at that site.
4. Sacral subluxation may only be evident during extension of the lumbosacral junction (Figure 5.217). When findings are equivocal in a standard lateral view, make an

A

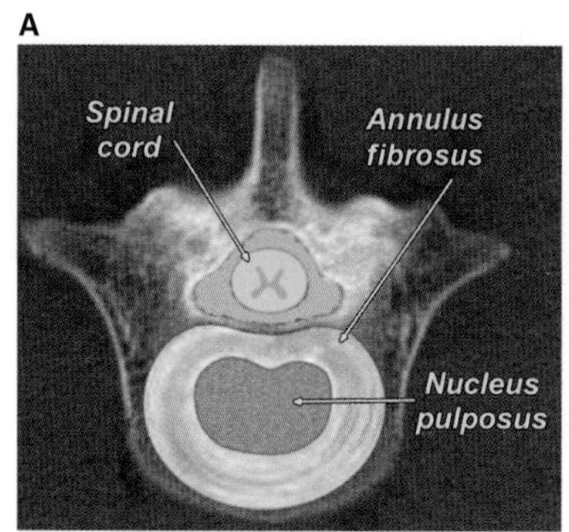

B

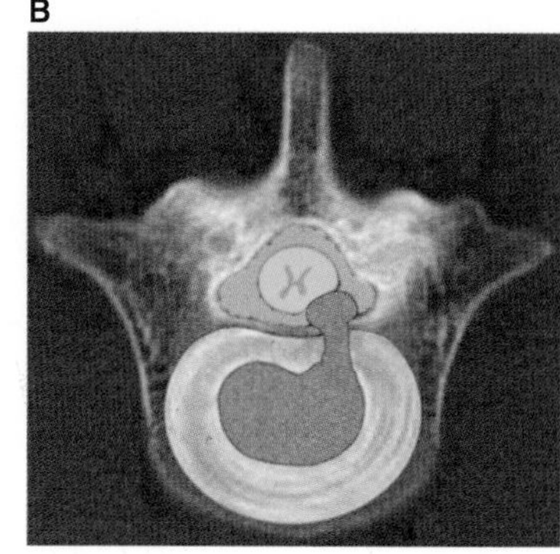

C

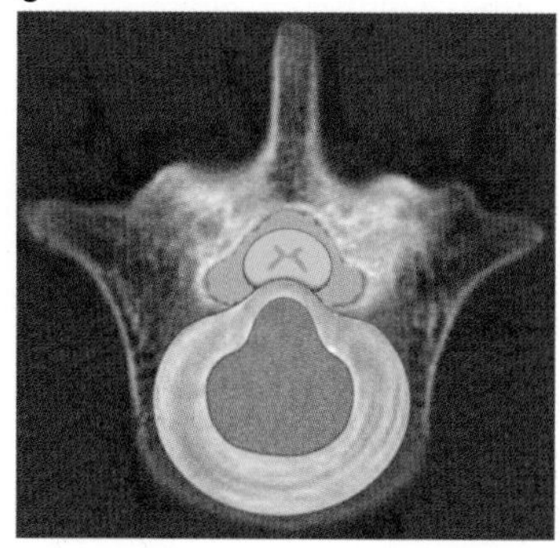

Figure 5.216 Intervertebral disc herniation. Cross-sectional CT images of a lumbar vertebra illustrating normal anatomy (**A**), an acute intervertebral disc rupture and herniation (**B**), and a chronic disc herniation (**C**).

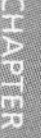

extended lateral view by pulling the pelvic limbs caudally. If there is a functional instability at the lumbosacral junction, the sacrum often will be displaced ventrally in relation to the last lumbar vertebra. If needed, a flexed lateral view can be made by pulling the pelvic limbs cranially to help document the degree of functional instability.

A

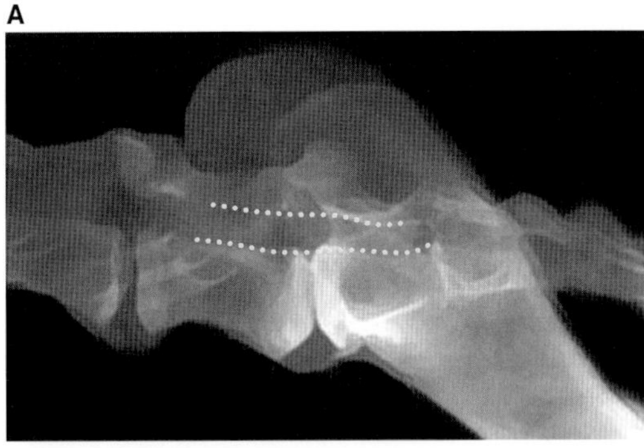

B

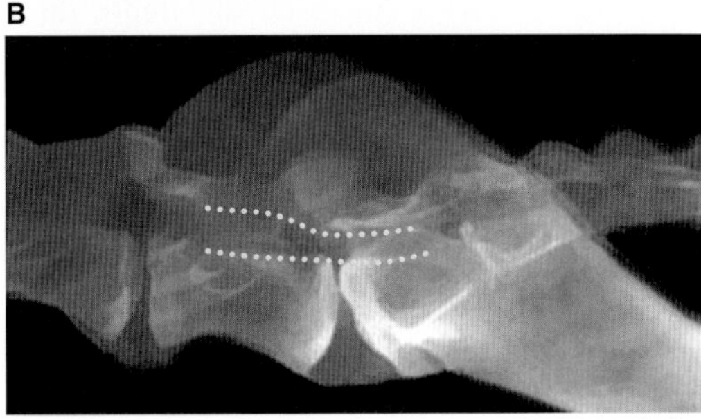

Figure 5.217 Lumbosacral instability. **A**. A standard lateral view of a dog lumbosacral junction depicts normal alignment of the sacrum and last lumbar vertebra and a uniform spinal canal (dotted lines). **B**. An extended lateral view of the same dog depicts slight ventral displacement of the sacrum in relation to the last lumbar vertebra, resulting in a "stair-step" narrowing of the spinal canal and dorsal wedging of the intervertebral disk space.

In radiographs of patients with lumbosacral disease or cauda equina syndrome, spondylosis deformans or/and transitional vertebrae often are present. These findings may or may not contribute to the severity of the clinical signs. Stenosis or instability at the the lumbosacral junction can occur in any dog or cat but is reported most often in large-breed dogs (e.g., German Shepherd Dog, Greyhound). Clinical signs vary with the severity and duration of nerve root compression and may be unilateral or bilateral. An acute onset of signs may be caused by fracture, discospondylitis, and others. Survey radiographs sometimes appear normal in patients with lumbosacral disease.

Contrast radiography of the lumbosacral junction is performed only if surgery is planned should a surgical lesion be identified. Myelography opacifies the subarachnoid space; however, in most dogs the space ends at about the fifth or sixth lumbar vertebra. That said, a myelogram may yield some useful information because the dural sac typically extends through the sacrum, but epidurography may be preferred over myelography. An epidurogram can reveal compression or displacement of the cauda equina. Lateral views made during extension and flexion of the pelvis may be needed, especially if the lesion is dynamic, functional, or caused by ligamentous hypertrophy. Discography has been used to identify rupture of the annulus and dorsal protrusion of the nucleus pulposus at the lumbosacral junction.

Discospondylitis

Inflammation in an intervertebral disc may not be visible in radiographs unless or until it involves the adjacent vertebral bodies. In many cases, the intervertebral disc space initially widens, but later narrows or collapses during healing. Vertebral lesions appear as irregular-shaped, ill-defined, osteolytic areas in one or both opposing endplates (Figure 5.218). In chronic cases the endplates become sclerotic. The vertebral bodies may or may not fuse during healing. Spondylosis frequently develops at the affected sites.

Discospondylitis most often is caused by a bacterial or mycotic infection. More than one intervertebral disc may be affected and they may not be adjacent. In general, radiographs of the entire spine are recommended when discospondylitis is suspected. Blood and urine cultures may help identify the causative agent, but sampling at an affected site often is more diagnostic. Brucellosis should be ruled out due to its zoonotic potential.

Serial radiographs aid in identifying new lesions and monitoring the patient's response to therapy. Lesions are considered inactive if no change is seen in two or more serial studies. The radiographic appearance of a lesion may initially increase in severity, even with appropriate treatment and clinical improvement, because radiographic signs tend to lag behind clinical signs.

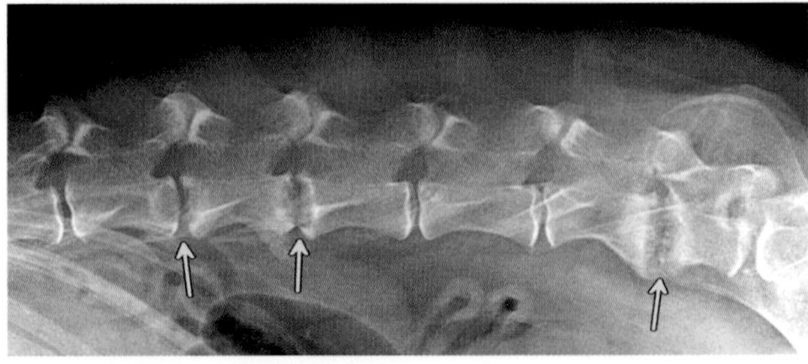

Figure 5.218 Discospondylitis. Lateral view of a dog lumbar spine depicting multiple sites of osteolysis in the vertebral body endplates with adjacent osteosclerosis and widening of the intervertebral disk spaces (arrows).

Schmorl's node

A Schmorl's node occurs when the nucleus pulposus herniates into the body of one or both adjacent vertebra. Schmorl's nodes typically are associated with trauma and weak vertebral endplates, the latter due to either incomplete ossification or metabolic bone disease. They may be associated with fibrocartilaginous emboli and ischemic myelopathy.

In radiographs, a Schmorl's node appears as a well-defined, concave defect in a vertebral body endplate (Figure 5.219). They are uncommon, most often reported in the lumbar and lumbosacral regions. The lesion may be centrally located in the endplate or more peripheral. Both opposing endplates sometimes are involved. Osteosclerosis frequently surrounds the defect. The intervertebral disc space commonly is narrowed and misshapen. A Schmorl's node may resemble early discospondylitis, but they are less active and less aggressive in serial radiographs. Schmorl's nodes most often are reported in large-breed dogs, particularly German Shepherds, and may or may not be symptomatic.

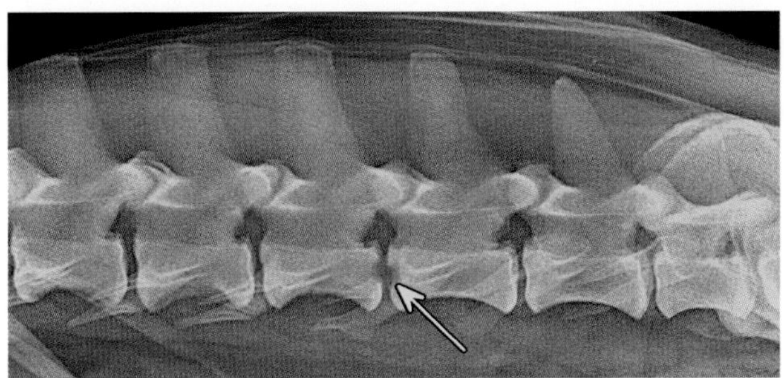

Figure 5.219 Schmorl's node. Lateral view of a dog lumbar spine depicting focal concave defects centrally located in the opposing endplates of L4 and L5 (arrow) due to herniation of disc material into the adjacent vertebrae.

Spinal cord disorders

Disorders of spinal cord rarely are evident in survey radiographs. Myelography may yield some diagnostic information, but most spinal cord disorders are best evaluated with cross-sectional imaging (e.g., MRI, CT).

Syringomyelia is characterized by fluid-filled cavities in the spinal cord called *syrinx*. In a myelogram, syrinx that communicate with the subarachnoid space appear as contrast-filled areas within the cord parenchyma. Syrinx can expand over time and progressively damage the spinal cord. Syringomyelia most often is reported in Cavalier King Charles Spaniels and Weimaraners and frequently is associated with occipital dysplasia or Chiari-like malformation. In addition to causing neck pain and neurologic signs, a characteristic clinical sign of syringomyelia is scratching the neck.

Hydromyelia is abnormal dilation of the central canal. It may be congenital or acquired. In a myelogram, the central canal fills with contrast medium. The canal may be evenly widened or more saccular in appearance. Neurologic signs may or may not be present. Hydromyelia may be associated with hydrocephalus.

Arachnoid cysts are "cyst-like" structures that develop in the subarachnoid space. They may form due to a congenital abnormality or secondary to trauma. In a myelogram, the "cysts" fill with contrast medium and produce abrupt dilations in the subarachnoid space. They most often are reported in the dorsal cervical region of young dogs and usually are asymptomatic.

Cervical spondylomyelopathy

Commonly called "wobbler syndrome," cervical spondylomyelopathy is a disorder in which one or more cervical vertebrae are malformed or malaligned, leading to compression of the spinal cord. Compression causes progressive demyelination and myelomalacia which lead to clinical signs of neck pain, ataxia, and a wobbly gait.

Classic radiographic findings include subluxation of the cervical vertebrae, flattening of the vertebral bodies, and spinal canal stenosis. **Vertebral subluxation** is recognized in radiographs as dorsal displacement of the cranial end of a vertebral body(s) in relation to the caudal end of the adjacent vertebra (Figure 5.220). The dorsal displacement creates a "stair-step" along the ventral spinal canal. Subluxation often is dynamic and may only be visible in radiographs made with the patient's neck flexed or extended (Figure 5.221). Note: use extreme caution when manipulating the neck because large movements can increase the severity of the patient's clinical signs, particularly if the animal is sedated or anesthetized. **Flattening** of a vertebral body typically is seen at the cranioventral border, most often involving C5, C6, or C7 (Figure 5.221). **Stenosis** of the spinal canal tends to be more severe at the cranial end of a malformed vertebra, resulting in a wedge-shaped appearance to the canal (Figure 5.222).

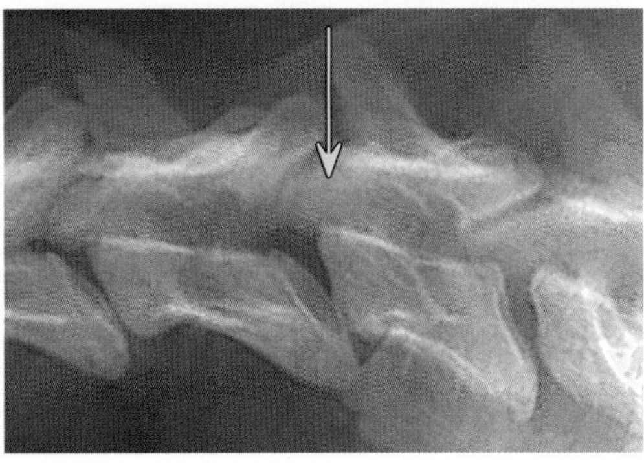

Figure 5.220 Cervical spondylomyelopathy. Lateral view of a dog cervical spine depicting subluxation at C5–6. The cranial end of C6 is dorsally displaced in relation to C5 (arrow), creating a "stair-step" along the ventral spinal canal.

Other less specific radiographic findings of wobbler syndrome include narrowed intervertebral disc spaces, mineralized intervertebral discs, and degenerative changes such as DJD, vertebral end-plate osteosclerosis, and spondylosis deformans (Figure 5.223). In many cases, however, survey radiographs are normal. Myelography may be useful to demonstrate the extra-dural compression of the spinal cord. The location of a lesion seen in a myelogram sometimes differs from what was suspected from survey radiographs.

A

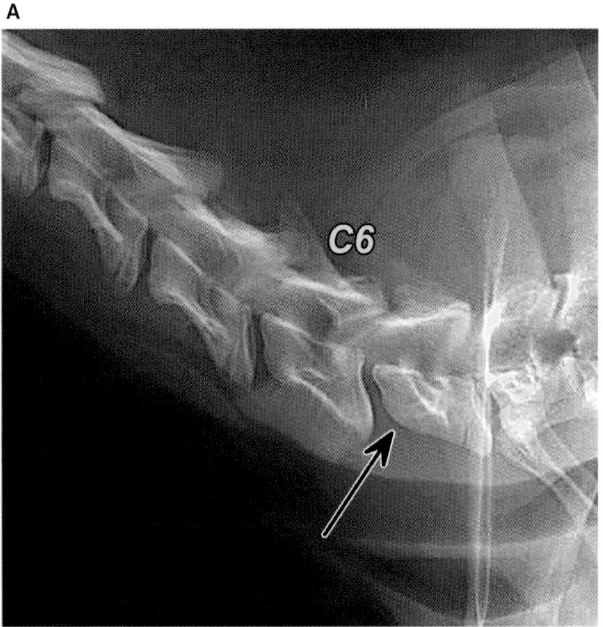

B

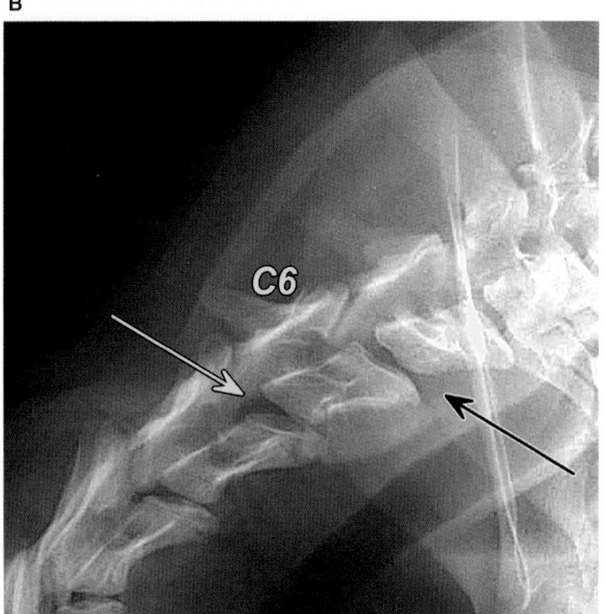

Figure 5.221 Cervical spondylopathy. **A**. Extended lateral view of a dog cervical spine. C6 is identified by its large ventral lamina. The cranioventral border of C7 is flattened (arrow). **B**. Flexed lateral view of the same dog. C6 is dorsally displaced in relation to C5 due to subluxation at C5–6 (yellow arrow). The black arrow points to the flattened area of C7.

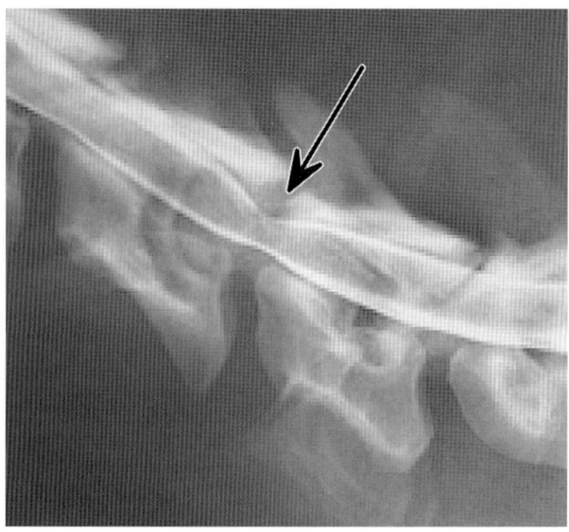

Figure 5.222 Cervical spondylomyelopathy. Lateral view of a dog cervical spine myelogram depicting dorsal compression of the spinal cord at C5–6 (arrow) caused by a malformation of C6 that narrows the spinal canal.

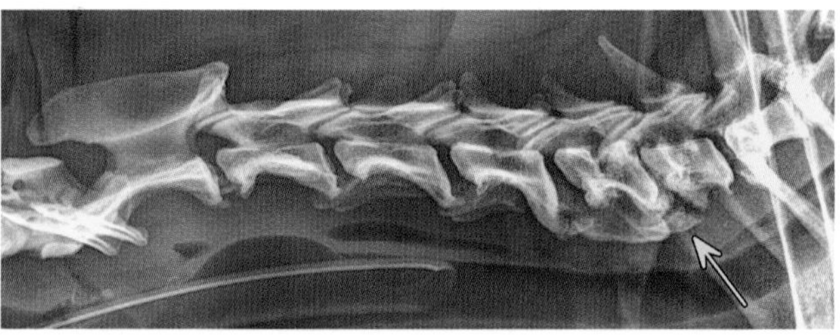

Figure 5.223 Cervical spondylomyelopathy. Lateral view of a dog cervical spine depicting a narrowed intervertebral disc space and degenerative changes at C6–7 (arrow) due to chronic vertebral instability and intervertebral disc disease.

There are several different mechanisms by which abnormal pressure is exerted on the spinal cord. All of them cause damage to the spinal cord and peripheral nerves. Four mechanisms are described below, ranked in order of decreasing probability that a successful treatment can be performed. They may or may not occur simultaneously.

1. Malformation of the vertebral body and formation of osteophytes on the articular processes that lead to narrowing of the spinal canal. This mechanism has been reported at C3–7. Narrowing is progressive and becomes more severe as the animal grows and DJD progresses. Clinical signs usually appear at 1–2 years of age.

2. Malformation of the vertebral arch results in instability between vertebrae and dynamic narrowing of the spinal canal. This mechanism has been reported at C4–7 and is seen most often in young Great Danes.
3. Vertebral instability leads to hypertrophy of the dorsal longitudinal ligament and compression of the spinal cord. Extension of the neck causes the thickened ligament to "bunch up," which increases cord compression. Flexion of the neck stretches the ligament and relieves compression.
4. Vertebral instability and chronic intervertebral disc disease. Protrusion of disc material into the spinal canal contributes to compression of the spinal cord. This mechanism is reported most often at C5–6 and C6–7 and in middle-aged or older Doberman pinchers.

Head and neck

Normal radiographic anatomy

Dog skulls differ more in size and shape than do the skulls of any other mammalian species. The shape of a dog's head commonly is grouped into one of three categories: *doliocephalic, mesaticephalic,* or *brachycephalic.*

Doliocephalic heads are long and narrow. The nasal cavity is longer than the cranium and the occipital crest is relatively large (e.g., Collie, Irish Setter).

Mesaticephalic heads exhibit a "medium" conformation with a nasal cavity that is approximately equal in length to the cranium (e.g., German Shepherd, Labrador Retriever).

Brachycephalic heads are short and wide with a nasal cavity that is considerably shorter than the cranium (e.g., Bulldog, Boston Terrier). In brachycephalic breeds, the maxilla is short and the mandible relatively long. The teeth often are crowded and sometimes displaced. The cranium usually is dome-shaped with a small occipital crest. The frontal sinuses often are small or absent. The soft palate may be thickened and the submandibular tissues relatively large, which can displace the hyoid bones caudally.

Cat skulls are less variable than dogs. Distinctive features in cats compared to dogs include a relatively large cranium and a large osseous tentorium. The tympanic bullae are relatively larger in cats than in dogs and each is divided by an inner bony shell. Dog and cat skull anatomy is illustrated in Figures 5.224–5.233.

Tympanic bullae are air-filled cavities associated with the middle ear. They form the ventral parts of the temporal bones. The tympanic bullae communicate with the nasopharynx via the auditory tube. Located medial and dorsal to the tympanic bullae is the most dense and opaque bone in the body, the *petrous temporal bone,* which houses the components of the inner ear.

At the base of the skull is the *foramen magnum,* an opening that allows the spinal cord to pass from the cranial vault into the vertebral column. The foramen magnum may be better visualized in a rostrocaudal view.

The **cranial vault** (cranial cavity) contains the brain and the organs of hearing and equilibrium. It is formed by the frontal, parietal, occipital, temporal, sphenoid, and basioccipital bones, and the cribriform plate of the ethmoid bone. The bones are joined together by fibrous joints called *sutures.* The upper portion ("roof" or "cap") of the cranial vault is the **calvarium**. The calvarium is formed by the dorsal parts of the frontal, parietal, and occipital bones. The bones of the cranial vault are relatively thicker in some breeds than others (e.g., Pit Bull Terrier).

The **temporomandibular joints (TMJ)** are synovial joints formed by the articulation of the condylar process of the mandible with the mandibular fossa of the temporal bone (Figure 5.254). Caudal to each TMJ is the *retroarticular process* of the temporal bone. This process is relatively larger in cats than in dogs and results in a tighter TMJ in cats.

The paired mandibles are joined rostrally by the *mandibular symphysis,* which is a cartilage joint. The symphysis allows the mandibular rami to move independently, which is why a TMJ can luxate without fracturing.

The **nasal cavity** extends from the external nares to the cribriform plate. Caudal to the cribriform plate is the brain (the cribriform plate separates the nasal cavity from the brain). The *nasal septum* divides the nasal cavity symmetrically into right and left sides. The nasal septum is made up of the vomer bone ventrally and cartilage dorsally. Only the ventral osseous part of the septum (the vomer bone) is seen in radiographs. It appears as a thin, linear bony separation between the nasal cavities (Figures 5.225 and 5.228). Damage to the dorsal cartilagenous part of the nasal septum may not be visible unless the ventral bony part also is damaged. In cats and brachycephalic dogs, the vomer bone may be slightly curved as a normal anatomic variation. The nasal cavities are filled with fine bony structures called *turbinates* or *conchae.* These appear in radiographs as thin, somewhat parallel, mineral opacity lines. The *maxillary* turbinates are more cranial and the *ethmoid* turbinates are more caudal.

There are **four primary air passages** or *meatuses* in the nasal cavity. The *dorsal meatus* is located between the nasal bone and the dorsal turbinates. The *middle meatus* is located between the dorsal and ventral turbinates. The *ventral meatus* is dorsal to the hard palate. The *common meatus* is on either side of the nasal septum.

There are two pairs of paranasal sinuses adjacent to the nasal cavity. The **frontal sinuses** are located dorsal to the orbits and communicate with the nasal cavity. They tend to be relatively larger in cats and large-breed dogs, particularly Saint Bernards. Frontal sinuses often are absent in brachycephalic breeds. The **maxillary sinuses** are located ventral to the orbits, but may be more accurately described as recesses rather than true sinuses. They are difficult to distinguish in radiographs.

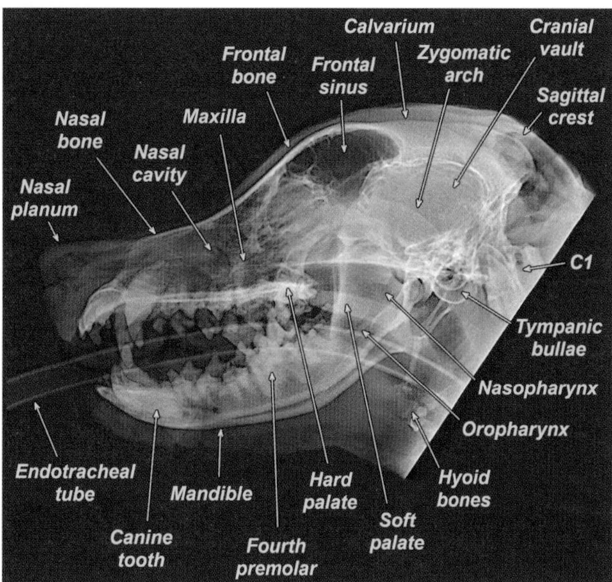

Figure 5.224 Normal dog skull. Lateral view of a dog head depicting normal anatomy. An endotracheal tube is present.

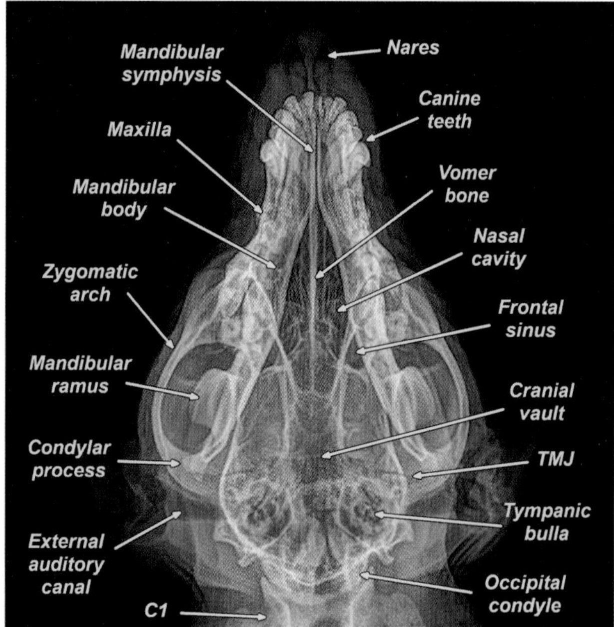

Figure 5.225 Normal dog skull. DV view of a dog head depicting normal anatomy. The vomer bone is the visible bony part of the nasal septum.

Teeth

All teeth are similar in structure but differ in size and shape (Figures 5.230 and 5.231). The **crown** is the exposed tooth, the part above the gumline. The **root** is below the gumline. The number of tooth roots varies from one to three. The **cervical** or neck region of a tooth is the area between the crown and the root. **Enamel** is the thin, hard, mineralized tissue that covers the crown. It is the hardest and most radiopaque part of the tooth. **Dentin** is the bone-like material that supports the enamel. It is slightly less opaque than enamel and makes up most of the substance of a tooth.

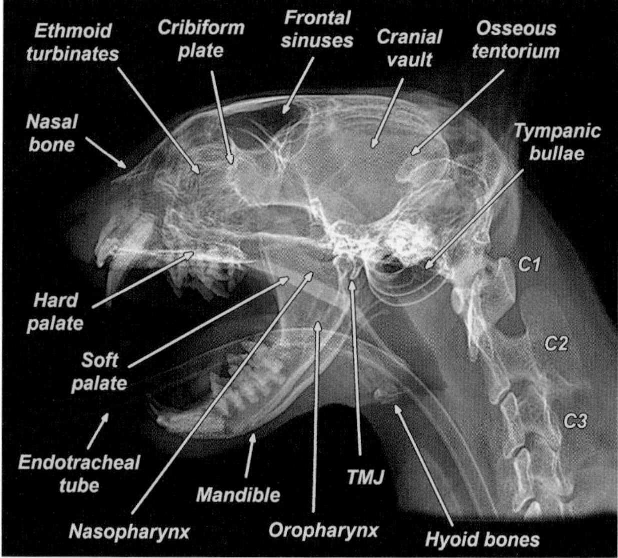

Figure 5.226 Normal cat skull. Lateral view of a cat head depicting normal anatomy. The ethmoid turbinates are in the nasal cavities surrounded by the maxillary bone. The very opaque bone at the dorsal aspect of the tympanic bullae is the petrous temporal bone.

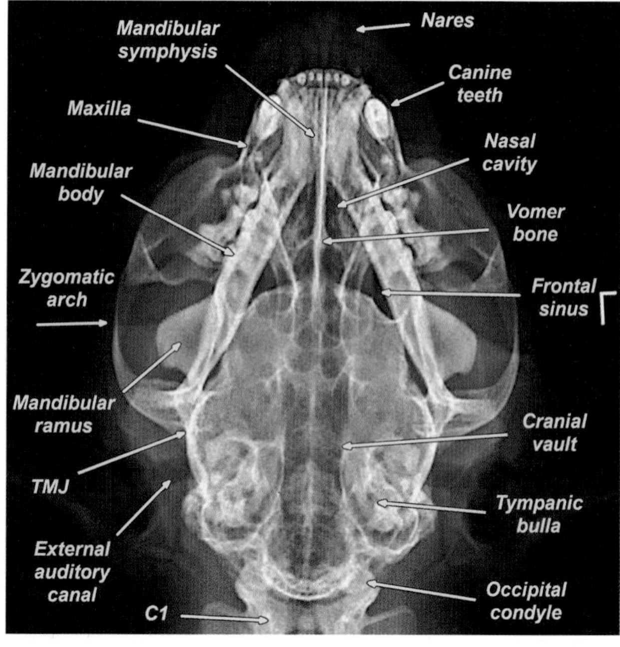

Figure 5.227 Normal skull. DV view of a cat skull depicting normal anatomy. The orbits are located just medial to zygomatic arches.

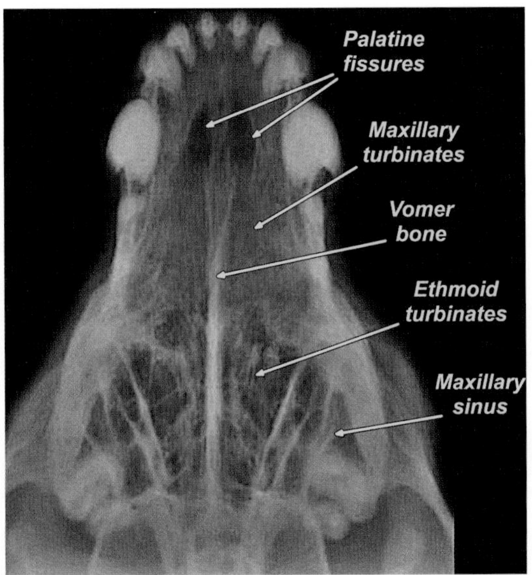

Figure 5.228 Normal dog maxilla. Open-mouth VD view of a dog head depicting normal anatomy.

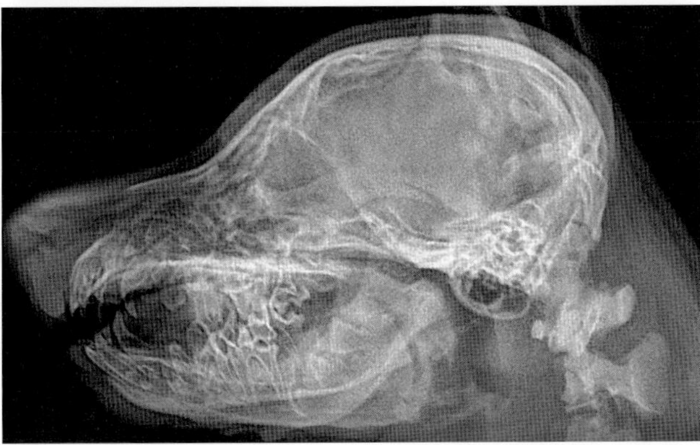

Figure 5.229 Normal immature dog skull. Lateral view of a 2-month-old puppy head.

The **pulp cavity** is located in the center of a tooth. It is less opaque than dentin and contains nerves, blood vessels, and connective tissue. Cementum is not distinguished in radiographs, but it covers roots of the teeth and serves as an attachment for the periodontal ligaments.

Periodontal ligaments fill the **periodontal space** and anchor the teeth to the underlying alveolar bone. The periodontal space appears as a thin, soft tissue opacity line surrounding the tooth roots. Adjacent to the periodontal space is a thin, well-defined, osteosclerotic line called the **lamina dura**. The lamina dura is a dense layer of alveolar bone that is a useful radiographic structure to assess osteopenia. **Alveolar bone** is the cancellous bone in the mandible and maxilla that supports the teeth. The *alveolar crest* is the surface bone that lies between the crowns of adjacent teeth. *Interradicular bone* is the deeper bone between adjacent teeth and *furcation bone* is between the tooth roots.

Deciduous teeth in dogs and cats usually erupt between 3 and 6 weeks of age and are naturally shed as the permanent teeth erupt (Figure 5.229). Deciduous teeth in large breed dogs tend to erupt earlier than in small breeds and teeth in female dogs often erupt earlier than in male dogs.

Permanent teeth begin to erupt at about 3 months of age and finish at about 7 months. The pulp cavities and root canals in permanent teeth initially are large with an open *apical foramen*. As the tooth root lengthens over the next several months, the apical foramen closes and the pulp cavity and root canal gradually narrow. In older animals, the pulp cavity and root canal may not be evident in radiographs. Also as an animal ages, the lamina dura tends to become less

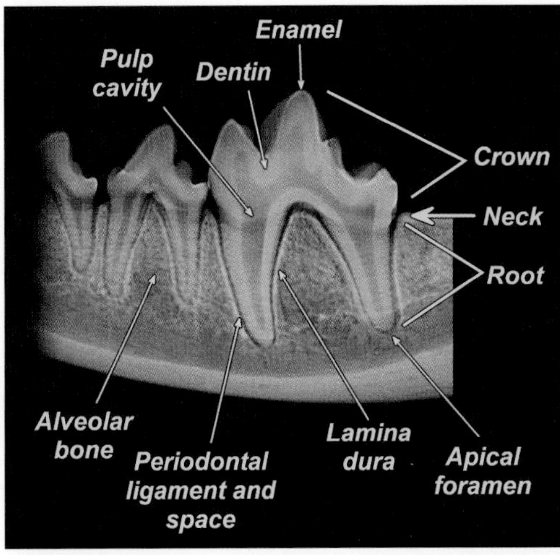

Figure 5.230 Normal tooth. Lateral view of a dog mandible depicting normal anatomy of the first molar tooth. The periodontal ligament fills the periodontal space.

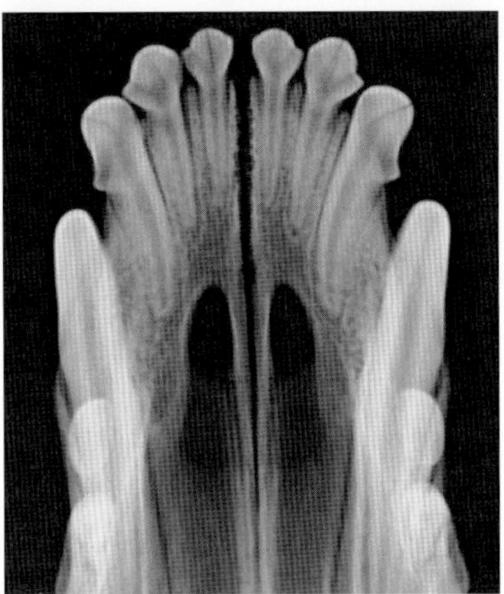

Figure 5.231 Normal teeth. Intraoral view of a dog rostral maxilla depicting normal incisor teeth.

A

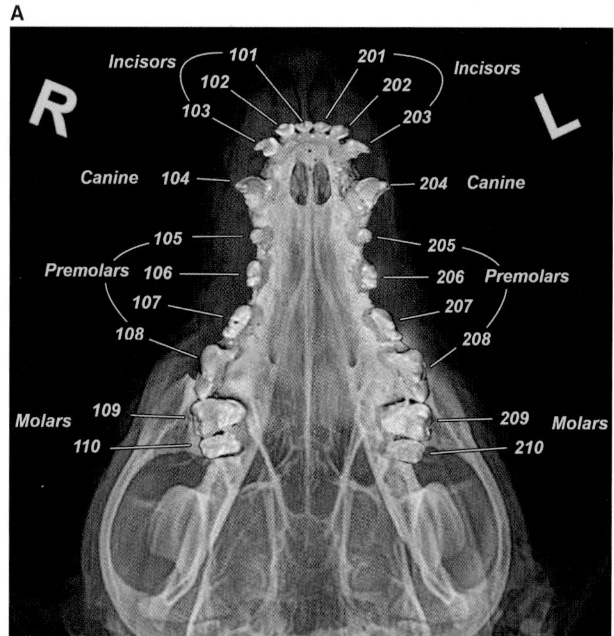

B

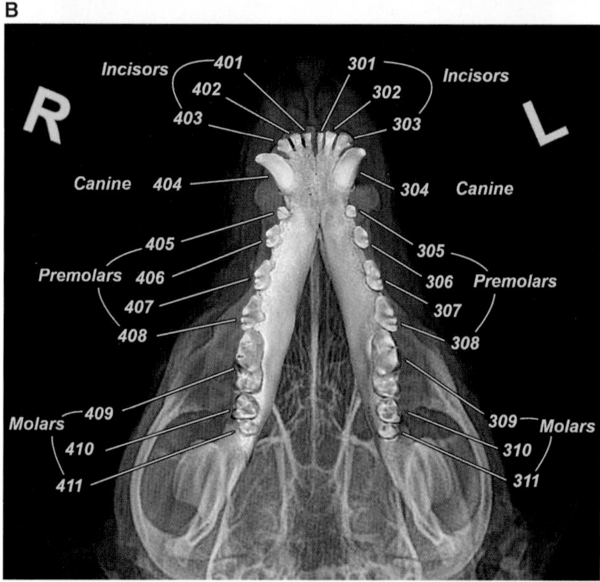

Figure 5.232 Modified Triadan numbering system. DV views of a normal dog head illustrating the maxillary teeth (**A**) and the mandibular teeth (**B**). Each tooth is identified by a three-digit number. The first digit indicates the quadrant: 1 is right maxillary, 2 is left maxillary, 3 is left mandibular, and 4 is right mandibular. The second and third digits denote the tooth position in that quadrant. Note: the numbering always begins on midline.

distinct due to the increased opacity and smaller trabeculae in the alveolar bone.

Dental formulas are commonly used to denote the normal number and type of teeth in an animal. Dental formulas for both immature and mature dogs and cats are listed in Box 5.5. The *modified Triadan numbering system* was designed to be a consistent method of identifying teeth across all animal species (Figures 5.232 and 5.233).

Salivary glands

Salivary glands are not visible in radiographs unless mineralized, enlarged, or opacified with contrast medium. There are four pairs of larger salivary glands in dogs and cats: *parotid, zygomatic, mandibular,* and *sublingual* (Figure 5.262). Multiple smaller salivary glands also are present, including the dorsal and ventral buccal glands.

A

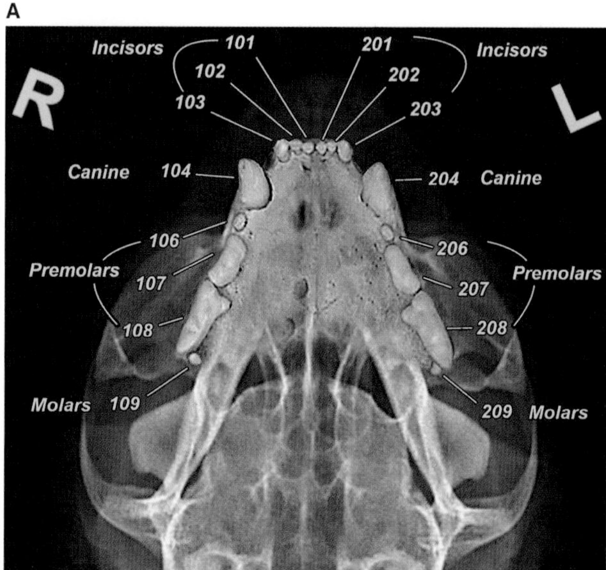

B

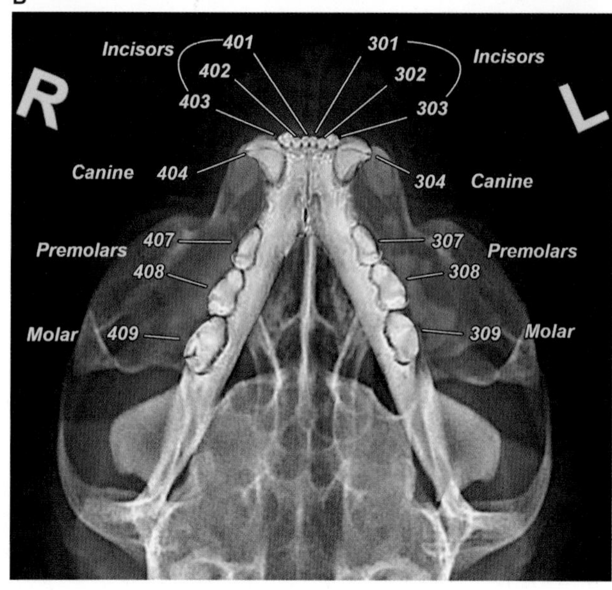

Figure 5.233 Modified Triadan numbering system. DV views of a normal cat skull illustrating the maxillary dental arcade (**A**) and the mandibular dental arcade (**B**). Each tooth is identified by a three-digit number as described in Figure 5.230.

Box 5.5 Dental formulas in dogs and cats

Dog

Deciduous: $2\times\frac{\overset{\text{I C P}}{3\ 1\ 3}}{3\ 1\ 3}=28$

(Some authors refer to the last upper and lower premolar teeth as the molars.)

Permanent: $2\times\frac{\overset{\text{I C P M}}{3\ 1\ 4\ 2}}{3\ 1\ 4\ 3}=42$

Cat

Deciduous: $2\times\frac{\overset{\text{I C P}}{3\ 1\ 3}}{3\ 1\ 2}=26$

Permanent: $2\times\frac{\overset{\text{I C P M}}{3\ 1\ 3\ 1}}{3\ 1\ 2\ 1}=30$

Pharynx and larynx normal radiographic anatomy

Radiographs of the head often include the pharynx and larynx. These structures can be evaluated when they contain gas (Figure 5.234). The **pharynx** extends from the level of the eyes to the level of C1–2. It is associated with both the respiratory and alimentary tracts. The **nasopharynx** is located caudal to the hard palate and dorsal to the soft palate. The **oropharynx** is located ventral to the soft palate and is bordered by the tongue, tonsils, and larynx. The **larynx** is located between the pharynx and the first tracheal ring. It is the passageway for air between the pharynx and the trachea. Extension of the head and neck pulls the larynx cranially and dorsally, whereas flexion pushes it caudally and ventrally. In brachycephalic dogs and in overweight dogs, excessive tissue (including fat) in the cervical and pharyngeal regions may obscure the pharynx and displace the larynx caudally and ventrally.

The larynx consists of five cartilagenous structures: the epiglottis, the paired arytenoid cartilages, the cricoid cartilage, and the thyroid cartilage. The **epiglottis** is the flexible, triangular-shaped structure that covers the opening to the trachea during swallowing to prevent aspiration. It is located a few millimeters caudal to the basihyoid bone. In radiographs, the cranial tip of the epiglottis is variable in position. It may be dorsal, ventral or level with the soft palate, depending on the stage of respiration and swallowing. At the base of the epiglottis are the vocal folds, which are not distinguished in radiographs. However, in dogs there are *lateral ventricles* (*lateral saccules*) adjacent to the vocal folds. The *lateral ventricles* often can be identified in radiographs as ellipsoid, gas-containing structures superimposed on the thyroid cartilage. In cats, *lateral ventricles* are reported not to exist. The epiglottis tends to be the most consistently visible laryngeal structure in cats.

The **laryngeal cartilages** are soft tissue opacity. In most dogs, the cartilages begin to mineralize by 2–3 years of age, often sooner in chondrodystrophic breeds. In cats, the

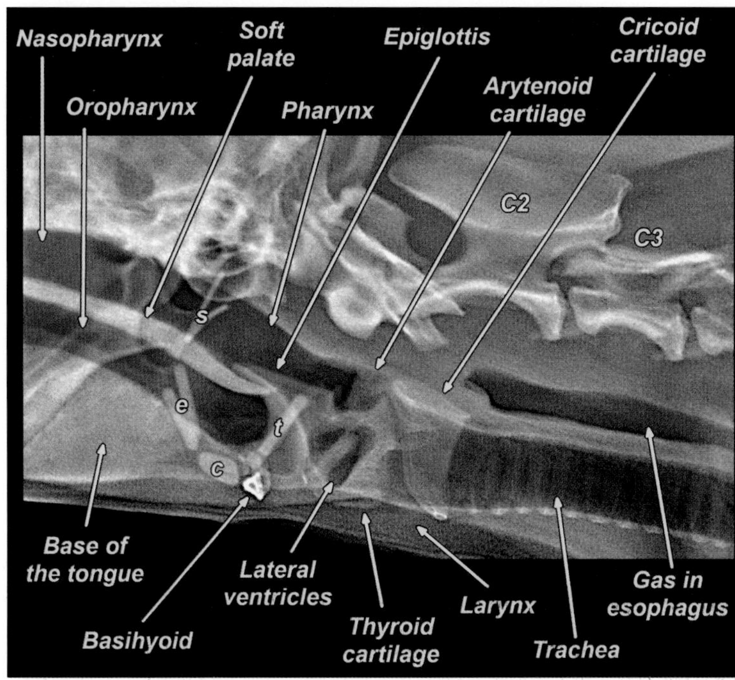

Figure 5.234 Normal pharynx and larynx. Lateral view of a dog cervical region depicting normal anatomy. The larynx includes the epiglottis, arytenoid cartilage, cricoid cartilage, and thyroid cartilage. The tip of the epiglottis lies just dorsal to the soft palate. The lateral ventricles are superimposed on the thyroid cartilage. The paired hyoid bones are labeled **s** = stylohyoid, **e** = epihyoid, **c** = ceratohyoid, and **t** = thyrohyoid. The basihyoid is unpaired and in the lateral view appears quite opaque because it is viewed end-on resulting in summation along the length of the bone. There is gas in the cranial esophagus; the gas outlines the caudal part of the cranial esophageal sphincter.

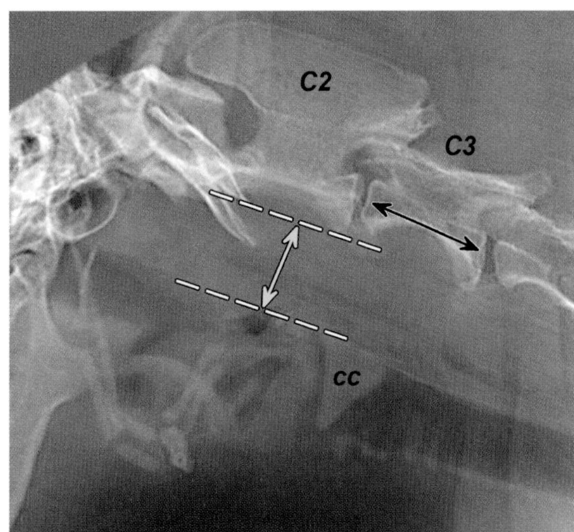

Figure 5.235 Retropharyngeal space. Lateral view of a dog cervical region illustrating the normal size of the retropharyngeal space. In general, with the head in a neutral position (about 135° with the neck), the width of the retropharyngeal space (yellow double-headed arrow) should not exceed the length of C3 (black double headed arrow). The width is measured from the dorsal edge of the cricoid cartilage (cc) to the ventral plane of C2.

cartilages rarely mineralize. Mineralization tends to progress with age and appears well-defined in radiographs and confined to the borders of the cartilage. Pathologic mineralization on the other hand tends to be excessive and more heterogeneous. The cricoid cartilage often is visible in dogs. It is wide dorsally, tapers ventrally, and is attached to the first tracheal ring. The thyroid cartilage is the largest laryngeal cartilage. It is attached to the cricoid cartilage dorsally and to the hyoid bones cranially.

The **hyoid bones** are the suspensory apparatus for the tongue and larynx. They often can be identified in lateral views that include the larynx. Named from cranial to caudal, the hyoid bones are *stylohyoid, epihyoid, ceratohyoid, basihyoid,* and *thyrohyoid*. All of the bones are paired except the basihyoid, which is transversely oriented in relation to the others. Because it is oriented transversely, the basihyoid bone is viewed end-on in a lateral view and its length is summated to create a rather opaque bony structure. Be careful not to mistake the basihyoid bone for a foreign object or fracture fragment. There is a cartilagenous attachment between the hyoid bones and the tympanic bullae. The positions and angulations of the hyoid bones vary with the position of the head and neck.

The **retropharyngeal space** is the soft tissue opacity area between the pharynx and the spine. It contains the retropharyngeal lymph nodes and should be examined for evidence of swelling or a mass (e.g., abscess, lymphadenomegaly, hematoma, tumor). In general, the dorsoventral dimension of retropharyngeal space should not exceed the length of C3 in a properly positioned lateral radiograph (Figure 5.235). Rotation of the head and neck can distort the appearance of the retropharyngeal space.

Skull radiographs

The skull is a complex structure that requires high-quality radiographs. Symmetrical positioning is important because one side usually is compared with the other. If correct positioning is not possible, take malpositioning into account when interpreting radiographic findings.

Measure the thickest (widest) part of head, typically midway between the eyes and the ears, and center the x-ray beam at the level of the eyes.

Collimate the field-of-view to include the entire head, from the tip of the nose to the first cervical vertebra. The smaller the field-of-view, the less scatter radiation and the better the radiographic detail and contrast.

Always include lateral and DV/VD views with any radiographic evaluation of the head. Additional views of the specific area of interest can then be added as needed:

1. **Lateral** view; position the side with the lesion closest to the image receptor (Figure 2.46). Pay attention to support the head so it is truly lateral in position.
2. **DV/VD** view; DV may be easier to position small dogs, brachycephalic breeds, and cats (Figure 2.47); VD may be easier with deep-chested dogs.
3. **Oblique** views: lateral view made with the head tilted to one side or the other to evaluate a frontal sinus, dental arcade, or to visualize a mass in profile (Figure 2.48).
4. **Open-mouth** views: lateral, lateral oblique, or VD view made with the mouth open to reduce superimposition artifacts (Figures 2.49, 2.50, 2.54):
   a. Lateral open-mouth view to examine the nasopharynx without superimposition of the vertical rami of the mandible.
   b. Lateral oblique open-mouth view to visualize one dental arcade without superimposition of the opposite arcade.
   c. VD open-mouth view to examine the nasal cavity and maxilla without a superimposed mandible.
5. **Rostrocaudal** views: VD views made with the nose pointed toward the x-ray tube to better visualize parts of the skull by eliminating superimposition of the maxilla or mandible (Figures 2.51–2.54):
   a. Rostrocaudal skyline view to examine the frontal sinuses, zygomatic bones, and orbits.
   b. Flexed rostrocaudal view to better visualize the foramen magnum.
   c. Extended rostrocaudal view to examine the feline tympanic bullae.
   d. Open-mouth rostrocaudal view to better visualize the odontoid process (dens) and the canine tympanic bullae.

6. **Intra-oral** views: the image receptor is placed inside the patient's mouth to isolate the mandible, maxilla, or a tooth without superimposition of the adjacent structures (Figures 2.55, 2.56, 2.58).
7. **Temporomandibular joint** (TMJ): lateral views made with the nose tilted up or down to better visualize an individual TMJ (Figure 2.57).
8. **Altered exposures**: with film radiography, the exposure settings may need to be adjusted to better visualize a specific skull bone or compartment or an adjacent soft tissue structure.

Due to superimposition of many bones and cavities, a systematic approach is essential when evaluating skull radiographs. Dividing the skull into regions may be useful to make sure you examine all parts of the head (Table 5.8).

Multilobular tumor of the skull

These are slow-growing primary bone tumors that develop from a focal area of abnormal periosteal activity in part of the skull. They are more common in young adult, medium-to-large breed dogs. Other names include: *multilobular osteoma, chondroma of the skull, chondroma rodens,* and *juvenile calcifying aponeurotic fibroma*. These tumors typically produce a well-defined, irregular or nodular-shaped bony mass that is 1–10 cm in size. The affected bone may be deformed, but there is no osteolysis and minimal soft tissue swelling. Very large tumors may extend into adjacent structures, such as a frontal sinus to cause rhinitis, or an orbit resulting in exophthalmia, or a temporal or zygomatic bone leading to difficulty opening the jaw, or the underlying brain to cause neurologic signs.

Craniomandibular osteopathy (CMO)

CMO is characterized by prolific new bone production on the mandible and cranium and occasionally involving the long bones. It is a self-limiting, non-inflammatory, non-neoplastic disease of unknown etiology that affects growing dogs.

Periosteal new bone production usually begins along the mandibles, near the angular processes (Figure 5.236). Bone production tends to be extensive and usually bilateral but may not be symmetrical. It frequently involves the petrous temporal bone and may lead to thickening of the tympanic bullae and calvarium. Bony proliferation adjacent to the temporomandibular joints can physically prevent opening the mouth.

Craniomandibular osteopathy most often is reported in certain terrier breeds (e.g., West Highland White, Scottish, Boston, Cairn). Clinical signs of mandibular pain and swelling with difficulty eating generally appear between 3 and 8 months of age. Bony proliferation usually ceases and signs regress at skeletal maturity.

Cranial hyperostosis is a condition reported in Bullmastiff puppies that may be a manifestation of craniomandibular osteopathy. Lesions associated with cranial hyperostosis include thickening and osteosclerosis in the frontal and parietal bones of the skull.

Cranial vault fractures

Many skull fractures are small, linear, and nondisplaced, making radiographic detection difficult. Oblique and tangential views may aid in visualizing fracture lines. Keep in mind that overlapping fractures may produce lines of increased opacity. Normal sutures and vascular channels are less opaque than bone and may be mistaken for fracture lines, especially in immature animals. These may be differentiated from fractures due to a lack of soft tissue swelling.

Soft tissue swelling usually is present at acute fracture sites. There may also subcutaneous emphysema if the fracture is open or involves the nasal cavity or a frontal sinus (Figure 5.237). Skull fractures may be simple or comminuted, and the fragment(s) sometimes are depressed; displaced into the associated cavity (Figures 5.238 and 5.239). Follow-up radiographs may document a periosteal response, which helps identify a fracture that was not apparent in the initial radiographs.

Hydrocephalus

Hydrocephalus is an excessive accumulation of fluid in the ventricular system of the brain. Radiographs are insensitive for diagnosing hydrocephalus unless there are significant secondary changes to the cranial vault. Secondary changes may include pressure remodeling that enlarges the cranial vault, making the calvarium appear thinner and more dome-shaped (Figure 5.240). The cranial cavity may appear hazy and indistinct in radiographs. The inner border of the calvarium may be more smooth and uniform because the convolutional markings created by a normal brain are diminished or lost due to pressure remodeling. In immature animals with hydrocephalus, the fontanelles often remain open and the sutures may remain visible for longer than expected periods of time.

Hydrocephalus may be congenital or acquired, obstructive or nonobstructive, and can occur in any dog or cat at any age. Chihuahuas and Yorkshire Terriers may be overrepresented. Congenital hydrocephalus tends to produce more alterations to the skull than the acquired forms. The skull may appear normal during the early stages of hydrocephalus and in animals in which it is acquired after ossification of the skull is complete.

Cranial vault neoplasia

Skull tumors are uncommon in dogs and cats. They may involve the nasal cavity, oral cavity, or cranial vault. Soft tissue tumors sometimes invade the skull by direct extension. Metastatic tumors rarely involve the skull, other than multiple myeloma, which typically produces numerous, focal, osteolytic lesions ("punched out" areas).

Table 5.8 Regions for systematic evaluation of lateral and DV views of the head

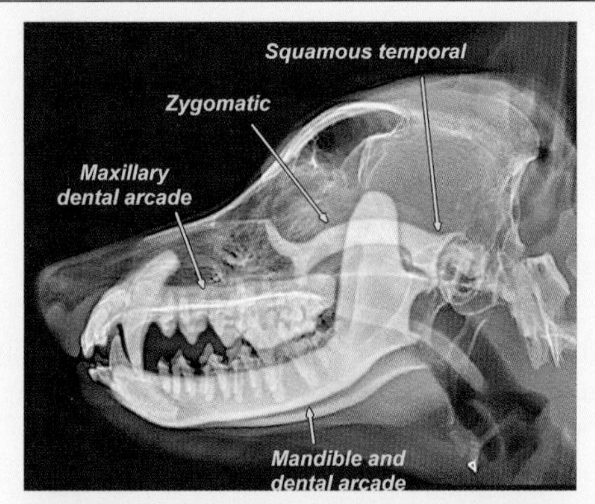	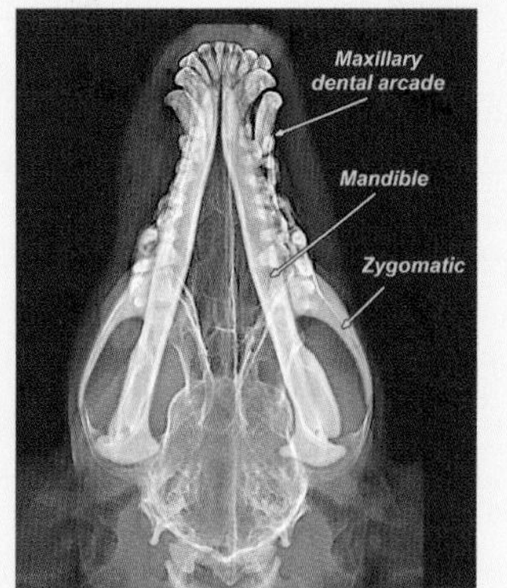	**Region I**. Structures to be evaluated include the mandibles (horizontal and vertical rami, condyloid process, TMJs, dental arcade, symphysis); maxillary dental arcade, zygomatic arch and squamous temporal bone.
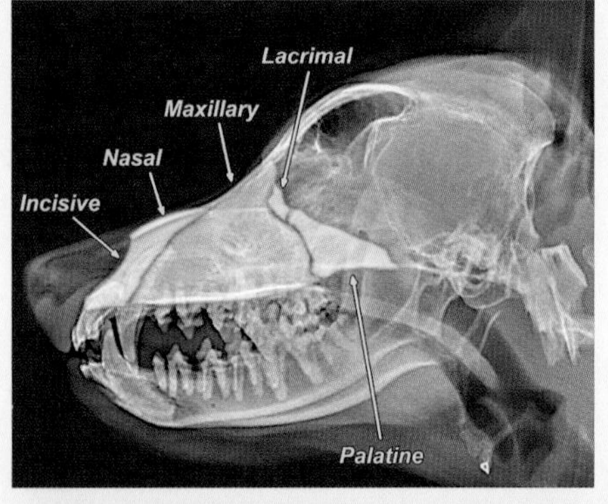	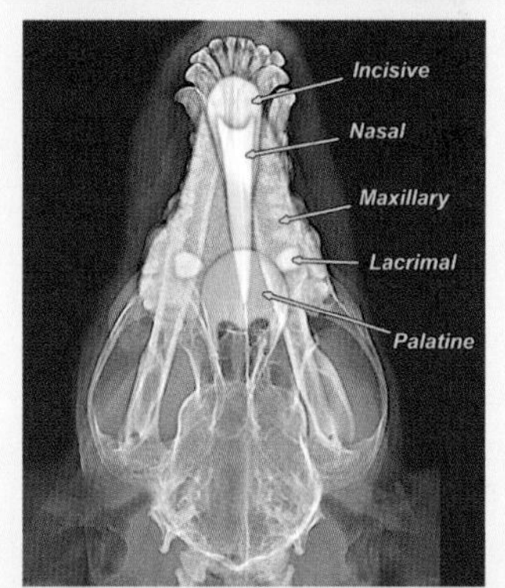	**Region II**. Structures to be evaluated include the maxilla, nasal cavity and turbinates; vomer bone (nasal septum); cribriform plate; hard palate; frontal sinuses and supraorbital process.
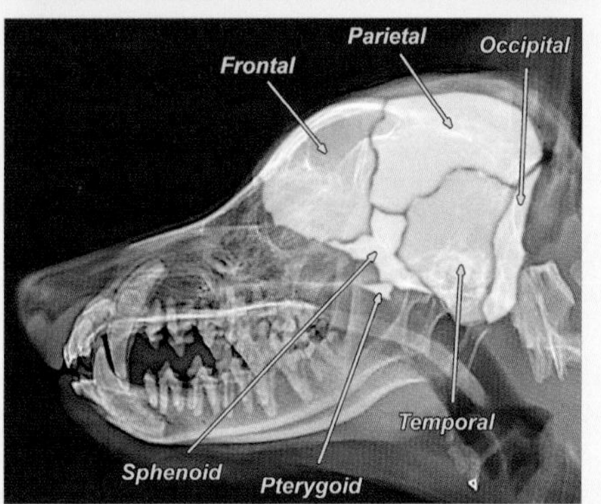	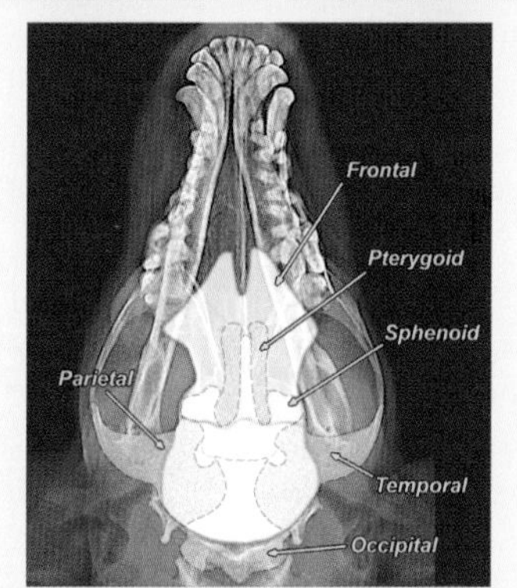	**Region III**. Structures to be evaluated include the cranial vault: frontal, parietal, occipital, temporal bones; petrous temporal bone (inner ear); tympanic bullae (middle ear); occipital condyles and foramen magnum.
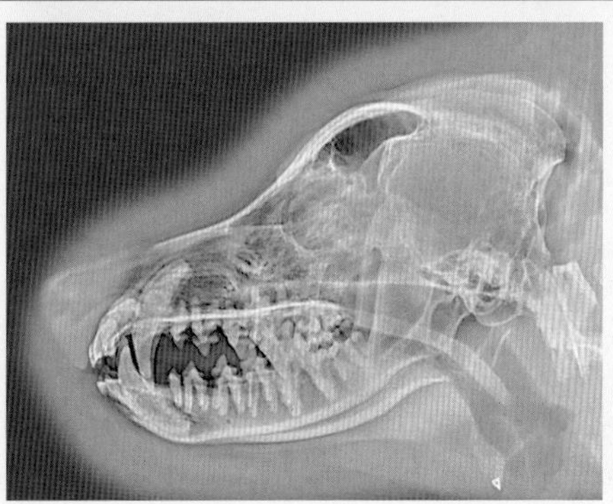	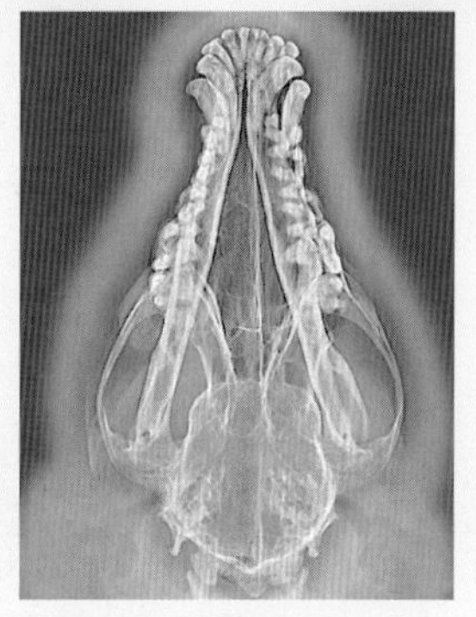	**Region IV**. Structures to be evaluated include the cutaneous and sub-cutaneous soft tissues; soft palate, nasopharynx, oropharynx, pharynx; retropharyngeal space; larynx, hyoid bones; external auditory canals; cervical spine.

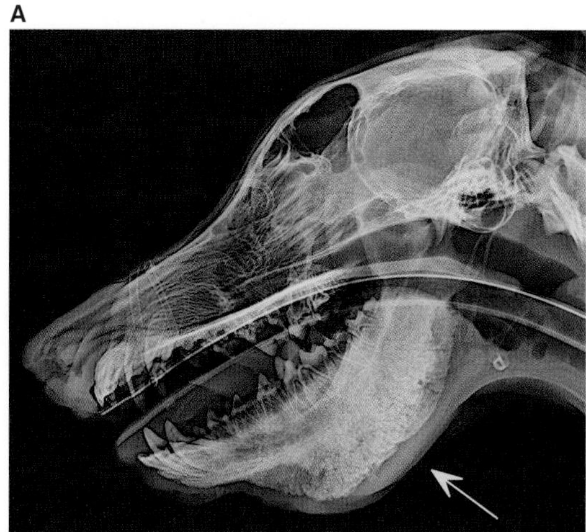

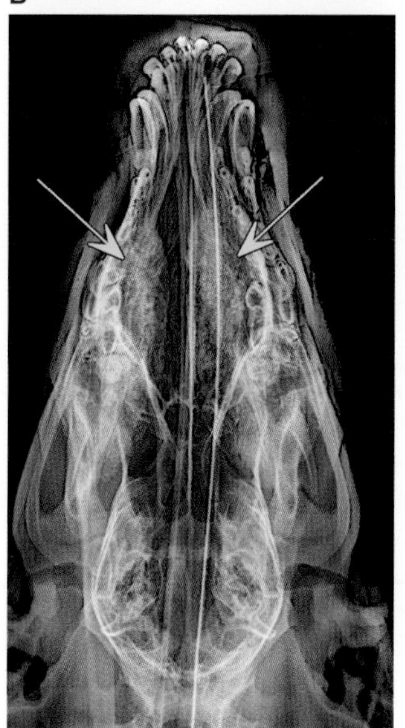

Figure 5.236 Craniomandibular osteopathy. Lateral view (**A**) and DV view (**B**) of a dog head depicting prolific new bone production along the right and left hemimandibles (arrows). Periosteal new bone is irregular but well-defined.

Osteosarcoma is the most common malignant tumor of the skull. In the calvarium, it tends to be more osteoproductive and better-defined than in the long bones, but in the facial bones it often is more osteolytic.

Osteoma is the most common benign tumor of the skull. It is a slow-growing neoplasm that more often arises in the mandible, cranial vault, or sinuses. The margins of an osteoma usually are smooth, well-defined, and sclerotic. Multilobular osteomas can produce a lobulated soft tissue opacity mass with diffuse amorphous or granular mineralization and a well-defined, localized area of osteolysis. They more often arise in the parietal crest, temporooccipital region, or zygomatic bone.

Soft tissue tumors that involve the maxilla or mandible tend to be primarily osteolytic with little or no periosteal response. They may cause osteolysis in the bone adjacent to the teeth and may displace the teeth, but the teeth themselves rarely are invaded or destroyed.

Brain tumors, whether primary or metastatic, seldom are visible in survey radiographs. Meningiomas occasionally will mineralize and may be visible near the calvarium as an area of increased opacity. Brain tumors that are located immediately adjacent to bone occasionally will produce a periosteal response, usually smooth and well-defined.

Occipital dysplasia

Occipital dysplasia refers to the incomplete ossification of the occipital bone that results in an enlarged foramen magnum. The foramen magnum may be better visualized in an overexposed rostrocaudal view, made with the x-ray beam angled rostrodorsal 20° caudoventral (Figure 2.70). Enlargement of the foramen magnum usually occurs in the dorsal direction and varies from slight to marked.

Occipital dysplasia most often is reported in toy and miniature dog breeds. It frequently is accompanied by other abnormalities (e.g., hydrocephalus, shortening of first cervical vertebra, atlantoaxial malformation, occipital hypoplasia). Clinical signs often are absent unless there is herniation of

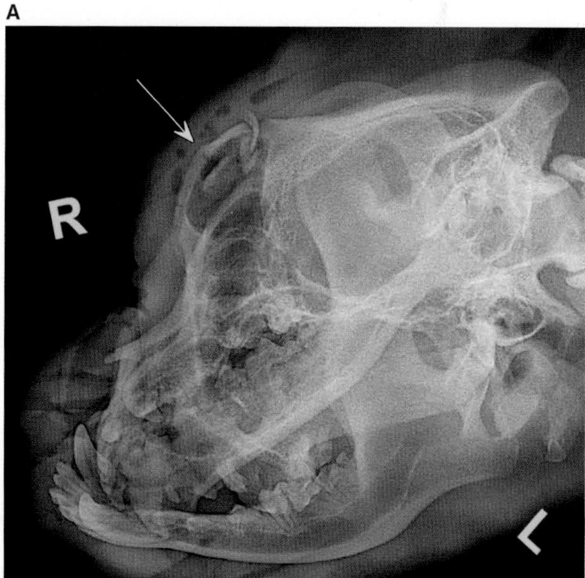

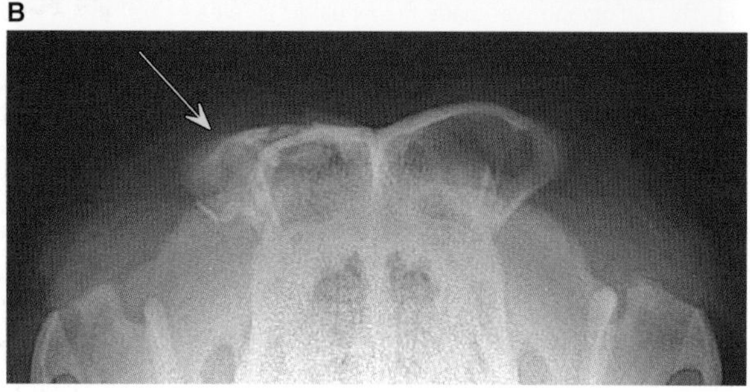

Figure 5.237 Skull fracture. Lateral oblique view (**A**) and skyline view (**B**) of a brachycephalic dog depicting a comminuted fracture in the right frontal bone (arrows) with mild soft tissue swelling and subcutaneous emphysema.

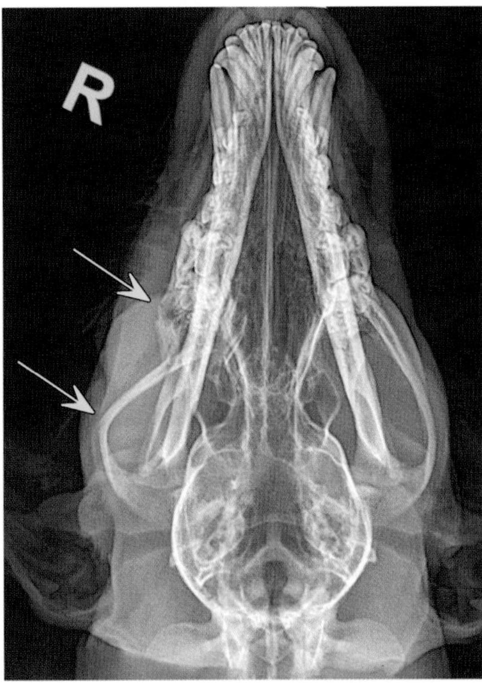

Figure 5.238 Skull fracture. DV view of a dog head depicting a medially displaced segmental fracture in the right zygomatic bone (arrows) and mild soft tissue swelling.

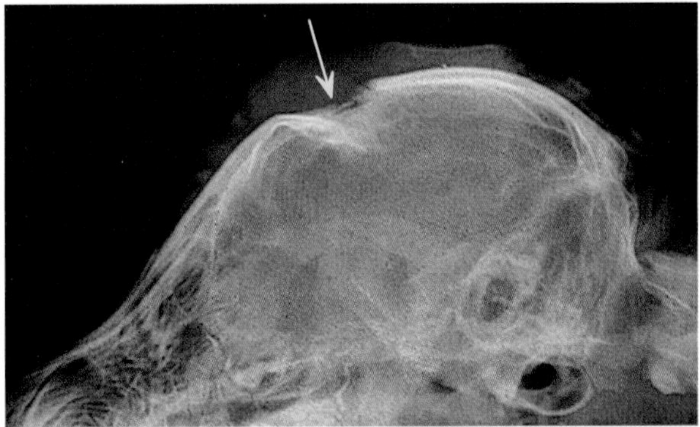

Figure 5.239 Skull fracture. Lateral oblique view of an immature dog head. The radiograph was made tangential to an area of soft tissue swelling to evaluate that part of the skull. The arrow points to a depressed fracture along the dosolateral calvarium.

the brain stem or cerebellum. Chiari-like malformation is another developmental abnormality of the occipital bone, usually accompanied by syringomyelia. It also is most often reported in small and toy breed dogs, particularly Cavalier King Charles Spaniels.

Otitis (externa, media, and interna)

Inflammation involving the external, middle, and/or inner ear most often is caused by a bacterial infection. Survey radiographs of patients with acute otitis typically are unremarkable. The external auditory canal may be narrowed or obscured due to soft tissue swelling or the presence of fluid, exudate, or debris in the lumen (Figure 5.241). Nonvisualization of an external auditory canal may also be due to congenital absence of the ear canal or a previous surgical procedure.

Chronic otitis can lead to mineralization of the external auditory canal. Incidental mineralization frequently is seen in the ear canals of older animals (probably a remnant of previous disease). Such "age-related" mineralization generally appears as thin, well-defined rings in the lumen of the ear canal.

Otitis can involve the ipsilateral tympanic bulla and increase the bulla opacity, either due to the presence of exudates, the formation of a polyp, or a periosteal response that thickens the bulla wall. Severe inflammation can lead to

A

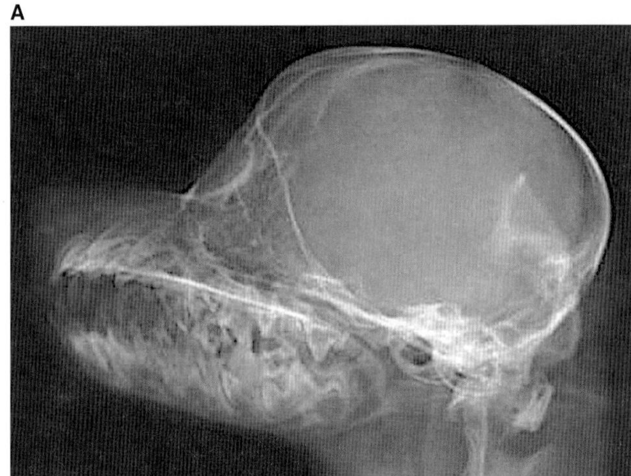

B

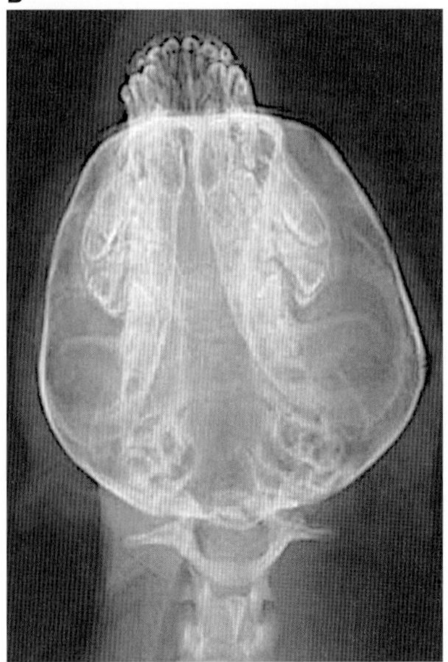

Figure 5.240 Hydrocephalus. Lateral view (**A**) and DV view (**B**) of a puppy with an expanded cranial vault and thinning of the calvarium. The cranial vault is homogeneous in appearance.

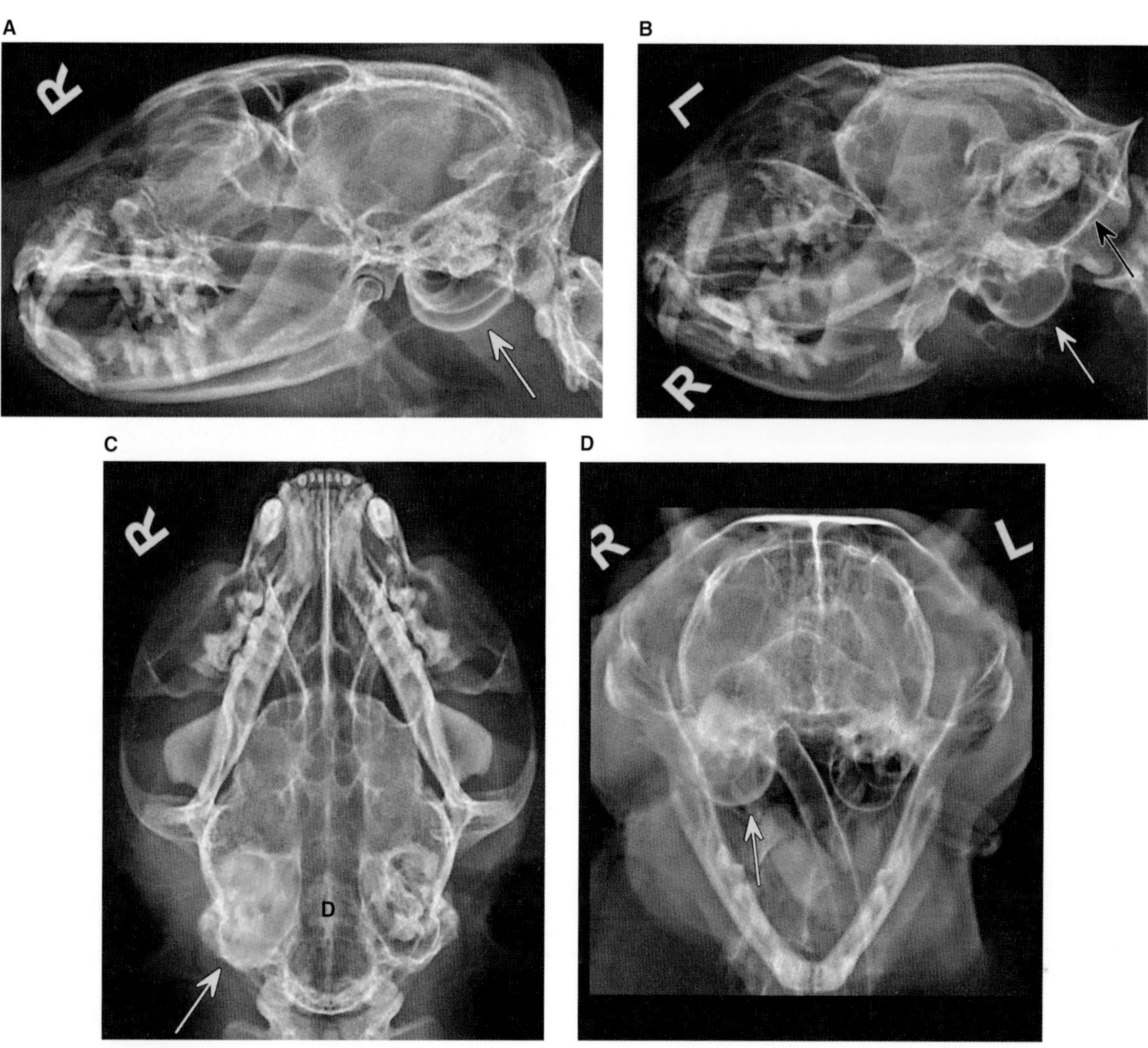

Figure 5.241 Chronic otitis. Lateral view (**A**), lateral oblique view (**B**), DV view (**C**) and open mouth rostrocaudal view (**D**) of a cat head depicting increased opacity in the right tympanic bulla and thickening of the right bulla wall (yellow arrows). The left bulla is normal. In the oblique view, the left bulla (black arrow) is positioned dorsal to the right. In the DV view, gas is absent from the right external auditory canal due to soft tissue swelling and there is faint linear mineralization in the canal.

osteolysis of the bulla, but bone loss is more likely to be caused by neoplasia.

Nasopharyngeal polyps sometimes are visible in a lateral radiograph as soft tissue opacity in the nasopharynx (Figure 5.242). Polyps are non-neoplastic and may precede or follow otitis. They are more common in cats than in dogs, especially younger animals. Polyps may be solitary or multiple and can arise from the auditory tube or middle ear. A polyp may extend into the external ear canal or tympanic bulla. Clinical signs that may be associated with a nasopharyngeal polyp include nasal discharge, sneezing, and stridor.

Nasal cavity and frontal sinus

The nasal cavity and frontal sinuses are evaluated for symmetry, opacity, and visibility of the turbinates. Gas adjacent to the turbinates makes them visible in radiographs. Fluid or abnormal soft tissue in the nasal cavity can efface much of the tubinates, but some of the fine bony structures often can still be discerned through the soft tissue opacity material (Figure 5.243). Complete loss of the fine bony structures often is due to osteolysis and destruction of the turbinates (Figure 5.244). Disease in the nasal cavity may extend into the adjacent structures (e.g., frontal sinuses, frontal bone, maxillary bone, cranial vault, teeth, soft tissues).

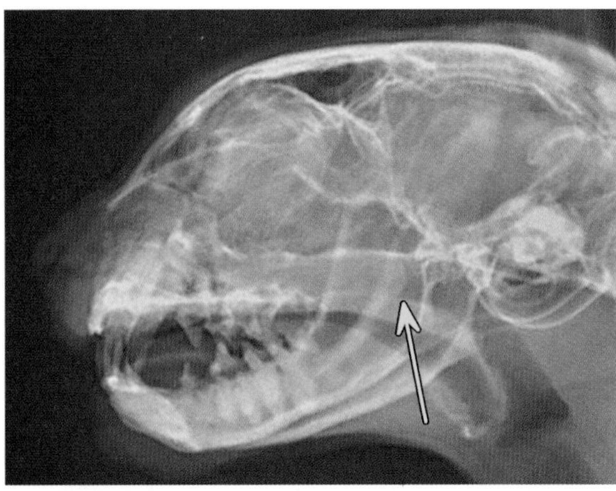

Figure 5.242 Nasopharyngeal mass. Lateral view of a cat head depicting soft tissue opacity in the rostral half of the nasopharynx. The arrow points to the caudal border of a soft tissue mass.

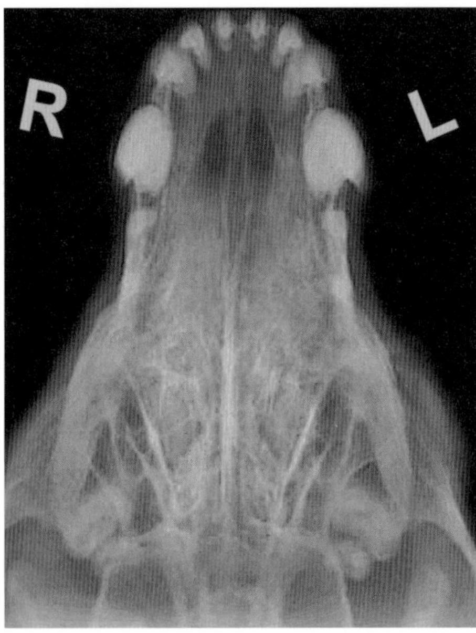

Figure 5.243 Rhinitis. Open-mouth VD view of a dog head depicting increased opacity in both nasal cavities. The turbinates are effaced, but still visible, without evidence of osteolysis at this time.

Radiographic findings often are nonspecific regarding the etiology of the nasal lesions, but they aid in determining the locations and extent of the lesions.

Aggressive lesions (e.g., tumors, severe osteomyelitis) frequently result in increased opacity and osteolysis in the nasal cavity (Figures 5.251 and 5.252). Lesions often are easier to see in an open mouth VD view (Figure 5.245). The nasal septum may be deviated by an expanding tumor (Figure 5.252) or other mass. In general, unilateral aggressive lesions are more likely to be neoplastic and bilateral lesions are more likely to be infection, but this is not always the case. Cytology or histopathology is required for definitive diagnosis.

Masses or foreign objects in the nasopharynx may be visible in a well-positioned lateral view. Carefully examine the nasopharynx just caudal to the last maxillary molar tooth (Figure 5.242). This area may be better visualized by increasing the x-ray exposure and opening the patient's mouth to rotate the mandibular ramus and eliminate its superimposition.

Inflammation/infection of nasal cavity

Rhinitis and/or sinusitis may be due to an infection (e.g., bacterial, viral, mycotic), inhaled irritant, foreign object, or allergy. Chronic infection often includes a bacterial component, which may be a secondary complication of a viral or mycotic infection.

Survey radiographs often are unremarkable in patients with acute nasal cavity infections. Supplemental views may aid in lesion detection (e.g., open-mouth VD, rostrocaudal, intraoral). A frequent but nonspecific radiographic finding of rhinitis is increased opacity in one or both sides of the nasal cavity (Figures 5.243 and 5.245). Note: superimposition of the tongue or an endotracheal tube may be mistaken for increased opacity in the nasal cavity. Rhinitis sometimes involves the paranasal sinuses, either unilaterally or bilaterally. However, the nasal septum often remains intact and external soft tissue swelling and facial deformity are rare. Osteolysis is more likely with neoplasia or advanced mycosis. Rarely, a chronic or severe bacterial infection can lead to osteolysis.

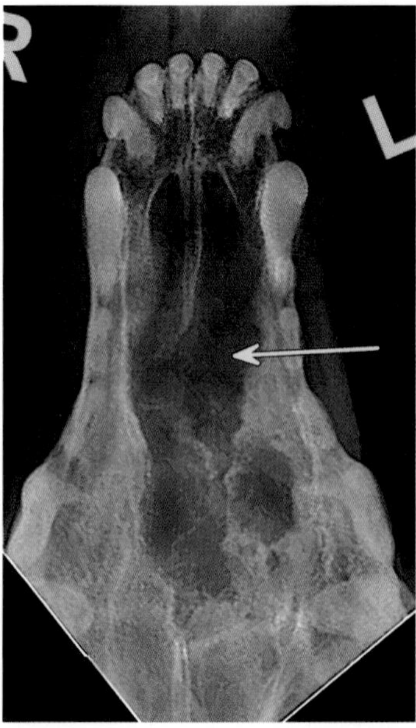

Figure 5.244 Aggressive lesion. Open mouth VD view of a dog head depicting geographic osteolysis that involves both nasal cavities. The arrow points to destruction of the vomer bone (nasal septum).

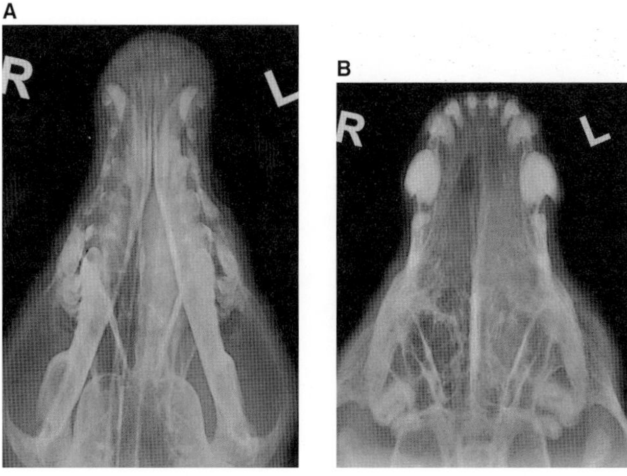

Figure 5.245 Nasal cavity lesions. VD view (**A**) and open-mouth VD view (**B**) of the same dog head depicting unilateral increased opacity in the left nasal cavity. The full extent of the is easier to see without superimposition of the mandible.

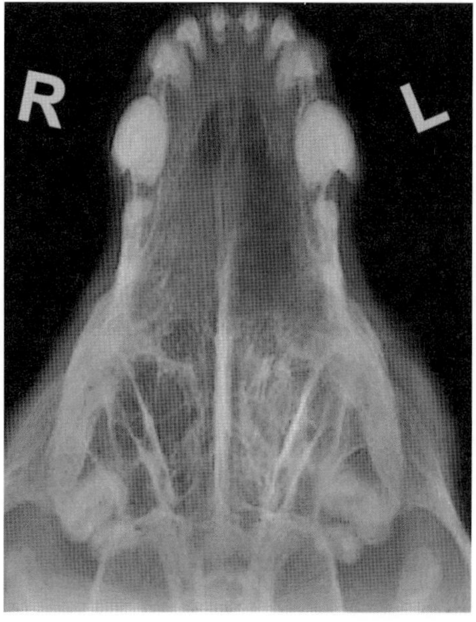

Figure 5.246 Rhinitis. Open-mouth VD view of a dog head depicting decreased opacity and osteolysis in the rostral portion of the left nasal cavity and increased opacity in the caudal portion. The rostral fine bony structures associated with the nasal turbinates are lost. The ethmoid turbinates are visible through the increased opacity and appear intact. The radiographic appearance is typical for a fungal infection but not diagnostic of a mycosis. Neoplasia or bacterial infection can produce similar findings. Laboratory testing is necessary for diagnosis.

Mycotic rhinitis tends to begin in the rostral third of the nasal cavity (Figure 5.246). Focal areas of osteolysis may be scattered in the turbinates, sometimes surrounded by thickened bone. *Cryptococcus* tends to produce a non-destructive, hyperplastic rhinitis. *Aspergillosis* often causes osteolysis, but rarely in the vomer bone (nasal septum).

Foreign objects can lodge anywhere in the nasal cavity or nasopharynx. Mineral or metal opacity objects often are visible in radiographs, but some may be obscured by overlying bone. Soft tissue opacity materials (e.g., plant awns) generally are not evident in survey radiographs. A soft tissue mass or localized fluid accumulation may create a detectable increase in opacity.

Neoplasia of nasal cavity

Most nasal tumors are slow growing and slow to metastasize. They more often are reported in dogs than in cats, with the highest incidence in dolichocephalic breeds. Adenocarcinoma and squamous cell carcinoma are most common in dogs and lymphosarcoma is most common in cats.

Early in the course of nasal neoplasia, radiographic findings often are nonspecific and may resemble infection. The affected side of the nasal cavity may be increased in opacity, usually unilateral but sometimes bilateral. Tumors tend to originate in the caudal or middle third of the nasal cavity; at about the level of a carnassial tooth. In radiographs, an irregular-shaped soft tissue opacity may be visible in the nasal cavity and/or frontal sinus. Osteolysis of nasal turbinates, septum, vomer bone, and/or cortical bone is common as the neoplasia progresses (Figure 5.247). The nasal septum

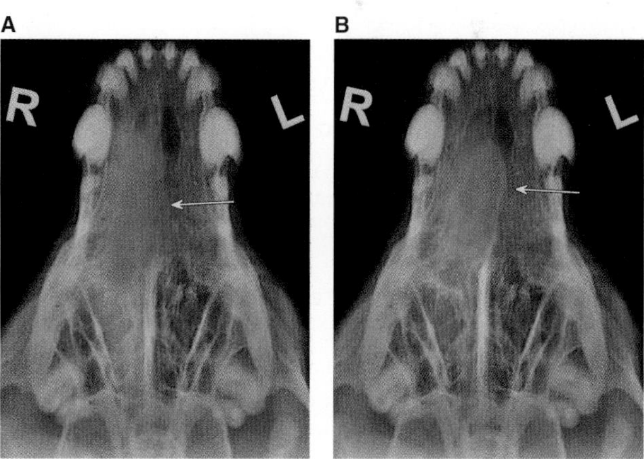

Figure 5.247 Nasal neoplasia. **A**. Open-mouth VD view of a dog head depicting increased opacity throughout the right nasal cavity with an indistinct nasal septum (arrow) and loss of fine bony structures. **B**. Open-mouth VD view of a dog head depicting a mass in the right nasal cavity resulting in osteolysis and left lateral deviation of the nasal septum (arrow).

may be displaced or deviate away from the neoplasm. Tumors can extend caudally through the cribriform plate and into the cranial vault. Again, a soft tissue mass may be visible in nasopharynx, immediately caudal to maxillary dental arcade (lateral radiograph). Tumors in the nasal cavity or frontal sinus sometimes enlarge, resulting in facial deformity, missing teeth, and external swelling.

Frontal sinus mucocele

A mucocele is a benign, cyst-like mass that can form in a frontal sinus of a patient with an obstructed draining duct. Obstruction may result from a fracture in the nasal or frontal bone, a mass in the caudal aspect of the nasal cavity, chronic inflammation, or a mucous plug. The mucocele increases the opacity in the frontal sinus, usually unilaterally (Figure 5.248). The associated frontal bone may be thinned due to expansion of the mucocele and pressure remodeling. Frontal sinus mucoceles are uncommon in dogs and cats.

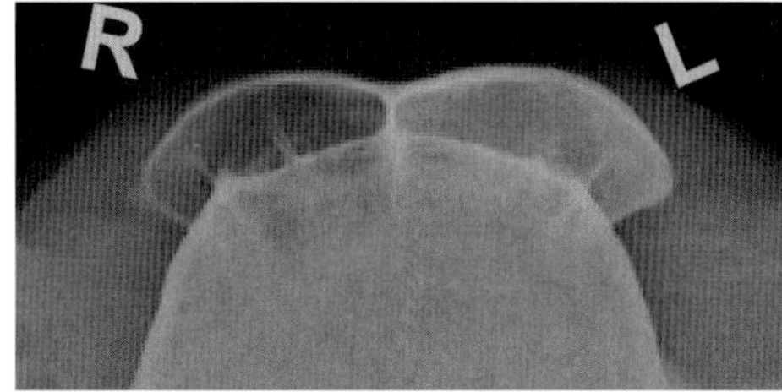

Figure 5.248 Frontal sinus mucocele. Rostrocaudal view of a dog head depicting increased opacity in the left frontal sinus without evidence of osteolysis. A similar appearance may result from neoplasia or inflammation in the sinus.

A

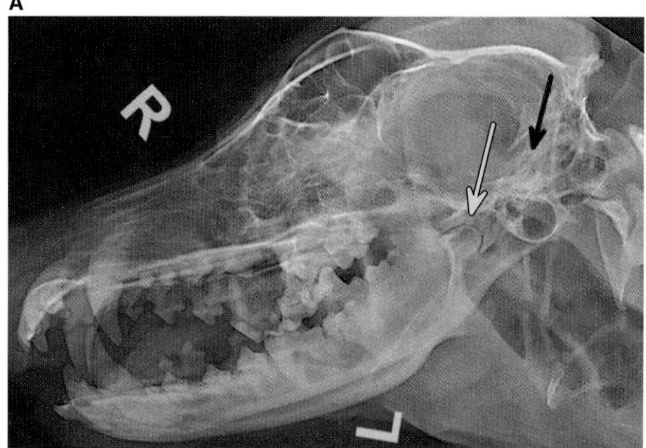

B

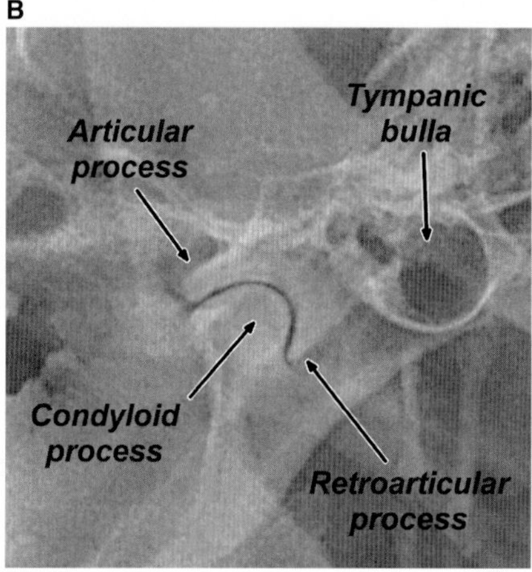

Figure 5.249 Normal temporomandibular joint. **A**. Lateral view of a dog head made with the nose tilted to image the left TMJ (yellow arrow). The right TMJ (black arrow) is not aligned with the x-ray beam and is not well visualized. **B**. Close-up of the left TMJ depicting the normal anatomy.

Temporomandibular joint (TMJ)

The normal radiographic appearance of a TMJ is depicted in Figure 5.249.

Temporomandibular joint dysplasia

Malformation of the TMJ is a rare congenital abnormality that typically presents as a flattened mandibular condyle with an abnormal slope. Other radiographic findings include a shallow mandibular fossa and an abrnormally shaped retroarticular process. The temporomandibular joint space usually is widened and the mandible may be shifted to one side. TMJ dysplasia can be unilateral or bilateral. The abnormal TMJ often is easiest to see in a well-positioned DV view. TMJ dysplasia is reported more often in certain dog breeds (e.g., Bassett Hounds, Dachshunds, Irish Setters, Spaniels, Pekingese). Affected dogs may or may not be symptomatic. Clinical signs include brief to extended periods of intermittent open-mouth locking of the mandible, usually after hyperextension of the jaw (as in yawning).

Subluxation/luxation of temporomandibular joint

In many patients with a dislocated TMJ, the mandibular condyle is displaced rostally and dorsally (Figure 5.250). Caudal or lateral luxations can occur, but they are less common. A concurrent fracture of the mandibular ramus or luxation of the mandibular symphysis may be present. Caudal luxations usually include a fracture of the retroglenoid process. TMJ luxations tend to occur more often in cats than in dogs. Malocclusion is a common finding during physical examination due to rostral and lateral displacement of the mandible. Malocclusion may not be evident with TMJ luxation if the mandibular body is fractured.

A

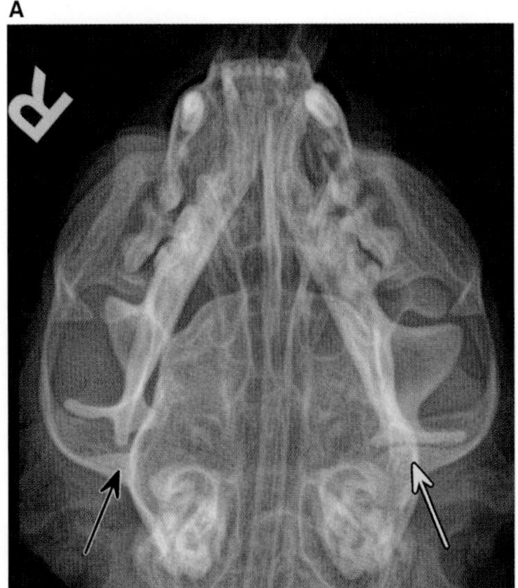

B

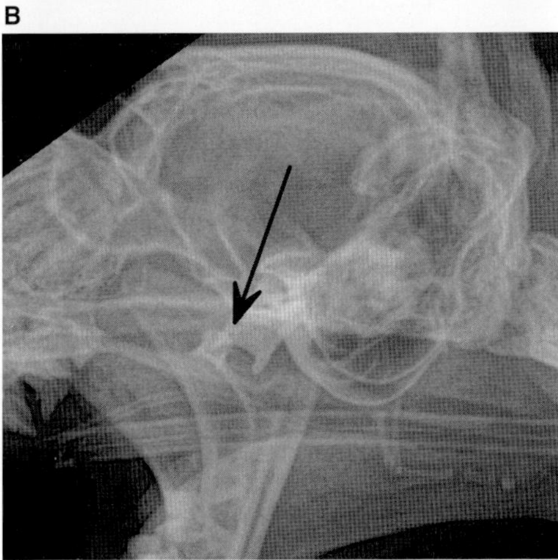

C

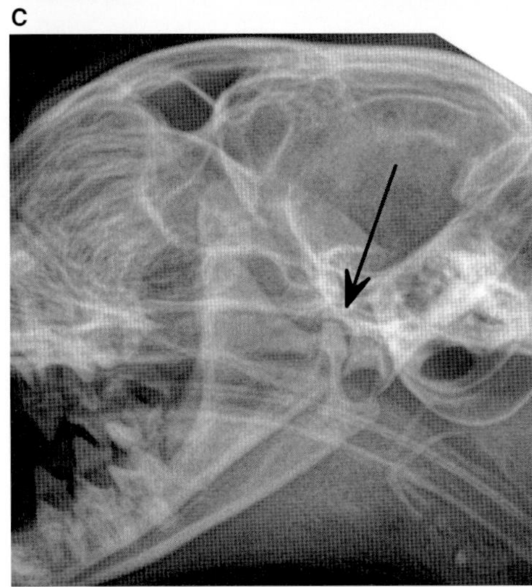

Figure 5.250 Temporomandibular joint luxation. DV view (**A**), open mouth lateral view (**B**), and standard lateral view (**C**) of a cat head depicting rostral luxation of the right TMJ (black arrow). The left TMJ (yellow arrow) is normal. The standard lateral view (C) was made following reduction of the TMJ luxation.

Teeth

Congenital and acquired abnormalities in the size, shape, or number of teeth are common in dogs and cats and may or may not be clinically significant. Congenital abnormalities are frequently seen in brachycephalic breeds. An abnormal number of teeth may be symmetric or asymmetric.

Dental calculus

The presence of hardened plaque or tartar on the teeth is a common finding in dogs and cats but may not be evident in radiographs. Dental calculus may make the tooth margin appear irregular. Mineralized plaque sometimes is visible above the gingival crest or on the tooth root.

Dental caries

Cavities in teeth may be visible in radiographs as less opaque areas or defects in the enamel or dentin. Dental decay can extend into the pulp cavity and adjacent bone, resulting in a tooth root abscess (Figure 5.251).

Feline tooth resorption

Resorptive lesions are common in the teeth of adult cats. The etiology is unknown, but the dentin is progressively destroyed by odontoclasts. Any and all teeth can be affected, but lesions are most common in the mandibular premolars. Type I lesions appear in radiographs as defects in the tooth crown and a normal-appearing periodontal space with easily recognized tooth roots. In radiographs of type II lesions, the periodontal space is absent and the tooth roots appear to blend with the alveolar bone. Both type I and type II lesions may be present at the same time.

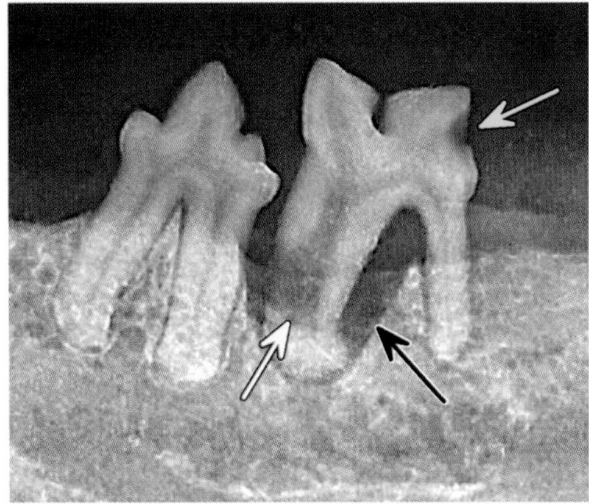

Figure 5.251 Dental disease. Lateral view of a mandible depicting widening of the periodontal space due to osteolysis (black arrow) and defects (cavities) in the tooth crown (yellow arrow) and tooth root (white arrow). The pulp cavity in the cranial root of the affected tooth is enlarged due to tooth decay.

Tooth fractures

Fractures in teeth may be caused by chewing on hard objects or other trauma. The canine teeth tend to be affected more often, followed by the carnassial teeth and the incisors. Exposure of the pulp cavity can lead to a tooth root abscess. Small, linear cracks or fissures sometimes are visible in radiographs of damaged teeth and sometimes a portion of the tooth is missing.

Periodontal disease

Inflammation surrounding the teeth is common in dogs and cats, but seldom is visible in radiographs until bony changes occur. In patients with chronic periodontal disease, the furcation bone (between the tooth roots) becomes less-defined and less opaque and the alveolar crest (surface bone) progressively regresses, becoming more irregular in margination. The periodontal space widens and the lamina dura becomes faint or disappears, usually beginning at the alveolar crest (Figures 5.251 and 5.253). Teeth may be absent. Severe or advanced periodontal disease can predispose to pathological fracture in a tooth or bone.

Tooth root abscess

The initial radiographic finding with most tooth root abscesses is widening of the periodontal space at the tip of a root due to osteolysis. A halo of decreased bone opacity may surround the root (Figures 5.252 and 5.254), sometimes with a rim of osteosclerosis. In chronic cases, parts of the tooth root may be resorbed allowing infection to enter and enlarge the pulp cavity, eventually killing the tooth. Infection can extend further into the adjacent bone to cause osteomyelitis and a bone abscess, weakening the bone and predisposing to pathological fracture. Infection in a tooth can lead to a periapical or radicular cyst, which may may be indistinguishable from a tooth root abscess.

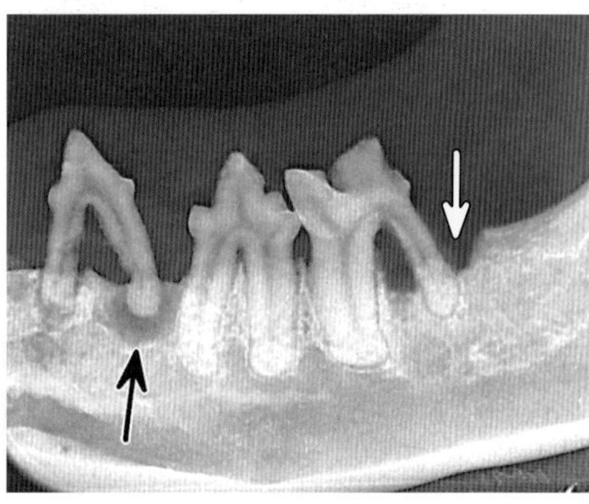

Figure 5.252 Dental disease. Lateral view of a mandible depicting a tooth root abscess (black arrow) and resorption of alveolar crest (white arrow).

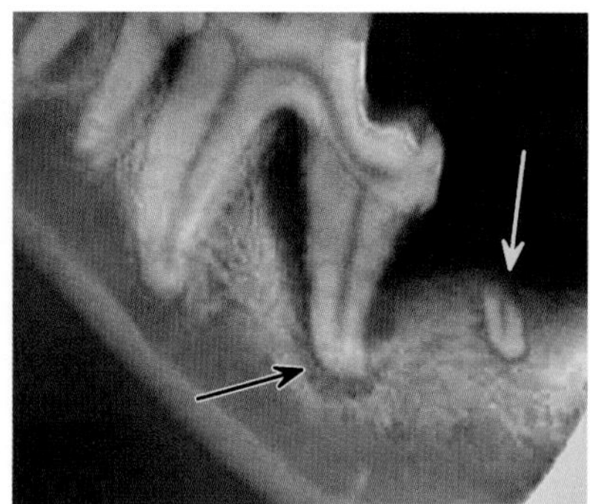

Figure 5.253 Dental disease. Lateral view of a mandible depicting a retained tooth root (yellow arrow) and periodontal disease (black arrow).

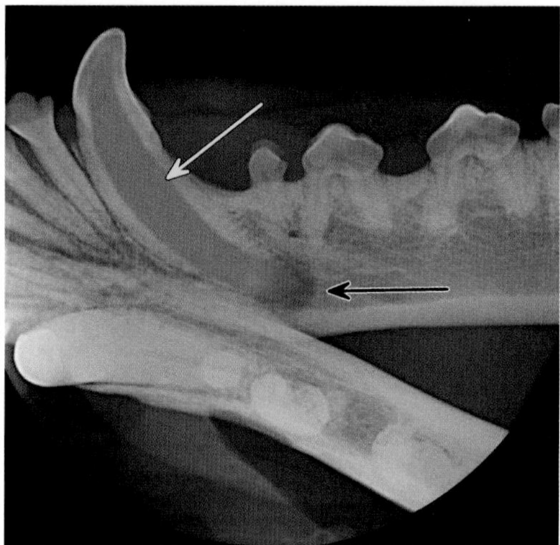

Figure 5.254 Tooth root abscess. Intraoral oblique view of a dog rostral mandible depicting osteolysis at the apical foramen of a canine tooth root (black arrow) and enlargement of the pulp cavity (yellow arrow).

Metabolic disease

Diseases that affect calcium metabolism can lead to demineralization of bone. Loss of the lamina dura often is the earliest radiographic finding. With progression there is a diffuse decrease in bone opacity and less bone-to-soft tissue contrast (Figure 5.255). The teeth, however, remain mineral opacity and may appear to "float" in soft tissue.

Hyperparathyroidism is a common cause of bone demineralization. Loss of minerals makes the mandible more flexible, commonly called "rubber jaw." With advanced disease there is generalized demineralization of the skeleton and softening of the skull, spine, and long bones.

Tooth neoplasia

Both malignant and benign tumors can arise in the oral cavities of dogs and cats. Tumors that involve the teeth may originate from dental elements, bone, or soft tissue. The type of tumor seldom can be determined from radiographs alone.

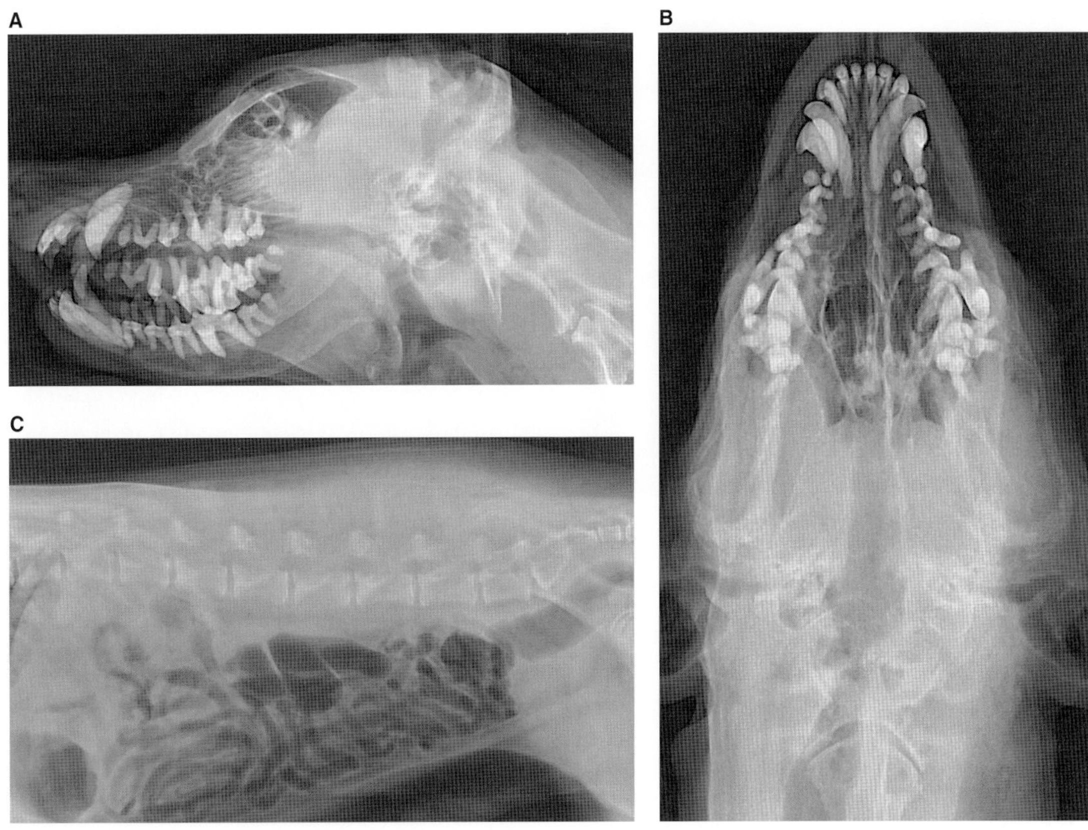

Figure 5.255 Hyperparathyroidism. Lateral view (**A**) and VD view (**B**) of a dog head and a lateral view (**C**) of the lumbar spine depicting severe demineralization of bone due to nutritional secondary hyperparathyroidism. The teeth appear to "float" in the soft tissue opacity mandible and maxilla.

Dental origin tumors (odontogenic tumors) may resemble osteomyelitis or a bone cyst (Figure 5.256). Many dental origin tumors (e.g., ameloblastoma, odontoma, fibroma) are benign and slow growing, but they can be locally aggressive and may invade bone.

Dentigerous cysts are not tumors, but produce similar signs. They form around unerupted teeth and may continue to grow, destroying the adjacent bone and teeth. Large cysts can predispose to pathologic fracture.

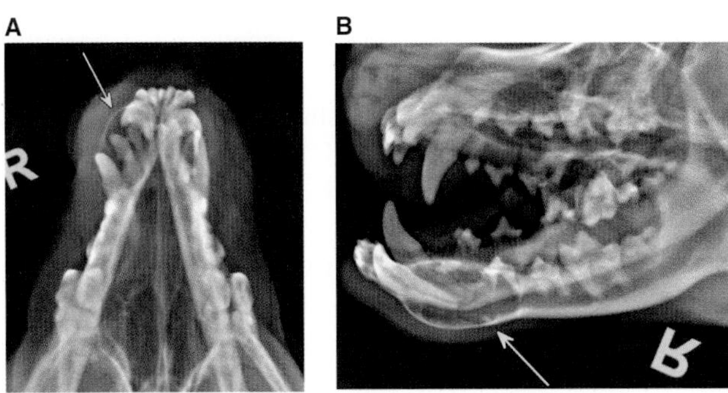

Figure 5.256 Dentigerous cyst. Lateral oblique view (**A**) and DV view (**B**) of a dog head depicting a well-defined expansile osteolytic lesion in the right rostral hemimandible (yellow arrows).

Nonodontogenic tumors often are malignant (e.g., malignant melanoma, squamous cell carcinoma, fibrosarcoma, osteosarcoma). Osteolysis tends to be aggressive, producing irregular and ill-defined margins. Pathologic fractures can occur. Periosteal responses range from not visible in radiographs to very active new bone formation. Squamous cell carcinomas frequently involve the rostral mandible in dogs.

Salivary glands and nasolacrimal duct

Normal salivary glands are not distinguished in radiographs. The locations of the salivary glands are illustrated in Figure 5.257.

Sialolithiasis

Salivary gland calculi are rare in dogs and cats. They may result from chronic inflammation and most often are reported in the ducts of the parotid and sublingual salivary glands. Sialoliths can completely obstruct a duct, leading to swelling of the gland and sometimes the formation of a sialocele. In radiographs, sialoliths appear as small, rounded or linear, mineral opacity structures in the area of

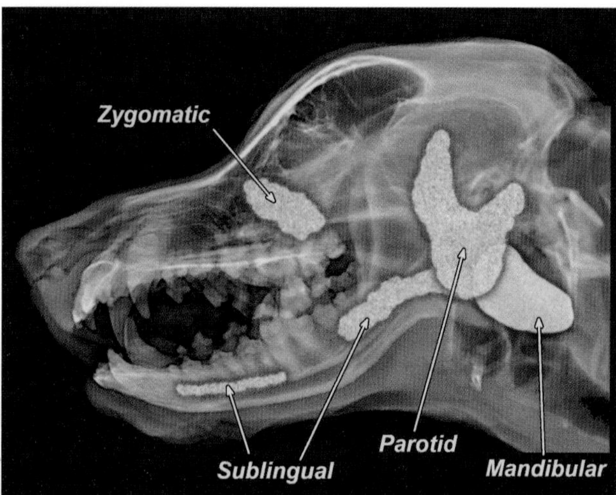

Figure 5.257 Salivary glands. Lateral view of a dog head illustrating the salivary glands.

a salivary gland or its duct. They may be solitary or multiple. Swelling or a mass effect may be present in the nearby soft tissues.

Sialocele

A sialocele is a sac filled with saliva from a leaking salivary gland or salivary duct. When large enough, a sialocele may be visible in radiographs as a non-specific soft tissue swelling, usually in the submandibular area. Large sialoceles (or salivary mucoceles) can displace the pharynx itself or just displace gas from the pharynx. A mineral opacity structure in or near the swelling may represent a sialolith (as described earlier) or dystrophic mineralization. A secondary infection in a sialocele may lead to a periosteal response or osteolysis in an adjacent bone.

Damage to a salivary gland or its duct may be caused by trauma, migrating foreign material, or an obstruction. The sublingual salivary glands are particularly susceptible to damage.

Sialoceles are reported more often in young male dogs, especially German Shepherds and toy breeds. They are rare in cats. Affected animals typically present with a slowly enlarging, nonpainful, fluctuant swelling in the ventral submandibular region. A sialocele adjacent to the tongue is called a *ranula*. Sialography may aid in identifying the site of a ruptured duct.

Salivary duct fistula

A fistula is an abnormal communication. Salivary duct fistulas are rare in dogs and cats. They most often involve the parotid salivary duct and may communicate with an external surface. Survey radiographs may reveal non-specific soft tissue swelling. Sialography aids in evaluating the patency of the salivary ducts and fistulography can be used to assess communication with a salivary duct. Salivary duct fistulas can result from trauma (e.g., bite wounds), previous surgery, tumor, or severe infection.

Salivary gland neoplasia

Salivary gland tumors are rare in dogs and cats, most often reported in the parotid and mandibular salivary glands of older animals. Large tumors may produce soft tissue swelling and occasionally they can cause osteolysis in the adjacent bones. Sialography may demonstrate displacement or infiltration of a salivary gland.

Carcinomas are the most common primary salivary gland tumors and can metastasize to regional lymph nodes or lung. Secondary tumors typically invade from the adjacent tissues (e.g., fibrosarcoma, lymphoma). Salivary gland tumors are reported more often in poodle and spaniel breeds. Clinical signs include firm, nonpainful, localized swelling. Large masses may cause dyspnea or dysphagia.

Nasolacrimal duct abnormalities

Abnormalities of the nasolacrimal ducts typically are associated with some degree of obstruction. Obstruction may be congenital due to absence of the punctum (*imperforate punctum*), atresia or stenosis of the duct, or facial malformations such as a shortened muzzle (e.g., American Cocker Spaniel, English Bulldog, Bedlington Terrier). Acquired obstruction may result from solidification of normal debris or from pathology such as inflammation, neoplasia, trauma, or a cyst.

Survey radiographs often are normal. There may be increased opacity in the maxilla, nasal cavity, or orbit. Osteolysis sometimes occurs due to pressure remodeling. Dacryocystorhinography can be used to evaluate the patency of a nasolacrimal duct and to identify sites of obstruction, displacement, dilation, or rupture.

Pharynx and larynx

The pharynx and larynx are evaluated for position, size, shape, and opacity. They are best examined in a well-positioned lateral view. Rotation or flexion of the patient's head and neck can displace the larynx and distort the apparent size and shape of the pharynx and retropharyngeal space. Suspected abnormalities should be carefully scrutinized for positioning artifacts.

Pharyngeal swelling

Swelling in the area of the pharynx may be diffuse or localized. Diffuse swelling may be due to edema, hemorrhage, or inflammation. Swelliing can displace pharyngeal gas, making the pharyngeal space appear smaller, narrower, or absent. Severe swelling may impair respiration or swallowing. Note: many patients with pharyngeal disease present with no radiographically visible abnormalities.

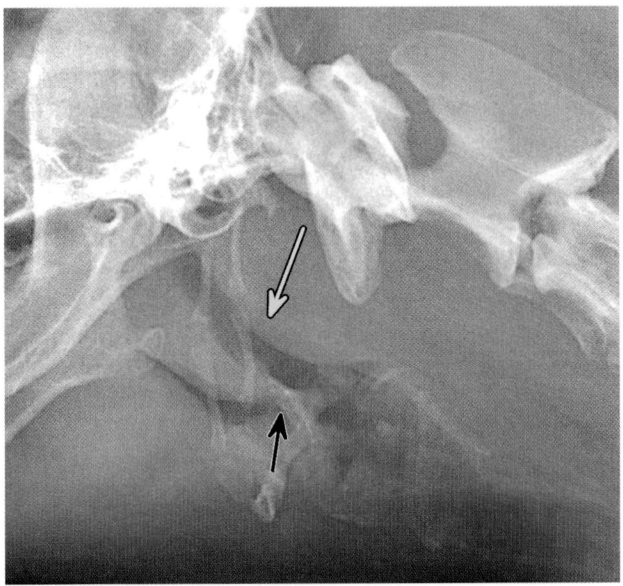

Figure 5.258 Retropharyngeal swelling. Lateral view of a dog cervical region depicting ventral displacement of the dorsal pharyngeal wall (yellow arrow) resulting in narrowing of the pharynx. There is incidental mineralization in the epiglottis (black arrow) and the soft palate is thickened.

Localized swelling usually is a mass (e.g., tumor, abscess, hematoma, lymphadenomegaly, cyst, polyp). Masses can arise within or adjacent to the nasopharynx or oropharynx. They may originate in a tonsil, lymph node, salivary gland, epiglottis, or soft palate. The type and origin of a mass seldom can be determined from radiographs.

Pharyngeal masses that displace gas from the pharynx may reduce its apparent size. They may or may not displace the pharynx itself. The margins of a mass may be visible if outlined by gas. Retropharyngeal masses often displace the pharynx and larynx ventrally (Figure 5.258).

Dysphagia and cricopharyngeal achalasia

Disorders that interfere with normal swallowing may or may not be evident in survey radiographs. A foreign object or a mass sometimes is identified in the pharynx or retropharyngeal region.

Cricopharyngeal achalasia most often is reported in young dogs, whereas other causes of dysphagia are more common in middle-aged and older animals. Achalasia is characterized by inadequate relaxation of the cricopharyngeal muscle during swallowing, which may be difficult to differentiate from pharyngeal dysfunction. The classic description of Cricopharyngeal achalasia is that swallowing is normal, but the esophagus is effectively obstructed at the cranial esophageal sphincter and the food immediately returns to the mouth.

Laryngeal disease

Laryngeal disease often leads to some degree of physical or functional obstruction and respiratory distress. Physical obstruction may be due to a mass that narrows the larynx. Functional obstruction results from weak or ineffective laryngeal muscles, either due to hypoplasia or loss of innervation (e.g., laryngeal paralysis). Laryngeal masses may be intraluminal, mural, or extramural. Gas in the larynx sometimes outlines the margin of a mass or foreign object. The laryngeal cartilage may be displaced or abnormal in shape. Laryngeal tumors are rare in dogs and cats, but usually advanced at the time of radiography. Congenital laryngeal cysts may involve the vocal cords, epiglottis, arytenoid cartilage, or thyroid cartilage. Granulomas and abscesses often are associated with foreign material. Hematomas and excessive granulation tissue may result from trauma or previous surgery. Laryngeal polyps may occur.

Laryngeal hypoplasia is congenital narrowing of the larynx due to abnormal development of the cartilage. It may be accompanied by weak abductor muscles. In a lateral view, the larynx typically is narrowed dorsoventrally and the pharynx is smaller than normal. The soft palate often is thickened and elongated. Laryngeal hypoplasia most often is reported in brachycephalic breeds (e.g., Bulldog, Boston Terrier).

Laryngeal paralysis results from loss of innervation to the intrinsic muscles of the larynx. The vocal folds and arytenoid cartilage are not abducted during inspiration. Radiographic findings often are non-specific. The pharynx may be dilated. The lateral ventricles may become more rounded or may not be visible at all. Severe inspiratory dyspnea due to upper airway obstruction may cause some degree of narrowing in the cervical trachea and widening of the thoracic trachea. In severe cases, radiographic findings may include hyperinflated lungs, inward bulging intercostal muscles, and neurogenic pulmonary edema. In chronic cases, the lungs may appear small and opaque due to compromised inspiration and failure to inflate. Laryngeal paralysis may be congenital or acquired. It most often is reported in large-breed dogs and may be heritable in some. It is rare in cats.

Hyoid bone diseases

Fractures and luxations are the most common hyoid bone pathologies, usually caused by trauma (e.g., leash injury, bite wound). One or more hyoid bones may be fractured, displaced, or malaligned. Osseous remodeling, including a periosteal response and osteolysis, may be present due to a nearby mass. Tumors are rare (e.g., osteosarcoma). Clinical signs are related to problems with breathing and swallowing.

Differential diagnoses for musculoskeleton

All areas of each radiograph should be scrutinized in a systematic manner. Each anatomic structure must be carefully examined for **position**, as well as **size**, **shape**, and **opacity**. Abnormalities caused by trauma are frequently accompanied by other signs of trauma (e.g., fractured ribs, subcutaneous emphysema, soft tissue swelling, free gas or fluid in the thoracic or abdominal cavity).

- Soft tissue abnormalities
- General bone abnormalities
- Abnormal opacity of bone
- Fractures:
  - Types of fractures
  - Fracture complications
  - Factors that affect fracture healing
- Abnormal shape of bone
- Chondrodysplasia (dwarfism)
- Joints
- Head and pharynx abnormalities

Abnormal position of limb

1. Improper radiographic positioning.
2. Bone fracture.
3. Joint dislocation.

Increased size of soft tissues

1. General increased size of soft tissues:
   - **a.** Obesity.
   - **b.** Subcutaneous fluid:
     - **1)** Edema (e.g., trauma).
     - **2)** Hemorrhage (e.g., trauma, neoplasia).
   - **c.** Inflammation (e.g., cellulitis, vasculitis).
2. Regional increased size of soft tissues:
   - **a.** Edema (e.g., lymphedema).
   - **b.** Hemorrhage (e.g., trauma, neoplasia).
   - **c.** Iatrogenic (e.g., fluid administration).
   - **d.** Large mass (e.g., lipoma).
   - **e.** Inflammation (e.g., cellulitis, vasculitis).
3. Localized or focal increased size of soft tissues:
   - **a.** Focal swelling away from a joint:
     - **1)** Bruise, hematoma.
     - **2)** Abscess, granuloma, seroma.
     - **3)** Cyst.
     - **4)** Neoplasia.
     - **5)** Hernia (e.g., umbilical hernia).
     - **6)** Arteriovenous fistula.
     - **7)** Iatrogenic (e.g., injection site).
   - **b.** Swelling at a single joint (may be bilateral):
     - **1)** Joint effusion:
       - **1)** Inflammation/infection.
       - **2)** Osteochondrosis.
       - **3)** Hemarthrosis (e.g., trauma, coagulopathy).
     - **2)** Synovial thickening; villonodular synovitis.
     - **3)** Synovial cyst.
     - **4)** Joint capsule fibrosis.
     - **5)** Neoplasia (e.g., synovial cell sarcoma).
   - **c.** Swelling at multiple or all joints:
     - **1)** Immune-mediated diseases (polyarthritis may begin in one joint).

Decreased size of soft tissues

1. General decreased size of soft tissues:
   - **a.** Emaciation.
2. Regional decreased size of soft tissues:
   - **a.** Disuse atrophy:
     - **1)** Pain (e.g., osteoarthritis, fracture).
     - **2)** Immobilization (e.g., splint, cast).
     - **3)** Paresis/paralysis.
3. Local decreased size of soft tissues:
   - **a.** Loss of tissue:
     - **1)** Trauma (e.g., bite wound, vehicular trauma).
     - **2)** Surgical removal.

Abnormal shape of soft tissues is usually related to focal enlargements or focal decreases in size

Increased opacity in soft tissues

1. General increased opacity in soft tissues:
   - **a.** Typically an artifact due to underexposed radiograph or superimposition of adjacent structure.
2. Regional or local increased opacity in soft tissues:
   - **a.** Foreign material.
   - **b.** Dystrophic mineralization:
     - **1)** Trauma.
     - **2)** Chronic inflammation/infection.
     - **3)** Long standing abscess, granuloma, hematoma.
     - **4)** Myositis ossificans; caused by trauma to muscle.
     - **5)** Ossifying tendonitis/enthesopathy; occurs at insertion sites of muscles due to chronic inflammation or repetitive trauma.
     - **6)** Meniscal calcification.
     - **7)** Osteochondrosis.
     - **8)** "Joint mouse"; mineralized fragment in a joint.
     - **9)** Iatrogenic:
       - **1)** Reaction to suture material.
       - **2)** Drug reaction (e.g., progesterone).
       - **3)** Tissue damage at a surgical or injection site.
     - **10)** Idiopathic.

Increased opacity in soft tissues (*continued*)

- **c.** Metastatic mineralization:
  - **1)** Metabolic disease/endocrine disease (e.g., hyperparathyroidism, Cushing's syndrome).
  - **2)** Vitamin D toxicosis.
  - **3)** Vascular mineralization.
- **d.** Neoplastic mineralization (bone producing tumor):
  - **1)** Osteosarcoma.
  - **2)** Osteochondroma.
  - **3)** Synovial osteochondroma.
- **e.** Iatrogenic:
  - **1)** Positive contrast medium (e.g., fistulogram, arthrogram).
  - **2)** Surgical implant (e.g., Penrose drain).

Conditions that mimic increased opacity in soft tissues

1. Underexposed radiograph.
2. Superimposed structure:
   - **a.** Wet or dirty hair coat; medication on skin.
   - **b.** Cutaneous nodule; nipple.
   - **c.** Positioning aid (e.g., sandbag, foam wedge).
   - **d.** Dirt or stain on or in the image receptor.

Decreased opacity in soft tissues

1. General or regional decreased opacity in soft tissues:
   - **a.** Emaciation, disuse atrophy.
   - **b.** Subcutaneous emphysema:
     - **1)** Trauma (e.g., open or penetrating wound).
     - **2)** Iatrogenic; recent surgery, recent injection or fluid administration.
     - **3)** Gas-producing bacterial infection.
     - **4)** Fistulous tract.
     - **5)** Leakage of gas from lung, trachea, or GI structure.
2. Local decreased opacity in soft tissues:
   - **a.** Fat:
     - **1)** Normal fascial plane.
     - **2)** Normal intra-articular fat (e.g., infrapatellar fat pad in stifle).
     - **3)** Fatty mass (e.g., lipoma, liposarcoma).
   - **b.** Gas:
     - **1)** Subcutaneous emphysema.
     - **2)** Intra-articular gas:
       - **1)** Post-arthrocentesis or post-arthroscopy.
       - **2)** Negative contrast arthrogram.
       - **3)** Vacuum phenomenon; sudden traction on joint releases nitrogen gas that was dissolved in joint fluid. Reported in shoulder, intervertebral disc space, and between sternebrae. More often seen with osteoarthritis or intervertebral disc disease.

Conditions that may mimic decreased opacity in soft tissues

1. Overexposed radiograph.
2. Decreased size of soft tissue that results in less than expected opacity in soft tissues (e.g., atrophy, surgical removal, loss of tissue due to severe trauma).

General bone abnormalities

Before discussing specific bone lesions, first consider the distribution and anatomic location of bone lesions.

Distribution of bone lesions

1. General or diffuse lesions (entire skeleton):
   - **a.** Metabolic/endocrine disease (e.g., hyperparathyroidism).
   - **b.** Nutritional deficiency or excess (e.g., vitamin A, vitamin D).
   - **c.** Chronic systemic disease.
   - **d.** Hereditary disease.
2. Regional or multifocal lesions; more than one bone (polyostotic), may be in one or more limbs; bilateral lesions may or may not be symmetrical:
   - **a.** Trauma.
   - **b.** Neoplasia (e.g., multiple myeloma, sarcoma, carcinoma).
   - **c.** Developmental anomaly (e.g., chondrodystrophy).
   - **d.** Systemic infection (e.g., hematogenous spread).
   - **e.** Disuse atrophy.
   - **f.** Panosteitis.
   - **g.** Hypertrophic osteodystrophy (HOD).
   - **h.** Hypertrophic osteopathy (HO).
3. Local or focal lesion; one bone (monostotic):
   - **a.** Trauma (e.g., fracture, bone bruise).
   - **b.** Neoplasia (malignant or benign tumor).
   - **c.** Focal infection/inflammation.
   - **d.** Developmental anomaly.
   - **e.** Cyst-like lesion (e.g., bone cyst, bone abscess).
   - **f.** Avascular necrosis.
   - **g.** Retained cartilaginous core.
4. Other terms used to describe the locations of bone lesions:
   - **a.** Periosteal.
   - **b.** Cortical.
   - **c.** Medullary.
   - **d.** Articular.
   - **e.** Epiphyseal, physeal, metaphyseal, or diaphyseal.

Abnormal position of bone

1. Poor patient positioning.
2. Bone fracture.
3. Joint luxation.

Abnormal opacity in bone

1. Bone is less opaque and more opaque than expected.
2. Bone may be less opaque than expected due to either a decrease in its mineral content (demineralization) or due to destruction of the bone (osteolysis).
3. Bone may be more opaque than expected due to either a summation of new bone (e.g., periosteal response, osteophytes) or an increase in its mineral content (osteosclerosis).

Abnormal opacity in bone (*continued*)

4. Abnormal bone opacity may be generalized (involving the entire skeleton), regional (involving one part of the skeleton or a limb), or localized (involving one bone).

Both increased opacity and/or decreased opacity in bone

1. Primary bone tumor:
   a. Osteosarcoma (most common).
   b. Fibrosarcoma (mandible, ribs, vertebrae).
   c. Chondrosarcoma (flat bones such as skull and ribs, less malignant than osteosarcoma).
   d. Hemangiosarcoma (more often in younger dogs).
   e. Malignant histiocytoma.
   f. Lymphosarcoma (more common in cats).
   g. Myeloma.
   h. Liposarcoma.
2. Secondary bone tumor:
   a. Any malignant neoplasm can spread to bone.
   b. Malignant soft tissue tumor can invade adjacent bone.
3. Bone infection (osteomyelitis):
   a. Bacterial (e.g., *Staphylococcus, Pseudomonas*).
   b. Mycotic (e.g., *Aspergillus, Blastomyces, Coccidioides, Cryptococcus, Histoplasma*).
   c. Protozoal (e.g., Hepatozoonosis, Leishmaniasis, Neosporosis).
4. Joint disease:
   a. Arthritis (e.g., immune mediated erosive arthritis, septic arthritis).
   b. Chronic hemarthrosis.
   c. Villonodular synovitis.

Decreased opacity in bone

1. General decreased opacity in bone (osteopenia):
   a. Hyperparathyroidism (primary, renal, nutritional).
   b. Chronic systemic disease (e.g., thyroid, liver, kidney, pancreas, toxins).
   c. Cushing's syndrome (iatrogenic, adrenal, pituitary).
   d. Hypervitaminosis A (especially cats).
   e. Vitamin D deficiency; traditionally called *rickets* in young animals and *osteomalacia* in older animals.
   f. Other nutritional deficiency (e.g., starvation, malabsorption syndrome, trace element deficiency).
   g. Pregnancy/lactation.
   h. Acromegaly (cats).
   i. Paraneoplastic syndrome, pseudohyperparathyroidism (multiple tumor types).
   j. Chronic drug therapy (e.g., corticosteroids, primidone, phenytoin, phenobarbital).
   k. Hereditary diseases (e.g., mucopolysaccharoidosis, fibrous osteodystrophy).
   l. Congenital hypothyroidism.
2. Regional decreased opacity in bone:
   a. Disuse atrophy in a limb:
      1) Chronic pain and lameness (e.g., fracture, osteoarthritis).
      2) Immobilization (e.g., cast, splint, rigid bone plate).
      3) Long-term paraplegia, tetraplegia, or paralysis.
3. Local decreased opacity in bone:
   a. Osteomyelitis (Table 5.9).
   b. Neoplasia.

Table 5.9 Causes of osteomyelitis

1. Bacterial osteomyelitis:
   a. *Brucella canis* (zoonotic potential).
   b. *Escherichia coli.*
   c. *Pasteurella.*
   d. *Proteus.*
   e. *Pseudomonas.*
   f. *Staphylococcus.*
   g. *Streptococcus.*
2. Mycotic osteomyelitis:
   a. *Coccidioides immitis* ("Valley fever"); endemic in the southwestern United States and northern Mexico. Bone lesions tend to involve the distal appendicular skeleton.
   b. *Blastomyces dermatiditis*; endemic in the mid-western United States and parts of Canada. Bone lesions tend to be solitary and located distal to the elbow or stifle; lesions may be multifocal.
   c. *Histoplasma capsulatum*; found worldwide; endemic in the Midwestern United States. Bone lesions are rare in dogs and cats.
   d. *Cryptococcus neoformans*; occurs worldwide; found throughout the United States. Typically a systemic disease with bone being one of the last tissues involved; lesions most often are reported in the head. Nasal cavity infections more common in cats; usually nondestructive, may cause hyperplastic rhinitis.
   e. *Aspergillosis* spp.; common throughout the United States. Bone lesions most often are reported in the head and spine. In the nasal cavity, often causes osteolysis with multiple punctate areas of decreased opacity that may be surrounded by thickened bone; osteolysis of the internasal septum (vomer bone) is uncommon.
3. Protozoal osteomyelitis:
   a. *Hepatozoonosis*; occurs worldwide. Infection tends to be lifelong with frequent relapses; can be fatal.
   b. *Leishmaniasis*; worldwide zoonotic disease; endemic in Central and South America, Africa, India, Southern Europe, and in parts of the United States and Canada. Lesions often in long bones, vertebrae, and pelvis. May see intramedullary sclerosis and osteolytic joint disease.
   c. *Neosporosis*; worldwide distribution. Bone lesions tend to be more severe in the pelvic limbs; may be unilateral or bilateral. Genu recurvatum may be present (stifle bends backwards) due to muscle contracture that leads to rigid hyperextension. Angular limb deformity and joint deformity may develop.

Decreased opacity in bone (*continued*)

- c. Pressure remodeling caused by an adjacent structure:
  - 1) Enchondroma of paired bone.
  - 2) Villonodular synovitis.
- d. Fracture (traumatic, pathologic).
- e. Cyst-like lesion:
  - 1) Bone cyst; may be single or multiple.
  - 2) Aneurysmal bone cyst (caused by a vascular abnormality in the bone).
  - 3) Intraosseous epidermoid cyst (reported in distal phalanges and in vertebrae).
  - 4) Bone abscess.
- f. Retained cartilaginous core.
- g. Osteochondrosis.
- h. Avascular necrosis of the femoral head and neck.
- i. Feline femoral neck metaphyseal osteopathy.
- j. Bone loss adjacent to an implant (e.g., loose implant, stress protection provided by the implant).
- k. Incomplete ossification (e.g., epiphyseal dysplasia, humeral condyle in Spaniels).
- l. Iatrogenic (e.g., bone biopsy).

<u>*Conditions that may mimic decreased opacity bone*</u>

1. Overexposed radiograph.
2. Superimposition of subcutaneous emphysema.
3. Less overlying soft tissues (e.g., atrophy, emaciation).
4. Immature animal with incomplete endochondral ossification.
5. Summation of adjacent new bone that creates the false appearance of less opacity in normal bone.

Increased opacity in bone

1. General increased opacity in bone:
   - a. Osteopetrosis; bones become thick, dense, and brittle; pathologic fractures are common; reported in Basenji.
   - b. Hypervitaminosis A (especially cats).
   - c. Para-neoplastic syndrome that leads to generalized osteosclerosis.
   - d. Immune mediated disease:
     - 1) Feline leukemia virus; can produce medullary sclerosis with a nonregenerative anemia in cats.
     - 2) Systemic lupus erythematosus (SLE).
2. Regional increased opacity in bone:
   - a. Hypertrophic osteopathy (HO); can begin as localized and may progress to generalized:
     - 1) Disease in thoracic cavity:
       - 1) Primary or metastatic pulmonary neoplasia (most common).
       - 2) Other pulmonary mass (e.g., abscess)
       - 3) Severe bronchopneumonia.
       - 4) Cardiomegaly (e.g., congestive heart failure, heartworm disease).
       - 5) Megaesophagus.
       - 6) Intrathoracic foreign object.
       - 7) Spirocercosis.
       - 8) Rib chondrosarcoma.
     - 2) Disease in abdominal cavity:
       - 1) Hepatic or renal mass.
       - 2) Urinary bladder mass.
       - 3) Large or numerous cystic calculi.
   - b. Panosteitis (may also produce a periosteal response).
   - c. Craniomandibular osteopathy.
   - d. Canine leukocyte adhesion disorder; reported in young Irish Setters.
   - e. Mucopolysaccharoidosis (cats).
   - f. Myelosclerosis.
   - g. Bone infarcts.
   - h. Lead poisoning.
   - i. Growth arrest lines.
   - j. Excess Vitamin D.
   - k. Metaphyseal condensation; reported in immature Newfoundland dogs.
3. Local increased opacity in bone:
   - a. Normal subchondral bone.
   - b. Periosteal response; elevation of periosteum due to trauma, surgery, inflammation, or tumor.
   - c. Degenerative disease:
     - 1) DJD; osteophytes, enthesophytes.
     - 2) Eburnation.
     - 3) Spondylosis.
     - 4) Disseminated skeletal hyperostosis (DISH).
   - d. Fracture with overlapping fragments; folding fracture, compression fracture.
   - e. Healing or healed fracture.
   - f. Hypertrophic osteodystrophy (HOD); later stages of the disease due to mineralized subperiosteal hemorrhage and periosteal new bone production.
   - g. Hypertrophic nonunion fracture.
   - h. Neoplastic mineralization (e.g., osteoma, parosteal osteosarcoma).
   - i. Osteochondromatosis.

<u>*Conditions that may mimic increased opacity in bone*</u>

1. Underexposed radiographs.
2. Increase in overlying soft tissues.
3. Debris on hair or skin.

Abnormal bone size and shape

1. Abnormal bone length:
   - a. Chondrodysplasia; normal variant in some breeds (e.g., Bassett Hound, Bulldog, Dachshund).
   - b. Fracture, compression fracture (traumatic, pathologic).
   - c. Premature closure of a physis; bone may become abnormally straight or develop abnormal bowing.
   - d. Tension on a bone due to asynchronous growth of paired bones (e.g., radius/ulna, tibia/fibula).
   - e. Dietary deficiency (e.g., rickets).

Abnormal bone size and shape (*continued*)

   f. Congenital hypothyroidism.
   g. Hemimelia (absence of one of a normally paired set of bones).
2. Abnormal bone angulation or alignment:
   a. Fracture (traumatic, pathologic).
   b. Soft tissue damage (luxation, subluxation).
   c. Healed malunion fracture.
3. Abnormal expansion in a bone:
   a. Malignant tumor (e.g., osteosarcoma, chondrosarcoma).
   b. Osteochondroma.
   c. Enchondroma.
   d. Bone cyst.
   e. Osteomyelitis.
   f. Hypertrophic osteodystrophy.

Chondrodysplasia (dwarfism)

1. When chondrodysplasia is not characteristic for the breed, it is commonly called **dwarfism**. Different types of dwarfism are described below.
2. Chondrodysplasia of Great Pyrenees presents with shortened limbs and shortened bodies, but a normal size skull. The thoracic limbs tend to be shorter than the pelvic limbs resulting in a forward slanting body.
3. Chondrodysplasia of Alaskan Malamutes produces short, bowed limbs, but normal sized body, spine, and skull.
4. Dwarfism of Norwegian Elkhound is similar to dwarfism of Alaskan Malamutes, but the body tends to be shorter.
5. Enchondrodystrophy is disproportionate dwarfism in English Pointers. The thoracic limbs tend to be more severely affected than pelvic limbs. Also called dysostosis, affected puppies may exhibit abnormal movements, such as a bunny-hopping gait. Mandibular prognathism may be present.
6. Feline osteodystrophy or chondrodysplasia of Scottish Fold Cats predominately affects the distal appendicular skeleton (tarsi, carpi, metatarsals, metacarpals, phalanges). The pelvic limbs tend to be more severely affected than the thoracic limbs. New bone production may be seen along the plantar and palmar aspects of the pes and manus, which occasionally leads to ankylosis. Osseous remodeling can appear aggressive in some cats, with punctate osteolysis in the tarsal and carpal bones. Affected cats typically exhibit short, deformed limbs, a short inflexible tail, overgrown nails, and partial deafness.
7. Multiple epiphyseal dysplasia (pseudo-chondrodysplasia); reported in Beagles and Miniature Poodles. Affected dogs present with shortened limbs, spinal kyphosis, and enlarged joints. Poor growth, difficulty standing, and abnormal gait usually are recognized by two to three weeks of age.
8. Ocular-skeletal dwarfism in Samoyeds tends to present with thoracic limbs shorter than pelvic limbs and a varus (inward) deformity at the elbows and a valgus (outward) deviation in the distal limbs. Affected dogs typically exhibit prominent doming of the forehead, lameness, retinal detachment, and cataracts.
9. Skeletal-retinal dysplasia in Labrador Retrievers or ocular chondrodysplasia leads to abnormally shortened limbs with a normal body length. Affected dogs exhibit impaired vision, valgus limb deformities, and hyperextended hind legs.
10. Tibial metaphyseal dysplasia is reported in Dachshunds and leads to abnormal development of the distal tibial metaphysis. It may be unilateral or bilateral. The affected tibia is abnormally shortened and curved, usually resulting in a secondary deformity of the fibula. The lateral trochlear groove in the distal tibia is shallow, which leads to subluxation of the tibiotarsal joint and pes varus, an inward curving of the foot (only the lateral part of the foot touches the ground). A pointed exostosis may be present on the medial aspect of the distal tibial metaphysis.

Fractures

Types of fractures

1. Incomplete fracture: cortex is broken on only one side, bone is not in complete discontinuity.
   a. Greenstick (hairline) fracture: on the convex side of the bone.
   b. Folding, torus, buckling fracture: on the concave side of the bone.
2. Complete fracture: extends through the entire bone.
   a. Simple: one fracture line and two fragments.
   b. Complex: multiple, non-continuous fracture lines and more than two fragments.
   c. Comminuted: all fracture lines communicate at a single point.
3. Closed fracture: overlying skin is intact.
4. Open (compound) fracture: overlying skin is perforated.
5. Avulsion fracture: occurs at the attachment point of a ligament, tendon, or joint capsule; a piece of bone is pulled away from the main bone.
6. Compression fracture: the ends of the bone fragments are jammed together resulting in a shortened or collapsed bone.
7. Chip fracture: "knock off a corner."
8. Slab fracture: "knock off a chunk."
9. Shearing (abrasion) fracture: open fracture created by severe friction or glancing trauma.
10. Pathologic fracture: weakened bone breaks under normal stresses.

Types of fractures (*continued*)

11. Physeal fracture: occurs in an immature bone:
    a. Trauma, most common cause.
    b. Chondrodysplasia.
    c. Retained cartilaginous core
    d. Hypertrophic osteodystrophy.
    e. Osteomyelitis.
    f. Internal fracture repair.

<u>Conditions that may mimic a fracture</u>

1. Normal physis (immature animal).
2. Nutrient foramen.
3. Superimposed structure:
    a. Fascial plane.
    b. Skin fold.
    c. Wet or dirty hair coat.
4. Grid lines.
5. Mark or scratch on viewbox or viewing screen.
6. Summation of adjacent new bone production creates the appearance of decreased opacity in normal bone.
7. Digital artifact (Überschwinger artifact).
8. Mach line (an optical illusion created by overlying structures).

Radiographic findings of a fracture complication

1. Absence of callus:
    a. Loss of blood supply.
    b. Note: primary bone healing may not produce a callus.
2. Excessive new bone production at the fracture site:
    a. Instability of the fragments.
    b. Osteomyelitis.
    c. Stripping of periosteum, either at the time of initial injury or during surgery.
    d. Presence of a bone graft.
3. Change in position of the fracture fragments due to inadequate stabilization.
4. Osteolysis at the fracture site:
    a. Osteomyelitis.
    b. Pathologic bone (e.g., neoplasia, bone cyst).
5. Widening of the gap between fracture fragments:
    a. Movement of the fragments.
    b. Loss of bone at the fracture site (e.g., osteomyelitis).
    c. A piece of soft tissue or fat is positioned between the fragments, increasing their separation.
6. Decreased opacity around a fixation device:
    a. Movement (loosening) of the implant.
    b. Osteomyelitis (typically an uneven, irregular zone of lysis).
    c. Bone necrosis (e.g., from a high-speed drill).
    d. Electrolysis or "metallosis"; an adverse reaction to a metallic implant.
7. Persistent soft tissue swelling (post-traumatic swelling typically resolves in 7–10 days):
    a. Infection.
    b. Hemorrhage.
    c. Edema.
8. Soft tissue atrophy (e.g., disuse, neurologic injury).
9. Mineralization in soft tissues (rule out a pre-existing condition and presence of a bone graft).
10. Narrowed joint space (e.g., chronic lack of movement and joint contracture).
11. Bone or limb deformity (e.g., physeal damage and premature closure of a growth plate).
12. Neoplastic transformation (rare); also called implant-associated sarcoma. Occurs at site of a bone implant or where complex healing has occurred. May not be evident until years later.

Factors that affect fracture healing.

1. Age; young animals tend to heal faster than older animals.
2. Nutrition; fracture healing requires adequate calcium, phosphorous and other nutrients.
3. Patient's general state of health; conditions such as obesity, diabetes mellitus, hypercortisolism, and others can delay fracture healing.
4. Blood supply; depends on the viability of the adjacent tissues. Reduction or removal of the hematoma can slow healing.
5. Fracture location; for example, metaphyseal fractures tend to heal faster than diaphyseal fractures. Some bones heal more slowly than others (e.g., distal radius and ulna, distal tibia).
6. Configuration of fracture fragments. At least 50% bone contact between fragments is desirable for efficient healing. Spiral and oblique fractures tend to heal faster than transverse fractures.
7. Soft tissue or fat between fragments can delay healing.
8. Loss or removal of a large bone fragment can delay healing.
9. Stability of fracture fragments; the less movement at the fracture site, the quicker it will heal. External forces pulling on the fragments can delay healing (e.g., tendons, ligaments).
10. Type of fixation. Intramedullary implants may disrupt endosteal blood supply and slow healing.
11. Healing may also be delayed by an adverse reaction to a metallic implant or due to loosening or premature removal of a fixation device.
12. Disease in the bone can lead to a delayed union, a nonunion, or failure to heal (e.g., infection, tumor).

Joints

Abnormal joint alignment

1. Tearing or stretching of supporting ligaments (luxation, subluxation).
2. Abnormal bone development (e.g., hip dysplasia, elbow dysplasia).
3. Arthritis (Table 5.10).

Conditions that may mimic abnormal joint alignment

1. Poor patient positioning (e.g., rotation).

Narrowed joint space

1. Loss of articular cartilage:
   a. Degenerative joint disease.
   b. Erosive arthritis (Table 5.10), septic arthritis.
2. Muscle contraction (e.g., infraspinatus at the shoulder, quadriceps at the stifle).
3. Periarticular fibrosis.

Conditions that may mimic narrowed joint space

1. Poor positioning; x-ray beam not aligned with joint space.

Table 5.10 Immune-mediated arthritis

There are multiple types of immune-mediated arthritis and numerous etiologies, some of which are listed below. The diagnosis seldom is made from radiographs alone; however, radiographs often are useful to differentiate nonerosive from erosive forms of arthritis.

Noninfectious, nonerosive, immune-mediated arthritis

1. Radiographic signs:
   a. Swelling at the affected joints, which may be periarticular and/or due to joint effusion
   b. Multiple joints usually are affected (polyarticular), often bilaterally
   c. No erosive lesions, no loss of articular cartilage, no active bone remodeling
   d. Degenerative joint disease is a common sequela
   e. Hepatosplenomegaly may be present
2. Idiopathic polyarthritis; etiology is unknown, but arthritis may be associated with disease in another part of the body (e.g., intestines, liver, tumor)
3. Vaccine-induced polyarthritis: associated with recent vaccination (e.g., canine distemper virus, calicivirus). Usually self-limiting; most cases resolve in less than a week
4. Drug-induced polyarthritis: caused by an adverse reaction to a medication, often an antibiotic. Joints become swollen and painful within a few days or weeks following drug exposure and tend to rapidly improve after drug withdrawal
5. Systemic lupus erythematosus (SLE): tends to affect the carpi, tarsi, metatarsi, stifles, and elbows most severely
6. Polyarthritis/polymyositis complex: polyarthritis is complicated with chronic myositis. Reported most often in Spaniel breeds. Bilateral joint swelling, muscle atrophy, and muscle contracture
7. Polyarthritis/meningitis syndrome: polyarthritis is complicated with spinal pain (neck pain) and sometimes neurologic signs
8. Sjogren syndrome: leukocytic destruction of exocrine glands (affects production of tears and saliva), may also cause an erosive polyarthritis (may resemble rheumatoid arthritis)
9. Chinese Shar-Pei fever syndrome: inherited disease, often with amyloidosis; recurring episodes of fever and swelling in one or both tarsi (may also affect other joints)
10. Heritable polyarthritis of the adolescent Akita: rare polyarthritis in young Akitas (less than 1 year old); often with peripheral lymphadenopathy and fever
11. Polyarteritis nodosa: multisystemic, inflammatory disease of unknown etiology, most often reported in Beagles; vasculitis of small and medium sized arteries can lead to polyarthritis

Erosive, non-infectious, immune-mediated arthritis

1. Radiographic findings:
   a. Often affects multiple joints
   b. Swelling at the joints, often both periarticular and intra-articular (joint effusion)
   c. Narrowed joint spaces due to loss of articular cartilage
   d. Osteolysis in adjacent bones
   e. Subluxation or luxation of one or more joints due to degradation of supporting structures
2. Feline noninfectious polyarthritis: may be erosive or non-erosive. Periosteal new bone production may be present and, in chronic cases, new bone can bridge the smaller joint spaces, leading to ankylosis. The carpi and tarsi most often are involved; occasionally the stifles, elbows, shoulders, and hips. most often reported in young, male cats (1–5 years of age)
3. Polyarthritis of greyhounds (Felty's syndrome); an uncommon, slowly progressive polyarthritis of unknown etiology; characterized by marked destruction of articular cartilage and narrowed joint spaces
4. Reiter's disease: a reactive polyarthritis that occurs secondary to disease in another part of the body (e.g., urogenital tract). Reported more often in cats than in dogs; characterized by a marked periosteal response that extends beyond the confines of the joint. Bone proliferation occurs at attachment sites of ligaments and tendons and usually is accompanied by osteolysis. Tends to be most severe in the tarsi and carpi and may involve the elbows and stifles
5. Rheumatoid arthritis, a severe, progressive, and destructive form of polyarthritis with an unknown etiology. The carpi and tarsi most often are affected, followed by the metacarpi and metatarsi. Uncommon in dogs and cats, most often reported in middle-aged, small-breed dogs

Widened joint space

1. Joint effusion:
   a. Arthritis (Table 5.10).
   b. Cruciate ligament or meniscal injury.
2. Hemarthrosis.
3. Synovial thickening.
4. Mass in joint (e.g., neoplasia).
5. Subluxation (ligamentous instability).
6. Epiphyseal dysplasia (e.g., chondrodysplasia).

Conditions that may mimic a widened joint space

1. Immature animal; incomplete ossification of the bones associated with the joint.
2. Traction on a joint, such as the hip or shoulder.

Shoulder mineral opacity structures

1. Normal sesamoid bone in the supraspinatus or infraspinatus muscle tendon; often bilateral; smooth bordered and well-defined (Table 5.11).
2. Normal caudal glenoid accessory ossification center.
3. Degenerative joint disease with osteophytes on the humeral head, distal scapula, or in the bicipital groove.
4. Osteochondrosis with mineralized free fragments in the caudoventral aspect of the joint.

Table 5.11 Sesamoid bones that may be visible in radiographs of dogs

Joint	Location
Shoulder	• Clavicle (brachiocephalicus tendon) • Supraspinatus tendon of insertion • Infraspinatus tendon of insertion
Elbow	• Supinator tendon of origin
Carpus	• Abductor pollicis longus tendon
Metacarpophalangeal and metatarsophalangeal	• Single dorsal sesamoid in extensor tendon • Paired palmar/plantar sesamoids in interosseous tendons
Coxofemoral	• Iliopubic cartilage cranial to iliopubic eminence
Stifle	• Quadriceps femoris tendon of insertion (patella) • Gastrocnemius tendon of origin (fabellae) • Popliteal tendon
Tarsus	• Lateral plantar tarsometatarsal sesamoid • Intraarticular tarsometatarsal sesamoid

5. Synovial osteochondroma with intra-capsular mineral opacity nodules.
6. Tendinopathy; focal or linear mineralization associated with the biceps, infraspinatus, or supraspinatus muscle tendon(s).
7. Avulsion fracture.

Elbow mineral opacity structures

1. Sesamoid bone (Table 5.11).
2. Degenerative joint disease.
3. Osteochondrosis.
4. Ununited anconeal process.
5. Fragmented medial coronoid process.
6. Tendon calcification.
7. Mineralized joint fragment.
8. Synovial osteochondroma.
9. Avulsion fracture.
10. Epicondylar spur.

Stifle mineral opacity structures

1. Intra-articular:
   a. Bone fragment (avulsion fracture, chip fracture).
   b. Dystrophic mineralization (involving meniscus, ligament, or infrapatellar fat pad).
   c. Osteochondritis dissecans (OCD).
   d. Synovial osteochondromatosis (especially in cats).
   e. Mineralized cartilage fragment ("joint mouse").
   f. Neoplasia (e.g., synovial sarcoma).
   g. Pseudogout.
2. Periarticular:
   a. Sesamoid bone (fabella, popliteal sesamoid).
   b. Multipartite fabella.
   c. Fracture fragment (avulsion, chip, or comminuted).
   d. Degenerative joint disease.
   e. Calcifying tendinopathy (e.g., quadriceps muscles, gastrocnemius muscle).
   f. Hypervitaminosis A.
   g. Dystrophic mineralization (e.g., tumor, chronic hematoma, abscess).

Spine

Abnormal spinal alignment

1. Scoliosis: lateral curvature (memory tips: Snakelike or Serpentine).
2. Lordosis: ventral curvature (memory tips: carrying a Load; rhymes with Low).
3. Kyphosis: dorsal curvature (memory tips: K2 mountain peak; rhymes with High).
4. Congenital malformation of vertebrae:
   a. Hemivertebrae.
   b. Transitional vertebrae.
   c. Block vertebrae.

Abnormal spinal alignment (*continued*)

5. Functional scoliosis (due to a spinal cord anomaly):
   a. Aplasia, hypoplasia, or myelodysplasia.
   b. Hydromyelia (fluid in an enlarged central canal).
   c. Syringomyelia (fluid in the spinal cord parenchyma).
   d. Cerebellar hypoplasia and hydrocephalus (Dandy-Walker Syndrome).
   e. Spinal dysraphism.
6. Acquired malalignment of vertebrae:
   a. Muscle contraction or spasm.
   b. Abdominal pain (cause arching of back or kyphosis).
   c. Back pain (e.g., intervertebral disc disease, discospondylitis).
   d. Weakening of fibrous tissues that support the vertebrae (usually causes lordosis):
      1) Old age.
      2) Overweight.
      3) Hypercortisolism (Cushing's syndrome).
   e. Trauma:
      1) Vertebral subluxation, luxation, or fracture.
      2) Healed malunion vertebral fracture.
   f. Neoplasia.
   g. Osteomyelitis.
   h. Cervical spondylomyelopathy (e.g., wobbler syndrome).
   i. Hyperparathyroidism.
   j. Atlantoaxial instability.
   k. Lumbosacral instability.
   l. Calcium phosphate deposition (Great Dane).
   m. Hypervitaminosis A (cats).
   n. Mucopolysaccharidosis.

Abnormal shape of vertebrae

1. Normal anatomic variation:
   a. C7 and L7 are shorter than the adjacent vertebrae.
   b. L7 is more variable in shape than other lumbar vertebrae.
   c. T11 is the anticlinal vertebra with a more perpendicular dorsal spinous process.
   d. L3 and L4: ventral margins are hazy due to normal anatomy.
2. Congenital and developmental abnormalities:
   a. Hemivertebrae.
   b. Transitional vertebrae.
   c. Block vertebrae (fused vertebrae).
   d. Sacrocaudal dysgenesis (cats).
   e. Spinal dysraphism; failure of parts of the vertebra to unite (e.g., spina bifida).
   f. Fused dorsal spinous processes.
   g. Abnormal dens (e.g., agenesis, dorsal angulation).
   h. Osteochondrosis.
   i. Cervical spondylomyelopathy (wobbler syndrome).
   j. Pituitary dwarfism.
   k. Congenital hypothyroidism.
3. Acquired abnormalities:
   a. Fracture (traumatic, pathologic).
   b. Prior surgery (e.g., laminectomy).
   c. Osteolysis (e.g., infection, neoplasia).
   d. Spondylosis deformans, DISH.
   e. Syndesmitis ossificans.
   f. Baastrup's disease (bony proliferation between the dorsal spinous processes).
   g. Bone cyst (aneurysmal).
   h. Schmorl's node.
   i. Hypervitaminosis A (cats).
   j. Mucopolysaccharidosis (cats).

Abnormal size of spinal canal

1. Wider than expected spinal canal:
   a. Normal at cervical and lumbar intumescence (C5–7 and L3–5).
   b. Neoplasia (e.g., astrocytoma, ependymoma, lymphoma).
   c. Hydromyelia (especially at C2).
   d. Syringomyelia (spinal arachnoid cyst).
2. Narrower than expected spinal canal:
   a. Congenital or developmental abnormality (e.g., hemivertebrae, thoracic or lumbosacral stenosis).
   b. Cervical spondylomyelopathy.
   c. Expansile lesions in the adjacent vertebrae.
   d. Healing vertebral fracture.
   e. Calcium phosphate deposition disease (Great Dane puppies).

Abnormal intervertebral disc space

1. Narrowed disc space:
   a. Absence of intervertebral disc:
      1) Prior surgery (e.g., laminectomy, fenestration).
      2) Protruded or extruded disc.
   b. Hemivertebra.
   c. Chronic discospondylitis.
   d. Cervical spondylomyelopathy (wobbler syndrome).
   e. Vertebral neoplasm.
   f. Fracture or luxation involving intervertebral space.
   g. Incomplete block vertebra.
   h. Schmorl's node.
2. Widened disc space:
   a. Hemivertebra.
   b. Acute discospondylitis.
   c. Neoplasia.
   d. Fracture or luxation involving intervertebral space.
   e. Schmorl's node.
3. Increased opacity of intervertebral disc space:
   a. Mineralized intervertebral disc (partial or complete).
   b. Presence of contrast medium (e.g., "discogram").
4. Decreased opacity of intervertebral disc space:
   a. Vacuum phenomenon: gas bubble develops in disc space due to traction on vertebral column.

Abnormal intervertebral disc space (*continued*)

5. Increased opacity of vertebral endplate:
   a. Chronic collapse of intervertebral disc space.
   b. Hemivertebrae.
   c. Osteochondrosis.
   d. Osteoporotic vertebral body.
6. Decreased opacity of vertebral endplate:
   a. Acute discospondylitis.
   b. Schmorl's node.
   c. Neoplasia.

Conditions that may mimic abnormal intervertebral space

1. Normal variations in disc space width:
   a. Narrowing at anticlinal space (T10–11).
   b. C2–3 often is narrower than the caudal spaces.
   c. Lumbar intervertebral disc spaces typically are wider than thoracic intervertebral disc spaces.
   d. Lumbosacral disc space often is wider than the cranial disc spaces.
2. Spine not parallel to image receptor.
3. Primary x-ray beam not perpendicular to disc space.
4. Positioning artifact (patient in traction).
5. Superimposed structure (e.g., spondylosis, rib, transverse process, wet or dirty hair coat).

Causes of lumbosacral disease

1. Congenital stenosis.
2. Vertebral malformation (e.g., spina bifida).
3. Thickening of vertebral arch and pedicles.
4. Subluxation, luxation, or fracture of a vertebra.
5. Intervertebral disc degeneration or protrusion.
6. Osteochondrosis.
7. Hypertrophy/hyperplasia of interarcuate ligament.
8. Discospondylitis.
9. Neoplasia (primary or metastatic).
10. Inflammation in spinal canal (e.g., neuritis, empyema).
11. Conditions that clinically mimic lumbosacral disease:
    a. Hip dysplasia.
    b. Stifle disease (e.g., cranial cruciate ligament injury).
    c. Polyarthropathy.
    d. Myopathy.
    e. Myasthenia gravis.
    f. Thrombosis in distal aorta or/and iliac arteries.
    g. Fibrocartilaginous emboli.

Myelogram lesions

1. Extradural lesion:
   a. Intervertebral disc protrusion or extrusion (most common).
   b. Hypertrophied ligaments:
      1) Cervical spondylomyelopathy.
      2) Lumbosacral instability.
   c. Neoplasia.
   d. Fracture.
   e. Luxation.
   f. Healing fracture.
   g. Osteophytes at vertebral articulations.
   h. Hemorrhage or hematoma (e.g., secondary to trauma, coagulopathy).
   i. Subarachnoid cyst.
   j. Discospondylitis.
   k. Epidural scarring (e.g., following laminectomy).
   l. Hypervitaminosis A and new bone production (cats).
   m. Calcinosis circumscripta.
   n. Migrating foreign object.
2. Intradural-extramedullary lesion:
   a. Tumor, primary or metastatic.
   b. Hemorrhage or hematoma.
   c. Subarachnoid cyst.
3. Intramedullary lesion:
   a. Spinal cord edema or hemorrhage:
      1) Trauma.
      2) Intervertebral disc herniation.
      3) Tumor.
      4) Coagulopathy.
      5) Parasite migration.
   b. Neoplasia (e.g., astrocytoma, glioma, lymphoma); most often reported at cervicothoracic and thoracolumbar junctions.
   c. Granulomatous meningoencephalitis.
   d. Ischemic myelopathy (may not be visible in a myelogram).
   e. Fibrocartilaginous embolization/infarct (rarely causes spinal cord swelling).
   f. Hydromyelia (especially in Chiari malformation).
   g. Syringomyelia.
   h. Dermoid or epidermoid cysts.

Conditions that can mimic a myelographic lesion

1. Air bubbles (iatrogenic).
2. Normal widening of spinal cord at cervical or lumbar intumescence.
3. Relatively larger spinal cord in cats and small dogs.

Skull

Cranium abnormalities

1. Decreased opacity of calvarium:
   a. Normal less opaque lines (e.g., sutures, vascular channels).
   b. Hyperparathyroidism.
   c. Fracture.
   d. Osteomyelitis.
   e. Neoplasia.
2. Increased opacity of cranium:
   a. Periosteal response (e.g., trauma, tumor, infection).
   b. Craniomandibular osteopathy.

Cranium abnormalities (*continued*)

- **c.** Foreign object.
- **d.** Overlap of fracture fragments.
- **e.** Meningioma (especially cats); increased opacity in cranium adjacent to tumor or mineralization of the tumor.

3. Mineralization in external auditory canal:
- **a.** Normal, age-related change (appears as thin, smooth-bordered, well-defined calcification that encircles the canal).
- **b.** Chronic inflammation.
- **c.** Neoplasia.
- **d.** Foreign material.
- **e.** Otolith.

4. Narrowing or absence of external auditory canal:
- **a.** Congenital absence of ear canal.
- **b.** Previous surgical ablation.
- **c.** Occlusion by wax, debris, or purulent material.
- **d.** Occlusion by polyp or neoplastic mass.
- **e.** Compression by adjacent soft tissue mass or swelling.

5. Increased opacity of tympanic bulla:
- **a.** Summation artifact.
- **b.** Otitis; bacterial infection is most common cause.
- **c.** Polyps; nasopharyngeal or auricular in origin.
- **d.** Neoplasia:
  - **1)** Osteosarcoma.
  - **2)** Squamous cell carcinoma.
  - **3)** Ceruminous carcinoma.
  - **4)** Adenocarcinoma.
  - **5)** Fibrosarcoma.
- **e.** Otolith.
- **f.** Granuloma.
- **g.** Cholesteatoma (benign growth associated with eardrum).
- **h.** Craniomandibular osteopathy (usually bilateral).

6. Decreased opacity of tympanic bulla:
- **a.** Previous bulla osteotomy.
- **b.** Neoplasia.
- **c.** Severe inflammation/infection.

Frontal sinus abnormalities

1. Frontal sinus not visualized:
- **a.** Normal breed variation (e.g., brachycephalic, small breed dog).
- **b.** Aplasia.
- **c.** Mucopolysaccharidosis (cats).

2. Increased opacity in frontal sinus:
- **a.** Iatrogenic (e.g., recent nasal flush).
- **b.** Inflammation/infection:
  - **1)** Bacterial.
  - **2)** Mycotic (e.g., cryptococcosis, aspergillosis).
  - **3)** Viral.
  - **4)** Allergic.
  - **5)** Dental disease.
- **c.** Foreign material (often unilateral).
- **d.** Neoplasia (soft tissue or osseous origin).
- **e.** Hemorrhage (e.g., trauma, coagulopathy).
- **f.** Kartagener's syndrome.
- **g.** Parasites; rare (e.g., capillariasis).
- **h.** Thickening of overlying bone:
  - **1)** Healing fracture.
  - **2)** Hyperparathyroidism.
  - **3)** Craniomandibular osteopathy.
  - **4)** Canine leukocyte adhesion disorder.
  - **5)** Acromegaly (cats).
- **i.** Mucocele.

3. Decreased opacity in frontal sinus:
- **a.** Osteolysis of overlying bone:
  - **1)** Neoplasia.
  - **2)** Osteomyelitis (e.g., bacterial, mycotic).
  - **3)** Chronic foreign material.

Nasal cavity abnormalities

1. Radiographic signs:
- **a.** Altered opacity in nasal cavity, focal or diffuse; may involve one or both sides of nasal cavity.
- **b.** Osteolysis may or may not be present; determine whether the nasal turbinates are visible (fine bony structures may be indistinct, but still visible).
- **c.** Deviation or osteolysis of internasal septum.

2. Increased opacity in nasal cavity:
- **a.** Neoplasia (e.g., adenocarcinoma [dogs], squamous cell carcinoma [dogs], lymphosarcoma [cats]).
- **b.** Foreign material; may lodge anywhere in the nasal cavity or nasopharynx.
- **c.** Hemorrhage (e.g., trauma, coagulopathy).
- **d.** Inflammation/infection:
  - **1)** Viral; most common cause of acute infection.
  - **2)** Fungal; endemic areas; tends to begin in the rostral third of the nasal cavity (e.g., *Aspergillus, Blastomycosis, Cryptococcus, Penicillium*).
  - **3)** Bacterial (e.g., *Bordatella, Pasteurella*).
  - **4)** Parasitic (e.g., *Cuterebra*).
  - **5)** Allergic (e.g., pollen, dust, mold).
  - **6)** Inhaled irritants (e.g., smoke, foreign body).
  - **7)** Lymphoplasmacytic rhinitis.
  - **8)** Dental disease (e.g., tooth root abscess).

3. Decreased opacity in nasal cavity:
- **a.** Neoplasia.
- **b.** Severe/advanced infection.
- **c.** Congenital defect of the hard palate.
- **d.** Previous rhinotomy.
- **e.** Viral rhinitis (cats).

Teeth abnormalities

1. Displacement of teeth:
- **a.** Fracture.
- **b.** Neoplasia.

Teeth abnormalities (*continued*)

   - **c.** Osteomyelitis.
   - **d.** Hyperparathyroidism ("rubber jaw").
   - **e.** Developmental anomaly.
- **2.** Decreased number of teeth:
   - **a.** Congenital/genetic:
      - **1)** Hypodontia (absence of one or a few teeth).
      - **2)** Oligodontia (absence of multiple teeth).
      - **3)** Anodontia (absence of all teeth, rare without other associated abnormalities).
   - **b.** Developmental (failure of tooth to erupt):
      - **1)** Mechanical obstruction (e.g., adjacent tooth blocks eruption).
      - **2)** Abnormal periodontal ligament.
      - **3)** Trauma that prevents tooth development.
   - **c.** Acquired loss of teeth:
      - **1)** Previous extraction.
      - **2)** Trauma.
      - **3)** Advanced periodontal disease.
      - **4)** Neoplasia.
      - **5)** Osteomyelitis.
      - **6)** Hyperparathyroidism.
- **3.** Increased number of teeth (polyodontia, supernumerary teeth):
   - **a.** Retained deciduous teeth.
- **4.** Abnormal tooth shape:
   - **a.** Developmental anomaly (Gemini tooth = tooth with a conjoined or divided crown).
   - **b.** Fracture.
   - **c.** Abnormal wear (e.g., chewing on rocks).
   - **d.** Partial extraction (e.g., crown removed, but roots remain).
   - **e.** Advanced periodontal disease.
   - **f.** Large teeth may cause crowding and periodontal disease later in life.
- **5.** Malocclusion of teeth:
   - **a.** Abnormal tooth or bone development.
   - **b.** Retained deciduous teeth.
   - **c.** Abnormal positions of teeth.
   - **d.** Temporomandibular luxation or dysplasia.
   - **e.** Fracture or callus of the mandible or maxilla.
   - **f.** Craniomandibular osteopathy.
   - **g.** Mass causing mechanical obstruction.
- **6.** Abnormal tooth opacity:
   - **a.** Fracture.
   - **b.** Dental caries.
   - **c.** Wide pulp cavity:
      - **1)** Immature tooth.
      - **2)** Dead tooth (notice that one or more of the pulp cavities in the affected tooth are wider than in the adjacent teeth).
      - **3)** Inflammation/infection.
   - **d.** Genetic malformation.
- **7.** Abnormal opacity adjacent to teeth:
   - **a.** Periodontal disease.
   - **b.** Neoplasia (e.g., epulis, odontogenic tumors).
   - **c.** Hyperparathyroidism (primary or secondary).
- **8.** Neoplasia associated with teeth:
   - **a.** Dental origin tumors (e.g., ameloblastoma, odontoma).
   - **b.** Non-odontogenic malignant tumors:
      - **1)** Squamous cell carcinoma (more common).
      - **2)** Fibrosarcoma (especially larger breed dogs; Golden Retriever)
      - **3)** Malignant melanoma (especially small-breed dogs, uncommon in cats).
      - **4)** Acanthomatous epulis.
   - **c.** Benign oral tumors:
      - **1)** Fibromatous epulis.
      - **2)** Ossifying epulis.
      - **3)** Viral-induced papilloma.
   - **d.** Cysts (benign, but can mimic tumors):
      - **1)** Periapical or radicular cyst.
      - **2)** Dentigerous cyst.
      - **3)** Odontogenic keratocyst.
      - **4)** Primordial cyst.

Temporomandibular joint (TMJ) abnormalities

- **1.** Poor visualization of TMJ:
   - **a.** Poor patient positioning.
   - **b.** Underexposed radiograph.
- **2.** Displaced TMJ (luxation/subluxation):
   - **a.** Fracture.
   - **b.** Dysplasia (unilateral or bilateral).
   - **c.** Contralateral mandibulectomy.
- **3.** Abnormal opacity at TMJ:
   - **a.** Healing fracture (e.g., zygomatic arch).
   - **b.** Degenerative joint disease.
   - **c.** Craniomandibular osteopathy (CMO).
   - **d.** Canine leukocyte adhesion disorder; reported in young Irish Setters.
   - **e.** Osteomyelitis (e.g., extension from ear).
   - **f.** Neoplasia.
   - **g.** Ankylosis: due to trauma, CMO, chronic otitis media.

Pharynx and larynx abnormalities

- **1.** Displacement of larynx:
   - **a.** Excessive tissue:
      - **1)** Obesity.
      - **2)** Brachycephalic breed.
   - **b.** Severe dyspnea (e.g., laryngeal paralysis).
   - **c.** Hyoid bone pathology.
   - **d.** Adjacent mass effect:
      - **1)** Lymphadenopathy.
      - **2)** Abscess.
      - **3)** Sialocele.

Pharynx and larynx abnormalities (*continued*)

- **4)** Tumor.
- **5)** Hematoma.
- **6)** Thyroid gland enlargement.
- **7)** Edema.
- **8)** Retropharyngeal swelling (causes ventral displacement):

2. Increased pharyngeal or laryngeal opacity:
- **a.** Excessive soft tissue; thickened soft palate (may be normal for brachycephalic breed).
- **b.** Diffuse increase in opacity:
  - **1)** Inflammation due to oral or systemic illness; often involves tonsils and regional tissues.
  - **2)** Hemorrhage due to trauma or coagulopathy.
  - **3)** Edema:
    - **1)** Trauma (e.g., ingested foreign material).
    - **2)** Allergic reaction (e.g., insect bite).
    - **3)** Severe dyspnea.
- **c.** Local increase in opacity (mass):
  - **1)** Pharyngeal tumor:
    - **1)** Soft palate: melanoma, fibrosarcoma.
    - **2)** Pharyngeal wall: sarcoma, extension of tonsillar carcinoma.
    - **3)** Tonsil: squamous cell carcinoma, lymphosarcoma.
  - **2)** Laryngeal tumor:
    - **1)** Squamous cell carcinoma (most common).
    - **2)** Lymphoma (more often in cats).
    - **3)** Leiomyoma.
    - **4)** Rhabdomyosarcoma.
    - **5)** Secondary invasion by thyroid or tonsillar carcinoma.
  - **3)** Nasopharyngeal polyp (originate in nasopharynx or middle ear); more common in cats.
  - **4)** Lymphadenomegaly:
    - **1)** Inflammation/infection.
    - **2)** Neoplasia (e.g., oral tumor, thyroid tumor, nasal tumor, lymphoma).
  - **5)** Mucous gland retention cysts; reported in oropharynx, near base of epiglottis.
  - **6)** Abscess or granuloma (e.g., foreign object); may involve pharynx, salivary glands, lymph nodes.

3. Mineralization in larynx:
- **a.** Normal, age-related change in laryngeal cartilages.
- **b.** Normal hyoid bones.
- **c.** Mineralized mass (long standing abscess, hematoma).
- **d.** Neoplastic mineralization; often extensive and heterogeneous.
- **e.** Foreign material.
- **f.** Sialolith.

4. Dilation of pharynx:
- **a.** Pharyngeal paralysis.
- **b.** Severe dyspnea (e.g., respiratory obstruction).

5. Narrowing of laryngeal airway:
- **a.** Hypoplasia.
- **b.** Neoplasia (carcinoma in dogs, lymphoma in cats).
- **c.** Cyst (rare congenital development).
- **d.** Adjacent mass effect (e.g., granuloma, abscess, tumor, hematoma, edema).

Glossary of Radiologic Terms

abscess An accumulation of purulent material in an abnormal cavity surrounded by a wall and typically associated with inflammation. May be caused by infection or presence of foreign material.

absorbed x-ray An x-ray that loses all of its energy inside the patient and completely disappears. Where x-rays are absorbed in radiography, the resultant image is more white (less black).

achondroplasia "Without cartilage formation"; a genetic disorder of bone growth that results in disproportionate dwarfism. Appendicular bones are short and thick, metaphyses are cupped and flared, and physes are irregular. Some dog breeds normally are classified as achondrodysplastic (e.g., Bulldog) (a term that often is used interchangeably with chondrodystrophic).

air bronchogram A radiographic sign that occurs during alveolar filling due to retention of air in a bronchus. It appears as a tubular, sometimes branching, gas opacity structure (bronchus) surrounded by soft tissue opacity lung parenchyma. The degree of contrast between the gas-filled bronchus and fluid-filled alveoli depends on the amount of alveolar filling; more complete filling = greater contrast. Air bronchograms only occur with alveolar filling, but alveolar filling can occur without air bronchograms. In most cases of alveolar filling, the bronchus also fills with fluid. Sometimes gas in the bronchus is resorbed. Air bronchograms rarely are seen in collapsed lungs. When present, there usually is some degree of alveolar filling in the collapsed lung.

air gap Distance between patient (subject or object) and image receptor; increasing the air gap allows scattered x-rays to dissipate but results in magnification of the image.

ALARA (**A**s **L**ow **A**s **R**easonably **A**chievable) The overriding principle of radiation safety. Understanding that some radiation exposure is necessary, it must be demonstrated that the medical benefit is worth the exposure risk when using radiation. Factors that influence the degree of radiation exposure include amount of shielding, distance from source of x-rays, time spent in presence of x-rays, and intensity of x-rays.

aliasing In digital radiographs, an artifact that appears as a series of repeating lines superimposed on the image.

alveolar filling Replacement of the air in the lung air spaces due to an influx of fluid (e.g., blood, edema) or cells (e.g., neoplasia, purulent material). Any solid area of soft tissue opacity in the lung that is not vessel, nodule, or mass is alveolar filling. The air bronchogram sign is characteristic of alveolar filling but is not necessary for diagnosis of alveolar filling. Common causes include pneumonia, hemorrhage, neoplasia, edema.

alveolar pulmonary pattern A radiographic appearance that occurs due to alveolar filling or collapse. Appears as soft tissue opacity in the lung that obscures the margins of adjacent soft tissue structures (e.g., blood vessels, pulmonary nodules, diaphragm, cardiac silhouette).

amyloidosis A rare disorder of protein metabolism that results in deposition of insoluble protein (*amyloid*) in glomeruli and interstitium of kidneys (and also in other organs). May be heritable (e.g., Shar-Pei, Abyssinian) or acquired (sequela to chronic inflammation/infection). Associated syndromes include Shar-Pei fever, Akita fever/polyarthropathy, Gray Collie. Some cat breeds are predisposed (e.g., Abyssinian, Asian shorthair, Siamese). Clinical signs vary with severity of disease and organs affected; many animals die shortly after onset of signs.

angiocardiography A radiographic contrast study of the heart and great vessels.

Radiography of the Dog and Cat: Guide to Making and Interpreting Radiographs, Second Edition. M.C. Muhlbauer and S.K. Kneller.

Companion website: www.wiley.com/go/muhlbauer/dog

angiography A radiographic contrast study of blood vessels.

Anode Positive terminal in an x-ray tube that attracts electrons from the cathode (negative terminal). Anode contains a target made of metal (tungsten) with a high melting point to withstand the intense heat generated by the electron beam bombardment.

anode heel effect See **heel effect**.

apophysis Essentially, a non-weight-bearing epiphysis; a normal bony projection that serves for the attachment of tendons or ligaments (e.g., greater trochanter, tibial tuberosity); a secondary ossification center that contributes to the shape of a bone but does not contribute to overall bone length.

appendicular Pertaining to the limbs.

arteriovenous fistula An abnormal communication between an artery and a vein.

arthritis Inflammation of a joint; may be caused by trauma, infection, or immune-mediated disease. Term often is erroneously used for degenerative joint disease.

arthrography A radiographic contrast study of a joint. Arthrogram.

artifact An erroneous finding. Artifacts may be caused by technical problems associated with film, screens, grid, development, exposure, cassettes, x-ray table, etc., or they may be patient-related issues such as debris on skin/haircoat, superimposed cutaneous or subcutaneous structures. Artifacts can mimic disease, impair image quality, and obscure abnormalities.

asynchronous growth Refers to the disproportionate rate of growth between paired bones (e.g., radius/ulna, tibia/fibula), typically caused by damage to a physis and commonly resulting in an angular limb deformity and joint subluxation.

atelectasis Incomplete expansion of part or all of a lung. Also used to describe partial or complete lung collapse. Atelectasis may result from disease of lung or pleural space. Common with animals positioned in lateral recumbency.

atresia ani A rare malformation of the anus. Radiographs sometimes are used to assess the severity of the condition, which varies from a stenosis to a complete blockage. Typically, the colon is largely distended with feces. A fistula can develop between the rectum and either the vagina, urinary bladder, or urethra, enabling the patient to defecate through the vagina or urethra. Gas must be in the rectum to visualize the abnormality in survey radiographs. Sometimes elevating the caudal end of the patient will allow gas in the descending colon to move into the rectum. Evaluate the distance between the rectum and the anal membrane using positive contrast medium (either oral or per-rectal dosing) or a radiopaque probe inserted into the anus. When possible, add a negative-contrast enema (pneumocolon) to identify the rectum. Infusion of iodinated contrast medium into the urethra, vagina, or rectum may document a fistula or other malformation.

avascular necrosis of the femoral head A loss of blood supply to the developing femoral head that results in bone necrosis and eventual collapse. Condition may be idiopathic, genetic, or traumatic. The eponym is "Legg-Calve-Perthes disease."

axial Pertains to the median line of the body, a limb, or other structure. Axial skeletal structures include vertebral column, skull, hyoid bones, ribs, and sternum.

barium sulfate A positive contrast medium with a high degree of opacity (atomic number of barium is 56). Barium is a white crystalline powder that is micro-pulverized and placed in suspension. It a Adheres well to suspending agents, enabling it to efficiently coat mucosal surfaces. Barium is not metabolized or absorbed. The word "barium" comes from the Greek word meaning "heavy."

barium enema A radiographic contrast study of the colon using barium sulfate.

beak sign Occurs when contrast medium fills only the entrance of the pyloric sphincter; commonly associated with pyloric stenosis.

beam direction Path of the x-rays as they enter and exit a structure (e.g., dorsoventral, dorsopalmar).

beam hardening Refers to increasing the average energy of the x-ray beam by using filters to remove lower energy x-rays. Filters commonly are made of aluminum and positioned in the path of the primary x-ray beam near the x-ray tube window.

bezoar A concretion of fibrous material commonly found in the stomach or intestine.

binary number A Base 2 numbering system used by computers. The position of each digit (bit) in a binary number represents an exponent of 2. In a base 10 numbering system (decimal system), the position of each digit represents an exponent of 10. This means that moving right to left in a decimal number, the value of each digit is 10^0, 10^1, 10^2, 10^3, 10^4, etc., whereas in a binary number the value of each digit (bit) is 2^0, 2^1, 2^2, 2^3, 2^4, etc. Each decimal digit can be any numeral 0–9, but each binary digit can only be 0 or 1. In both numbering systems, adding more digits to the number makes the total value of the number grow exponentially, either by factors of 2 or 10. The value of a binary number or a decimal number is the sum of all of its digits as shown below.

The number 29 as expressed in decimal and binary numbering systems				
Position of digit				
5	4	3	2	1
Decimal value of digit position				
10^4 10,000	10^3 1000	10^2 100	10^1 10	10^0 1
Binary value of digit position				
2^4 16	2^3 8	2^2 4	2^1 2	2^0 1
Decimal number 29				
0	0	0	2	9
(0 × 1000) + (0 × 100) + (1 × 10) + (3 × 1) = 29				
Binary number 29				
1	1	1	0	1
(1 × 16) + (1 × 8) + (1 × 4) + (0 × 2) + (1 × 1) = 29				

How to read decimal and binary numbers:

The decimal number "1101" is read as follows:

- "1" is the digit in the thousand position (10^3)
- "1" is the digit in the hundred position (10^2)
- "0" is the digit in the ten position (10^1)
- "1" is the digit in the one position (10^0).

Add the digits, each multiplied by its base exponent, to determine the value of the number:

(1 × 1000) + (1 × 100) + (0 × 10) + (1 × 1) =
1000 + 100 + 0 + 1 =
1101

The binary number "1101" is read as follows:

- "1" is the digit in the eight position (2^3)
- "1" is the digit in the four position (2^2)
- "0" is the digit in the two position (2^1)
- "1" is the digit in the one position (2^0)

Add the digits, each multiplied by its base exponent, to determine the value of the number:

(1 × 8) + (1 × 4) + (0 × 2) + (1 × 1) =
8 + 4 + 0 + 1 = **13**

bit The smallest unit of digital data. A bit is a digit in a binary number ("bit" is short for **Bi**nary Digi**t**).

bit depth The number of unique shades of gray available to display a radiograph. Not every gray shade will necessarily be used in the radiograph, but the shades can be displayed with that level of precision.

Bit depth (N)	Number of bytes	Shades of gray (2^N)	Common name
1	0.125	2	Bit
4	0.5	16	Nibble
8	1	256	Byte
16	2	65,536	Word
32	4	4,294,967,296	Double word
64	8	Big number	Quad word
2^{10}	1024	Bigger number	Kilobyte (Kb)
2^{20}	1,048,546	. . .	Megabyte (Mb)
2^{30}	1,073,741,824	. . .	Gigabyte (Gb)
2^{40}	Big number. . .	. . .	Terabyte (Tb)

block vertebra A congenital defect caused by failure of one or more vertebral bodies to segment normally during development. Vertebrae appear fused, but each vertebral body maintains normal length.

bone cyst A cavity within bone, often filled with fluid. Usually, well-defined margins and may be septated.

bone infarcts Foci of necrosis caused by decreased blood supply to intramedullary bone; appear as multiple small areas of increased medullary opacity.

bone sclerosis An increase in opacity of bone; eburnation is a type of bone sclerosis.

bone spur A well-defined bony projection. Term is used to describe osteophytes (occur along non-weight-bearing articular margins) and enthesophytes (occur at sites of attachment to bone, e.g., ligaments, tendons, joint capsules).

border effacement Occurs when two structures of same opacity are in contact and their individual margins are no longer distinguishable where they touch. The margin of a structure is only visible when it is adjacent to a different opacity (i.e., opacity interface). Other names: edge effacement, silhouette sign/effect. Erroneously called "loss of detail."

brachycephalic Refers to the shape of a skull in which the nasal cavity is considerably shorter than the cranium. Also, the cranium commonly is more dome shaped, frontal sinuses tend to be small or absent, and the occipital protuberance often is small. Examples: English Bulldog, Pug.

Bremsstrahlung x-ray An x-ray that is produced from the loss of kinetic energy that occurs when a speeding electron from the x-ray tube cathode nears the nucleus of a target atom in the anode, causing the electron to slow down and change direction; bremsstrahlung = "braking radiation."

bronchial blood vessels Part of the systemic circulation that provides blood for lung nutrition. Bronchial arteries and veins are too small to be seen in radiographs. They contribute only about 1% of the total blood volume in the lungs (the pulmonary blood vessels supply the remaining 99%).

bronchial cuffing Thickened soft tissue opacity around a bronchus due to accumulation of fluid, cells, or fibrosis; a sign of bronchial disease or peribronchial accumulation; also peribronchial cuffing, peribronchial infiltrates.

bronchial pulmonary pattern A radiographic appearance in which bronchial walls appear thickened and/or increased in opacity (latter includes mineralization of bronchial walls). Commonly caused by proliferation or infiltration of collagenous and cartilaginous tissues and associated mucous glands. May also result from accumulation of peribronchial interstitial fluid or cellular material. The size and shape of the bronchial lumen may be altered.

bronchiectasis Abnormal and permanent dilation of bronchi or bronchioles with loss of normal branching and tapering.

bronchitis Inflammation of the bronchi.

bronchography A radiographic contrast study of the major airways.

bronchopneumonia Inflammation of the lungs that usually begins in the terminal bronchioles.

brown fat Present in juvenile animals to help with thermoregulation. Brown fat is composed of smaller lipids and receives a larger blood supply than mature fat. It is higher in water content and therefore more opaque than adult fat.

brush border The edge or margin resembles the bristles of a brush.

buccal On the side that faces the cheek; used to describe lesions associated with the mouth.

Bucky A device that holds a grid within the x-ray table. The Bucky moves the grid rapidly during exposure to blur the grid lines. Modern grid lines are very thin and only faintly visible; therefore, a Bucky may not be necessary with modern equipment. First introduced by Dr. Hollis Potter and often called a Potter-Bucky diaphragm.

Bucky factor See **grid factor**.

calcification The normal or abnormal deposition of calcium salts in soft tissues.

calcinosis Abnormal deposition of calcium salts in various tissues.

- *calcinosis cutis:* Calcium deposits in the skin, often secondary to hypercortisolism.
- *calcinosis circumscripta (tumoral calcinosis):* Deposits of calcium in subcutaneous, tendinous, ligamentous, or muscular tissues as firm, well-circumscribed, tumor-like nodules; typically occurring on limbs, over bony prominences, and under foot pads.

calculus A stone or concretion of material, usually mineral salts, that forms in an organ or duct of the body (pl. *calculi*). Other names for renal calculi include *nephroliths, uroliths,* and *kidney stones.*

calvarium The upper, domelike part of the skull, formed by the frontal, parietal, and occipital bones; the encasement for the brain.

cancellous bone The trabeculated, spongy, or porous bone found in ends of long bones, in vertebrae, and in flat bones.

canine leukocyte adhesion disorder (CLAD) Rare inherited condition of abnormal granulocytes resulting in mandibular periosteal response and metaphyseal flaring.

carcinomatosis Widespread distribution of neoplasia throughout a body cavity; commonly used to describe diffuse implantation of tumor nodules within the peritoneal space (e.g., pancreatic carcinoma).

cardiac silhouette Outline of the pericardial sac and its contents as seen in a thoracic radiograph.

carnassial teeth Relatively large teeth that are adapted for shearing; includes the maxillary fourth premolar teeth and the mandibular first molar teeth.

cartilage joint Two or more bones united by hyaline cartilage or fibrocartilage (e.g., costochondral junctions, pelvic symphysis).

cassette A light-tight, semi-rigid container used to house and protect either x-ray film and screens or a phosphor-coated imaging plate during exposure and transport to processing.

cathode The negative terminal in the x-ray tube. Cathode filament emits electrons, which are attracted to the anode (positive terminal). Current (electrons) flows from cathode to anode. In x-ray tubes, the cathode commonly consists of a helical tungsten filament, behind which is a molybdenum reflector cup used to focus the electron emission toward the anode target.

caudal Toward the tail or hind part of the body. Also used to designate the flexor side of a limb proximal to the carpus and tarsus.

caudocranial Refers to the path of the x-ray beam (x-rays enter the caudal aspect of the body part and exit the cranial aspect).

cecal inversion Also called cecocolic intussusception. Prolapse of the cecum into the ascending colon is uncommon in dogs and cats. It typically affects young animals (less than 4 years) but can occur at any age. Cecal inversion usually is associated with hypermotility due to inflammation or parasitism. It may be predisposed in animals with a weak ileocecocolic ligament. Clinical signs vary with severity and duration of the obstruction (hematochezia, tenesmus, vomiting).

celiography A radiographic contrast study of the peritoneal space.

central beam Refers to the x-ray photons in the middle of the x-ray beam.

cervical spondylopathy Syndrome that may include deformity of vertebral bodies, narrowing of the vertebral canal, vertebral instability, and/or malarticulation with varying degrees of spinal cord compression in the neck.

characteristic x-ray An x-ray that is produced when an outer shell electron gives up energy as it drops to fill a void created by a lost inner shell electron; x-ray energy corresponds to the difference in binding energy between the outer shell and inner shell electrons, which is characteristic of the type of atom.

characteristic curve A graphic representation of the dynamic range of an image receptor. Characteristic curves are also known as *H & D curves*, named for the two chemists who developed them in 1890, Hurter and Driffield.

cholangiography A radiographic contrast study of the bile ducts.

cholecystocholangiography A radiographic contrast study of the gall bladder and bile ducts.

cholecystography A radiographic contrast study of the gall bladder.

cholelith A calculus or concretion in the gall bladder.

choledocolith A calculus or concretion in a bile duct.

chondrodysplasia Inherited deformities of the bony skeleton caused by abnormal cartilage development. Affected animals are characterized by a normal-sized trunk with abnormally shortened limbs.

chondrodystrophic Refers to an animal exhibiting chondrodysplasia (e.g., Dachshund, Bassett Hound). Term often is used interchangeably with achondrodysplastic.

chondroma A benign, slow-growing tumor of cartilage, more often occurring in flat bones (e.g., scapula, pelvis, ribs) and appearing as a well-defined, expansile mass that is less opaque than surrounding bone. A chondroma may contain mineralized components.

chylothorax Accumulation of chyle in the pleural space, often secondary to rupture of the thoracic duct.

chylous effusion Accumulation of chylous fluid in the pleural space, may be associated with heart failure, mediastinal neoplasia, or mediastinitis.

cineradiography (cineflurography) The making of a video record directly from a fluorescent screen (i.e., recording of real-time radiographic imaging.)

cirrhosis of the liver Hepatic cirrhosis is scarring and fibrosis of liver that is caused by chronic inflammation that eventually leads to liver failure. Many animals with hepatic cirrhosis are asymptomatic until liver failure; regenerative nodules may develop in damaged liver. Clinical signs vary with severity of disease, but may include polyuria, polydipsia, GI signs, neurologic signs (hepatoencephalopathy). Causes of hepatic cirrhosis include infection (e.g., viral, leptospirosis), toxins, copper storage disease, immune-mediated diseases, and idiopathic.

clock face analogy Technique used to approximate the locations of major components of the cardiac shadow by mentally superimposing the numbers of a clock face over the cardiac silhouette on a lateral or ventrodorsal/dorsoventral thoracic radiograph.

Codman's triangle Occurs when aggressive soft tissue opacity material wedges between a mineralized periosteal response and the underlying cortex. The periosteal response may appear solid, well-defined, and homogeneous in this area, giving the erroneous appearance of a benign, inactive lesion (which is not the true nature of the disease process). Codman's triangle develops at the periphery of a rapidly growing disease process, usually on the diaphyseal side.

coin lesion A descriptive term referring to a pulmonary nodule approximately 1 cm in diameter.

collimation Process of restricting the size and shape of the x-ray beam to the area of interest. Collimation helps reduce scatter radiation, which improves image quality and reduces radiation exposure to nearby personnel.

collimator An adjustable device used to restrict the size and shape of the x-ray beam and which is attached near the x-ray tube.

comparison radiographs Images made of the side opposite to the one being investigated or images of a similar subject (e.g., littermate) or known normal subject, used to aid in distinguishing normal from abnormal.

compartmentalization (of the stomach) A classic radiographic finding in patients with gastric dilatation and volvulus (GDV). It appears as two large, gas-filled "bubbles" in the cranial abdomen. The "compartments" or "bubbles" represent the gastric pylorus and body of the stomach, separated by a fold or band of soft tissue (sometimes called a "shelf" of soft tissue). Compartmentalization usually is easiest to see in a right lateral view, but it is not present in all cases of GDV. Colloquial nicknames include "reverse C," "boxing glove," "double bubble," "Popeye's arm," and "Smurf hat."

compression radoigraphy Technique used to improve visualization of a structure(s) by displacing the adjacent structures to eliminate superimposition (e.g., displace overlying intestine to better visualize kidney, urinary bladder, uterus, etc. or to separate the digits during radiography of a foot). A low-density plastic paddle or wooden spoon is used to gently compress the abdomen or foot. Abdominal compression is contraindicated in animals with pain, tense abdomen, or peritoneal effusion. X-ray exposure usually is decreased to accommodate thinner body thickness. During the performance of an excretory urogram, caudal abdominal compression is used to deliberately obstruct the flow of urine for a short period of time to dilate the renal collecting system and enhance filling and opacification.

computed tomography (CT) A diagnostic imaging modality that creates cross-sectional views of a body part using x-rays and computers. The source of x-rays rotates around the patient, transmitting a thin x-ray beam through the body part to detectors on the opposite side. CT images have inherent high contrast and eliminate superimposition of overlying structures.

consolidation Refers to pathology of the lung in which alveolar air has been replaced by organized cellular exudate or by invasion of neoplastic cells.

constipation Infrequent or difficult passage of feces.

contralateral Pertaining to the opposite side.

contrast media Compounds or materials used to increase or decrease opacity to create an opacity interface between an examined structure and the adjacent tissues.

contrast study A radiographic procedure using a positive or negative contrast agent to enhance visualization of an organ or structure that is inadequately seen on survey radiographs. A contrast study is indicated only if it will provide information not available on survey radiographs and will assist the clinician in managing the case or in developing a diagnosis without harming the patient.

contusion A local area of hemorrhage or bruising.

cortical bone The dense, homogeneous bone that forms the shaft of long bones and the outer layer of small and cuboidal bones.

costophrenic angle Junction of the thoracic wall (rib cage) and diaphragm at the caudolateral aspect of the thoracic cavity on a ventrodorsal or dorsoventral radiograph. Angle normally is sharp and well-defined, but it becomes rounded when pleural fluid is present.

cranial Toward the head; opposite is **caudal**.

craniocaudal Refers to the path of the x-ray beam (x-rays enter the cranial aspect of the body part and exit the caudal aspect).

cretinism (congenital hypothyroidism) Disproportionate dwarfism caused by abnormal development of the thyroid gland, defective thyroid hormone synthesis, or iodine deficiency. Most often is reported in Boxers and sometimes in other breeds (e.g., Affenpinscher, Giant Schnauzer, Great Dane, Scottish Deerhound).

crus The part of pelvic limb between femur and tarsus, the shank; also a part of the diaphragm that anchors the cupula to the spine, so named because its shape was thought to resemble a leg.

cut back zone Refers to the area in a long bone where the wider metaphysis is actively remodeling to become the more-narrow diaphysis. The bony margins in the cut back zone normally appear indistinct and may be mistaken for pathology (e.g., hypertrophic osteodystrophy, osteomyelitis, trauma).

cystography A radiographic contrast study of the urinary bladder. Cystogram. Pneumocystogram.

dacryocystorhinography A radiographic contrast study of the nasolacrimal duct.

decubitus Position assumed when lying down. Opposed to erect or standing.

degenerative joint disease (DJD) The most common joint disorder in dogs and cats, characterized by degradation of articular cartilage and subchondral bone (also called osteoarthritis and osteoarthrosis). May result from trauma, infection, age-related wear, overuse, developmental anomalies, immune-mediated disease, and other causes. The most common radiographic sign is osteophyte formation.

definition Refers to the sharpness of the margins of a lesion. Definition should not be confused with detail (the quality of the radiograph) or the shape of the structure (which may be smooth or irregular) or the opacity interfaces (which are affected by body condition, the type of disease process, and others). Definition is affected by the level of activity and the aggressiveness of a disease process. Poor definition is due to lack of a physical border. For example:

- A well-defined periosteal response is inactive; an ill-defined periosteal response is active.
- Well-defined osteolysis is less aggressive; ill-defined osteolysis is more aggressive.
- A well-defined pulmonary nodule is more likely to be a tumor; an ill-defined lung nodule is more typical of an abscess or mycotic granuloma.

delayed union fracture The bone fragments do not unite within the expected period of time, but healing is believed to eventually occur.

density *Radiographic density* refers to the degree of blackening of a radiograph. *Physical density* refers to the characteristic of a material to block x-rays. Previously, the term *density* was used synonymously with *opacity*. *Density* is still used to describe opacity on CT images.

detail Refers to the quality of the radiograph; detail is affected by technical factors such as exposure settings, motion artifact, type of image receptor, focal spot size, and others. It is one of the four characteristics of radiographic quality: density, detail, distortion, contrast. Detail has nothing to do with the patient and everything to do with how the radiograph was created. Detail should not be confused with definition (described above) or the opacity interfaces in the subject (patient). Detail is enhanced by using a small focal spot, tight collimation, larger distance between the focal spot and image receptor, and a shorter distance between subject and image receptor. Other factors that increase detail include using a grid to reduce scatter radiation and avoiding patient motion.

detector See **image receptor**.

development of x-ray film Refers to the chemical process that converts activated silver halide crystals to metallic silver particles. Silver particles blacken the film to create the final image. Development may be accomplished manually or using an automatic film processor.

dextrocardia Condition in which most of heart is positioned in right hemithorax with the cardiac apex right of midline.

diaphysis "Between physes"; the middle portion or shaft of a long bone; the area between the metaphyses; a primary center of ossification of a long bone.

DICOM (Digital Imaging and Communication in Medicine) A specific file format (such as jpeg or tif) used to store digital images and which contains information specific to the patient, type of digital equipment used, image transmission, and pixel data. DICOM files are safeguarded to prevent permanent altering of images and can only be viewed with a DICOM viewer.

distinction Refers to the visibility of margins in parts of the radiograph. An indistinct margin may be caused by a weak opacity interface (e.g., fluid next to a soft tissue opacity structure) or the absence of a physical border (e.g., aggressive osteolysis, alveolar filling).

dirty lungs Refers to an interstitial lung pattern in which vascular and bronchial margins are partially obscured and appear hazy due to increased opacity in the lung interstitium.

discography A radiographic contrast study of the central portion of an intervertebral disc.

discospondylitis Inflammation or infection of an intervertebral disc (other names: intradiscal osteomyelitis, diskitis).

disproportionate dwarfism Chondrodysplasia that affects certain parts of the skeleton.

- **chondrodysplasia of Great Pyrenees** presents with shortened limbs and shortened bodies, but a normal size skull. The thoracic limbs tend to be shorter than pelvic limbs resulting in a forward slanting body.
- **chondrodysplasia of Alaskan Malamutes** produces short, bowed limbs, but normal-sized body, spine, and skull. Macrocytic, hemolytic anemia is associated with disproportionate dwarfism.
- **dwarfism of Norwegian Elkhound** is similar to dwarfism of Alaskan Malamutes, but the body tends to be shorter.
- **enchondrodystrophy** disproportionate dwarfism in English Pointers. The thoracic limbs tend to be more severely affected than pelvic limbs. Also called dysostosis. Affected puppies may exhibit abnormal movements, such as a bunny-hopping gait. Mandibular prognathism may be present.
- **feline osteodystrophy** or **chondrodysplasia of Scottish Fold Cats** predominately affects the distal appendicular skeleton of fold-ear cats (tarsi, carpi, metatarsals, metacarpals, phalanges). The pelvic limbs tend to be more severely affected than the thoracic limbs. New bone production may be seen along the plantar and palmar aspects of the pes and manus. New bone occasionally leads to ankylosis. Osseous remodeling can appear aggressive in some cats, with punctate osteolysis in the tarsal and carpal bones. Affected cats typically exhibit short, deformed limbs, a short inflexible tail, overgrown nails, and partial deafness. They may have difficulty standing, an abnormal gait, and lameness.
- **multiple epiphyseal dysplasia**, also called pseudochondrodysplasia, has been reported in Beagles and Miniature Poodles. Affected dogs present with shortened limbs, spinal kyphosis, and enlarged joints. Poor growth,

difficulty standing, and abnormal gait usually are recognized by 2–3 weeks of age.

- **ocular-skeletal dwarfism in Samoyeds** Affected dogs present with thoracic limbs shorter than pelvic limbs, a varus (inward) deformity at the elbows, and a valgus (outward) deviation in the distal limbs. Affected dogs typically exhibit prominent doming of the forehead, lameness, retinal detachment, and cataracts.
- **skeletal-retinal dysplasia in Labrador Retrievers** or ocular chondrodysplasia. Leads to abnormally shortened limbs with a normal body length. Affected dogs exhibit impaired vision, valgus limb deformities, and hyperextended hind legs.
- **tibial metaphyseal dysplasia** reported in Dachshunds and leads to abnormal development of the distal tibial metaphysis. It may be unilateral or bilateral. The affected tibia is abnormally shortened and curved, usually resulting in a secondary deformity of the fibula. The lateral trochlear groove in the distal tibia is shallow, which leads to subluxation of the tibiotarsal joint and pes varus, an inward curving of the foot (only the lateral part of the foot touches the ground). A pointed exostosis may be present on the medial aspect of the distal tibial metaphysis.

disseminated idiopathic skeletal hyperostosis (DISH) Flowing mineralization along contiguous vertebral bodies. DISH resembles severe spondylosis deformans. Forestier's disease is a similar condition in humans.

distal Away from the trunk of the body; away from the center of the body; or away from the point of origin of a body structure (e.g., intestines, bronchi, ureters, etc.). Opposite is **proximal**.

distortion *Geometric distortion* occurs when one part of the patient (subject or object) is positioned further from the image receptor than other parts, creating uneven magnification. *Positional distortion* refers to errors in positioning, such as rotation of the sternum in a ventrodorsal radiograph or placing a structure of interest at the periphery of the field of view, which can falsely alter the normal appearance.

diverticulum A pouch or sac extending outward from a hollow organ or structure (e.g., stomach, intestine, esophagus, urinary bladder).

donut sign Refers to the end-on visualization of a bronchus with either a thickened wall, increased endobronchial secretions, or peribronchial infiltrate. "Donuts" sometimes are called "cheerios."

dolichocephalic Refers to the shape of a skull in which the nasal cavity is longer than the cranium. The occipital crest tends to be prominent in animals with this type of skull. Examples: Collie, Greyhound.

dorsal Toward the back or spine. Opposed to ventral. Also refers to the top, front, or extensor surface of limbs (at or below the carpus and tarsus) and the top of the head.

dorsal recumbency Animal is positioned lying on its back.

dorsopalmar/plantar Describes the path of the x-ray beam (x-rays enter the dorsum of the limb and exit the palmar/plantar surface).

dorsoventral (DV) radiograph The x-ray beam enters the dorsal surface of a body part and exits the ventral surface.

dose The recommended quantity of an agent required for therapy or a specific procedure.

double contrast A radiographic contrast study using negative (e.g., gas) and positive contrast media (e.g., barium, iodinated agents).

double physis sign Refers to the line of decreased opacity within the metaphysis parallel to the physis in animals suffering from hypertrophic osteodystrophy.

dural ossification A degenerative condition of unknown clinical significance in the dog, characterized by osseous metaplasia of the dura mater.

dysplasia Refers to the abnormal development or growth of a structure (e.g., hip dysplasia, elbow dysplasia).

dystrophic mineralization The abnormal, localized precipitation of inorganic material in damaged, degenerating, or dead tissue.

eburnation Subchondral osteosclerosis, commonly occurs after articular cartilage has been lost.

ectopic ureter A congenital defect in which one or both ureters empties abnormally into the urethra or vagina. It is more common in dogs than in cats. Females more often are affected than males. Ectopic ureter may be intramural or extramural. With an intramural defect, the ureter enters the bladder in the normal location but tunnels through the bladder wall to bypass the trigone. This is the most common form of ectopic ureter in dogs. An extramural defect is more common in cats. In these cases, the ureter completely bypasses the bladder to enter the urethra directly. Clinical signs include continuous or intermittent incontinence, urine scalding, vaginitis. Possible complications include ascending infection or ureteral obstruction leading to hydronephrosis.

ectrodactyly A congenital malformation in which one or more central digits are absent or reduced in size.

edge enhancement See **Mach band**.

effusion An escape of fluid into a body cavity; an abnormal collection of fluid in hollow spaces of the body.

Ehler-Danlos syndrome An inherited disorder resulting in greater elasticity of connective tissues and increased joint laxity.

elbow incongruity A distinct disorder in which the distal humerus and trochlear notch of the ulna do not fit properly due to abnormal development of the proximal ulna or humeral condyle; elbow incongruity is associated with elbow dysplasia and often erroneously included in the description of asynchronous growth of the radius and ulna.

emphysema The abnormal accumulation of gas in a tissue (e.g., subcutaneous emphysema, emphysematous cystitis). Also, the overinflation of a lung(s) (see **pulmonary emphysema**).

enchondroma A benign cartilaginous tumor that develops from displaced growth cartilage. Tumor continues to grow and expand but fails to ossify. Appears in radiographs as an expansile, well-defined area of decreased opacity in the medullary cavity of a long bone (usually in the metaphysis or diaphysis).

endochondral ossification The formation of bone in a cartilaginous framework.

endosteum Similar to the periosteum but lines the medullary cavities of bones.

enteral The administration of a substance to a patient that involves the alimentary tract (i.e., esophagus, stomach, and intestines). Methods of administration include oral, sublingual, and rectal.

enthesophyte A bony growth or spur projecting outward from a site of joint capsule, tendinous or ligamentous attachment; mineralization of said attachments.

epidurography A radiographic contrast study of the cauda equina and associated nerve roots.

epiphysis "Upon the physis." The rounded end of a long bone that supports the articular cartilage. The epiphysis forms from a secondary ossification center at the proximal or distal end of most long bones. In immature animals, the epiphysis is separated from the metaphysis by the physis.

epithelial Relating to the thin tissue forming the outer layer of a body's surface and lining the alimentary canal and other hollow structures.

erect Position in which the animal is vertical (frequently held upright and usually standing on its hind legs); x-ray beam commonly is directed horizontally.

esophagography A radiographic contrast study of the esophagus. Esophagram.

excretory urography (EU) A radiographic contrast study of the kidney and ureters. Other names: intravenous urography (old term: intravenous pyelogram or IVP).

exostosis A bony growth that projects outward from the surface of a bone. The term is nondescript, and any exostosis should be investigated and further described as to origin (e.g., periosteal response, osteophyte, enthesophyte).

extension The straightening of a limb or other body part; opposite is **flexion**.

extrapleural sign Refers to lesions arising outside the parietal or mediastinal pleura; commonly originating from the thoracic wall, diaphragm, or mediastinum. Presents as a mass bulging into the thoracic cavity, displacing (indenting) the adjacent lung. Margins of the mass taper cranially and caudally to blend with the thoracic wall, diaphragm, or mediastinum.

Fanconi syndrome Congenital or acquired renal tubular dysfunction; Hereditary in Basenji; idiopathic in Norwegian Elk-hound, Shetland Sheepdog, Miniature Schnauzer. May be acquired secondary to cystic disease, adverse drug reaction, heavy metal toxins, or multiple myeloma. Affected animals are unable to concentrate urine and cannot resorb glucose, electrolytes, protein, or uric acid. Glucosuria with normal blood glucose is highly suggestive of Fanconi syndrome. Clinical signs of renal disease are progressive, typically beginning at 3–8 years of age and lead to renal failure. Survey and contrast radiographs usually are normal.

feline polyarthritis A progressive, noninfectious, erosive or nonerosive inflammation of multiple joints with or without bone proliferation.

feline capital physeal dysplasia syndrome A condition of unknown etiology in which osteonecrosis of the femoral neck leads to pathologic fracture at the capital physis. May be unilateral or bilateral (if unilateral, the contralateral limb often is affected within 6–12 months).

fibrous joint A bony union with little mobility and lacking a joint cavity (e.g., sutures of the skull, attachment of hyoid bones to petrous temporal bone, attachment of tooth to alveolar bone). Other names: synarthrodial joint, synarthrosis.

field of view Area of the body through which the primary x-ray beam passes. Field of view should be restricted to the area of interest by collimating the x-ray beam. Restriction of the field of view helps maximize image quality, minimize scatter radiation, and decrease distortion.

filament A thin, threadlike conducting wire with a high melting point that is part of the cathode (the negative side of the x-ray tube). The filament is the source of electrons.

filling defect Anything that prevents contrast medium from occupying a hollow organ or space. Appears as a less opaque area(s) on a positive contrast study and a more opaque area(s) on a negative contrast study. May be caused by pathology or artifact.

film:screen system Refers to a conventional radiography set up with a piece of x-ray film sandwiched between two intensifying screens and housed in a light-proof cassette.

fissure line See **pleural fissure line**.

fistulography A radiographic contrast study used to investigate a fistulous tract or draining wound. Fistulogram.

flail chest Refers to instability of the thoracic wall caused by sequential, segmental rib fractures that result in a portion of the chest wall becoming functionally detached. Flail chest is an emergency situation because it results in paradoxical respiratory movements (detached portion is pulled inward during inspiration and pushed outward during expiration).

flexion The bending of a limb or body part; opposite is **extension**.

fluoroscopy A radiologic procedure using x-rays and a fluorescent screen to create real-time radiographic movies of anatomic structures. Fluoroscopy commonly is used to evaluate swallowing, GI motility, dynamic respiratory diseases, movements of the diaphragm, and for interventional studies. Patient and nearby personnel are exposed to relatively high levels of radiation. Modern fluoroscopy systems allow images to be viewed via electronic intensification, which enhances visibility and decreases exposure.

fluid level The interface between fluid and gas, demonstrated by using a horizontal x-ray beam (e.g., standing lateral radiograph, erect ventrodorsal radiograph). Gas must be present to document the fluid level (need to see gas-fluid interface).

focal spot The area on the anode target of an x-ray tube that is struck by electrons and from which x-rays are emitted.

focal film distance (FFD) The distance from the focal spot to the film or image receptor. Other names: source-to-image distance (SID), focal-receptor distance (FRD).

fogging Refers to the nondiagnostic blackening (or graying) of a film radiograph. May be caused by scatter radiation, visible light, pressure, heat, or chemicals.

foreign material Any object or matter that is not normal to the place where it is found. Sometimes the term *foreign body* is used; however, a *body* is the physical structure of an organism.

fracture A break or discontinuity in bone caused by a physical force that exceeds the structural capacity of the bone or by a disease that weakens the bone.

- *articular fracture:* A break in a bone that extends to a joint surface.
- *avulsion fracture:* A break in a bone that occurs at an attachment site (e.g., ligament, tendon) and results in a piece of bone being pulled away from the main bone.
- *chip fracture:* A corner or edge of a bone is broken.
- *closed fracture:* The overlying skin and soft tissues are intact.
- *comminuted fracture:* Multiple breaks in a bone that communicate at a single point; results in three or more fragments.
- *complete fracture:* A break in a bone that extends through the entire bone.
- *compression fracture:* The ends of the bone fragments are impacted into each other, resulting in a shortened or collapsed bone.
- *depression fracture:* A fragment of a broken bone is located below the normal bone surface.
- *fissure fracture:* An incomplete break in a bone that extends from another fracture.
- *folding fracture (torus or buckling fracture):* The cortex is broken on the concave side.
- *greenstick fracture (hairline fracture):* An incomplete linear break on the convex side of a bone.
- *incomplete fracture:* A partial break in a bone; the bone is not in complete discontinuity; appears in radiographs as a break in only one side of the cortex.
- *open fracture:* The overlying skin and soft tissues are perforated.
- *physeal fracture:* A break in bone that involves a physis (occurs in immature animals); see physeal fracture.
- *segmental fracture:* Multiple breaks in a long bone that do not communicate; results in an isolated segment or fragment.
- *simple fracture:* A single break in a bone, resulting in two fragments.
- *stress fracture (fatigue fracture):* A break in a bone caused by damage from repetitive cycling.
- *pathologic fracture:* A break in a bone that has been weakened by underlying disease or a developmental defect.
- *Shearing fracture (abrasion fracture):* An open break or loss of bone secondary to severe friction or glancing trauma.
- *slab fracture:* The edge of a bone is broken and the fracture line extends from one articular surface to the other.

gas-producing bacteria Organisms include *E. coli, Proteus, Aerobacter*; animals with diabetes mellitus are predisposed infection and emphysematous cystitis due to glucosuria.

gastric dilatation and volvulus (GDV) A potentially life threatening, emergency situation that occurs when the stomach rotates around its axis (predominately its longitudinal or mesenteric axis). Rotation displaces the pylorus dorsally and to the left, which results in the duodenum wrapping around the esophagus. Gastric volvulus most often occurs in the clockwise direction (viewing the patient from caudal to cranial). Rotation greater than 180° twists the gastroesophageal junction to prevent eructation and obstructs the pyloric outflow. Gastric dilation can precede or follow gastric volvulus. Transient, intermittent volvulus can occur without dilation. Clinical signs of GDV include a distended and painful abdomen, non-productive retching, hypersalivation, dyspnea, and shock.

gastric ulcer Open sores or holes in the lining of stomach. Gastric ulcers vary from small, superficial erosions to deep, indurated depressions in the gastric mucosa. They often are difficult to see in radiographs. To be reliably diagnosed, the radiographic signs of an ulcer must persist in multiple images. When viewed from the side (x-ray beam is tangential to the ulcer), an ulcer typically appears as a barium-filled outpouching that extends away from the stomach lumen. Larger, more chronic ulcers often are surrounded by thickened mucosa, which may project into the stomach lumen. The edges of an ulcer may taper smoothly, appear irregular, or they may be shaped like a square, the latter similar in appearance to pseudoulcers in the duodenum. When viewed *en face* (the x-ray beam is perpendicular to the ulcer), an ulcer may resemble a bullseye target (⊙). This is because barium fills the central crater in the ulcer and the surrounding thickened wall creates a circular filling defect. A double-contrast gastrogram tends to be more sensitive than barium alone for detecting gastric ulcers. A barium-filled stomach can mask small mucosal lesions.

gastrography A radiographic contrast study of the stomach. Gastrogram.

geographic osteolysis A relatively large area of bone loss.

gout Disease caused by defective metabolism of uric acid. Rare in dogs, most often reported in Dalmatians. High levels of uric acid may lead to formation of cystic calculi and mineral deposits in joints.

gram Years ago, radiographs were also called radiograms. Currently, *gram* is used to describe contrast studies (e.g., esophagram, cystogram); for example, cystography is performed to produce a cystogram.

granuloma A mass or nodule of chronically inflamed tissue with granulations (small, rounded masses of tissue that form during healing), usually associated with an infectious process.

graph In imaging terminology, this term refers to an image. Practically the term has come to mean a survey image ("plain" or non-contrast image): a radiograph.

gravel sign The sedimentation and accumulation of tiny, sand-like mineral opacity objects immediately proximal to the site of a gastric or intestinal obstruction. Stasis allows heavier particles to precipitate.

grid A device designed to block scatter x-rays from reaching the image receptor while allowing transmitted x-rays to pass through. Grids consist of alternate strips of an x-ray absorbing material (usually lead) interspaced with a relatively non-absorbing material such as carbon fiber or aluminum. The grid is positioned between the subject (patient) and the image receptor.

grid cutoff A radiographic artifact caused by incorrect use of a grid that results in unwanted absorption of transmitted x-rays, most often seen with parallel grids.

grid factor The amount of transmitted x-rays absorbed by the grid. A grid factor may be 2, 3, or 4 meaning that the exposure must be increased 2, 3, or 4 times compared to the exposure used with no grid. This calls for more output from the x-ray tube and delivers more exposure to the patient. If the grid factor is 2, then the grid would block 1/2 of the primary rays. Also called "bucky factor" or "dose penalty."

grid lines A series of parallel, less opaque (white) lines across the entire radiograph caused by the undesirable absorption of transmitted x-rays by the lead strips in a grid; a negative density artifact.

grid ratio The ratio of the height of the lead strips to the distance between them. In most grids, the strip height is 2–5 mm and the distance between strips is 0.25–0.4 mm. Grid ratios range from 5 : 1 to 16 : 1.

ground-glass appearance A homogenous, hazy, or somewhat mottled appearing structure that resembles looking at it through semi-opaque glass or "bathroom glass."

growth arrest lines Thin, well-defined, horizontal lines of increased opacity in a long bone diaphysis (most common in femur). May be caused by dietary changes or systemic illness during growth.

heel effect Refers to the variation in intensity of the x-ray beam between cathode and anode sides of the x-ray tube. Because the target is angled, the bottom or "heel" of the anode focal spot absorbs some of the x-rays. Absorption on the anode side results in more x-rays being emitted from the cathode side of the x-ray tube. Therefore, the thicker part of the subject should be positioned on the cathode side to take advantage of the heel effect. The heel effects occurs because x-rays originate not only from the surface of the anode target but also from deep inside. X-rays produced inside the target have to travel back out to join the x-ray beam, and some of these will be attenuated. Some of the x-rays that have to pass through the thicker heel part of the anode will be absorbed, which means fewer x-rays will be emitted from the anode side of the x-ray tube than from the cathode side. The difference between the two sides can be as much as 40%.

hematoma A localized accumulation of blood within tissues outside of the vessels. Other names: bruise, contusion.

hemimelia Congenital partial or complete absence of a normally paired bone (e.g., radius/ulna, tibia/fibula).

hemivertebra Congenital defect resulting in only partial development of a vertebral body.

hemothorax Accumulation of blood within the pleural space.

hernia Abnormal protrusion of an organ or portion of an organ through an opening (commonly in a structure that normally contains it).

herringbone pattern In an esophagram of a cat, this is the appearance of the distal esophagus created by the transverse or oblique mucosal folds in the distal third of the feline esophagus.

heterotopic bone formation Focal ossification in an abnormal location; typically refers to small (less than 3 mm), well-defined and slightly irregular-shaped mineral opacity structures in the lung, which also are called *pulmonary osteomas* or *pulmonary microlithiasis*.

hiatus/hiatal An opening, gap, or cleft; term usually is associated with the diaphragm (e.g., *hiatal hernia*).

high-frequency x-ray machine Type of equipment in which the electric current to the x-ray tube is manipulated to produce nearly constant potential voltage. Constant voltage results in a more uniform production of x-rays with an average energy closer to the selected kVp. With standard x-ray machines (fully rectified, single phase), the voltage rises to peak and falls to zero 120 times per second, which produces an average energy of the x-ray beam equal to only about two-thirds that of the kVp selected on the control panel.

HIS (hospital information system) Term to include all aspects of hospital information (e.g., administration, financial, clinical).

horizontal beam radiography Technique in which the x-ray beam is directed horizontally (i.e., across the x-ray table) to make a radiograph. Animal typically is standing or in lateral recumbency. Technique may be used to document presence of free fluid or gas in a body space, to reposition fluid to better visualize obscured structures, or when minimal movement of the patient is required.

hydrocephalus An excessive accumulation of fluid in the ventricular system of the brain. Obstructive or noncommunicating hydrocephalus is the more common form. It is caused by a ventricular obstruction, which can result from a congenital abnormality, trauma, infection, parasite migration, or neoplasia. Nonobstructive or communicating hydrocephalus is less common and is caused by failure of arachnoid villi to absorb cerebral spinal fluid at an adequate rate. Congenital hydrocephalus is more often reported in small, toy, and brachycephalic dogs (e.g., Yorkshire Terrier, Chihuahua, Maltese, Toy Poodle, Boston Terrier, English Bulldog, Pekingese, Lhasa Apso, Pug, Pomeranian, Cairn Terrier). In cats, hydrocephalus is less common than in dogs (may be hereditary in Siamese cats), and it may be associated with feline infectious peritonitis. Clinical signs of hydrocephalus include an enlarged, dome-shaped cranium with open fontanelles; visual and auditory deficits; vocalization; and an abnormal gait.

hydrocolpos Cystic dilation and accumulation of fluid in the vagina with expansion of the vaginal lumen.

hydronephrosis Dilation of the renal collecting system secondary to a congenital or acquired obstruction to urine outflow. Clinical signs vary with the degree and duration of the obstruction. Acute obstruction often is very painful, and the kidneys may appear normal in radiographs during early/mild obstruction. Chronic partial obstructions may be relatively asymptomatic until the animal is in renal failure. Progressive hydronephrosis leads to unilateral or bilateral renomegaly, usually with smooth margins. Complete obstruction can destroy kidney function within a few days. Telangiectasia can lead to a congenital urinary outflow problem, which may be evident during the vascular phase of an excretory urogram as anomalous vasculature.

hydroureter Dilation of the ureter, most often due to obstruction. Caudal abdominal compression is used to deliberately dilate the renal collecting system to enhance filling and opacification.

hyperostosis Widening of cortical bone due to appositional growth of osseous tissue at endosteum or periosteum.

hyperparathyroidism A systemic condition in which excessive production of parathyroid hormone by overactive parathyroid glands leads to abnormal loss of mineral from bone. May be *primary* caused by parathyroid gland disease (e.g., adenoma, carcinoma, adenomatous hyperplasia) or *secondary* due to nutritional deficiency or chronic renal disease.

hypertrophic osteodystrophy (HOD) A systemic disease of unknown etiology that results in subperiosteal hemorrhage and transient defects in metaphyseal mineralization. Appears in radiographs as line of decreased opacity parallel to physis and mineralization along the metaphysis. May be associated with canine distemper.

hypertrophic osteopathy (HO) A periosteal response that occurs secondary to a mass-effect in the thoracic or abdominal cavity. HO is also called *secondary hypertrophic pulmonary osteopathy* or *Marie's disease*, the latter named for the French pathologist who in 1890 first associated abnormal bone growth with lung disease. It most often is reported in middle-aged to older dogs, but can occur in any age, breed, or gender. The most common cause of HO is intra-thoracic disease (e.g., large lung tumors, infection, severe cardiomegaly), but it can result from certain intra-abdominal infections, tumors, and large masses. The mechanism is unknown, but it likely is associated with periosteal blood flow.

hydrothorax Accumulation of fluid within the pleural space.

iatrogenic Pathology caused by medical examination or treatment.

idiopathic Of unknown etiology; occurring without known cause.

ileus Partial or complete obstruction due to hypomotility or physical blockage. May be associated with intestine, esophagus, ureter, or bile duct.

ill-defined The margin of a structure is not well visualized. A simple test is whether or not you can easily trace the edges of the structure with a pencil or stylus. When used to describe bone lesions, ill-defined osteolysis is more aggressive; an ill-defined periosteal response is more active. *Ill-defined* is not the same as *irregular*. *Well-defined* is not the same as *smooth*.

image detector See **image receptor**.

image receptor The part of an imaging system that captures the image. An imaging receptor may be a film (conventional radiography) or a phosphor plate (digital radiography). X-rays that pass through the patient to the image receptor form the latent image. Other names: detector, image detector.

indistinct See ill-defined, definition, distinction.

infiltrate Accumulation of abnormal cells in a tissue; typically describes diffuse lesions in bone or lung.

intensifying screen A plastic sheet coated with rare earth phosphorous and used to convert x-rays to visible light. Intensifying screens are mounted inside a light-proof cassette, and a piece of x-ray film is placed between two screens in the cassette. Purpose of intensifying screens is to reduce x-ray exposure by enhancing the effect of x-rays on film.

intensity of the x-ray beam The number of x-rays arriving per unit time over a specific area. Beam intensity is controlled by the quality and quantity of x-rays, the size of the field-of-view (amount of collimation), and the distance from the focal spot.

interlobar fissure line See **pleural fissure line**.

International Elbow Working Group Formed in 1989; the IEWG established a grading scale to help classify elbow dysplasia. The severity of the disease is based on the size (thickness) of new bone on the proximal, non-articular border of the anconeal process:

1. Grade 0 (normal): no evidence of new bone production; smooth, well-defined anconeal margin.
2. Grade 1 (mild): anconeal new bone is less than 3 mm thick.
3. Grade 2 (moderate): anconeal new bone is 3–5 mm thick, subchondral osteosclerosis may be present along with the ulnar trochlear notch.
4. Grade 3 (severe): anconeal new bone is greater than 5 mm thick, osteophytes and enthesophytes often are present on the distal humerus and proximal radius.

interstitial pulmonary pattern A radiographic appearance caused by increased amount of tissue, fluid, or cellular material in the non-air-containing lung parenchyma. Increased opacity is within the lung but not involving vessels, bronchi, or alveoli. This is the least specific lung pattern and a frequently overused term. Rarely is a true interstitial lung pattern visible in radiographs without some degree of alveolar filling.

intervertebral disc disease (IVDD) Protrusion or extrusion of disc material into the spinal canal which compress the spinal cord or nerve roots and leads to neurological symptoms. IVDD can occur in any disc and most often results from degeneration of the disc. Dehydration of nucleus pulposus leads to replacement of gelatinous material with cartilage or fibrous tissue, resulting in loss of disc pliability. The nucleus may mineralize, resulting in further loss of compressibility. The annulus fibrosis also degenerates and weakens, allowing disc material to protrude or extrude into spinal canal. The dorsal part of the annulus is the thinnest. Disc material may be gelatinous, fibrous, or mineralized and can damage the spinal cord.

- **Hansen type I disc herniation** Complete extrusion of nucleus pulposus into spinal canal; an acute condition that tends to be clinically more severe than type II and is more common in chondrodystrophic breeds.
- **Hansen type II disc herniation** Protrusion (or bulging) of disc into spinal canal without rupture of annulus; often a more gradual and progressive disease process; more common in older non-chondrodystrophic breeds; also associated with cervical spondylopathy and lumbosacral instability.

intramembranous ossification Refers to the formation of bone in sheets of connective tissue (e.g., bones of the skull).

intravenous urography (IVU) See **excretory urography**.

intussusception A segment of intestine slides or "telescopes" into the lumen of an adjacent segment leading to a partial or complete bowel obstruction. The invaginated segment is called the *intussusceptum* and it is displaced into the receiving segment which is called the *intussuscipiens*. Intussusceptions occur most often either in the jejunum or at the ileocolic junction. An ileocolic intussusception may prevent gas from entering the cecum and ascending colon.

iodinated contrast media Positive contrast agents that contain iodine (atomic number 53). Non-ionic agents are preferred. Ionic agents are hyperosmolar (hypertonic), rapidly absorbed, quickly diluted, and can be irritating to tissues.

ionization Process by which an atom acquires a negative or positive charge by losing or gaining electrons; x-rays contain sufficient energy to cause ionization and can alter molecules, break chemical bonds, and damage or destroy living cells.

ipsilateral On or pertaining to the same side.

irregular A descriptive term that refers only to the shape of a structure or lesion. The term *irregular* should not be confused with *ill-defined*. *Irregular* does not indicate cause, activity, or aggressiveness of a lesion.

kVp (kilovolt peak) The maximum voltage applied across the x-ray tube. Determines the kinetic energy of the electrons and therefore, the highest energy in the x-ray beam. Determines the quality and penetrating ability of the x-ray beam. Influences the radiographic contrast (degree of difference between black and white in a radiograph). 1 kilovolt = 1000 volts.

kyphosis Dorsal curvature of the spine.

labial On the side that faces the lips; used to describe lesions associated with the mouth.

lateral Toward the side; away from the midline plane. Opposite is **medial**.

lateral recumbency Animal is positioned lying on its side.

lateral radiograph The x-ray beam enters the right or left side of a body part and exits the opposite side.

lesion A detected radiographic abnormality.

levocardia The normal left side position of the heart.

lingual On the side that faces the tongue.

lordosis Ventral curvature of the spine.

lumbophrenic angle Junction of the diaphragm and lumbar spine at the dorsocaudal aspect of the thoracic cavity on a lateral radiograph.

lumbosacral instability Abnormal movement between last lumbar and first sacral vertebrae due to a congenital or acquired disorder. Radiographically characterized by narrowing of the vertebral canal or intervertebral foramina (which causes compression of the nerve roots that form the cauda equina in the lumbosacral region). Other names: cauda equina syndrome, lumbosacral stenosis, lumbosacral malarticulation.

lung collapse Partial or complete loss of lung volume due to reduced size of the alveoli and loss of alveolar air. Lung collapse (atelectasis) may appear as alveolar filling and can only be distinguished due to decreased lung size. A mediatinal shift often is present, toward the smaller lung. Common causes include bronchial obstruction, prolonged recumbency.

lung consolidation Increased opacity in lung parenchyma without loss of lung volume. Consolidation is due to alveolar filling. Common causes include pneumonia, hemorrhage, neoplasia, and edema.

lung markings Refers to the radiographically visible bronchial walls and pulmonary vessels.

luxation Complete loss of contact between articular surfaces.

lymphadenopathy Abnormal lymph node; term generally is used to describe lymph node enlargement (more correct term is *lymphadenomegaly*).

lymphography (lymphangiography) A radiographic contrast study of the lymphatic vessels.

Mach band An optical illusion in which a false black line or false white line occurs at the boundary between two different opacities. A negative Mach band (black line) occurs along the edge of a convex structure (e.g., outer margin of bone cortex). A positive Mach band (white line) occurs at the edge of a concave structure (e.g., acetabulum and under femoral head on a ventrodorsal pelvic radiograph), which may be mistaken for osteophytes (i.e., on the femoral neck). Mach bands cannot be eliminated by knowledge of their existence; the illusion occurs in the retina, and the brain actually sees it. Mach bands were described in 1865 by physicist Ernst Mach. Other names: Mach line, edge enhancement.

magnetic resonance imaging (MRI) A diagnostic imaging procedure that creates cross-sectional images of a body part using powerful magnetic fields. The magnetic field temporarily alters the positions of protons in the patient. As these protons return to their normal positions, they emit radio waves that are detected by computers to create images with superior anatomic detail. The patient is not exposed to harmful radiation during an MRI procedure.

magnification Process of enlarging the radiographic appearance of a structure(s) by increasing the object to image receptor distance (OID). Using a small focal spot will aid in maintaining definition that is lost by the change in beam geometry.

malunion fracture The bone has healed, but there is abnormal bone geometry (i.e., bone is abnormally shortened, malaligned, angled, or rotated).

manus Distal part of a thoracic limb; includes carpus, metacarpus, and digits.

mAs (milliampere seconds) Product of the strength of the current through the x-ray tube (milliamperes) and the length of time the current is on (seconds). Determines the number of electrons emitted and, therefore, the number of x-rays produced (quantity of x-ray beam). Influences radiographic density (degree of blackness in a radiograph).

mass effect Displacement of viscera or other structures away from their normal positions without distinct visualization of the borders of a mass.

mass lesion A solitary lesion larger than 3 cm in diameter.

median Pertaining to the middle of the body.

medial Toward the midline of the body or on the inner (axial) surface of an extremity. Along the median. Opposite is **lateral**.

mediastinal shift Displacement of the heart and/or other mediastinal structures toward the right or left side. May be caused by alteration in lung volume, an intra-thoracic mass, unilateral fluid or gas in pleural space, or congenital defect (e.g., pectus excavatum).

meningocele Neural defect in which the meninges protrude through a dorsal spinal defect.

meningomyelocele Neural defect in which the spinal cord, meninges, or nerve roots protrude through a dorsal spinal defect.

mesenchymal Refers to cells that develop into connective tissue, blood vessels, and lymphatic tissue.

metaphysis "Next to the physis". The wider portion of a long bone between the diaphysis and the physis. The area in a long bone where growth cartilage is transformed into cortical bone.

metastatic calcification The deposition of calcium salts in tissues away from a disease site, most often due to abnormal calcium/phosphorus metabolism.

microlithiasis Focal areas of mineralization (less than 3 mm in size) in an organ, usually the lung. (Other names: heterotopic bone formation, pulmonary osteomas).

miliary nodules Small in size, like a millet seed (1–2 mm). Other names: micronodules.

mineralization The abnormal bioprecipitation of inorganic substances (such as calcium) in organic tissue; includes petrification and fossilization. *Calcification* is the normal or abnormal deposition of calcium salts. A type of normal calcification is ossification, which is the deposition of calcium to create new bone. Calcification occurs during ossification, but the reverse is not true. *Heterotopic ossification* produces extra-skeletal bone, which is bone in soft tissues where bone normally does not exist. *Petrification* and *fossilization* are additional types of mineralization.

mixed pulmonary pattern Two or more lung patterns are visible concurrently (i.e., bronchointerstitial, interstitial, and alveolar).

monoarticular One joint (i.e., all lesions in the same joint).

monostotic In the same bone.

moth-eaten osteolysis Multiple areas of bone loss, smaller and less distinct than geographic osteolysis.

mucopolysaccharidosis A group of inherited diseases characterized by accumulations of mucopolysaccharides, which can lead to permanent damage in musculoskeletal, ocular, neurologic, and circulatory systems.

myelocele Neural defect in which the spinal cord protrudes through a dorsal spinal defect.

myelography A radiographic contrast study of the spinal cord involving injection of positive contrast medium into the spinal subarachnoid space. Myelogram.

myelosclerosis Increased opacity in the medullary cavity of bone, fibrosis of the bone marrow

myositis ossificans The deposition of inorganic materials in muscle, usually secondary to trauma.

mural Pertaining to or occurring in the wall of a body cavity.

negative contrast agent A contrast medium that absorbs very few x-rays and is less opaque than soft tissue or fat (i.e., a gas such as room air, carbon dioxide, nitrous oxide, or oxygen).

nephrogram The phase in excretory urography during which the kidneys are opacified by positive contrast medium.

niche A recess in the wall of a hollow organ that retains contrast. Ulcers and diverticuli are examples.

nodular lesion A spherical lesion measuring up to 30 mm in diameter.

nodular pulmonary pattern One or more small, rounded lesions in the lung (i.e., a structured interstitial pulmonary pattern).

nonionic iodinated contrast media Positive contrast agents that are water-soluble but not converted into ions, similar in osmolality to plasma, and cause fewer adverse reactions compared with ionic contrast media.

nonunion fracture Fracture healing ceases before a complete union has occurred.

Norberg angle A numerical assessment of coxofemoral joint subluxation made on an extended ventrodorsal pelvic radiograph. Measurement is made by drawing a line connecting the centers of the two femoral heads and another line extending from the center of each femoral head to the cranial edge of the corresponding acetabular rim. Norberg angle greater than 105 is normal, between 90 and 105 is borderline, and less than 90 is abnormal.

object The thing or item being radiographed (i.e., patient or body part). Other names: subject, patient.

object-film distance (OFD) The distance between the patient and the film or image receptor. In digital radiography, object-receptor distance.

object-receptor distance (ORD) The distance between the patient and the image receptor or receptor.

oblique radiograph Animal or body part is slightly rotated from true lateral or true ventrodorsal/dorsoventral positioning to displace overlying structures from area of interest or to view a structure in profile. Oblique radiography may also be accomplished by changing the angle of the x-ray beam.

obstipation Inability to pass feces.

OFA Orthopedic Foundation for Animals, established in 1966.

oligocephalic Shape of skull in which the nasal cavity is approximately equal in length to the cranium. Other names: mesaticephalic.

opacity (radiopacity) Characteristic of a material to block (attenuate or absorb) x-rays. The more opaque a material, the more x-rays are blocked and the whiter the material appears in a radiograph. One of five basic opacities is assigned to a material; gas, fat, soft tissue, bone, or metal. The inherent opacity of a material is related to its density (atomic number and degree of compaction). Overall opacity of a material relates to its thickness.

opacity interface The visible difference in shades of gray between two adjacent structures which allows them to be differentiated in a radiograph. Without opacity interfaces, a radiography would be homogenous, with no visible structures (see **relative opacity**). Opacity interfaces are affected by body condition (e.g., emaciation, immature age) and disease processes (e.g., effusion) and should not be confused with detail (affected by technical factors) or definition (refers to margination of a lesion).

opaque Not clear or transparent; impenetrable, not allowing light, radiation, sound, heat, etc. to pass through; not transmitting any of these.

organic iodinated compounds Positive contrast agents commonly used to study intravascular, intrathecal, intraarticular, and soft tissue structures. High atomic number and mass of iodine result in high opacity in these agents, which are available as ionic (hypertonic) and nonionic (isotonic) preparations.

orthogonal radiographs Radiographs made at right angles (perpendicular or 90 degrees) to each other. Radiographs are two-dimensional images of three-dimensional subjects and orthogonal projections are required for meaningful evaluation.

ossification The process of creating new bone by osteoblasts, usually in a cartilaginous or fibrous tissue matrix. Calcification occurs during ossification, but the reverse is not true.

ossification center A site of bone formation; primary centers of ossification develop in the diaphyses, secondary centers develop in the epiphyses and apophyses, and accessory centers form sesamoid bones.

osteoblasts Cells that deposit bony matrix and are responsible for ossification.

osteoclasts Cells that dissolve bone mineral and matrix; an osteoclast can resorb eight times amount of bone produced by an osteoblast.

osteocytes Cells in bone that help maintain calcium homeostasis and mechanical properties of bone.

osteochondritis dissecans (OCD) A developmental condition in which abnormal blood supply to epiphyseal bone disturbs endochondral ossification, resulting in thickening, softening, necrosis, and eventual collapse of cartilage.

osteochondroma A benign bony mass caused by abnormal location of physeal cartilage. Mass usually stops growing at skeletal maturity, but malignant transformation to chondrosarcoma or osteosarcoma can occur. Appears as an expansile, inhomogeneous, osseous mass extending away from bone, typically with irregular borders and well-defined margins. Multiple osteochondroma is called osteochondromatosis or multiple cartilaginous exostoses.

osteogenesis imperfecta Rare in dogs and cats, it is a generalized condition caused by a defect in collagen production and resulting in fragile bones. May be confused with hyperparathyroidism.

osteolysis An abnormal area of active bone resorption caused by disease. The pattern of osteolysis reflects the aggressiveness of the disease process. The more aggressive the disease process, the less distinct the bony margins, the longer the zone of transition between normal and abnormal bone, and the more rapid the rate of change in serial radiographs. Patterns of osteolysis include geographic, moth-eaten, and permeative.

osteoma A rare, benign, slow-growing, osseous neoplasm that protrudes from the surface of a bone, usually on the skull.

osteomalacia Softening of bones due to faulty mineralization of available osteoid; may result from nutritional deficiency, chronic renal or intestinal disease. The ratio of mineral to osteoid is low (bone is "bad quality, good quantity").

osteomyelitis Inflammation of bone; usually caused by an acute or chronic infection (e.g., bacterial, fungal, protozoal organisms). Technically, bone and medullary cavity.

osteopenia "Too little bone"; there is a decrease in bone mass due to osteolysis, osteoporosis, or osteomalacia.

osteopetrosis Uncommon congenital disease leading to a generalized increase in bone thickness and opacity. Other names: marble bone.

osteophyte A well-defined bony growth or bone spur projecting outward from a periarticular margin. Results from degeneration and mineralization of proliferating articular cartilage in non-weight-bearing areas. The common true sign of degenerative joint disease.

osteoporosis "Porous bones"; loss of bone mass leading to weak and brittle bones with decreased opacity; may result from disuse or metabolic disease. The ratio of mineral to osteoid is normal, but both are diminished (bone is "good quality, bad quantity"). Other names: bone atrophy.

osteosclerosis (sclerosis) Increased bone opacity; an area of bone with elevated density (more mineral is present in the bone). Radiographically more opaque.

otic canalography A radiographic contrast study of the external auditory canal.

PACS (picture archiving and communication system) A network of computers used to accomplish many of the services required in digital radiography:

P: Pictures made available for viewing, interpretation, reporting, and consultation from multiple modalities (radiology, ultrasound, CT, MRI, etc.).

A: Archiving and storage of imaging studies for both short and long terms.

C: Communication with local and remote computers, professionals, and consultants to manage workflow and share information.

S: System coordination and integration to works with radiology information systems (RIS), hospital information systems (HIS), and others to enable a paperless environment.

palmar Associated with the palm of the hand; refers to the bottom surface of a distal thoracic limb or manus. Opposed to dorsal.

panosteitis A self-limiting bone disorder of unknown etiology that causes an acute onset of pain in one or more bones. Multiple bones may be affected either simultaneously or sequentially. Lameness commonly shifts between legs. Lesions usually are asymmetrical in distribution. Appears in radiographs as areas of increased medullary opacity, typically near a nutrient foramen and sometimes with a periosteal response.

parenteral Any means of administering a substance to a patient that does not involve the alimentary tract (e.g., injecting directly into the body, transcutaneous, inhaled).

parosteal osteosarcoma A rare, slow-growing bone tumor that arises from the surface of the bone instead of the intramedullary region. Commonly appears as a smooth-bordered, nonaggressive bony mass arising from the surface of the bone.

patchy Refers to multiple, indistinct, irregularly shaped lesions; commonly used to describe amorphous areas of increased opacity in the lungs.

pathologic fracture A loss of continuity in a bone that has been weakened by an underlying disease process or developmental defect; typically caused by neoplasia or metabolic bone disease.

penumbra The partial outer shadows that blur the edges of structures and decrease radiographic detail. Occurs due to the fact that x-rays do not originate from a single point but are generated over a small area. Penumbra can be minimized by using a small focal spot, a longer distance between the focal spot and image receptor, and a shorter distance between the patient (subject or object) and image receptor. Other names: geometric unsharpness.

peribronchial cuffing or infiltrates Thickened soft tissue opacity around a bronchus due to accumulation of fluid, cells, or fibrosis; a sign of bronchial disease or peribronchial accumulation; also bronchial cuffing.

perineal hernia Weakening of the muscles that support the rectum (i.e., the pelvic diaphragm) allows displacement of fat and organs from the pelvis and abdominal cavity (e.g., rectum, prostate gland, urinary bladder). Rectal displacement or diverticulum leads to partial or complete obstruction and colon largely distended with fecal material (fecal impaction). Soft tissue swelling often is visible in the perineal region, located ventral and lateral to the base of the tail. The rectum may be deviated laterally (VD view). The urinary bladder may or may not be recognized (may need retrograde urethrocystogram for identification). Barium enema: may document rectal deviation or rectal diverticulum. The inflated bulb of the rectal catheter can obscure lesions in the anal canal and distal rectum. Pneumocolon can help identify colon location and shape.

periosteal response Formation of new bone to fill the space created when the periosteum is separated from the cortex. New bone forms perpendicular to the periosteum. The appearance of the margin of the periosteal new bone formation reflects the activity of the disease process (the less distinct the margin, the more active the disease process).

periosteum Outer covering of bones; covers exterior of all bones except at the joint surfaces. Periosteum consists of two layers; a tough outer layer of fibrous connective tissue for protection and an inner cambium layer for bone production. The cambium produces new bone for circumferential growth in immature bones and healing when bone is damaged and periosteum is separated from cortex.

permeative osteolysis Numerous tiny areas of bone loss, sometimes difficult to distinguish from normal bone.

pes Distal part of a pelvic limb; includes tarsus, metatarsus, and digits.

phosphor A rare-earth compound that emits an instantaneous flash of light after interaction with an x-ray. The light is phosphorescence rather than fluorescence (latter glows for a longer period of time).

physis The cartilaginous growth plate located between the metaphysis and the epiphysis of an immature long bone. Other names: epiphyseal plate, growth plate.

physeal fracture A break in bone that occurs through a physis (occurs in immature animals). Fracture commonly is described using Salter–Harris classification. The physis affected and the age at which the damage occurred are important because the percentage of growth at the proximal and distal ends of a long bone varies over time. The greatest difference between proximal and distal physeal growth occurs in the ulna, where the distal physis contributes approximately 90% to overall growth. The distal ulnar physis is particularly susceptible to damage due to its unique conical shape.

phytobezoar An accumulation or concretion of plant material (fruit, vegetable, or grass fibers) within the alimentary tract (usually stomach or intestine).

plantar Associated with the sole of the foot; refers to the bottom surface of a distal pelvic limb or pes. Opposite of dorsal when referring to a hindlimb.

pleural fissure line Linear increased opacity between lung lobes. May represent pleural thickening (line is uniform in thickness and does not taper), pleural effusion (line widens peripherally and tapers toward the hilus), or interlobar fat (line is wider centrally and tapers peripherally). Other names: interlobar fissure line, fissure line.

pleural thickening Increased width and opacity of parietal or visceral pleura due to deposits of fibrin or mineral.

pleurography A radiographic contrast study of the parietal and visceral pleural surfaces made by instilling contrast medium into the pleural space.

plication Abnormal bunching of small intestine with tight turns and irregular pockets of gas, commonly caused by linear foreign material. Other names: pleating, accordion pleating.

pneumatocoele An air-filled cyst in a lung; usually results from trauma.

pneumomediastinum Presence of free gas in the mediastinum; results in visualization of mediastinal structures not normally seen.

pneumopericardiography A radiographic contrast study of the pericardial space; used to evaluate the pericardial sac, epicardial surface of the heart, and origin of the aorta and pulmonary arteries. Typically performed by instilling gas in the pericardial sac.

pneumoperitoneum Free gas in the peritoneal space.

pneumoperitoneography A radiographic contrast study of the peritoneal space; gas is instilled into the peritoneal space.

pneumothorax Presence of free gas in the pleural space.

- *Simple* pneumothorax: air in pleural space is less than or equal to atmospheric pressure.
- *Closed* pneumothorax: a simple pneumothorax caused by either a ruptured lung, ruptured airway, or ruptured esophagus, the latter as an extension of a pneumomediastinum. The thoracic wall remains intact and the pleural gas originates from inside the body. In patients with small lung ruptures that seal rapidly, pleural gas usually is resorbed within 48 hours.
- *Open* pneumothorax: a simple pneumothorax caused by a penetrating wound that creates an opening in the thoracic wall that allows air (gas) to enter the pleural space. Pleural pressure is similar to atmospheric pressure.
- *spontaneous* pneumothorax occurs acutely with no history of trauma. Gas may leak into the pleural space from a ruptured lung bulla or an eroded airway, the latter due to a tumor, abscess, or parasite migration.
- *Tension* pneumothorax: a closed pneumothorax in which pressure within the pleural space is greater than atmospheric pressure, resulting in compression atelectasis of the lung(s).

pollakiuria Increased frequency of urination.

polyarticular Associated with multiple joints.

polyarthritis Inflammation affecting multiple joints.

polydactyly Congenital abnormality in which one or more extra digits are present.

polyostotic Associated with multiple bones.

poorly-defined Similar meaning to *ill-defined*, but sometimes used as a qualifier when making a decision between *well-defined* and *ill-defined*. Such a lesion should be reevaluated in a week or so, especially if the lesion margins are becoming better-defined on serial radiographs but not quite well-defined.

portography A radiographic contrast study of the portal venous system. Contrast agent is injected into a mesenteric vein (venous portography) or the spleen (splenoportography).

portosystemic vascular shunt (PSS) An abnormal communication between the portal vascular system and the systemic circulation. PSS may be congenital or acquired, intra-hepatic or extrahepatic. Congenital intra-hepatic shunts are more common in large-breed dogs (e.g., Irish Wolfhound, Golden Retriever) and often include a persistent ductus venosus. Congenital extra-hepatic shunts are more common in cats and small-breed dogs (e.g., Miniature Schnauzer, Yorkshire Terrier) and usually involve azygous vein or caudal vena cava. Congenital PSS can result from microvascular dysplasia, an inherited abnormality in small breed dogs (e.g., Cairn Terrier) in which tiny blood vessels in liver are absent or underdeveloped. Acquired PSS more often are reported in older animals with chronic liver disease that leads to portal hypertension (multiple shunts often are present).

positive contrast agent A contrast medium that absorbs many x-rays and is more opaque than soft tissue or bone (e.g., barium sulfate, organic iodinated compounds).

pronate To rotate a limb inward so that the palmar or plantar surface faces downward (or lateral) and the dorsal or cranial surface faces upward (or medial).

proportionate dwarfism Chondrodysplasia that affects all parts of the skeleton equally, usually due to inadequate growth hormone caused by a pituitary problem. Most often is reported in German Shepherds, Miniature Pinschers, Spitzes, and Covelian Bear Dogs. Concurrent anomalies may be present, including hypothyroidism, patent ductus arteriosus, and megaesophagus.

proximal Anatomical term that means nearest the trunk or point of origin. Proximal is used to describe the part of a limb nearest its attachment to the body or the part of a body structure that is closer to its origin (trachea, bronchi, intestines, ureters, etc.). Opposite is **distal**.

pseudoarthrosis "False joint"; a fibrous capsule filled with serum that may form at the site of a long-term nonunion fracture, chronic dislocation, or developmental abnormality.

pseudo-nodule A discrete soft tissue or mineral opacity that mimics a pulmonary nodule (e.g., end-on visualization of a pulmonary vessel, superimposed nipple, costochondral junction, heterotopic bone formation).

pseudogout Also called *chondrocalcinosis* or *calcium pyrophosphate deposition disease*, is a rare condition of unknown etiology that can cause soft tissue mineralization near or in a joint.

pulmonary emphysema Refers to increased size of lung air spaces due to air trapping secondary to severe bronchial disease and inability to expire trapped air.

pyelogram The phase in excretory urography during which contrast medium opacifies the renal collecting system (e.g., renal pelvis, pelvic recesses).

pyothorax Accumulation of purulent exudate in the pleural space.

pyruvate kinase deficiency An inherited deficit in an erythrocyte enzyme that can lead to hemolytic anemia. Radiographs may reveal increased medullary opacity in all parts of the appendicular and axial skeleton. The disease has been reported in certain dog breeds (e.g., Basenji, West Highland White Terriers) and in cats. Affected animals typically exhibit clinical signs of anemia, including lethargy and exercise intolerance.

quantum (plural *quanta*) A unit of electromagnetic energy that is the smallest quantity that can exist on its own. A quantum acts both like a particle and a wave.

Quantum mottle The "noise" in a radiograph caused by the random manner in which x-rays strike an image receptor. It gives the image a grainy or sand-like appearance and reduces radiographic detail. This is the fluctuation in the number of x-rays (quanta) per unit of x-ray beam that are recorded by the image receptor.

radiograph The image produced by passing x-rays through an object onto a radiosensitive image receptor. Other names: radiogram, Roentgenogram.

radiographic density Refers to the amount of blackness in a radiograph. Increased radiographic density = increased blackness.

radiographic finding An abnormality in a radiograph; a radiographic sign that is detected and reported.

radiographic sign An abnormality or the unexpected appearance of a structure in a radiograph, also radiographic finding.

radiography The science and art of making radiographs. Other names: Roentgenography.

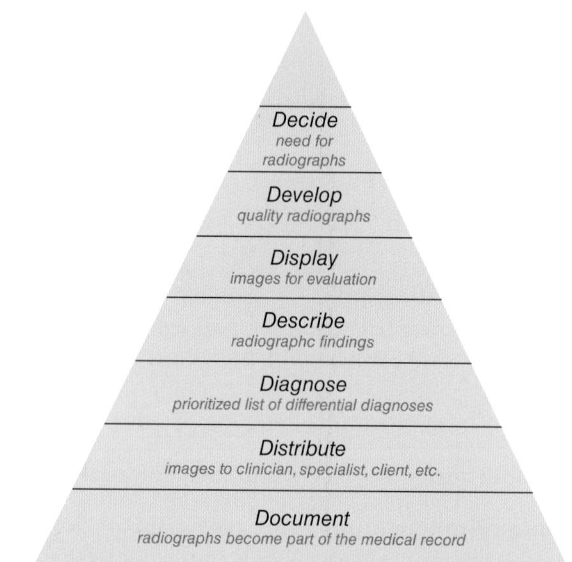

This illustration depicts the basic steps in radiography. All radiographs are processed, displayed, interpreted, distributed, and stored. Film radiography provides a single product for all of these, whereas digital radiography separates them into individual steps.

radiologist A specialist trained in the diagnostic and therapeutic uses of x-rays, radionuclides, radiation physics, and radiation biology. Other names: Roentgenologist.

radiology The scientific discipline of medical imaging using ionizing radiation, radionuclides, nuclear magnetic resonance, and ultrasound.

radiolucent/radiopaque Classically, these terms are used to label materials that block few or many x-rays or to indicated parts of a radiograph that appear lighter or darker than expected. These are subjective terms that convey less useful information than simply describing the relative opacity. For example, soft tissue opacity cystic calculi might commonly be labeled "radiolucent." These calculi would not be visible in a bladder filled with urine, yet they are labeled "radiolucent." The same calculi would be labeled "radiopaque" in a negative contrast cystogram. They would again be labeled "radiolucent" in a double contrast cystogram. It is much more useful to simply describe the calculi as "soft tissue opacity."

radiopacity See **opacity** (in a radiography text, *radio-* is a given and the radiopacity can be shortened to *opacity*).

recumbent (recumbency) Lying down; used to describe the position of a patient during radiography; e.g., lateral recumbency = lying on its side, sternal recumbency = lying on its ventrum, dorsal recumbency = lying on its back.

receptor See **image receptor**.

reflux Reversed flow, such as flow of gastric content into the esophagus, flow of esophageal content into the mouth, flow of contrast medium from urinary bladder into ureters.

regurgitation: Reflux of undigested food from the esophagus into the pharynx or nasal cavity (differentiate from vomiting).

relative opacity Refers to the differences in x-ray absorption by various materials. Every material absorbs x-rays in a characteristic manner, depending on the physical composition of that material. It is the variation in x-ray absorption that allows various materials to be differentiated on radiographs. Relative opacity of a material is described as it compares to (i) one of the five basic opacities (gas, fat, fluid, mineral, or metal), (ii) the opacity of adjacent structures (i.e., relatively increased or decreased in opacity), or (iii) the opacity of a known normal structure. Overall opacity of a material is also affected by its thickness.

retained cartilaginous core A temporary or permanent presence of cartilage in the distal portion of a long bone, most commonly in the distal ulna. Cartilage is soft tissue opacity. Core typically is shaped like a triangle, cone, or "candle flame."

reticular pattern Refers to a fine interlacing pattern of lines; usually used to describe appearance of an interstitial pulmonary pattern.

rheumatoid arthritis A severe, progressive, and destructive polyarthritis caused by circulating autoantibodies against IgG.

rhinography A radiographic contrast study of the nasal cavity.

rickets Vitamin D deficiency in young animals resulting in softening and weakening of bones.

RIS (radiology information system) Used to coordinate, manipulate, distribute, and store diagnostic imaging data.

Roentgen Wilhelm Conrad Roentgen, a German physicist who discovered x-rays in 1895 and won the first Nobel Prize in physics for his discovery.

Roentgenography Synonym for radiography.

rostral Toward the nose when discussing the head. Opposite is **caudal**.

Radiography Rules of Two

- **Two views** orthogonal radiographs are needed for complete interpretation.
- **Two opacities** a structure is visible only if it is adjacent to a structure with a different opacity.
- **Two occurrences** radiographic signs usually are visible in more than one view; if not, rule out artifact.
- **Two lesions** after finding an abnormality do not stop searching, always look for a second.
- **Two joints** include joints above and below a long bone.
- **Two tissues** if bone appears abnormal, examine the adjacent soft tissues; if soft tissue looks abnormal, examine the nearby bones.
- **Two sides** compare the opposite side or limb with suspected abnormality to opposite side or limb.
- **Two examples** compare radiographic findings with known normal radiographs.
- **Two occasions** compare current radiographs with previous radiographs (sometimes the old radiograph is the most important one).
- **Two visits** make follow-up radiographs to assess progress and response to therapy.
- **Two reads** evaluate radiographs again in light of patient history and results of laboratory testing.

sacrocaudal dysgenesis Developmental abnormality in which one or more sacral or caudal vertebrae is absent (e.g., Manx cats). Affected cats have been referred to as "stumpies" or "rumpies," depending on severity.

sail sign Refers to the normal thymus in an immature animal as seen on a ventrodorsal or dorsoventral radiograph; appears as a triangular-shaped soft tissue opacity structure in the cranial mediastinum, projecting toward the left. Sail sign is abnormal in adults.

sagittal Associated with the long axis or ventrodorsal plane of the body; ventrodorsal plane extends from head to tail and divides the body into right and left halves. Comes from Latin word meaning "arrow."

Salter–Harris type of fracture A classification scheme to describe fractures in immature bones according to degree of epiphyseal, physeal, and metaphyseal involvement and ranked by increasing probability of a gross deformity during healing.

- **type I** Fracture involves physis only.
- **type II** Fracture involves physis and metaphysis.
- **type III** Fracture involves physis and epiphysis.

- **type IV** Fracture involves physis, metaphysis, and epiphysis.
- **type V** A compression fracture of the physis.
- **type VI** A compression fracture involving only part of the physis.

scalloping Refers to the shape of a border which appears as a series of curved indentations. Used to describe lung margins during pleural effusion or cranial edge of caudally displaced diaphragm during severe pulmonary overinflation (latter is also called tenting of the diaphragm).

scatter radiation Secondary x-rays created by interactions of primary x-rays with the materials in their paths. Scatter x-rays travel in unpredictable directions and do not provide any useful information in the radiograph. They degrade image quality and expose patient and nearby personnel to unnecessary radiation. The amount of scatter increases as the volume of tissue irradiated increases. The larger the field-of-view and the thicker the body part, the more scatter radiation. Scatter is reduced using tight collimation and a grid or air gap.

scintigraphy A radiologic procedure involving the use of radioisotopes to provide functional information about an organ or body part. Scintigraphy is very sensitive in the detection of disease but not very specific as to etiology.

sclerosis See **osteosclerosis**.

scoliosis Lateral curvature of the spine; an "S"-shaped spine.

serial radiographs Images made in sequence either during a single study (e.g., gastrointestinal series, excretory urography) or over longer intervals of time (days or weeks) as follow-up evaluations to monitor progress and response to therapy of a disease or disorder.

sequestrum A fragment of bone that has lost its blood supply and is no longer viable. A sequestrum may be located in a less opaque area of bone called a *lacuna* and surrounded by an envelope of bone called an *involucrum*.

sialography A radiographic contrast study of the salivary ducts and glands.

skyline radiograph Primary x-ray beam is tangential to area of interest. Frequently involves flexion or extension of a body part.

source-to–image distance (SID) Distance between the focal spot (source of x-rays) and the image receptor. In film radiography, it is the focal-film distance.

signet ring sign Used to describe the radiographic appearance of a structure that resembles the shape of a finger ring with an insignia on the front. For example, a paragonimus lesion in which gas is present in a cyst along with a fluke. Also used to describe end-on visualization of a bronchus and adjacent pulmonary artery.

silhouette sign See **border effacement**.

source-to-object distance (SOD) Distance between the focal spot (source of x-rays) and the object being radiographed (i.e., subject or patient). Other names: focal-object distance (FOD).

specific gravity The ratio of the physical density (mass per unit volume) of a material relative to water.

speed A measure of the sensitivity of a film:screen system to x-rays and light.

spina bifida Congenital abnormality in which failure of the lateral vertebral arches to fuse dorsally results in incomplete development of the dorsal spinal process(es); also called "split spine" or "cleft spine." *Spina bifida occulta* is characterized by a small, asymptomatic split in a vertebra with a normal spinal cord. *Spina bifida manifesta* presents with a larger vertebral defect and a saclike protrusion (herniation) that contains spinal cord, meninges, or both: *myelocele*: sac contains spinal cord; *meningocele*: sac contains meninges; *meningomyelocele*: sac contains meninges and spinal cord or nerve roots. Cross-sectional imaging (e.g., CT, MRI) and myelography provide a more detailed evaluation.

spondylitis Inflammation of a vertebral body, usually caused by infection (e.g., migrating foreign material).

spondylosis deformans A noninflammatory degenerative disorder associated with the vertebral bodies and characterized by complete or incomplete bony bridging of ventral and lateral margins of vertebrae. NOT osteophytes.

static fog Radiographic artifact caused by static electricity; appears as blackened areas with irregularly branching patterns (resembles a picture of lightning) or as multiple foci (black dots) in a radiograph. Occurs more often in areas with low humidity (in some hospitals, antistatic strips are installed to discharge personnel prior to opening cassettes or handling film).

stenosing tenosynovitis involving the tendon of the abductor pollicis longus A chronic inflammation caused by overuse. Inflammation leads to fibrosis and enthesophyte formation on the dorsomedial aspect of the distal radius, and restriction of tendon movement.

stress fracture A break in bone caused by repetitive stress. The micro-damage to the bone occurs at a greater rate than can be offset by the reparative process.

stress radiography Technique used to investigate joint instability or subluxation. The bones proximal and distal to a joint are stabilized and a medial-to-lateral, lateral-to-medial, or orthogonal force is applied to document abnormal widening of the joint space or displacement of bones.

string sign Used to describe the radiographic appearance of a narrowed GI structure in a positive contrast study, such as bowel or pyloric outflow tract in a gastrogram or upper GI study. May or may not be due to disease; string sign may occur with peristalsis.

subluxation Partial loss of contact between articular surfaces.

summation Overlap of tissues in different planes which results in greater blockage of x-rays due to addition of attenuating characteristics of each tissue. Produces a whiter area on the radiograph at the site of overlap.

supinate To rotate a limb outward so that the palmar or plantar surface faces upward or medial and the dorsal or cranial surface faces downward or lateral.

survey radiographs A standard radiographic study of an area of the body (e.g., thorax, abdomen, head, extremity) made without the use of contrast medium. Also plain radiographs, flat plate radiographs.

syndactyly Congenital abnormality in which two are more digits are fused.

synostosis Fusion of normally separate bones. Other names: bony ankylosis.

synovial joint A freely movable articulation with a joint cavity, joint capsule, synovial fluid, and articular cartilage. Other names: diarthrodial joint, diarthrosis.

synovial osteochondroma Benign nodular proliferation of synovial membrane (primary form) or as a sequela to damaged cartilage (secondary form). Secondary form is more common and may result in mineralized fragments in the joint. A cartilage flap that breaks off and is nourished by synovial fluid may grow and mineralize; especially in the shoulders.

systematic approach An organized and deliberate method of examining a radiograph to avoid overlooking diagnostic information.

table top technique Image receptor (e.g., film, cassette) is placed on top of the table without an interposed grid between x-ray tube and receptor. Animal is positioned on top of the receptor. Because in most configurations, the grid is in a Bucky tray within the table, techniques using a grid may be called Bucky technique and without a grid, tabletop technique.

target Anode (positive) part of x-ray tube and site of x-ray production; composed of metal alloy with high melting point which is able to withstand the high temperatures generated by interaction with electron beam.

teat sign Describes the appearance of the pyloric antrum during a barium contrast study in which a relatively sharp, pointed, out-pouching of the pyloric antrum develops along the lesser curvature as a peristaltic wave pushes the contrast medium up against a mass-like or stenotic lesion around the pylorus.

technique chart A table of reliable x-ray exposures based on body part and thickness. Chart may be kVp variable or mAs variable. If a technique chart is not available, here are some quick tips to estimate mAs and kVp:

- Estimate mAs: multiply the patient's body weight in pounds by 0.1 and add 1 (mAs = (body wt. × 0.1) + 1). For example: to make an abdominal radiograph of a 22 pound dog, the mAs should be 3.2; (22 × 0.1) + 1 = 3.2. For thorax radiographs use 1/2 the mAs and for orthopedic images double it.
- Estimate mAs: another method is to estimate mAs based on patient body weight. For patients less than 10 kg, use 2.5–5 mAs; patients that weigh 10–25 kg, use 5–10 mAs, and for patients over 25 kg, sue 10–15 mAs.
- Estimate kVp: multiply the body part thickness in centimeters by 2 and add the SID in inches (kVp = (thickness × 2) + SID). For example: to make an abdominal radiograph of a body part that measures 14 cm thick and using a 35 inch SID, the kVp should be 63; (14 × 2) + 35 = 63.

telangiectasia A congenital vascular malformation that leads to dilation of ducts; can affect kidneys and other organs and may lead to thromboembolic disease, hydronephrosis; has been reported in Welsh Terriers and other dog breeds.

tenting Describes the appearance of an extremely caudally displaced diaphragm in which the diaphragmatic attachments become visible as cranially directed, pointed projections on a ventrodorsal or dorsoventral radiograph. May result from tension pneumothorax or severe overinflation of lungs.

thoracic inlet The cranial opening into the thoracic cavity, bounded bilaterally by the first pair of ribs, dorsally by the first thoracic vertebra, and ventrally by the manubrium.

tissue density Refers to the physical property of a body structure to attenuate x-rays based on the mass or specific gravity of that structure. Also called subject density and in modern radiography opacity. Bone and teeth are most dense; gas is least dense. Increased tissue density is increased opacity and leads to increased x-ray attenuation and whiter areas in a radiograph. Radiographic density is the blacker areas in a radiograph.

tracheal ratio Technique used to objectively measure the size of the tracheal lumen by comparing the width of the trachea to the width of the thoracic inlet. Measurements are made on a lateral view at the level of a line connecting the first sternebra and first thoracic vertebra.

tracheal stripe sign Occurs when the esophagus contains gas and the ventral esophageal wall blends with the dorsal tracheal wall to mimic false thickening of the tracheal wall (sign indicates presence of gas in the esophagus). Other name; tracheoesophageal stripe sign.

tracheography A radiographic contrast study of the lumen of the trachea.

tram lines Parallel soft tissue or mineral opacity lines representing abnormal bronchial walls (walls are thickened and/or increased in opacity and do not taper normally). Characteristic of a bronchial pulmonary pattern, but not as reliable for identifying thickened bronchi as donut signs (paired pulmonary vessels are often mistaken for thickened bronchial walls and confused with tram lines). Other names: railroad tracks.

transitional vertebra A developmental abnormality in which a vertebra has anatomic characteristics of two adjacent vertebral regions. (e.g., sacralization of L7, lumbarization of S1).

transmitted x-rays X-rays that pass through a patient unchanged. In an average abdominal study, only 1% of the primary x-rays (those emitted by the x-ray tube) that reach the patient are transmitted through the body. The rest are either scattered or absorbed, mostly scattered. Of the 1% transmitted x-rays, only 0.5% actually interact with the image receptor to form an image.

Triadan system A numbering system that provides a consistent method of identifying teeth across all animal species.

trichobezoar An accumulation or concretion of hair in the alimentary tract (usually stomach or intestine).

trichophytobezoar A concretion of hair and plant materials in the alimentary tract (usually stomach or intestine).

tungsten An element that is advantageous in the production of x-rays. Its high atomic number ($Z = 74$) gives more efficient Bremsstrahlung production compared to lower atomic number materials. Tungsten has a high melting point (3422°) and a low rate of evaporation, which makes it capable of high thermionic emission. Tungsten is highly malleable, so it can be formed into thin wire for the cathode filament.

typhlitis Inflammation of the cecum.

ultrasonography An imaging procedure that uses high-frequency sound waves to noninvasively examine soft tissue architecture and function with real-time dynamic imaging. No ionizing radiation or other known safety hazard is encountered with diagnostic ultrasonography. Value of ultrasonography is highly user dependent, relying on the sonographer's patience, skill, and experience.

ununited anconeal process Failure of the ossification center to fuse with the proximal ulna before 22 weeks of age (24 weeks in German shepherd dog).

upper gastrointestinal study A radiographic contrast study of the stomach and small intestine.

urachus A fetal embryologic canal or tube allowing communication between the fetal urinary bladder and the umbilical cord placenta.

ureterocele A congenital abnormality resulting in an abnormal, focal, cyst-like dilation of a terminal ureter.

urethrography A radiographic contrast study of the urethra. Urethrogram.

urography A radiographic contrast study of the kidneys and ureters. Other names: excretory urography, intravenous urography (old term: intravenous pyelogram or IVP).

vacuum phenomenon In a joint, a collection of gas that results when traction is applied creating negative intra-articular pressure, which allows nitrogen in the synovial fluid to escape and leak into the joint.

vaginography A radiographic contrast study of the vagina, cervix, and urethra.

vascular pulmonary pattern Pulmonary arteries or/and veins are larger or smaller than normal.

ventral Toward the belly or sternum. Contrast **dorsal**.

ventral recumbency Animal is positioned lying on its sternum.

ventrodorsal (VD) radiograph The x-ray beam enters the ventral surface of a body part and exits the dorsal surface.

vertebral heart size (VHS) An objective measurement of the size of the cardiac silhouette made on a lateral view thoracic radiograph using the lengths of thoracic vertebral bodies as units of measure. Technique is based on a study performed by Buchanan and Bucheler in 1995. Also called vertebral heart score, vertebral heart sum.

vertical beam The x-ray beam is directed vertically.

visual acuity The ability to resolve a spatial pattern in an image.

vomit Forceful expulsion of gastric or intestinal content through the mouth due to reflex contractions of stomach and abdominal muscles and preceded by nausea; usually caused by a problem caudal to the diaphragm (differentiate from regurgitation).

well-defined A distinct margin. A simple test to determine whether a margin is well defined or not is to attempt to accurately draw a line around the lesion or border. If you can easily trace the edges, it is well-defined. "Well-defined" often is incorrectly described as "smooth"; but *smooth* is a shape, whereas *well-defined* is a description of the margin.

Wolff's Law "Bone is deposited and removed according to the stresses placed on the frame."

x-rays A type of electromagnetic radiation (a form of energy with wave-like behavior that travels at the speed of light). The short wavelength and high frequency of x-rays allows them to penetrate many objects and to be useful for medical imaging. X-rays are a form of ionizing radiation and are carcinogenic; exposure to x-rays should always be "as low as reasonably achievable" (ALARA).

x-ray film Consists of a transparent sheet (base) coated with an emulsion containing silver halide crystals, which are sensitive to x-rays, visible light, heat, and pressure.

Index

Radiography of the Dog and Cat: Guide to Making and Interpreting Radiographs, Second Edition. M.C. Muhlbauer and S.K. Kneller.

Companion website: www.wiley.com/go/muhlbauer/dog